CHARNOLO
in
Health and Disease
With Special Reference to Nanotheranostics

T0239713

Sushil Sharma
American International School of Medicine
Georgetown, Guyana, South America
1755 East Park Place Blvd
Stone Mountain, Georgia, USA

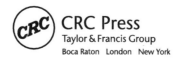

CRC Press
Taylor & Francis Group
Boca Raton London New York

CRC Press is an imprint of the
Taylor & Francis Group, an **informa** business

A SCIENCE PUBLISHERS BOOK

Cover Credit: Cover illustration reproduced by kind courtesy of the author, Dr. Sushil Sharma.

First edition published 2021
by CRC Press
6000 Broken Sound Parkway NW, Suite 300, Boca Raton, FL 33487-2742

and by CRC Press
4 Park Square, Milton Park, Abingdon, Oxon OX14 4RN

© 2021 Taylor & Francis Group, LLC
CRC Press is an imprint of Taylor & Francis Group, an Informa business

Library of Congress Cataloging-in-Publication Data
Names: Sharma, Sushil, Ph. D., D.M.R.I.T., author.
Title: Charnolophagy in health and disease : (with special reference to
    nanotheranostics) / Sushil Sharma.
Description: First edition. | Boca Raton : CRC Press, Taylor & Francis
    Group, 2021. | Includes bibliographical references and index.
Identifiers: LCCN 2020044926 | ISBN 9780367407902 (hardcover)
Subjects: LCSH: Biochemical markers--Diagnostic use. | Autophagic
    vacuoles--Therapeutic use. | Mitochondrial membranes--Abnormalities. |
    Nanomedicine.
Classification: LCC RB43.7 .S37 2021 | DDC 616.07/56--dc23
LC record available at https://lccn.loc.gov/2020044926

ISBN: 978-0-367-40790-2 (hbk)
ISBN: 978-0-367-67986-6 (pbk)
ISBN: 978-0-367-80909-6 (ebk)

Typeset in Times New Roman
by Shubham Creation

Preface

DNA recombinant technology, omics analysis, *in vivo* molecular imaging of gene-manipulated animals, and cell culture models of diseases, organoids, and functional genomics employing correlative and combinatorial bioinformatics were just beginning to evolve during the early 1970s when the Nobel Laureate Christian de Duve discovered lysosomes, peroxisomes, and autophagy. Biochemical and morphological studies were the primary focus of medical research in those days. It was difficult to precisely distinguish which particular intracellular organelle and associated gene(s) and/or biomarker(s) were implicated in disease progression or regression and its spatiotemporal relationship with autophagy (ATG). However, with the development of fluorescently labeled mitochondrial, ER, lysosomal, paroxisomal, genetic, epigenetic biomarkers, mtDNA, nDNA, miRNA, and mtmiRNA, we can now quantitatively estimate organelle or inclusion-specific ATGs in real time.

Recent discoveries have conferred unique opportunities to determine the exact molecular mechanism of MR, IMD, MQC, and ICD during the acute phase and CBMP during the chronic phase of disease progression in response to DPCI-induced free radical injury through the transcriptional activation of NRF-2 and PGC-1α. Mitochondria are the most susceptible to participate in pleomorphic CB formation, CP dysregulation, CS destabilization, and CBMP, implicated in apoptosis/necrosis in chronic MDR diseases. CBMP is triggered by DPCI-mediated free radical-induced CMB and mitochondrial degeneration characterized by CB formation, CP induction, CS destabilization, and CS exocytosis/endocytosis. Thus, CB formation is a highly intricate and orchestrated primary molecular mechanism of mitochondrial remodeling (MR), whereas CP involves Akt-ubiqitination and ATP-driven lysosomal-dependent phagocytosis of CB as a secondary molecular mechanism of MQC and ICD. CP regulates genes involved in the CB life cycle in health and CBMP in disease. Studying CP helps researchers to share and elucidate several aspects of generalized ATG in order to better understand the disease process and its theranostic significance. Endogenous, natural, and synthetic antioxidants regulate CP as well as ATG at the transcriptional and translational level by modulating similar genomic and proteomic profiles. Since, organelle-specific CP is the initial and early event involved in executing general ATG, I have used the term CP/ATG in this manuscript. DPCI induce initially organelle-specific CP (CB-ATG) to sustain MQC and ICD for NCF, followed by generalized ATG involving CBMP and apoptotic/necrotic cell death.

CB is a pleomorphic, quasi-crystalline, electron-dense stack of degenerated mitochondria, ER, and associated macromolecules and is formed in the most vulnerable cell in response to malnutrition, environmental pollution (NPs), heavy metal ions, ionizing radiation, and microbial (bacteria, virus, and fungus) infection-induced free radical overproduction. It contains toxic metabolites and prevents their dissemination through ATP-driven, lysosomal-dependent ATG (CP) and charnolosome (CS) exocytosis for NCF during the acute phase. CBMP is triggered by defective CP through the upregulation of DRP-1 and downregulation of mitofusin (Mfn), argyrophilic nucleolar organizer (AgNOR), mtDNA, and mtmiRNA during the chronic phase of disease progression in the most vulnerable cell. Dysregulated CP is involved in numerous NDDs, CVDs, systemic inflammations, chronic infections, and MDR malignancies. CP can be regulated at the transcriptional and translational levels by dietary restriction, intake of antioxidants, moderate exercise, controlled sex and sleep (*DRESS*) habits to improve mitochondrial bioenergetics and promote CP regulation and CS stabilization and its exocytosis for ICD and NCF to enjoy good health, longevity, and BQL. However, defective genes, a hostile environment, and hazardous life style (*GELS*) modifications result in early morbidity and mortality as described systematically in this edition. In addition, a byproduct of CP, charnolosome (CS) (and its metabolites), can be used for the early detection of microbial (including COVID-19*)* infections in biological fluids and macrophages. Although, fruits, vegetables, and nuts are excellent source of naturally-available antioxidants, they have reduced potency; hence, free radical scavenging NPs-loaded synthetic antioxidants can be developed as novel disease-specific spatio-temporal, targeted, safe, effective, and potent evidence-based personalized theranostic chranolopharmacotherapeutics (DSST-TSE-EBPT-CPTs) to improve drug delivery, MB, IMD, and ICD for NCF to remain healthy and enjoy BQL.

An organelle-specific ATG (such as CP, MTG, pexophagy, ERphagy, and nucleophagy) is exceedingly important to sustain a specific cellular function. CP is a dynamic recycling process that eliminates damaged organelles (particularly mitochondria) and proteins to maintain intracellular homeostasis. Hence, any genetic, epigenetic, physiological, biochemical, and/or pharmacological intervention to regulate CP will facilitate the TSE-EBPT of chronic MDR diseases with currently limited treatment options. Particularly, microbial (Zika, Ebola, Rubella, Corona, Hanta, Adeno, CMV, Influenza and Toxoplasma) infections and drugs of abuse (Caffeine, Nicotine, and Ethanol) suppress the pluripotency of stem cells by CP dysregulation to cause life-threatening anomalies as described in my book, *Zika Virus Disease: Prevention and Cure* ("Fetal Alcohol Spectrum Disorders'; and 'Nicotinism and Emerging Role of Electronic Cigarettes") (Vol. 1–4) by Nova Science Publishers, New York, U.S.A.

This edition illustrates the theranostic significance of antioxidants as CP regulators/ modulators in chronic MDR diseases and is an extension of my featured book, *The Charnoly Body: A Novel Biomarker of Mitochondrial Bioenergetics*, published by CRC Press, Taylor & Francis Group, in Florida, in the U.S.A. Functionally defective CP triggers CBMP, involving oil drop formation, CS destabilization, CS exocytosis/endocytosis inhibition, in severe malnutrition and MDR diseases. CP/ATG is transcriptionally regulated by a complex molecular machinery of ~30 ATG-related proteins and ~50 lysosomal enzymes those are downregulated in chronic diseases and aging. CP/ATG is induced by Parkin and DRP-1 upregulation, and mitofusin (Mfn-1, Mfn-2) and Opa-1, mtDNA, and mtmiRNA downregulation.

The mitochondria are highly vulnerable to CBMP in response to DPCI because of labile PUFA, omega-3 fatty acid-rich membranes, and naked, intron-less, GC-rich DNA, which is readily oxidized to 2,3 dihydroxy nonenal, and 8-OH-2dG, respectively, in response to a free radical attack. Such an attack disrupts mtmiRNA, miRNA, and epigenetics implicated in regulating protein synthesis, cell proliferation, inflammation, apoptosis, and necrosis.

These transcriptionally-regulated events are significantly impaired due to DPCI-induced, CBMP-mediated compromised CP. In general, CP represents highly intricate, ATP-driven, lysosomal-dependent molecular mechanism of MQC and ICD. It occurs initially to prevent the generalized ATG of other organelles and replace old nonfunctional, undesired, and fragmented mitochondria with new ones for constant and adequate ATP synthesis and intracellular homeostasis (which is highly crucial during aging). CP plays a pivotal role in ameliorating ERS, AgNOR, protein-synthesizing machinery, and nDNA to prevent proteostasis and sustain ICD and cell survival. Protein calorie malnutrition triggers CBMP, whereas nutritional rehabilitation regulates CP by inducing Beclin-1 and LC3-II, and reducing ataxin-3 and p62 in the most vulnerable stem cells.

It is important to emphasize that dysregulated CP, particularly during the first trimester (gastrulation phase) of pregnancy is involved in deleterious neurological, cardiovascular, musculoskeletal, respiratory, GIT, hepatic, renal, reproductive, and skin disorders in congenital diseases because the development of these organs requires zero-defective CP for ICD and NCF. As CP occurs earlier than ATG, it can serve as a gold-standard and sensitive biomarker to monitor environmental safety, theranostic potential of newly-discovered pharmaceuticals, and potential toxicity of microbes and NPs. Although, *C. elegans*, yeast, *Drosophila*, zebra fish, and genetically-engineered murine model of diseases have been used employing omics technology, functional genomics, and molecular imaging to investigate the cellular, molecular, genetic, and epigenetics of generalized ATG and its theranostic significance, limited studies are currently available to learn the exact role of CP in ATG regulation and CBMP in human health and disease, which forms the rationale of introducing this interesting book. Since CP is an energy (ATP)-driven, lysosomal-dependent, highly sensitive, transcriptional regulated, immediate and early, sequential prerequisite to trigger generalized ATG, particularly when it is dysregulated during the chronic phase of CBMP, and shares numerous common pathophysiological characteristics and biomarkers, I have written CP/ATG to emphasize the TSE-EBPT significance of organelle-specific ATG in NDDs, CVDs, microbial infections, drug addiction, and MDR malignancies in this manuscript.

This book consists of five parts: Part-1 Charnolophagy (General Topics); Part-2 Charnolophagy in Metabolic Disorders; Part-3 Charnolophagy in Systemic Disorders; Part-4 Charnolophagy in Inflammation, Cancer, Microbial Diseases, and Aging; Part-5 Charnolophagy in Nanomedicine. Chapters on NDDs, cancer, and nanotheranostics are sub-divided in two sections because the knowledge about these topics is expanding by almost every moment. The theranostic significance of CP in CQ-modified NPs drug delivery is also described briefly. The book helps the reader to better understand the intricate roles of CP/ATG in health and disease and motivate them to discover novel MB-based drugs to cure chronic MDR diseases. The currently available CP inhibitors and inducers pose serious adverse effects; hence, NPs as DSST-CP regulators/modulators minimize these adverse effects. CB agonists/antagonists, CP agonists/antagonists, CS stabilizers/destabilizers, and CS exocytosis/endocytosis agonists/antagonists are proposed to emphasize the clinical importance of natural and synthetic antioxidants. As potent free radical scavengers, antioxidants, prevent CB formation and CBMP as prophylactic agents during acute phase, and as CB inhibitors, CP regulators, CS stabilizers, CS exocytosis enhancers, and CBMP antagonists during the chronic phase. Curcumin, Resveratrol, CoQ_{10}, Melatonin, Queresteine, Berberine, Catechin, Lycopene as free-radical-scavenging antioxidants regulate CP and curb CBMP. Although, natural antioxidants can pass through the blood-brain barrier without adverse effects, they have low potency and require bulk consumption. Hence, ROS-scavenging antioxidant-loaded NPs, pegylagtion, and EPR are described elegantly to enhance drug delivery as unique theransotic strategy to remain healthy, enjoy BQL, and longevity.

Sushil Sharma
Ph.D; D.M.R.I.T

Acknowledgements

I extend sincere thanks and gratitude to my late mother "Charnoly", mentors, guides, teachers, and professional colleagues who encouraged and motivated me to discover charnolophagy (CP).

My respected teacher Professor Christian De Duve from Belgium was awarded a Nobel Prize in 1974. He was the one who discovered lysosomes and autophagy (ATG). Recently, Professor Yoshinori Ohsumi from Japan was awarded a Nobel Prize for discovering the basic molecular mechanism of autophagy (ATG). I have been following the footsteps of these legends during my doctoral and postdoctoral research career in several labs in India, Canada, and U.S.A.

I discovered "Charnoly body" (CB) as a pre-apoptotic biomarker of mitochondrial bioenergetics (MB) and charnolophagy (CP) to evaluate intracellular detoxification of the most vulnerable cells derived from pluripotent stem cells in the developing rat cerebellum and from the mice hippocampal CA-3 and dentate gyrus neurons in response to protein calorie malnutrition and intrauterine domoic acid exposure, respectively.

The concepts, mechanisms, and hypotheses in this book are original and based on my several years of research experience in biomedical sciences.

My sincere thanks and appreciation to the CRC Press, Taylor & Francis Group, Boca Raton, FL, U.S.A., Google, and the global scientific community for recognizing my original discovery of CP as an inclusion (CB)-specific ATG, which opens a new era for developing safe and effective therapeutics based on mitochondrial bioenergetics (MB), mitochondrial quality control (MQC), mitochondrial remodeling (MR), intramitochondrial detoxification (IMD) and intracellular detoxification (ICD) to remain healthy.

Respectfully submitted

Sushil Sharma, Ph.D; D.M.R.I.T
Academic Dean
American International School of Medicine
89 Middleton and Sandy Babb Kitty Street
Georgetown, Guyana, South America
H.Q.; 1755 East Park Place Blvd
Stone Mountain, Georgia, U.S.A.

Abbreviations

2-DG:	2-Deoxy-D-Glucose
3MA:	3-Methyladenine
4-HNE:	4-Hydroxynonenal
6-OH-DA:	6-Hydroxy Dopamine
8-OH, 2dG:	8-Hydroxy-2′-Deoxyguanosine
AAA:	ATPases Associated with Diverse Cellular Activities
AD:	Alzheimer's Disease
ADHD:	Attention Deficit Hyperactivity Disorder
AEC:	Airway Epithelial Cells
AHR:	Aryl Hydrocarbon Receptor
AIS:	Acute Ischmic Stroke
Akt:	Akt Serine/Threonine Kinase
Alpha-Syn:	Alpha Synuclein
Alpha-SynMTtko:	Alpha-Syn-Metallothionein Triple knockout
ALR:	Autophagic Lysosomal Reformation
ALS:	Amyotrophic Lateral Sclerosis
AMPs:	Antimicrobial peptides
AMPK:	Adenosine Monophosphate (AMP)-Activated Protein Kinase
ANDS:	Alternative Nicotine Delivery Systems
ANOVA:	Analysis of Variance
APS:	Autophagosome
ATF6:	Activating Transcription Factor 6
ATG:	Autophagy
ATG7:	ATG Related 7
ATG14:	ATG related 14
ATM:	Ataxia-telangiectasia mutated
$A\beta$:	Amyloid-β
BafA:	Bafilomycin A1
BALF:	Bronchoalveolar Lavage Fluid
BAX:	BCL2 Associated X, Apoptosis Regulator
BBB:	Blood Brain Barrier
BC:	Breast Cancer
BCL2:	B Cell Leukemia/Lymphoma 2

BDNF:	Brain Derived Growth Factor
BECN1:	Beclin-1
BECN1:	Beclin-1 (ATG Related)
BMI:	Basal Metabolic Index
BNIP3L:	Bcl-2/Adenovirus E1B 19 kDa protein-interacting protein 3-like
CCCP:	Carbonyl cyanidem-chlorophenyl hydrazone
CDA:	Cell Death-induced ATG
CGAS:	Cyclic GMP-AMP Synthase
CHD:	Congenital Heart Disease
ChoPL:	Choline Phospholipid
CLEM:	Correlative Light and Electron Microscopy
CMB:	Compromised Mitochondrial Bioenergetics
CML:	Chronic Myelogenous Leukemia
CMV:	Cytomegalovirus
CO:	Carbon Monoxide
Complex-1:	Ubiquinone NADH-Oxidoreductase
COPD:	Chronic Obstructive Pulmonary Disease
COVID-19:	Corona Virus with ID-2019
CP:	Charnolophagy
CPs:	Charnolopharmaceutics
CPS:	Charnolophagosome
CQ:	Chloroquine
CR:	Calorie Restriction
CR:	Chemoresistance
Cre:	Cre-Recombinase
CS:	Charnolosome
CS:	Cigarette Smoke
CSE:	Cigarette Smoke Exposure
CSDSF:	Charnolosome Destabilizaion Factor
CSE:	Cigarette Smoke Extract
CSF:	Cerebrospinal Fluid
CSF2/GM-CSF:	Colony Stimulating Factor 2
CSMF:	Charnolosome Membrane Fragmentation
CSMP:	Charnolosome Membrane Permabilization
CSMS:	Charnolosome Membrane Sequestration
CSS:	Charnolosome Stress
CSSF:	Charnolosome Stabilization Factor
CSSI:	Charnolsome Stability Index (CSSF/CSDSF)
CTSB:	Cathepsin B
CTSD:	Cathepsin D
Cu:	Copper
CVDs:	Cardiovascular Diseases
CXCL1:	C-X-C Motif Chemokine Ligand 1
DA:	Dopamine
DAergic:	Dopaminergic
DAF-2:	Dauer Formation-2
DAMPs:	Mitochondria-derived damage/or danger-associated molecular patterns.
DAPI:	4',6-Diamidino-2-Phenylindole
DAPK1:	Death Associated Protein Kinase 1
DC:	Diabetic Charnolopathy

DCs:	Dendritic Cells
DDIT3:	DNA-Damage Inducible Transcript 3
DDR1:	Discoidin Domain Receptor TK 1
DE:	Diabetic Embryopathy
DeepPhagy:	Deep Learning for ATG
DIP-EI/MS:	Electron Ionization Mass Spectrometry by Using a Direct Insertion Probe
DLB:	Dementia with Lewy Body
DMD:	Duchenne muscular dystrophy
DMSO:	Dimethyl Sulfoxide
DOM:	Domoic Acid
DPCI:	Diversified Physico-Chemical Injuries/insults
DSST-CS:	Disease-Specific Spatiotemporal Charnolosome
DSST-CPTs:	Disease-Specific Spatio-Temporal Charnolopharmaceuticals
EBPM:	Evidence-based Personalized Medicine
EBPT:	Evidence-based Personalized Theranostics
EBSS:	Earle's Balanced Salt Solution;
ECM:	Extracellular Matrix
eGFP:	Enhanced Green Fluorescent Protein
EIF2A:	Eukaryotic Translation Initiation Factor 2A
EIF2AK:	Eukaryotic Translation Initiation Factor 2 Alpha Kinase
EIF2AK3/PERK:	Eukaryotic Translation Initiation Factor 2 Alpha Kinase 3
Elavl3:	ELAV Like Neuron-Specific RNA Binding Protein 3
ELISA:	Enzyme-Linked Immunosorbent Assay
EPR:	Emergency preservation and resuscitation
ER:	Endoplasmic Reticulum
ERN1/IRE1:	Endoplasmic Reticulum to Nucleus Signaling 1
ERQC:	ER Quality Control;
ERS:	Endoplasmic Reticulum Stress
ERT:	Enzyme Replacement Therapy
ESCRT:	Endosomal Sorting Complexes Required for Transport; Gastroc/G: Gastrocnemius
FAO:	Fatty Acid Oxidation
FDA:	Food and Drug Administration
FFSS:	Flow Fluid Shear Stress
FG:	Folliculogenesis
FISH:	Fluorescence *In-Situ* Hybridization
FLIM:	Fluorescence Lifetime Imaging Microscopy
FMT:	Fecal Microbiota Transplantation
Foxos:	Forkhead transcription factors of the O class
^{18}F-DOPA:	^{18}F-Dihydroxyphenylaldehyde
GBM:	Glioblastoma multiforme
GFP:	Green Fluorescent Protein
GPC:	Glycerophosphorylcholine
GSD:	Geometric Standard Deviations
GSH:	Reduced Glutathione
GSK3B:	Glycogen Synthase Kinase 3 Beta
GWAS:	Genome Wide Association Studies
H&E:	Hematoxylin and Eosin
HMGB1:	High-mobility Group Box 1 Protein
H_2O_2:	Hydrogen Peroxide

HAT:	Histone Acetyltransferase
HAND:	HIV-associated Neurocognitive Disorders
HBEC:	Human Bronchial Epithelial Cells
HBSS:	Hanks Balanced Salt Solution
HBV:	Hepatitis B Virus
HCA:	High-content analysis
HCC:	Hepatocellular Carcinoma
HD:	Huntington's Disease
HDL:	High Density Lipoprotein
HDL-C:	High Density Lipoprotein-Cholesterol
HFD:	High Fat Diet
HIF-1α:	Hypoxia-Inducible Factor-1α
HO-1:	Heme Oxygenase-1
Hp:	Helicobacter Pylori
HPF:	Heriditary Periodic Fevers
HSP:	Heat Shock Protein
HSP-70:	Heat Shock Protein-70
HSPA5/GRP78/BiP:	Heat Shock Protein 5
HSPA5/GRP78:	Heat Shock Protein Family A (Hsp70) Member 5
HIF-1A:	Hypoxia-inducible Transcription Factor 1-alpha
i.p.:	Intraperitoneal
IBD:	Inflammatory Bowel Disease
ICD:	Intracellular Detoxification
IEM:	Inborn Errors of Metabolism
IFN:	Interferon
IGF1:	Insulin-Like Growth Factor 1
IL:	Interleukin
IL-10:	Interleukin-10
IL10R:	Interleukin 10 Receptor
IMD:	Intramitochondrial Detoxification
ING-4:	Inhibitor of Growth 4
IRGM:	Immunity Related GTPase M
IS:	Inflammasome
JNK:	c-Jun N-terminal kinase
KA:	Kainic Acid
KEGG:	Kyoto Encyclopedia of Genes and Genomes
LAP:	LC3-associated phagocytosis
LAMP1/2:	Lysosomal-Associated Membrane Protein 1/2
LAMP1:	Lysosomal-Associated Membrane Protein 1
LAMP2:	Lysosomal-Associated Membrane Protein 2
LAP:	LC3-Associated Phagocytosis
LBs:	Lewy Body
LBs:	Lamellar Bodies
LC3:	Microtubule Associated Protein 1 Light Chain 3
LC-MS:	Liquid Chromatography-Tandem Mass Spectrometry
LD:	Lipid Droplet
LD:	Lafora Disease
LDL:	Low Density Lipoprotein
L.m:	Listeria Monocytogen
LMP:	Lysosomal Membrane Permeabilization

LPS:	Lipopolysaccharides
LQC:	Lysosomal Quality Control
LRP:	Lung Resistance Related Protein
LRRK2:	Leucine-Rich Repeat Kinase 2
LSD:	LSD
MAM:	Mitochndrial Associated Membrane
MAP1LC3/LC3:	Microtubule Associated Protein 1 Light Chain 3
MAP1LC3B:	Microtubule-Associated Protein 1 Light Chain 3 Beta
MAPK:	Mitogen-Activated Protein Kinase
MB:	Mitochondrial Bioenergetics
MCAO:	Middle Cerebral Artery Occlusion
MCI:	Mild Cognitive Impairment
MDD:	Major Depressive Disorder
MDMA:	Methylene Deoxy Methamphetamine
MDR:	Multi Drug Resistance
MEFs:	Mouse Embryonic Fibroblasts
MHC:	Major Histocompatibility Complex
MicroPET:	Micro-Positron Emission Tomography
MIF:	Macrophage Migration Inhibitory Factor
miRNA:	microRNA
MMPs:	Matrix Metalloproteinases
MNCs:	Mononuclear Cells
MPP^+:	1-Methyl, 4-Phenyl, Pyridinium Ion
MPS:	Mitophagosome
MPTP:	1-Methyl, 2-Phenyl, 1, 2, 3, 6-Tetrahydropyridine
MQC:	Mitochondrial Quality Control
MRI:	Magnet Resonance Imaging
MRS:	Magnetic Resonance Spectroscopy
MS:	Multiple Sclerosis
MSA:	Multiple System Atrophy
MT:	Metallothionein
MT_{dko}:	Metallothionein Double Gene Knockout
MTG:	MitoTracker Green
MTG:	Mitophagy
MTG:	Streptomyces mobaraensis
MTOR:	Mechanistic Target of Rapamycin Kinase
MTORC1:	Mechanistic Target of Rapamycin Kinase Complex 1
MTT:	3-(4,5-dimethylthiazol-2-yl)-2,5-diphenyltetrazolium bromide
MTS:	Mitochondrial Targeting Sequence
MTS:	Mitochondrial Stress
MT_{trans}:	Metallothionein Transgenic
MVB:	Multivesicular Body
MYD88:	Myeloid Differentiation Primary Response Gene 88
nAChR:	Alpha-4 Nicotinic Acetylcholine Receptor
NAF-1:	Nutrient-deprivation ATG Factor-1
NAFLD:	Nonalcoholic Fatty Liver Disease
NASH:	Non-Alcoholic Steatohepatitis
NDCs:	Neurodegenerative Charnolopathies
NDDs:	Neurodegenerative Disorders
NLRP3:	NLR Family, Pyrin Domain Containing 3

NMR: Nuclear Magnetic Resonance
NO: Nitric Oxide
NOD2:   Nucleotide-binding Oligomerization Domain Containing 2
NOS: Nitric Oxide Synthase
NPs: Nanoparticles
NPC: Niemann-Pick Disease Type C
NPCs: Neurodegenerative Charnolopathies
Nrf-1:   Nuclear respiratory factor-1
Nrf-2:   Nuclear factor-erythroid 2-related factor-2
Nrip-1:   Nuclear receptor interacting protein-1
OA: Osteoarthritis
OGD: Oxygen and Glucose Deprivation
ONOO⁻:   Peroxynitrite Ion
OPTN: Optineurin
OSHA: Occupational Safety and Health Administration
PAH: Polycyclic Aromatic Hydrocarbons
PBMC: Peripheral Blood Mononuclear Cells
PBS: Phosphate-Buffered Saline
PC: Pancreatic cancer
PCD: Programmed Cell Death
PCR: Polymerase Chain Reaction
PCYT: Choline Phosphate Cytidylyltransferase
PCYT1A: Phosphate Cytidylyltransferase 1 Choline, Alpha
PD: Parkinson's Disease
PDGFR: Platelet Derived Growth Factor Receptor
PEG: Poly Ethylene Glycol
Pegylation: Covalent Conjugation of Drug with PEG
PGC-1α: Peroxisome Proliferator-activated Receptor Gamma Coactivator-1α
PET: Positron Emission Tomography
PI3K: Phosphoinositide-3-Kinase
PIK3C: Phosphatidylinositol-4:5-Bisphosphate 3-Kinase Catalytic Subunit
PKs: Pharmacokinetics
PLA2:   Phospholipase A2
PLD: Phospholipase D
PNPLA1:   Patatin-Like Phospholipase Domain-Containing Protein-1
PNS: Peripheral Nervous System
PRKN: Parkin RBR E3 Ubiquitin Protein Ligase
PRR: Pattern-Recognition Receptor
PT: Personalized Theranostics
PTEN-L: Phosphatase and Tensin Homolog (PTEN)-long
PtdCho: Phosphatidylcholine
PtdIns3P: Phosphatidylinositol-3-Phosphate
PTEN: Phosphatase and Tensin Homolog
PTSD: Post-Traumatic Stress Disorder
PTX: Paclitaxel
PUFA: Polyunsaturated Fatty Acids
PYCARD/ASC: PYD and CARD Domain Containing
RA: Rheumatoid Arthritis
RAAS: Renin-Angiotensin-Aldosterone System
Rapa: Rapamycin

RCD:	Regulated Cell Death
rER:	Rough Endoplasmatic Reticulum
RES:	Reticulo Endothelial System
RFP:	Red Fluorescent Protein
rhCTSD:	Human Recombinant CTSD
RHEB:	Ras Homolog, mTORC1 Binding
RhO$_{mgko}$:	Mitochondial Genome Knockout
RNAi:	RNA Interference
RNS:	Reactive Nitrogen Species
RONS:	Reactive Oxygen and Nitrogen Species
ROS:	Reactive Oxygen Species
RPE:	Retinal Pigment Epithelium
RPs:	Radiopharmaceuticals
RPTOR:	Regulatory Associated Protein of MTOR complex 1
RPS6:	Ribosomal Protein S6
RPS6KB1/p70S6K1:	Ribosomal Protein S6 Kinase Polypeptide 1
SASP:	Senescence-Associated Secretory Phenotype
shRNA:	Short Hairpin RNA
SI:	α-Syn Index (Nitrated α-Syn/Native α-Syn)
SIN-1:	3-Morpholinosydnonimine
siRNA:	Small Interfering RNA
SLE:	Systemic Lupus Erythematosus
SNCA:	Synuclein Alpha
SNP:	Single Nucleotide Polymorphism
SOD:	Superoxide Dismutase
SPECT:	Single Photon Emission Computerized Tomography
SQSTM1:	Sequestosome 1
SQSTM1/p62:	Sequestosome 1/p62
STAT3:	Signal Transducer and Activator of Transcription 3
α-Syn:	α-Synculein;
α-SynMTtko Mice:	α-Syn Metallothioneins Triple Knockout Mice
TBI:	Traumatic Brain Injury
TFAM:	Mitochondrial Transcription Factor A
TEM:	Transmission Electron Microscopy
TFEB:	Transcription Factor EB
TK:	Tyrosine kinase
TLR:	Toll-Like Receptor
TMRE:	Tetramethylrhodamine Ethyl Ester
TNF:	Tumor Necrosis Factor
TNFα:	Tumor Necrosis Factor-α
Tom40:	Translocase of Outer Membrane 40
TSC1/2:	Tuberous Sclerosis Complex 1/2
TTC:	2,3,5-triphenyltetrazolium chloride
TUNEL:	Terminal Deoxynucleotidyl Transferase dUTP Nick End Labelling
UC:	Ulcerative Colitis
ULK1:	Unc-51 Like ATG Activating Kinase 1
UN:	Undernutrition
UPR:	Unfolded Protein Response
VaD:	Vascular Dementia
VCP:	Valosin Containing Protein

VEGF:	Vasoendothelial Derived Growth Factor
wv/wv Mice:	Homozygous Weaver Mutant Mice
wv/wv-MTs:	Metallothioneins Over-Expressing Weaver Mice
XIAP:	X-linked Inhibitor of Apoptosis

Definitions

Anoikis   A programmed cell death which occurs in anchorage-dependent cells when they detach from the surrounding extracellular matrix. Cancer cells are anoikis-resistant, a prerequisite for their malignancy.

Antioxidants   Antioxidants are chemical compounds available from natural and synthetic sources. Antioxidants are endogenously synthesized in the mitochondria to prevent a direct free radical attack. Free radicals (OH, NO) are generated as a byproduct of oxidative phosphorylation (O/P) during ATP synthesis in the electron transport chain. Antioxidants, as free radical scavengers, prevent lipid peroxidation and DNA oxidation.

Apoptotic Body   A blebbing on the surface of plasma membrane following a chronic free radical attack. The fusion of CS body with the plasma membrane releases toxic mitochondrial metabolites to cause phosphatidyl serine externalization and release of intracellular constituents to induce chronic MDR diseases.

CB Epigenetics   Methylation of mitochondrial DNA at the N-3 position of cytosine and acetylation of histones at lysine residues.

Charnologenetics   Genetically-linked CB formation.

Charnolopharmacogenomics   Genomic changes associated with pharmacological induction or inhibition of CB.

CB-PET RPs   RPs to detect CB, CPS, CS, CP, and CS exocytosis/endocytosis. Disease-specific CB-PET radioligands will be clinically significant for the early differential diagnosis of NDDs, CVDs, and cancer.

Charnolopathy   Occurs in chronic degenerative diseases involving CB-specific proteinopathy due to CP dysregulation involving CB molecular pathogenesis (CBMP).

Charnolophagosome   A lysosome containing phagocytosed CB.

Charnolosome   An organelle following hydrolysis of CB by lysosomal enzymes.

Charnolopharmacotherapeutics   Therapeutics to control CB formation, CP induction, CS stabilization, and CS exocytosis for a NCF.

Charnolophagy (CP)   CP is CB-specific ATG. It is a mechanism that protects and maintains cellular function by sequestering harmful or dysfunctional mitochondria to lysosomes for degradation through CS formation. CP is a highly-specialized disease-specific spatiotemporal event which involves ATP-driven, lysosomal-dependent Akt-ubiquinated CB-ATG in response to DPCI-induced free radical (OH, NO: RONS) attack in the most vulnerable PPCs or in any vulnerable cell in the biological system as a mechanism of MQC and ICD to sustain NCF.

MR in response to DPCI-induced free radical generation triggers CB formation, CP induction, and CS destabilization resulting in CBMP in NDDs, CVDs, and MDR malignancies.

Charnolophagy Index   A ratio of CP versus ATG.

Charnolophagosome (CPS)   A highly unstable and functionally labile intracellular organelle which is formed following CP. It is electron-dense and ~2.5X larger than the size of a lysosome.

Charnolopharmaceuticals   CB-targeted pharmaceuticals for the safe and effective EBPT of chronic MDR diseases such as malignancies.

Charnolopharmacology   CB-targeted MB-based chemotherapeutics with well-established pharmacokinetics (PKs), pharmacodynamics (PDs), pharmacogenomics, beneficial effects, and adverse effects.

Charnoloscopy   A microscopic (usually confocal, atomic force, SEM, and TEM) evaluation of CB, CP, CPS, and CS, and their exocytosis/endocytosis.

Charnolosome (CS)   A CS is CB-specific autophagolysosome. It is formed when the phagocytosed CB in the CPS is hydrolyzed by the lysosomal enzymes. It is a single layered, highly unstable, and functionally labile organelle containing toxic mitochondrial metabolites.

Charnolosomics   A bioinformatics approach to analyze CB, CS, and CP biomarkers employing omics biotechnologies to evaluate MB, MR, IMD, and ICD for NCF to accomplish the TSE-EBPT of chronic MDR diseases.

Charnolostatic   An agent which inhibits CB formation.

Charnolocidal   An agent which eliminates CB in a physicochemically injured cell.

Charnolomimetic   An agent which augments CB formation.

Charnolotherapy   Therapeutic interventions of various diseases with novel CPTs.

Charnoly Body (CB)   It is a pleomorphic, multi-lamellar, electron-dense, quasi-crystalline, inclusion body generated in the most vulnerable cell due to free radical-induced degeneration and condensation of mitochondrial membranes. Free radicals are generated as a byproduct of mitochondrial O/P in the ETC and their production is augmented in DPCI. The energy requirement is increased during DPCI to eliminate CB as a mechanism of IMD. Free radicals cause degeneration of the mitochondrial membranes, which condense to form electron-dense penta or hepta-lamellar structures as an initial attempt to contain highly toxic mitochondrial metabolites such as Cyt-C, 2,3 dihydroxy nonenal, 8-OH 2dG, acetaldehyde, H_2O_2, ammonia, GAPDH, monoamine oxidases (MAOs), and TSPO (which serves as a cholesterol transport channel for the synthesis of steroid hormones to stabilize the mitochondrial and other intracellular membranes), calcium channel (TRPC) proteins, and microorganisms. These proteins are delocalized and denatured due to the RONS attack during CB formation which disrupts mitochondrial homeostasis to initiate cellular demise by induction of CBMP. Hence, CB can serve as a universal pre-apoptotic biomarker of CMB.

Crinophagy   Intracellular elimination of granular material for ICD.

CS Body   A blebbing on the surface of CS following a secondary or tertiary free radical attack due to lipid peroxidation during mitochondrial oxidative and ER stress. CS body pinches off from the CS and fuses with the plasma membrane to synthesize the apoptotic body.

Detection of CS   A CS can be detected by employing two fluorescent imaging probes: (i) Mitotracker, and (ii) Lysotracker. The Mitotracker determines the number of mitochondria and the Lysotracker determines the number of lysosomes. The mitochondria and lysosomes can be distinguished based on the red and green fluorescence respectively. These digital images are merged to localize yellow fluorescence-labeled CS. A CS exhibits yellow fluorescence because it has both lysosomal enzymes as well as mitochondrial metabolites. Moreover, CS is rich in the mtDNA oxidation product, 8-OH 2dG, and plasma membrane oxidation product, 2, 3 dihydroxy nonenal, which can be determined by labeling cells with fluorescently labelled specific antibodies. In addition to tissues and cultured cells, circulating CS biomarkers including 8-OH, 2dG, and 2, 3 dihydroxy nonenal can be estimated from the saliva, serum, plasma, blood, urine, hair, and toenail samples to quantitatively assess CB-based MB and CBMP. Various biomarkers of CS can also be determined by multiplex ELISA, SPR spectroscopy, antibody microarrays, cDNA microarray, and microRNA microarrays.

Diversified Physicochemical Injury (DPCI) Physicochemical injury can occur due to severe malnutrition, toxic environmental exposure, and in response to microbial (bacteria, viral, fungal, ameobic, and parasitic) infection to cause mitochondrial oxidative and nitrative stress and trigger CB formation in the most vulnerable cell.
Note: The term "diversified physicochemical injury (DPCI)" has been used to represent malnutrition, toxic environmental exposure, and/or microbial (bacteria, viral and fungal) infection in the most vulnerable cell in this edition.

Free Radicals Free radicals are highly unstable, reactive oxygen, nitrogen, and carbon species (RONS: $\cdot$OH, NO$\cdot$, CO$\cdot$) formed in the mitochondria as a byproduct to O/P in the ETC. Free radicals trigger lipid peroxidation of cellular membranes by inducing the structural and functional breakdown of polyunsaturated fatty acids (PUFA: linoic acid, linolenic acid, and arachidonic acid).

Mitophagy (MTG) It is a specialized form of organelle (mitochondria)-specific ATG.

Personalized Theranostics Individualized diagnosis and simultaneous treatment. It is significant for highly proliferative malignant carcinomas where there is a limited time window for the diagnosis and treatment.

Senotherapy A research area to develop novel theranostics for the TSE-EBPT of cellular senescence and age-related diseases. Senotherapy involves the use of anti-aging drugs to slow down "senescence".

Stages of Free Radical Attack There are primarily four stages of free radical attack: (i) Primary free radical attack (PFA), (ii) secondary free radical attack (SFA), (iii) tertiary free radial attack (TFA), and (iv) quaternary free radical attack (QFA). (i) PFA is attenuated by endogenously-synthesized antioxidants such as glutathione, MTs, HSPs, HIF α, thioredoxin, SOD, and catalase. (ii) SFA requires endogenously synthesized antioxidants as well as naturally produced antioxidants such as polyphenols (Resveratrol), Lycopene, Sirtuins, Rutins, Catechin, and Flavonoids to sustain IMD and ICD. (iii) TFA requires endogenously synthesized antioxidants, naturally synthesized antioxidants, and pharmacological antioxidants such as B Vitamins, Vitamin-A, D, E, Probucol, Edaravone, statins (Simvastatin, Atorvastatin), Vildaglipitin, and several others. (iv) QFA is difficult to attenuate and/or prevent by the above three sources of antioxidants. In general, QFA is associated with degenerative and proinflammatory apoptosis which triggers chronic MDR diseases.

Vulnerable Cells The cells derived from pluripotent stem cells and mesenchymal stem cells (such as neural progenitor cells, cardiac progenitor cells, endothelial progenitor cells, hepatic progenitor cells, renal progenitor cells, pulmonary progenitor cells, osteogenic progenitor cells, and germinal progenitor cells) from the developing embryo are the most vulnerable to physicochemical injury.

α-Synuclein Index A ratio of nitrated α-Syn versus native α-Syn as an early biomarker of NDDs.
Note: The reader may find terms such as lysosphagosome, phagolysosome, mitophagosome, phagomitosome, mito-auto-phagosomes (MAPS), charnolophagosome, phagocharnolosome, charnolosome, aggresome, aggregosome, and mitochondrial–derived vesicles, in the literature relevant to energy (ATP)-driven, lysosomal-dependent autophagy of primarily nonfunctional, undesired, and/or degenerated mitochondria which exist in numerous pleomorphic forms (CBs) following DPCI-induced free radical injury in the most vulnerable cell. Similarly, the nomenclature of different ATGs is provided in this edition.

Contents

Preface   *iii*

Acknowledgements   *vii*

Abbreviations   *ix*

Definitions   *xvii*

Introduction   1

Concluding Remarks   78

Part-1 Charnolophagy (General Topics)

Chapter-1 Charnolophagy as Immediate and Early ATG   83

Chapter-2 Charnolophagy in Intramitochondrial and Intracellular Detoxification   87

Chapter-3 Charnolophagy as a Biomarker of Novel Drug Discovery   102

Chapter-4 Organ and Disease-specific Charnolophagy   106

Chapter-5 Charnolophagy in Pressure Ulcers   116

Chapter-6 Charnolophagy in Toxicology   128

Part-2 Charnolophagy in Metabolic Disorders

Chapter-7 Charnolophagy in Congenital Diseases   139

Chapter-8 Charnolophagy in Inborn Errors of Metabolism *(Recent Update)*   157

Chapter-9 Charnolophagy in Malnutrition   180

Chapter-10 Charnolophagy in Diet Restriction   196

Chapter-11 Charnolophagy in Gastrointestinal Diseases   202

Chapter-12 Charnolophagy in Liver Diseases   209

Chapter-13 Charnolophagy in Diabetes   231

Chapter-14 Charnolophagy in Obesity   242

Chapter-15 Charnolophagy in Hyperlipidemia   249

Part-3 Charnolophagy in Systemic Disorders

Chapter-16 Charnolophagy in Skin and Hair Diseases   257

Chapter-17 Charnolophagy in Musculoskeletal Diseases   268

Chapter-18 Charnolophagy in Pulmonary Diseases   286

Chapter-19 Charnolophagy in Cardiovascular Diseases   298

Chapter-20 Charnolophagy in Renal Diseases   320

Chapter-21 Charnolophagy in Reproductive Diseases   325
Chapter-22 Charnolophagy in Ophthalmic Diseases   338
Chapter-23 Charnolophagy in Neurodegenerative Diseases (Part 1)   347
Chapter-24 Charnolophagy in Neurodegenerative Diseases (Part 2)   356
Chapter-25 Charnolophagy in Parkinson's Disease   366
Chapter-26 Charnolophagy in Alzheimer's Disease   385
Chapter-27 Charnolophagy in Stroke   392

Part-4 Charnolophagy in Inflammation, Cancer, Microbial Infections, and Aging

Chapter-28 Charnolophagy in Inflammatory Diseases   401
Chapter-29 Charnolophagy in Cancer (A)   417
Chapter-30 Charnolophagy in Cancer (B)   441
Chapter-31 Charnolophagy in Microbial Infections   468
Chapter-32 Charnolophagy in Aging   503

Part-5 Charnolophagy in Nanomedicine

Chapter-33 Charnolophagy in Nanotheranostics (Part 1)   527
Chapter-34 Charnolophagy in Nanotheranostics (Part 2)   567

Index   *581*

Introduction

A mitochondrion is the cell organelle of prokaryotic origin with generally an ovoid or elliptical shape and is the major source of ATP synthesis (the word ATP and energy are used synonymously). Mitochondria are present in all living cells except erythrocytes and euglena. Mitochondria can migrate and change their shape, size, organization, geometry, and topography depending on the metabolic needs of a cell. They contain specific enzymes for oxidative phosphorylation (O/P), the tricarboxylic acid (TCA) cycle (for glucose metabolism), and the β-oxidation of fatty acids. Usually mitochondria are abundant at locations where energy requirements are high, such as cardiomyocytes, skeletal myocytes, osteocytes, hepatocytes, neurons, nephrons, enteric cells, and oocytes. Congenital, postnatal, and other diseases of adult life primarily involve the CNS, musculoskeletal, hepatic, pulmonary, skin, and/or renal system due to the dysregulation of charnolophagy (CP), charnolosome (CS) destabilization, and Charnoly body molecular pathogenesis (CBMP). Patients with childhood myopathy have abnormally giant mitochondria with para-crystalline inclusions, which are also observed in mitochondrial encephalomyopathy, lactic acidosis, stroke-like episodes (MELAS), and myoclonic epilepsy with ragged red fibers (MERRF).

Charnolophagy (CP), a term coined to describe autophagy (ATG) that targets CBs, has emerged as an important cellular process to maintain mitochondrial homeostasis and is regulated by various nutrients and nutritional stresses. The multifaceted contribution of mitochondria evolved with their role in energy production, $[Ca^{2+}]_i$ homeostasis, metabolic control, anti-inflammation, growth, survival, proliferation, differentiation, development, and apoptosis. The mitochondrial growth, fission, fusion, CP, and mitophagy (MTG) are transcriptionally regulated by the mtDNA, mtmiRNA, and nDNA. Molecular events that regulate the mitochondrial life cycle involve CB formation and CP induction during the acute phase, and CS destabilization and CBMP during the chronic phase of disease progression. Mitochondria are the key determinants of intracellular detoxification (ICD), intracellular toxicity (ICT), and normal cellular function (NCF), depending on the inducers and microenvironment. Free radicals are generated in the mitochondria as a byproduct of O/P, when energy requirements are elevated. Proteins that participate in the mitochondrial dynamics and ATG, also regulate their destruction through CP dysregulation, which confers a unique platform to develop the DSST-TSE-EBPT-CPTs for human health and happiness.

The author discovered lipid droplets (LDs) in the developing UN rat cerebellar Purkinje neurons as a doctoral student at the All India Institute of Medical Sciences New Delhi in 1982. LD is formed in patients undergoing undernutrition, diabetes, hyperlipidemia, obesity, aging, and in autosomal recessive congenital ichthyosis (ARCI) patients with PNPLA1 mutations in the most vulnerable cell due to CMB and dysregulated CP as described in this manuscript. Recently, Cohen (2018) demonstrated that fatty acids stored in LDs are delivered to mitochondria when the cells are starved, which requires lipases and mitochondrial fusion, where these are replenished with FAs supplied by ATG, having a theranostic significance for cancer. They discussed the life cycle of LDs compared to mitochondria, peroxisomes, and autophagosomes (more specifically CPS). LDs are organelles because these are composed of proteins and lipids, and undergo biogenesis, maturation, turnover, and interactions with other organelles. Kong et al. (2018) reported about the enzymes and regulatory proteins during lipolysis and peroxisomal β-oxidation and lipid degradation in microalgae. They elaborated upon the biotechnological applications of the acetyl-CoA products via glyoxylate cycle and gluconeogenesis, vesicle trafficking, cell cycle, and ATG in the lipid turnover and catabolism. Lipid degradation is also important in microalgae because their survival in the changing environment requires remodeling and the mobilization of lipids, comprising lipolysis, to release fatty acids and be catalyzed by LDs lipases. Although degradation of fatty acids to acetyl-CoA occurs in the peroxisomes through β-oxidation, it may occur in mitochondria as well.

The identification of lipoproteins that determine mitochondrial pleomorphism including CB formation and MR are still evolving. CB is a nonfunctional intracellular inclusion which is phagocytosed by ATP-driven lysosomal activation following Akt-ubiquitination. The lysosomes confer surveillance for ICD. The mitochondria are rich in alkaline phosphatase, whereas, the lysosomes are rich in acid phosphatase as biomarkers for their identification and characterization. The mitochondria are involved in redox balance, whereas the lysosomes are involved in acid-base balance. The lysosomes phagocytose CBs through ATP-driven ATG (classified as CB-ATG or CP) to eliminate nonfunctional mitochondria from the erythroblasts before they become erythrocytes. Any delay or defect in CP may cause reticulocytosis, elliptocytosis, ovalocytocytosis, spherocytosis, sickle cell anemia, thalacemia, anemia, and leukemia, involving CBMP; which is a step forward to learn senotherapy. The mitochondrial metabolites such as Cyt-C, caspases, apoptotic-inducing factor (AIF), 8-OH, 2dG, 2, 3 dihydroxy nonenal, 4-hydroxy nonenal, lactate, acetate, acetaldehyde, acetone, ammonia, H_2O_2, GAPDH, MAOs, TRPCs, XO, COX, and TSPO are highly toxic, when delocalized. In particular, Cyt-C is loosely and non-covalently attached to the IMM and is delocalized in response to DPCI. It is toxic to membranes, mtDNA, mtRNA, mtmiRNA, and nDNA and triggers apoptosis through caspase-3 activation and poly (ADP) polymerase (PARP) cleavage, as noticed in cerebral and cardiovascular atherosclerotic plaques. Due to the vulnerability of reactive oxygen and nitrogen species (RONS) induced lipid peroxidation and labile genetic and epigenetics of the mtDNA, CP occurs much earlier than ATG as an early response to DPCI in the most vulnerable cell. All other organelles are spared from the immediate and direct RONS attack except mitochondria, ER, lysosomes, and CS. Although, increased lysosomal activity triggers a pro-inflammatory cascade due to TSPO (18 kDa: a cholesterol channel protein) delocalization during the acute phase, enhanced production and CS destabilization induces MDR malignancies involving inflammasomes activation during the chronic phase. The ultrastructure of adrenal cortical cells which synthesize LDs reflects the synthesis of steroid hormones. The steroid precursor, cholesterol, is stored in LDs as esters along with fatty acids. With tubular cristae, the surface area of the IMM is increased, where steroid biosynthesis occurs (that is, cholesterol>pregnenolone). Stimulation by ACTH augments steroid hormone synthesis as a function of increase in SER and mitochondrial cristae. However, energy production and the anti-inflammatory role of the mitochondria are compromised when CBMP is triggered in response to DPCI-induced free radical overproduction. Since the past three decades, we have been investigating the cellular, molecular, genetic, and epigenetic basis of CBMP and its theranostic significance in health and disease, employing gene-manipulated cellular and murine models of NDDs, CVDs, and MDR malignancies with a primary focus on PD, AD, drug addiction, stroke, and aging. A brief list of the theranostic significance of mitochondria is illustrated in Fig. 1.

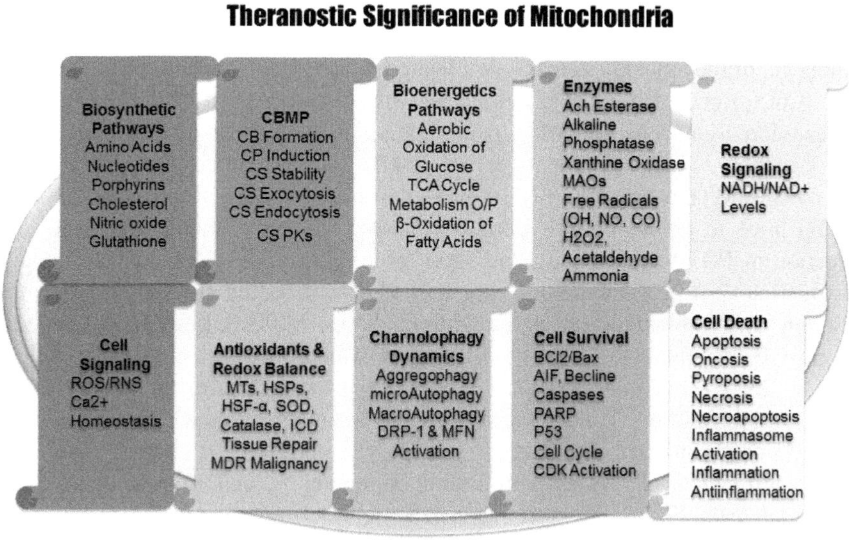

Theranostic Significance of Mitochondria

Figure 1

Compromised CP in Disease Progression

The CNS is highly susceptible to even minor free-radical injury as noticed in acute ischemic stroke. CB, as a pleomorphic, multi-lamellar, electron-dense membrane stack of degenerated mitochondrial and ER membranes is formed in response to DPCI in the most vulnerable stem cells of the developing embryo. Viral (Ebola, Rubella virus, CMV, and Zika) infections during intrauterine life compromise stem-cell pluripotency and induces charnolopathies, characterized by arthrogryposis, microcephaly, and musculoskeletal anomalies with life-long consequences. Influenza, SARS, MERS, and COVID-19 also highjack CP in the pulmonary macrophages to cause fever, xerostomia, fatigue, rhinitis, bronchitis, pharyngitis, pneumonia, and even fatalities, particularly among aging immunocompromised individuals with preexisting conditions. During the acute phase, CB formation (as an adaptive response) attempts to contain the spread of toxic pathogens and metabolites and is eliminated by lysosomal-dependent ATP-driven phagocytosis as CP to sustain MQC and ICD for NCF. Any delay or defect in CP at the transcriptional or translational level can trigger CVDs, NDDs, and MDR malignancies.

Original Discoveries

I have been investigating the cellular, molecular, genetic, and epigenetic mechanisms of mitochondrial bioenergetics in health and disease. I discovered CB, CP, CS, and CBMP in the Purkinje neurons of the developing undernourished rat cerebellar cortex as a doctoral student in India (Sharma et al. 1986, 1987, Sharma 1988) and in the hippocampal CA-3 and dentate gyrus regions of intrauterine Domoic acid and Kainic acid-exposed mice and rats, respectively as a postdoctoral scientist in Canada and U.S.A. (Sharma et al. 1993, Dakshinamurti et al. 1993). Kainic acid and Domoic acid-induced seizure thresholds were significantly reduced in protein malnourished (Sharma et al. 1990) and in Pyridoxine (Vitamin-B6)-deficient adult rats (Sharma and Dakshinamurti 1992). A specific 5-HT-1A receptor agonist, 8-OH-DPAT increased Domoic acid-induced seizure thresholds, suggesting that Pyridoxine-mediated 5-HT synthesis confers mitochondrial neuroprotection by inhibiting CB formation by regulating CP and by inhibiting CBMP (Sharma and Dakshinamurti 1993). A specific monoamine oxidase-B

(MAO-B) inhibitor, Selegiline also provided mitochondrial neuroprotection in human dopaminergic (SK–N–SH) neurons by preventing 1-methyl, 4-phenyl 1,2,3,6 pyridinium (MPP$^+$)-induced mitochondrial damage implicated in CBMP (Sharma et al. 2003), whereas ubiquinone (CoQ$_{10}$) provided neuroprotection in 1-methyl, 4-phenyl- 1,2,3,6 tetrahydropyridine (MPTP)-treated α-Synuclein and MTs gene-manipulated mice *in vivo* and in MPP$^+$-treated SK–N–SH neurons *in vitro* (Sharma et al. 2004). We developed α-Synuclein MTs-triple knock out (α-Syn-MTtko) mice and MTs-over-expressed homozygous weaver (wv/wv) mutant (wv/wv-MTs) mice to confirm the hypothesis that MTs provide ubiquinone (CoQ$_{10}$)-mediated neuroprotection in PD, AD, and drug addiction by inhibiting CB formation, by regulating CP, and by preventing CBMP (Sharma et al. 2013a). We reported the clinical significance of MTs in cell therapy and Nanomedicine and highlighted that MTs as potent CB antagonists, CP agonists, and CBMP attenuators can be utilized to evaluate neutral, protective and toxic NPs (Sharma et al. 2013b), major depressive disorders (Sharma 2014a, b) and stress of the soldier and civilian (Sharma 2014c). We also described the theranostic significance of antioxidants as CB and CBMP antagonists and CP regulators in various NDDs (Sharma and Ebadi 2014a) and clinical significance of CB as a universal biomarker of cell injury (Sharma and Ebadi 2014b), in novel drug discovery (Sharma 2014d, e), in developing CPTs for the TSE-EBPT of NDDs, CVDs, and MDR malignancies (Sharma 2014f), in developing mitochondrially-targeted Nanomedicines (Sharma 2014g) and in evidence-based personalized nanotheranostics (Sharma 2014h). As an invited speaker, international scientific consultant, and chairperson, I presented the theranostic significance of CB in novel drug discovery of PD, AD, and drug addiction (Sharma 2014h) and MTs as potent free radical scavengers in aging (Sharma and Ebadi 2014b); to evaluate psychology of craving (Sharma et al. 2014); in drug addiction (Sharma 2015); in vascular dementia (Jagtap et al. 2015); in fetal alcohol syndrome (Chabenne et al. 2014, Sharma et al. 2015); to assess environmental toxicity (Sharma 2014d); to assess the theranostic potential of newly-developed MAO inhibitors (Sharma 2015a), as biomarkers of nutritional stress in AD (Sharma et al. 2016a); in early diagnosis of drug addiction and other proinflammatory diseases (Sharma 2016c); in personalized medicine (Sharma 2016d); in developing novel PET radiopharmaceuticals (Sharma 2016e); in prenatal diagnosis of fetal alcohol spectrum and other genetic disorders by amniocentesis, chorionic villous sampling, and umbilical cord blood sampling by estimating 8-OH 2dG and 4-hydroxynonenal as early molecular indicators of CB formation, CP dysregulation, and CBMP in the amniotic fluid and chorionic villous cells (Sharma 2017a). Furthermore, we can utilize CB and CP as mitochondrial-targeted *inclusionopathy* and *inclusionophagy*, respectively for better understanding of translational multimodality neuroimaging (Sharma 2017b), Zika virus microcephaly during intrauterine life (Sharma 2017c); and assess the deleterious consequences of Nicotinism particularly in young adolescent population (Sharma 2018a,b,c,d). Recently, I consolidated afore-mentioned original discoveries in a book "The Charnoly Body: A Novel Biomarker of Mitochondrial Bioenergetics, CRC Press, Taylor & Francis Science Group, Boca Raton, FL, U.S.A. (Sharma 2019) to elucidate the theranostic significance of CP in this edition. Hence, going through "The Charnoly Body" and "Charnolophagy in Health & Disease" simultaneously will provide better understanding of mitochondrial inclusion-specific ATGs in chronic MDR diseases and their TSE-EBPT.

CP and MQC

Almost all cells have an efficient system of MQC and ICD through lysosomal-driven ATP-dependent CP system, with the exception of neurons, muscles, and spermatocytes, as these are highly specialized terminally differentiated cells. Both mitochondria as well as lysosomes participate in CP to sustain MQC. Although CP can occur in the neurons, MQC and ICD are inefficient because nonfunctional or degenerated organelles or macromolecules go on accumulating to form inclusions in these non-dividing cells. Also, though spermatocytes have mitochondria, they lack lysosomes to execute CP, MTG, or ATG for ICD and MQC autonomously. Hence, oocyte mitochondria and lysosomes execute paternal CP during prezygotic phase because it is a highly crucial spatiotemporally regulated event during fertilization. A slight perturbation in CP execution following conception can have deleterious consequences and trigger diversified congenital anomalies such as microcephaly, craniofacial abnormalities, arthrogryposis, musculoskeletal anomalies, cardiovascular problems, renal impairments, skin disorders, and reproductive diseases.

Mitochondrial Fusion and Fission

Mitochondria play a crucial role in stress regulation, lipid synthesis, Ca^{2+} storage, CP/ATG induction, membrane fusion/fission, and cellular demise through apoptosis and/or necrosis. Long and fused mitochondria are optimal for ATP synthesis, whereas their fission facilitates CP induction and cell division. So far, only a single mitochondrial fission protein (DRP-1) has been identified. Farmer et al. (2018) reviewed the GTPases in mitochondrial fusion and fission, and their mechanisms of regulation. They focused on linking endocytic regulatory proteins with the VPS35 cargo selection complex for their homeostasis. The mitochondria enter cycles of fission and fusion which led to them being organize into two distinct states: the 'individual state' and the 'network state'. When compromised with DPCI, these are subjected to degradation. The elimination pathway relies on CP, which plays crucial role in numerous cellular activities. Defective CP accumulates nonfunctional CBs, which if they remain persistent, are associated with NDDs. Liu and Okamoto (2018) reviewed a link between mitochondria and ATG in yeast and multicellular eukaryotes. They emphasized the principles underlying CP and MQC. There is now evidence to suggest generalized ATG in the management of MQC. Mitochondria serve as platforms for regulating CP-mediated ATG. These interdependent relationships coordinate metabolic plasticity in the cell (Okamoto and Kondo-Okamoto 2012). Mitochondria and ATG act in response to changes in cellular energy, nutrients, and stress. The interaction between mitochondria and ATG is evolutionarily conserved because defects in one of them could impair the other, resulting in the risk of vulnerability to various diseases. Lee et al. (2012) explored redox signaling in the regulation of ATG to evaluate the mechanisms of CP induction. Dysfunction in mitochondria and ATG play a pivotal role in disease progression through CP dysregulation. RONS at low levels behave as signaling molecules, and at high levels may damage organelles. Oxidative damage and mitochondrial dysfunction result in ATP depletion, accumulation of cytotoxic metabolites, and apoptosis. Hence, the interface between stress adaptation and cell death is important for learning redox biology and disease pathogenesis. Autophagosomes form membrane structures, sequester damaged, oxidized, or dysfunctional macromolecules and organelles, and direct them to the lysosomes for degradation. Hence, CP/ATG dysfunction results in abnormal mitochondrial activity and RONS stress.

Lipid peroxidation is characterized by a free-radical-induced structural and functional break-down of PUFA in the plasma membrane. A lysosome containing a phagocytosed CB is named as charnolophagosome (CPS). A CPS is transformed to CS, when the phagocytosed CB is hydrolyzed by the proteolytic and lipolytic enzymes. A CPS is almost 2.5 times larger than the actual size of a lysosome (250 µm to 2.5 µm). A CS is a highly susceptible and has a half-life of 4–5 hrs. A subsequent free radical attack can induce blebbing to form CS bodies, which pinch off from the parent CS and fuse with the plasma membrane to release toxic mitochondrial metabolites, resulting in phosphatidyl serine (Annexin) externalization and eventually, non-DNA-dependent apoptosis through leaky apoptotic bodies, which are degraded in a hostile microenvironment of free radicals. The OH and NO radicals in the presence of iron (Fe) participate in the Fenton reaction to synthesize deleterious $ONOO^-$ ions, which induce oxidative as well as nitrative stress to cause further degeneration in a physico-chemically injured cell. The $ONOO^-$ ions induce lipid peroxidation of labile CS membranes and oxidation of mtDNA to synthesize 8-OG 2dG, which can be estimated from tears, nasal discharge, saliva, serum, plasma, CSF, synovial fluid, semen, vaginal fluid, urine, hair, and toe nail samples of a patient to evaluate mtDNA integrity. The mtDNA resides in a hostile microenvironment of free radicals generated as a byproduct of O/P. Hence, various genetic and epigenetic changes occur more readily in the mtDNA as compared to the nDNA. Methionine from the cytosol enters in the mitochondria to synthesize S-methyl adenosine (SAM) in the presence of ATP and methyl transferase. The SAM causes methylation of the mtDNA at the N-3 position of the cytosine. Thus, epigenetic changes can occur more readily and frequently in the mtDNA as compared to the nDNA.

The mitochondrial membranes are labile because these are rich in omega-3 (docosatrienoic acid, docosatetraenoic acid, docosapentaenoic acid, docohexanoic acid, and eicopentanoic acid) fatty acids. The omega-3 fatty acids are abundant in the CNS and are involved in myelination, which is impaired in NDDs. Thus, mitochondria are readily destroyed to trigger CBMP in the CNS. The nDNA remains protected from free radicals because it is surrounded by the nuclear wall and nucleoplasm and does not exist in direct vicinity of RONS as the mtDNA. The formation of methyl cytosine or hydroxymethyl cytosine occurs rarely in the nDNA. The structural and functional integrity and super helicity of nDNA is maintained by the topoisomerases and helicases, in addition to histones and protamines. Hence, the determination of 8-OH, 2dG and 2, 3 dihydroxy nonenal can provide an accurate estimate of CMB, mitochondrial degeneration, CP induction, and CBMP. The mitochondrial metabolites can induce structural and functional degradation of even nDNA to cause inter-nucleosomal fragmentation, apoptosis, and random DNA fragmentation, leading to necrosis. Both apoptosis as well as necrosis are implicated in NDDs in the developing and aging brain.

Mitochondria are maintained in an organelle network by intricately balanced fission and fusion pathways, which play a crucial role in sensing cellular stress. Recently, Gilkerson (2018) explored mitochondrial dynamics involved in sensing cellular stress in the organelle network and highlighted that fission/fusion is highly sensitive to CMB, oxidative stress, other stimuli, and may contribute to inflammation, ATG, and apoptosis. The overlapping activity with *m*-AAA protease 1 (OMA1) metallopeptidase, a stress-sensitive modulator of mitochondrial fusion, and Drp-1 modify mitochondrial dynamics in response to DPCI. Hence, OMA1 and Drp-1 are critical factors in cellular stress-response involving CB formation, CP induction, CS destabilization, and CBMP.

Mitochondrial Dynamics in Stress

Mitochondria move along cytoskeleton and interact with each other by membrane tethering, fusion, and fission. Zemirli et al. (2018) correlated the mitochondrial dynamics with their role in nutrient deprivation, pathogen attack, diseases, fusion/fission, and CP/ATG. Mitochondrial dysfunction represents an important cellular stressor and when intense and persistent, the cells unleash an adaptive response to prevent their extinction. Mitochondria can influence nuclear transcription and DNA methylation to modulate cellular stress. Mayorga et al. (2019) hypothesized that mitochondrial dysfunction triggers an epigenetically mediated adaptive response through DNA methylation. They studied cellular stress responses (that is, CP/ATG and apoptosis) in mitochondrial dysfunction and explored nDNA methylation in cell survival. The experiments on myoblasts revealed that mitochondrial dysfunction triggers a methylation-dependent pro-survival response. The assays done on mitochondrial disease patient tissues showed increased CP/ATG and the enhanced DNA methylation of tumor suppressor genes in cell survival, confirming that mitochondrial dysfunction triggers a "pro-survival" adaptive state by the methylation of nuclear genes. The components of the fission and fusion machinery, including Drp-1, Mfn-1/2, and OPA1 in mitochondrial pleomorphism, are indispensable for CP/ATG, apoptosis, and necroptosis. Xie et al. (2018) examined the mitochondrial network in 3 types of cell death, including CP/ATG, apoptosis, and necroptosis. Cancers often exhibit a fragmented mitochondrial phenotype involving CBMP. Thus, the fragmented ratio can reflect prognosis and a theranostic response. They also emphasized how Drp-1, involved in mitochondrial fission, could be a novel theranostic target for cancer.

Computational Mitochondrial Swelling

The swelling of mitochondria plays an important role in the disease pathogenesis by stimulating CP, MTG, ATG, apoptosis, and/or necrosis. Changes in the permeability of the IMM to ions and other substances induce osmotic pressure, leading to matrix swelling. The modeling of mitochondrial swelling is important for the simulation and prediction of *in vivo* events during a RONS attack. Makarov et al. (2018) developed a computational model to determine the mechanism of mitochondrial swelling based on osmosis, rigidity of the IMM, and dynamics of ionic/neutral species, as a biophysical approach, where osmotic pressure was compensated by the rigidity of the IMM. The occurrence of mitochondrial membrane deformations compensated for osmotic pressure effect. This effect was linear and reversible at small membrane deformations and could restore normal mitochondrial morphology. The membrane rigidity dropped to zero at large deformations, and swelling became irreversible, suggesting that increased dysfunctional mitochondria induces CP and cell death. Mitochondrial dysfunction is the cause of many diseases. The functioning of mitochondria is impossible without interaction with other cellular compartments. Retrograde signaling pathways connect mitochondria and the nucleus. The signal transducers in the yeast retrograde response are Rtg1p, Rtg2p, and Rtg3p proteins, as well as four negative regulatory factors—Mks1p, Lst8p, and two 14-3-3 proteins (Bmh1/2p). Trendeleva and Zvyagilskaya (2018**)** analyzed retrograde signaling as a stress or homeostatic response to changes in metabolic and biosynthetic activities during mitochondrial dysfunction. Moreover, MQC is under surveillance by ATG, a cell recycling process which degrades and removes damaged mitochondria implicated in CBMP. Inadequate CP/ATG results in compromised MQC, MB, and metabolic stress. Redmann et al. (2018) described a workflow to assess morphology, function, mtDNA, protein denaturation, metabolism, and CP/ATG for the assessment of MQC. They tested a protocol to studies when cell numbers are limited to explore the CB life cycle where MQC is compromised. The clinically significant mitochondrial disorders involving CBMP are illustrated in Fig. 2.

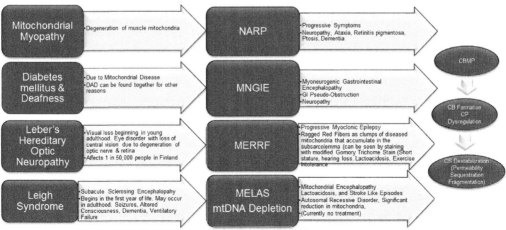

Friedreich's ataxia affects the mitochondria but is not associated with mitochondrial proteins

Figure 2

Organelle Zones in Mitochondria and CBMP

Recent developments in molecular imaging have identified organelle functions (Shimizu 2018). Most of these functions are performed in limited areas within organelles classified as 'zones'. In mitochondria, we find the apoptosis zone, necrosis zone, ATG zone, mitochondrial-derived vesicle budding zone, and innate immunity zone. The membrane contact site between mitochondria and the ER, referred to as MAM, is also a zone for lipid transfer, sterol exchange, Ca^{2+} transfer, CP, ATG, and NDDs. I have introduced CP-dependent the CS regulatory (CPR) zone, which determines the cell survival or CBMP in response to DPCI. Hence, the elucidation of organelle zones is essential to better understand mitochondrial functions in health and disease (Fig. 3).

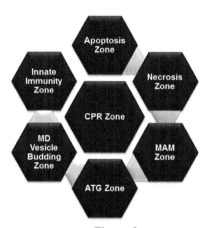

Figure 3

Development in Hymenoptera

Gonçalves et al. (2018) verified cellular events of the Malpighian tubule renewal during the metamorphosis of Hymenoptera (honeybee) to determine cell remodeling, and their roles in the excretory activity. The cells of the larval Malpighian tubules degenerate by apoptosis and ATG, and the new Malpighian tubules are formed by cell proliferation. The cellular remodeling occurred from dark-brown-eyed pupae, indicating the onset of excretion in Malpighian tubules. In adult forager workers, there were two cell types: one with an abundance of mitochondria, vacuoles, microvilli, and a narrow basal labyrinth for urine production, and the other with a dilated basal labyrinth, long microvilli, and the absence of sphero-crystals. This highlighted their role in urine re-absorption. During metamorphosis, the tubules remained non-functional until the light-brown-eyed pupae were formed. Hence, this organism is highly vulnerable to CBMP following toxic exposure during early pupal stages.

Triple "I" Hypothesis

The ICD following DPCI-induced free radical injury is transcriptionally and translationally regulated by the triple "I" hypothesis, comprising: (i) identify (ii) inform, and (iii) isolate or eliminate. The nonfunctional and/or degenerated mitochondria are first *identified* by the mitochondrial network. This event is *informed/transmitted* to other normally functioning mitochondria at the mtDNA and nDNA levels. The nDNA enhances genes involved in

CB formation and CP induction for the *isolation/elimination* of unhealthy and/or nonfunctional CBs by ATP-driven mitochondrial regeneration, rejuvenation, repair, or replacement to sustain IMD and ICD for NCF. Although nonfunctional or damaged mitochondria involved in CB formation have a similar chemical composition, these remain nonfunctional yet highly toxic; hence, they participate in CBMP, whereas the remaining functional mitochondria establish new network to sustain MQC. CB is subsequently Akt-ubiquinated and phagocytosed by ATP-driven lysosomal-dependent CP and eliminated by exocytosis. These molecular events are compromised in NDDs, CVDs, MDR malignancies, chronic infections, and aging due to CBMP. Hence, the intervention to regulate triple "I" will go a long way in the theranostic management of chronic MDR diseases.

Transcriptional Regulation of CSexoR and CSendoR

The rate of CS exocytosis (CSexoR) and CS endocytosis (CSendoR) are highly intricate energy-driven transcriptional events. The CS is formed when CB is Akt-ubiquinated, phagocytosed, and hydrolyzed by the lysosomes. Since CS is a structurally labile organelle containing toxic mitochondrial metabolites, it is efficiently exocytosed to sustain ICD. The rate of CS exocytosis is retarded in chronic MDR diseases and aging, which enhances ICT, whereas the rate of CS endocytosis is accelerated in MDR malignancies to induce cell transformation and hyper-proliferation. The severity of illness, invasiveness, and/or metastasis are governed by the cancer- stem-cell-specific CSendoR. Hence, novel CPTs can be developed to regulate CSexoR and CSendoR to accomplish the TSE-EBPT of chronic MDR diseases.

CB Formation and CP Induction (Hypothesis)

The Purkinje neurons of the developing rat cerebellar cortex possess a highly susceptible network of 1000 mitochondria. In response to DPCI, a considerable fraction of them are destroyed. A mitochondrion loses contact from its network when it becomes either nonfunctional, undesirable, or degenerated. Hence, mitochondrial degeneration is not simply a random or uncontrolled event, because fragmentation of even a single mitochondrion is sufficient to destroy the other cellular organelles (including normal mitochondria, ER membranes, ribosomes, peroxisomes, Golgi bodies, lysosomes, CS, and nucleus). Its like having a patient with a viral flu or infection where 1000 persons are sitting in a hall. If this patient sneezes just once, all of them will be infected. However, this does not occur when the mitochondria are destroyed during toxic, nutritional, or environmental insult. Depending on the intensity and frequency of RONS and $[Ca^{2+}]_m$, the mitochondria initially alter their shape, become elongated, flask-like, and/or swollen with inclusions due to the denaturation of labile proteins. Hence, before fragmentation, the nonfunctional and/or degenerating mitochondrial membranes (along with attached ER membranes) fuse to form pleomorphic electron-dense multi-lamellar stacks (identified as CBs) to contain toxic metabolites. These CBs are subsequently Akt-ubiquinated and recognized by the lysosomes for CP. Thus, CB formation and CP induction are the most economical, fundamental, and highly efficient mechanisms of ICD and MQC to prevent disease progression.

Several rationales for CB formation and CP induction in response to DPCI in the most vulnerable cell can be proposed: (i) The mitochondrial membranes and non-helical, GC-rich, intron-less mtDNA are most susceptible to DPCI-induced free radical injury/insult as compared to other intracellular organelles; (ii) mitochondrial stress generates deleterious RONS, which induce ERS to cause further degenerative changes; (iii) ATP requirements are elevated during DPCI as a mechanism of ICD and MQC; (iv) free radicals (OH, NO) synthesis is increased as a byproduct of O/P in the ETC during RONS stress; (v) free radicals induce the lipid peroxidation of PUFA and omega-3 fatty acids to cause the structural and functional breakdown of mitochondrial membranes; (vi) CB formation occurs as an immediate and early response to prevent the dissemination of toxic metabolites from the degenerating mitochondria; (vii) CB formation prevents the dissemination of 18 kDa proteins (TSPO), MAOs, XOs, HOs, acetyl choline esterase, alkaline phosphatase, TRPCs, 8-OH, 2dG, 2, 3 dihydroxy nonenal, acetate, lactate, acetone, ammonia, H_2O_2, Ca^{2+} and, particularly Cyt-C (which is loosely and non-covalently attached within the IMM and is readily delocalized during free radical attack); (viii) formation of CBs restricts the uncontrolled dissemination of toxic metabolites to sustain ICD during the acute phase, (ix) CB is recognized as a nonfunctional inclusion during the chronic phase and hence, it is Akt-ubiquinated and eliminated by lysosomal-dependent ATP-driven CP; (x) transcriptionally as well as translationally-regulated CP is involved in ICD, MQC, and NCF, whereas dysregulated CP is involved in chronic MDR diseases; (xi) CB formation in response to DPCI and its phagocytosis through lysosomal-dependent ATP-driven process is the most efficient and economical mechanism of the elimination of nonfunctional and degenerating mitochondria, because at any given time the mitochondrial mass remains significantly high compared to lysosomes, which are increased in response to DPCI. Moreover, the Akt-ubiquitination of CB, associated ER membranes, and macromolecules is highly crucial for phagocytosis, which can occur more efficiently through CP as compared to the elimination of randomly scattered degenerated mitochondria or ER membranes during this process. The mitochondrial size may vary from 0.5 μm to 10 μm, whereas a lysosomal size varies from 0.25 μm to 2.5 μm, rendering them incapable of complete phagocytosis during nutritional stress, when mitochondria fragmentation is increased and regeneration is compromised due to the downregulation of Drp-1 and Mfns. Hence, CB formation during the acute phase is an early attempt to prevent the contamination of the healthy mitochondrial network and other organelles. During aging, CBMP is augmented due to the downregulation of CP, and the compromised synthesis of lysosomal enzymes and MQC, rendering a cell highly susceptible to LSDs (observed in the form of lipofuscin granules). Thus, MQC, IMD, ICD, and LQC are highly crucial events for the normal growth, proliferation, differentiation, development, and survival of a cell. Efficient CP is highly crucial to control brain regional cybernetics at the synaptic terminals to release neurotransmitters through CP regulation and CS stabilization. These intricate events at the synaptic terminals are impaired in drug addiction (smoking, alcoholism), diabetes, AD, and

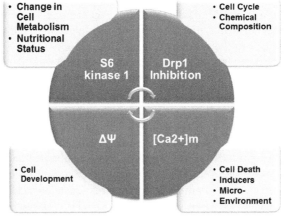

Figure 4

aging, which induce MCI during the acute phase and early morbidity and mortality during the chronic phase of the disease progression.

CB Pleomorphism

Cellular processes, including apoptosis/necrosis, depend on changes in mitochondrial shape, size, organization, geometry, topography, and ultrastructure. The ultrastructural phenotype of CB depends on the intensity and frequency of the free radical attack. CB may exist in numerous pleomorphic forms depending on the composition of mitochondrial membranes, the nature of physicochemical injury, and whether Ca^{+2} translocated from the ER membranes to mitochondria. A CB may exist as a LD, a loose lamellar, dense-lamellar, quasi-crystalline, or pure crystalline ultrastructure, depending on its chemical composition, with differential susceptibility to Akt-ubiquitination and ATP-driven lysosomal-dependent CP to prevent or enhance CBMP. CB pleomorphism was observed in developing UN rat cerebellar Purkinje neurons as these are highly vulnerable and have the maximum number of mitochondria. As Purkinje neurons develop postnatally, a minor physicochemical insult may readily trigger CBMP involving nucleolar AgNOR inactivation and the inhibition of the protein-synthesizing machinery to determine the structural and functional integrity of their membranes. CB pleomorphism occurs depending on the level and nature of proteins and lipids in these inclusions. All immature or developmentally defective mitochondria devoid of cristae condense to participate in CB formation during nutritional stress. CB remains loosely packed if there is inadequate or no protein in the mitochondria. Some of the mitochondria lose their cristae and contain dense inclusions as denatured proteins. Thus, CB pleomorphism is governed by the level of lipoproteins and glycoproteins, intensity and frequency of RONS, $[Ca^{2+}]_i$, antioxidants, drug exposure, inducers, and microenvironment. Their phagocytosis by lysosomal enzymes depends on the levels of soluble and insoluble proteins. Denatured proteins remain un-hydrolyzed and form a major bulk of intra-neuronal inclusions. For example, the conformational change of Prion proteins from an α-helical structure to the β-pleated sheets is involved in the spongiform leukoencephalopathies, dementia, and sudden death.

Usually, a mature CB appears as electron-dense, penta or heptalemallar stack of fragmented membranes to contain and prevent the dissemination of toxic metabolites or microbial toxins. We may have the following pleomorphic forms: (i) electron-dense LD, (ii) loosely-packed multi-tubular structure, (iii) loosely-packed multi-tubular lamellar stack, (iv) electron-dense penta or hepta-lamellar stack, and (v) electron-dense multi-lamellar stack. CB appears as LD, when it is completely devoid of proteins (which provide structural and functional stability to the plasma membranes) and as a loosely-packed multi-tubular structure, when the mtDNA is downregulated to compromise the synthesis of 34 proteins for the formation of cristae and enzymes of the ETC in addition to >1300 proteins encoded by the nDNA. A loosely-packed-tubular CB is formed from immature and defective mitochondria devoid of cristae and ETC. These inclusions are incapable of O/P and compromise the MB. A CB exists as a loosely packed multi-lamellar stack when some of the mitochondria are elongated to form tube or flask-like structures. Ligia et al. (2011) showed that mitochondrial morphology determines the cellular response to macroATG. When ATG is triggered, mitochondria elongate. During starvation, cAMP is increased to activate protein kinase A (PKA), which phosphorylates Drp-1, leading to mitochondrial fusion and CB formation. Elongated mitochondria are spared from CB/ATG degradation, possess more cristae, increased dimerization and ATP synthase, and ATP synthesis. When elongation is genetically or pharmacologically blocked, mitochondria consume excessive ATP, augmenting starvation-induced death. Thus, changes in mitochondrial morphology determine the fate of the cell during CP/ATG. Electron-dense inclusions were noticed in the defective mitochondria due to protein denaturation (Sharma 1984; Sharma et al 1986; Sharma et al 1987). A loosely packed multilamellar CB (*cis-form*) was transformed to condense-packed electron-dense penta or hepta-lamellar structure (*Trans form*) to contain toxic metabolites and prevent their dissemination in the cytoplasm (Sharma 1984). CB may exist as electron-dense multi-lamellar (>20) stacks of degenerated membranes during the chronic phase of disease progression. Nemani et al. (2018) reported that mitochondria undergo $[Ca^{2+}]_i$-induced shape change that is distinct from fission and swelling. Mitochondria change their shape depending on $[Ca^{2+}]_c$ and $[Ca^{2+}]_m$ to sustain their bioenergetics. Dysregulated $[Ca^{2+}]_c$ causes $[Ca^{2+}]_m$ overload, induces permeability transition pore, and cell death. Ablation of MCU-mediated Ca^{2+} uptake increases $[Ca^{2+}]_c$ and fails to prevent stress-induced cell death. $[Ca^{2+}]_c$ elevation is essential for the mitochondrial shape transition (MiST), which is mediated by the protein Miro1 through its EF-hand domain. Ca^{2+}-dependent disruption of Miro1/KIF5B/tubulin complex is determined by the Miro1 EF1 domain. Hence, Miro1-dependent MiST is essential for CP, and is attenuated in Miro1 EF1 mutants, suggesting that the cytosolic Ca^{2+} sensor determines Ca^{2+} signals as MiST. The factors affecting CB pleomorphism are presented in Fig. 4.

CP Dysregulation Triggers CBMP

CP dysregulation was induced in developing postnatal rats by nutritional deprivation, which triggered mitochondrial remodeling, causing CB formation, CP dysregulation, and CBMP. The mitochondria were elongated and enlarged due to a lack of energy (ATP) to execute fission. Intra-mitochondrial dense inclusions were noticed in these remodeled mitochondria within 10 days of postnatal undernutrition due to CMB. A progressive degeneration was characterized by tube and flask-like mitochondria in the intrauterine Domoic acid (IUD)-exposed mice hippocampal CA-3 and dentate gurus regions in vivo, and in the mitochondrial genome knock out (RhO_{mgko}) primary cortical and hippocampal mouse cultured neurons *in vitro*. DPCI induced inhibition in the pluripotency of germinal pluripotent stem cells to cause congenital anomalies. The membrane fragments were loosely packed as observed in 10–20 days developing postnatal UN rats. The multi-lamellar stacks were condense-packed and remained persistent even after nutritional rehabilitation. The aggregation of mature CBs ran concomitantly with caspase-3 activation and PARP cleavage to cause time-dependent apoptosis. Within the first 10–20 days, efficient CP was noticed, whereas 30 days of severe undernutrition induced lysosomal-resistant CB to participate in CBMP and induce apoptotsis followed by necrotic cell death as confirmed by an increase in inter-nucleosomal DNA fragmentation and sub-G1 peak (Fig. 5).

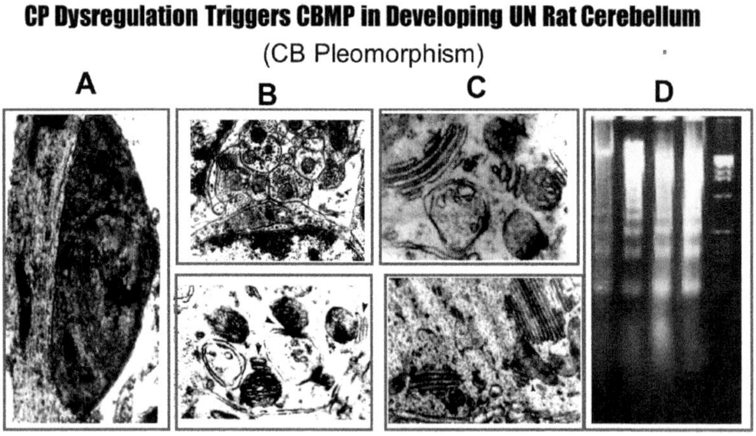

CP Dysregulation Triggers CBMP in Developing UN Rat Cerebellum
(CB Pleomorphism)

Figure 5

A pictorial diagram of CBMP is illustrated in Fig. 6.

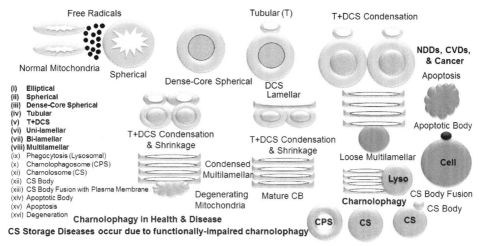

Figure 6

The release of toxic CS metabolites induced the dysfunction of other organelles including the nucleus, ER, peroxisomes, and Golgi body to cause ubiquitination and eventually generalized ATG, suggesting that CP regulates generalized ATG as illustrated in Fig. 7.

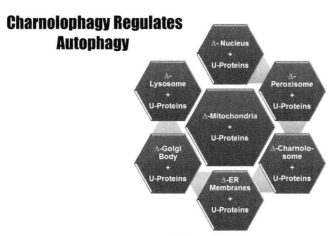

Figure 7

Recently, Tran et al. (2018) discovered that S6 kinase 1 (S6K1) contributes to mitochondrial dynamics, homeostasis, and function. Mouse embryo fibroblasts lacking S6K1 (S6K1-KO MEFs) exhibited fragmented mitochondria and an increase of Drp-1 and its active form, pS616, in both whole cell extracts and mitochondrial fractions. There was no evidence of ATG or MTG in the S6K1 depleted cells. Glycolysis and mitochondrial respiratory activity were higher in the S6K1-KO MEFs, whereas ATP synthesis remained unaltered. The inhibition of Drp-1 by Mdivi1 (Drp-1 inhibitor) induced ATP production and $\Delta\Psi$ collapse. The depletion of S6K1 increased Drp-1-mediated fission, leading to enhanced glycolysis. The fission form of mitochondria compromised ATP synthesis and $\Delta\Psi$, suggesting a crucial role of S6K1 in mitochondria remodeling (MR) and energy metabolism by modulating O/P. The sequential events of CBMP are presented in Table 1.

Table 1   Different Stages of CBMP

Stage	Clinical Condition	Mitochondrial Phenotype	Consequence
1.	Normal	Elliptical	NCF, ICD
2.	Minor PCM and/or other stress	Spherical	$\Delta\Psi$ Collapse, Mega-pore Formation, (*Reversible*) [ICD]
3.	Moderate PCM and/or other stress	Elongated	Increased ROS, Reduced O/P & ATP (*Reversible*) [ICD]
4.	Severe PCM and/or other stress	Loose lamellar Stack	CMB, Neuronal Dysfunction (CP) & MTS, Akt-Ubiquitination (*Irreversible*) [ICD]
5.	Highly severe PCM and/or other stress	Dense lamellar Stack	Progressive NDDs, MTS, & ERS (CBMP) Loss of MAMs, LAMPs & mitochondrial network, Drp-1 induction, Opa-1 & Mfn (1,2) inhibition, (*Irreversible*) [ICT]
6.	Highly severe PCM and DPCI	Oil Drop Formation	Developmental Charnolopathies (MTS, ERS, & LS) (*Irreversible*) [ICT]

PCM: Protein calorie malnutrition, DPCI: Diverse physicochemical injury/insult, MTS: Mitochondrial stress, ERS: ER stress, MAMs: Mitochondrial-associated membranes, LAMPs: Lysosome-associated membrane proteins, LS: Lysosomal stress, ICD: Intracellular detoxification, ICT: Intracellular toxicity. The sequential events in CP and CBMP under normal and pathological conditions are presented in Table 2.

Table 2   The Sequential Events in CP and CBMP under Normal and Pathological Conditions

Normal:M-PFA-**MR**-SFA-**MF**-TFA-**CB**-Lyso/ATP-**CP**-CPS-CS-**CSexo**-IMD/ICD-**NCF**
Path:CB--QFA---**CSD**--CSP-CSS-CSF--Toxins Rel-PARP/Casp--**CBMP**-Apopt- **MDR Dis**

M: Mitochondria; PFA: Primary free radical attack; MR: Mitochondrial remodeling; SFA: Secondary free radical attack; MF: Mitochondrial fragmentation; TFA: Tertiary free radical attack; CB: Charnoly body; Lyso: Lysosomes; ATP: Adenosine triphosphate; CP: Charnolophagy; CPS: Charnolophagosome; CS: Charnolosome; CSexo: Charnolosome exocytosis; IMD: Intramitochondrial detoxification; ICD: Intracellular detoxification: NCF: NCF; QFA: Quaternary free radical attack; CSD: Charnolosome detoxification; CSP: CS permeabilization; CSS: Charnolosome sequestration; CSF: Charnolosome fragmentation; Rel: Release; PARP: Poly (ADP) robosyl polymerase; Casp: Caspases; CBMP: Charnoly body molecular pathogenesis; APO: Apoptosis; MDR Dis: Multidrug resistant diseases. CBMP in response to DPCI in the most vulnerable cell is presented in Fig. 8.

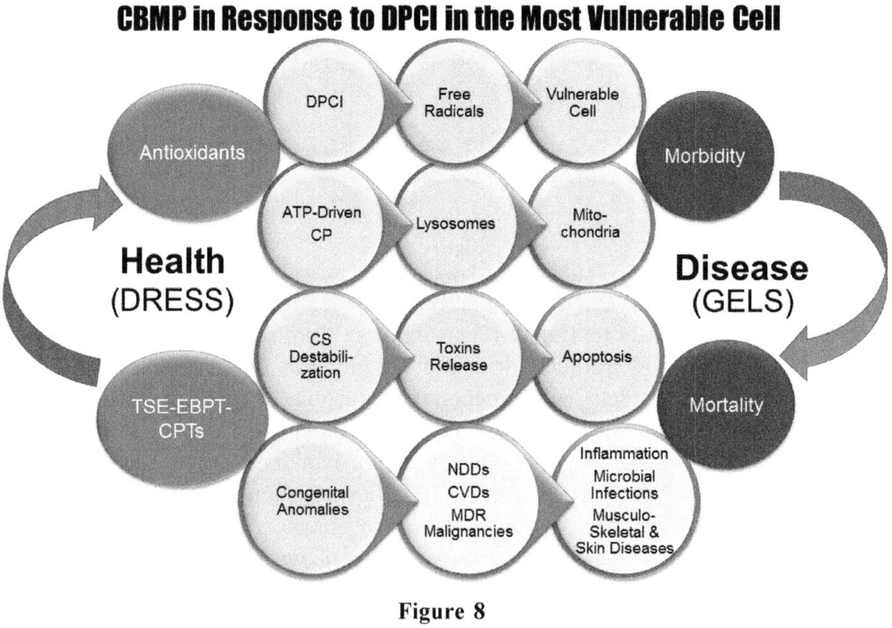

CBMP in Response to DPCI in the Most Vulnerable Cell

Figure 8

Organ and Disease-Specific Induction, Expression, Inhibition, and Elimination of CB

CP can occur in both healthy and diseased individuals as a mechanism of ICD. The induction, expression, inhibition, and elimination of CB occurs in a disease-specific spatiotemporal manner. Many cells in our body are eliminated and replaced every day by CB formation and CP induction. During brain development, CB formation as well elimination is highly efficient; that is why children learn as well as forget frequently as compared to the slow learning and forgetting process of adults. As a function of aging, lysosomal enzymes involved in CP are reduced along with CMB, which delays or impairs CP. The delayed clearance of CB is responsible for the accumulation of protein aggregates such as amyloid-β (1–42) plaques in AD, Lewy bodies in PD, SOD in ALS, huntingtin in HD, fradrictin in Fredrick ataxia, and prion proteins in Crufeldt-Jacob's disease. The accumulation of protein aggregates occurs due to overwhelming mitochondrial degeneration while the accumulation of pleomorphic CB in the perinuclear region impairs the normal transcriptional and translational activity of genes and miRNA involved in regulating protein synthesis and nucleocytoplasmic interactions. The accumulation of CB and/or destabilized CS due to defective CP in the dendritic region inhibits neuritogenesis at the junction of the axon hillock. This inhibits the normal axoplasmic transport of enzymes, proteins, neurotransmitters, hormones, growth factors, neurotrophic factors such as IGF-1, BDNF, and NGF to cause delayed sensorimotor learning in the synaptic region and induces impaired transmission to cause defective neurocybernetics and cognitive performance such as learning, intelligence, memory, and behavioral deficits in progressive NDDs and aging. (*Sequence of CBMP: DPCI-Free Radicals-MRS-Akt-Ubi-Lysosome Induction-CBMP-ERS-ATG-CVDs, NDDs, Cancer*).

CB Formation and CP Induction

DPCI-induced free radical injury destroys the most susceptible mitochondria from a cell. Mitochondria proliferate and degenerate exponentially; hence, they require spatiotemporally-efficient QC mechanisms through CP regulation for ICD. CBMP is triggered by uncontrolled CB formation, CP dysregulation, and CS destabilization in MDR diseases (particularly in aging) when the MQC mechanisms are compromised and lysosomal enzymes are inactivated to execute efficient CP. All mitochondria are not destroyed simultaneously. If it happens, the cell will undergo immediate apoptosis and/or necrosis. Hence, CB formation is an immediate and early event of MQC, IMD, and ICD, restricting the dissemination of toxic metabolites and infectious pathogens. In highly invasive MDR malignancies, cell proliferation, apoptosis, necrosis, inflammation, CP, and ATG occur simultaneously. These simultaneous events render resistance to conventional chemotherapy and pose a significant challenge in their radical elimination. Since mitochondrial membranes, mtDNA, and mtmiRNAs are the most vulnerable to the deleterious attack of free radicals and their own metabolites, these are sacrificed to protect nDNA for cell survival. Since CP is an ATP-driven lysosomal-dependent process, we need to have constant regeneration, rejuvenation, repair, and QC of mitochondria for NCF. Particularly, we need structurally and functionally intact coronary arteries for normal myocardial function which is impaired in aging due to increased ICT and pro-inflammatory cytokines, resulting in early morbidity and mortality. Depending on the spatiotemporal intensity and frequency of DPCI; CP is triggered as an immediate and early event of ICD, whereas CS destabilization (permeabilization, sequestration, and fragmentation) and CBMP (CMB, lysosomal dysfunction, CP dysregulation, inflammasome activation, apoptosis, and necrosis), and CS endocytosis/exocytosis occur in chronic MDR diseases. Hence, CP regulation induces MQC, ERQC, and LQC to inhibit MTS, ERS, and LS for NCF.

CB Formation for NCF

CB accumulation at the junction of the axon hillock may impair the axoplasmic transport of ions, neurotransmitters, neurotropic factors, and enzymes at the synaptic terminals. Therefore, drugs may be developed to inhibit CB formation in NDDs and CVDs (Sharma and Ebadi 2014a,b,c). The nonspecific induction of CB in hyper-proliferating cells causes alopecia, myelosuppression, GIT symptoms, cardiovascular toxicity, and infertility during cancer chemotherapy. Hence, drugs may be developed to induce cancer stem cell-specific CB formation to cure MDR malignancies and chronic infections. The natural abundance of mitochondria and the genetic susceptibility of mtDNA qualify CB as an early, unique, and sensitive universal biomarker of theranostic significance. Nutritional rehabilitation, physiological zinc supplementation, and/or metallothioneins (MTs) prevent CB formation, particularly during early neuronal development and aging so that a healthy young life and aging may be enjoyed. By contrast, unhealthy lifestyle choices such as alcohol intake, cigarette smoking, a high-fat and salt-rich diet, or malnutrition because of ignorance and poverty may cause early morbidity and mortality due to the induction of CBMP. MTs can be induced by diet-restriction and moderate exercise to circumvent free radical overproduction, prevent CB formation, and progressive NDDs, including chronic drug addiction. Hence, drugs may be targeted to inhibit CB formation and regulate CP to prevent or treat NDDs and CVDs, and enhance cancer-stem-cell-specific CB formation for the eradication of MDR malignancies. Mitochondrial dysfunction plays a crucial role in the CP/ATG cascade due to $\Delta\Psi$ collapse. The interaction of the triphenylphosphonium (TPP)-based cation, 10-(6′-ubiquinonyl) decyltriphenylphosphonium, (MitoQ) with HepG2 cells suggests that it is adsorbed on the IMM with its cationic moiety, augmenting positive charge and "pseudo-$\Delta\Psi$," which inhibits ATP synthase. Lyamzaev et al. (2018) emphasized that "pseudo-$\Delta\Psi$" contradicts electrophoretic displacements of cations through phospholipid membranes. They provided evidence that TPP-cations dissipate $\Delta\Psi$ in HepG2 cells and that the ATG induction correlated with the uncoupling of O/P. Hence, O/P uncoupling through mitochondrial penetrating cations may have theranostic significance in MDR malignancies.

CP and CS Membrane Destabilization

Transcriptionally regulated CP promotes CS stabilization and CS exocytosis; whereas transcriptionally dysregulated CP promotes ICT due to CS destabilization to induce NDDs, CVDs, and MDR malignancies. The CS membrane is destabilized in response to free radical-induced DPCI in the most vulnerable cell. There are primarily three types of CS destabilizations depending on the frequency and intensity of free radical attack: (a) CS membrane permeabilization (CSMP), (b) CS membrane sequestration (CSMS), and (c) CS membrane fragmentation (CSMF). A primary free radical attack induces CSMP; a secondary free radical attack induces CSMS; whereas, a tertiary free radical attack induces CSMF. CSMP at the synaptic terminal impairs neurotransmission to cause MCI due to defective brain regional neurocybernetics, represented by learning, intelligence, memory, and behavior deficits; CSMS induces morbidity; whereas CSMF induces mortality. CS destabilization is augmented by genetic defects, microbial infections, and drugs of abuse (including tobacco and alcohol). However, endogenous and exogenous antioxidants stabilize CS to prevent early morbidity and mortality.

Stem Cells as CP Regulators

CP, the process by which damaged mitochondria undergo ATG, has emerged as a key regulator of cell metabolism. Recently, I described the theranostic potential of stem cells as CB inhibitors, CP regulators, CS stabilizers, CS exocytosis enhancers for the TSE-EBPT of chronic MDR diseases (Sharma 2019). ATG is a catabolic pathway by which cellular components are delivered to the lysosome for degradation and recycling as a repair mechanism; it is also involved in cell remodeling during development and differentiation. Recent studies revealed the role of CP and ATG in the regulation of stem cells during embryonic and postnatal development, tissue homeostasis, and repair in adult life. Boya et al. (2018) focused on the QC, MR, and metabolic functions of ATG during activation, self-renewal, and differentiation of embryonic, adult, and cancer stem cells. I introduced "CP" in relation to a group of disorders in which mutations in mitochondrial proteins or their molecular partners lead to deleterious consequences in brain development, particularly fetal alcohol syndrome and Zika virus-induced microcephaly. Similarly, the Golgi apparatus (GA) is involved in lipid biosynthesis, membrane secretion, post-translational processing, trafficking of proteins, and control of mitosis, cell polarity, migration, and morphogenesis, and stress responses including CP, ATG, and apoptosis. Mutations in GA proteins can lead to syndromes with multisystem involvement. >40% of the GA-related genes associated with disease affect the central or peripheral nervous system, emphasizing its significance for NCF. Rasika et al. (2018) proposed the term "Golgipathies" to describe a group of disorders in which mutations in GA proteins lead to impaired brain development, particularly microcephaly, white-matter defects, and intellectual disability. They included other disorders whose symptoms may be indicative of altered neurodevelopment, from neurogenesis to neuronal migration and hypothalamo-pituitary-adrenal axis has secretory function for the maturation of post mitotic neurons and myelin.

CP: A Double-Edged Sword?

Although CP is an acute response to DPCI and has a pro-survival role, it may be implicated in CS destabilization and CBMP during the chronic phase of disease progression. CP eradicates DPCI-mediated free radical-induced CB through ATG by regulating kinases and phosphatases-linked signal transduction at the transcriptional and translation level during the acute phase. If a cell fails to execute aforementioned housekeeping events, CBMP is triggered to cause generalized ATG in MDR diseases due to the uncontrolled release of toxic metabolites from the destabilized CS, causing concomitant inflammation, apoptosis, and necrosis. In this defensive process, even normal functioning cells, mitochondria, and other organelles may be destroyed when a generalized ATG is triggered. Hence, CP does not seem to be a double-edged sword. In fact, it is a primary molecular event to prevent or inhibit disease development and toxic metabolites, pro-inflammatory cytokines, microbial pathogens, and malignant transformation. Hence, CP can be employed as the most sensitive mitochondrially-targeted biomarker for the TSE-EBPT of MDR diseases, assessment of disease prognosis, environmental protection, biosafety of NPs, and almost all aspects of health and disease.

IMD vs ICD

IMD is maintained by endogenously synthesized antioxidants by scavenging free radicals generated as a byproduct of O/P in the ETC. Structurally and functionally intact mitochondria synthesize ATP through O/P, the TCA cycle, and the β oxidation of fatty acids. The energy requirements are elevated during DPCI, resulting in free radical overproduction compromising IMD. Exogenously administered natural or synthetic antioxidants ameliorate mitochondrial redox stress to sustain IMD. However, during chronic exposure to free radicals, PUFA-rich membranes and mtDNA are downregulated to trigger CBMP. Although CB is recognized as a nonfunctional inclusion, it is an immediate and early attempt to contain toxic mitochondrial metabolites to prevent the dissemination of toxic metabolites and protect remaining mitochondrial network during intracellular housekeeping. The nonfunctional degenerating mitochondria are pulled out of the functional mitochondrial network. CB is Akt-ubiquinated and recognized by the lysosomes for ATP-driven phagocytosis to induce CP and sustain ICD. Both IMD as well as ICD are highly crucial to sustain intracellular homeostasis to prevent MR, CS destabilization, and CBMP during RONS-mediated MTS, ERS, and LS.

Alpha-Synuclein (α-Syn) and CBMP

Alpha-Synuclein (α-Syn) controls mitochondrial function during physiological and pathological conditions. Impaired CP/ATG, CMB, $[Ca^{2+}]_i$ dyshomeostasis, and alteration in mitochondrial morphology involving CBMP are involved in PD progression. Vicario et al. (2018) focused on the role of α-Syn within mitochondria and its targets for PD theranostics. α-Syn is the major component of amyloid fibrils in Lewy bodies.The mutations and/or duplication/triplication in its gene cause familial autosomal dominant PD. A fraction of α-Syn is localized to mitochondria upon specific stimuli, highlighting its mechanism of action. Cyt-C release, $[Ca^{2+}]_i$ homeostasis, $\Delta\Psi$ control, and ATP synthesis are influenced by α-Syn. α-Syn localization within mitochondria may account for its aggregation, making the α-Syn-mitochondrial relationship highly significant to our understanding of PD pathogenesis. I discovered α-Syn index as a function of MPP$^+$-induced mitochondrial and ERS involving CB formation and CBMP and its inhibition with a specific MAO-B inhibitor, Selegiline, in cultured human DAergic (SK-N-SH) cells (Sharma et al. 2003). α-Syn toxicity was associated with cell cycle alterations, DNA-damage responses (DDR), and the deregulation of ATG. Sampaio-Marques et al. (2019) demonstrated that α-Syn expression induces Ras2-dependent growth signaling, cell cycle re-entry, DDR activation, and degradation of ribonucleotide reductase 1 (Rnr1) for the dNTP synthesis which leads to cell death and aging; it is abrogated by deleting RAS2, inhibiting DDR or ATG, or overexpressing RNR1 in a yeast model. α-Syn expression in H4 neuroglioma cells induced cell cycle re-entry and S-phase arrest, ATG, and the downregulation of RRM1, RNR1, and the inhibition of the ATG degradation of RRM1-rescued cell death. These findings represented a model of α-Syn toxicity that has implications for understanding α-synucleinopathies and other age-related NDDs. Various neurodegenetative charnolopathies are induced in response to the oxidative and nitrative stress of ONOO$^-$ ions which cause the α-Syn Index to participate in CBMP-induced NDDs such as PD, AD, and ALS.

Nomenclature of Organelle-specific ATG

Organelle-specific ATG is currently the most interesting and highly fascinating area in the biomedical field. Knowledge and wisdom regarding mitochondria-specific ATG (CP) is expanding due to the remarkable evolution of disease- and organ-specific DNA recombinant, omics, and molecular imaging technologies. Because CP is involved in almost all aspects of acute and chronic diseases, any physiological and/or pharmacological intervention in its regulation will go a long way towards the clinical management of chronic MDR diseases. Recently, several investigators assigned different names to further expand our knowledge and wisdom: (i) organelle-specific ATG, (ii) mitochondrial ATG, (iii) mitochondrial-specific ATG, (iv) nonfunctional mitochondrial ATG, (v) degenerated mitochondrial ATG, (vi) macro ATG, (vii) bulk ATG, (viii) CP, (ix) mito-lyso-ATG, (x) aggrephagy, (xi) lyso-apoptophagy, (xii) MTG, and (xiii) CB-autophagy. When we do not know the exact nature and origin of ATG cargo, it is immaterial whether we use the term ATG or aggrephagy. However, CP is a CB-specific ATG; hence, it needs biochemical, EM, and fluorescence microscopic authentication as we now have CP-specific fluorochromes and proteomic and genomic biomarkers to distinguish CB, CP, and CS to assess their structural and functional stability. Irrespective of the terminology used to describe ATG, the entire concept revolves around the mitochondria, ER, lysosomes, and their QC. Mitochondrial membranes, mtDNA, mtmiRNA, peroxysomes, and nDNA are promising family members of CP, implicated in highly intricate life and death decisions in response to DPCI. This edition offers a systematic description of CP to accomplish the TSE-EBPT of chronic MDR diseases. I sincerely hope that it will enhance the existing knowledge and wisdom on MQC and ICD for NCF. The nomenclature of ATG is presented in Fig. 9.

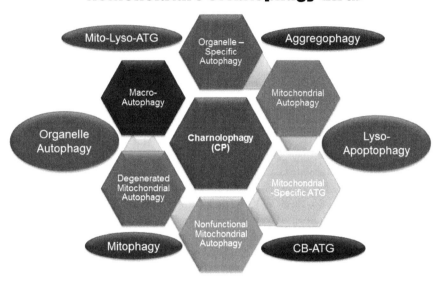

Figure 9

CP/ATG is a highly regulated, evolutionary-conserved, transcriptionally as well as translationally regulated process which serves as a defense mechanism and eliminates microorganisms from the host cell. CP may or may not be associated with apoptosis if it occurs soon after DPCI; however, delayed or defective CP is accompanied with CBMP, implicated in apoptosis/necrosis and disease progression. As CP occurs earlier than generalized ATG as a mechanism of MQC and ICD for NCF, all biomarkers of ATG may not be present in a cell undergoing CP; however, all the CP biomarkers can be detected in a cell undergoing generalized ATG. A CP can be classified in three broad categories: (i) basal or physiological CP, (ii) delayed or metabolic CP, and (iii) defective or pathological CP. (i) Basal CP occurs in normal health as a mechanism of IMD and ICD; (ii) metabolic CP occurs during malnutrition and can be regulated by nutritional rehabilitation; (iii) defective CP occurs in chronic NDDs, CVDs, and MDR malignancies and requires novel DSST-TSE-EBPT-CPTs, in addition to endogenous and naturally available antioxidants as free radical scavengers. Some natural or synthetic antioxidants have poor solubility and reduced penetration through the BBB such as curcumin; hence, ROS-scavenging antioxidant-loaded NPs may be developed to improve their delivery in the CNS. Recently, Pan et al. (2019) proposed two types of CP/ATG, that is, (i) mild CP/ATG and (ii) excessive CP/ATG. Mild CP/ATG inhibits apoptosis, whereas excessive CP/ATG promotes apoptosis, based on their experiments on the anticancer effect of Se on HepG2 cells by regulating HMGB1 protein under hypoxia. The reduced HMGB1 outside the cell stimulates CP/ATG by inhibiting the Akt/mTOR axis, implicated in CP/ATG regulation.

Lysosomes and CP

Lysosomes are pivotal in regulating metabolism, endocytosis, CP, and ATG and are implicated in cancer. The lysosomal V-ATPase induces apoptosis and interferes with lipid metabolism in cancer. As a major hub for metabolic signaling pathways, lysosomes are multifunctional organelles with roles in plasma membrane repair, CP, ATG, MTG, nutrient sensing, and pathogen elimination. Lamming and Bar-Peled (2019) highlighted that the growth regulators (including mTOR) reside at the lysosomal surface to accomplish their key role in nutrient sensing and cellular homeostasis. The transcriptional networks required for lysosomal maintenance and function are now being unraveled and their connection to signaling pathways revealed. The catabolic and anabolic pathways that converge on the lysosome link this organelle with multiple facets of cellular functions. When these pathways are dysregulated, they underlie multiple diseases, and promote cellular and organismal aging. Thus, learning how lysosome-based signaling pathways function will elucidate their theranostic potential in chronic MDR diseases. A wide range of lysosomal storage diseases (LSDs) show defects in both CP/ATG and Ca^{2+} homeostasis. Liu et al. (2019) discussed the role of ER and lysosomal Ca^{2+} in CP/ATG regulation and Ca^{2+} homeostasis in Niemann-Pick type-C disease and Gaucher disease. Hence, Ca^{2+} serves as a key regulator of CP/ATG. The crosstalk between these pathways in the LSD pathogenesis is yet to be established. Further understanding of this relationship will reveal TSE-EBPT strategies for these devastating syndromes. The LSDs encompass a group of >50 inherited diseases characterized by the accumulation of lysosomal substrates. Two-thirds of patients experience neurological symptoms. Recently, Bajaj et al. (2019) focused on the pathways that regulate lysosomal biogenesis and their implications for LSDs and late-onset NDDs. Lysosomal proteins are synthesized in the ER and transported to the endo-lysosomes. Several receptors execute post-Golgi trafficking of lysosomal proteins. Some of them recognize their cargo proteins based on specific amino acid signatures, others based on a glycan in lysosomal proteins. All receptors involved in lysosomal biogenesis are under the control of TFEB, which coordinates the expression of lysosomal hydrolases, membrane proteins, and ATG proteins in response to lysosomal and nutritional stress. TFEB is primed for activation in LSDs but its function is impaired in NDDs like AD, PD, and ALS, because of the interactions that limit TFEB expression or activation. Thus, disrupted TFEB function is implicated in the pathogenesis of these diseases.

Studies in animal models have shown that exogenous expression of TFEB and its activation attenuate disease phenotypes. TFEB-mediated lysosomal biogenesis and function counteract the progression of these diseases. Leung et al. (2019) studied lysosomes using a DNA-based combination reporter that images pH and chloride simultaneously in the live cells. They called this technology two-ion measurement or 2-IM. It shows two lysosomal populations, one of which was absent in primary cells derived from patients with Niemann-Pick disease. When these cells were treated with therapeutics, the second population re-emerged. Hence, resolving lysosomes by 2-IM could enable researchers to understand the molecular mechanisms of LSDs, monitoring disease progression, and evaluating theranostic response. Imanikia et al. (2019) reported that expressing the UPRER transcription factor xbp-1s in the neurons or intestine of *C. elegans* extends lifespan, upregulates lysosomal genes and activates lysosomes in the intestine and their function is crucial for xbp-1s-mediated increase in proteostasis and longevity. They reported that the UPR of the ER (UPRER) is a mediator of secretory pathway homeostasis. The expression of the spliced and active form of the UPRER transcription factor XBP-1, XBP-1s triggered activation of the UPRER in the intestine through release of a secretory signal, leading to longevity. The expression of XBP-1s in the neurons or intestine improved proteostasis through clearance of toxic proteins. Intestine-specific RNA-seq analysis was conducted to identify genes upregulated when XBP-1s was expressed in neurons to demonstrate that neuronal XBP-1 increases the expression of genes involved in lysosomal function. Lysosomes in the intestine expressing neuronal XBP-1s were more acidic, with increased protease activity. Hence, the intestinal lysosomal function was necessary for increased lifespan suggesting that activation of the UPRER in the intestine can increase the lysosomal activity, leading to longevity and improved proteostasis in tissues. Sun et al. (2017) used the gene knockdown experimental model to discover the role of Numb, an endocytic adaptor protein, in regulating ATG. Numb depletion induced the accumulation of ATG vacuoles, as verified by RFP-LC3 staining combined with TEM. Numb depletion impaired ATG through inhibiting lysosomal enzymes (Cathepsin D, β-glucuronidase, and β-glucosidase) and elevated lysosomal pH and decreased glycosylated lysosomal-associated membrane proteins (LAMPs). Rab7 activity was inhibited in Numb-depleted cells, suggesting a novel function of Numb in ATG regulation. However, it remains unknown whether NUMB also regulates CP and CBMP. Mutations in the CLN7/MFSD8 gene encoding the lysosomal membrane protein CLN7 are causative of CLN7 disease, an inherited NDD that affects children. To gain insight into the mechanisms of CLN7 disease, von Kleist et al. (2019) developed an immortalized cell line based on cerebellar (Cb) granule neuron precursors isolated from $Cln7^{-/-}$ mice and demonstrated that Cln7-deficient neuron-derived Cb cells display an abnormal phenotype that includes increased size and defective outward movement of endosomes and lysosomes as well as impaired lysosomal exocytosis. Whereas $Cln7^{-/-}$ Cb cells were CP/ATG-competent, the loss of Cln7 enhanced cell death during chronic nutritional deprivation. The Reduced cell survival of Cln7-deficient cells was accompanied by impaired protein kinase B/Akt phosphorylation at Ser473 during long-term starvation, suggesting that the lysosomal transporter CLN7 is involved in their motility and plays an important role in neuronal survival during starvation. Bartel et al. (2019) performed an LC-MS/MS analysis to investigate lipid distribution in cells. Interfering with lysosomal function changed the composition and subcellular localization of triacylglycerids, accompanied by an upregulation of PGC1α and PPARα expression (major regulators of energy and the lipid metabolism). Cardiolipin was reduced, driving mitochondria into fission, accompanied by $\Delta\Psi$ collapse and reduction in O/P, resulting in ROS deregulation and the induction of mitochondria-driven apoptosis involving CBMP. Additionally, cells underwent a metabolic shift to glutamine dependency, correlated with the fission and sensitivity to lysosomal inhibition in Ras mutated cells. A study elucidated on the interaction between lysosomes, lipid metabolism, and mitochondrial function and provided an association between Ras mutations and sensitivity towards lysosomal inhibitors. Elliott et al. (2019) discovered that replication stress response (RSR) inhibitors were lethal while interacting with CQ in PDAC cells. CQ reduced nucleotide biosynthesis, induced replication stress, mitochondrial dysfunction, and depletion of aspartate, a precursor for nucleotide synthesis. Supplementation with aspartate rescued the phenotypes induced by CQ. The synergy of CQ and the RSR inhibitor VE-822 was validated in both the 2D and 3D cultures of PDAC cell lines, a heterotypic spheroid culture with cancer-associated fibroblasts, and in *in vivo* xenograft and syngeneic PDAC mouse models, indicating a co-dependency on functional lysosomes and RSR in PDAC and the translational potential of the combination of CQ and RSR inhibitors. In autoimmunity, as in other chronic inflammatory disorders, the metabolism of immune cells may be remodeled, impairing sensitive tolerance mechanisms. Bendorius et al. (2018) examined the distribution and therapeutic effects of the 21-mer peptide called P140, which demonstrated excellent immune response modulation in inflammation. They measured the effect of P140 and control peptide on isolated mitochondria, the distribution of peptides, and their influence on the ATG regulators in live cells. While P140 targeted macro- and chaperone-mediated ATG, it had little effect on CP. However, it suppressed NET release from neutrophils exposed to immobilized NET-anti-DNA IgG complexes, suggesting that in the mitochondrial-lysosome axis, the P140 peptide does not operate by affecting mitochondria directly.

It is known that mutation in LAMP-2 gene is associated with Danon disease, which leads to cardiomyopathy/heart failure. Chi et al. (2019) identified the LAMP-2 isoform B (LAMP-2B) for a lysosome fusion in cardiomyocytes (CMs) and reported that LAMP-2B functions independently of syntaxin 17 (STX17) for autophagosome-lysosome fusion in non-CMs. LAMP-2B interacted with CP/ATG-related 14 (ATG14) and vesicle-associated membrane protein 8 (VAMP8) through its C-terminal coiled coil domain (CCD) to promote CP/ATG fusion. CMs derived from hiPSC-CMs from Danon patients exhibited reduced co-localization between ATG14 and VAMP8, defects in CP/ATG fusion, as well as mitochondrial and contractile abnormalities. This phenotype was recapitulated by LAMP-2B knockout in non-Danon hiPSC-CMs. The gene correction of the LAMP-2 mutation rescued the Danon phenotype, suggesting STX17-independent CP/ATG fusion in CMs, as a mechanism for cardiomyopathy and targeting defective LAMP-2B-mediated CP/ATG for the TSE-EBPT of Danon disease.

CS Stability Determines Cellular Fate

DPCI-induced free radical overproduction increases ATP requirements in the mitochondria, which enhances free radical overproduction as a byproduct of O/P. The mitochondria either becomes nonfunctional and/or destroyed or fuses to trigger CB formation. CB is phagocytosed by lysosomes through ATP-driven Akt-ubiquitination. The resultant CPS is transformed to CS when the phagocytosed CB is hydrolyzed by the lysosomal enzymes. Usually, PFA does not induce CS destabilization. The CS is efficiently exocytosed for phase-1 and phase-2 metabolism in the liver through hepatoporal circulation. SFA causes CS destabilization during a disease's chronic phase to induce the release toxic metabolites and cause the degeneration of other intracellular organelles (that is, ER, Golgi, peroxysomes, ribosomes, nucleus etc.) resulting in generalized ATG and apoptotic and/or necrotic cell death triggered by GELS and attenuated by DRESS. Apoptotic and/or necrotic cell death occurs in various NDDS, CVDs, and MDR malignancies with currently limited TSE-EBPT options. Thus, CS stability determines cellular fate, as illustrated in Fig. 10.

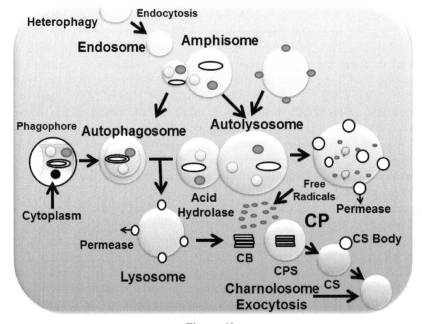

Figure 10

CS Analysis of Chronic MDR Diseases

CS analysis provides a direct estimate of CP regulation, MQC, and ICD in acute and chronic MDR diseases. We can estimate primarily five major CS metabolites (8-OH, 2dG, 2,3 dihydroxy nonenal, lactate, N-acetyl aspartate (NAA), and Cyt-C) in addition to acetaldehyde, H_2O_2, and ammonia, and Cr/PCR ratio from the biological fluids by standard biochemical methods or through high-resolution magic angle spinning nanoNMR spectroscopy to determine the CS stability index (Table 5). Subsequently, advanced omics (genomic, proteomic, lipidomic, metallomic, glycomic, and metabolomic) microRNA, mtmicroRNA, and epigenetic analysis can be performed employing LC-MASS for the proteomic analysis, multiple fluorochrome and monoclonal-Ab-labeled probes by flow cytometry, ELISA, micro-Arrays, molecular imaging, FERT, SPR spectroscopy, TEM, SEM, and atomic force microscopy. Furthermore, *in vivo* multimodality molecular imaging can be performed with CT/SPECT/MR/PET depending on the patient's need, time, accessible technology, personal knowledge, wisdom, expertise and resources available (Table 3).

Table 3 A Quantitative Analysis of the CS Stability Index for the TSE-EBPT of Chronic MDR Diseases

S.No.	*Biological Sample*	*Clinical Significance*
1.	Skin, Hair, Toe Nails	Skin Disorders, SAPHO, Eczema, Psoriasis, Infections, Cancer
2.	Burn Papules	Severity and Degree of Burns
3.	Acne Fluid	SAPHO, Cause and Severity of Acne
4.	Tears, Aqueous Humor, Vitreous Humor	Ophthalmic Diseases, Xero-ophthalmia, Retinal Degeneration, Macular Degeneration
5.	Saliva	Diseases of Oral Cavity, Sojourn's Disease, Xerostomia, Oral Infections, Infections, Oral Cancer
6.	Sputum	Pulmonary Diseases, Microbial Infections, ARDS, Pneumonia, CF, Lung Carcinoma
7.	Urine	Renal Disorders, Drug Metabolism, Nephrolithiasis, UTI, Nephrotic Syndrome, Renal Carcinoma
8.	Feces	GIT Disorders, Duodenal Ulcers, H, Pylori Infection, Crohn' Disease, Ulcerative Colitis, IBD
9.	Bile	Jaundice, Cholelithiasis, Hydrophobic Drug Metabolism
10.	CSF	CNS Disorders, NDDs, Aging
11.	Vaginal Discharge, Menstrual Fluid	Urinogenital Disorders, UTI Infections, Infertility Issues, & UT Cancers
12.	Semen	Genitourinary Disorders, UTI (Prostate) Cancer, & Infertility
13.	Blood, Serum, Plasma	Diseases of internal organs (Lungs, Liver, Heart, Muscle, Kidney
14.	Bone Marrow (Smear)	Hematopoietic Diseases, Leukemia, Anemias, & Lymphomas
15.	Pus	Severity of Abscess and Clinical Prognosis after Surgery
16.	Synovial Fluid	Detection of Osteoarthritis, Rheumatoid Arthritis, & Gout
17.	Fluid from Pulmonary Edema & Effusions	Congestive Heart Failure, CF, COPD, & ARDS
18.	Amniotic Fluid (US-Guided Amniocentesis)	Gynecological Disorders, Congenital Diseases, IEM, Genetic Counseling, Karyotyping, Chromosomal Disorders (Down Syndrome, Turner Syndrome, Klinefelter Syndrome, Cushing's Syndrome), Cerebral Palsy, Autism, Microbial (Bacteria, Virus, Fungus, and Parasite) Infections, IUD Drug Abuse

Invasive procedures (such as biopsies, amniocentesis, synovial fluid, aqueous and vitreous humor, pleural effusions, edematous fluids, and CSF lumber puncture etc.) may be avoided provided it is highly essential for the patient and given his/her willingness and consent. CT, MRI, and US-guided interventions are currently available for the patient's safety and comfort to provide an early detection of congenital disorders. Potential CS biomarkers are presented in Fig. 11.

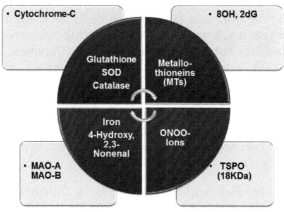

Potential Charnolosome Biomarkers

Figure 11

CP-ATG Interaction (Recent Update)

Mitochondria remain in a constant dynamic of fusion and fission in response to cellular cues. Fusion generates healthy mitochondria, whereas fission results in the removal of non-functional organelles. Changes in mitochondrial dynamics are implicated in several human diseases. Angelika et al. (2011) highlighted that CP/ATG interaction is a cellular survival pathway that recycles components to compensate nutrient depletion and ensures the appropriate degradation of organelles. Mitochondrial number and their health are regulated by CP, a process by which excessive or damaged mitochondria participating in CBMP are subjected to ATG elimination. CP malfunction contributes to neuronal loss in PD. In addition to ATGs, mitochondrial integrity can also influence the ATG and vice-versa. Yi et al. (2018) found that Mec1/ATR, as a sensor of DNA damage, is essential for glucose starvation-induced ATG. Mec1 is recruited to mitochondria where it is phosphorylated by Snf1 in response to glucose starvation. Phosphorylation of Mec1 leads to the assembly of a Snf1-Mec1-ATG1 on mitochondria, which promotes the association of ATG1 with ATG13. Mitochondrial respiration is required for glucose starvation-induced ATG. The Snf1-Mec1-ATG1 module is essential for maintaining mitochondrial respiration and regulating glucose starvation-induced CP/ATG, which is a key determinant for mitochondrial health and NCF. The mitochondria's ability to influence and be influenced by CP/ATG places both mitochondria and CP/ATG in a unique position where defects in one or the other could increase the risk to various metabolic and CP/ATG-related diseases. CP/ATG is thus a key determinant for MQC and NCF. Hence, I have used combined CP/ATG in this edition. Both CP as well as ATG have similar as well as distinct physicochemical characteristics as described in this edition.

CP/ATG in Infectious, Non-infectious, and Lifestyle Diseases

ATG is a cellular degradation process that plays an important role in maintaining homeostasis and preventing nutritional, metabolic, and infection-induced stresses. Although some molecules in budding yeast, such as ATG32p, Uth1p, and Aup1p, have been identified, the mechanistic and regulatory features of CP have yielded conflicting results (Kissová et al. 2004).

Alexander et al. (2012) suggested that differences in experimental conditions may have contributed to these discrepancies. Understanding these differences may help place the mechanism and regulation of CP in context, and indicate the intricate role CP/ATG play in the life and death decisions. ATG dysfunction can have pathological consequences, including tumor progression, pathogen virulence, and ND. ATG has both positive and negative roles in infection, cancer, neural development, metabolism, cardiovascular health, immunity, and iron homeostasis. Khandia et al. (2019) described the mechanisms of ATG and its associations with other cell death mechanisms, including apoptosis, necrosis, necroptosis, and autosis. Genetic defects in ATG can cause childhood encephalopathy with NDDs in adulthood, Crohn's disease, hereditary spastic para-paresis, Danon disease, X-linked myopathy, and inclusion body myositis. Further studies on ATG in microbial infections could help to develop novel theranostic strategies in pathogenic microbes. These investigators highlighted various inducers and suppressors of ATG to design novel theranostics strategies and develop CP/ATG-targeted drugs in numerous diseases.

CP/ATG Dysregulation in the Corona Virus Infection

Coronavirus (primarily from camel, cat, cattle, and bat origin) causes respiratory syndrome and has currently affected 219 countries, >202 million individuals, and >2.8 million fatalities especially in the U.S.A., India, Mexico, Brazil, Wuhan State (China). South Korea, Japan, Italy, and France have also been heavily impacted by this novel virus. "If genes are the loaded guns, does the environment serve as a trigger" This phrase holds true even for Corona viral infection because age, environmental pollution, cigarette smoking, eating habits. and pre-existing medical conditions are all risk factors which determine the health of an individual. Certain microbial infections such as infectious mononucleosis, Helicobacter pylori, and now the Corona virus infection can spread easily through deep (mouth to mouth) kissing and even by a simple sneeze. The frequent washing of hands with detergent and/or using hand sanitizer, and wearing a face mask can help but can't completely prevent its spread. We definitely need a vaccine to prevent any future outbreak as a prophylaxis. As an intracellular pathogen, this virus remains confined to mitochondria, can utilize lipoproteins to synthesis its coat proteins, and escape from the direct exposure of an antiviral drug. Typical clinical symptoms of Corona viral infection are fever, fatigue, diarrhea, and flu-like symptoms (cough, cold, and rhinorrhea). Initially it triggers inflammation to cause nostrilitis, followed by bronchitis, bronchiolitis, and eventually pneumonia. Similar to severe acute respiratory distress syndrome (SARS) and middle east respiratory distress syndrome (MERS), the virus hijacks the macrophage-induced CP/ATG system and is not easily eliminated, resulting in impaired lysosome-mitochondrial crosstalk, CMB, and ICD for NCF. Hence, we need to develop a mitochondrial-targeted vaccine and anti-inflammatory disease-specific CB antagonists, CP agonists, and CBMP antagonist as novel CPTs for its elimination from the bronchial airways epithelial progenitor cells, and macrophages to stay healthy. Meanwhile. natural and/or synthetic antioxidants and fluid intake can facilitate ICD and boost MB as free radical scavengers for NCF. How COVID-19 highjacks the CP/ATG of cells in the pulmonary system to cause flu like symptoms, pneumonia, and eventually mortality is yet to be established. Further studies in this direction will confer unique opportunity to develop a MB-targeted-vaccine for its prophylaxis and novel CPTs to cure its infection. Corona or any other virus can infect macrophages to compromise CP at various sites such as ER membranes, mitochondria, CBs, CPS, CS, and in the nucleus. The virus can reside in the CB, CPS, or CS to escape lysosomal hydrolytic enzymes, and phagocytosis, and cause a compromised exocytosis and CS destabilization and triggers CBMP implicated in apoptotic cell death. A pictorial diagram illustrating potential intracellular sites of viral infection are presented in Fig. 12. (For more details please refer to Chapter 31). Chen et al. (2014) reported that corona virus induces ATG through its papaine-like protease activity.

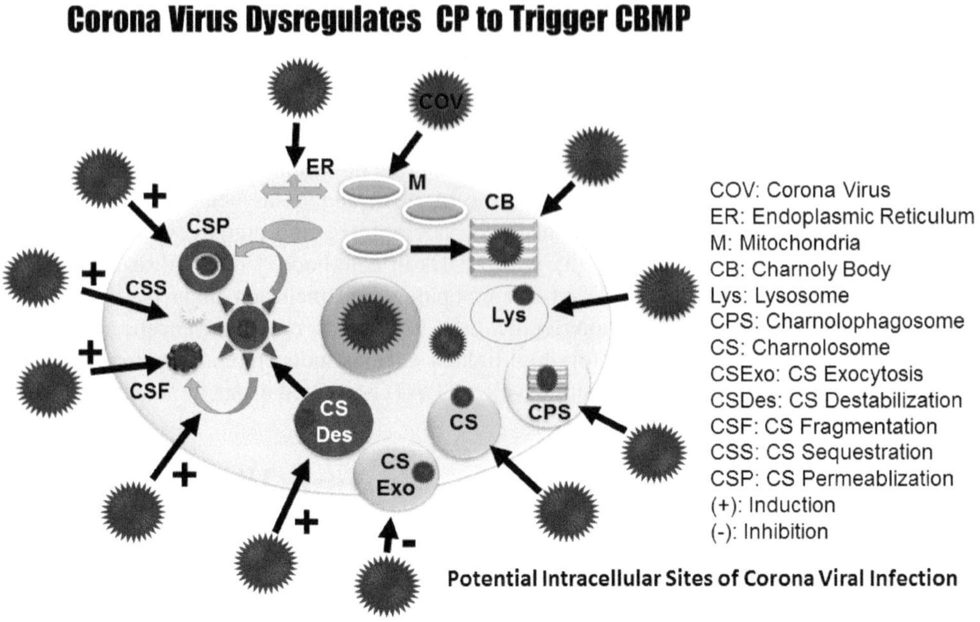

Corona Virus Dysregulates CP to Trigger CBMP

COV: Corona Virus
ER: Endoplasmic Reticulum
M: Mitochondria
CB: Charnoly Body
Lys: Lysosome
CPS: Charnolophagosome
CS: Charnolosome
CSExo: CS Exocytosis
CSDes: CS Destabilization
CSF: CS Fragmentation
CSS: CS Sequestration
CSP: CS Permeablization
(+): Induction
(-): Inhibition

Potential Intracellular Sites of Corona Viral Infection

Figure 12

Virulence of COVID-19 Infected CS

Usually COVID-19 does not stay as a free entity in the biological system. It is recognized as a foreign and undesired entity and is immediately phagocytosed by macrophages, where it may be trapped in the CBs, CPS, and CS, and remain stable for about 2–3 weeks as illustrated in the figure. Hence, COVID-19 infected CS (COVID-19-CS) can be detected from the bronchio-alveolar fluid and fecal matter by RT-PCR or ELISA using RNA-specific primers and a viral coat protein (viroporine)-specific antibody, respectively, during active phase of infection. The virus causes fever and fatigue by compromising the systemic mitochondrial bioenergetics (MB) and prevents the synthesis of anti-inflammatory steroid hormones from the macrophages and epithelial cell mitochondria due to TSPO (18 KDa cholestrerol transporting protein)-delocalization to enhance inflammasome activation and hyper-cytokinemia. The IL-1 overproduction is implicated in hyperthermia which downregulates the hypothalamic thermoregulatory centers to cause hyperpyrexia, leading to xerostomia and fatal pneumonia. In the pulmonary system, COVID-19-CS causes mast cell, basophil, and plasma cell activation to release histamine and other mediators to cause broncho-constriction, inflammation, and mucus accumulation as seen in COPD patients suffering from asthma, emphysema, bronchitis, rhinorrhea, and cystic fibrosis with breathing difficulty. COVID-19 causes a cardiorespiratory arrest and fatality, particularly in old immunocompromised patients with pre-existing conditions, where CP is compromised and CS is not properly exocytosed or detoxified due to non-functional lysosomal hydrolytic enzymes. Through systemic circulation, COVID-19-CS infects hyper-proliferating GIT cells to trigger dysregulated CP and enhance CBMP to cause diarrhea, dehydration, alkalosis, paralysis, and death. Hence, we need to develop a vaccine to inhibit Corona virus-induced CBMP and to regulate CP to minimize the viral load from the bronchio-alveolar and GIT system (two primary centers of its organotropism and virulence) and novel CPTs to curb aforementioned clinical symptomatology. The viral infection renders enhanced susceptibility to bacterial or fungal infections in HIV patients, who die primarily due to opportunistic infections.

CP/ATG-regulatory Domain in HCLS1-associated Protein X-1

HCLS1-associated protein X-1 (HAX1) promotes cell survival through attenuation of the damaged signals from ER and mitochondria, known as targets for CP/ATG during stress. Li et al. (2018) investigated whether CP/ATG can be upregulated in response to HAX1 overexpression and identified the functional motif in HAX1 for CP/ATG induction. Autophagosome accumulation, $\Delta\psi$, and apoptosis were analyzed in HEK293 cells with full-length or truncated HAX1-encoding genes, while empty vector-transduced cells served as control. Upon the oxidative stress, CP/ATG induction was observed in HAX1-overexpressing cells, as well as HAX1-truncated cells that encoded peptide segments (AA127-180). Oxidative stress-induced $\Delta\psi$ collapse and apoptosis were suppressed in HAX1-overexpressing cells, represented by reduced DNA fragmentation and decreased caspase-9 cleavage. The HAX1-induced CP/ATG response was abrogated when AA127-180 was removed, compromising the anti-apoptotic effects, indicating that CP/ATG is involved in HAX1-induced cyto-protection, and AA127-180 serves as the CP/ATG-regulatory domain of this anti-apoptotic protein.

CP/ATG and UPS

Recently, Kocaturk and Gozuacik (2018) reported that ATG and the UPS are the two major QC and recycling mechanisms for cellular homeostasis in eukaryotes. Ubiquitination is utilized as a degradation signal by both systems, yet, through different mechanisms. The UPS is responsible for the degradation of short-lived and soluble misfolded proteins whereas ATG eliminates long-lived insoluble protein aggregates and even whole organelles (for example, mitochondria, peroxisomes) and intracellular parasites (for example, bacteria, virus). Both the UPS and CP recognize their targets through ubiquitin tags. In addition to an indirect connection between the two systems through ubiquitylated proteins, other connections and reciprocal regulatory mechanisms between these degradation pathways were also indicated.

CP/ATG-apoptosis Interaction

Cooper (2018) highlighted the interaction between CP/ATG and apoptosis with a primary emphasis on the role of ROS. These investigators reported that both act by eliminating aberrant or unnecessary cytoplasmic material, such as misfolded proteins, supernumerary and defective organelles. CP/ATG is triggered by ROS, and by clearing the defective organelles, ROS levels are lowered thereby restoring MQC and ICD. If cellular homeostasis cannot be accomplished, the cells can choose an apoptotic pathway. Both CP/ATG and cell-death mechanisms respond to the same stresses and share key regulatory proteins, suggesting that these pathways are interlinked. Recently, Onishi et al. (2018) demonstrated that during prolonged respiratory growth, CP is impaired in yeast cells lacking Get1/2, a transmembrane complex mediating the insertion of tail-anchored (TA) proteins into the ER membrane. The loss of Get1/2 caused only slight defects in selective and generalized ATG. CP and other ATG-related processes remained normal in cells lacking Get3, an ATP-driven chaperone that promotes the delivery of TA proteins to the Get1/2 complex. The Get1/2-deficient cells exhibited induction and mitochondrial localization of ATG32 for CP/ATG. Get1/2 was important for ATG32-independent, promoted CP, suggesting that Get1/2-dependent TA protein(s) and/or the Get1/2 complex may serve in CP induction. A workshop took place at Delphi Greece where Charonis et al. (2017) elaborated on calreticulin and calnexin and the role of Ca^{2+} in cellular signaling and in CP/ATG, ERS, UPR, and in immune responses. These presentations were focused on hemophilia, obesity, diabetes, Sjogren's syndrome, Chagas diseases, MS, ALS, neurological malignancies (especially glioblastoma), hematological malignancies (thrombocythemia and myelofibrosis), lung adenocarcinoma, and renal pathology with an emphasis on fibrosis and drug toxicity. In addition, the role of calreticulin and calnexin in growth and wound healing, and the use of extracellular calreticulin as a biomarker for certain diseases was discussed with a primary emphasis on CP/ATG.

Generally, axonopathies are NDDs caused by axonal degeneration, affecting the longest neurons, and are caused by genetic defects in proteins involved in the dynamics of the ER. Liu et al. (2019) highlighted the defects in ATG and Ca^{2+} homeostasis in Niemann-Pick type C disease and Gaucher's disease. A wide range of LSDs show defects in both ATG and Ca^{2+} homeostasis, as Ca^{2+} is a key regulator of ATG. Krols et al. (2019) indicated that ER is a pivotal player in inter-organelle communication. Defects in the ER fusion protein, ATL3, identified in patients suffering from hereditary sensory and autonomic neuropathy, resulted in an increased number of ER-mitochondrial contacts both in HeLa cells and in patient-derived fibroblasts, which in turn resulted in higher phospholipid metabolism, ATG induction, and augmented Ca^{2+} crosstalk between both organelles. The mitochondria in these cells displayed reduced motility and the number of axonal mitochondria expressing disease-causing mutations in ATL3 was decreased, indicating the interdependence of subcellular organelles.

Recently, Senft and Ronai (2015) summarized the crosstalk among the processes regulating ERS responses. Cellular stress, induced by external or internal cues, activated systematic processes aimed at either restoring cellular homeostasis or committing cell death, including the UPR, CP/ATG, hypoxia, and mitochondrial function, as part of the global ERS response. When one of the ERS elements was impaired, the overall cellular homeostasis was perturbed. Activation of the UPR triggered changes in mitochondrial function or CP/ATG, which could modulate the UPR crosstalk. Yoshimori et al. (2018) highlighted that protein aggregates and damaged or superfluous organelles such as mitochondria, ER, peroxisomes, endosomes ,and lysosomes can be degraded by ATG in a highly selective manner. CP plays an important role in controlling intracellular pathogens. Although altering the CP/ATG level has become a theranostic target for various diseases, the exact molecular mechanism of CP/ATG induction/repression remains uncertain.

CP/ATG in Plants

It is generally held that plant cells do not have lysosomes. Some scientists believe that it is matter of terminology. The lysosomal abundance is maximum in phagocytes, such as macrophages, but almost all cells contain lysosomes. The lysosomes contain ~60 enzymes to break down cellular and non-cellular components. Upon nutritional starvation, the lysosomal number is reduced to <50 per cell, and their size is increased to 500–1,500 nm as a result of membrane fusion. If lysosomes burst, or the other organelles like peroxisomes burst, the deleterious changes resulting in cascade failure. The necrotic cell's enzymes spill into the cytoplasm and cause the necrosis of adjacent cells. Lysosomes contain hydrolytic (proteases, lipases, and nucleases) enzymes which destroy foreign bodies, microbes, or toxic substances entering the cell. Vacuoles in the plant cells have these hydrolytic enzymes that function as lysosomes. But the vacuoles cannot undergo self-catalysis as observed in the lysosomes (hence they are called as 'suicidal bags') as described in the Wikipedia article "Controversies in Botany" (https://www.reddit.com/r/botany/comments/d3v0mb/controversies_in_botany/).

NEET Protein Clusters

In humans, three genes encode for NEET proteins: cisd1 encodes mitoNEET (mNT), cisd2 encodes the nutrient-deprivation ATG factor-1 (NAF-1), and cisd3 encodes MiNT (Miner2). Karmi et al. (2018) reported that these proteins play key roles in processes related to normal metabolism and disease. NEET proteins are involved in iron, Fe–S, and ROS homeostasis and regulate ATG and apoptosis. MNT and NAF-1 are homo-dimeric and reside on the OMM. NAF-1 also resides in the membranes of the ER-associated mitochondrial membranes (MAM). MiNT is a monomer with distinct asymmetry in the molecular surfaces surrounding the clusters, and resides within the mitochondria. NAF-1 and mNT share similar backbone folds to the plant homodimeric NEET protein (At-NEET), while MiNT's fold resembles bacterial MiNT protein. Despite the variation of amino acid sequence, all NEET proteins retain their CDGSH domain and possess 3Cys: 1His [2Fe–2S] cluster coordination as NEET protein [2Fe-2S] clusters.

Syntaxin 17 Regulates PGAM5 in Mitochondrial Division

PGAM5, a mitochondrial protein phosphatase that is linked to PINK1, facilitates mitochondrial division by dephosphorylating Drp-1. At the onset of CP, PGAM5 is cleaved by PARL, which degrades PINK1 in healthy cells, and its cleaved form facilitates the engulfment of CBs by dephosphorylating the CP receptor, FUNDC1. Sugo et al. (2018) showed that the function and localization of PGAM5 are regulated by syntaxin 17 (Stx17), a MAM protein implicated in mitochondrial dynamics. The loss of Stx17 causes PGAM5 aggregation and failure of the de-phosphorylation of Drp-1, leading to mitochondrial elongation. In Parkin-mediated CP, Stx17 is a prerequisite for PGAM5 to interact with FUNDC1, indicating that Stx17-PGAM5 plays a pivotal role in mitochondrial division and PINK1/Parkin-mediated CP.

A Pseudo-receiver Domain in ATG32 for CP

In yeast, CP is dependent on the ATG receptor, ATG32, an OMM protein. Once activated, ATG32 recruits the ATG machinery, facilitating mitochondrial capture in phagophores, the precursors to autophagosomes. To investigate CP regulation, Xia et al. (2018) examined the structure of ATG32. They identified a domain for CP induction, and for the proteolysis of the C-terminal domain of ATG2 and recruitment of ATG11. The solution structure of this domain (as determined by NMR spectroscopy) revealed that ATG32 contains a pseudo-receiver (PsR) domain and the PsR domain of ATG32 regulates ATG32 and CP induction.

USP30 in Pexophagy and CP

USP30 is an integral protein of the OMM that counteracts PINK1 and Parkin-dependent CP following mitochondrial depolarization. Marcassa et al. (2018) used two CP reporters to reveal suppression by USP30, a PINK1-dependent component of basal CP in cells lacking Parkin, and proposed that USP30 acts upstream of PINK1 (through modulation of the PINK1-substrate) and determines CP initiation. A fraction of endogenous USP30 was targeted to peroxisomes where it regulates basal pexophagy in a PINK1- and Parkin-independent manner, suggesting the critical role of USP30 in scavenging ROS and in the regulation of the PINK1-dependent and PINK1-independent CP pathway.

ARL3 in ATG

ADP-ribosylation factor-like3 (ARL3) is a member of the ADP-ribosylation factor family of GTP-binding proteins and plays a crucial role in regulating ciliary trafficking. Luo et al. (2018) explored ARL3 subcellular localization in HEK293T, Neuro-2A, and U251 cells by density gradient centrifugation and immunofluorescence. ARL3 was expressed in most of the organelles. An iodixonal step gradient confirmed that ARL3 is localized to the mitochondria, endosomes, lysosomes, and proteasome. ARL3 promoted aggregation of GFP-LC3, upregulation of LC3-II/LC3-I and downregulation of SQSMT1/BECN1. Knocking down of ARL3 inhibited ATG, suggesting that it is necessary for ATG.

MQC by Thyroid Hormone Receptor and ERRα

Thyroid hormone receptor β1 (THRB1) and estrogen-related receptor α (ESRRA; also known as ERRα), play crucial roles in mitochondrial dynamics. Singh et al. (2018) performed transcriptome and ChIP-seq analyses and found that genes that were co-regulated by THRB1 and ESRRA were involved in metabolic pathways, including O/P, the TCA cycle, and the β-oxidation of fatty acids. TH increased ESRRA expression in a THRB1-dependent manner through the induction of PPARGC1A (also known as PGC1α). TH induced MB, fission, and CP in an ESRRA-dependent manner. TH also induced the expression of the ATG-regulating kinase ULK1 through ESRRA, which promoted Drp-1-mediated mitochondrial fission. ULK1 activated the docking receptor protein FUNDC1 and its interaction with the MAP1LC3B-II to induce CP/ATG. The siRNA knockdown of ESRRA, ULK1, Drp-1, or FUNDC1 inhibited TH-induced clearance of CBs through CP and decreased O/P, suggesting that the various mitochondrial actions of TH are mediated through the stimulation of ESRRA expression, while the regulation of mitochondrial turnover through PPARGC1A-ESRRA-ULK1 is mediated by mitochondrial fission and CP, suggesting that hormonal or pharmacologic induction of ESRRA could improve MQC in metabolic disorders. Furthermore, Lonardo et al. (2019) discussed the pathogenic mechanisms in hypothyroidism-induced NAFLD and the protective role of thyroid hormone (TH) in NFALD. They investigated whether hypothyroid rats may develop NAFLD via hyper-phagia; whether mitochondria become energetically more efficient; the overall energy balance if diversion of fatty substrates occurs; and the molecular pathogenesis of NFALD by metabolomics, cell imaging, lipophagy, ATG, and genetically engineered mouse models. They also described the pathogenic role of TH, metabolic syndrome, and other risk factors in hypothyroidism-related NAFLD and the development of NAFLD-related HCC in hypothyroidism.

Phagophore from Recycling Endosomes

The earliest recognizable structure in CP/ATG is the double-membraned cup-shaped phagophore. Newly formed PtdIns3P are destined to become phagophores recruits WIPI2, which bind together ATG16L1 to define the sites of autophagosome formation. Puri et al. (2018) showed that the membrane recruitment of WIPI2 requires PtdIns3P and RAB11A to mark recycling endosomes. Multiple core ATG proteins are associated with the recycling endosomes as opposed to being recruited to the ER-mitochondrial contact sites. Isolation of the recycling endosomes confirmed that they recruit CP/ATG proteins. Imaging data revealed that recycling endosomes engulf ATG substrates. The sequestration of CB depends on early CP/ATG regulators, suggesting that autophagosomes evolve from the RAB11A compartment.

mRNP Proteins and Mitochondrial tRNAs

Cytoplasmic localization, stability, and the translation of mRNAs are controlled by their association with mRNA-binding proteins (mRNP), including cold shock domain (CSD)-containing proteins, heterogeneous nuclear ribonucleoproteins (hnRNPs), and serine/arginine-rich(SR) proteins. Jády et al. (2018) demonstrated that the most abundant mRNP protein, the CSD-containing Y-box-binding protein 1 (YBX1), the closely related YBX3 protein and other mRNP proteins, such as SRSF1, SRSF2, SRSF3, hnRNP A1 and H, specifically interact with mt tRNAs. YBX1 recognizes the D- and/or T-stem-loop regions of mt TRNAs by relying on the RNA-binding capacity of its CSD. YBX1 and YBX3 interact with mt tRNAs in the cytosol. CP promotes the release of mt tRNAs from the mitochondria into the cytoplasm. The association of mRNP with mt tRNAs was increased upon transcriptional inhibition and decreased during apoptosis. Hence, the interaction of mt tRNAs with mRNA-binding proteins may influence cytoplasmic mRNA stability and/or translation.

CP in MQC and CBMP

Recently, Gustafsson and Dorn (2019) provided a comprehensive overview of CP/ATG in cellular homeostasis and disease and concepts in these areas. They highlighted that CP and non-CP pathways play crucial roles in MQC. They also mention the important functions fulfilled by mitochondria as both energy generators for tissue homeostasis and gateways to apoptotic and necrotic cell death. Non-CP MQC mechanisms and IMD are also important in maintaining NCF whereas CP is an acute cell stress response. CP's regulation of MQC, metabolic reprogramming, and cell differentiation suggest that the mechanisms linking genetic or acquired defects in CP to NDDs and CVDs or cancer are more complex than the simple failure of MQC. Described below is a list of potential CP biomarkers for developing the TSE-EBPT of chronic MDR diseases (Table 4).

Table 4   Potential CP Biomarkers

S.No	Biomarker	Characteristics
1.	DRP-1	A protein involved in mitochondrial fission.
2.	Mitofusin (Mfn) Mfn-1, Mfn-2, Opa-1.	A protein involved in mitochondrial fusion.
3.	CP stabilizing factor	A mitochondrial polypeptide implicated in CP regulation.
4.	CP destabilizing factor	A mitochondrial polypeptide implicated in CP dysregulation and induced in MDR malignancies.
5.	CS stabilizing factor	A mitochondrial polypeptide implicated in CS regulation and downregulated in MDDs, CVDs, and NDDs.
6.	CS destabilizing factor	A mitochondrial polypeptide implicated in CS dysregulation and downregulated in MDDs, CVDs, and NDDs and upregulated in MDR malignancies.
7.	2,3 dihydroxy nonenal & 4 hydroxy nonenal	An oxidation product of the mitochondrial membrane.
8.	8-OH, 2dG	An oxidation product of mtDNA.
9.	Ubiquinone-(NADH) oxidoreductase (Complex-1)	The rate-limiting complex-1 enzyme system of O/P.
10.	Superoxide dismutase (SOD)	Dismutatases super anions
11.	Catalase	Converts H_2O_2 in to water.
12.	TSPO (18 k DA)	A cholesterol-transporting channel.
13.	Heat shock proteins (70–8)	Mitochondrial stress molecules
14.	Heat shock factor	Mitochondrial stress molecule
15.	Hypoxia-inducible factor-α	A factor induced in high altitudes and downregulated in chronic kidney failure.
16.	MT1, MT2, MT3, MT4	A free radical scavenging metal(Zinc)-binding metalloproteins induced in infections, inflammations, MDR malignancies and downregulated in MDDs, CVDs, and NDDs.
17.	Monoamine oxidases (A & B)	Enzymes on the OMM for the oxidation of NE, 5-HT, and DA.
18.	Xanthine oxidase	Enzymes involved in purine metabolism and induced in gout.
19.	Alkaline phosphatase	A biomarker mitochondrial enzyme induced in MDR malignancies (osteosarcoma).
20.	Glutathione	A tripeptide antioxidant in free radical scavenging.
21.	Cytochrome-C	Non-covalently attached O/P enzyme on the IMM in the ETC.
22.	Apoptosis-inducing factor (AIF)	A mitochondrial factor involved in apoptotic cell death.
23.	Poly-ADP-ribosyl polymerase (PARP)	Enzyme involved in DNA polymerization and repair and is cleaved by caspases.

Table 4   (*Contd...*)

Table 4 (contd.)   Potential CP Biomarkers

S.No	Biomarker	Characteristics
24.	Caspases	Cysteine-aspartate proteases involved in PARP cleavage and apoptosis.
25.	Hydroxy-methyl transferase	Enzyme involved in epigenetic modification by converting cytosine at position N-3 to methyl cytosine and hydroxyl-methyl cytosine.
26.	Lactate dehydrogenase	An enzyme involved in lactate production during anaerobic condition and catalyzes the conversion of lactate to pyruvate during ATP synthesis in cells. Organs relatively rich in LDH are the heart, kidney, liver, and muscle.
27.	Alanine aminotransferase (ALT)	Mitochondrial enzymes induced by hepatotoxicity and infection, inflammation, drug abuse.
28.	Aspartate aminotransferase	Mitochondrial enzymes induced by hepatotoxicity infection, inflammation, drug abuse.
29.	mtDNA polymerase-γ	An enzyme involved in mtDNA synthesis.
30.	Peroxisome proliferator-activated receptors (PPARs)	A ligand-activated transcription factors of the nuclear hormone receptor superfamily: (PPARα, PPARγ, and PPARβ/δ). Activation of PPAR-α reduces triglyceride level, involved in regulation of MB, IMD, and MQC.
31.	Mitochondrial miRNA (miR-2392)	Regulates mitochondrial transcription and provide rationale for the use of mitomiRNA and mtDNA-encoded genes to predict chemo-sensitivity and clinical prognosis in cancer.
32.	N-Acetyl aspartate (NAA)	A biomarker of mitochondrial injury in CBMP.
33.	Cr/PCR Ratio	A biomarker of MB and IMD.
34.	α-Syn Index (Nitrated α-Syn/Native α-Syn)	A biomarker of neurodegenerative α-Synopathies and charnolopathies (PD, PDD, MSA, ALS, AD).
35.	Thioredoxine	A free radical scavenging protein in the mitochondria.
36.	Acetyl choline esterase	An enzyme involved in the structural breakdown of Ach for synaptic transmission.
37.	Succinic dehydrogenase	A key enzyme in intermediary metabolism and aerobic energy production, which catalyzes the oxidation of succinate into fumarate in the TCA cycle and derives electrons fed to the respiratory chain complex III to reduce oxygen and form water.
38.	Nicotinamide Adenine Dinucleotide Phosphate Hydrogen (NADPH)	A product of the first stage of photosynthesis and is used to help fuel the reactions that take place in the second stage of photosynthesis. Plant cells need light energy, water, and CO_2 to carry out the steps of photosynthesis. NADPH and reduced glutathione-dependent enzymes are involved in the modulation of NE-induced, ATP-driven hepatic microsomal calcium pump.
39.	Glyceraldehyde 3-phosphate dehydrogenase (GAPDH)	An enzyme involved in breaking down glucose to obtain ATP. In eukaryotes, it catalyzes the sixth step in glycolysis, converting glyceraldehyde 3-phosphate to D-glycerate 1, 3-bisphosphate (1,3-BPG).
40.	Heme Oxygenase	A mitochondrial antioxidant enzyme.
41.	p53	A tumor-suppressor gene. Mutation in this gene is involved in cancer induction, which occurs during I/R injury. Also known as TP53 or tumor protein (EC: 2.7. 1.37), it is a gene that codes for a protein that regulates the cell cycle and functions as a tumor suppressor.
42.	Beclin	A protein that in humans is encoded by the BECN1 gene. It is a mammalian ortholog of the yeast autophagy-related gene 6 (ATG6) and BEC-1.

Table 4   (*Contd...*)

Table 4 Potential CP Biomarkers

S. No	Biomarker	Characteristics
43.	p62	A classical receptor of ATG, it is a multifunctional protein involved in signal transduction pathways, including the Keap1–Nrf2 pathway. It is also involved in the proteasomal degradation of ubiquitinated proteins the Keap1–Nrf2 pathway in the proteasomal degradation of ubqiuitinated proteins. When the cellular p62 level is manipulated, the quantity and location of ubiquitinated proteins change, having a considerable impact on cell survival. Altered p62 can lead to some diseases. The proteotoxic stress imposed by proteasome inhibition can activate ATG through p62 phosphorylation. A deficiency in ATG may compromise the ubiquitin–proteasome system, since overabundant p62 delays the delivery of the proteasomal substrate to the proteasome, despite its catalytic activity being unchanged. p62 and the proteasome can modulate the activity of HDAC6 deacetylase, influencing the ATG degradation.
44.	mtDNA	It is a non-invasive cancer diagnostic biomarker. The rest of the mitochondria genes are made up of 22 tRNAs and 2 rRNA.
45.	mtmiRNA	It is involved in mitochondrial damage and biogenesis (miR-122, miR-202-3p), regulation of ATP synthesis, abolishing O/P, causing $\Delta\Psi$ collapse due to increased ROS production (miR-338-5p, miR-546, miR-34c); and inducing mtDNA damage and depletion (miR-546). miRNAs may be sensitive biomarkers for the early detection of mitochondrial toxicity involving CP dysregulation, CS destabilization, and CBMP.
46.	Apo-E4	Individuals carrying the $\varepsilon4$ allele of apolipoprotein E (Apo- E4) are at an increased risk of AD in later life. It is an established biomarker for *ER* mitochondrial communication. Apo E allele $\varepsilon4$ (Apo-E4) is a risk factor for AD. It remains uncertain how the ApoE fragment associates with mitochondria and causes their dysfunction.

The positive and negative roles of CP-ATG are presented in Fig. 13.

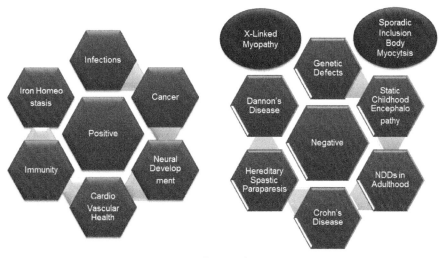

Figure 13

CP/ATG Regulation

In yeast, the phosphorylation of the CP receptor ATG32 by casein kinase 2 (CK2) upon induction of CP is a prerequisite for the interaction of ATG32 with ATG11 (an adaptor protein for selective ATG), following the delivery of mitochondria to the vacuole for degradation. Because CK2 is constitutively active, ATG32 phosphorylation is precisely regulated to prevent undesired CP. Furukawa et al. (2018) found that the protein phosphatase 2A (PP2A)-like protein, phosphatase Ppg1, was essential for the de-phosphorylation of ATG32 and CP inhibition. They identified the Far3, Far7, Far8, Far9, Far10, and Far11, as Ppg1-binding proteins. The deletion of Ppg1 or Far proteins accelerated CP. The deletion of a cytoplasmic region (amino acid residues 151–200) of ATG32 caused the same phenotypes as in ppg1Δ cells, suggesting that the de-phosphorylation of ATG32 by Ppg1 is required in this region. Hence, Ppg1 and the Far complex dephosphorylate ATG32 to prevent dysregulated CP. Liu and Okamoto (2018) showed that the TORC1-signaling pathway regulates CP in budding yeast via SEACIT (Seh1-associated complex inhibiting TORC1), which consists of Iml1, Npr2, and Npr3. Cells lacking SEACIT displayed reductions in CP during prolonged respiratory growth, while the other selective ATGs were less affected. CP defects were rescued in the SEACIT mutants (1) treated with Rapamycin, a specific TOR kinase inhibitor, (2) lacking Gtr1, a TORC1-stimulating Rag family GTPase downstream of SEACIT, and (3) devoid of Pib2, a PI-3-phosphate-binding TORC1 activator. The loss of Npr2 exacerbated CP defects in cells lacking ATG13, a TORC1 effector crucial for the activation of ATG-related processes, suggesting the requirement for additional CP-specific regulator(s) of TORC1. The npr2-null cells failed to stabilize the interaction of ATG32 with ATG11, a scaffold protein essential for CP, suggesting the SEACIT-mediated inactivation of TORC1 signaling to promote respiration-induced CP. Wible and Bratton (2018) described the mechanisms by which ROS activates ATG, and CP suppresses the formation of ROS. They also highlighted examples in which ROS suppress, rather than activate, ATG; and CP promotes, rather than inhibits, ROS production, thereby contributing to cell death. CP promotes generalized ATG to induce inflammasome activation and apoptosis when CS exocytosis is impaired or delayed during the chronic phase of disease progression. Thus, CS stability determines cell survival or cell death in a physicochemically-injured cell. Given that ROS are implicated in cancer, diabetes, atherosclerosis, NDDs and I/R injury, a further understanding of the association between ROS and CP/ATG is needed.

Quantitative Assessment of CP

CP can be quantitatively assessed by biochemical, morphological, molecular imaging, omics, digital fluorescence imaging, confocal microscopy, flow cytometry, TEM, SEM, atomic force microscopy, LC-MASS, and SPR analysis. Herrington et al. (2019) described topics of pathology related to CP/ATG to accomplish the TSE-EBPT of various diseases. These topics ranged from the impacts of the microbiome through ATG and cell death to advances in immunity and the use of functional genomics for understanding, classifying, and treating cancer and to provide updates in specific areas of pathology including: ARDS CD44; DAMP; DNA damage response; EndoPredict (EPclin); Epstein-Barr virus; Foxo3a; GATA3; Group 2 innate lymphoid cells; ILC2; KRT5; MLKL; MammaPrint; MapQuantDx; NanoString; OncotypeDX; PAMP; PD-1; PD-L1; PPAR-γ; RB1; TGF-β; TP53; VUS; abscopal response; acral; acute kidney injury, transplantation; adaptive immunity; alveolarization; apoptosis; autoimmunity; ATG; basal-like bladder cancer; biobank; bioinformatics; biomarkers; BC; BC index; bronchopulmonary dysplasia; cancer genes; cancer predisposition; cancer stem cell; cancer syndromes; caspase-3; checkpoint inhibitors; chemokine; chemoprevention; chronic inflammation; circulating tumor DNA (ctDNA); cutaneous; desmoplastic; dormancy; driver genes; drug resistance; dysbiosis; extracellular matrix; familial adenomatous polyposis; ferroptosis; fibroblasts; gasdermin; genomic signatures; hedgehog; hereditary colorectal cancer; hypoxia; imaging mass cytometry; immune-oncology; *in situ* hybridization; inflammation; innate immunity; interferon; interleukin; leukotriene; liquid biopsy; lung cancer, small cell lung cancer, pathology, molecular genetics, *in vitro* models; lung development; lymphatic system; lynch syndrome; macrophages; parallel sequencing; matrix metalloproteinase; melanoma; metastasis; microbiota; mismatch repair, microsatellite instability; mitochondria; mucosal; multiplexed immunohistochemistry; multiplexed ion beam imaging; muscle-invasive bladder cancer; mutations; myeloid-derived suppressor cells; nasopharyngeal carcinoma; necroptosis; neutrophil extracellular traps; neutrophils; polyposis; population health science; postnatal development; predictive; prognostic; prognostic signatures; prosigna; protease; pyroptosis; quiescence; radiation; ROS; respiratory infection; screening; severe inflammatory response syndrome; size-based diagnostics; statistics; stem cells; tissue biomarkers; toll-like receptor; translational research; triple negative BC; tumor invasion; tumor microenvironment; tumor progression; tumor-infiltrating lymphocytes; type 2 immunity; urothelial carcinoma; uveal; variants of uncertain significance. In September 2018, the 5th FASEB Meeting was held on the topic, *Small GTPases in Membrane Processes: Trafficking, ATG and Disease* in Leesburg, Virginia (Turn et al. 2019). A broad spectrum of topics was covered, including the biophysical and structural properties of small GTPases and their regulators to determine their exact role in ciliary function, cell motility, cell cycle, development, and CP/ATG, to evaluate disease pathology.

A key protein used to study ATG is the microtubule-associated protein 1 light chain 3 (LC3B). This protein is recruited from the cytosol, and matured and bound to the membrane for monitoring ATG. ATG can also be monitored by employing chimeric proteins LC3B when they are fused to GFP and RFP. Autophagosomes marked by an RFP: GFP:LC3 show both RFP and GFP signals. After fusion with lysosomes, the GFP signals are reduced due to acidic conditions, while RFP signals remain stable. New et al. (2019) described an imaging-based high-throughput screen for endogenous ATG evaluation, which used a genome-wide siRNA library to identify ATG regulators in mammalian cells. Genetic tools have been developed to study NDDs in zebrafish. In addition to optical clarity and fast *ex utero* development, the zebrafish brain is relatively small and has structures similar to its mammalian counterparts. Khuansuwan et al. (2019) developed a transgenic zebrafish that expresses eGFP-Map1lc3b under the elavl3 promoter to monitor ATG in neurons and screen CP/ATG-modulating compounds. They determined the applicability of this transgenic line by quantifying autophagosomes via treatment with a CP/ATG inducer (Rapamycin) and inhibitors (3-MA) and proposed a method for quantifying CPS accumulation and CP/ATG induction. They found that Isradipine did not modulate CP/ATG, whereas Nilotinib induced both CPS and CP/ATG, which could be used to identify CP/ATG modulators to halt NDDs progression.

Biochemical Methods of CP Estimation

CP induction/repression can be quantitatively assessed by estimating the lipid peroxidation product, 2, 3 dihydroxy nonenal, and the mtDNA oxidation product, 8-OH, 2dG, as basic CP biomarkers from the biological fluids of a patient to accomplish the TSE-EBPT of MDR diseases.

Molecular Imaging of CP

Fluorescent Probes

CP can be quantitatively estimated by employing two flourochromes, that is, *MitoTracker* and *LysoTracker*, and their co-localization by digital fluorescence microscopy. Their co-localization can be determined by merging the fluorescence images and regression analysis to determine the line of best fit at a 45° angle with a positive correlation coefficient >0.8. Hypoxia, iron depletion, and nitrogen starvation induce mild MTG, which is difficult to detect through decreased mitochondrial mass. Ishikawa et al. (2018) described a CP-detection method, which can be used from human iPS cells to neurons, followed by an image-based assay. Recently, Yamashita and Kanki (2018) detected MTG using mito-Keima and described protocols for its induction and detection of using mito-Keima-expressed cells which can be used for the quantitation of CP and CBMP as well.

The emphasis in this field of research has been geared towards the real-time visualization of molecular events to gain insights into the pathogenesis of diseases. Lu et al. (2019) highlighted that since many signal transduction and molecular events are implicated in CVDs, neuropsychiatric disorders, and cancers, a novel method to investigate their basic mechanisms is required for drug discovery. They developed probes for imaging pathological events to learn PDs and toxicity of pharmacological agents. Monitoring ATG can provide valuable insights into understanding human pathological mechanisms, developing novel drugs, and exploring CP/ATG regulation in health and disease. Chen et al. (2019) proposed a strategy to monitor ATG by lighting up the G-quadruplex structures entering autolysosomes by designing a fluorescent probe. Tian et al. (2019) developed a dual-site controlled fluorescent probe for the detection of pH in the cytoplasm and lysosomes. With this probe, the downregulation of pH in the lysosomes and cytoplasm during ATG can be detected. The detection of the GFP-ATG8 vacuolar delivery is one of the most useful methods for monitoring yeast CP/ATG. Zhang et al. (2019a) conducted a real-time analysis of nitrogen starvation-induced ATG in wild-type and knockout mutants of 35 ATG-related (*ATG*) genes in yeast and obtained 1,944 confocal images containing >200,000 cells. They labelled 8,078 ATG and 18,493 non-ATG cells and developed DeepPhagy, which offered better accuracy in identifying cells undergoing ATG. DeepPhagy was used to analyze and classify ATG phenotypes of the 35 *ATG* knockout mutants into three classes. It was also used to analyze three additional types of ATG phenotypes, including the targeting of ATG1-GFP to the vacuole, the vacuolar delivery of GFP-ATG19, and the disintegration of ATG bodies by GFP-ATG8. DeepPhagy could be applied to estimate organelle and inclusion-specific ATGs including CP.

Detection of Mitochondrial pH

Intracellular pH is an important parameter in various pathophysiological processes such as CP and CBMP. Niu et al. (2018) presented a hemicyanine-based probe (HcPH) for the detection of pH changes during CP/ATP. HcP-H exhibited reversible and ratiometric fluorescence of pH fluctuation during deprotonation/protonation, exhibiting orange fluorescence (λ_{em} = 557 nm) in basic media (pH 8.0) and green fluorescence (λ_{em} = 530 nm) in acidic media (pH 6.2), respectively. In HeLa, cells this probe accumulated in mitochondria, and co-localized with Mito-Tracker Green FM. The fluorescence imaging of HcP-H in HeLa cells subjected to nutritional deprivation demonstrated that it can monitor the pH changes during mitochondria-associated CP to sequentially evaluate CBMP in living cells.

Viscosity Estimation

Intracellular viscosity is related to many functional disorders and diseases. Abnormal viscosity changes are the indications of metabolite diffusion in the mitochondria. Zhang et al. (2019) reported a fluorescent (NI-VIS) probe, which uses quinolone, as an acceptor group and a twisted intramolecular charge transfer (TICT) to detect viscosity, mitochondrial targeting, and near-infrared emission. The NI-VIS probe had a sensitive response to viscosity changes in an aqueous environment. As the viscosity of a DPBS-glycerol system increased from 1.0 to 999 cP, NI-VIS exhibited a 100X increase in fluorescence. This method confirmed variation in mitochondrial viscosity of HeLa cells and its decrease during starvation-induced CP/ATG.The NI-VIS probe was also employed to visualize the viscosity variation in human cirrhotic liver. Experiments with zebrafish suggested that this probe can map micro-viscosity and aid in estimating CP molecular dynamics of biological samples.

CP Estimation by Flow Cytometry

Close links have been established between defective CP and diseases, including NDDs, CVDs, cancer, diabetes, and other metabolic diseases. Um et al. (2018) described a method for assessing CP by flow cytometry using the mitochondria-targeted fluorescent protein Keima (mt-Keima), which can analyze CP more efficiently than conventional microscopy or immunoblotting-based methods. Yamashita and Kanti (2018) described the protocols for induction and detection of iron depletion and hypoxia-induced CP using mito-Keima-expressing cells. Although several stimuli can induce CP, iron depletion, hypoxia, and nitrogen starvation induce mild CP, which is difficult to detect by measuring the decrease in mitochondrial mass.

CP Estimation by MitoPho8Δ60

Yao et al. (2018) developed a "mitoPho8Δ60" assay to study CP in budding yeast. Pho8, a vacuolar phosphatase protein, was genetically engineered to be targeted to mitochondria. When CP was induced, the phosphatase protein, along with mitochondria, was conveyed to the vacuole, where its C-terminal peptide was removed and the phosphatase was activated. The mitoPho8Δ60 activity was correlated with the amount of mitochondria delivered to the vacuole. Thus, this assay served as a tool to quantitatively estimate CP in yeast and other biological samples.

Ubiquitination in Mammalian Cells

The covalent modification of proteins with ubiquitin is essential for biological processes in mammalian cells. Van Wijk et al. (2019) reported that proteins are conjugated with single or multiple ubiquitin molecules in a dynamic fashion, which determine their half-lives, localization, or function. Ubiquitination was studied by a genetic and biochemical analysis of enzyme structure-function relationships, reaction mechanisms, and physiological relevance. The researchers provided microscopy-based imaging of differentially-linked ubiquitin using confocal and super-resolution microscopy, to illustrate the role of ubiquitin in antibacterial CP/ATG and pro-inflammatory signaling. Using an ubiquitin-dependent CP inducer, the lactone ivermectin, Zachari et al. (2019) combined genetic and imaging experiments. Ubiquitination of mitochondrial fragments was the earliest event, followed by auto-phosphorylation of TBK1, ATG proteins FIP200, and ATG13, whereas ULK1 and ULK2 were dispensable. Receptors acted upstream of ATG13 and downstream of FIP200. The VPS34 complex served at the omega-some step. ATG13 and optineurin targeted mitochondria in an oscillatory manner, suggesting multiple initiation steps in the CP/ATG execution. The targeted ubiquitinated mitochondria were held by ER strands even without functional ATG machinery and CP adaptors, suggesting that CP is ubiquitinated and encased in ER strands during CP induction and CS formation.

CP Imaging in *Drosophila*

Studies on the *Drosophila* model of NDDs revealed that the loss of Park/Parkin and PINK1 causes mitochondrial pathology in flight muscles and in the DAergic neurons. Studies in cultured cells discovered a crucial role of PRKN/PARK2 and PINK1 in CP. Recently, Cornelissen et al. (2018) engineered *Drosophila* that expressed the CP reporter, mt-Keima, and demonstrated that it occurs in flight muscle cells and DAergic neurons *in vivo* and increases with aging, depending on

PARK and PINK1, suggesting that the mitochondrial phenotypes of PARK- and PINK1-deficient flies are independent of the CP defect, and that these proteins may have multiple functions in the regulation of these organelles. Brazill et al. (2018) developed a fluorescence-based imaging method to examine *Drosophila* by using Fiji/ImageJ to analyze cellular processes and quantified protein aggregates in the *Drosophila* optic lobe using fluorescent-tagged mutant huntingtin. They assessed the CP/ATG-lysosome flux with the ratiometric-based quantification of a fluorescent reporter of CP/ATG, which included a segmentation step to minimize selection bias and to increase resolution. This approach could be extended for the analysis of other cell structures and processes implicated in NDD, such as proteinaceous puncta (stress granules and synaptic complexes), as well as membrane-bound compartments (mitochondria and membrane-trafficking vesicles). This method could facilitate an understanding of NDD through CB formation and CP induction implicated in CBMP.

DCF1 in Mitochondria

Dendritic Cell Factor 1 (DCF1) is a transmembrane protein that regulates neural stem cell differentiation and dendritic spine formation. DCF1 plays a role in ATG during the regulation of amyloid precursor proteins. Chen et al. (2018) used DCF1 tagged with GFP expressed in HelaS3 and HEK293T cells. DCF1 was expressed in the mitochondria, Golgi apparatus, ER, endosomes, lysosomes, and proteosomes. An iodixanol step gradient confirmed that DCF1 is localized in these organelles. In addition, DCF1 affected the expression and localization of MGST1.

Detection of Mitochondria-ER Contact Sites

Yang et al. (2018) designed a genetically encoded reporter using a split GFP protein for labeling MERCs. They analyzed its distribution during the cell cycle, starvation, ERS, and apoptosis, and found that MERCs are dynamic structures that undergo remodeling within minutes. Mitochondrial morphology affected the distribution of MERCs while the CCCP and Oligomycin-A enhanced MERC formation. Any physiological or pharmacological intervention that led to ATG or apoptosis increased the MERC signal. However, increasing cellular LD load did not change MERCs.

CP Dynamics in *C. elegans*

Distinct cell types display different requirements for mitochondrial turnover depending on their metabolic status, differentiation state, and environmental cues, indicating the necessity of developing novel tools for the spatiotemporal assessment of CP. *C. elegans* is highly suitable for the kind of analysis which provides the simultaneous monitoring of CP *in vivo* in different tissues and cell types, during development, stress conditions, and/or throughout the life span. Palikaras et al. (2019) described methods for monitoring early and late CP in the muscles and neurons of *C. elegans*, so as to provide insights into the generation of imaging methods to investigate the exact role of CP under normal and pathological conditions.

Primary Fetal RPE Cultures

The daily shedding and renewal of photoreceptor outer segments (OS) is critical for maintaining vision, which relies on the efficient uptake, degradation, and sorting of OS by the retinal pigmented epithelium (RPE). Poor OS degradation has been linked to retinal degenerations such as Stargardt disease and macular degeneration. Zhang et al. (2019b) established a method in fetal culture cells which facilitated the studies of RPE secretion in response to OS ingestion and preserved RPE differentiation and polarization during the imaging of OS phagocytosis. They optimized Mer TK-dependent OS phagocytosis, which was then studied to measure total OS phagocytosis by the RPE and chemical transfection, dextran labeling, and immunocytochemistry; and thus, evaluate players in OS degradation, such as lysosomes and ATG proteins. They developed image analysis macros in the Fiji/Image-J software to determine the exact fate of OS in the pathogenesis of retinal diseases.

ATG in Murine Skeletal Muscle

In addition to the currently available lysosomotropic drugs and ATG, whole-body knockout mouse models provide alternative methods to modulate and detect ATG *in vivo* (König et al. 2019). These investigators injected Colchicine, an autophagosome-lysosome fusion inhibitor, into the skeletal muscles of ATG-related (Atg5-shRNA) mouse models to evaluate temporal regulation and down-regulation of ATG *in vivo*. Methods to quantify ATG, such as CP transgenic reporters, *in situ* immunofluorescent staining, and flow cytometry, in mature skeletal muscle and cells were determined. The Atg5-shRNA mice provided insight into the potential implications of ATG inhibition.

Autophagosome Formation in ATG

By employing ^{13}C-labeled choline, ^{13}C-magnetic resonance spectroscopy, and immunoblotting, Andrejeva et al. (2019) showed increased choline phospholipid (ChoPL) production and the activation of PCYT1A (phosphate cytidylyltransferase 1, choline, α), the rate-limiting enzyme of phosphatidylcholine (PtdCho) synthesis, during ATG. The loss of PCYT1A compromised autophagosome formation in ATG cells. The direct tracing of ChoPLs with fluorescence and immunogold labeling revealed the incorporation of ChoPLs into autophagosomal membranes, ER, and mitochondria during the anticancer treatment. The localization of fluorescence signals from ChoPLs and mCherry-MAP1LC3/LC3 was also identified in autophagosomes accumulating in cells treated with ATG-modulating compounds. Cells undergoing ATG had an altered ChoPL profile, with longer and more unsaturated fatty acid/alcohol chains, suggesting that a *de novo* synthesis may be required to enhance ChoPL and alter its composition, together with replacing phospholipids from other organelles during autophagosome formation and turnover. This *de novo* ChoPL synthesis and PCYT1A may lead to the development of agents targeting CP/ATG-induced MDR.

INS-IGF1 Signal in Aging

Aging is associated with a gradual decline in cellular proteostasis, resulting in protein mis-folding diseases, such as AD, PD or ALS, which exhibit a complex pathology involving proteotoxicity. Using *C. elegans,* Sandhof et al. (2019) investigated how misfolded PD-associated SNCA/α-Syn accumulates in endo-lysosomal vesicles. Irrespective of whether they were being expressed in myocytes or DAergic neurons, accumulated proteins were transmitted into the hypodermis as the subject's age increased, indicating that epithelial cells might play a role in degradation when the endo-lysosomal degradation was overloaded. The inter-tissue dissemination of SNCA was regulated by endo- and exocytosis (neuron/muscle to hypodermis) and basement membrane remodeling (muscle to hypodermis). The transferred SNCA conformers were improperly cleared and induced endo-lysosomal membrane permeabilization. Reducing INS (insulin)-IGF1 signaling provided protection by maintaining endo-lysosomal integrity, suggesting that the degradation of lysosomal substrates is coordinated across different tissues. The chronic dissemination of poorly degradable proteins into neighboring tissues exerted toxicity, suggesting that restoring endo-lysosomal function with pathological inclusions in unaffected cell types might halt disease progression.

CP/ATG and MRI in MS

Castellazi et al (2019) investigated Atg5 and Parkin as biomarkers of ATG and CP, respectively, and estimated lactate levels in the CSF and serum samples of MS patients. CSF and serum samples from 60 MS patients were analyzed: 30 with MRI evidence of disease, Gd-based contrast agent positive (Gd+), and 30 without MRI evidence of disease (Gd–). Atg5, Parkin, and lactate were measured. Serum Atg5, Parkin, and lactate were more elevated in Gd+ than in Gd– MS patients, and CSF Atg5 and Parkin were greater in Gd+ than in Gd– MS. These findings suggested that molecular markers of ATG and CP were increased in the CSF of MS patients during the active phase of the disease and that these markers, together with lactate, were also increased in the blood, implicating their role in MS pathogenesis and prognosis.

Regulation of ULK1 by NDP52 and TBK1

Vargas et al. (2018) used chemically induced dimerization (CID) along with CRISPR KO lines to analyze the molecular basis of autophagosome biogenesis. The ectopic placement of NDP52 on mitochondria or peroxisomes initiated MTG by activating the ULK1 complex. NDP52-induced MTG was dependent on interaction with the FIP200/ULK1 complex, which was facilitated by TBK1. Ectopically tethering ULK1 to cargo bypassed the requirement for ATG receptors and TBK1. The focal activation of ULK1 occurred independently of AMPK and mTOR, which highlighted the coordination of the ULK1 complex localization by the ATG receptors and TBK1 (which acted as a driver of targeted autophagosome biogenesis).

GABARAP Fluorescence Imaging

Simons et al. (2019) developed an ATG-related antibody that targeted the GABA type A receptor-associated protein (GABARAP). By fluorescence protein tagging, and genetic and orthogonal strategies, they characterized the anti-GABARAP (8H5) antibody by confocal microscopy and compared it with fluorescence-protein-tagged GABARAP, GABARAPL1, or GABARAPL2 expressed in GABARAP knockout cells. This antibody demonstrated a high specificity for GABARAP without cross-reactivity to other mATG8 family members. Möckel et al. (2019) determined the depolarization and diffusion of GABARAP to elucidate its dynamics on the pico- to nanosecond time scale and its diffusion for protein concentrations spanning nine orders of magnitude. They compared the GABARAP dynamics by monitoring the ^{15}N spin relaxation of the backbone amide groups, fluorescence anisotropy decays, and fluorescence correlation spectroscopy of side chains labeled with BODIPY FL, and molecular movies of the protein by MD simulations. These parameters were correlated and confirmed with various techniques. A method that compared the parameters of the backbone and side chains to identify hinges for large-scale, functionally relevant intra-domain motions, such as residues 27/28 at the interface between the two subdomains of GABARAP, was proposed. This technique provided a quantitative picture of multiscale protein dynamics and solvation which allowed the researchers to study the functional dynamics of GABARAP or other proteins involved in CP/ATG.

CS Stability Index (CSI)

The CS stabilization factors (CSSF) and CS destabilization factors (CSDSF) can be determined *in vitro* in cultured cells, and *in vivo* in a tissue autopsy or biopsy sample by differential centrifugation, and characterized by omics biotechnology, immunoblotting, RT-PCR, digital fluorescence confocal imaging, flow cytometry, FRET, TEM, atomic force microscopy, LC-Mass spectroscopy, cDNA microArrays, multiple antibody ELISA, and SPR spectroscopy. The CS stability index (CSSI) can be determined by estimating the intracellular concentration of

CSSF and CSDSF. The ratio of CSSF vs CSDF provides a CS stability index (*CSSI = CSSF/CSDSF*) as a direct measure of CP regulation/dysregulation. The CSSI was reduced in RhO_{mgko} cells, as an *in vitro* model of PD, AD, and aging, and in MPTP-treated MT_{dko}, wv/wv, and α-SynMT$_{tko}$ mice *in vivo* (Sharma et al. 2004, Sharma et al. 2013). The ratio of CS stabilization factor vs CS destabilization factor can be used as a direct measure of CP regulation in the most vulnerable cell. (*CSI = CSSF/CSDF*). It is a ratio of stable CSs divided by stable CSs + permeable CS (CSperm) + sequestered CS (CSseq) + fragmented CS (CSfrag). A positive linear correlation between CSSI and α-Syn Index (SI = Nitrated α-Syn/Native α-Syn) with a correlation coefficient of 0.95, indicated that CSSI can be utilized as a specific biomarker of CP regulation/deregulation for the development of the TSE-EBPT-CPTs of chronic MDR diseases (Sharma et al. 2003). CS permabilization in the synaptic region is involved in synaptic silence to cause confabulations during Wernicke-Kereskoff's syndrome in alcoholics, which is ameliorated by Thiamine (vitamin-B1) because it serves as a cofactor of thiamine pyrophosphatase, which is involved in the activation of transketolase in the TCA cycle for ATP synthesis. Thiamine stabilizes the CS membrane to prevent its permeabilization by augmenting hippocampal MB. CS sequestration releases toxic metabolites to induce impaired synaptic transmission due to inhibition in the adequate release of neurotransmitter(s) required for the depolarization of the post-synaptic membrane for electrical conduction. Thus, CS sequestration can trigger early clinical manifestations of MCI in chronic alcoholism, schizophrenia, AD, Down's syndrome, Autism, and progeria.

CP As a Mechanism of IMD and ICD

Different types of CP-mediated detoxification include: (a) environmental detoxification, (b) physical detoxification, (c) systemic detoxification, (d) extracellular detoxification, (e) intracellular detoxification, (f) peri-mitochondrial detoxification, (g) intra-mitochondrial detoxification, (h) perinuclear detoxification, (i) intra-nuclear detoxification, and (j) detoxification of other intracellular organelles. CP can be broadly classified in two distinct categories: (i) Regulated CP and (ii) Dysregulated CP depending on the physico-chemical characteristics of CS inducers. CS is destabilized in response to free radical-induced DPCI in the stem cells

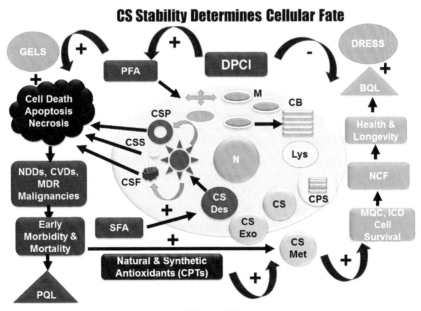

Figure 14

involving CBMP. Natural or synthetic antioxidants as free radical scavengers stabilize CS, whereas drugs of abuse and microbial infections destabilize CS to release toxic metabolites and induce apoptosome, inflammasome, metallosome, and necroapoptosome to trigger NDDs, CVDs, and MDR malignancies implicated in early morbidity and mortality. Clinically-significant DRESS habits including dietary restriction, moderate exercise, controlled sex and sleep improve MB and promote CP regulation, CS stabilization and its exocytosis to sustain IMD, ICD, and NCF to enjoy good health, longevity, and better quality of life (*BQL*); whereas GELS modifications including defective genes, hostile environment, and unhealthy life style triggers early morbidity, mortality, and poor quality of life (*PQL*). CP and ICD are presented in Fig. 14.

ATG Theranostics

ATG Modulators for MDR Diseases

Medical conditions including cancer, NDDs, infections and immune system disorders, and IBD could benefit from the theranostic modulation of ATG. Recently, Panda et al. (2019) used chemical screening in mammalian cells and the key ATG modulators, and highlighted the theranostic potential of these compounds in specific disease contexts. Various chemical screening approaches were established for the drug discovery of ATG modulators based on the perturbations of ATG reporters or the clearance of ATG substrates. Several pharmacological modulators of ATG act either via the classical mTOR pathway or independently of mTOR. Many of these have beneficial effects in transgenic models of NDDs, CVDs, myopathies, hepatic diseases, renal diseases, diabetes, cancer, infectious diseases, and in aging. *Drosophila* represents an excellent model to study disease mechanisms owing to its simple genetics, and the conservation of human disease genes and ATG processes. Bhattacharjee et al. (2019) described various ATG pathways in flies and human cells *(CP, macroATG, microATG and chaperone-mediated ATG)*, and *Drosophila* models of diseases to learn how defects in ATG genes and pathways contribute to CBMP.

Ca^{2+} Regulates ATG

Bootman et al. (2018) highlighted the roles of Ca^{2+} signals, Ca^{2+} channels, and Ca^{2+} sources in controlling ATG, which is initiated via vesicular engulfment of cellular materials and degraded via lysosomal hydrolases, with the 'autophagic flux'. ATG is a multi-step pathway requiring an interaction of scaffolding and signaling molecules. In particular, orthologs of the family of ~30 ATG-regulating (ATG) proteins that were first characterized in yeast play crucial roles in the initiation of autophagic vesicles in mammalian cells. The serine/threonine kinase, mTOR, is a major regulator of the ATG response of cells to nutrient starvation. In addition, AMPK, which is a key sensor of cellular energy status, can trigger ATG by inhibiting mTOR, or by phosphorylating other downstream targets. Ca^{2+} is implicated in ATG-signaling pathways (encompassing both mTOR and AMPK), as well as in ATG, when it is not involved with these kinases. Chelator to prevent cytosolic Ca^{2+} signals inhibited ATG in response to different stimuli, suggesting that buffering Ca^{2+} affects ATG, and that Ca^{2+} plays an essential role as a pro-ATG signal. However, Ca^{2+} signals can exert anti-ATG actions as well. Ca^{2+} channel blockers induce ATG due to the loss of ATG-suppressing Ca^{2+} signals and sequestration of Ca^{2+} by mitochondria to maintain MB and suppress AMPK-dependent ATG.

Transcriptional Regulation of ATG

Macro-ATG is a catabolic process that relies on the function of the lysosome and the autophagosome. The recent discovery of a transcriptional gene network that co-regulates the biogenesis and function of these two organelles, the transcription factors, miRNAs, and epigenetic regulators of ATG, demonstrated that this catabolic process is controlled by both transcriptional and post-transcriptional mechanisms. Di Malta et al. (2019) discussed the nuclear events that control ATG, focusing on the role of the MiT/TFE transcription factor. They suggested that the transcriptional regulation of ATG could be targeted for the treatment of genetic diseases, such as LSDs and NDDs. Zhao and Zhang (2019) focused on genetic disorders caused by hypomorphic or regulatory mutations in early acting ATG genes or by mutations in genes acting at autophagosome maturation. Protein aggregates assembled via liquid-liquid phase separation (LLPS) exhibited biophysical properties that were modulated by disease-related mutations. The abnormal phase transition of protein aggregates affected their removal and was associated with the pathogenesis of various NDDs.

ATG Inhibitors

The primary step in inducing ATG involves membrane nucleation, controlled by the ULK complex and Beclin-1. Inhibitors of positive regulators of the ULK complex and Beclin-1 block ATG, including inhibitors to the MAP kinases, JNK1, ERK, and p38. The induction of ATG and LC3 is required for vesicle expansion and formation. Inhibitors of the class III PI3 kinases can block ATG. Subsequently, molecules that inhibit lysosome acidification block the formation of autophagosome and autophagic degradation. *InvivoGen* in San Diego, U.S.A. provides inhibitors that target molecules that can impact ATG and can be used to study ATG including: Inhibitors of Beclin-1: SP600125 MAP Kinase Inhibitor – ATG Inhibitor – JNK inhibitor U0126 MAPK Kinase Inhibitor – ATG Inhibitor – MEK1 and MEK2 Inhibitor Inhibitors of autophagosome/autophagolysosome formation. 3-MA. PI3K inhibitor: ATG inhibitor: Bafilomycin A1 endosomal acidification inhibitor – ATG inhibitor LY294002 PI3K inhibitor – ATG Inhibitor SB202190 MAP Kinase Inhibitor – p38/RK MAP Kinase Inhibitor – ATG inducer SB203580 MAP Kinase Inhibitor – p38 MAP Kinase Inhibitor – ATG inducer Wortmannin.

PGAM5 in Mitochondria

Recently, Yamaguchi et al. (2018) reported that PGAM5 is a phosphatase that exists in the IMM through its transmembrane domain and is cleaved upon mitochondrial dysfunction. PGAM5 localizes to the OMM based on the findings that PGAM5 is associated with cytoplasmic proteins. Cleaved PGAM5 was released from mitochondria during CP, which was inhibited by proteasome inhibitors in HeLa cells stably expressing the E3 ubiquitin ligase Parkin. However, treatment of HeLa cells lacking Parkin with CP-inducing agents caused PGAM5 cleavage but did not cause its release from mitochondria. Thus, cleaved PGAM5 released depending on the proteasome-mediated rupture of the OMM during CP, which preceded the ATG-mediated degradation of mitochondria. This suggested that PGAM5 senses mitochondrial dysfunction in the IMM, and acting as a signaling molecule, regulates the cellular response to stress upon its cleavage and release from mitochondria.

ATG during Hypoxic Stress in HDPCs

Park et al. (2018) investigated the role of ATG in hypoxia-induced apoptosis of human dental pulp cells (HDPCs). $CoCl_2$ treated HDPCs were used to mimic hypoxic conditions, which decreased cell viability. Apoptosis-related signal molecules, cleaved caspase-3 and PARP, were enhanced in $CoCl_2$-treated HDPCs. HDPCs exposed to $CoCl_2$ also promoted ATG, showing upregulated p62 and LC3-II levels, typical ATG markers, and increased acidic auto-phago-lysosomal vacuoles. ATG inhibition by 3MA or RNA interference of LC3B enhanced caspase-3 activation and PARP cleavage, and the release of Cyt-C from mitochondria into cytosol in the $CoCl_2$-treated HDPCs.

However, ATG activation by Rapamycin enhanced the p62 and LC3-II, whereas PARP and caspase-3 cleavage was reduced, indicating that $CoCl_2$ activated ATG survival effects in $CoCl_2$-induced apoptosis. $CoCl_2$ upregulated HIF-1α and decreased mTOR/p70S6K phosphorylation. The HIF-1α inhibitor, YC-1, decreased p62 and LC3-II, and augmented caspase-3 activation and PARP cleavage in response to $CoCl_2$. YC-1 enhanced the phosphorylation of mTOR and p70S6K, suggesting that $CoCl_2$-induced ATG via mTOR/p70S6K is mediated by HIF-1α, and that $CoCl_2$-induced ATG through the mTOR/p70S6K pathway plays a protective role in HDPCs' hypoxic stress.

CP/ATG Modulators in Mammalian Cell

The reporters and assays for monitoring CP/ATG are currently becoming more sensitive in measuring CP/ATG flux with a potential for drug discovery. Seranova et al. (2019) described *in vitro* screening platforms to identify ATG modulators in mammalian cells using fluorescence and high-content imaging, flow cytometry, fluorescence and luminescence detection by microplate reader, immunoblotting, and immunofluorescence. The ATG reporters in these screening platforms were either based on CP/ATG markers like LC3 or ATG substrates such as aggregation-prone proteins or p62/SQSTM1. These investigators highlighted ATG assays for characterizing CP/ATG modulators from primary screening. Since CP/ATG is implicated in diverse pathophysiological conditions, these will enable identifying novel chemical modulators or genetic regulators with theranostic significance in chronic MDR diseases.

ATG, CP, and MTG Genes

CP/ATG is primarily a lysosomal degradation pathway for survival, differentiation, development, and homeostasis, and plays a crucial role in diverse pathologies, including microbial infections, cancer, NDDs, and aging, as well as in heart, liver and kidney diseases as described in this edition. Several selective ATG substrates and receptors are enhancing our knowledge regarding cellular functions of ATG. We need to regulate ATG at different stages of disease progression or regression. We can manipulate various ATG pathways to learn various disease processes. The Human ATG database (HADb), developed in Dr. Guy-Berchem's labs, provides an up-to-date list of genes and proteins involved in ATG. HADb provides different tools for the analysis, search, and visualization to facilitate predictions. To accomplish this goal, several updates are made. (Abdul Rahim et al. 2017, Goodwin et al. 2017, Galluzi et al. 2017). The HADb is the first human ATG-related database which provides updated information regarding human genes involved in ATG, which similar to CP, is a lysosomal degradation pathway implicated in cell survival, growth, differentiation, development, intracellular homeostasis, and plays a pivotal role in health and disease. Currently, its pathophysiological role in diversified CBMPs include microbial (bacteria, viral, fungal, and parasitic) infctions, cancer, CVDs, hepatic, renal, and NDDs is being investigated. HADb confers a comprehensive and updated list of human genes and proteins involved in ATG. General information, comments and genomic annotations is used to describe genes. The annotations and the navigation of genome can be performed by using internal *GBrowse* or link to *Ensembl*. There is also a provision to browse the entire database entries. For proteins, HADb has proposed general, structural and functional information to access various properties of a protein (family, post transcriptional modification, interaction, function, cell location, features, and isoforms). A subsection clustering of proteins presents different motifs, sites and domains on the ATG proteins. We can also go to *"Look for Gene"* section through HADb query's interface and search gene using symbol or synonym, chromosome location, keywords (a protein function) or external database accessions. In addition to ATG informatory, HADb will provide different tools for analysis, search and visualization to facilitate explorations, predictions and studies in near future. To achieve this goal, several updates will be made available. This database is as comprehensive as possible and open to any suggestion and submission. For example, there are ~20 evolutionarily conserved ATG-related genes (ATG), characterized in yeast. These genes have been compiled by FlyBase curators using publications (Kourtis and Tavernarakis 2009, Zirin and Perrimon 2010, Érdi et al. 2012). These studies have increased the number of CP/ATG related genes and proteins. Although many proteins are involved in CP/ATG, Beclin-1, Atg5, ATG7, LC3, ATG12 and ATG16L1 have been studied extensively as these are implicated in nucleation and autophagosome elongation. However, ATG6 or BECN1 gene expression is unspecific. ATG8 proteins induce membrane fusion, which is an important process in ATG. mTOR is a negative regulator of ATG and its direct inhibitors induce ATG. Beclin-1 is negatively regulated by caspases, the inhibitors of which promote Beclin-1 to trigger ATG. In addition, inhibitors of the 26S proteasome and the epigenetic regulators, histone deacetylases and DNMTs, increase ATG, while LC3 proteins process ATG. *InvivoGen* provides >1,800 full-length sequenced genes, primarily involved in immunity and cancer. All ATG gene sequences are available online on the gene page. Human & mouse genes in pUNO1 are provided as open reading frames (ORFs) from the ATG to the Stop codon, excluding introns and untranslated regions. As the ORFs are amplified from cDNA libraries, a variant form (*allele*) is sometimes obtained. Most of the variations have been reported in Gene bank. Genes for naturally secreted proteins include the native signal sequence. Engineered proteins meant to be secreted (such as particular fragments of longer proteins, like angiostatic proteins) may include the signal sequence of the human suitable for expression in mammalian cells. Each ORF is cloned in a mammalian expression cassette consisting of a potent and ubiquitous composite promoter (hEF1α-HTLV) and the SV40 polyadenylation signal. Each ORF is flanked by a unique restriction site at the 5' and 3' ends to facilitate its subcloning into another vector. Genes are supplied in pUNO1, a plasmid selectable in both bacterial and mammalian cells with HYPERLINK "https://www.invivogen.com/blasticidin" blasticidin. Some genes are also provided in pUNO2 (HYPERLINK "https://www.invivogen.com/zeocin" zeocin selection) or pUNO3 (HYPERLINK "https://www.invivogen.com/hygromycin" hygromycin selection). Fusion genes (ie. HYPERLINK "https://www.invivogen.com/puno-il12elasti-p40-p35" IL12, HYPERLINK "https://www.invivogen.com/puno-il39elasti" IL39, HYPERLINK "https://www.invivogen.com/puno-endo18-angio" ENDO:ANGIO) with the 'elasti' linker (VPGVG). Genes with selected modifications (gain/loss of function mutations, dominant-negative versions, disease-related variations, interesting alleles). HA-tagged genes (such as TLR and TLR-related genes) that allow efficient and specific detection by immunoblotting using the anti-HA tag antibody. For further details, please refer to: https://www.invivogen.com/genes. These include: Inhibitors of mTOR activation: Metformin AMPK activator – ATG inducer, Perifosine Akt inhibitor – Autophagy inducer, Rapamycin mTOR inhibitor – TLR signaling inhibitor – ATG inducer Everolimus mTOR inhibitor – ATG inducer Resverator, NF-κB inhibitor – mTOR inhibitor – ATG inducer. Activators of Autophagosome Formation: MG-132 26S proteasome inhibitor SAHA Pan-Histone deacetylase inhibitor, Trichostatin A Reprogramming Enhancer – Epigenetic Inhibitor – Histone deacetylase inhibitor as described in Table 5.

ATG Genes

The exact role of ATG in inflammatory diseases such as Crohn disease was first identified by GWAS and in multiple mechanistic studies. In particular, ATG16L1 is well studied in knockout and hypomorph settings as well as while recapitulating the Crohn disease-associated T300A polymorphism. ATG16L1 has a homolog, ATG16L2, which is involved in Crohn disease and systemic lupus erythematosus (SLE). To understand the contribution of ATG16L2 to ATG pathways and other cellular functions, Khor et al. (2019) analyzed an ATG16L2 knockout mouse. The researchers found that ATG16L1 and ATG16L2 contributed to ATG and ontogeny in myeloid, lymphoid, and epithelial lineages. Dysregulation of these lineages could contribute to Crohn disease and SLE, highlighting the significance of evaluating cell-specific effects. A novel genetic interaction between ATG16L2 and epithelial ATG16L1 was established highlighting how these genes may contribute to disease.

Table 5   ATG-Related Pharmacological Agents and Genes

S.No	Characteristics	Pharmaceuticals & Genes
1.	Inhibitors of mTOR Activation	Metformin, Perifosine, Rapamycin, Everolimus, Resveratrol
2.	Activators of Autophagosome Formation	MG-132, SAHA, Trichostatin, Z-VAD-FMK
3.	Autophagy Inhibitors	Inhibitors of Beclin-1: SP600125, U0126
4.	Inhibitors of Autophagosome/ Autophagolysosome Formation	3-Methyladenine, Bafilomycin-A, Chloroquine, LY294002, SB202190, SB203580, Wortmanin
5.	Autophagy-related Genes	ANXA-1, ATG3, ATG4A, ATG4B, Atg5, ATG7, ATG10, ATG12, ATG13, ATG14, ATG16L, BECN1, FIP200 (RB1CC1), GABARAPL1, HSPB-8, IRGM, LAMP2, LC3A, LC3B, LC3B-GFP, LRSAM1, Pellino3, RAB7A, TFEB, TRIM13, TRIM21, ULK2, UVRAG, VSP15, VSP34
6.	Autophagy Reporter Cells	HelaDiFluTMhLC3 Cells, RAW-Difluo™ mLC3 Cells: THP1- DiFluTM hLC3 Cells

ATG E2 ATG3 Mediates Allosteric Regulation

ATG depends on the E2 enzyme, ATG3, which functions in a conserved E1-E2-E3 trienzyme cascade that catalyzes the lipidation of ATG8-family ubiquitin-like proteins (UBLs). Molecular mechanisms underlying ATG8 lipidation remain poorly understood despite its association with ATG3, the E1 ATG7, and the composite E3 ATG12-Atg5-ATG16 and pathologies including cancers, infections, and NDDs. Zheng et al. (2019) reported that an ATG3 element E123IR (E1, E2, and E3-interacting region) serves as an allosteric switch. NMR, biochemical, crystallographic, and genetic data indicated that in the absence of the enzymatic cascade, the ATG3^{E123IR} constructs intramolecular interactions restraining ATG3's catalytic loop, while E1 and E3 enzymes remove this brace to activate ATG3 and elicit ATG8 lipidation. ATG3's E123IR protects the E2~UBL thioester bond from reactivity toward aberrant nucleophiles, while ATG8 lipidation cascade enzymes induce E2 active site remodeling through a specific mechanism to drive ATG. The ATG-related genes and studies on them are shown in (Table 6).

Role of p62/SQSTM1

SQSTM1/p62 is a stress-induced, scaffold protein involved in multiple cellular processes including ATG, regulation of inflammatory responses, and redox homeostasis. Its altered function is associated with NDDs, metabolic and bone diseases (downregulation), and carcinogenesis (upregulation). Alegre et al. (2018) evaluated the expression of p62 in cultured Hep3B cells and their derived ρ° cells (lacking mitochondria), along with markers of ATG and mitochondrial dysfunction. The effect of Efavirenz was compared with known pharmacological stressors, Rotenone, Thapsigargin, and CCCP, and with transient siRNA and p62 overexpression. In Hep3B cells, Efavirenz augmented p62 protein content, an effect not observed in the corresponding ρ° cells. p62 upregulation followed enhanced SQSTM1 expression mediated through CHOP/DDIT3, while other regulators (NF-κB and Nrf2) were not involved. The inhibition of ATG with 3MA or with the transient silencing of Atg5 did not affect SQSTM1 expression in Efavirenz-treated cells while p62 overexpression ameliorated the deleterious effect of Efavirenz on cell viability. p62 exerted a specific, ATG-independent role and protected Efavirenz-induced ROS generation and activation of the NLRP3 inflammasome, suggesting a multifunctional role of p62 which may help understanding the off-target effects of theranostically significant drugs.

Table 6 ATG-related Genes with References

S.No	Name	Application	References
1.	ATG1	Autophagy-specific gene 1, unc-51, DK-4, dATG1	Érdi et al. 2012, Zirin and Perrimon, 2010, Kourtis and Tavernarakis 2009
2.	ATG2	Autophagy-specific gene 2	Érdi et al. 2012, Kourtis and Tavernarakis 2009
3.	ATG3	Autophagy-specific gene 3	Érdi et al. 2012, Zirin and Perrimon, 2010, Kourtis and Tavernarakis 2009
4.	ATG4a	Autophagy-specific gene4a	Érdi et al. 2012, Zirin and Perrimon, 2010, Kourtis and Tavernarakis 2009
5.	ATG4b	Autophagy-specific gene4b	Érdi et al. 2012, Zirin and Perrimon, 2010, Kourtis and Tavernarakis 2009
6.	Atg5	Autophagy-related 5, Autophagy-specific gene 5,	Érdi et al. 2012, Zirin and Perrimon, 2010, Kourtis and Tavernarakis 2009
7.	ATG6	Autophagy-specific gene6. Beclin, Beclin-1, Beclin-1, Autophagy-specific gene 6	Érdi et al. 2012, Zirin and Perrimon, 2010, Kourtis and Tavernarakis 2009
8.	ATG7	Autophagy-related protein 7, Autophagy-related gene 7, Autophagy-specific gene 7, ATG-7	Érdi et al. 2012, Zirin and Perrimon, 2010, Kourtis and Tavernarakis 2009
9.	ATG8a	Autophagy-related 8a ATG8, LC3, Autophagy-specific gene 8a, DrATG8a	Érdi et al. 2012, Zirin and Perrimon 2010
10.	ATG9	Autophagy-related 9	Érdi et al. 2012, Kourtis and Tavernarakis 2009
11.	ATG10	Autophagy-related 10	Érdi et al. 2012, Zirin and Perrimon 2010, Kourtis and Tavernarakis 2009
12.	ATG12	Autophagy-specific gene 12	Érdi et al. 2012, Zirin and Perrimon, 2010, Kourtis and Tavernarakis 2009
13.	ATG13	Autophagy-related 13	Érdi et al. 2012, Zirin and Perrimon 2010
14.	ATG14	Autophagy-related 14	Érdi et al. 2012, Zirin and Perrimon 2010
15.	ATG16	Autophagy-related 16	Érdi et al. 2012, Zirin and Perrimon 2010
16.	ATG17	Autophagy-related 17 FIP200	Érdi et al. 2012, Zirin and Perrimon 2010
17.	ATG18a	Autophagy-related 18a ATG18, Autophagy-specific gene 18	Érdi et al. 2012
18.	ATG18b	Autophagy-related 18b ATG18, l(2)k09410	Érdi et al. 2012
19.	ATG101	Autophagy-related 101	Érdi et al. 2012, Zirin and Perrimon 2010

Mitochondrial Dynamics and Mitophagy (MTG)

Under normal physiological conditions, mitochondria undergo cycles of fission and fusion, which help preserve MQC through matrix contents and IMD. An imbalance in the fission/fusion equilibrium or mitochondrial damage can lead to degradation of mitochondria by MTG. MTG induction, mitochondrial dynamics (fission and fusion), modulation of MTG by targeting individual components, and crosstalk with other modes of ATG including CP and MB form a complex interacting network that governs mitochondrial degradation and thereby, mitochondrial function and cellular integrity. We need to determine how the molecular mechanisms of these factors regulate MTG and develop strategies where CP/MTG interventions will lead to theranostically-useful outcomes. The mitochondrion-ligand-receptor-scaffold associates with the mitophagosomal membrane and interacts with the ATG machinery. The functional counterpart of ATG8 is LC3 and while the counterpart of ATG32 is yet to be discovered, evidence exists for proteins that function as receptors to link mitochondria with the ATG, depending on the cell type. BNIP3L, also called Nix, is a member of the Bcl-2 family of apoptotic regulators, which translocates to the mitochondria and is required for MTG during erythroid differentiation. The ectopic expression of BNIP3L causes activation of MTG even in normoxia (Novak and Dikic 2011). The phosphorylation in yeast MTG and de-phosphorylation of FUN14 domain containing 1 (FUNDC1), an OMM protein, enhances interaction with LC3, via LC3 interacting (LIR) motif to induce MTG. FUNDC1 is phosphorylated by Src kinase at Tyr18, which is located within the LIR motif to inhibit MTG. Although both Nix and FUNDC1 are involved in MTG induced by hypoxia, their roles in the induction of MTG appear different (Liu et al. 2012). The OMM proteins are ubiquitinated in depolarization-induced MTG. SQSTM1 (sequestosome 1/p62) contains an LIR motif that links LC3 to ubiquitinated proteins associated with the OMM and to the proteins of the ATG machinery (Jin and Youle 2013).

Zhu et al. (2014) highlighted that no single parameter is adequate to document MTG. This is because many of its molecules, such as Parkin, p62, ULK1, and MTG receptors, including FUNDC1, Bcl-2/E1B19kDa-interacting protein3-like (NIX/BNIP3L), BCL2/adenovirus E1B 19kDa interacting protein 3 (BNIP3), and ATG32, are phosphorylated in response to MTG stimuli. The phosphorylation status of these molecules could be used by developing antibodies to detect specific phosphorylation sites. Ceramide and mitochondrial toxins are used to induce MTG. These compounds are useful for studying MTG in cultured cells and may have off-target effects in addition to MTG. Compounds that target MTG receptors or regulators are important to study for drug development. Physiologically relevant stimuli, such as hypoxia, are recommended. Future studies should address whether there are common pathway(s) to mediate MTG in response to diversified mitochondrial stresses.

ATG32 confers selective mitochondrial sequestration as cargo for ATG. Aviva et al. (2014) highlighted that MTG is distinct from general ATG in that in the latter, mitochondria are engulfed by autophagosomes nonspecifically along with other cytoplasmic organelles, for example in the livers of rats treated with glucagon (Ashford and Porter 1962). Hence, for the proper execution of MTG, mitochondria need to display a specific tag that is activated so that those destined for ATG are distinguished, which can be accomplished if we systematically follow the CB life cycle and CBMP. Specific mitochondrial tags have now been identified in both yeast and metzoans, and the mechanisms of MTG have been clarified. Still lagging behind is the pathophysiological relevance of MTG, given that ATG can also degrade mitochondria non-selectively, and other pathways like CP can remove nonfunctional, undesired, and/or degenerated mitochondria, or selective mitochondrial components, via proteases, proteasomes, or lysosomes involved in CBMP (Soubannier et al. 2012; Vincow et al. 2013, Sharma et al. 2013). Although ATG32, the mitochondrial MTG tag in yeast, has no exact sequence homology to the mammalian tag proteins PINK1, FUNDC1, NIX, and BNIP3, similar mechanisms demonstrate common principles underlying CP and MTG in all eukaryotic cells. Esteban-Martinez et al. (2017) described a flow cytometry-based method using *MitoTracker* Deep Red for MTG assessment and demonstrated that when used in conjunction with lysosomal inhibitors, this method confers a novel means of assessing MTG. Sauvat and Kepp (2017) reported that MTG ensures cellular homeostasis, as it fosters the disposal of aged and damaged mitochondria that would be prone to produce ROS and hence endanger genomic stability. The ATG clearance of depolarized mitochondria plays a role in homeostasis as a link between the impaired function of the MTG-mediating proteins PINK1 and Parkin in PD. The researchers developed an image-based approach for the quantification of mitochondrial Parkin translocation for the initiation of MTG. Yang and Dondong (2018) highlighted that MB requires nuclear-and mitochondrial-encoded genes regulated by the PPARγ coactivator-1α (PGC-1α) which contributes to increased mitochondria content allowing efficient thermogenesis in response to cold and ATP synthesis to meet excercise demands. PGC-1α expression can also be modulated by upstream signaling pathways at both the transcriptional and posttranslational levels, such as Ca^{2+}/calmodulin-dependent protein kinase (CAMK) and calcineurin, AMPK, MAPK, etc. Upon activation, PGC-1α controls the expression of downstream genes, including estrogen-related receptors (ERRs), PPARs, and nuclear respiratory factors (NRFs), which determines MB and function, mediates a shift in fuel usage, and modulates ROS homeostasis in the heart. ERRs control mitochondrial O/P, whereas PPARs induce the β-oxidation of fatty acids. NRFs induce the expression of mitochondrial transcription factor A (TFAM) for mtDNA replication, transcription, and maintenance, which confirm the crucial role of PGC-1α in the regulation of MB. SIRT1, induced by an increase in the NAD^+ in the presence of reduced cellular energy stores, can regulate both MTG and MB by de-acetylating and activating ATG proteins and PGC-1α, respectively. Upregulation of MTG increases the activity of the MTG-inducer Parkin and then degrades the Parkin-interacting substrate (PARIS) for Parkin degradation through the UPS, which inhibits PGC-1α transcription by binding to the PGC-1α promoter, suggesting that promoting MTG relieves the suppression of MB. However, the relationship of Parkin, PARIS, and PGC-1α has been identified only in neuronal models. PGC-1α induces the expression of the transcription factor EB (TFEB), the major regulator of lysosome biogenesis and the ATG pathway, suggesting that MB and MTG are interconnected in both directions. mTOR also participates in the coordination of MTG and MB, suggesting that there exists a network that connects MTG with MB, which needs further investigation.

The power of genetics and the conservation of fundamental cellular processes among eukaryotes make a yeast suitable model for understanding the mechanism, regulation, and function of MTG. In budding yeast, ATG32, serves as a receptor for MTG that interacts with ATG11, an adaptor protein for selective ATG, and ATG8, an ubiquitin-like protein localized on the OMM. ATG32 is regulated transcriptionally and post-translationally to control MTG. As ATG32 is a MTG-specific protein, analysis of its deficient mutant enables investigation of the physiological roles of MTG. Kurihara et al. (2014) described that MTG is rarely induced in yeast under normal culture conditions or even if it is induced, it cannot be detected. MTG is induced by nitrogen starvation after pre-culturing yeast in a non-fermentable medium that facilitates the proliferation of mitochondria (for example, where lactate or glycerol is the sole carbon source). MTG is induced during the stationary phase when yeast cells are cultured in a non-fermentable medium (Kanki and Klionsky 2009, Kissova et al. 2004, Tal et al. 2007). Although macroautophagy is also activated under MTG-inducing conditions, mitochondria are selected and degraded by MTG via ATG11–ATG32 interactions (Narendra et al. 2009, Twig et al. 2008). Interference with F_0F_1-ATPase biogenesis in a temperature-sensitive fmc1 deletion mutant, or osmotic swelling of mitochondria caused by depletion of the mitochondrial K^+/H^+ exchanger Mdm38 induced MTG (Nowikovsky et al. 2007, Priault et al. 2005), while mitochondrial depolarization caused by carbonyl cyanide m-chlorophenyl hydrazone (CCCP) did not induce MTG in yeast (Kanki et al. 2009a, Kissova et al. 2004). Yoo et al. (2018) described the mechanism of MTG and the factors that play a role in this process. They focused on the roles of MTG adapters and receptors in the recognition of damaged mitochondria by autophagosomes and the functional association of MTG through the interaction of the MTG adaptor and receptor proteins with mitochondrial fusion and fission proteins. Arakawa et al. (2018) described methods to assess Atg5-independent MTG in mammalian cells. There is an Atg5-dependent conventional pathway and an Atg5-independent pathway; the latter is involved in the erythrocyte MTG. Rodger et al. (2018) summarized the current understanding of MTG in mammals and reported that MTG plays a significant role in maintaining the health of the mitochondrial network as well as the organism as a whole. Although, various molecular components of MTG have been discovered by *in vitro* work and cell line characterization, the exact pathophysiological significance of these findings remains uncertain. Moreover, mouse models revealed significant variation in MTG even under normal physiological conditions. They focused on programmed MTG and recent understanding of why, how, and where this takes place in mammals. In addition, Furuya et al. (2018) summarized the mechanism of MTG and its related proteins. These researchers emphasized that Parkin-mediated MTG is a quality control pathway that selectively removes damaged mitochondria *via* the ATG machinery. ATG receptors, which interact with ubiquitin and Atg8 family proteins, contribute to the recognition of damaged mitochondria by autophagosomes. NDP52, an ATG receptor, is required for ATG engulfment of damaged mitochondria during mitochondrial uncoupler treatment. The N-terminal SKICH domain and C-terminal zinc finger motif of NDP52 are required for its function in MTG. While the zinc finger motif contributes to poly-ubiquitin binding, the function of the SKICH domain remains unclear. These researchers reported that NDP52 interacts with mtRNA poly(A) polymerase (MTPAP) via the SKICH domain. During MTG, NDP52 invades depolarized mitochondria and interacts with MTPAP dependent on the proteasome but independent of ubiquitin binding. Loss of MTPAP reduced NDP52-mediated MTG, and the NDP52–MTPAP complex attracted more LC3 than NDP52 alone, indicating that NDP52 and MTPAP form an ATG receptor complex, which enhances ATG elimination of damaged mitochondria implicated in CB formation, CP induction, and CBMP. Furthermore, ubiquitin binding domain and Atg8 interacting motif (AIM)/LC3 interacting region (LIR) bind to the ATG-related protein 8 (Atg8) family (LC3 and GABARAP) proteins. These molecular events initiate ubiquitylated (damaged) mitochondria for their selective removal to sustain IMD and ICD. On the other hand, some specific OMM-anchored proteins containAIM/LIR motif as another type of ATG adaptor/receptor proteins.

MTG in yeast was first identified following the discovery of yeast mitochondrial escape genes (yme), particularly yme1, which showed the escape of mtDNA, but increased mitochondrial degradation. This gene mediates the escape of mtDNA, and the mitochondrial turnover was triggered by proteins (Tolkovsky 2009). In the ΔUTH1 strains, there was an inhibition of MTG. Uth1p was necessary to translocate mitochondria to the vacuole. AUP1 was investigated as a mitochondrial phosphatase that marks mitochondria for elimination. Another yeast protein, Mdm38p/Mkh1p, exchanges K^+/H^+ ions across the IMM, induces deletions which causes swelling, leads to ΔΨ collapse, and mitochondrial fragmentation implicated in CB formation, CP induction, CS destabilization and eventually CBMP, causing apoptosis/necrosis. Mitochondria-localized ATG32 plays a crucial role in yeast MTG. Once MTG is initiated, ATG32 binds to ATG11 and mitochondria are transported to the vacuole. ATG32 silencing stops the recruitment of ATG and mitochondrial degradation (Kanki et al 2009a and b, Vives-Bauza and Przedborski 2011). These proteins play a crucial role in MQC, but mutations in their genes induce dysregulation and selective degradation of mitochondria, triggering CBMP.

MTG Biomarkers

The LC3 is known as a biomarker of MTG regulation. The initiation of MTG causes the conversion of LC3-I to LC3-II, associated with the formation of autophagosomes. Factors Influencing MTG include: (a) MTG induction, (b) mitochondrial dynamics, (c) modulation of MTG mechanisms, and (d) crosstalk with other models of ATG including CP. Idiopathic pulmonary fibrosis (IPF) is a chronic interstitial lung disease with a poor prognosis and limited theranostic options. Rheumatoid arthritis (RA) is a chronic inflammatory autoimmune disease complicated by the development of interstitial lung disease (ILD), leading to early morbidity and mortality. A role of ATG and mitochondrial dysfunction in the development of IPF has been suggested, associated with lung fibroblasts and epithelial cells. Vasarmidi et al. (2018) examined the mRNA levels of molecules involved in the ATG pathway in broncho-alveolar lavage fluid

(BALF) derived cells from patients with IPF in comparison to patients with RA having ILD by RT-qPCR. The upregulation of Beclin-1 was observed in patients with RA-ILD compared with those with IPF. Unc-51 like ATG activating kinase 1 (ULK1), Bnip-3, and p62 did not show any difference in their mRNA expression. Similarly PINK1, and Parkin; E3 ubiquitin ligase (PRKN) expression, as well as PINK1 protein levels, were observed, demonstrating an increased expression of Beclin-1 in BALF cells from patients with RA-ILD, while similar levels in other key molecules implicated in the ATG pathway were observed. Sica and Maiuri (2016) reported that bulk MTG can lead to the removal of mitochondria in erythrocytes during their formation as well as in sperm-oocytes after fertilization or physiological adaptation to hypoxia. Mutations in PINK1 or Parkin occur in PD and AD. The discovery of Bnip-3, FUNDC1, and SMURF1 points out the complexity of the pathway and encourages researchers to achieve a better understanding of the pathophysiology of selective mitochondrial removal and pathogenesis of diseases caused by a dysfunction of mitochondrial-based CP, MTG, and ATG machinery.

Quantitative Estimation of MTG

MTG can be quantified by the loss of expression of mitochondrial proteins using immunoblotting or immunostaining. Although this technique is used to confirm the elimination of mitochondria, changes in protein levels can be influenced by proteasome degradation and alterations in biogenesis. Hence, MTG may be underestimated when extensive mitochondrial biosynthesis is occurring simultaneously. The measurement of mitochondrial content utilizes biomarkers of mitochondrial proteins or quantification of mtDNA. Early studies of MTG used the degradation of the TOM20 protein as a biomarker of mitochondrial mass. In addition to regulation of MTG, Parkin also mediates proteosome-dependent degradation of OMM proteins. However, loss of OMM proteins alone is inadequate to induce MTG. Intermembrane space proteins can be released after permeability transition and the turnover rate of inner membrane proteins can be variable, even within the same respiratory complex. Hence, these assays should utilize proteins from different mitochondrial compartments for the precise measurement of MTG. Similarly, the loss of mtDNA can be measured using qRT-PCR or by immunostaining using mtDNA antibodies. Although, assessing MTG through the use of mitochondrial markers is a simple method to determine the degradation of mitochondria, this assay quantifies the net change in mitochondrial content and therefore is unable to distinguish between MTG and degradation by other mechanisms that may occur simultaneously, such as CB formation, CP induction, CS destabilization and CBMP. However, CP as well as MTG utilize the same core ATG machinery (encoded by *ATG-related* genes) as do other forms of ATG (Jin et al. 2013), whether induced by different intrinsic cues (for example, genetically programmed versus damaged by cellular metabolism) or extrinsic factors (for example, environmental stimuli) (Bhatia-Kiššová and Camougrand 2013, Ding and Yin 2012, Jin and Youle 2013, Taylor and Goldman 2011). A cargo-ligand-receptor-scaffold model has been proposed to account for how cells can select between different cargo such as the mitochondria for elimination (Jin and Youle 2013, Mijaljica et al. 2012). The identity of each of the ligand-receptor-scaffold components differ depending on the organism, cell-type, and nature of stimulus. In yeast, MTG can be associated with the cellular remodeling that occurs upon the transition of cell growth and metabolism to a preferred carbon source. When yeast cells are shifted from lactate to glucose, excess mitochondria are destroyed. The MOM protein ATG32 functions as a receptor for MTG and interacts with ATG11 (scaffold protein) and ATG8 (autophagosome membrane-anchored protein) (Jin and Youle 2013). Although ATG32 is the sole receptor for MTG in yeast, ATG33 may facilitate this process. Phosphorylation plays a key role in the regulation of MTG. A kinase phosphorylates Ser114 and Ser119 on ATG32 to mediate the ATG11–ATG32 interaction (Hirota et al. 2012). Recently, Yamashita and Kanki (2018) a reported that mitochondrial quality and quantity are not only regulated by mitochondrial fusion and fission but also by mitochondria degradation. MTG, an ATG specific for damaged or unnecessary mitochondria is an important pathway for mitochondrial homeostasis. Several stimuli can induce MTG. Some of these stimuli, however, including hypoxia, iron depletion, and nitrogen starvation, induce mild MTG, which is difficult to detect through decreased mitochondrial mass. These investigators detected MTG induced under these conditions using mito-Keima as a reporter and described the protocols for induction and detection of hypoxia and iron depletion-induced MTG using mito-Keima-expressed cells.

Molecular Imaging of MTG

Similar to CP and ATG, MTG is a progressing sub-microscopic event, and thus live cell image-based detection tools with high spatial and temporal resolution are preferred over end-stage assays to study it. Indira et al. (2018) described two methods for measuring MTG using stable cells expressing EGFP-LC3 – Mito-DsRed to mark the early phase of MTG and mitochondria-EGFP-LAMP1-RFP stable cells for late events, which showed good spatiotemporal resolution in wide-field, confocal, and super-resolution microscopy. The fluorescent biomarkers, mito-Keima or mito-QC determined the direct delivery of mitochondrial components to the lysosome in real time with quantification of monoclonal cells expressing both probes. This platform could be used both for siRNA screening and to identify key MTG regulators for theranostic applications. Sato et al. (2019) described the methods for the induction of PINK1/Parkin-mediated MTG in cell lines, which is a key mechanism of MQC, and its defects, which cause PD onset. Upon $\Delta\Psi$ collapse, PINK1 and Parkin are activated to promote the proteasomal degradation of OMM proteins and selective elimination of damaged mitochondria by CP/ATG. Fukuda and Kanki (2018) highlighted the importance of MTG in yeast. In addition, Harper et al. (2018) discussed the biochemical steps and regulatory mechanisms that promote the conjugation of ubiquitin to damaged mitochondria via the PINK1 and the E3 ubiquitin-protein ligase Parkin and how ubiquitin chains promote autophagosomal capture. The recently discovered roles for Parkin and PINK1 in the suppression of mitochondrial antigen presentation confer alternative models for how this pathway promotes the survival of neurons. A deeper understanding of these processes has major implications for NDDs, including PD, where defects in CP and MTG are prominent (Sharma et al. 2013). The critical event in MTG is the translocation of cytosolic Parkin, an ubiquitin ligase, to the defective mitochondria. Kumar and Saha (2018) and Kumar et al. (2018) elucidated on the role of SESN2/Sestrin2, a stress inducible protein, in the mitochondrial translocation of PARK2/Parkin during MTG. SESN2 downregulation inhibited BECN1/Beclin-1 and Parkin interaction, thereby preventing mitochondrial accumulation of Parkin. SESN2 interacts with ULK1 (unc-51 like kinase 1) and assists ULK1 mediated phosphorylation of Beclin-1 at serine-14 for binding with Parkin prior to mitochondrial translocation. The trigger for the SESN2 activation and regulation of Parkin translocation was the generation of mitochondrial superoxide. The scavenging of superoxide reduced SESN2, resulting in retardation of Parkin translocation in the mitochondria. The SESN2-mediated cytosolic interaction of Parkin and Beclin-1 is PINK1-independent but mitochondrial translocation of Parkin is PINK1-dependent, suggesting the role of SESN2 as a regulator of Parkin-mediated MTG. Jimenez-Orgaz et al. (2018) found that RAB7 decorates late endosomes or lysosomes and its presence on the ER, trans-Golgi network, and mitochondrial membranes is regulated by retromer and RAB7-specific GAP TBC1D5. In the absence of either TBC1D5 or retromer, RAB7 activity and localization are no longer controlled and hyperactivated RAB7 expands over the entire lysosomal domain, resulting in a loss of RAB7 mobility and depletion of the inactive RAB7 pool on endomembranes. The control of RAB7 is not required for the recycling of retromer-dependent cargo, but enables the correct sorting of ATG9a and autophagosome formation around damaged mitochondria during Parkin-mediated MTG. Cummins et al. (2018) described the PINK1/Parkin MTG pathway in neurons, and in disease models of flies and mice. New mouse models that employ fluorescent biosensors to monitor MTG *in vivo* will facilitate understanding the role of the various clearance mechanisms in the brain in pathophysiological conditions involving CP dysregulation and CBMP. Recently, Williams and Ding (2018) updated information regarding MTG in different organisms and its pathophysiological significance. They also discussed the advantage and limitations of current methods for quantifying MTG in cultured cells and *in vivo* mouse models.

Similarities and Differences in ATG, CP, and MTG

ATG is transcriptionally-regulated process, and its dysregulation can contribute to cancer, immune diseases, and NDDs. ATG occurs primarily during the mass-scale elimination of nonfunctional or degenerated organelles or macromolecules in response to DPCI-induced free-radical injury in the most vulnerable cell, whereas MTG involves the removal of nonfunctional or undesired mitochondria, and CP involves the specific, efficient, and economical removal of CBs, formed due to the aggregation and condensation of degenerated mitochondrial membranes. CBs appear as pleomorphic degenerated mitochondrial-derived intracellular inclusions to contain toxic substances and sustain IMD, ICD, and MQC for NCF. CP is a specific ATG for the selective elimination of damaged mitochondria participating in CB formation during the acute phase and CBMP during the chronic phase. The frequency of CP is reduced and ATG is increased due to functionally impaired CP in aging, resulting in chronic MDR diseases, which can be estimated by measuring the CP index (CP Index = CP Flux/ATG Flux) utilizing multiple fluorochrome analysis with *MitoTracker* and *Lysotracker* and digital fluorescence imaging and merging the fluorescence images to distinguish between CP vs ATG puncta and by using 8-OH, 2dG and 2,3 dihydroxy nonenal as two specific biomarkers of CP. LC-3-IIB, p62, Becline, Drp-1, and Mfn are markers of MTG; whereas LAMP-1 and acid phosphatase can be used as lysosomal biomarkers for real time imaging of generalized ATG. CP, MTG, and ATG may occur independently or concomitantly in the most vulnerable cell in response to DPCI as a mechanism of MQC, IMD, and ICD, depending on the intensity and frequency of the free radical attack. In all these modes of nonfunctional or undesired mitochondrial elimination, ATP-driven, lysosomal-dependent phagocytosis occurs as a common event. However, CP and MTG are specialized forms of organelle (mitochondria)-specific ATGs, which occur as an early response to DPCI. Although ATG and MTG may not specify whether functional or nonfunctional or normal or abnormal mitochondria are eliminated, CP involves the specific elimination of CBs, generated by the condensation of immature, nonfunctional, degenerated, defective, and/or undesired mitochondrial membranes, associated ER membranes, and molecules involving specifically pleomorphic CB formation as an immediate and early attempt to contain toxic metabolites to sustain intracellular homeostasis. In LSDs, malnutrition, PD, AD, and aging the phagocytosed CBs are inadequately hydrolyzed due to the deficiency of specific lysosomal enzymes and the oxidative and nitrative denaturation of proteins, resulting in the formation of insoluble inclusion bodies. The free-radical-induced oxidation of –SH moieties at the cysteine residues and functionally-impaired long-range and short range forces of electrostatic attraction and repulsion, Vander Waal forces, breakdown of hydrogen bonds, ionic bonds, and covalent bonds trigger the denaturation of proteins (that is, DRP-1, Mfns, α-Syn), rendering them insoluble and incapable of elimination via CP, MTG, and ATG (particularly from the neurons and muscles), causing NDDs, CVDs, and musculoskeletal diseases.

There seems to be a cellular, molecular, genetic, and epigenetic overlap between different types of ATGs, which needs to be adequately addressed before IMD and ICD mechanisms can be effectively executed for the TSE-EBPT of chronic MDR diseases. This can be accomplished by employing correlative and combinatorial bioinformatics and by developing novel organelle-specific molecular probes. Specific biomarker labeled fluorescence or radiolabeled probes could be utilized to precisely determine the contribution of various ATGs (including CP and MTG). CP is the most efficient, highly orchestrated, and economical process of eliminating nonfunctional and/or degenerated mitochondria, associated ER fragments, and molecules to sustain MQC, IMD, and MB in response to DPCI-induced free radical injury in the most vulnerable cell. It involves CB formation, which contains toxic metabolites that can destroy plasma membranes, GC-rich, intron-less, uncoiled mtDNA, mtmiRNA, and nDNA, causing apoptotic and/or necrotic cell death. Spatiotemporally regulated CP sustains MQC, ICD, nDNA, NCF, cell survival, mitochondrial regeneration, rejuvenation, proliferation, and elimination of degenerated mitochondria in chronic MDR disease and aging. The transcriptional and translational activity of a DPCI-exposed vulnerable cell remains structurally and functionally-intact as a result of CB formation and CP induction because these events remain localized. Moreover, the nonfunctional and /or undesirable mitochondria lose their contact from the remaining functionally significant and transcriptionally-regulated mitochondrial network. Hence, the mitochondrial network remains structurally and functionally preserved during CB formation, and to a certain extent during CBMP, as compared to MTG and generalized ATG. Although biomarkers of both CP and MTG are similar, MTG may not require sequential CB formation, CP induction, and CS stabilization/destabilization, CS exocytosis/endocytosis, and CBMP. CP follows these sequential steps of CB elimination during the acute phase and CBMP during the chronic phase of disease progression. Although, CP, ATG and MTG involve the elimination of defective mitochondria following DPCI in the most vulnerable (iPPCs) cell, molecular footprints and ultrastructural characteristics of these subcellular events are distinct and strive to elucidate several currently unknown mechanisms of mitochondrial dynamics in health and disease.

MTG was first described by Lewis and Lewis (1915). TEM was used to observe mitochondrial fragments in liver lysosomes (Ashford and Porter 1962). It was suggested that mitochondria develop functional alterations which would activate ATG (Beaulaton and Lockshin 1977). The term "mitophagy' was in use by 1998 (Scott and Klionsky 1988, Scott and Youle 2010). MTG is regulated by ATG32 in yeast, whereas NIX and Bnip-3 are regulated by PINK1 and Parkin in mammalian MTG. MTG adjusts the mitochondrial number to changing cellular metabolic needs, for steady-state mitochondrial turnover, and during developmental stages, like the differentiation of erythrocytes (Youle and Narendra 2011). Organelles and cytoplasmic remnants are sequestered and targeted to the lysosome for hydrolytic digestion by ATG. Mitochondrial metabolism creates by-products that lead to DNA damage and mutations. Hence, a healthy population of mitochondria is critical for the well-being of cells. It was believed that the targeted degradation of mitochondria is a stochastic event, but recent studies suggest that MTG is a selective process (Kim et al. 2007). ROS in the mitochondria is a byproduct of O/P, which leads to cytotoxicity and cell death. Because of their role in the metabolism, mitochondria are highly susceptible to RON's damage and become incapable of generating ATP efficiently; they become permeable to release Cyt-C, which leads to caspases activation and PARP cleavage, inducing apoptosis. Mitochondrial damage is not caused solely by oxidative stress or disease processes; normal mitochondria may also accumulate oxidative damage as a function of time which may be deleterious for NCF, particularly in aging. The faulty mitochondria can also deplete cellular energy. To avoid the uncontrolled dissemination of degenerating mitochondrial toxins, CBs are formed and eliminated through ATP-driven lysosomal-dependent CP, MTG, and/or ATG. This turnover process of MR consists of sequestration and hydrolytic degradation by the lysosome. A comparative analysis of ATG, CP, and MTG is provided in Table 7.

Table 7 The Comparative Analysis of ATG, CP, and MTG

Characteristic Features	*ATG*	*CP*	*MTG*
Cell Specificity	Cell-specific	Cell-specific	Cell-specific
Organelle-specificity	NO	Yes (Mitochondria)	Yes (Mitochondria)
Energy (ATP) Driven	Yes	Yes	Yes
Lysosomal-Dependence	Yes	Yes	Yes
CB-specificity	No (Generalized)	Yes (CB-specific)	No (Mitochondrial-specific)
Characteristic Morphological Features	Not established	Pleomorphic, loose, or compact electron-dense, multi-lamellar, quasi-crystalline membrane stacks.	Not established
Chemical Signature	ATG-related biomarkers & genes	CP-related biomarkers & genes	Mitophagy-related biomarkers & genes
Phagocytosis	Yes	Yes	Yes
Post-Phagocytic Organelles	Autophagosome	Charnophagosome & charnolosome	Mitophagosome
Number of Genes Involved	>30	To be established.	To be established.
Number of Proteins Involved	>50	To be established.	To be established.
Sequence of Occurrence	Delayed	Immediate and early	Immediate
Intracellular Detoxification	Yes	Yes	Yes
MQC	May or may not	Yes	Yes
Transcriptional Regulation	Yes	Yes	Yes
Translational Regulation	Yes	Yes	Yes
Physiological Consequences	Cell death may occur	Usually cell death does not occur if it is transcriptionally and translationally regulated.	Usually cell death does not occur if it is transcriptionally and translationally regulated.
Acute Phase	May or may not be protective	Usually protective	Usually protective
Chronic Phase	Generally destructive	Generally destructive	Generally destructive
Incidence of Occurrence	Unspecific	Occurs in mitochondrial-rich cell population.	Occurs in mitochondrial-ich cell population.
Biomarker Availability	Yes	Yes	Yes
Cell-secificity	Unspecific	Occurs in spermatocytes during the postzygotic phase and in the developing neurons, hepatocytes, cardiomyocytes, erythrocytes, and skeletal muscle during severe malnutrition.	Unspecific
Characteristic Feature	Irreversible	Reversible & recycles	Irreversible & recycles

Table 7 (Contd...)

Table 7 (contd...) The Comparative Analysis of ATG, CP, and MTG

Characteristic Features	ATG	CP	MTG
Clinical Implications	Acute & chronic diseases	Acute & chronic diseases	Acute & chronic diseases
Pathological Feature	Chronic MDR diseases	Chronic MDR diseases	Chronic MDR diseases
Theranostic Significance	Yes	Yes	Yes
Lysosomal Storage Diseases	Yes	Yes	Yes
ER Stress	Uncertain	Implicated in ERS due to MTS-induced RONS overproduction.	Implicated in ERS due to MTS-induced RONS overproduction.
Genetic & Epigenetic Modification	Yes	Yes	Yes
PKs	Ill-defined	Well-defined	Well-defined
PDs	Ill-defined	Well-defined	Well-defined
Morphological Identification	Ill-defined due to biomarker un-specificity	Well-defined due to biomarker specificity.	Well-defined due to biomarker specificity.
Primary Biomarker(s)	ATG-related genes p62, Beclin	CP-related genes 8-OH, 2dG, 2,3 dihydroxy nonenal	Mitotophagy-related genes LC-3
Detection	Biochemical (lysosomal enzymes)	Fluorescence (*MitoTracker, LysoTracker*)	Fluorescence (*MitoTracker, LysoTracker*)
Epigenetic Biomarkers	Uncertain	Methyl cytosine and Hydroxymethyl cytosine in biological fluids	Methyl cytosine and Hydroxymethyl cytosine in biological fluids
Detection Accuracy, Sensitivity, & Reproducibility	Uncertain	Highly accurate, sensitive, and reproducible	Highly accurate, sensitive, and reproducible
In Vivo Molecular Imaging (Future Prospect)	Uncertain & Unspecific	By employing ^{18}F, ^{15}O, ^{13}N, and ^{11}C-labeled CB, CP, and CS biomarkers and 5D molecular imaging with real-time multimodality high-resolution PET, MRI, CT, and SPECT and accurately developed fusion algorithms.	By employing ^{18}F, ^{15}O, ^{13}N, and ^{11}C-labeled mitophagy-specific biomarkers and 5D molecular imaging with real-time multimo-dality high-resolution PET, MRI, CT, SPECT and accurately developed fusion algorithms.
Number of Lysosomal Enzymes Involved	Lysosomes are filled with >60 hydrolases. They mediate the degradation of extracellular particles from endocytosis and intracellular components.	To be established.	To be established.

Amount of Energy Consumption	To be established.	To be established.
Duration Required	There are no exact rules, but extended fasting—for 36, 48, or even 72 hrs without food.	To be established.
Number of Mitochondrial Involved	To be established.	To be established. Mitochondrial number and health is regulated by MTG.
Organ Specificity	To be established.	To be established.
Disease Specificity	To be established	To be established.
Genetic Specificity	To be established	To be established.
Molecular Specificity	To be established	To be established.
Ethnic Specificity	To be established	To be established.
Genetic Susceptibility	ATG16L1	To be established.
Gender Susceptibility	Lower basal levels may predispose women to develop greater pathology.	To be established.
Age Susceptibility	Declines with age and impaired ATG predisposes the individual towards age-related diseases (CVDs NDDs, and MDR malignancies).	To be established.
Environmental Susceptibility	Environmental Pollutants and allergens induce oxidative stress and mitochondrial dysregulation, and senescence, promoting COPDs.	To be established.
Temperature Susceptibility	*The cellular processes that break down cellular components during senescence, starvation, and stress. Susceptibility of plant pollen to temperature stress, is yet to be established.*	To be established.
Most Susceptible Age Group	Age-related decline in chaperone-mediated ATG.	To be established.

Table 7 *(Contd...)*

Table 7 (contd...) The Comparative Analysis of ATG, CP, and MTG

Characteristic Features	ATG	CP	MTG
Influence of Body Composition	Impaired ATG contributes to muscle dysfunction in obesity and the damage is muscle-fiber dependent. A chronic high-fat high-sucrose diet increases body weight, tissue mass, and muscle function changes.	To be established.	To be established.
Influence of Exercise	Affects CVDs risk factors, endothelial function, and body fat composition.	Exercise enhances CP and CS exocytosis for ICD.	To be established.
Influence of Sex	Lower basal ATG in women may predispose to developing greater differences in the expression of LC3 and p62 in the skeletal muscles and spinal cord.	To be established.	To be established.
Influence of Sleep	The acute disruption of sleep rhythm in healthy individuals results in decreased ATG, suggesting an effect on circadian ATG sleep quality. Regulating ATG may have anti-aging and rejuvenating.	To be established.	To be established.
Influence of Drugs of Abuse	METH, *cocaine*, morphine, nicotine, and alcohol are risk factors for the progression of HIV-1. During drug-induced toxicity, ATG is altered in various cell types.	To be established.	To be established.
Biomarker Genes	Ataxin-3, p62, Belin 1, Atg5, ATG7, , ATG12 and ATGI6Ll, ATG1, ATG2, ATG3II,ATG4a, ATG4b, Atg5, ATG6, ATG7, ATG8a, ATG9, ATG10, ATG12, ATG13, ATGI4, ATGI6, ATGI7, ATGl8a, ATGl8b, ATGl0I	DRP-1, Mfn, TSPO (18kDa), MAO (a,b), XO, HO, HSP-70, HIF-1α, MTs, SOD, Catalase, Ubiquinone-NADH Oxido-reductase (Complex-1)	Beclin-1, LC-3II, Ataxin-3, p62 Parkin, p62, ULK1, and MTG receptors, including Parkin, FUNDC1, Bcl-2/ E1B19kDa-interacting protein3-like(NIX/ BNIP-3L), BCL2/adenovirus E1B-19kDa interacting protein 3 (Bnip-3), ATG32, DRP-1, Mfn-1

Most Susceptible Organ	Almost all organs but liver, brain, and skeletal muscles during severe malnutrition.	Almost all organs but liver, brain, and skeletal muscles during severe malnutrition.	Almost all organs but liver brain, and skeletal muscles during severe malnutrition.
Molecular Imaging	Available ($\Delta\Psi$, ROS, 8-OH, 2dG, 2,3, Dihydroxy nonenal, Lactate)	Available ($\Delta\Psi$, ROS, 8-OH, 2dG, 2,3, Dihydroxy nonenal, Lactate)	Available ($\Delta\Psi$, ROS, 8-OH, 2dG, 2,3, Dihydroxy nonenal, Lactate)
Primary role	Generalized ICD	MR, IMD, MQC, MB, ICD	MR, IMD, MQC, MB, ICD
Circulating Biomarker(s)	Available mtDNA, miRNAs	Available mtDNA, miRNAs, & mtmiRNAs	Available mtDNA, miRNAs, & mtmiRNAs
$\Delta\Psi$ & mtDNA	Downregulated	Downregulated	Downregulated
Most Common Stressor(s)	Starvation Tunicamycine, DPCI: microbial infection, ionizing radiation, environmental toxins, heavy metal ions (RONS)	Starvation (PCM) DPCI: infection, ionizing radiation, environmental toxins, heavy metal ions (oxidative & nitrative stress)	Starvation, Dinitrophenol, DPCI: microbial infection, environmental toxins, ionizing radiation, heavy metal ions (RONS)
Theranostic Target	Ubiquitin proteosomal pathways (to be established)	TSPO (18 KDa), 8-OH, 2dG, 2, 3 Dihydroxy Nonenal, MAOs, XO, HO, HSPs, HIF-1α, Ubiquitin proteosomal Pathway, Beclin-1, LC-3II, Ataxin-3, p62	Ubiquitin proteosomal pathway, Interferon-stimulated gene (ISG-15) Beclin-1, LC-3II, Ataxin-3, p62
nDNA	May be destroyed.	Usually remains intact and may regulate functionally impaired transcription.	Usually remains intact and may regulate functionally impaired transcription.
Unique Characteristics	Unspecific	Inclusion (CB)-specific ATG implicated in CBMP	Mitochondrial (organelle)-specific ATG

The above table indicates that ATG is characterized by relatively unspecific, uncertain, and generalized features of ICD due to the phagocytosis of almost any organelle, whereas CP and MTG are highly intricate, orchestrated, and mitochondrial-specific events possessing several common molecular, genetic, and epigenetic features.

Mitochondrial depletion reduces senescence effectors and phenotypes while preserving ATP production via enhanced glycolysis (Correia-Melo et al. 2016). There are several pathways by which MTG is induced in mammalian cells. The PINK1 and Parkin pathway is the best characterized, and is initiated by deciphering the difference between healthy and damaged mitochondria participating in CBMP. A 64-kDa protein, PINK1 can be utilized to detect MQC. PINK1 contains MTS and is recruited to the mitochondria. PINK1 is imported to the OMM via the TOM complex, and partially through the IMM via the TIM complex to span the IMM. The import into the IMM is associated with the cleavage of PINK1 from 64-kDa into 60-kDa. PINK1 is then cleaved by PARL into 52-kDa protein, which is degraded to keep the concentration of PINK1 under control (Jin and Youle 2012). In unhealthy mitochondria, the IMM is depolarized due to free radical overproduction. The $\Delta\Psi$ is necessary for the TIM-mediated protein import. In depolarized mitochondria, PINK1 is not imported into the IMM, is not cleaved by PARL, and increases in the OMM, recruiting Parkin (Lazarou 2015, Kane et al. 2014). Parkin is a cytosolic E3 ubiquitin ligase (Kitada et al. 1998). PINK1 phosphorylates Parkin at S65, homologs to the site where ubiquitin is phosphorylated, which activates Parkin by inducing dimerization. This allows the Parkin-mediated ubiquitination on other proteins. Because of the PINK1-mediated recruitment to the mitochondrial surface, Parkin can ubiquitylate proteins in the OMM, such as Mfn-1/Mfn-2 and mitoNEET. The ubiquitylation of mitochondrial surface proteins brings in MTG-initiating factors. Parkin promotes ubiquitin chain linkages on both K63 and K48. K48 ubiquitination initiates degradation of the proteins, and initiates mitochondrial degradation. K63 ubiquitination recruits ATG adaptors LC3/GABARAP, which induce MTG. Other pathways that can induce MTG include MTG receptors on the OMM. These receptors include NIX1, Bnip-3 and FUNDC1, which contain LIR sequences that bind LC3/GABARAP and lead to the degradation of the mitochondria. In hypoxic conditions, Bnip-3 is upregulated by HIF-1α and phosphorylated at serine residues near the LIR, which promotes LC3 binding. FUNDCI is also hypoxia-sensitive and is present at the OMM during normal physiological conditions.

In neurons, mitochondria are distributed heterogeneously throughout the cell to areas where energy demands are high, such as synapses and Nodes of Ranvier. The mitochondrial distribution is maintained primarily by motor protein-mediated transport along the axon. While neuronal MTG occurs primarily in the cell body, it may also occur in the axon at sites distant from the cell body via the PINK1-Parkin pathway (Narendra et al. 2009, Saxton and Hollenback 2012, Ashrafi et al. 2014). MTG in the CNS may also occur transcellularly, where damaged mitochondria in retinal ganglion cell axons may be passed to neighboring astrocytes for degradation through *trans*MTG (Davis et al. 2014).

Mitochondrial membrane proteins are encoded by both the nuclear and mitochondrial genomes. Nuclear-encoded proteins pass through OMM via translocase of the OM TOM complex which contains the SAM complex for the biogenesis of OM proteins. The insertion of proteins with internal signal sequences to the IMM is mediated by the translocase of the IM (TIM22 complex). Matrix-targeted and inner membrane-sorted pre-proteins with cleavable N-terminal pre-sequences are directed to the TIM23 complex which requires the ATP-driven pre-sequence translocase-associated motor (PAM). A small number of IM proteins are encoded by mtDNA. Oxa1 is the main insertase and, together with Mdm38 and Mba1, binds ribosomes and inserts proteins into the IM. Intermembrane space proteins (IMS) with cysteine motifs require the machinery for import and assembly (MIA) in the IMS. Mitochondria exist in a dynamic network, undergoing fusion and fission, which facilitate IM and OM fusion and the exchange of organelle contents within living cells. Mitochondrial fusion depends on the action of three GTPases: mitofusions (Mfn-1 and Mfn-2) mediating the membrane fusion on the OM, and Opa1 for IMM fusion. Mitochondrial fission requires the local organization of Fis1 and the recruitment of GTPase Drp-1 for the fission that leads to membrane scission. Different Parkin substrates have been identified in mitochondria: the mitofusin mitochondrial assembly regulatory factor (MARF), mitofusin 1, mitofusin 2, and voltage dependent anion-selective channel protein 1 (VDAC1), all of which are embedded in the OMM. Parkin promotes the recruitment of p62, an ubiquitin-binding adaptor also known as sequestosome 1, which can aggregate ubiquitinated proteins by polymerizing with other p62 molecules and recruit ubiquitinated cargo into autophagosomes by binding to LC3. P62 accumulates on mitochondria, binds to Parkin-ubiquitinated substrates, mediates clumping of mitochondria, and links ubiquitinated substrates to LC3 to facilitate ATG degradation of ubiquitinated proteins. The histone deacetylase HDAC6 also binds ubiquitinated substrates, accumulates on mitochondria following Parkin translocation, and is required for Parkin-mediated MTG. LC3 is synthesized as proLC3 in the cytosol. Soon after its translation, proLC3 is cleaved by ATG4B to expose the carboxyterminal Gly of LC3 (LC3-l), which is activated by the same E1-like enzyme, ATG7, transferred to ATG3, and conjugated to phosphatidyl-ethanolamine (PE)). The LC3-PE conjugate is known as LC3-II, an autophagosome membrane bound form of LC3. The ATG12-Atg5 conjugate functions such as an E3-like ligase for LC3 lipidation. Following the formation of the isolation membrane, it elongates to engulf mitochondria. During elongation of the isolation membrane, the Atg5-ATG12-ATG16L complex forms a cup-shaped structure. LC3-II localizes to the isolation membrane, while the Atg5-ATG1-ATG16L complex dissociates from it. Soon after autophosome formation, its outer membrane fuses with lysosomes to form autolyosomes. The lysosomal hydrolases, including cathespins and lipases, degrade the intra-autophoagosomal contents, whereas cathepsins degrade LC3-II on the intra-autophagosomal surface.

ER-Mitochondrial Interaction in CP Regulation

The mitochondrial translocase of the outer membrane (TOM) is a protein complex that is essential for the post-translational import of nuclear-encoded mitochondrial proteins. Among its subunits, TOM70 and TOM20 are associated with the core complex, shedding light on their roles within the OMM. By using mammalian cell lines, Filadi et al. (2018) demonstrated that TOM70 clusters in distinct OMM foci, overlapping with sites in which the ER contacts mitochondria. TOM70 depletion impairs IP3-linked ER to mitochondrial Ca^{2+} transfer, which is dependent on the capacity of TOM70 to interact with IP3-receptors and favors their functional recruitment close to mitochondria. The reduced Ca^{2+} transfer to mitochondria, observed in TOM70-depleted cells, attenuates mitochondrial respiration, induces CMB and ATG, and inhibits proliferation, suggesting a role of TOM70 in pro-survival ER-mitochondria communication, and ER-mitochondrial signaling as a key regulator of cell fate. Generally, ERS occurs due to excessive exposure to free radicals released from the mitochondria as a byproduct of O/P whereas CB formation inhibits ERS. The mitochondrial-ER contacts (MERCs) as the mitochondria-associated membrane (MAM), were discovered in the early 1950s (Simmen and Herrera-Cruz 2018). The two organelles exchange Ca^{2+} and lipids. ER and mitochondria move closer to enhance contacts during ERS, hypoxia, or nutrient deprivation, favoring CB formation and CBMP, while over nutrition lessens these contacts. Signaling associated with these intracellular events modulates the contact site during ATG, apoptosis, and the alterations in the mitochondrial metabolism. Tethering complexes, as well as key MAM proteins including chaperones of the ER and mitochondria, control the plasticity of MERC, which is impaired during CBMP. Hence, MAM composition and its plasticity are critical for the development of metabolic syndrome, NDDs, CVDs, and cancer. ERS is induced in response to mitochondrial RONS stress. A mitochondrion loses its structural and functional contacts from rest of its network and ER before participating in CBMP. Initially, redox imbalance causes swelling due to $\Delta\Psi$ collapse, formation of megapores, increased permeability, and translocation of intraluminal as well as cytosolic Ca^{2+} to the mitochondria. The opening of mega-pore allows the entry of water and electrolytes to cause mega-mitochondrio-genesis (Sharma et al. 2003). Some of the ER membranes still remain attached and fuse with the mega-mitochondria (Size: 1–10 μm: with reduced cristae) to prevent their fragmentation. All swollen mitochondria condense along with the fused ER membranes and become elongated to remain incapable of fission due the downregulation and delocalization of MFN and AgNOR, DRP-1, XO, HO-1, HIF-1α, P^{53}, MAOs, TRPCs, and TSPO. The condensed mitochondria sequester water to form electron-dense, multi-lamellar stacks as a sieve to prevent the dissemination of toxic metabolites. Hence, the pleomorphic phenotype of CB depends on the intensity and frequency of free radicals, chemical composition of membranes, and Ca^{2+} within the mitochondria, intraluminal ER, and cytoplasm. CB is Akt-ubiquinated and recognized by the lysosomes for phagocytosis and involves ATP-driven phagocytosis as a secondary mechanism of ICD to sustain MQC and ICD to prevent CBMP. Due to the downregulation of AgNOR, ribosomes, RER, ATP depletion, and compromised protein (MFN and DRP-1)-synthesizing machinery during DPCI, mitochondria can neither divide nor function properly. The fusion of ER membranes and increased $[Ca^{2+}]_i$ contribute to their enlarged size, rendering them incapable of fission. The persistent lack of nutrients also contributes to this lack of fission. Ca^{2+} also facilitates ER membrane fusion with the mitochondrial membranes to confer CB pleomorphism during CBMP.

Recently, Tao et al. (2019) showed that miR-4465 inhibited the expression of PTEN, upregulated phosphorylated Akt, and attenuated ATG by activating mTOR in HEK293, HeLa, and SH-SY5Y cells. MiR-4465 reduced PTEN mRNA via targeting the 3′UTR, elucidating the molecular mechanism of miRNA-regulated PTEN-related ATG which may provide novel strategies for the treatment of PTEN-related diseases. The ER forms contacts with other endo-membranes to exchange materials (for example, Ca^{2+} and lipids) to modulate fission, cargo sorting, and movement. During autophagosome formation, contacts between the ER and the phagophore are crucial for the expansion and closure. ERS triggers the UPR, which restores the normal function of the ER. Guo et al. (2018) demonstrated that miR-346, which is induced under ERS, modulates ATG in HeLa cells. By regulating ATG, miR-346 reduced the ROS level in the cells, thus protecting them from death following ERS. GSK3B is the target of miR-346 and participates in ERS-related ATG. MiR-346 activates ATG by interrupting the association between BCL2 and BECN1 in a GSK3B-dependent manner. This study shed new light on the role of miRNAs during ERS and suggested a novel mechanism of ATG induction during ERS.

Zhao et al. (2018) found that the ER-localized ATG protein EPG-3/VMP1 plays an essential role in controlling ER-phagophore dissociation and the disassembly of ER contacts with LDs, mitochondria, and endolysosomes. VMP1 regulates the ER contact by activating the ER Ca^{2+} channel ATPase sarcoplasmic/ER Ca^{2+} transporting (ATP2A/SERCA). Calmodulin (CALM) acts as one of the downstream Ca^{2+} effectors that controls the PIK3C3/VPS34-PtdIns3K to maintain these contacts. This study provided insights into the molecular mechanisms which regulate ER contacts and generate auto-phagosomes. Multiple molecular mechanisms contribute to pathological changes in neurons. A large fraction of these alterations can be linked to dysfunction in the ER and mitochondria, affecting the metabolism and secretion of lipids and proteins, Ca^{2+} homeostasis, and energy production. These organelles interact with each other at domains on the ER called as MAMs, which rely on the interaction of proteins localized either at the mitochondria or at the ER interface for exchange of Ca^{2+}, metabolites, and lipids. MAMs also play a crucial role in the control of mitochondria dynamics and CP/ATG and have emerged as a key element in connecting changes observed in NDDs. Bernard-Marissal et al. (2018) focused on the role of MAMs in ALS and hereditary motor and sensory neuropathy, and how they affected neurons with long projecting axons. They discussed how defects in MAM signaling may impair $[Ca^{2+}]_i$ homeostasis, mitochondrial dynamics, ER function, and ATG, resulting in axonal degeneration. The impact of MAM dysfunction in glial cells affect the latter's capacity to support neurons and/or axons. They emphasized the role of MAMs as a promising biomarker for the TSE-EBPT of NDDs.

Crosstalk between Organelles-specific ATGs

Although overlapping omics biomarkers, signaling mechanisms, and functional characteristics exist among ATG, CP, and MTG, these have distinct features in their presentation and impact on the biological system in health and disease. ATG is a cytosolic QC process that recognizes substrates through receptor-mediated mechanisms. Procollagens, the most abundant gene products in Metazoa, are synthesized in the ER, and a fraction that fails to attain the native structure is cleared by ATG. Forrester et al. (2019) performed siRNA interference and CRISPR-Cas9 or knockout-mediated gene deletion of candidate ATG and ER proteins in collagen producing cells. The ER-resident lectin chaperone Calnexin (CANX) and the ER-phagy receptor FAM134B were required for the ATG-mediated QC of endogenous procollagens. CANX, as co-receptor, recognized ER luminal misfolded pro-collagens and interacted with the ER-phagy receptor, FAM134B. In turn, FAM134B bound the autophagosome membrane-associated protein LC3 and delivered a portion of ER containing both CANX and pro-collagen to the lysosome for degradation. Thus, a crosstalk between the ER-QC machinery and the ATG pathway selectively disposes proteasome-resistant misfolded components from the ER.

Pexophagy, Mitochondria, and CP

Pexophagy is selective ATG that targets peroxisomes and is essential for the maintenance of the homeostasis of peroxisomes for the prevention of peroxisome-related disorders. Peroxisomes are highly dynamic intracellular organelles in the metabolism of long-chain fatty acids, d-amino acids, and polyamines. Peroxisomes are also connected to mitochondria, and both organelles regulate redox signaling. Peroxisome dysregulation is implicated in several metabolic diseases, and evidence highlights the important role of diminished peroxisomal functions in aging. Cho et al. (2018) focused on the induction and regulation of pexophagy, and the adaptors involved in mediating pexophagy. They described the roles of pexophagy in various pathophysiological responses, providing insight into the clinical relevance of pexophagy regulation. Understanding how pexophagy interacts with biological functions will facilitate the development of novel therapeutics in peroxisomal dysfunction-related diseases. Walker et al. (2018) reported that a byproduct of peroxisomal metabolism is the generation and detoxification of RONS, particularly H_2O_2. Because of its relatively low reactivity, H_2O_2 has a longer half-life and a high diffusion rate, which makes H_2O_2 an efficient signaling molecule. Peroxisomal proteins are also subject to oxidative modification and inactivation by the RONS they generate, but the LonP2 protease can remove such oxidatively-damaged proteins involved in CBMP to prolong their lifespan. Peroxisomal homeostasis must adapt to the metabolic state of the cell, by a combination of their proliferation, the removal of excess or damaged organelles by pexophagy, as well as by peroxisome inheritance and motility. The tumor suppressors ATM and TSC, which regulate mTORC1 signaling, regulated pexophagy in response to RONS. Hence, impaired peroxisome homeostasis can impair CP to cause physiological consequences.

Estimation of Organelle-specific ATGs and Their Theranostic Significance

Some investigators have used the term micro-autophagy to describe the elimination of a small portion of a cell without any specific description of intracellular organelle (ICO) and whether the cell survived or lost its structural and functional integrity. Similarly, macrophagy, bulk autophagy, and agrephagy have been used to describe a massive elimination process without any description of a mechanism of specific ICO. However, CP, MTG, ER-phagy, Golgiphagy, pexophagy, and nucleophagy represent the elimination of specific ICOs and can be detected by using organelle-specific fluorochromes, digital fluorescence imaging microscopy, and flow cytometry. Although, we can acquire real time *in vivo* images of ICOs in cultured cells, their inherent limitations include a precise sequence, localization, resolution, and quantitation. Although, high-resolution TEM and SEM can provide precise localization and identification of organelles, their structural and functional integrity is compromised during fixation and staining. Generally, we obtain TEM and SEM images of the dead material. Moreover, these methods are costly, time-consuming, and cumbersome when longitudinal studies are performed. Hence, we need to develop efficient, sensitive, and *in vivo* DSST biomarkers for the identification and characterization of organelle-specific ATGs in real time and *in vivo* to establish their exact pathophysiological significance in health and disease. Nevertheless, we should not be carried away with the impression that TEM and SEM are not important. In fact, the original discoveries of mitochondria, ER membranes, ribosomes, lysosomes, peroxisomes, CBs, CS, and intracellular events (including ATG, MTG, and CP) were discovered only by classical TEM and SEM analyses. Progress in *in vivo* and *in vitro* quantitative molecular imaging and omics technology employing correlative and combinatorial bioinformatics has improved our knowledge and wisdom regarding the exact TSE-EBPT of ICO and inclusion-specific ATGs such as CP. Thus, CP can be recognized as an original discovery of mitochondrial inclusion-specific ATG. Henceforth, we need to use these terms more carefully to describe the disease process. For example, I have described CP index and CS index to quantitatively estimate the loss and gain of mitochondria in a biological system. Hence, the cell survival may or may not be affected seriously during phagocytosis of nonfunctional mitochondria, ER membranes, lysosomes, and peroxisomes. Although, a cell may survive under stressful situations, it may contribute to chronic MDR diseases. In addition, nucleophagy is a process of downregulation of nDNA which usually occurs in response to severe DPCI and may induce irreversible intracellular injury to cause apoptosis in the most venerable cell.

CP Detection by Flow Cytometery and Other Methods

All forms of ATGs can be distinguished and quantitatively estimated by a flow cytometer with cell sorting facility employing organelle-specific fluorescently labeled biomarkers. The cells can be sorted and enriched using specific florochrome-labeled probes to quantitatively estimate the intensity and frequency of CP in health and disease. The sorted cells can be subjected to cDNA microarray analysis to further confirm and differentiate characteristic signatures (feature selection) from the heat maps and CP/ATG/MTG-linked genetic network analysis. These data can be correlated and confirmed by immunoblotting, RT-PCR, LC-MASS proteome analysis, FRET, pathway-specific ELISA, and SPR spectroscopy to correlate and confirm the results and accomplish the TSE-EBPT of chronic MDR diseases. These results can be further confirmed by sequencing representative biomarker gene(s) and/or protein(s). Recently, Beclin-1, LC-3II, ataxin-3, and p62 were used for the evaluation of MTG.

Theranostic Potential of CP/CS Regulators

I have proposed to develop CP regulators as novel DSST-TSE-EBPT-CPTs, as CP modulators, CP modifiers; CP inducers/CP agonists, and CP inhibitors/CP antagonists, depending on the physicochemical characteristics of the disease (Sharma 2019). We can utilize disease-specific CP *in vitro* in cell culture and *in vivo* in animal models for the preclinical screening of theranostic agents. CP-targeted drugs will revolutionize the conventional wisdom of chemotherapy and routine clinical practice because these agents will be based primarily on MQC, IMD, MB, and ICD with minimum or no adverse effects, which will improve our immune system, general health, productivity, longevity, and QOL. Based on these strategies, we can develop CS stabilizers/destabilizers, CS agonists/CS antagonists, CS modulators/CS regulators, CS exocytosis enhancers/CS exocytosis inhibitors, and CS endocytosis inhibitors to authenticate the theranostic potential of CP modulators/regulators for the TSE-EBPT of NDDs, CVDs, and MDR malignancies as described in this edition.

Through proper genetic selection, diet restriction, moderate exercise, sex, and sleep (DRESS) habits and by selecting a safe environment and lifestyle (GELS), we can enjoy BQL and longevity. Increased physical and sexual activity and drugs of abuse, indiscriminate use of contraceptive pills, repeated pregnancies, repeated abortions, microbial infections, environmental pollutants, heavy metal ions, MDR malignancies, increased consumption of saturated fat, salt, sugar, tobacco and alcohol, a sedentary life-style, repeated surgeries, organ transplantation, severe bodily injuries, and lack of exercise, and microbial infections compromise MB and cause CNS, cardiovascular, musculoskeletal, hepatic, GIT, and renal malfunctions resulting in fatigue, lethargy, somnolence, obesity, early morbidity, and morality. Hurries, worries, curries, and forced physical and sexual activity enhance sympathetic activity to release NE and opioid peptides (endorphins and encephalines), which induce intestinal immobilzation, resulting in constipation. Persistent constipation promotes ICT and pro-inflammatory septicemia. Moreover, the buildup of tyramines by consuming smoked meat, processed tofu, cheese, and ethanol increases BP, which in turn enhances the risk of HTN, micro-angiopathies, CVDs, renal failure, and even fatal sub-arachnoid hemorrhage. Hence, a Mediterranean diet rich in vitamins and antioxidant (fruits, vegetables, nuts) olive oil (rich in PUFA and omega-3 fatty acids), in addition to moderate exercise is recommended for general health and well-being.

The unique feature of CP is that it primarily involves the phagocytosis of pleomorphic mitochondrial-inclusion-specific CBs which can be easily detected by modern bioanalytical and molecular imaging procedures. In addition to cultured cells, tissues, and disease-specific 3D organoids, we can detect and follow the CB lifecycle, CP induction, CS destabilization, and CBMP in real time *in vitro* by time-lapse cinematography, digital fluorescence imaging, and *in vivo* by PET molecular imaging of live gene-manipulated animal model of diseases to determine the clinical significance of newly-developed theranostic agents. Particularly, ^{18}F, ^{15}O, ^{13}N, ^{11}C-labelled CB, CP, and CS biomarkers can be employed to reconstruct noninvasive multimodality (5D) molecular images of human body with high-resolution PET, MRI, CT, and SPECT *in vivo*. We can also develop fusion algorithms and co-registration protocols to detect intricate CP events in real time to discover novel CPTs and evaluate their exact theranostic significance in health and disease. Hence, the future of CP is promising as well as challenging. Although certain genes and proteins exhibit an overlap between ATG, CP and MTG, with further improvement in biotechnology, we will be more precise, accurate, and reproducible in distinguishing theranostically significant genes and proteins involved in various types of ATGs in health and disease.

The Theranostic Significance of Antioxidants as CP Regulators

Various natural and synthetic antioxidants prevent CB formation by maintaining the MQC, ICD, and by preventing MR as these may serve as CP regulators, CS stabilizers, and CBMP antagonists to confer theranostic benefit in various diseases, including NDDs, CVDs, diabetes, cancer, and aging as free radical scavengers by improving MB. There are primarily three types of antioxidants:

(i) Endogenous antioxidants: Superoxide dismutase, Catalase, Glutathione, Metallothioneins, Heat shock proteins, Hypoxia inducible factor-1α (HIF-1α), Carnitine. Chemerin, BCl-2, Beclin-1.

(ii) Natural antioxidants: Resveratrol, Melatonin, Curcumin, Lycopene, Catechin, Cyanidin, Quercetin, Ginsenoside Rb1, Protocatcchuic acid, Caffcic acid, Fucoxanthine, Kaempferol, Formononetin, Betaine, Zeaxanthin dipalmitate, Akebia Saponin D, Tanshinone IIA, Ginsenoside Rb1, Carnosic Acid, Sesemin, Indole-3-Carbinol, CoQ$_{10}$, Thymoquinone, Raffinose, Apigenin, Quercetogetin, Irisin, Gastrodin, Empagliflozin, Humanin, H2S, Estrogen, Oleuropein aglycone (OLE), and various other polyphenol and flavonoids, Thioredoxin, Lycium barbarum polysaccharide (LBP), Morusin, Melatonin, Salidroside, Trifolium Pratens L, Fucoxanthine, Torins, Lycium barbarum polysaccharide (LBP), and Salvia miltiorrhiza ('Danshen' in Chinese), Xiao-Xu-Ming decoction, Naringin, URB597, Tetrahydrocurcumin, Calretinine, Sirtuins, Rutins, Mitofusin, Cardiolipin, Atrial Natriuretic Factor (ANF), Arhalofenate acid, Quercetin.

(iii) Synthetic antioxidants: C(60) Fullerene-Derived (PEG-C(60)-3), PEG-C(60)-3, and PTX-C(60)-2 Nanomaterials (as free-radical sponges), Hydrogen, NaHS, N-acetyl Cystine (NAC), Acetyl-L-carnitine, H2Se, CO, Metformin, Glibenclamide, Statins, Vildagliptin, Edoravone, Probucol, Fenofibrate, Liproxstatin1 PPARγ Agonists, Vitamins A, D, and E, as CB antagonists, CP agonists, and CS stabilizers confer protection in CVDs, NDDs, and MDR malignancies. Fruits, vegetables, and nuts are a rich source of antioxidants as illustrated in this edition and in Table 8.

Table 8 The Health Benefits of Antioxidants as CP Regulators

S.No	Active Principal	Biological Source	Health Impact
1.	Sulphur Compounds	Garlic, Leeks, Onions, Ginger	Fights common cold, reduce BP, improves cholesterol, lower risk of heart attack, blood, sugar, bone density, antibacterial, digestion.
2.	Anthocyanins	Berries, Eggplant, Grapes	Anti-inflammatory, anti-carcinogenic, anti-viral, fights common cold, reduce BP, battles UTI.
3.	β-Carotene	Apricot, Carrot, Mango, Parsley, Pumpkin, Spinach,	Skin, mucus membrane, eye health, vision, immune system.
4.	Catechins	Green Tea, Red Grapes	Prevent cell damage, disease fighting.
5.	Copper (Cu)	Milk, Lean Meat, Nuts, Sea Food	Formation of RBCs, bone, BV, CNS, CVDs, osteoporosis.
6.	Cryptoxanthins	Red capsicum, Mangoes, Pumpkin	Inhibits bone resorption, prevents cell and DNA damage, lung cancer, colon cancer.
7.	Flavinoids	Tea, Green Tea, Citrus Fruits, Onion, Grapes, Apple	Prevent cancer, CVDs, stroke, asthma.

Table 8   *Contd...*

Table 8 (Contd.)   The Health Benefits of Antioxidants as CP Regulators

S.No	Active Principal	Biological Source	Health Impact
8.	Indoles	Crucifers Vegetables (Broccoli, Cabbage, Cauliflower)	Reduce the risk of cervical and BC.
9.	Isoflavinoids	Lentils, Milk Peas, Tofu, Soy Bean	Prevents cardiovascular disease, osteoporosis, hormone-dependent cancer and loss of cognitive function.
10.	Lignans	Sesame Seed, Bran, Whole Grain, Bran	Immune system, hormone balance.
11.	Luteins	Green Leafy Vegetables, Spinach, Corn	Protects and maintains healthy cells in the eyes.
12.	Lycopene	Tomato, PINK Grapefruit, Watermelon	Sun protection, improved. heart health, and a lower risk of certain types of cancers.
13.	Manganese	Seafood, Lean Meat, Milk, Nuts	Reduce disease, inflammation, in combination with glucosamine and chondroitin, blood sugar regulation, lower incidences of epileptic seizures.
14.	Polyphenols	Thyme, Oregano	Help treat digestion issues, weight management, fight diabetes, NDDs, CVDs.
15.	Selenium	Seafood, Offal, Lean Meat, Whole Grains	Prevent CVDs, thyroid problems, cognitive decline, cancer.
16.	Vitamin A	Liver, Sweet Potato, Carrot, Milk, Egg Yolk	Protects eyes from night blindness and age-related decline, lowers risk of certain cancers, supports a healthy immune system, reduces risk of acne, supports bone health, promotes healthy growth and reproduction.
17.	Vitamin C	Orange, Black Currants, Kiwi Fruit, Mangoes, Broccoli, Spinach, Capsicum, Blueberry, Strawberry	Formation of collagen, absorption of iron, strengthening the immune system, wound healing, and the main-tenance of cartilage, bones, and teeth.
18.	Vitamin E	Vegetable oil, Wheat germ oil, Avocado, Nuts, Seeds, Whole grains	Prevent coronary heart disease, supports immune function, prevent inflammation, promotes eye health, and lower the risk of cancer.
19.	Zinc	Seafood, Milk, Nuts	Regulating immune function, treating diarrhea. Effects learning and memory, battles the common cold, encourages wound healing, provides a decreased risk of age-related chronic disease.
20.	Zoochemicals	Red Meat, Offal, Fish, Plants	CVDs and cancer.

Modified from: Carlsen et al. 2010. The total antioxidant content of more than 3100 foods, beverages, spices, herbs and supplements used worldwide. Nutr J 9:3.

The Theranostic Significance of CPI

The CP index (CPI) is a ratio of CP vs ATG. Inflammation, infection, and/or traumatic injuries are associated with compromised CPI and chronic MDR diseases in aging. Based on MB, CPI, and ICD, we can arbitrarily divide a human life span in five major phases as illustrated in Table 9.

Table 9   CPI, Life Cycle, and Disease Risk

S.No	Phase	Age (Years)	CPI	Physiological Consequences
1	Energy Production	0–25	Linear increase	Growth & development of body (vulnerable O/P, CP, and lysosomal ICD)
2	Energy Dissipation	25–50	Plateau	Reproduction, fertility, fecundity (efficient O/P,CP & lysosomal ICD)
3	Energy Restoration	50–60	Gradual decline	Minor to moderate risk of infections & inflammations (compromised O/P, CP, and lysosomal-ICD)
4	Energy Conservation	60–75	Further decline	Major risk of infections, inflammations (compromised O/P, CP, and lysosomal ICD)
5	Energy Depletion	75–100	A sharp decline	+Anemia, fatigue, morbidity, & mortality (lack of O/P, CP, IMD, and lysosomal ICD), increased risk of microbial (bacteria, virus, fungus, parasite) infections, NDDs, CVDs, and chronic MDR malignancies, morbidity & mortality

CPI follows a normal distribution pattern. The risk of CVDs, NDDs, and MDR malignancies increases when CPI declines due to CMB and impaired MQC as a function of aging. CPI is compromised due to impaired lysosomal activity, defective ubiquitination, O/P, and free-radical-induced MR and CBMP, implicated in CB formation, dysregulated CP, CS destabilization, and CBMP. CPI is directly proportional to IMD, ICD, and MB. Hence, compromised MB, IMD, and ICD are responsible for chronic illnesses. Genes, environment, and lifestyle play a pivotal role in determining MB, MR, CB formation, CP induction, CPI, IMD, and ICD; hence, explaining an individual's predisposition to an increased or decreased life span, microbial infection, inflammation, immunity, chronic MDR diseases, early or delayed morbidity, mortality, and longevity. CS can serve as a primary biomarkers of early viral detection in the biological fluids and macrophages. Different phases of the life cycle described in the above table are synonymous to sequential events of ATG described by Nobel Laureate Professor Yoshinori Ohsumi in 2016 in yeast and plants.

Note: The list of items presented in the tables is far from complete, may have several limitations, and might have been omitted due to lack of my own knowledge and limited space allocated to write this manuscript. Please accept my apologies.

CONCLUSION

This edition highlights the theranostic significance of CP as a basic molecular mechanism of IMD, ICD, and MQC for NCF to remain healthy. Since CP is an immediate and early pre-requisite for the induction of generalized ATG, the author has written CP/ATG to systematically elucidate the disease process for theranostic applications in this edition. In general, CP is dysregulated in severe malnutrition (over nutrition or undernutrition), anemia, vitamin deficiencies NDDs, stroke, CVDs (ischemic heart disease), endocrine abnormalities, diabetes, dehydration, over-hydration, water and electrolyte imbalance, MDR malignancies, microbial (bacterial, viral, fungal, and parasite) infections, HIV/AIDS, environmental toxins, inorganic and organic poisons, road and flight accidents, burns, ionizing radiation injuries, surgical and accidental injuries, pressure ulcers, and numerous congenital, genetic, epigenetic disorders, and aging due to compromised MB, IMD, MQC, and ICD of stem cells and other vulnerable cells. Particularly, astronauts, organ-transplanted, and severely war-wounded persons experience these devastating changes in CP dynamics due to isolation, immobility, and severe malnutrition; hence, they are subjected to cachexia and sarcopenia. This vulnerable group is provided a specialized radapertized or radurized diet to boost their MB and immune system and prevent CBMP accompanied with compromised CP. The rationale of CP induction and inhibition in health and disease is described in this edition with a primary objective to develop DSST-TSE-EBPT-CPTs to cure chronic MDR diseases. ROS-scavenging antioxidant-loaded NPs for enhanced CNS delivery of CPTs for the effective treatment of NDDs, CVDs, inflammatory diseases, and aging, and vice versa for the treatment of chronic MDR malignancies are proposed in this edition. It will be promising to learn the exact spatiotemporal sequence of events in (i) generalized, (ii) organelle, (iii) and inclusion (CB)-specific ATGs (CP) to establish their exact overlap and theranostic significance in acute and chronic inflammatory and non-inflammatory diseases. Hence, it is highly prudent to discover novel TSE-EBPT strategies for the successful clinical management of various MDR diseases. Meanwhile, we can follow *DRESS* and *GELS* principles to stay healthy and be productive. Furthermore, novel CPTs and MB-targeted pharmaceuticals such as CB agonists/ antagonists, CP agonists/antagonists, CS stabilizers/destabilizers, and CS exocytosis enhancers/ inhibitors can be developed for the treatment of chronic MDR diseases for longevity and BQL.

REFERENCES

Abdul Rahim, S.A., A. Dirkse, A. Oudin, A. Schuster, et al. 2017. Regulation of hypoxia-induced autophagy in glioblastoma involves ATG9A. Br J Cancer 117: 813–825.

Alegre, F., A.B. Moragrega, M. Polo and A. Marti-Rodrigo. 2018. Role of p62/SQSTM1 beyond ATG: A lesson learned from drug-induced toxicity in vitro. Br J Pharmacol 175: 440–455.

Alexander, I., R. May, J. Devenish and M. Prescott. 2012. The many faces of mitochondrial autophagy: Making sense of contrasting observations in recent research. International Journal of Cell Biology 2012: 1–18. Article ID 431684.

Andrejeva, G., S. Gowan., G, Lin., A.-C. LF Wong Te Fong, et al. 2019. De novo phosphatidylcholine synthesis is required for autophagosome membrane formation and maintenance during autophagy. Autophagy 16(6): 1044–1060.—Please check reference

Angelika, S.R. and J. Lippincott-Schwartz. 2011. Mechanisms of mitochondria and ATG crosstalk. Cell Cycle 10: 4032–4038.

Arakawa, S., S. Honda, S. Torii, M. Tsujioka, et al. 2018. Monitoring of Atg5-Independent MTG, Methods Mol Biol 1759: 125–132.

Ashford, T.P. and K.R. Porter. 1962. Cytoplasmic components of hepatic cell lysosomes. The Journal of Cell Biology 12: 198–202.

Ashrafi, G., J.S. Schlehe, M.J. Lavoie and T.L. Schwartz. 2014. MTG of damaged mitochondria occurs locally in distal neuronal axons and requires PINK1 and Parkin. J Cell Biol. 206: 655–70.

Aviva, M. and K.T. Tolkovsky. 2014. Tieu in Autophagy: Cancer, Other Pathologies, Inflammation, Immunity, Infection, and Aging: Volume 4.

Bajaj, L., P. Lotfi, R. Pal, A.D. Ronza, et al. 2019. Lysosome biogenesis in health and disease. J Neurochem 148: 573–589.

Bartel, K., H. Pein, B. Popper, S. Schmitt, et al. 2019. Connecting lysosomes and mitochondria – A novel role for lipid metabolism in cancer cell death. Cell Commun Signal 17: 87.

Beaulaton, J. and K.R. Lockshin. 1977. Ultrastructural study of the normal degeneration of the intersegmental muscles of Antheraea polyphemus and Manduca sexta (Insecta, Lepidoptera) with particular reference of cellular ATG. Journal of Morphology 154: 39–57.

Bendorius, M., I. Neeli, F. Wang, S.R. Bonam, et al. 2018. The mitochondrion-lysosome axis in adaptive and innate immunity: Effect of lupus regulator peptide P140 on mitochondria autophagy and NETosis. Front Immunol 9: 2158.

Bernard-Marissal, N., R. Chrast and B.L. Schneider. 2018. Endoplasmic reticulum and mitochondria in diseases of motor and sensory neurons: A broken relationship? Cell Death Dis. 9: 333.

Bhatia-Kiššová, I. and N. Camougrand. 2013. Mitophagy: A process that adapts to the cell physiology. Int J Biochem Cell Biol. 45(1): 30–33.

Bhattacharjee, A., A. Szabó, T. Csizmadia, H. Laczkó-Dobos, et al. 2019. Understanding the importance of ATG in human diseases using *Drosophila*. J Genet Genomics 46: 157–169.

Bootman, M.D., T. Chehab, G. Bultynck, J.B. Parys, et al. 2018. The regulation of ATG by calcium signals: Do we have a consensus? Cell Calcium 70: 32–46.

Boya, P., P. Codogno and N. Rodriguez-Muela. 2018. Autophagy in stem cells: Repair, remodelling and metabolic reprogramming. Development 145(4): dev146506.

Brazill, J.M., Y. Zhu, C. Li and R.G. Zhai. 2018. Quantitative cell biology of neurodegeneration in *Drosophila* through unbiased analysis of fluorescently tagged proteins using imageJ. J Vis Exp (138): e58041.

Carlsen, M.H., B.L. Halvorsen, K. Holte, S.K. Bohn, et al. 2010. The total oxidant content of more than 3100 foods, beverages, spices, herbs, and supplements used worldwide. Nutr. J. 9: 3.

Castellazzi, M., S. Patergnani, M. Donadio, C. Giorgi, et al. 2019. Correlation between auto/mitophagic processes and magnetic resonance imaging activity in multiple sclerosis patients. J Neuroinflammation 16: 131. https://doi.org/10.1186/s12974-019-1526-0.

Chabenne, A., C. Moon, C. Ojo, A. Khogali, et al. 2014. Biomarkers in fetal alcohol syndrome (Recent Update). Biomarkers and Genomic Medicine 6: 12–22.

Charonis, A.S., M. Michalak, J. Groenendyk, L.B. Agellon, et al. 2017. Endoplasmic reticulum in health and disease: The 12th International Calreticulin Workshop, Delphi, Greece. J Cell Mol Med 21: 3141–3149.

Chen, X., K. Wang, Y. Xing, J. Tu, et al. 2014. Coronavirus membrane-associated papain-like proteases induce autophagy through interacting with Beclin1 to negatively regulate antiviral innate immunity. Protein Cell 5(12): 912–927.

Chen, Y., R. Feng, G. Luo, J. Guo, et al. 2018. DCF1 subcellular localization and its function in mitochondria. Biochimie 144: 50–55.

Chen, H., H. Sun, S. Zhang, W. Yan, et al. 2019. Monitoring ATG in live cells with a fluorescent light-up probe for G-quadruplex structures. Chem Commun (Camb) 55: 5060–5063.

Chi., C., A. Leonard, W.E. Knight, K.M. Beussman, et al. 2019. LAMP-2B regulates human cardiomyocyte function by mediating autophagosome–lysosome fusion. PNAS 116: 556–565.

Cho, D,H., Y.S. Kim, D.S. Jo, S.K. Choe, et al. 2018. Pexophagy: Molecular mechanisms and implications for health and diseases. Mol Cells 41: 55–64.

Cohen, S. 2018. Lipid droplets as organelles. Int Rev Cell Mol Biol 337: 83–110.

Cooper, K.F. 2018. Till death do us part: The marriage of autophagy and apoptosis. Oxid Med Cell Longev 2018: Article ID 4701275.

Cornelissen, T., P. Verstreken, W. Vandenberghe. 2018. Imaging MTG in the fruit fly. Autophagy 14: 1656–1657.

Correia-Melo, C., F.D. Marques, R. Anderson, G. Hewitt, et al. 2016. Mitochondria are required for pro-ageing features of the senescent phenotype. The EMBO Journal 35: 724–42.

Cummins, N. and J. Götz. 2018. Shedding light on MTG in neurons: What is the evidence for PINK1/Parkin MTG in vivo? Cell Mol Life Sci 75: 1151–1162.

Dakshinamurti, K., S.K. Sharma, M. Sundaram and T. Watanabe. 1993. Hippocampal changes in developing postnatal mice following intrauterine exposure to domoic acid. J Neurosc 13(10): 4486–4495.

Davis, C.H., K.Y. Kim, E.A. Bushong, E.A. Mills, et al. 2014. Transcellular degradation of axonal mitochondria. PNAS 111: 9633–9638.

Di Malta, C., L. Cinque and C. Settembre. 2019. Transcriptional regulation of autophagy: Mechanisms and diseases. Front Cell Dev Biol 7: 114.

Ding, W.X and X.M. Yin. 2012. Mitophagy: mechanisms, pathophysiological roles, and analysis. Biol Chem 393: 547–564

Elliott, I.A., A.M. Dann, S. Xu, S.S. Kim, et al. 2019. Lysosome inhibition sensitizes PC to replication stress by aspartate depletion. PNAS 116: 6842–6847.

Erdi, B., P. Nagy, A. Zvara, A. Varga, et al. 2012. Loss of the starvation-induced gene Rack1 leads to glycogen deficiency and impaired autophagic responses in *Drosophila*. Autophagy 8(7): 1124–1135

Esteban-Martinez, L., B. Villarejo-Zori and P. Boya. 2017. Cytofluorometric assessment of mitophagic flux in mammalian cells and tissues. Methods Enzymol 588: 209–217.

Farmer, T., N. Naslavsky and S. Caplan. 2018. Tying trafficking to fusion and fission at the mighty mitochondria. Traffic 19: 569–577.

Filadi, R., N.S. Leal, B. Schreiner, A. Rossi, et al. 2018. TOM70 sustains cell bioenergetics by promoting IP3R3-mediated ER to mitochondria Ca^{2+} Transfer. Curr Biol 28: 369–382.

Forrester, A., C. De Leonibus, P. Grumati, E. Fasana, et al. 2019. A selective ER-phagy exerts procollagen quality control via a Calnexin-FAM134B complex. EMBO J 38(2): e99847.

Fukuda, T. and T. Kanki. 2018. Mechanisms and physiological roles of MTG in yeast. Mol Cells 41: 35–44.

Furukawa, K., T. Fukuda, S.I. Yamashita, T. Saigusa, et al. 2018. The PP2A-like protein phosphatase Ppg1 and the far complex cooperatively counteract CK2-mediated phosphorylation of Atg32 to inhibit mitophagy. Cell Rep 23(12): 3579–3590.

Furuya, N., S. Kakuta, K. Sumiyoshi, M. Ando, et al. 2018. NDP52 interacts with mitochondrial RNA poly(A) polymerase to promote mitophagy. EMBO Rep 19(12): e46363.

Galluzzi, L., J.M. Bravo-San Pedro, B. Levine, D.R. Green, et al. 2017. Pharmacological modulation of autophagy: Therapeutic potential and persisting obstacles. Nat Rev Drug Discov 16: 487–511.

Gilkerson, R. 2018. A disturbance in the force: Cellular stress sensing by the mitochondrial network. Antioxidants (Basel) 7(10): 126.

Gonçalves, W.G., K.M. Fernandes, W.C. Santana, G.F. Martins, et al. 2018. Post-embryonic development of the Malpighian tubules in Apis mellifera (Hymenoptera) workers: morphology, remodeling, apoptosis, and cell proliferation. Protoplasma 255: 585–599.

Goodwin, J.N., W.E. Dowdle, R. DeJesus, Z. Wang, et al. 2017. Autophagy-independent lysosomal targeting regulated by ULK1/2-FIP200 and ATG9. Cell Rep 20: 2341–2356.

Guo, J., Z. Yang, X. Yang, T. Li, et al. 2018. miR-346 functions as a pro-survival factor under ER stress by activating mitophagy. Cancer Lett 413: 69–81.

Gustafsson, Å.B and G.W. Dorn, II. 2019. Evolving and expanding the roles of mitophagy as a homeostatic and pathogenic process. Physiol Rev 99: 853–892.

Harper, J.W., A. Ordureau and J.M. Heo. 2018. Building and decoding ubiquitin chains for mitophagy. Nat Rev Mol Cell Biol 19: 93–108.

Herrington, C.S., R. Poulsom and P.J. Coates. 2019. Recent advances in pathology: The 2019 Annual Review Issue of The Journal of Pathology. J Pathol 247: 535–538.

Hirota, Y., D. Kang and T. Kanki. 2012. The physiological role of mitophagy: New insights into phosphorylation events. Int J Cell Biol 2012: Article ID 354914.

Imanikia, S., N.P. Özbey, C. Krueger, M.O. Casanueva, et al. 2019. Neuronal XBP-1 activates intestinal lysosomes to improve proteostasis in C. elegans. Curr Biol 29: 2322–2338.

Indira, D., S.N. Varadarajan, S.S. Lupitha, A. Lekshmi, et al. 2018. Strategies for imaging MTG in high-resolution and high-throughput. Eur J Cell Biol 97: 1–14.

Ishikawa, K.I., A. Yamaguchi, H. Okano and W. Akamatsu. 2018. Assessment of mitophagy in iPS cell-derived neurons. Methods Mol Biol 1759: 59–67.

Jády, B., A. Ketele and T. Kiss. 2018. Dynamic association of human mRNP proteins with mitochondrial tRNAs in the cytosol. RNA (12): 1706–1720. doi: 10.1261/rna.066738.118.

Jagtap, A., S. Gawande and S. Sharma. 2015. Biomarkers in vascular dementia. (A Recent Update). Biomarkers and Genomic Medicine 7: 43–56.

Jimenez-Orgaz, A., A. Kvainickas, H. Nägele, J. Denner, et al. 2018. Control of RAB7 activity and localization through the retromer-TBC1D5 complex enables RAB7-dependent mitophagy. EMBO J 37: 235–254.

Jin, S.M. and R.J. Youle. 2012. PINK1- and Parkin-mediated mitophagy at a glance. J Cell Sci 125: 795–799.

Jin, S.M. and R.J. Youle. 2013. The accumulation of misfolded proteins in the mitochondrial matrix is sensed by PINK1 to induce PARK2/Parkin-mediated mitophagy of polarized mitochondria. Autophagy 9: 1750–1757.

Kane, L.A., M. Lazarou, A.I. Fogel, K. Yamano, et al. 2014. PINK1 phosphorylates ubiquitin to activate Parkin E3 ubiquitin ligase activity. J Cell Biol 205: 143–53.

Kanki, T and D.J. Klionsky. 2008. Mitophagy in yeast occurs through a selective mechanism. J Biol Chem. 283: 32386–32393.

Kanki, T. and D.J. Klionsky. 2009. Atg32 is a tag for mitochondria degradation in yeast. Autophagy 5(8): 1201–1202.

Kanki, T., D. Kang, D.J. Klionsky. 2009a. Monitoring mitophagy in yeast: the Om45-GFP processing assay. Autophagy 5(8): 1186–1189.

Kanki, T., K. Wang, M. Baba, C.R. Bartholomew, et al. 2009b. A genomic screen for yeast mutants defective in selective mitochondria autophagy. Mol Biol Cell 20(22): 4629–4870.

Karmi, O., H.B. Marjault, L. Pesce, P. Carloni, et al. 2018. The unique fold and lability of the [2Fe-2S] clusters of NEET proteins mediate their key functions in health and disease. J Biol Inorg Chem 23: 599–612.

Khandia, R., M. Dadar, A, Munjal, K. Dhama, et al. 2019. A comprehensive review of autophagy and its various roles in infectious, non-infectious, and lifestyle diseases: Current knowledge and prospects for disease prevention, novel drug design, and therapy. Cells 8(7): 674.

Khor, B., K.L. Conway, A.S. Omar, M. Biton, et al. 2019. Distinct tissue-specific roles for the disease-associated autophagy genes ATG16L2 and ATG16L1. J Immunol 203: 1820–1829.

Khuansuwan, S., L.M. Barnhill, S. Cheng and J.M. Bronstein. 2019. A novel transgenic zebrafish line allows for in vivo quantification of autophagic activity in neurons. Autophagy 15: 1322–1332.

Kim, I., S. Rodriguez-Enriquez and J.J. Lemasters. 2007. Selective degradation of mitochondria by mitophagy. Archives of Biochemistry and Biophysics 462: 245–253.

Kissová, I., M. Deffieu, S. Manon, N. Camougrand. 2004. Uth1p is involved in the autophagic degradation of mitochondria. J Biol Chem 279: 39068–39074.

Kitada, T., S. Asakawa, N. Hattori, H. Matsumine, et al. 1998. Mutations in the Parkin gene cause autosomal recessive juvenile Parkinsonism. Nature 392: 605–608.

Kocaturk, N.M. and D. Gozuacik. 2018. Crosstalk between mammalian autophagy and the ubiquitin-proteasome system. Front Cell Dev Biol 6: 128. doi: 10.3389/fcell.2018.00128

Kong, F., I.T. Romero, J. Warakanont and Y. Li-Beisson. 2018. Lipid catabolism in microalgae. New Phytol. 218: 1340–1348. doi:10.1111/nph.15047

König, J., T. Grune and C. Ott. 2019. Assessing ATG in murine skeletal muscle: Current findings to modulate and quantify the autophagic flux. Curr Opin Clin Nutr Metab Care 22: 355–362.

Kourtis, N. and N. Tavernarakis. 2009. Autophagy and cell death in model organisms. Cell Death Differ 16: 21–30.

Krols, M., B. Asselbergh, R. De Rycke, V. De Winter, et al. 2019. Sensory neuropathy-causing mutations in ATL3 affect ER-mitochondria contact sites and impair axonal mitochondrial distribution. Hum Mol Genet 28: 615–627.

Kumar, A. and C. Shaha. 2018. SESN2 facilitates mitophagy by helping Parkin translocation through ULK1 mediated Beclin1 phosphorylation. Sci Rep 8(1): 615.

Kumar, A., A. Dhawan, A. Kadam and A. Shinde. 2018. Autophagy and mitochondria: Targets in neurodegenerative disorders. CNS Neurol Disord Drug Targets 17: 696–705.

Kurihara, Y. and K. Tomotake. 2014. Mitophagy induction in yeast. *In*: M. Hyatt (ed.), Autophagy: Cancer, Other Pathologies, Inflammation, Immunity, Infection, and Aging, Vol. 4. Academic Press, Elsevier, UK, pp. 1–304.

Lamming, D.W. and L. Bar-Peled. 2019. Lysosome: The metabolic signaling hub. Traffic 20: 27–38.

Lazarou, M. 2015. Keeping the immune system in check: a role for mitophagy. Immunol Cell Biol 93: 3–10.

Lee, J., S. Giodano and J. Zhang. 2012. ATG, mitochondria and oxidative stress: Cross-talk and redox signaling. Biochem J 441: 523–540.

Leung, K., K. Chakraborty, A. Saminathan and Y. Krishnan. 2019. A DNA nanomachine chemically resolves lysosomes in live cells. Nat Nanotechnol 14: 176–183.

Lewis, M.R. and W.H. Lewis. 1915. Mitochondria (and other cytoplamic structures) in tissue cultures. American Journal of Anatomy 17: 339–401.

Li, Y.L., W.F. Cai, L. Wang, G.S. Liu, et al. 2018. Identification of the functional autophagy-regulatory domain in HCLS1-associated protein X-1 that resists against oxidative stress. DNA Cell Biol 37: 432–441.

Ligia, C., L.C. Gomes, G. De Benedetto., L. Scorrano L. 2011. During autophagy mitochondria elongate, are spared from degradation and sustain cell viability. Nature Cell Biology 13: 589–598.

Liu, L., D. Feng, G. Chen, M. Chen, et al. 2012. Mitochondrial outer-membrane protein FUNDC1 mediates hypoxia-induced mitophagy in mammalian cells. Nat Cell Biol 14: 177–185.

Liu, Y. and K. Okamoto. 2018. The TORC1 signaling pathway regulates respiration-induced MTG in yeast. Biochem Biophys Res Commun 502: 76–83.

Liu, S.W., J.C. Chang, S.F. Chuang, K.H. Liu, et al. 2019. Far-infrared radiation improves motor dysfunction and neuropathology in spinocerebellar ataxia type 3 mice. Cerebellum 18: 22–32.

Lonardo, A., S. Ballestri, A. Mantovani, F. Nascimbeni, et al. 2019. Pathogenesis of hypothyroidism-induced NAFLD: Evidence for a distinct disease entity? Dig Liver Dis 51: 462–470.

Lu, L., Z.Y. Wu, X. Li and F. Han. 2019. State-of-the-art: Functional fluorescent probes for bioimaging and pharmacological research. Acta Pharmacol Sin 40: 717–723.

Luo, G., Y. Sun, R. Feng, Q. Zhao, et al. 2018. ARL3 subcellular localization and its suspected role in ATG. Biochimie 154: 187–193.

Lyamzaev, K.G., A.V. Tokarchuk, A.A. Panteleeva, A.Y. Mulkidjanian, et al. 2018. Induction of ATG by depolarization of mitochondria. Autophagy 14: 921–924.

Makarov, V.I., I. Khmelinskii and S. Javadov. 2018. Computational modeling of in vitro swelling of mitochondria: A biophysical approach. Molecules 23: 783.

Marcassa, E., A. Kallinos, J. Jardine and E.V. Rusilowicz-Jones. 2018. Dual role of USP30 in controlling basal pexophagy and mitophagy. EMBO Rep 19: e45595.

Mayorga, L., B.N. Salassa, D.M. Marzese, M.A. Loos, et al. 2019. Mitochondrial stress triggers a pro-survival response through epigenetic modifications of nuclear DNA. Cell Mol Life Sci 76: 1397–1417.

Mijaljica, D., T.Y. Nazarko, J.H. Brumell, W.P. Huang, et al. 2012. Receptor protein complexes are in control of autophagy. Autophagy 8(11): 1701–1705

Möckel, C., J. Kubiak, Q. Schillinger, R. Kühnemuth, et al. 2019. Integrated NMR, fluorescence, and molecular dynamics benchmark study of protein mechanics and hydrodynamics. J Phys Chem B 123: 1453–1480.

Narendra, D., A. Tanaka, D.F. Suen and R.J. Youle. 2009. Parkin-induced mitophagy in the pathogenesis of Parkinson disease. Autophagy 5: 706–708.

Nemani, N., E. Carvalho, D. Tomar, Z. Dong, et al. 2018. MIRO-1 determines mitochondrial shape transition upon GPCR activation and Ca^{2+} stress. Cell Rep 23: 1005–1019.

New, M., T. Van Acker, M. Jiang, R. Saunders, et al. 2019. Identification and validation of novel autophagy regulators using an endogenous readout siGENOME screen. *In*: N. Ktistakis and O. Florey (eds), Autophagy: Methods in Molecular Biology, Vol 1880. Humana Press, New York, NY, pp. 359–374.

Niu, L.Q., J. Huang, Z.H. Yan, Y.H. Men, et al. 2018 Fluorescence detection of intracellular pH changes in the mitochondria-associated process of MTG using a hemicyanine-based fluorescent probe. Spectrochim Acta A Mol Biomol Spectrosc 207: 123–131.

Novak, I. and I. Dikic. 2011. Autophagy receptors in developmental clearance of mitochondria. Autophagy 7(3): 301–303.

Nowikovsky, K., S. Reipert, R.J. Devenish and R.J. Schweyen. 2007. Mdm38 protein depletion causes loss of mitochondrial K^+/H^+ exchange activity, osmotic swelling and mitophagy. Cell Death Differ 14(9): 1647–1656.

Okamoto, K. and N. Kondo-Okamoto 2012. Mitochondria and ATG: Critical interplay between the two homeostats. Biochim Biophys Acta 820: 595–600.

Onishi, M., S. Nagumo, S. Iwashita and K. Okamoto. 2018. The ER membrane insertase Get1/2 is required for efficient mitophagy in yeast. Biochem Biophys Res Commun 503: 14–20.

Palikaras, K., E. Lionaki and N. Tavernarakis. 2019. Mitophagy dynamics in *Caenorhabditis elegans*. *In*: N. Ktistakis and O. Florey (eds), Autophagy: Methods in Molecular Biology, Vol 1880. Humana Press, New York, NY, pp. 655–668.

Pan, X., Z. Song, C. Wang, T. Cheng, et al. 2019. H$_2$Se induces reductive stress in HepG2 cells and activates cell autophagy by regulating the redox of HMGB1 protein under Hypoxia. Theranostics 9: 1794–1808.

Panda, P.K., A. Fahrner, S. Vats, E. Seranova, et al. 2019. Chemical screening approaches enabling drug discovery of autophagy modulators for biomedical applications in human diseases. Front Cell Dev Biol 7: 38. doi: 10.3389/fcell.2019.00038

Park, S.Y., E.G. Sun, Y. Lee, M.S Kim, et al. 2018. ATG induction plays a protective role against hypoxic stress in human dental pulp cells. J Cell Biochem 119: 1992–2002.

Priault, M., B. Salin, J. Schaeffer, F.M. Vallette, et al. 2005. Impairing the bioenergetic status and the biogenesis of mitochondria triggers mitophagy in yeast. Cell Death Differ 12: 1613–1621.

Puri, C., M. Vicinanza and D.C. Rubinsztein. 2018. Phagophores evolve from recycling endosomes. Autophagy 14: 1475–1477.

Rasika, S., S. Passemard, A. Verloes, P. Gressens, et al. 2018. Golgipathies in neurodevelopment: A new view of old defects. Dev Neurosci 40: 396–416.

Redmann, M., G.A. Benavides, W.Y. Wani, T.F. Berryhill, et al. 2018. Methods for assessing mitochondrial quality control mechanisms and cellular consequences in cell culture. Redox Biol 17: 59–69.

Rodger, C.E., T.G. McWilliams and I.G. Ganley. 2018. Mammalian mitophagy – from *in vitro* molecules to *in vivo* models. FEBS J 285: 1185–1202.

Sampaio-Marques, B., A. Guedes, I. Vasilevskiy, S. Gonçalves, et al. 2019. α-Syn toxicity in yeast and human cells is caused by cell cycle re-entry and ATG degradation of ribonucleotide reductase 1. Aging Cell 18: e12922.

Sandhof, C.A., S.O. Hoppe, S. Druffel-Augustin, C. Gallrein, et al. 2019. Reducing INS-IGF1 signaling protects against non-cell autonomous vesicle rupture caused by SNCA spreading. Autophagy 29: 878–899.

Sato, S., T. Norikura and Y. Mukai. 2019. Maternal quercetin intake during lactation attenuates renal inflammation and modulates autophagy flux in high-fructose-diet-fed female rat offspring exposed to maternal malnutrition. Food Funct 10: 5018–5031.

Sauvat, A. and O. Kepp. 2017. Molecular characterization of autophagic responses, part B edited by Lorenzo Galluzzi, José Manuel Bravo-San Pedro, Guido Kroemer. 588: 2–576.

Saxton, W.M. and P.J. Hollenbeck. 2012. The axonal transport of mitochondria. Journal of Cell Science 125: 2095–2104.

Scott, S.V. and D.J. Klionsky. 1988. Delivery of Proteins and organelles to the vacuole from the cytoplasm. Current Opinion in Cell Biology 10: 523–529.

Scott, I. and R.J. Youle. 2010. Mitochondrial fission and fusion. Essays Biochem 47: 85–98.

Senft, D. and Z.A. Ronai. 2015. UPR, autophagy, and mitochondria crosstalk underlies the ER stress response. Trends Biochem Sci 40: 141–148.

Seranova, E., C. Ward, M. Chipara, T.R. Rosenstock, et al. 2019. In vitro screening platforms for identifying ATG modulators in mammalian cells. Methods Mol Biol 1880: 389–428.

Sharma, S.K., U. Nayar, M.C. Maheshwari, et al. 1986. Ultrastructural studies of P-cell morphology in developing normal and undernourished rat cerebellar cortex. Electrophysiological Correlates Neurology 34: 323–327.

Sharma, S.K., U. Nayar, M.C. Maheshwari and B. Singh. 1987. Effect of undernutrition on developing rat cerebellum: Some electrophysiological and neuromorphological correlates. J. Neurol. Sciences. 78: 261–272.

Sharma, S.K. 1988. Nutrition and Brain Development. *In*: Proceedings of the First World Congress of Clinical Nutrition. New Delhi, India, p. 5–8.

Sharma, S.K., W. Selvamurthy, M.C. Maheshwari and T.P. Singh. 1990. Kainic acid induced epileptogenesis in developing normal and undernourished rats -A computerized EEG analysis. Ind Jr Med Res 92: 456–466.

Sharma, S.K. and K. Dakshinamurti. 1992. Seizure activity in Pyridoxine-deficient adult rats. Epilepsia 33: 235–247.

Sharma, S.K., U. Nayar, M.C. Maheshwari and B. Singh. 1993. Purkinje cell evoked unit activity in developing undernourished rats. J Neurol Sci 116: 212–219.

Sharma, S.K., W. Selvamurthy and K. Dakshinamurti. 1993. Effect of environmental neurotoxins in the developing brain. Biometeorology 2: 447–455.

Sharma, S.K. and K. Dakshinamurti. 1993. Suppression of domoic acid-induced seizures by 8-(OH)-DPAT. J Neural Transmission 93: 87–89.

Sharma, S., E. Carlson and M. Ebadi. 2003. The neuroprotective actions of selegiline in inhibiting 1-Methyl, 4-Phenyl, pyridinium ion (MPP+)-induced apoptosis in dopaminergic neurons. J Neurocytol 32: 329–343.

Sharma, S., M. Kheradpezhou, S. Shavali, H.El-Refaey, et al. 2004. Neuroprotective actions of coenzyme Q_{10} in Parkinson's Disease. Methods Enzymol 382: 488–509.

Sharma, S. and M. Ebadi. 2013. Antioxidant targeting in neurodegenerative disorders. *In*: I. Laher (ed.). Springer Verlag, Germany, pp. 1–30.

Sharma, S., C.S. Moon, A. Khogali, A. Haidous, et al. 2013a. Biomarkers of Parkinson's disease (Recent Update). Neurochem Int 63: 201–229.

Sharma, S., A. Rais, R. Sandhu, W. Nel, et al. 2013b. Clinical significance of metallothioneins in cell therapy and nanomedicine. Int J Nanomed 8: 1477–1488.

Sharma, S. 2014a Beyond Diet and Depression, Vol. 1. Nova Sciences Publishers, New York, U.S.A.

Sharma, S 2014b Beyond Diet and Depression, Vol. 2. Nova Sciences Publishers, New York, U.S.A.

Sharma, S. 2014c Nanotheranostics in evidence based personalized medicine. Curr Drug Targets 15: 915–930.

Sharma, S. 2014d. Molecular pharmacology of environmental neurotoxins. *In*: E. Leone (ed.), Kainic Acid: Neurotoxic Properties, Biological Sources, and Clinical Applications. Nova Science Publishers, New York, pp. 1–47.

Sharma, S. and M. Ebadi. 2014a Significance of metallothioneins in aging brain. Neurochemistry International 2014: 65: 40–48.

Sharma, S. and M. Ebadi. 2014b. Charnoly body as a universal biomarker of cell injury. Biomarkers and Genomic Medicine 6: 89–98.

Sharma, S., B. Nepal, C.S. Moon, A. Chabenne, et al. 2014. Psychology of craving. Open Jr of Medical Psychology. 3: 120–125.

Sharma, S., S. Gawande, A. Jagtap, R. Aboulela, et al. 2015. Fetal alcohol syndrome; prevention, diagnosis, and treatment. Journal of Drug Addiction, Education, and Eradication 11(2): 127–166.

Sharma, S. 2015a. Monoamine Oxidase Inhibitors: Clinical Pharmacology, Benefits, and Adverse Effects. Nova Science Publishers, New York. U.S.A.

Sharma, S. 2015b. Alleviating Stress of the Soldier and Civilian. Nova Science Publishers, New York. U.S.A.

Sharma, S., J. Choga, V. Gupta, P. Doghor, et al. 2016. Charnoly body as novel biomarker of nutritional stress in Alzheimer's disease. Functional Foods in Health and Disease. 6(6): 344–377.

Sharma, S. 2016a. Progress in PET Radiopharmaceuticals (Quality Control & Theranostics). Nova Science Publishers, New York. U.S.A.

Sharma, S. 2016b. Personalized Medicine (Beyond PET Biomarkers). Nova Science Publishers, New York. U.S.A.

Sharma, S. 2016c. PET radiopharmaceuticals for personalized medicine. Curr Drug Targets 17: 1894–1907.

Sharma, S. and W. Lippincott. 2017. Emerging biomarkers in Alzheimer's disease (Recent Update). Current Alzheimer Research 14 (in press)

Sharma, S. 2017a. Translational multimodality neuroimaging. Curr Drug Targets 18: 1039–1050.

Sharma, S. 2017b. Zika Virus Disease (Prevention and Cure). Nova Science Publishers, New York, U.S.A.

Sharma, S. 2017c. Fetal Alcohol Spectrum Disorders: Concepts, Mechanisms, and Cure. Nova Science Publishers, New York U.S.A.

Sharma, S. 2018a. Nicotinism and the Emerging Role of E-Cigarettes (With Special Reference to Adolescents), Vol. 1: Concepts, Mechanisms, and Clinical Management. Nova Science Publishers, New York, U.S.A.

Sharma, S. 2018b. Nicotinism and the Emerging Role of E-Cigarettes (With Special Reference to Adolescents), Vol. 2: Concepts, Mechanisms, and Clinical Management. Nova Science Publishers, New York, U.S.A.

Sharma, S. 2018c. Nicotinism and the Emerging Role of E-Cigarettes (With Special Reference to Adolescents), Vol. 3: Concepts, Mechanisms, and Clinical Management. Nova Science Publishers, New York, U.S.A.

Sharma, S. 2018d. Nicotinism and the Emerging Role of E-Cigarettes (With Special Reference to Adolescents), Vol. 4: Concepts, Mechanisms, and Clinical Management. Nova Science Publishers, New York, U.S.A.

Shimizu, S. 2018. Organelle zones in mitochondria. J Biochem 165: 101–107.

Sica, V. and M.C. Maiuri. 2016. *In*: M. Hyatt (ed.), Autophagy: Cancer, Other Pathologies, Inflammation, Immunity, Infection, and Aging, Vol. 9. Elsevier Publishers, pp 343–357.

Simmen, T. and M.S. Herrera-Cruz. 2018. Plastic mitochondria-endoplasmic reticulum (ER) contacts use chaperones and tethers to mould their structure and signaling. Curr Opin Cell Biol 53: 61–69.

Simons, I.M., J. Mohrlüder, R. Feederle, E. Kremmer, et al. 2019. The highly GABARAP specific rat monoclonal antibody 8H5 visualizes GABARAP in immunofluorescence imaging at endogenous levels. Sci Rep 9: 526.

Singh, B.K., R.A. Sinha, M. Tripathi, A. Mendoza, et al. 2018. Thyroid hormone receptor and ERRα coordinately regulate mitochondrial fission, mitophagy, biogenesis, and function. Sci Signal 11(536): eaam5855.

Soubannier, V., G.L. McLelland, R. Zunino, E. Braschi, et al. 2012. A vesicular transport pathway shuttles cargo from mitochondria to lysosomes. Curr Biol 22: 135–141.

Sugo, M., H. Kimura, K. Arasaki, T. Amemiya, et al. 2018. Syntaxin 17 regulates the localization and function of PGAM5 in mitochondrial division and mitophagy. EMBO J 37(21): e98899.

Sun, H., Y. Liu, L. Zhang, X. Shao, et, al. 2017. Numb positively regulates autophagic flux via regulating lysosomal function. Biochem Biophys Res Commun 491: 780–786.

Tal, R., G. Winter, N. Ecker, D.J. Klionsky, et al. 2007. Aup1p, a yeast mitochondrial protein phosphatase homolog, is required for efficient stationary phase mitophagy and cell survival. J Biol Chem 282: 5617–5624.

Tao, Z., C. Feng, C. Mao, J. Ren, et al. 2019. MiR-4465 directly targets PTEN to inhibit Akt/mTOR pathway–mediated autophagy. Cell Stress Chaperones 24: 105–113.

Taylor, R. and S.J. Goldman. 2011. Mitophagy and disease: New avenues for pharmacological intervention. Curr Pharm Des 17(20): 2056–2073.

Tian, M., C. Liu, B. Dong, Y. Zuo, et al. 2019. A dual-site controlled ratiometric probe revealing the simultaneous down-regulation of pH in lysosomes and cytoplasm during autophagy. Chem Commun (Camb) 55: 10440–10443.

Tolkovsky, A.M. 2009. Mitophagy. Biochimica et Biophysica Acta 1793: 1508–1515.

Tran, Q., J.H. Jung, J. Park, H. Lee, et al. 2018. S6 kinase 1 plays a key role in mitochondrial morphology and cellular energy flow. Cell Signal 48: 13–24.

Trendeleva, T.A. and R.A. Zvyagilskaya. 2018. Retrograde signaling as a mechanism of yeast adaptation to unfavorable factors. Biochemistry 83: 98–106.

Turn, R.E., R.S. D'Souza and A.A. Wall. 2019. Meeting report-small GTPases in membrane processes: FASEB summer research conference. Traffic 20: 259–262.

Twig, G., B. Hyde, O.S. Shirihai. 2008. MMitochondrial fusion, fission and autophagy as a quality control axis: The bioenergetic view. Biochem Biophys Acta 1777: 1092–1097.

Um, J.H., Y.Y. Kim, T. Finkel and J. Yun. 2018. Sensitive measurement of mitophagy by flow cytometry using the pH-dependent fluorescent reporter mt-Keima. J Vis Exp (138): e58099.

van Wijk, S.J, S. Fulda, I. Dikic and M. Heilemann. 2019. Visualizing ubiquitination in mammalian cells. EMBO Rep 20: e46520.

Vargas, J.N.S., C. Wang, E. Bunker, L. Hao, et al. 2019. Spatiotemporal control of ULK1 activation by NDP52 and TBK1 during selective ATG. Mol Cell 74: 347–362.

Vasarmidi, E., S. Sarantoulaki, A. Trachalaki, G. Margaritopoulos, et al. 2018. Investigation of key autophagy-and mitophagy-related proteins and gene expression in BALF cells from patients with IPF and RA-ILD. Mol Med Rep 18: 3891–3897.

Vicario, M., D. Cieri, M, Brini and T. Calì. 2018. The close encounter between alpha-synuclein and mitochondria. Front Neurosci 12: 388.

Vincow, E.S., G. Merrihew, R.E. Thomas, N.J. Shulman, et al. 2013. The PINK1-Parkin pathway promotes both mitophagy and selective respiratory chain turnover *in vivo*. PNAS 110(16): 6400–6405.

Vives-Bauza, C. and S. Prezedborski. 2011. Mitophagy: the latest problem for Parkinson's disease. Trends Mol Med 17: 158–165.

von Kleist, L., K. Ariunbat, I. Braren, T. Stauber, et al. 2019. A newly generated neuronal cell model of CLN7 disease reveals aberrant lysosome motility and impaired cell survival. Mol Genet Metab 126: 196–205.

Walker, C.L., L.C.D. Pomatto, D.N. Tripathi and K.J.A. 2018. Davies. Redox regulation of homeostasis and proteostasis in peroxisomes. Physiol Rev 98: 89–115.

Wible, D.J. and S.B. Bratton. 2018. Reciprocity in ROS and autophagic signaling. Curr Opin Toxicol 7: 28–36.

Williams, J.A. and W.X. Ding. 2018. Mechanisms, pathophysiological roles and methods for analyzing MTG- recent insights. Biol Chem 399: 147–178.

Xia, X., S. Katzenell, E.F. Reinhart, K.M. Bauer, et al. 2018. A pseudo-receiver domain in ATG32 is required for mitophagy. Autophagy 14: 1620–1628.

Xie, L.L., F. Shi, Z. Tan, Y. Li, et al. 2018. Mitochondrial network structure homeostasis and cell death. Cancer Sci 109: 3686–3694.

Yamaguchi, A., H. Ishikawa, M. Furuoka, M. Yokozeki, et al. 2018. Cleaved PGAM5 is released from mitochondria depending on proteasome-mediated rupture of the outer mitochondrial membrane during mitophagy. J Biochem 165: 19–25.

Yamashita, S.I. and T. Kanki. 2018. Detection of iron depletion- and hypoxia-induced MTG in mammalian cells. Methods Mol Biol 1782: 315–324.

Yang, Z., X. Zhao, J. Xu, W. Shang, et al. 2018. A novel fluorescent reporter detects plastic remodeling of mitochondria-ER contact sites. J Cell Sci 131: jcs208686.

Yang, Z. and S. Dondong. 2018. Mechanism and Regulation of Selective MTG in Cardiometabolic Disease in Autophagy and Cardiometabolic Diseases. Ed. R. Jun Elsevier Publishers. p 1–340.

Yao, Z., X. Liu and D.J. Klionsky. 2018. MitoPho8Δ60 assay as a tool to quantitatively measure mitophagy activity. Methods Mol Biol 1759: 85–93.

Yi, C., J.J. Tong and L. Yu. 2018. Mitochondria: The hub of energy deprivation-induced autophagy. Autophagy 14: 1084–1085.

Yoo, S.M. and Y.K. Jung. 2018. A molecular approach to mitophagy and mitochondrial dynamics. Mol Cells 41: 18–26.

Yoshimori, T., H. Zhang and A. Simonsen. 2018. Selective autophagy (Z2). April 22—26, 2018 Westin Miyako Kyoto • Kyoto, Japan

Youle, R.J. and D.P. Narenda. 2011. Mechanisms of mitophagy. Nat Rev Mol Cell Biol 12: 9–14.

Zachari, M., S.R. Gudmundsson, Z. Li, M. Manifava, et al. 2019. Selective ATG of mitochondria on a ubiquitin-endoplasmic-reticulum platform. Dev Cell 50: 627–643.

Zemirli, N., E. Morel and D. Molino. 2018. Mitochondrial dynamics in basal and stressful conditions. Int J Mol Sci 19(2): 564.

Zhang. Y., Y. Xie, W. Liu, W. Deng, et al. 2019a. DeepPhagy: A deep learning framework for quantitatively measuring autophagy activity in *Saccharomyces cerevisiae*. Autophagy 16(4): 626–640.

Zhang, Q., F. Presswalla, K. Feathers, X. Cao, et al. 2019b. A platform for assessing outer segment fate in primary human fetal RPE cultures. Exp Eye Res 178: 212–222.

Zhao, Y.G. and H. Zhang. 2018. The ER-localized ATG protein EPG-3/VMP1 regulates ER contacts with other organelles by modulating ATP2A/SERCA activity. Autophagy 14: 362–363.

Zhao, Y.G. and H. Zhang. 2019. Core ATG genes and human diseases. Curr Opin Cell Biol 61: 117–125.

Zheng, Y., Y. Qiu, C.R.R. Grace, X. Liu, et al. 2019. A switch element in the autophagy E2 Atg3 mediates allosteric regulation across the lipidation cascade. Nat Commun 10: 3600.

Zhu, Y., G. Chen, L. Chen, W. Zhang, et al. 2014. Monitoring mitophagy in mammalian cells. Methods Enzymol 547: 39–55.

Zirin, J. and N. Perrimon. 2010. *Drosophila* as a model system to study autophagy. Semin Immunopathol 32: 363–372.

Concluding Remarks

This edition introduces the systematic description of inclusion (CB)–specific ATG as CP and its relationship and overlap with organelle-specific ATG and generalized ATG for the TSE-EBPT of chronic diseases. CP seems to be first original discovery of inclusion-specific ATG of clinical significance. Although, the theranostic potential of CP in MB, MR, IMD, and ICD has been described, we need to learn more regarding its exact spatio-temporal transcriptional and translational regulation for the safe and effective treatment of chronic NDDs, CVDs, infectious diseases, drug addiction, and belligerent MDR malignancies. Many issues, questions, overlapping observations, and concerns remain unresolved in this emerging topic of medicine. Currently, we know very little regarding inclusion-specific ATGs and their exact cellular, molecular, genetic, and epigenetic significance and functional relationship with generalized ATG in health and disease. Hence, these have been described using various names as discussed earlier. With further improvement in biotechnology, we will have integrated knowledge about these specialized forms ATGs and their exact functional relationship with generalized ATG. Further studies in this direction will provide their exact significance in evidence-based nanotheranostics. Mitochondrial remodeling (MR) during free radical-induced CB formation occurs as a primary event of IMD and ICD to contain toxic substances within the cell, whereas CP is a secondary event to sustain intracellular homeostasis. Further studies on CP, MTG, and ATG interaction will go a long way in the clinical management of chronic diseases. Although, ER-phagy and LD formation occur concomitantly during CP induction in the developing UN rat cerebellar Purkinje neurons, only limited studies are as yet available in this direction. The selective vulnerability of certain mitochondria and their transcriptional regulation particularly within a terminally differentiated, non-dividing (neurons and myocytes) cells in response to DPCI remains enigmatic. Other organelle-specific ATGs including pexophagy, ER phagy, and nucleophagy might be interlinked to CP and their exact theranostic significance is yet to be established. Although several questions and concerns are well-established in ATG, these need to be resolved more precisely and systematically for CP to elucidate its exact pathophysiology and personalized theranostics as described in my book. *Personalized Medicine: Beyond PET Biomarkers* by Nova Sciences Publishers in New York, U.S.A. (Sharma 2017). Various CP/ATG regulators/inhibitors/modulators including CQ, 3-MA, Tunicamycin, Rapamycin, and Doxorubicin are described to establish their exact theranostic significance in health and disease. In addition to adopting dietary restriction, moderate exercise, controlled sex and sleep (*DRESS*) and modifying genes, environment, and life style (*GELS*) principles, the theranostic potential of antioxidants, such as CoQ_{10}, Resveratrol, Melatonin, Curcumin, Catechin, Querestine, Berbarine,

Lycopene, Carotene, Spirulina, Vildaglipitin, Statins, Edaravone, Probucol, Leucovorin, and NAC used routinely as free radical scavengers, CP regulators, and boosters of MB is briefly described. Further research on CP-targeted drugs, molecular imaging, omics technology, and functional genomics, employing correlative and combinatorial bioinformatics and *in vivo* multimodality real time molecular imaging with PET, SPECT, CT, and MRI using properly designed fusion algorithms with disease-specific radiolabeled and/or NPs-labeled biomarkers or receptor ligands and novel discoveries of DSST-TSE-EBPT-CPTs will revolutionize our existing knowledge and wisdom regarding the routine clinical management of genetic and acquired diseases, eventually leading to improved human productivity, fecundity, longevity, and BQL.

REFERENCE

Sharma, S. 2017. Personalized Medicine: Beyond PET Biomarkers. Nova Science Publishers, New York, U.S.A.

Part-1
Charnolophagy
(General Topics)

1

Charnolophagy as Immediate and Early ATG

INTRODUCTION

"Auto" means self and "phagy" means digestion. Hence, the literal meaning of ATG is "self-digestion" and CP is the most sensitive, immediate, and early process of inclusion-(CB)-specific ATG. CP is a highly intricate mechanism, which eliminates nonfunctional or damaged mitochondria to sustain MQC and IMD for NCF. Although, DPCI-induced free radical overproduction jeopardizes IMD to trigger CBMP, other nonfunctional, defective, and/or degenerating intracellular organelles including nucleus, lysosomes, peroxisomes, charnolosome (CS), Golgi body, and E.R membranes may be subjected to organelle-specific ATG. CP occurs more frequently in response to DPCIs in the most vulnerable neural progenitor cells, cardiac progenitor cells, pulmonary epithelial progenitor cells, hepatocyte progenitor cells, gastro-epithelial progenitor cells, renal progenitor cells, and germinal progenitor cells, derived from iPPCs during embryonic development to trigger diversified congenital syndromes and other developmental anomalies in the CNS, cardiovascular system, musculoskeletal system, GIT, renal system, and integumentary system, broadly classified as developmental charnolopathies. DPCI induce mitochondrial oxidative and nitrative stress to enhance free radical overproduction to induce lipid peroxidation, characterized by structural and functional breakdown of polyunsaturated fatty acids (PUFA: linoeic acid, linolenic acid, and arachidonic acid) in the plasma membrane and mtDNA oxidation. The mitochondrial membranes are highly rich in PUFA and omega-3 fatty acids (docosahexanoic acid, icosapentanoic acid), which render them highly susceptible to free radical attack and trigger degenerative changes characterized by CP dysregulation and CBMP in chronic multidrug-resistant (MDR) diseases.

This chapter highlights CP as a highly orchestrated, sensitive, organelle (mitochondrial inclusion: CB)-specific immediate and early ATG which occurs in the most vulnerable cell in response to DPCI in health and disease.

Original Discovery of CB and CP

CB was discovered as a pleomorphic, multi-lamellar, electron-dense, quasi-crystalline stack of condensed and degenerated mitochondrial membranes in the developing UN rat Purkinje neuronal dendrites, hippocampal neural progenitor cells, and in the cardiac progenitor cells (derived from pluripotent stem cells) in response to the environmental neurotoxins, Kainic acid and Domoic acid. CB appears as a nonfunctional intracellular inclusion and is phagocytosed by the lysosomes through ATP-driven CP to sustain ICD. The lysosomes are involved in cell surveillance for maintaining intracellular homeostasis and NCF. CB formation and hence, CP induction, occur frequently due to the structural and functional vulnerability of mitochondrial membranes to free radical-induced lipid peroxidation (as these are highly rich in PUFA) and genetic and epigenetic vulnerability of mtDNA (as it is GC-rich and easily oxidized to form 8-OH, 2dG and methylated at the cytosine residues) as compared to nDNA which is double helical, condensed, and remains protected by histones and protamines. Hence, CP can be utilized as the most sensitive immediate and early biomarker of CB-ATG in any physico-chemically-injured cell. Other organelles including nucleus, lysosomes, peroxisomes, proteasome, and Golgi body, are not phagocytosed as frequently and are spared from the immediate, early, and direct attack of free radicals. The mtDNA is intron-less and remains in a hostile microenvironment of free radicals generated as a byproduct of O/P in the mitochondrial matrix. Moreover, mtDNA is naked, non-helical, devoid of histones and protamines, which render it highly susceptible to genetic and epigenetic modifications. The cytosine is readily methylated by S-adenosyl methionine (SAM) at position N-3 on the naked mtDNA to trigger CBMP. Hence, early detection of 2, 3 dihydroxy nonenal, 4-OH, nonenal and 8-OH, 2dG from the biological fluids can provide a quantitative estimate of mitochondrial bioenergetics (MB) of a patient. On the other hand, the nDNA is supercoiled, double helical, compact, and remains protected by the nuclear wall and nucleoplasm. Histones, protamines, and topoisomerases provide structural and functional stability to gyrases to maintain its helicity. Hence, genetic and epigenetic changes occur rarely in the nDNA because histone acetylation at the lysine moieties has to occur first to open the super helical structure to expose the cytosine residues for their methylation.

Mitochondrial Susceptibility to CBMP

CBMP is involved in almost all cell possessing mitochondria. As CB is a nonfunctional mitochondrial inclusion, it is phagocytosed upon ubiquitination by ATP-driven lysosomal activation. CP is the most sensitive, immediate and early event of CMB to form a CPS. The CPS is transformed to CS, when the phagocytosed CB is hydrolyzed by the lysosomal enzymes. Secondary free radical attack (SFA) causes CS destabilization.

Depending on the intensity and frequency of free radical attack, a CS is permeabilized, sequestered, or fragmented to release toxic metabolites to induce further activation of lysosomes, which can phagocytose other nonfunctional or degenerated organelle or ubiquitinated and denatured proteins as a final attempt of ICD through generalized ATG. No other organelle is as cytotoxic and generates free radicals as compared to CS (a byproduct of CB). Hence, it is logical to propose that CP is the immediate and early event that controls ATG of other defective, nonfunctional, and/or degenerating organelles and denatured ubiquitinated and aggregated proteins for ICD. In addition, mitochondria synthesize anti-inflammatory and membrane stabilizing steroid hormones (that is, testosterone, estrogen, and progesterone) by transport of cholesterol through the 18 kDa TSPO channel protein localized on the outer mitochondria membrane (OMM). The steroid hormone synthesis is compromised due to TSPO, BCl_2-Becline, Bax, xanthine oxidase (XO), heme oxygenase (HO), and monoamine oxidases (MAOs) delocalization during CBMP. The delocalized MAOs translocate to the nucleus to induce TGF-β gene which augments mitochondrial damage triggering CBMP and inflammation due to the induction of Drp-1 and inflammasomes and downregulation of mitofusin (MFN) in the absence of anti-inflammatory steroid hormones. These molecular events trigger carcinogenesis, which can be prevented by developing stem cell specific CS antagonists because the endocytosis of stem cell-specific CS is involved in malignant transformation of nonproliferative cells and induce metaplasia, dysplasia, invasion, and metastasis. CBMP is involved in the transformation of erythroblasts to myloblasts (which cause myeloid leukemia), columnar epithelial cells to squamous epithelial cells (which cause Barret's esophagus), and pulmonary epithelial cells to squamous epithelial cells (which cause small cell lung carcinoma).

Free Radical-induced CBMP

In vivo as well as *in vitro* experimental data suggest that mitochondria in the most vulnerable cell exhibit differential susceptibility to free radical-induced CBMP in response to endogenous or exogenous DPCI. Depending on the metabolic and physiological needs, a cell may possess anywhere between 22–1000 mitochondria. For example, a sperm has 22–75 spirally-arranged compact mitochondria in the middle piece for motility and fertilization, whereas a neuron may have between 750–1000 mitochondria (Purkinje neurons). Terminally differentiated cells (including skeletal muscle, cardiac, hepatocytes, osteocytes, and CNS neurons) have a fixed number of mitochondria. An oocyte has the maximum mitochondria (250,000–600,000) because it needs sufficient energy to execute paternal CP as well as CS exocytosis during the pre-zygotic phase soon after fertilization, and during the development of the embryo in the post-zygotic phase for the normal growth of the fetus. Osteoblasts also possess a high number of mitochondria for osteogenesis. About 40% of the myocardial and skeletal muscles, 20% of the liver tissue, and 15% of the CNS is composed exclusively of mitochondria as these are metabolically high-energy-demanding tissues. Although, it depends primarily on the frequency and intensity of free radical attack, all mitochondria are not destroyed at any given time in response to DPCI. The exact molecular mechanism of differential and selective vulnerability of mitochondria to free radical-induced CBMP remains enigmatic.

It was discovered in the developing UN rat cerebellar Purkinje neurons that numerous mitochondria remain small in size, single layered, with only few cristae (2–4), devoid of mtDNA. Occasionally, these immature mitochondria contained electron-dense lipoprotein aggregates as inclusion bodies in the form of LDs. Immature and physiologically-inactive mitochondria directly incorporated with the electron-dense, degenerated membranes to initially form pleomorphic multi-tubular loose CB (*cis*-CB), followed by multi-lamellar condensed membrane stacks forming mature quasi-crystaline CB (*trans*-CB); Trans-CBs were subsequently phagocytosed by lysosomes following Akt-ubiquitination. Developmentally-immature and nonfunctional mitochondria devoid of cristae and mtDNA are frequently destroyed by free radicals as these are unable to synthesize ATP due to the downregulation of ETC, O/P, and a lack of steroid hormones. A physico-chemically-injured cell may have between 7–8 mature CBs at any given time because other pleomorphic CB phenotypes existing in immature primordial and in different developmental stages are readily phagocytosed by the activated lysosomes upon Akt-ubiquitination. CB is variable and exhibits differential phenotypes and vulnerability, depending on the cellular, molecular, genetic predisposition, biochemical composition, inducers, and microenvironment. CBMP is highly complex and intricate in MDR malignancies, because inflammation, apoptosis, necrosis, proliferation, infection, immortalization, CP, MTG, and ATG occur concomitantly in these cells. Hence, it will be highly prudent to discover immediate and early molecular events of CBMP of particular cancer stem cells involved in MDR malignancies for their timely eradication. It will be promising to develop specific CPTs for the eradication of stem cell-specific CS (CSscs) in MDR malignancies.

CP vs ATG

Although both CP and ATG require (i) Akt-ubiquitination of nonfunctional organelles and associated proteins in response to DPCI-induced free radical attack on the most vulnerable stem cell and ATP-driven lysosomal activation, CP involves predominantly phagocytosis of CB during mitochondrial remodeling (MR) and degeneration. Generally, ATG is nonspecific and can phagocytose any nonfunctional, degenerated, and/or undesired intracellular organelle. CP can selectively influence cell death, inflammation, immune response, and exert both adaptive and maladaptive roles in disease pathogenesis. CBMP involving CB formation, CP induction, and CS destabilization are deleterious events as these are implicated in chronic MDR diseases. Although, increased lysosomal activity triggers pro-inflammatory cascade in a physicochemical-injured cell during the acute phase; enhanced CP increases the incidence of CS destabilization which triggers inflammasome to cause MDR diseases during chronic phase. Hence, CP-mediated CB elimination is highly prudent to sustain IMD and ICD for NCF.

There are primarily three major stages of IMD and ICD: (a) CB formation (b) CP induction, and (c) CS exocytosis. CP involves Akt-ubiquitination of CB for lysosomal recognition followed by energy (ATP)-driven phagocytosis for CB elimination, whereas, ATG is an intracellular homeostatic mechanism for the turnover of various cellular organelles and proteins, in which double-membraned autophagosomes sequester cytoplasmic cargos, delivered to the lysosome for degradation. ATG as an important modulator of human disease including acute kidney injury, which can arise in response to nephrotoxins, sepsis, I/R, and in chronic renal diseases, including comorbidities (diabetes and kidney injury). Roles of ATG in polycystic kidney disease and renal carcinoma have been described. Hence, targeting both CP and ATG pathway may confer the TSE-EBPT of diabetes and associated comorbidities as described in this edition.

CONCLUSION

This chapter presented an introduction to generalized ATG and inclusion (CB)-specific ATG (also named as CP). Differential susceptibility of RONS-induced CBMP in the most vulnerable iPPCs and the basic difference between CP and ATG to accomplish the TSE-EBPT of chronic MDR diseases were also highlighted.

2

Charnolophagy in Intramitochondrial and Intracellular Detoxification

INTRODUCTION

CP is an immediate and early event as it occurs initially when the cell undergoes degenerative changes due to free radical-induced toxic insult. Free radicals are reactive oxygen, nitrogen, and carbonyl (OH, NO, CO) species with a half-life of 10^{-13} to 10^{-14} seconds and possess a highly reactive and unstable lone pair of electrons which induce lipid peroxidation of plasma membranes. Since the mitochondrial membranes are constantly exposed to free radicals, these are degenerated more readily during DPCI in the most vulnerable cell as compared to other cellular organelles. Thus, CP occurs earlier than ATG as a mechanism of ICD.

CP-mediated IMD and ICD are highly crucial events which occur throughout our lives to replace damaged and nonfunctional (particularly mitochondria) organelles. Certain intracellular organelles are highly susceptible to CP as compared to generalized ATG for disease progression or remission. When IMD and ICD of the liver, kidney and lymphatics are optimized, the macrophages from these key organs function more efficiently to remove toxins from the rest of body to prevent septicemia, toxemia, and lethal shock. This makes IMD and ICD the most important components of systemic detoxification.

Although CP is similar to ATG in several fundamental aspects, it has unique characteristics as it involves free radical-induced degeneration of highly labile mitochondrial membranes, mtDNA, and mtmiRNA. DPCI trigger CB formation, CP induction, and CPS formation to contain toxic mitochondrial metabolites in the cytoplasm. The CPS is converted to CS, when the phagocytosed CB is hydrolyzed by the lysosomal enzymes. CP is thus an ATP-driven, lysosome-dependent process and occurs efficiently in normal cells, while it is impaired in LSDs and diseased, cancerous, or aging cells.

This chapter highlights the theranostic significance of CB as a universal biomarker of cell injury and the protective role of nutritional rehabilitation, physiological Zn^{2+}, and MTs which can independently serve as CP agonists, CBMP antagonists, and intracellular detoxifiers.

Adverse effects of MDR malignancies due to non-specific CB formation and CP dysregulation are associated with GIT stress (abdominal pain, nausea, and vomiting), cardiotoxicity, hepatoxicity, nephrotoxicity, dermatitis, alopecia, myelosuppression (anemia, neutropenia, and thrombocytopenia), neurotoxicity (visual and auditory impairments), and infertility. Nutritional rehabilitation, physiological zinc, and/or MTs prevent CB formation, augment CP and stabilize CS during early neuronal development and aging. By contrast, alcohol intake, cigarette smoking, a high-fat and salt-rich diet, or malnutrition because of ignorance and poverty cause early morbidity and mortality. The MTs can be induced by regular diet and moderate exercise to circumvent free radical overproduction, prevent CB formation, regulate CP, and hence progressive NDDs, including drug addiction (Sharma and Ebadi 2011a,b; Sharma and Ebadi 2014a-c). Downregulation of CP may lead to progressive NDDs and CVDs accompanied with intracellular inclusions (Sharma 2014). Hence, drugs may be developed to inhibit CBMP to prevent or treat NDDs, CVDs, and enhance cancer-stem-cell-specific CB formation to inhibit CP for the theranostic management of MDR malignancies.

A spermatocyte having defective or no mitochondria remains immotile and cannot fertilize the oocyte. Artificial fertilization is successful in only 40% cases, due to induction of CBMP in unsuccessful cases. During fertilization, the tail is left behind, whereas the head and middle piece penetrate in the oocyte and the paternal nDNA fuses with the maternal nDNA. However, the paternal CB in the oocyte is recognized as a nonfunctional inclusion and is phagocytosed by CP. CS is subsequently exocytosed to sustain ICD for normal postzygotic development. Hence, physiologically and metabolically active CP and CS exocytosis are highly crucial for the growth and development of the fetus. Any impairment in CP and/CS exocytosis during first trimester (gastrulation phase) of pregnancy can induce charnolophathies represented by craniofacial abnormalities, still birth, abortion, anencephaly, mesencephalic, microcephaly, as noticed in fetuses exposed to nicotine addiction, alcoholism, other drugs of abuse, antidepressants, antipsychotics, antiepileptic, anesthetics, and microbial (bacteria, virus, and fungal) infections during pregnancy. Particularly, Zika virus, cytomegalovirus, and rubella virus induce developmental charnolopathies. Hence, CP has a highly crucial theranostic significance in normal embryonic development.

The multi-lamellar, electron-dense membrane stacks were discovered in developing UN rat Purkinje neurons (Sharma et al. 1986, Sharma et al. 1987, Sharma et al. 1993, Dakshinamurti et al. 1993), which were subsequently identified in the hippocampal CA-3 and dentate gyrus neurons of Kainic acid and Domoic acid (DA)-exposed mice, and were named as "Charnoly bodies" (CB; Charnoly is the nickname of author's late mother) (Sharma 2013). Domoic acid-induced seizure discharge activity significantly enhanced CBMP in pyridoxine (Vitamin-B_6) deficient adult rats (Sharma and Dakshinamurti 1992). Subsequently, sequential events involved in the CB life cycle and CBMP were discovered (Sharma et al. 1993a). A Purkinje cell evoked unit activity in response to peripheral electrical stimulation, exhibited increased incidence of electrical fatigue and increased after hyperpolarization duration in the developing UN rat cerebellar Purkinje neurons due to increased $[Ca^{2+}]_i$, CB formation, dysregulated CP, and induction of CBMP (Sharma et al. 1993b). An intra-hippocampal microinjection of 5-HT_{1A} receptor agonist, 8-hydroxy-2-(di-n-propylamino)tetralin (8-hydroxy-DPAT), into the dentate gyrus inhibited DA-induced seizure activity in male adult rats, suggesting that 5-HT provides mitochondrial neuroprotection by inhibiting CBMP (Sharma and Dakshinamurti 1993).

Stress-induced overproduction of free radicals may cause CB formation in the most vulnerable hippocampal neurons because of the degeneration of the mitochondria due to AD, PD, drug addiction, infections, and depression (Sharma et al. 2014). However, nutritional rehabilitation, physiological Zn^{2+}, and MTs inhibited CB formation in the rat brain. As MTs regulate Zn^{2+}-mediated transcriptional activation of genes involved in cell growth, proliferation, and differentiation; they serve as early and sensitive biomarkers of NDDs, CVDs, and MDR malignancies (Sharma et al. 2013a,b,c). MTs inhibit CB formation and confer ubiquinone (CoQ_{10})-mediated neuroprotection as free-radical scavengers in the aging brain (Sharma and Ebadi 2014). MTs are low-molecular weight, cysteine-rich, zinc-binding proteins and are induced in nutritional stress and in response to environmental neurotoxins: Kainic acid (KA), Domoic acid (DA), acromelic acid, polychlorinated biphenyls (PCBs), and heavy metals such as mercury, lead, cadmium, and arsenic), and NPs (Sharma 2014).

Elimination of Toxic CS Metabolites

Highly toxic CS metabolites are eliminated from our body through tears, nasal discharge, sputum, saliva, serum, plasma, sweat, tear, blood, CSF, urine, menstrual fluid, pleural effusions, fecal matter, pus, toenails, and hairs. The detection and nature of CS metabolites depends on the age, sex, disease status, genetic makeup, and ethnic origin. Physical exercise eliminates CS metabolites through sweat from almost all parts of our body. A balanced diet, salt, fat restriction, and moderate exercise facilitate intracellular, extracellular, and systematic CS detoxification.

Undernutrition vs Calorie Restriction

MB is significantly impaired in the developing UN brain. However, CR boosts MB by preventing CB formation and by augmenting CP during acute phase, and by stabilizing CS and its exocytosis during chronic phase. Clinical manifestations of the deleterious effects of nutritional stress in UN children motivated the author to discover the physiological and pharmacological significance of CBMP in developing UN rats. This led to the discovery of CB, CP, and CS as theranostic biomarkers. Typical clinical manifestations of a 2.5-month old female child, who was undernourished because of lactation failure in the mother, were folded skin, loss of muscle tone, neuromuscular degeneration, peripheral edema, loss of hair, sarcopenia, persistent diarrhea, dehydration, and face like an old person. The same child after 25 days of nutritional rehabilitation with cow's milk formula exhibited coordination of muscular activity, reappearance of muscle tone, and hair growth, confirming that nutritional stress compromises MB which can be restored by nutritional rehabilitation. Usually body weight and chest to encephalic ratios (that is, circumference) are calculated to assess the severity of nutritional stress in developing UN children. However, on moral and ethical grounds, CBMP cannot be studied in developing UN children. Hence, CBMP in experimental animals and the brain to body weight ratio in humans can be used as biomarkers of nutritional status.

Brain to Body Weight Ratio

The ratios of brain weight versus body weight were determined in 5- to 30-days-old postnatal developing N and UN rats. At any given age, this ratio was higher in the UN rats than in the N rats and reduced as a function of nutritional rehabilitation. Because this ratio in experimental animals was not significantly affected during postnatal undernutrition, some investigators proposed a brain-sparing hypothesis, which was subsequently challenged when the brain regional neurochemistry, electrophysiology, and ultrastructural studied were conducted. The original discovery of CBMP in developing UN Purkinje neurons further challenged the brain-sparing hypothesis. Postnatal undernutrition was induced by increasing the litter size of the lactating mother and by reducing the protein casein to 50% in the daily diet of the lactating mother, as described by Widdowson and McCance (1956). Cerebellar tissue was processed for TEM analysis (Sharma and Ebadi 2014). The data were analyzed by a two-way multiple measure analysis of variance (ANOVA). *F* values were calculated by taking ratios of SD sequars. These values were used to calculate *p* values to determine the level of significance between N and UN brain weights and body weights. One-way ANOVA was performed on rats that were undernourished for 30 days to determine the rate of CB elimination as a function of nutritional rehabilitation of 80 days. CB formation was practically eliminated in rats, which were undernourished for

30 days and subsequently rehabilitated for 80 days due to CB inhibition and CP induction, indicating CB recycling in the developing brain.

Original Hypothesis

The following hypothesis was proposed: "*MTs provide ubiquinone (CoQ$_{10}$)-mediated protection by inhibiting CBMP.*" (Sharma et al. 2013a,b,c). Several experiments on mitochondrial genome knockout (RhO$_{mgko}$) cells in an *in vitro* cellular model of PD, AD, and aging in cell culture and in MT gene-manipulated mice were performed to confirm this hypothesis.

MTs conferred neuroprotection in response to MPP$^+$ ions and rotenone in cultured human dopaminergic SK-N-SH and SH-SY5Y cells and in MTs gene-manipulated mice in response to MPTP (Sharma et al. 2004). Brain regional CoQ$_{10}$ was significantly reduced in MT$_{dko}$ mice and increased in MT$_{rans}$ mice. A specific MAO-B inhibitor, Selegiline, attenuated MPP$^+$-induced apoptosis through MTs-mediated mitochondrial protection (Sharma et al. 2003). Since brain regional CoQ$_{10}$ levels were significantly reduced in genetic and experimental models of PD, a sensitive method was developed to determine brain regional CoQ$_{10}$ (Sharma and Ebadi 2004). CoQ$_{10}$ boosted mitochondrial complex-1 activity and inhibited proinflammatory NF-$\kappa\beta$ when overexpressed in homozygous wv/wv mice (Ebadi et al. 2004). A potent ONOO-donor 3-morpholinosydnonimone (SIN-1)-induced oxidative and nitrative stress implicated in CBMP was attenuated in MTs overexpressed DAergic neurons and in MTtrans mice (Sharma and Ebadi 2003, Ebadi and Sharma 2003).

A potent ONOO$^-$ ion generator 3-morpholinosydnonimine (SIN-1)–induced neurotoxicity was evaluated in control wild-type (control$_{wt}$) mice, MTs double knockout (MT$_{dko}$) mice, MTs-transgenic (MT$_{trans}$) mice, and in cultured SK-N-SH neurons to determine the neuroprotective potential of MTs against ONOO$^-$ induced neurodegeneration in PD. SIN-1–induced lipid peroxidation, ROS, caspase-3 activation, and apoptosis were attenuated by MTs gene overexpression and augmented by MTs gene downregulation (Ebadi et al. 2005). A progressive NS-DA-ergic degeneration in wv/wv mice was associated with enhanced nitrite ion synthesis, downregulation of MTs, and significantly reduced dopamine and ^{18}F-DOPA uptake as determined by high resolution microPET neuroimaging. The striatal ^{18}F-DOPA and ^{18}FdG uptakes were significantly higher in MT$_{trans}$ mice than in MT$_{dko}$ and α-Syn$_{ko}$ and wv/wv mice. MTs' overexpression in wv/wv mice attenuated brain regional CBMP, and restored ^{18}F-DOPA and ^{18}FdG uptakes to normalcy. These observations confirmed that NOS activation and ONOO$^-$ synthesis is involved in CBMP-mediated etiopathogenesis of PD, and that MTs' gene induction may provide neuroprotection (Ebadi and Sharma 2003; Ebadi 2004; Ebadi et al. 2005; Ebadi and Sharma 2006). MTs conferred anti-inflammatory action in poly-substance abuse (Sharma and Ebadi 2011a, b), in aging (Sharma and Ebadi 2014a), in cell therapy and nanomedicine (Sharma et al. 2013a), and in many other NDDs (Sharma and Ebadi 2014c; Sharma et al. 2016).

The CB Life Cycle

The CB life cycle was explored in N and on UN rat cerebellar Purkinje neurons employing LM and TEM analyses (Sharma 2013a,b,c). The structurally-intact synaptic terminal appeared round and dense, but the degenerated synaptic terminals appeared swollen, club-shaped, and cloudy due to destabilization of labile CS membranes. Synaptic degeneration in the Purkinje neurons may be responsible for impaired and/or delayed motor learning in nutritionally-stressed children and delayed eye blinking in intrauterine fetal alcohol-exposed developing children (Kang and Gleason 2013, Pipatpiboon et al. 2013). Similar ND changes in Purkinje neurons were implicated in impaired eye blinking and in an animal model of fetal alcohol syndrome (Jacobson et al. 2011, Chabenne et al. 2014). Normal rat cerebellar Purkinje neuron dendrites revealed Golgi apparatus, rough ER, and elliptical mitochondria with well-defined cristae during 15 days of postnatal life. The mitochondria and Golgi body became swollen and aggregated in 15-days-old UN rats. The mitochondrial membranes were degenerated, fragmented, and transformed into electron-dense stacks. At the basal portion of the electron-dense membrane stacks, the mitochondria were fused to maintain the function of these stacks. The CB translocated to the damaged region of the plasma membrane to repair desmosomes and preserve the structural and functional integrity of the plasma membrane. The swollen mitochondria fused with the immature CBs. The electron-dense membrane stacks became independent penta or heptalamellar units (*mature CB*), which served as a membrane reserves during nutritional stress, prevented further neurotoxicity and uncontrolled neuro-inflammation. A fully mature CB appeared electron-dense multi-lamellar (usually penta-lamellar or hepta-lamellar) independent units. These multi-lamellar inclusions were eliminated by CP during minor to moderate undernutrition. CB formation appeared to form a bridge between apoptosis and neurodegeneration. It was a transitory phase since nutritional rehabilitation eliminated CBs. During severe nutritional stress, CBs were agglomerated with other synaptic proteins such as α-Syn to form persistent inclusions at an early stage of NDD in aging. In permanently damaged neurons CBs induced neurodegeneration. Whether CBs can synthesize ATP by O/P and possess structurally and functionally intact ETS and O/P to synthesize ATP remains uncertain. CB may be transformed to functional mitochondria during nutritional rehabilitation. Further research will resolve this intriguing yet highly significant issue.

CB Formation and CP Induction

Hippocampal atrophy occurs in AD, schizophrenia, alcoholism, progeria, Pick disease, Down's syndrome, ALS, and depression. In AD, CB formation and CP inhibition occurs in the zinc-containing hippocampal neurons, because of MT-3 deficiency (Sharma and Ebadi 2014). CB formation in these neurons may also cause depression which can be prevented by MTs' induction, physiological Zn^{2+}, and nutritional rehabilitation. MT-3 inhibits CBMP by augmenting CP, thereby preventing hippocampal damage in AD by serving as potent free radical scavengers. MTs prevent senile dementia by boosting MB. Hence, drugs or antioxidants may be developed to inhibit CBMP in the hippocampal region to prevent progressive neurodegeneration in AD, PD, ALS, and MDDs. In particular, depression is the comorbid factor in NDDs, CVDs, chronic inflammatory diseases, postoperative patients, PTSD, war-wounded, space explorers, hypothyroidism, and in cancer patients. Hippocampal neurons may be destroyed in MDDs because of CB formation and compromised CP; however, PUFA and omega-3 fatty acids may attenuate CBMP and augment mitochondrial regeneration to enhance neurogenesis, thereby promoting an antidepressant action by alleviating symptoms of ADHDs in young adolescents. Inhibiting CBMP and augmenting CP by nutritional rehabilitation, physiological Zn^{2+}, and MTs can prevent various NDDs such as PD, AD, drug addiction, and depression. MTs may be induced by diet and moderate exercise to prevent hippocampal CB formation implicated in the pathogenesis of ADHD. The fat-1 transgenic mouse had enriched levels of DHA in the brain because transformation of omega-6 to omega-3 fatty acids, was implicated in enhanced hippocampal neurogenesis, suggesting a mechanism by which omega-3 fatty acids could ameliorate depression and mood. Omega-3 fatty acids such as EPA and DHA may prevent and treat depression by inhibiting CB formation and by promoting CP and neurogenesis in the hippocampus. Because DHA can be obtained through diet, its intake by depressed patients or people at risk for depression may facilitate managing the disease and aid individuals who cannot achieve remission via conventional pharmacological interventions. CP molecular dynamics in health and disease is presented in Fig. 15.

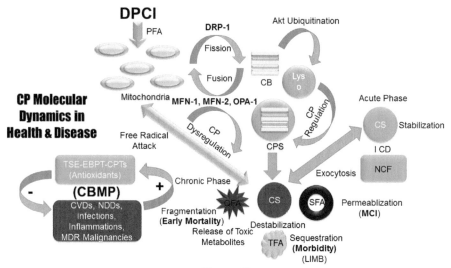

Figure 15

CP Induction and CS PKs

A CS is exocytosed and enters in the systemic circulation through hepato-portal circulation to be metabolized in the liver. Cyt-P450 system is involved in the detoxification of toxic CS metabolites. Water-soluble (hydrophilic) CS metabolites are excreted through the kidney, whereas water-insoluble (hydrophobic) metabolites like lipids are emulsified by the bile and excreted through intestinal route in fecal matter. CP and CS-PKs in ICD are presented in Fig. 16.

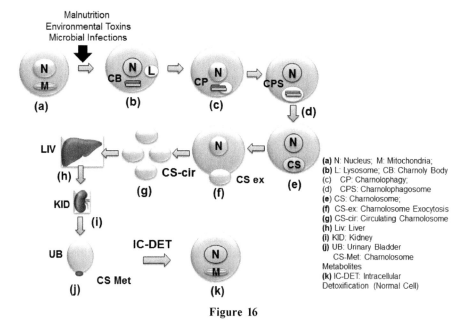

Figure 16

CBMP and CP Dysregulation

DPCI increase the requirement of ATP in the most vulnerable cell which enhances mitochondrial oxidative and nitrative stress. Free radical-induced degeneration of mitochondria is triggered by mega-pore formation, translocation of Ca^{2+} from the ER to the mitochondria, and $\Delta\Psi$ collapse to trigger CB formation to contain toxic metabolites. Physiological and/or pharmacological dysregulation of CP and CBMP is involved in progressive NDDs, CVDs, and MDR malignancies. A CS is a structurally and functionally labile single-layered intracellular organelle, which forms CS bodies in response to the secondary exposure to a free radical attack. CS bodies are permeablized, sequestered, or degraded depending on the physicochemical injury to cause morbidity represented by cognitive (learning, memory, intelligence, and behavior) impairments, followed by early morality, particularly in the immunocompromised aging subject.

Electrophysiological Correlates of CBMP

CB formation increased significantly from 5 days to 30 days of postnatal UN as a function of nutritional stress. A maximum incidence of CB formation occurred in the apical dendrite, followed by BD and OBD. To establish an electrophysiological deficit due to CB formation in the developing UN brain, Purkinje neuron-intracellular-evoked unit activity was recorded. Significantly reduced unit activity in UN rats was represented by the increased latency of response, reduced number and amplitude of spikes, increased incidence of fatigue in response to peripheral electrical stimulation, increased after-hyperpolarization duration, and increased $[Ca^{2+}]_i$ due to CBMP. Differences in the duration of Purkinje neuron-evoked-unit activity and ^{14}C-glucose uptake in the cerebellar cortex of N and UN rats were estimated to evaluate CBMP. The mean duration of Purkinje neuron-evoked-unit activity was recorded from N and UN rats and subtracted to determine the difference in the duration, Δ-T, which was plotted as a function of the difference in the rate of ^{14}C-glucose uptake in the cerebellar cortex to determine difference in the energy, Δ-E. The quantitative estimates of Δ-E determined the difference in the MB between the N and UN rats. The regression analysis revealed a positive linear correlation between Δ-T and Δ-E in N and UN rats (that is, $\Delta T = k \Delta E$, where k is a constant and depends on the nature of a cell under investigation). The Δ-E and Δ-T tended to zero during nutritional rehabilitation. (Source: Sharma's original findings.)

Parkinsonian Neurotoxins Induce CBMP

Free radical-induced CB formation and CP dysregulation results in CS destabilization which can release toxic metabolites in the intracellular as well as extracellular compartment. The release of toxic metabolites such as Cyt-C, GAPDH, 2, 3 dihydroxy nonenal, and 8-OH, 2dG is involved in MAOs-mediated TGF-β activation and its translocation to the nucleus to trigger genes involved in apoptosis. The epigenetic changes are also induced by free radical-induced histone acetylation and DNA methylation, which induce altered gene expression in chronic illnesses. Parkinsonian neurotoxins (Salsolinol, 1-Benzyl-tetrahydroisoquinoline), and Rotenone, and drugs of abuse (MPTP, Cocaine, Methamphetamine, and Methylene deoxymethamphetamine (MDMA) trigger CBMP by downregulating ubiquinone dinucleotide hydrogen (NADH)-oxidoreductase (complex-1; a rate limiting enzyme) in O/P and ATP synthesis-induced CP inhibition in cultured DA-ergic (SK-N-SII) neurons; by contrast, the MAO-B inhibitor, Selegiline prevented MPP^+-induced mitochondrial degeneration and CBMP by augmenting MT induction (Sharma and Ebadi 2003). Although MT_{dko} mice did not exhibit any overt clinical symptoms of Parkinsonism, they were highly susceptible and were completely immobilized. By contrast, MT_{trans} mice could walk with stiff legs and an erect tail after seven days of 10 mg/kg i.p. MPTP treatment, which induced Parkinsonism, suggesting the therapeutic potential of MTs as CBMP inhibitors, IMDs, and MB rejuvenators (Sharma et al. 2004). The CoQ_{10} levels were also significantly higher in the striatum of MT_{trans} mice than in the normal control (C57Bl/6J) mice or in the MT_{dko} mice, confirming the hypothesis that MTs provide CoQ_{10}-mediated neuroprotection by inhibiting CBMP. Mitochondrial genome knockout (RhO_{mgko}) neurons were highly susceptible to MPP^+-induced apoptosis, which was attenuated when these aging neurons were transfected with a mitochondrial genome encoding complex-1. Furthermore, a calcium regulatory protein—transient receptor potential channel 1 (TRPC),–prevented MPP^+-induced complex-1 inhibition and apoptosis in cultured SH-S-Y5Y neurons, suggesting its theranostic potential as a CBMP inhibitor in NDDs (Bollimuntha et al. 2005).

CB and CP in RhO_{mgko} Cells

RhO_{mgko} cells were prepared by selectively knocking out the mitochondrial genome to mimic the cellular model of aging. The RhO_{mgko} cells were highly susceptible to MPP^+, Rotenone, and Salsolinol-induced degeneration, and augmented CBMP, without any significant effect on the nDNA. Depending on the metabolic activity, a cell may possess 1000 mitochondria or more each having its own 34 Kb, double-stranded, intron-less highly sensitive, naked DNA. The mtDNA damage occurs at an earlier stage of NDDs or CVDs because it remains constantly under the direct influence of free radicals (Sharma et al. 2004). Mitochondrial CoQ_{10} and complex-1 were significantly reduced in the RhO_{mgko} cells, as observed in AD, PD, and aging. Transfection of RhO_{mgko} cells with the complex-1 gene increased CoQ_{10} and ATP synthesis, supporting that NDDs occur because of CBMP due to the downregulation of the mitochondrial genome. The fluorochrome (JC-1)-stained digital fluorescence microscopic picture of a cell demonstrated crimson-colored mitochondria in the intracytoplasmic region. RhO_{mgko} neurons exhibited a club-shaped appearance without any neurites, dendrites, axons, and synaptic terminals. RhO_{mgko} neuron upon complex-1 gene transfection exhibited neurite and axonal growth, confirming the pivotal role of MB in cell differentiation, development, and maturation.

MTs and other Antioxidants Inhibit CBMP

MTs are significantly reduced in the hippocampal regions; an event which induces ND by synthesizing amyloid-β plaques in AD and Lewy body (LB) formation in PD. Translocation of MTs in the mitochondria and nucleus during oxidative and/or nitrative stress occurs as a mechanism of cellular defense. MTs attenuate $ONOO^-$-induced DNA damage, whereas α-Syn nitration facilitates LB formation during PD progression (Sharma and Ebadi 2003). SI was discovered as the ratio of nitrated α-Syn versus native α-Syn (Sharma et al. 2003) which may be utilized as a sensitive biomarker of CB and LB pathogenesis in the submandibular gland of PD patients. The accumulation of CBs at the junction of axon hillock may inhibit the axoplasmic transport of ions, enzymes, neurotransmitters, growth factors, and mitochondria at the presynaptic region, thereby resulting in sensory-motor impairments in PD, AD, and depression. Therefore, drugs may be developed to inhibit CBMP and induce CP in the hippocampal neurons. Initially, $\Delta\Psi$, 8-OH-2dG synthesis, and the SI may be determined by confocal microscopy, flow cytometry, and Comet assay as initial triggers of CBMP to evaluate the theranostic potential of drugs in cell culture. TEM studies may be performed subsequently to authenticate CBMP attenuation *in vivo*. This unique approach could save lot of time, money, and energy of pharmaceutical industries interested in developing novel drugs for the TSE-EBPT of NDDs, CVDs, infectious diseases, and MDR malignancies. CB formation may also serve as an early and sensitive biomarker in drug addiction, depression, diabetes, obesity, inflammation, and pain. The biological effects of MTs' induction are presented in Fig. 17.

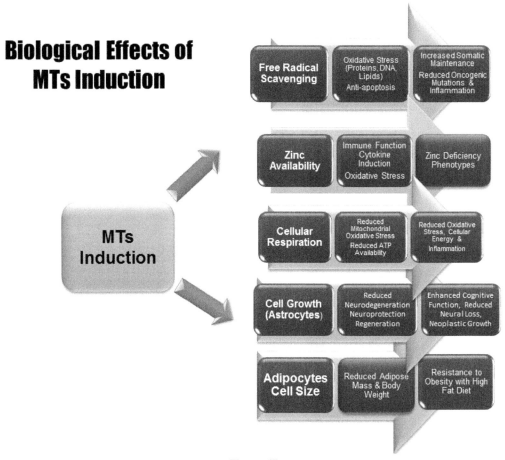

Figure 17

CBMP in MDR Malignancies

Cancer stem cells remain in their niches and induce malignancies on stimulation. In MDR malignancies, the MTs are induced because of the inhibition of CB formation and CP induction. Presently-available anticancer and anti-infective drugs cause alopecia, myelosuppression, and GIT symptoms because of nonspecific induction of CBMP and CP inhibition in highly proliferating cells. Therefore, drugs may be developed to augment cancer-stem-cell-specific localized CBMP and inhibit CP for the effective treatment of MDR malignancies with minimal or no adverse effects.

MTs Protection

MTs enhance CP and stabilize CS as a mechanism of IMD and ICD in the most vulnerable cell in response to DPCI. MTs stabilize CS to provide mitochondrial defense involved in ATP synthesis and cellular protection. MTs-induced mitochondrial protection inhibits CBMP to prevent NDDs and CVDs and augments MDR malignancies. MTs as CP enhancers and CS stabilizers are illustrated in Fig. 18.

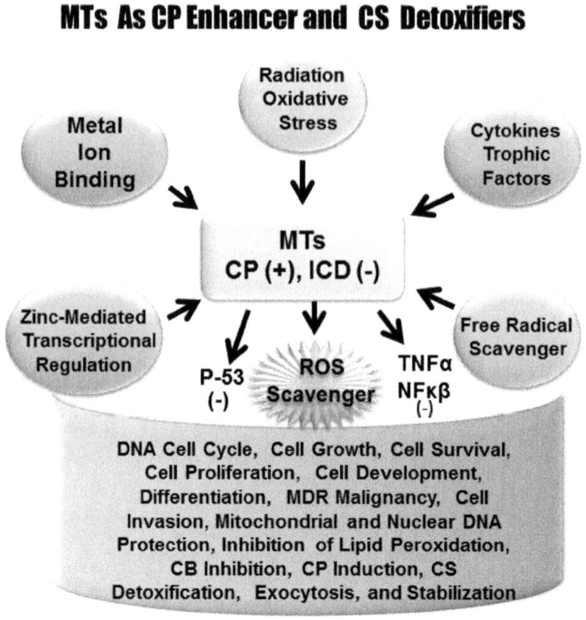

MTs As CP Enhancer and CS Detoxifiers

Radiation Oxidative Stress

Metal Ion Binding

Cytokines Trophic Factors

MTs CP (+), ICD (-)

Zinc-Mediated Transcriptional Regulation

Free Radical Scavenger

P-53 (-)   **ROS Scavenger**   **TNFα NFκβ (-)**

DNA Cell Cycle, Cell Growth, Cell Survival, Cell Proliferation, Cell Development, Differentiation, MDR Malignancy, Cell Invasion, Mitochondrial and Nuclear DNA Protection, Inhibition of Lipid Peroxidation, CB Inhibition, CP Induction, CS Detoxification, Exocytosis, and Stabilization

Figure 18

Free radical overproduction trigger CBMP to form CS bodies, which pinch off and fuse with the plasma membranes to form apoptotic bodies. The apoptotic bodies burst to release all the intracytoplasmic components to cause chronic MDR diseases such as CVDs and NDDs. MTs provide structural and functional stability to prevent CVDs by inhibiting CBMP. MTs Boost MB as illustrated in Fig. 19.

MTs Boost MB, Prevent CB, Enhance CP and Stabilize CS in Health & Disease

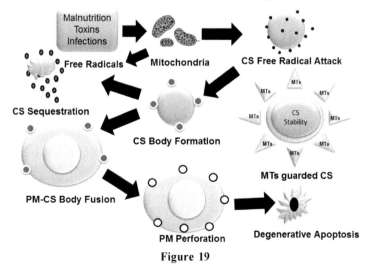

Malnutrition Toxins Infections

Free Radicals   **Mitochondria**   **CS Free Radical Attack**

CS Sequestration

CS Body Formation   **CS Stability**   **MTs**

MTs guarded CS

PM-CS Body Fusion

PM Perforation   **Degenerative Apoptosis**

Figure 19

MTs have numerous other protective roles. MTs confer protection in the most vulnerable, metabolically-active stem cell. MTs also provide protection in radiation-induced oxidative stress, cytokine trophic factors release, scavenge free radicals through their cysteine-rich –SH moieties, and enhance Zn-mediated transcriptional regulation of genes involved in growth, development, cell division, differentiation, and metal ion binding. MTs confer mitochondrial protection by preventing or inhibiting CB formation and by inhibiting mitochondrial degeneration during the acute phase. MTs scavenge free radicals during the chronic phase to prevent CS destabilization to inhibit CBMP and apoptosis. MTs-mediated free radical elimination, mitochondrial protection, CP induction, and CS stabilization are implicated in chronic MDR malignancies. Hence, we need to develop DSST-TSE-EBPT-CPTs for the clinical management of currently incurable diseases. MTs enhance CP and stabilize CS to prevent apoptosis and render immortalization to cancer stem cells in MDR malignancies. MTs prevent CBMP by inhibiting CB formation and enhance CP during the acute phase. During chronic phase, MTs stabilize CS membranes and their exocytosis as a mechanism of ICD for NCF by four categories of CS: (i) MTs normal CS, (ii) MTs inadequate CS, (c) MTs deficient CS, and (d) MTs overexpressing CS. MTs-normal CS exists in a metabolically-active and physiologically-significant cell; MTs-inadequate CS is involved in acute recoverable diseases, and MTs-deficient CS is involved in chronic diseases such as NDDs and CVDs; whereas MTs-overexpressing CS is involved in MDR malignances. CP occurs efficiently in a cell containing MTs-overexpressing CS and is involved in MDR malignancies. Free radicals are scavenged by MTs to provide mitochondrial protection. MTs also stabilize CS membranes to prevent CS body formation which fuses with the plasma membrane to form highly unstable apoptotic bodies. ROS generated in the most vulnerable cell in response to DPCI are scavenged by glutathione, SOD, and catalase during the acute phase. MTs are at least 30X more potent as compared to glutathione and serve as potent free radical scavengers, through –SH moieties on the cysteine residues. In addition to CS, MTs stabilize lysosomes to confer protection. MTs confer zinc-mediated transcriptional regulation of genes is involved in the proliferation of cancer stem-cell specific MDR malignant cells. Various protein synthesis inhibitors in anticancer drugs inhibit AgNOR and the protein synthesizing machinery in the RER membranes to prevent carcinogenesis and malignant transformation. The cancer stem cells are highly rich in MTs and synthesize MTs overexpressing CS in response to anticancer chemotherapy to sustain MDR malignancies. In addition, MTs protect cancer stem cell-mediated protein synthesis, required for their growth and proliferation in MDR malignancies. Hence, we need to develop novel CPTs as specific cancer-stem-cell CS antagonists to successfully cure MDR malignancies as illustrated in Fig. 20.

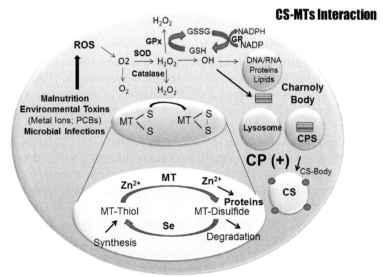

MTs Prevent CB Formation, enhance CP, and stabilize CS as Free Radicals Scavengers
and Versatile Cellular and Molecular Detoxifiers in Human Body

Figure 20

MTs Gene-Manipulated Mice

α-Syn-MT$_{tko}$ mice were developed to confirm the protective role of MTs in PD, AD, and drug addiction. These genotypes exhibit 40% mortality, body tremors, and typical Parkinsonian symptoms. Homozygous weaver (wv/wv) mutant mice exhibited nigrostriatal, hippocampal, and cerebellar damage as noticed in PD, AD, and drug addiction, respectively. MTs were downregulated and they exhibited typical symptoms of multiple drug addiction, morbidity, and mortality. MTs overexpressing weaver (wv/wv-MTs) mutant mice were developed by crossbreeding MTs transgenic males with wv/wv females because male wv/wv mice were sterile. The MTs overexpressing weaver (wv/wv-MTs) mice exhibited attenuation of body tremors and served as an animal model of drug rehabilitation. By performing in vivo micro-PET neuroimaging with [^{18}F] FdG and [^{18}F]DOPA and by estimating CoQ$_{10}$ and complex-1 activity, we established that MB was significantly improved in wv/wv-MTs mice as compared to the control (C57BL/6J) mice; which further supported the above hypothesis (Sharma et al. 2013; Sharma and Ebadi 2014). The importance of MTs, ubiquinone, $\Delta\Psi$, mtDNA oxidation product, 8-OH-2dG, and α-Syn index (SI) as novel theranostic biomarkers was highlighted for the early detection of CBMP and neurodegenerative charnolopathies. Hence, these mitochondrial inclusion-specific (CBMP) biomarkers may facilitate exploring the TSE-EBPT of CB formation and CP induction/repression in health and disease (Sharma et al. 2013).

Complex I Activity

Cells adapt to nutrient and energy deprivation by inducing ATG, which is regulated by the mTOR and AMPKs. Thomas et al. (2018) found that cell metabolism influences the ability to induce ATG, with complex I function being an important factor in the initiation, amplitude, and duration of response. Phenformin or genetic defects in complex I suppressed ATG induced by mTOR inhibitors, whereas ATG was induced by increased mitochondrial metabolism. mTOR inhibitors increased phospholipids and mitochondrial-associated membranes (MAMs) in a complex I-dependent manner. The complex I ATG defect led to the inability to increase MAMs, limiting phosphatidylserine decarboxylase activity and mitochondrial phosphatidylethanolamine, which support ATG, indicating the dynamic and metabolic regulation of ATG.

Melatonin

Neurons contain a high number of mitochondria, and produce oxidative stress and live for a long time without proliferation; therefore, mitochondrial homeostasis is highly crucial to their health. Mitochondrial fission is necessary for the transmission of mitochondria to daughter cells during mitosis. Mitochondrial fragmentation has been used as an indicator of their dysfunction and CBMP. Oxidative stress induces changes in the mitochondrial network. Cesarini et al. (2018) determined the effects of melatonin on the mitochondrial network in HT22 serum-deprived cells, which increased ROS, activated plasma membrane voltage-dependent anion channels (VDACs), and affected the expression of pDRP1 and Drp-1 fission proteins. Parallel increases in ATG and apoptosis were observed. Damaged and dysfunctional mitochondria participated in CBMP and were deleterious to the cell; hence, their elimination through CP is crucial to cell survival. Melatonin reduced cell death and restored MB by regulating CP/ATG and by preventing free-radical-induced CBMP to confer neuroprotection.

CONCLUSION

This chapter described the original discovery of CB, theranostic significance of CP as an immediate and early biomarker of ICD, and the hypothesis that MTs confer CoQ_{10}-mediated protection by inhibiting CBMP as confirmed in cell culture and RhO_{mgko} neurons as an *in vitro* model of aging and in MT gene-manipulated mice in addition to elimination of toxic CS metabolites in undernutrition vs CR, and brain to body weight ratio to evaluate CBMP. The CB life cycle, inhibition of CBMP by MTs through CP regulation and its PKs in ICD, CB formation, and CP dysregulation in NDDs and chronic MDR diseases, environmental toxins, and regulation of CP, CS, and free radical hypothesis of disease progression, MTs defense, augmentation of MB, and prevention of CBMP were also described. MTs, as CP enhancers, CS stabilizer, and CS detoxifiers conferred protection in NDDs, CVDs, and MDR malignancies. MTs as CP agonists and scavengers of RONS protect mitochondria, whereas CS-MTs interaction is involved in CP regulation and ICD. MTs-induced zinc-mediated transcriptional regulation of genes is involved in growth, proliferation, differentiation, and development in NDDs, CVDs, and MDR malignancies. Electrophysiological correlates of CBMP, MPTP-induced CBMP, complex I activity, protection of hippocampal HT22 cells by melatonin in serum deprivation, attenuation of CBMP in gene-manipulated mice, and CP to evaluate ICD were described. MTs prevented CBMP by augmenting disease prevention and health promotion.

REFERENCES

Bollimuntha, S., B. Singh, S. Shavali, S.K. Sharma, et al. 2005. TRPC1-mediated inhibition of 1-Methyl-4-phenylpyridinium ion neurotoxicity in human SH-SY5Y neuroblastoma cells. J Biol Chem 280: 2132–2140.

Cesarini, E., L. Cerioni, B. Canonico, G. Di Sario, et al. 2018. Melatonin protects hippocampal HT22 cells from the effects of serum deprivation specifically targeting mitochondria. PLoS One 13(8): e0203001.

Chabenne, A., C. Moon, C. Ojo, A. Khogali, et al. 2014. Biomarkers in fetal alcohol syndrome. Biomarkers and Genomic Medicine 6: 12–22.

Dakshinamurti, K., S.K. Sharma, M. Sundaram and T. Watanabe 1993. Hippocampal changes in developing postnatal mice following intrauterine exposure to domoic acid. J Neurosci 13: 4486–4495.

Ebadi, M., S. Sharma, S. Shavali and H. El Refaey. 2002. Neuroprotective actions of selegiline. J Neurosci Res 67: 285–289.

Ebadi, M. and S. Sharma. 2003. Peroxynitrite and mitochondrial dysfunction in the pathogenesis of Parkinson's disease. Antioxid Redox Signal 5: 319–335.

Ebadi, M., S. Sharma, S. Wanpen and A. Amornpan. 2004. Coenzyme Q10 inhibits mitochondrial complex-1 down-regulation and nuclear factor-kappa B activation. J Cell Mol Med 8: 213–222.

Ebadi, M., H. Brown-Borg, H. El Refaey, B. Singh, et al. 2005. Metallothionein-mediated neuroprotection in genetically engineered mice models of Parkinson's disease. Mol Brain Res 134: 67–75.

Ebadi, M., S. Sharma, P. Ghafourifar, H. Brown-Borg, et al. 2005. Peroxynitrite in the pathogenesis of Parkinson's disease and the neuroprotective role of metallothioneins. Methods Enzymol 396: 276–298.

Ebadi, M. and S. Sharma. 2006. Metallothioneins 1 and 2 attenuate peroxynitrite-induced oxidative stress in Parkinson disease. Exp Biol Med (Maywood) 231(9): 1576–1583.

Jacobson, S.W., M.E. Stanton, N.C. Dodge, M. Pianar, et al. 2011. Impaired delay and trace eye blink conditioning in school-age children with fetal alcohol syndrome. Alcohol Clin Exp Res 35: 250–264.

Kang, J.X. and E.D. Gleason. 2013. Omega-3 fatty acids and hippocampal neurogenesis in depression. CNS Neurol Disord Drug Targets 12: 460–465.

Pipatpiboon, N., H. Pintana, W. Pratchayasakul, N. Chattipakorn, et al. 2013. DPP4-inhibitor improves neuronal insulin receptor function, brain mitochondrial function and cognitive function in rats with insulin resistance induced by high-fat diet consumption. Eur J Neurosci 37: 839–849.

Sharma, S.K., U. Nayar, M.C. Maheshwari, B.G. Gopinath, et al. 1986. Ultrastructural studies of P-cell morphology in developing normal and undernourished rat cerebellar cortex. Neuromorphological correlates. Neurol India 34: 323–327.

Sharma, S.K., U. Nayar, M.C. Maheshwari, B. Singh. 1987. Effect of undernutrition on developing rat cerebellum: some electrophysiological and neuromorphological correlates. J Neurol Sci 78: 261–272.

Sharma, S.K and K. Dakshinamurti. 1992. Seizure activity in pyridoxine-deficient adult rats. Epilepsia 33: 235–247.

Sharma, S.K., W. Selvamurthy and K. Dakshinamurti. 1993a. Effect of environmental neurotoxins in the developing brain. Biometeorology 2: 447–455.

Sharma, S. K., U. Nayar, M.C. Maheshwari, B. Singh. 1993b. Purkinje cell evoked unit activity in developing undernourished rats. J Neurol Sci 116: 212–219.

Sharma, S.K. and K. Dakshinamurti. 1993. Suppression of domoic acid-induced seizures by 8-(OH)-DPAT. J Neural Transm 93: 87–89.

Sharma, S. and M. Ebadi. 2003. Metallothionein attenuates 3-morpholinosydnonimone (SIN-1)-induced oxidative and nitrative stress in dopaminergic neurons. Antioxid Redox Signal 5: 251–264.

Sharma, S.K., E.C. Carlson and M. Ebadi. 2003. Neuroprotective actions of selegiline in inhibiting 1-methyl, 4-phenyl, pyridinium ion (MPP+)-induced apoptosis in SK-N-SH neurons. J Neurocytol 32: 329–343.

Sharma, S.K. and M. Ebadi. 2004. An improved method for analyzing coenzyme Q homologues and multiple detection of rare biological samples. J Neurosci Methods 137: 1–8.

Sharma, S., M. Kheradpezhou, S. Shavali, H. El Refaey, et al. 2004. Neuroprotective actions of coenzyme Q10 in Parkinson's disease. Methods Enzymol 382: 488–509.

Sharma, S. and M. Ebadi. 2011a. Therapeutic potential of metallothioneins as anti-inflammatory agents in polysubstance abuse. IIOAB Journal 2: 50–61.

Sharma, S. and M. Ebadi. 2011b. Metallothioneins as early and sensitive biomarkers of redox signaling in neurodegenerative disorders. IIOAB Journal 2: 98–106.

Sharma, S., C.S. Moon, A. Khogali, A. Haidous, et al. 2013. Biomarkers in Parkinson's disease (recent update). Neurochem Int 63(3): 201–229.

Sharma, S. 2013. Charnoly body as a sensitive biomarker in nanomedicine. Proceedings of the International Translational Nonomedicine Conference. Boston, MA: North Eastern University. (July 26–28, 2013). [Invited Speaker].

Sharma, S., A. Rais, R. Sandhu, W. Nel, et al. 2013. Clinical significance of metallothioneins in cell therapy and nanomedicine. Int J Nanomed 8: 1477–1488.

Sharma, S., B. Nepal, C.S. Moon, A. Chabennes, et al. 2014. Psychology of craving. Open J Med Psychol. 3: 120–125.

Sharma, S and M. Ebadi. 2014a. Charnoly body as a universal biomarker of cell injury. Biomarkers & Genomic Medicine. 6: 89–98.

Sharma, S. and M. Ebadi. 2014b. Significance of metallothioneins in aging brain. Neurochem Int 65: 40–48.

Sharma, S. and M. Ebadi. 2014c. Antioxidants as potential therapeutics in neurodegeneration. *In*: I. Laher (ed.), System Biology of Free Radicals and Antioxidants. Springer Verlag, Heidelberg, pp. 2191–2273. https: //doi.org/10.1007/978-3-642-30018-9_85

Sharma, S. 2014. Charnoly body as a universal biomarker of novel drug discovery in nanomedicine. Conference: BIT's 12th International Drug Discovery Conference, August 2014. Suzhou, China.

Sharma, S. 2014a. Novel biomarkers in Parkinson's disease. Conference: BIT's 4th International Conference in Molecular Medicine, November 2014. Haikou, China.

Sharma, S. 2014b. Charnolo-pharmacon-therapeutics of multi drug resistant diseases. Conference: BIT's 5th International MediChem Conference, November 2014. Suzhou, China.

Sharma, S. 2014c. Charnoly body as a universal biomarker of novel drug discovery in nanomedicine. Conference: BIT's 12th International Drug Discovery Conference, August 2014. Suzhou, China.

Sharma, S. 2014d. Charnoly body as a universal biomarker of novel drug discovery in nanomedicine. Conference: BIT's 12th International Drug Discovery Conference, August 2014. Suzhou, China.

Sharma, S. 2014e. Charnoly body as universal biomarker in nanomedicine. Conference: 2nd International Conference on Translational Nanomedicine, July 2014. Boston, MASS, U.S.A.

Sharma, S. 2014f. Mitochondrially-targeted nanomedicines. Conference: BIT's 5th World Gene Conference (WGC-2014), November 2014. Haikou, China.

Sharma, S. 2014g. Nanotheranostics in evidence based personalized medicine. Curr Drug Targets 15: 915–930.

Sharma, S. 2014h. Molecular pharmacology of environmental neurotoxins. *In*: E. Leone (ed.), Kainic Acid: Neurotoxic Properties, Biological Sources, and Clinical Applications. Nova Science Publishers, New York, NY, pp. 47–94.

Sharma, S. 2016. Conference: Drug Discovery and Therapy World Congress. Wyne memorial Convention Center, Boston, Mass, U.S.A.

Sharma, S. 2016a. Charnoly body as a novel biomarker of zika virus induced microcephaly. Conference: Drug Discovery & Therapy World Congress-2016 (Track: CNS Drug Discovery & Therapy). John B. Hynes Veterans Memorial Convention Center, Boston, U.S.A.

Sharma, S. 2016b. Charnoly body as a novel biomarker of zika virus induced microcephaly. Conference: Drug Discovery & Therapy World Congress-2016 (Track: CNS Drug Discovery & Therapy). John B. Hynes Veterans Memorial Convention Center, Boston, U.S.A.

Sharma, S. 2016c. Conference: Drug Discovery & Therapy World Congress-2016 (Track: CNS Drug Discovery & Therapy), Sep 21, 2016. John B. Hynes Veterans Memorial Convention Center, Boston, U.S.A. (Invited Lecture).

Sharma, S. 2016d. Disease-specific charnoly body formation in neurodegenerative and other diseases. Conference: Drug Discovery and Therapy World Congress, August 2016. Wyne memorial Convention Center, Boston, Mass, U.S.A.

Sharma, S.K., J. Choga, P. Doghor, J. Renteria, et al. 2016. Charnoly body as a novel biomarker of nutritional stress in Alzheimer's disease. Functional Foods in Health and Disease 6: 344–378.

Sharma, S. and W. Lippincott. 2017. Biomarkers in Alzheimer's disease-recent update. Curr Alzheimer Res 14(999).

Sharma S. 2017a. PET radiopharmaceuticals for personalized medicine. Curr Drug Targets 17(999): 1894–1907.

Sharma, S. 2017b. Translational multimodality neuroimaging. Curr Drug Targets 18: 1039–1050.

Sharma, S. 2017c. Charnolosome-antioxidants interaction in health and disease. Conference: 22nd International Conference on Functional Foods, September 2017. Harvard Medical School, Boston, Mass, U.S.A. (Invited Lecture).

Thomas, H.E., Y. Zhang, J.A. Stefely, S.R. Veiga, et al. 2018. Mitochondrial complex I activity is required for maximal ATG. Cell Rep 24: 2404–2417.

Widdowson, E.M. and R.A. McCance. 1956. The effects of chronic undernutrition and of total starvation on growing and adult rats. Br J Nutr 10: 363–373.

3

Charnolophagy as a Biomarker of Novel Drug Discovery

INTRODUCTION

Identification of the key ATG targets is highly crucial for developing novel TSE-EBPT-CPTs for the clinical management of NDDs, CVDs, and MDR malignancies. CP represents a novel and promising target for future drug development and theranostic applications. CP is important to the novel discovery of CPTs, particularly in chronic MDR diseases and aging where it is inadequately accomplished. CP occurs in health to sustain normal transcription, translation, and post-translation of physiologically-significant molecules including nucleic acids, proteins, lipids, and carbohydrates, whereas, spatio-temporally dysregulated CP participates in the induction of CBMP, implicated in chronic MDR diseases. Induction of CB is an immediate and early attempt to contain toxic mitochondrial metabolites in a physico-chemically injured cell. CB is a pleomorphic intracellular inclusion, which requires efficient spatiotemporal elimination through CP. Any delay and/or impairment in CP execution can induce inflammation, apoptosis, and/or necrosis, associated with chronic diseases such as NDDs and CVDs, as well as MDR malignancies. Hence, CP regulation is highly crucial to remain healthy. A delayed CP can impair normal biochemical and physiological homeostasis of a cell.

This chapter describes the clinical significance of CP as a novel biomarker of drug discovery and the TSE-EBPT-CPTs of MDR diseases.

MDR Malignancies

The role of circulating cancer-stem-cell-specific CS bodies and their involvement in malignancy was recently highlighted (Sharma 2017a, b, c). Their fusion with the normal non-proliferative cell can induce immortalization and malignant transformation to invade other body organs during metastasis. Hence, spatiotemporal induction and expression of CP is highly crucial for IMD and ICD. The human lifespan also depends on the cell-specific spatiotemporal induction and expression of CP. Various drugs of abuse including caffeine, tobacco smoking, alcohol, cocaine, amphetamine, methamphetamines, and opioids (morphine and heroin) trigger CBMP in a normal cell by inducing CB sequestration, impaired CP, and CS exocytosis. Drugs of abuse impair ICD process by disrupting CP to cause poor prognosis in NDDs, CVDs, infectious diseases, and MDR malignancies (Sharma 2018). Hence, chronic drug addicts encounter frequent early morbidity or mortality due to immunocompromised CBMP. Various oncogenes are triggered during malignant transformation due to impaired CP and CS exocytosis. Drugs of abuse as such may not induce carcinogenesis, but they may trigger CBMP by inducing oxidative and nitrative stress involving free radical overproduction. Hence, the prognosis of NDDs, CVDs, and anticancer treatment remains poor in drug addicts. The drugs of abuse also induce CBMP in progenitor cells to trigger NDDs, CVDs, and MDR malignancies.

Atherosclerosis

The basic molecular mechanism of atherosclerotic plaque rupture in hyper-proliferating smooth muscle cells (involving vascular neointimal hyperplasia) was described in response to Cyt-C release due to CB sequestration and CS destabilization (when CP is either delayed or impaired). This release causes ventricular thinning and rupture in extreme clinical conditions following myocardial infarction and volume or pressure overload in ischemic heart disease due to HTN and congestive heart failure. Hence, spatiotemporal CB elimination, CP induction, and CS exocytosis are highly crucial to prevent CBMP. Various antioxidants (SOD, catalase, glutathione, MTs, and HSPs), as free radical scavengers, protect highly vulnerable proteins (enzymes, hormones, growth factors, trophic factors, cytokines) during oxidative and nitrative stress by inhibiting CBMP cascade. The antioxidants inhibit CB formation and enhance CP during the acute phase and stabilize CS and enhance its exocytosis during the chronic phase. The cells in our body have their own in-built system of spatiotemporal CP, ICD, growth, proliferation, differentiation, development, and death which is governed by the transcriptional regulation of genes and microRNAs. Any endogenous and/or exogenous toxic exposure can disturb these orchestrated events and cause acute and chronic diseases, early morbidity, and mortality. Although endogenously synthesized antioxidants (such as glutathione, MTs, SOD, catalase, and HSPs) are involved in inhibiting CBMP, they may play a deleterious role in MDR malignancies, when a cancer cell becomes highly proliferative and remains undifferentiated or de-differentiated. Hence, induction and expression of these antioxidants may inhibit or enhance CBMP to sustain hyper-proliferation during malignant transformation.

AD vs Gout

Gout develops generally in individuals who frequently consume highly protein-rich seafood, beef, pork, goat meat, poultry, eggs, milk, and cheese. Currently, we have limited choice to either suffer from the sheer pain of gout or develop AD. The incidence of AD is lower among gouty patients because uric acid as an antioxidant serves as a free radical scavenger in the CNS and prevents CBMP. In AD, increased acetyl choline esterase activity causes degradation of the neurotransmitter, ACh, which is involved in memory consolidation in the hippocampal CA-3 and dentate gyrus neurons; whereas, in gout patients, xanthine oxidase is increased, which converts hypoxanthine to uric acid. Uric acid crystalizes at a low temperature (35.6°C) and forms needle-shaped yellow birefringent crystals in the joints which can be detected in the synovial fluid by polarizing microscopy. In addition to prescribing xanthine oxidase inhibitor (Allopurinol), physicians advice gout patients to keep their joints warm by wearing woollen pads to alleviate pain. These clinical findings confirm free radical theory of mitochondrial degeneration and CBMP in progressive NDDs. Colchicine may be prescribed to gout patients to prevent lymphocyte proliferation and activation; however, it causes severe gastric pain and abdominal discomfort because GIT cells are highly proliferative and are destroyed during Colchicine treatment. That is why it is currently not recommended as an anti-micro tubular drug even for cancer patients and those suffering from other proinflammatory conditions. Colchicine inhibits tubulin assembly to prevent spindle formation during mitosis. Other anticancer drugs, Podophyllotoxin, Vinblastine, and Vincristine induce selective depolymerization of microtubules and targeted action on the cancer cells in BC, ovarian cancer, uterine cancer, and prostate cancer. On the other hand, Paclitaxel hyper-polymerizes the mitotic spindle to prevent its division and halts cancer cell proliferation. The inhibition of mitotic spindle or its division trigger tumor-specific CBMP to cause apoptosis and/or necrosis, which halts cancer cell proliferation. However, both tubulin assemblers as well as deassemblers during mitosis require efficient MB (Sharma et al. 2013a,b; Sharma 2014; Sharma and Ebadi 2014; Sharma 2015; Sharma et al. 2016; Sharma 2017a,b,c). Hence, development of DSST-CP agonists/antagonists as novel CPTs will have great TSE-EBPT potential in chronic NDDs, CVDs, and MDR malignancies (Sharma 2018, 2019).

Mitochondrial Steroid Hormones Synthesis

Although the exact function of steroid hormones in the adrenal cortex is well-established, the precise role of their biosynthesis in the mitochondria remains enigmatic. There are three types of steroid hormones: (a) glucocorticoids (cortisol), (b) mineralocorticoids (aldosterone), and (c) sex steroid hormones (testosterone, estrogen, and progesterone). The primary precursor for the synthesis of steroid hormones, cholesterol, enters mitochondria through a specific cholesterol transporter channel (TSPO), which is the 18 kDa transmembrane protein that is located on the OMM, and regulates cholesterol entry in the mitochondria. Steroid hormones are constantly needed for the structural and functional integrity of IMM which remains in a hostile microenvironment of free radicals synthesized constantly during ATP synthesis in the ETC. Mitochondria not only synthesize steroid hormones for the structural and functional integrity of their own membranes, but also other organelles for NCF. DPCI delocalize TSPO to trigger a proinflammatory response. The synthesis of TSPO is impaired and it is delocalized during severe malnutrition due to free radical overproduction. Uncontrolled transport of cholesterol in the mitochondria forms crystals which aggravate syndrome X personality (characterized by hyperlipidemia, hypercholesterolemia, hypertriglyceridemia, central obesity, increased body mass index, insulin-resistance, and pumpkin-shaped body due to inadequate CP in the adipocytes (also identified as lipophagy). Impaired or absence of steroid hormone synthesis in the mitochondria renders other organellar membranes highly susceptible to free radical-induced lipid peroxidation. These deleterious changes trigger CBMP to cause either noninflammatory apoptosis or proinflammatory necrosis. Accumulation of cholesterol in the adipocytes is prevented by statins (Simvastatin, Atorvastatin, and Pitavastatin). Statins inhibit the rate-limiting cholesterol synthesizing enzyme, HMG-COA-reductase. However, their indiscriminate use causes rhabdomyolysis involving pelvic muscle degeneration, pain, and myoglobinuria characterized by chocolate-colored urine. In severe cases, even kidney damage may occur by degeneration of nephrons due to the release of myoglobin. Rhabdomyolysis and myopathies can occur in hyper-lipidemic patients, who consume statins indiscriminately with a futile attempt to reduce their body weight. Cholesterol forms a major ingredient of plasma membranes in addition to phospholipids (phosphatidyl choline and phosphatidyl ethanolamine). Phosphatidyl ethanolamine and phosphatidyl serine along with PUFA (linoic acid, linoleic acid, and arachidonic acid) provide structural fluidity, whereas cholesterol provides structural stability to the plasma membrane. Thus, absolute absence or impaired cholesterol synthesis is involved in muscle wastage in the pelvic region, with severe pain, and walking difficulty. Abnormal accumulation of Ca^{2+} in the mitochondria due to TRPC delocalization in response to DPCI can cause Ca^{2+} crystallization and induction of CBMP to cause atherosclerotic plaque formation. Various Ca^{2+} channel antagonists, including phenyl alkyl amines (Verapamil), dihydropyridines (Nifedipine, Nicardipine, Nitrendipine, Nisoldipine), and benzodiazepines (Diltiazem), prevent Ca^{2+} crystallization in the vascular smooth muscle cells and endothelial cells to prevent arterial stiffening and thickening implicated in hypertension, ischemic cardiovascular or cerebrovascular injury, atherosclerosis heart failure, and acute ischemic stroke. With moderate exercise, we mobilize the cholesterol from the intracellular compartment to the mitochondria through the TSPO channel to augment steroid hormones synthesis for membrane stability. Moderate exercise also depletes the white adipocytes involved in obesity and increases the synthesis of brown adipose tissue (BAT) which contains mitochondrial-rich adipocytes to increase muscle strength, whereas white adipose tissue (WAT) is devoid of mitochondria and compromises the muscle bioenergetics and is the primary cause of fatigue and generalized weakness in obese hyperlipidemia patients. Regular exercise and reduced fat intake can prevent complications of syndrome X. Hence, any physiological and/or pharmacological intervention to inhibit synaptic CB formation and CP induction during the acute phase and stabilize CS membranes, preventing CS blebbing, and augmenting CS exocytosis as a mechanism of synaptic detoxification and normal neuro-cybernatics during the chronic phase will be beneficial for the clinical management of many NDDs, CVDs, musculo-skeletal disorders, and MDR malignancies. Hence, CB prevention/inhibition, CP induction, and CS exocytosis to prevent CBMP at the synaptic regions are highly crucial events for IMD and synaptic detoxification to sustain cognitive performance in AD.

CONCLUSION

This chapter described free radical theory of atherosclerosis, gout, and AD and the significance of mitochondrial steroid hormones to prevent CBMP implicated in chronic NDDs, CVDs, and MDR malignancies. Hence, quantitative assessment of CP can be used as a biomarker of novel drug discovery. It will be promising to sustain IMD and ICD for normal neuro-cybernetics and cognitive performance which is impaired in PD, AD, and ALS. Moreover, calcium channel antagonists, and statins alleviate diabetes, CVDs, and obesity to a certain extent by regulating CP and by preventing CBMP.

REFERENCES

Sharma, S., C.S. Moon, A. Khogali, A. Haidous, et al. 2013a. Biomarkers in Parkinson's disease (recent update). Neurochemistry International 63: 201–229.

Sharma, S., A. Rais, W. Nel, R. Sandhu, et al. 2013b. Clinical significance of metallothioneins in cell therapy and nanomedicine. Int J Nanomedicine 8: 1477–1488.

Sharma, S. 2014. Nanotheranostics in evidence based personalized medicine. Current Drug Targets 15: 915–930.

Sharma, S. and M. Ebadi. 2014. Charnoly body as a universal biomarker of cell injury. Biomarkers & Genomic Medicine 6: 89–98.

Sharma, S., J. Choga, V. Gupta, P. Doghor, et al. 2016. Charnoly body as a novel biomarker of nutritional stress in Alzheimer's disease. Functional Foods in Health and Disease 6: 344–378.

Sharma, S. 2017a. Charnolosome-antioxidants interaction in health and disease. Conference: 22nd International Conference on Functional Foods at Harvard Medical School, Sep 21–23. Boston, Mass, U.S.A. (Invited Speaker).

Sharma, S. 2017b. Fetal Alcohol Spectrum Disorders: Concepts, Mechanisms, and Cure (Neurology-Laboratory and Clinical Research Developments). Nova Science Publishers, New York, U.S.A.

Sharma, S. 2017c. Zika Virus Disease: Prevention and Cure. Nova Science Publishers, New York, U.S.A.

Sharma, S. 2018. Nicotinism and Emerging Role of eCigarettes (with special reference to adolescents), Vol 1-4. Nova Science Publishers, New York, U.S.A.

Sharma, S. 2019. The Charnoly Body: A Novel Biomarker of Mitochondrial Bioenergetics. Taylor and Francis, CRC Press, Boca Raton, Florida. U.S.A.

4

Organ and Disease-specific Charnolophagy

INTRODUCTION

CP is an adaptive detoxification response to attenuate pathological conditions, including NDDs, CVDs, infections, aging, and MDR malignancies. The energy requirements are significantly elevated during oxidative and nitrative stress, resulting in extensive structural and functional degradation of mitochondria in the most vulnerable cell. CB originates from the degenerated mitochondrial membranes due to DPCI-induced free radical overproduction during O/P in the ETC; whereas, the condensation of fragmented mitochondrial membranes is an immediate and early attempt to contain toxic metabolites such as Cyt-C, acetaldehyde, H_2O_2, lactate, GAPDH, AIF, Caspase-3, 8-OH, 2dG, 2,3 dihydroxy nonenal, and ammonia in a restricted microenvironment within the cell. Each degenerated mitochondrial fragment serves as a CB primordium. A CB can be classified based on the level of its maturation. An immature CB is called as *cis-CB* whereas a mature CB is called as *trans-CB*. A *cis-CB* consists of loosely packed mitochondrial membranes and may exist in numerous pleomorphic forms depending on its physico-chemical characteristics. The lamellae in *cis-CB* are usually swollen, less electron-dense, and smaller in size compared to compactly packed, electron-dense, quasi-crystalline, thin lamellae in the mature *trans-CB*. *cis-CBs* as well as *trans-CBs* are eliminated via ATP-driven, lysosomal-dependent CP for survival, differentiation, development, intracellular homeostasis, and ICD. CP occurs more efficiently during the acute (*cis-CB*) phase as an immediate and early attempt of IMD and ICD for NCF. Lysosomes can also phagocytose mature CB (*trans-CB*) during the intermediate phase. However, during the chronic phase, lysosomal-resistant CB is formed due to denaturation of mitochondrial proteins (mitofusin, P[53], AIF, MTs, and BCl$_2$); these are partially eliminated by CP. A *trans-CB* and/or CS during chronic phase is destabilized to release toxic metabolites. Translocation of these metabolites in the nucleus impairs gene expression at the post-transcriptional level by inducing microRNAs and mtmiRNA epigenetic changes, apoptosis, and/or necrosis in CVDs, NDDs, and MDR malignancies. We have been focused since last >3 decades primarily on the mitochondrial-targeted CB biomarkers and the theranostic significance of various endogenous, natural, and synthetic antioxidants as free radical scavengers in UN, PD, AD, and drug addiction (Sharma et al. 2013a, Sharma et al. 2013b, Sharma and Ebadi 2014, Jagtap et al. 2014). As a scientific consultant, chairperson, plenary speaker, he highlighted the theranostic significance of disease-specific CP in NDDs, CVDs, and MDR malignancies in various national and international conferences, symposia, and workshops, and published several books on organ and disease-specific CB (Sharma 2014a–g, Sharma 2016a–e, Sharma 2017a). This chapter describes the theranostic significance of disease-specific CP for the development of novel TSE-EBPT-CPTs in chronic MDR diseases.

The shape, size, organization, geometry, topography, number, and arrangement of mitochondria depend on its physiological activity in a cell. For example, mitochondrial are compactly arranged in cells involved in movement including: (i) *cardiomyocytes,* (ii) *skeletal muscle sarcomeres, and* (iii) *spermatocytes,* because cells involved in movement require higher amount of energy (ATP) which is generated in the mitochondria during Kreb's cycle, oxidative phosphorylation, and glycolysis. In these highly specialized, terminally differentiated cells, other organelles such as ER membranes, Golgi membranes, peroxisomes, and even lysosomes, were hardly noticed. Hence, upon loss of energy due to DPCI, the mitochondria readily compromise their bioenergetics and are directly transformed to densely-packed multi-membranous *trans-CB* and are destroyed during the chronic phase by the release of their own toxins to cause myocardial infarction, ventricular thinning, and eventually, ventricular rupture due to volume or pressure overload due to HTN and congestive heart failure. The atherosclerotic plaque rupture in blood vessels occurs due to CS sequestration during the chronic phase. Metabolically active immotile cells such as neurons, neuroglia (astrocytes, oligodendrocytes, and microglia), hepatocytes, GIT epithelial cells, pulmonary epithelial cells, pancreatic cells, nephrons, and osteocytes possess randomly localized mitochondrial network. DPCI increase the requirement of ATP to sustain IMD and ICD in these cells. Free radical-induced lipid peroxidation occurs more readily in the brain during acute ischemic stroke because it is highly rich in lipids. The CS is a single-layered highly unstable organelle, which is exocytosed to prevent the release of toxic metabolites. Any delay or disruption in the CS exocytosis can trigger deleterious inflammation, apoptosis, and/or necrosis as early events in CBMP. Endogenous antioxidants (glutathione, MTs, HSPs, HSF-α, HIF-1, BCl_2, SOD, catalase, and P^{53}), naturally-occurring antioxidants (Resveatrol, Curcumin, Sirtuins, Rutins, Catechins, Kycopenes, and LSDs) stabilize CS membranes as free radical scavengers, whereas, synthetic antioxidants (Melatonin, Vitamin-A, D, E, and K, Probucol, Edaravon, and statins) prevent CBMP by stabilizing CS membranes during DPCI-induced primary, secondary, and tertiary free radical attack. However, the quaternary free radical attack is deleterious as it destabilizes the CS membranes to form CS bodies, which are pinched off to fuse with the plasma membrane to release toxic metabolites and cause phosphatidyl serine externalization and membrane blebbing to form apoptotic bodies. The apoptotic bodies are labile and burst to release intracellular constituents and cause non-DNA dependent cellular demise. Hence, drugs may be developed to prevent CB formation and augment CP during the acute phase. It enhances CS stabilization and its exocytosis during the chronic phase of disease progression. Although, curcumin possesses antioxidant, anti-inflammatory, and anti-apoptotic properties, it is inadequately soluble in water and does not cross the BBB efficiently. Hence, we need to develop ROS-scavenging-antioxidant-loaded NPs for efficient brain delivery of drugs to accomplish their full TSE-EBPT potential. CP is triggered primarily by downregulation of mtDNA, whereas ATG is triggered by both mtDNA as well as nDNA downregulation. MicroArray analysis revealed alteration in genes involved in ATG, whereas CP involves primarily downregulation of mtDNA, mtRNA, and mtmiRNA, which can directly or indirectly influence the transcriptional activity of nuclear genes involved in cell proliferation, differentiation, and development. The theranostic significance of disease-specific CP in chronic MDR diseases is described below:

CP in Drug Addiction

Recently, the author was invited to present a lecture on CB as a novel biomarker in drug addiction in Orlando, Florida (2015) to highlight CB as a pre-apoptotic biomarker of CMB, which is formed in the most vulnerable cell in response to nutritional stress, environmental toxins, or drug of abuse due to free radical-induced mtDNA downregulation. It is detected as a pleomorphic multi-lamellar, electron-dense, membrane stack of degenerated mitochondrial membranes in the hippocampal CA-3 and dentate gyrus neurons, hypothalamic neurons, and cerebellar Purkinje neurons in animal models of FAS, PD, AD, vascular dementia, and drug addiction. MTs inhibit CB formation and augment CP by regulating Zn^{2+}-mediated transcriptional regulation of genes involved in growth, proliferation, and differentiation in gene-manipulated DAergic (SK-N-SH and SHY5Y) cells and in genetically engineered mouse models of multiple drug abuse. Hence, drugs may be developed to prevent CB formation and induce CP during the acute phase and by developing CB antagonists and CS stabilizers to avert the chronic phase to detect, prevent, and treat drug addiction (Sharma 2015a).

CP in Nicotinism

Tobacco addiction (also known as nicotinism) remains a preventable healthcare challenge in the entire world and is the most significant cause of loss pertaining to national and international economy and productivity. Nicotinism poses a significant challenge to the general health and well-being of adolescents, pregnant women, and developing infants. Adolescents are highly vulnerable to nicotine addiction and suffer from PQL, early morbidity, and mortality. Nicotine exposure during intrauterine life can induce degenerative charnolopathies (such as abortion, stillbirth, sudden infant death syndrome, microcephaly, growth retardation, ADHD, autism, and craniofacial abnormalities) in developing infants; likewise, asthma, COPD, cancer, and infertility can develop in adults. Tobacco smoking kills ~6 million people each year, and 5 million of these deaths are the result of direct tobacco use, while ~600,000 are the result of non-smokers being exposed to secondhand smoke. Nearly 80% of the world's one billion smokers live in low- and middle-income countries. Some tobacco smoking-related health risks include: lung cancer, COPD, CVDs, stroke, asthma, reproductive anomalies, premature low birth weight infants, diabetes, blindness, cataracts, macular degeneration, and nearly 10 types of cancer, including colon, cervix, liver, stomach and pancreatic cancer (PC). There are ~7,000 toxic chemicals in tobacco which can directly or indirectly cause cancer, stroke, and heart attack to induce early morbidity and mortality involving CBMP. At least 70 chemicals have been implicated in inducing cancer. A person's life span is reduced by at least 10 years because of smoking tobacco. Nicotine is the primary ingredient in tobacco, possessing a highly addictive potential which causes physical tolerance and psychological dependence, with severe withdrawal symptoms and frequent for relapse. Chronic smokers find it difficult to quit smoking as the success rate is only 33%. Although several preventive and therapeutic measures have been implemented to minimize the risks of illnesses associated with tobacco smoking, a considerable amount of research is needed to further minimize this devastating, yet preventable addiction from the entire world. Recent trends in the reduction of smoking in several countries including the US, Canada, and Australia seems quite encouraging; yet smoking in several other countries such as Serbia, Slovenia, Russia, China, and India, remains a significant challenge. Recent outbreak of COVID-19 pandemic fatalities particularly included aging individuals who had a chronic tobacco smoking history and pre-existing conditions such as COPDs, and CVDs. Recently, electronic cigarettes (e-cigarettes) emerged as the next generation of nicotine products with different brand names in the market. Although their popularity has increased particularly among adolescents in the Western world, the extent of psychiatric comorbidity with e-cigarettes use and dual use of conventional (combustible) vs e-cigarettes remains uncertain. As many as 460 new brands of e-cigarettes have been introduced. Older brands tend to highlight their merits over conventional (incinerating) cigarettes while newer brands emphasize consumer choice in multiple flavors and product versatility. Public awareness and proper education (particularly for young adolescents) will go a long way in early prevention and successful clinical management of nicotinism. Please refer to the author's books on nicotinism (four volumes) (Sharma 2018)(released by Nova Science Publishers, New York, U.S.A.) for learning more about the basic molecular biology, molecular genetics, emerging biotechnology, diseases linked to nicotinism, and their possible prevention and cure. These books present the basic pharmacogenomics of nicotinism and the emerging role of e-cigarettes as an alternative to reduce tobacco cravings and related health risks, and to prevent secondhand smoking-related health risks. These books illustrate the novel concept of MB-based CPTs for the clinical management of nicotinism with future prospects to minimize tobacco-smoking behavior, and/or quit smoking with minimum withdrawal symptoms. The primary objective is to minimize nicotine-induced early morbidity and mortality due to asthma, emphysema, cancer, heart attack, diabetes, obesity, infertility, major depressive disorders, schizophrenia, AD, and several other neurological and neuropsychiatric disorders involving functionally impaired CP and deleterious CBMPs. These books confer recent knowledge and wisdom regarding the harmful and therapeutic benefits of tobacco smoking by incineration or by vaping through e-cigarettes. In addition, novel DSST charnolosomics and conventional omics (genomics, proteomics, metabolomics, lipidomics, and metallomics) with correlative and combinatorial bioinformatics are proposed to accomplish TSE-EBPT of nicotinism for a BQL.

CP in Fetal Alcohol Syndrome

Alcoholism exerts a genetic as well as epigenetic load and may be regarded as one of the most prevalent, identifiable, and preventable neuropsychiatric illnesses afflicting modern society today. Alcohol constituted 3.2% of all worldwide deaths in the year 2006 and is associated with >60 diseases, including FASD, cancers, CVDs, liver cirrhosis, neuropsychiatric disorders, and life-threatening injuries as described in the author's book, *Fetal Alcohol Spectrum Disorder: Concepts, Mechanisms, and Cure* (Nova Science Publishers, New York, U.S.A.) (Sharma 2017b). FASD is a collective term representing fetal abnormalities associated with maternal alcohol abuse. FASD is a devastating developmental disorder resulting from alcohol exposure during fetal development. Children with FASD become a serious and persistent socioeconomic burden to society, as they require specialized healthcare liabilities throughout their entire lives as a consequence of their parents' irresponsible drinking behavior. The primary aim of the inter-disciplinary and integrated genome research network (consisting of molecular biologists, psycho-pharmacologists, system biologists with mathematicians, human geneticists, and clinicians) is to better understand the genetics and epigenetics of alcohol addiction by identifying candidate genes and molecular mechanisms involved in the etiopathogenesis of FASD, and to provide recommendations to the government and scientific community for global dissemination of emerging knowledge and implementation of FASD interventions. A novel concept of charnolopharmacology involving CBMP is presented, which plays a crucial role in determining the life and death of the fetus during intrauterine fetal alcohol exposure. More specifically, MB-based CPTs for personalized theranostics of FASD, involving diversified charnolopathies, embryopathies, and infertility resulting in PQL can be developed. CPTs, based on ethanol-induced CBMP and the induction of charnolopathies initially in the spermatocyte and oocyte during the prezygotic phase, and subsequently, in the neural progenitor cells (NPCs) during the post-zygotic phase of fetal development are proposed. Hence, drugs inhibiting CB formation and/or augmenting CP during the acute phase, and stabilizing CPS and preventing CS sequestration and budding during the chronic phase, will have theranostic potential in FASD-associated charnolopathies. This book also introduces original concepts of MB, genomics, and epigenomics to successfully manage FASD. Particularly, MB-based CB prevention/inhibition, CP induction, and CPS and CS stabilizers are novel TSE-EBPT CPTs for the clinical management of FASD.

CP in Zika Virus Disease

The author was motivated to write a book on the subject called, *Zika Virus Disease: Prevention and Cure*, which has been recently released by Nova Science Publishers, New York, U.S.A. (Sharma 2017c) because currently there is no systematically-written document on the ZIKV virus or even COVID-19 disease, which could serve as a textbook for medical students, physicians, nurses, and other healthcare providers as well as a reference book for basic researchers, professors, and the general public to help develop a vaccine or specific cure. The author has highlighted ZIKV-induced CB formation and CP dysregulation due to CMB in the most vulnerable (neural progenitor cells, spermatocytes, and oocytes etc.) cells and their amelioration by physiological and/or pharmacological interventions. This book describes unique organ and disease-specific CB inhibitors, CP regulators, CB sequestration inhibitors, and CPS stabilizers as promising CPTs to aid in the prevention and treatment of the ZIKV or other virus-linked diversified spectrum of developmental charnolopathies in newborn infants and Guillain Barre Syndrome (GBS) in adults. The clinical management of ZIKV-induced GBS employing IV immunoglobulin and plasmapheresis is also described. Hence, vaccine and TSE-EBPTs can be developed based on disease-specific CP and CBMP-targeted CPTs for the complete eradication of viral infections (including COVID-19) as described in a chapter on CP and microbial infections in this edition.

CP in Depression

Depression is a complex global health challenge posing a considerable economical and psychological burden. Women, adolescents, and aging subjects are highly vulnerable to suffer from depression. Depression is linked to numerous modifiable and non-modifiable risk factors. Its effective treatment involves both psychotherapy and/or chemotherapy. Depression is the major comorbidity associated with obesity, metabolic syndrome (MetS), diabetes, aging, progressive NDDs including PD, AD, ALS, MS, migraine, drugs addiction. It is also a comorbidity in anemic female patients with hypothyroidism and postpartum syndrome, malnourished patients with eating disorders including bulimia and anorexia nervosa, early life stressful experiences, in injured soldiers and their families with PTSD, patients with severe chronic cancer and rheumatoid arthritis pain, coeliac disease, chronic kidney disease and hemodialysis patients with end-stage renal failure. Hence it is logical to initiate risk-free nonpharmacological interventions by selecting proper dietary regimens, moderate exercise, and by refraining from drug abuse (including coffee, cigarette smoking and alcohol) to remain healthy and productive throughout life by preventing CBMP. The novel dietary interventions are highly significant for the adolescent population, young women in their reproductive life, and the aging population of either sex. Currently available therapeutic agents have a low margin of safety and reduced therapeutic index with deleterious adverse effects including osteoporosis, obesity, hypertension, diabetes, CVDs, infertility and even fatalities if abused. A healthy lifestyle and consuming diets rich in mediterranean components can ameliorate minor to moderate symptoms of depression by preventing CBMP. In this regard, tryptophan-rich diets, diets rich in omega-3 fatty acids such as fish, olive oil, and flax seed oil, whole grains, soy bean, vitamin B_1, vitamin B_6, folate, and vitamin B_{12} along with iron and vitamin D_3 are highly significant as CP agonists and CS stabilizers to prevent CBMP for alleviating symptoms of depression. The author published a book on this topic, *Beyond Diet and Depression* (Nova Science Publishers, New York, U.S.A.) (Sharma 2014h–i) in two volumes. Vol. 1 provides basic knowledge of depression and the therapeutic potential of healthy dietary interventions including tryptophan-rich diet and the diet rich in omega-3 and PUFA. It provides basic guideline for the clinical theranostics of depression. In particular, the book describes various dietary interventions alone or in combination with pharmacological, and electroconvulsive therapy for the treatment of MDDs. Vol. 2 is devoted to important diets and their impact on depression. It covers various aspects of disease-specific depression and its alleviation by developing CP agonists. This volume focuses on the prevention and/or treatment of depression with specific dietary interventions and highlights disease-specific biomarkers for the early clinical diagnosis and TSE-EBPT of depression. Dietary interventions early in the course of depression might be beneficial to provide neuroprotection by inhibiting hippocampal and hypothalamic CBMP in depression and progressive NDDs as a consequence of free radicals-induced CMB. There are numerous anti-inflammatory, anti-apoptotic, and growth-promoting antioxidants which function as CP regulators in our diet, including flavonoids and polyphenols, which can enter CNS without any allergic reaction, about which very limited knowledge is yet available. This volume provides further insight on this subject and emphasizes the importance of antidepressant dietary regimens for healthy living at any age, particularly for aging, obese subjects, drug addicts, and female patients with hypothyroidism, eating disorders, post-traumatic stress disorder, chronic diseases and pain experience severe depression. A chapter is written on novel biomarkers and therapeutic strategies using the theranostic potential of CP for the differential diagnosis and TSE-EBPT of depression. A detailed description of CB formation and its prevention and/or inhibition by antioxidants and/or pharmacological agents via CP regulation is provided for the effective treatment of MDDs.

CP and Monoamine Oxidase Inhibitors

In his book, *Monoamine Oxidase Inhibitors: Clinical Pharmacology, Benefits, and Potential Health Risks* (Nova Science Publishers, New York, U.S.A.) (Sharma 2015b), the author has provided basic and applied knowledge about MAOIs, their classification, and clinical application as neuroprotective CBMP antagonists. He has also provided new information on this subject for doctors, patients, medical students, teachers, researchers, and basic biomedical scientists interested in learning the appropriate clinical application of MAOIs with proper understanding of the prevention and/or treatment of neurological and neuropsychiatric disorders. The book particularly engages with MAO-A and MAO-B-specific CBs in neurological disorders and their alleviation by CP induction. It is a book that will be of interest to patients suffering from PD, AD, PTSD, panic disorders, ADHD, and MDDs. Hence, specific CB-targeted MAOIs will have superior pharmacogenomics profiles, an enhanced margin of safety, maximum therapeutic index, and minimum or no adverse effects.

CP in Stress Alleviation

PTSD is a stress-related mental disorder which occurs following exposure to traumatic events. Neuroimaging studies have revealed that PTSD patients have reduced volume and abnormal functions in the hippocampus and the amygdala. A single prolonged stress (SPS) model revealed that apoptosis in certain brain regions, including the hippocampus, the amygdala, and the medial prefrontal cortex (mPFC) are associated with emotion and cognition. Jia et al. (2018) studied molecular mechanism of apoptosis in SPS rats, including ER and the mitochondrial pathways. For the ER pathway, PERK, IRE1, and ATF6 exhibited differential effect on apoptosis and neuroprotection. Three key factors were identified in the mitochondrial pathway and PTSD-induced apoptosis: corticosteroid receptors, apoptosis-related factors, and anti-apoptosis factors. These highlight the role of ATG and the basic differences between ATG and apoptosis in SPS rats and PERK inhibitors, IRE1 inhibitors, and Metformin as potential anti-apoptotic treatments for PTSD.

In his book, *Alleviating Stress of the Soldier and Civilian* (Nova Science Publishers, New York, U.S.A.) (Sharma 2015c), the author has highlighted that both soldiers as well as civilians have experienced the deleterious consequences of war. However, a soldier and his/her family face unexpected and unpredictable stresses requiring: physical and mental fitness, character, dedication, commitment, communication, mutual understanding, adjustment, discipline, tolerance, patience, isolation, resilience, hypervigilance, minimum vulnerability, sanitation, nutritional stress, sleep deprivation, patriotism, and sacrifice. In addition to the general public, this book is of interest to soldiers and their families serving in the Army, Navy, and Air force as they face diversified stressful situations for the sake of national and international defense during war and peace. Furthermore, agricultural scientists, farmers, policy planners, athletes, film actors, and those engaged in diversified physical, mental, economical, and a psychologically stressful environment will find this book interesting and informative with regard to selecting healthy diets for overall improved performance in life. Especially adolescents, young women, and old patients suffering from cancer, anemia, osteoporosis, rheumatoid arthritis and other chronic pains, CVDs, NDDs, and GIT, diabetes, and obesity suffer from diversified charnolopathies involving CBMP. Hence this book is informative, interesting, and helpful for a BQL of soldiers as well as for civilians. This book: (i) confers basic knowledge of diversified stresses; (ii) prepares readers to face stresses with patience, endurance, and resilience; (iii) and presents novel strategies of alleviating physical, psychological, and physiological stresses of war-wounded soldiers, prisoners of war (POWs), and veterans. The book guides the soldiers of the Army, Navy, Air Force, SEALS (sea, air, and land), POWs, and civilians to handle their professional and family stresses without having to suffer from combat stress reaction (CSR) or PTSD before, during, and/or after the war or conflict by preventing CBMP. It also guides those who experienced early childhood neglect, physical and/or sexual abuse, and other stresses of diversified origin. This book is devoted to the soldier's family members, their spouses, children, parents, relatives, and friends because of its motivational messages, immediate demand, and versatility. This unique manuscript encourages, motivates, excites, and guides young soldiers, civilians, and their families to tackle stresses with courage, patience, and resilience to successfully accomplish their training, pursue their adventurous professional career, and experience a fulfilling married life.

CP Targeted PET-RPs

In his book, *PET Radiopharmaceuticals. Quality Control & Theranostics* (Nova Sciences, New York, U.S.A.) (Sharma 2017d), the author described classical and potential PET-RPs which can provide high-resolution 5D images *in vivo* to simultaneously diagnose and treat the patient. This novel (theranostic) approach avoids futile therapies, unnecessary radiation exposure, and saves a lot of time, money, and energy. This informative book serves as a helpful guide for basic biomedical students, scientists, researchers, teachers, doctors, administrators, and affiliated staff involved in current and future development of novel PET-RPs to accomplish TSE-EBPT of chronic MDR diseases by developing CBMP-targeted novel CPTs as CB antagonists, CP agonists, and CS stabilizers. Existing books offer insufficient knowledge to accomplish the full potential of these highly specialized, expansive, and sophisticated labs, demanding in-depth knowledge, confidence, cooperation, mutual understanding, adjustment, time management, team effort, patience, resilience, and dedication. A systematic approach is provided to integrate cyclotron and PET-RPS labs, run the cyclotron properly, resolve technical problems efficiently, and maintain QC without being exposed to an unnecessary radiation hazard due to repetitive run failure, innocence, ignorance, negligence, misconception, misunderstanding, and/or overconfidence. The contents provided are thought provoking and motivate cyclotron engineers, basic scientists, radiopharmaceutical scientists, radiopharmacists, and physicians to develop novel CB-based PET-RPs in presently challenging era of nanotheranostics. The most recent knowledge of potential PET-RPs in the early theranostics of cancer, CVDs, NDDs, drug addiction, obesity, neurobehavioral disorders, rheumatoid arthritis, and chronic inflammatory illnesses is provided with currently limited theranostic options by highlighting the TSE-EBPT significance of disease-specific CPTs as CP regulators and CBMP modulators (Sharma 2017e).

Personalized Theranostics

The author has recently written a book, *Personalized Medicine: Beyond PET Biomarkers (Biotechnology in Agriculture, Industry and Medicine)* (Nova Sciences Publishers, New York, U.S.A.) (Sharma 2016f) which describes the theranostic significance of disease-specific CP-targeted CPTs for the TSE-EBPT of NDDs, CVDs, and MDR malignancies.

CP and Apoptosis by TFDP3 in Breast Cancer (BC)

Cancer/testis antigen TFDP3 belongs to the transcription factor DP (TFDP) family, which can bind to E2F family molecules to form a heterodimeric transcription factor E2F/TFDP complex, as an activator of cell cycle, involved in the regulation of cell proliferation, differentiation, apoptosis, and other physiological activities. TFDP3 is a tumor-associated antigen that expresses in malignant tumors and normal testicular tissue. Ding et al. (2018) investigated TFDP3 expression in mononuclear cell samples from tissue-derived malignant tumors, BC, and benign breast lesions and found that TFDP3 is expressed in the malignant form of tissues. They focused on the ability of TFDP3 to influence the MDR and apoptosis of tumor cells and examined the expression of TFDP3 and ATG regulation to cope with metabolic stress (such as malnutrition, growth factor depletion, or hypoxia) which removes erroneously folded proteins or defective organelles to prevent CBMP and intracellular pathogens. TFDP3 expression induced CP/ATG by upregulating LC3 (MAP1LC3) expression and by increasing autophagosomes during chemotherapy of malignant tumors. Since, DNA and organelles damage caused by the chemotherapy were repaired, TFDP3 contributed to tumor cell MDR. Treatment with siRNA inhibited TFDP3 expression, reduced ATG, and improved the sensitivity of tumor cells to chemotherapeutic drugs.

Stem Cell Theranostics and CP in Hematological Diseases

Recently, Ito et al. (2018), highlighted that hematopoietic stem cell divisions results in either self-renewal or differentiation to balance hematopoietic homeostasis; however, the heterogeneity of hematopoietic-stem-cell-enriched fractions has hindered the analysis. Advances in genetic

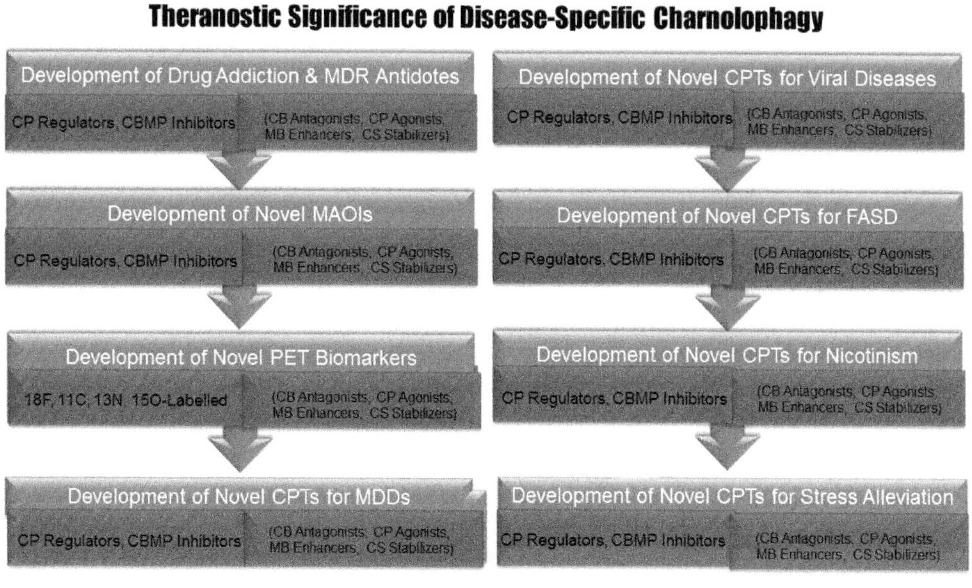

Theranostic Significance of Disease-Specific Charnolophagy

Development of Drug Addiction & MDR Antidotes — CP Regulators, CBMP Inhibitors (CB Antagonists, CP Agonists, MB Enhancers, CS Stabilizers)

Development of Novel MAOIs — CP Regulators, CBMP Inhibitors (CB Antagonists, CP Agonists, MB Enhancers, CS Stabilizers)

Development of Novel PET Biomarkers — 18F, 11C, 13N, 15O-Labelled (CB Antagonists, CP Agonists, MB Enhancers, CS Stabilizers)

Development of Novel CPTs for MDDs — CP Regulators, CBMP Inhibitors (CB Antagonists, CP Agonists, MB Enhancers, CS Stabilizers)

Development of Novel CPTs for Viral Diseases — CP Regulators, CBMP Inhibitors (CB Antagonists, CP Agonists, MB Enhancers, CS Stabilizers)

Development of Novel CPTs for FASD — CP Regulators, CBMP Inhibitors (CB Antagonists, CP Agonists, MB Enhancers, CS Stabilizers)

Development of Novel CPTs for Nicotinism — CP Regulators, CBMP Inhibitors (CB Antagonists, CP Agonists, MB Enhancers, CS Stabilizers)

Development of Novel CPTs for Stress Alleviation — CP Regulators, CBMP Inhibitors (CB Antagonists, CP Agonists, MB Enhancers, CS Stabilizers)

Figure 21

models, metabolomics, and single-cell approaches have explored hematopoietic stem cell self-renewal by metabolic cues, MB, CP/ATG, and MQC as key factors in evaluating their theranostic potential. A deeper understanding of how metabolism controls hematopoietic-stem-cells' fate is highly significant to confer better theranostics of hematological diseases. Theranostic significance of disease-specific CP is summarized in Fig. 21.

CONCLUSION

The theranostic significance of disease-specific CP for the treatment of chronic MDR diseases including major depressive disorders, drug addiction, nicotinism, fetal alcohol spectrum disorders, Zika virus, and novel COVID-19 disease is described in this chapter. The chapter also highlights the theranostic significance of CP in chronic MDR diseases. A brief description of MAO inhibitors, as CP agonists to alleviate PTSD, development of CP targeted PET-RPs, transcriptional regulation of CP/ATG and apoptosis by TFDP3 in BC and hematological diseases for personalized theranostics is provided. In addition, the significance of CP to accomplish TSE-EBPT of MDR diseases is emphasized.

REFERENCES

Ding, L.Y., M. Chu, Y.S. Jiao, Q. Hao, et al. 2018. TFDP3 regulates the apoptosis and ATG in BC cell line MDA-MB-231. PLoS One 13: e0203833.

Ito, K. and K. Ito. 2018. Hematopoietic stem cell fate through metabolic control. Exp Hematol 64: 1–11.

Jagtap, A., S. Gwande and S. Sharma. 2014. Biomarkers in vascular dementia: A recent update. Biomarkers and Genomic Medicine 7: 43–56.

Jia, Y., Y. Han, X. Wang and F. Han. 2018. Role of apoptosis in the Post-traumatic stress disorder model-single prolonged stressed rats. Psychoneuroendocrinology 95: 97–105.

Sharma, S., C.S. Moon, A. Khogali, A. Haidous, et al. 2013a. Biomarkers in Parkinson's disease (recent update). Neurochem Int 63(3): 201–229.

Sharma, S., A. Rais, R. Sandhu, W. Nel, et al. 2013b. Clinical significance of metallothioneins in cell therapy and nanomedicine. Int J Nanomed 8: 1477–1488.

Sharma, S. and M. Ebadi. 2014. Antioxidants as potential therapeutics in neurodegeneration. *In*: I. Laher (ed.), System Biology of Free Radicals and Antioxidants. Springer Verlag, Heidelberg, pp. 2191–2273. https: //doi.org/10.1007/978-3-642-30018-9_85

Sharma, S. 2014a. Charnolo-pharmacon-therapeutics of multi drug resistant diseases. Conference: BIT's 5th International MediChem Conference, November 2014. Suzhou, China.

Sharma, S. 2014b. Charnoly body as a universal biomarker of novel drug discovery in nanomedicine. Conference: BIT's 12th International Drug Discovery Conference, August 2014. Suzhou, China.

Sharma, S. 2014c. Nanotheranostics in evidence based personalized medicine. Curr Drug Targets 15: 915–930.

Sharma, S. 2014d. Novel biomarkers in Parkinson's disease. Conference: BIT's 4th International Conference in Molecular Medicine, November 2014. Haikou, China.

Sharma, S. 2014e. Charnoly body as a universal biomarker of novel drug discovery in nanomedicine. Conference: BIT's 12th International Drug Discovery Conference, August 2014. Suzhou, China.

Sharma, S. 2014f. Charnoly body as universal biomarker in nanomedicine. Conference: 2nd International Conference on Translational Nanomedicine, July 2014. Boston, MASS, U.S.A.

Sharma, S. 2014g. Mitochondrially-targeted nanomedicines. Conference: BIT's 5th World Gene Conference (WGC-2014), November 2014. Haikou, China.

Sharma, S. 2014h. Beyond Diet and Depression: Basic Knowledge, Clinical Symptoms and Treatment of Depression, Vol. 1. Nova Science Publishers, New York, U.S.A.

Sharma, S. 2014i. Beyond Diet and Depression: Disease-Specific Depression and Biomarkers, Vol. 2. Nova Science Publishers, New York, U.S.A.

Sharma, S. 2015a. Charnoly body as a novel biomarker in drug addiction. 4th International Conference & Exhibition on Addiction Research & Therapy. J. Addiction Res. 6:3.

Sharma, S.K. 2015b. Monoamine Oxidase Inhibitors: Clinical Pharmacology, Benefits, and Potential Health Risks. Nova Science Publishers, New York, U.S.A.

Sharma, S. 2015c. Alleviating Stress of the Soldier and Civilian. Nova Sciences Publishers, New York, U.S.A.

Sharma, S.K., J. Choga, P. Doghor, J. Renteria, et al. 2016. Charnoly body as a novel biomarker of nutritional stress in Alzheimer's disease. Functional Foods in Health and Disease 6: 344–378.

Sharma, S. 2016a. Charnoly body as a novel biomarker of zika virus induced microcephaly. Conference: Drug Discovery & Therapy World Congress-2016 (Track: CNS Drug Discovery & Therapy), John B. Hynes Veterans Memorial Convention Center, Boston, U.S.A.

Sharma, S.K. 2016b. Charnoly body as a novel biomarker of nutritional stress in Alzheimer's disease. Conference: 20th International Conference of FFC, 8th Functional & Medical Foods For Chronic Diseases, Sep 21–23. The Joseph B Martin Conference Center, Harvard Medical School, Boston, Mass, U.S.A.

Sharma, S. 2016c. Conference: Drug Discovery & Therapy World Congress-2016 (Track: CNS Drug Discovery & Therapy). At: John B. Hynes Veterans Memorial Convention Center, Boston, U.S.A.

Sharma, S. 2016d. Conference: Drug Discovery and Therapy World Congress, Wyne memorial Convention Center, Boston, Mass, U.S.A.

Sharma, S. 2016e. Disease-specific charnoly body formation in neurodegenerative and other diseases. Conference: Drug Discovery and Therapy World Congress, August 2016. Wyne Memorial Convention Center, Boston, Mass, U.S.A.

Sharma, S. 2016f. Personalized Medicine (Beyond PET Biomarkers). Nova Science Publishers, New York, U.S.A.

Sharma S. 2016g. PET radiopharmaceuticals for personalized medicine. Curr Drug Targets 17(999): 1894–1907.

Sharma, S. and W. Lippincott. 2017. Biomarkers in Alzheimer's disease-recent update. Curr Alzheimer Res 14(999).

Sharma, S. 2017a. Charnolosome-antioxidants interaction in health and disease. Conference: 22nd International Conference on Functional Foods, September 2017. Harvard Medical School, Boston, Mass, U.S.A (Invited Lecture).

Sharma S. 2017b. Fetal Alcohol Spectrum Disorders: Concepts, Mechanisms, and Cure. Series: Neurology – Laboratory and Clinical Research Developments. Nova Sciences Publishers, New York, U.S.A.

Sharma, S. 2017c. Zika Virus Disease: Prevention and Cure. Nova Science Publishers, New York, U.S.A.

Sharma, S. 2017d. Progress in PET Radiopharmaceuticals (Quality Control & Theranostics). Nova Science Publishers, New York, U.S.A.

Sharma, S. 2017e. Translational multimodality neuroimaging. Curr Drug Targets 18: 1039–1050.

Sharma, S. 2018. Nicotinism and Emerging Role of eCigarettes (with special reference to adolescents). Vol 1-4, Nova Science Publishers. New York, U.S.A.

Sharma, S. 2019. The Charnoly Body: A Novel Biomarker of Mitochondrial Bioenergetics. CRC Press, Taylor & Francis Group, Boca Raton, FL, U.S.A.

5

Charnolophagy in Pressure Ulcers

INTRODUCTION

Pressure ulcer (PU) is an injury to skin and its underlying tissue such as skeletal muscle. Compression, composed of mechanical deformation of muscle and external load, leads to localized ischemia, unloading reperfusion and, hence, a PU in bedbound patients. Sustained pressure can cut off blood circulation to vulnerable parts of the body. Without an adequate supply of blood, body tissues can die. Common PU sites include the skin over the ischial tuberosity, the sacrum, the heels of the feet, over the heads of the long bones of the foot, buttocks, over the shoulder, and over the back of the head (Bhat 2013). An ulcer is a sore on the skin or a mucous membrane, accompanied by the disintegration of tissue which can result in the complete loss of the epidermis, portions of the dermis, and even s.c. Ulcers are most common on the skin of the lower extremities and in the GIT tract. An ulcer on the skin appears as an inflamed tissue with an area of reddened skin. A skin ulcer is often visible in the event of exposure to heat or cold, irritation, or a problem with blood circulation. PU can also be caused due to a lack of mobility, which causes prolonged pressure on the tissues. The stress in the blood circulation is transformed to a skin ulcer, known as bedsores or decubitus ulcers (Kumar et al. 2004). Ulcers may become infected and transform to abscess containing pus. Skin ulcers appear as open craters, often round, with layers of skin that have eroded. The skin around the ulcer may be red, swollen, and tender. Patients may feel pain around the ulcer, and fluid may ooze from the ulcer. In some cases, ulcers can bleed and, rarely, patients experience fever. Sometimes, ulcers seem not to heal or healing tends to be slow. Ulcers that heal within 12 weeks are classified as acute, and long-lasting ones as chronic. Ulcers develop in stages involving CBMP. In stage-1 the skin is red with soft underlying tissue. In stage-2, the redness of the skin becomes more pronounced, swelling appears, and there may be blisters and loss of outer skin layers. As a function of time, the skin may become necrotic through the deep layers of skin, and the fat beneath the skin may become visible. In stage-4, deeper necrosis occurs, the fat underneath the skin and the muscle may also become exposed. In the last two stages, the sore may cause a further loss of fat and necrosis of the muscle; in severe cases it can extend down to bone, destruction of the bone may begin, and there may be sepsis of joints. Chronic ulcer symptoms include pain, friable granulation tissue, foul odor, and wound breakdown instead of healing. Symptoms tend to worsen once the wound is infected. Venous skin ulcers that may appear on the lower leg, above the calf or on the lower ankle cause achy and swollen legs. If these ulcers become infected, they may develop increased tenderness and redness. Before the ulcer establishes, there may be a dark red or purple skin over the affected area as well as a thickening, drying, and itchy skin. PU may be serious especially in people suffering from diabetes as they are at increased risk of developing diabetic neuropathy. Ulcers on the cheeks, soft palate, the tongue, and on the lower lip, usually last from 7–14 days. PU is also called as decubiti, decubitus, or decubitus ulcers, pressure injuries, pressure sores, and bedsores. Stage IV decubitus can display tuberosity of the ischium protruding through the tissue, and onset of osteomyelitis. The clinical management of PU may require plastic surgery. The main complication of PU is microbial infections, particularly in chronically-ill old and immunocompromised patients on dialysis and organ transplants.

Each year, more than 2.5 million people in the U.S.A. develop PU. The Agency for Healthcare Research and Quality (AHRQ) reported that ~2.5 million individuals are affected by PU and more than 60,000 patients die *each year* as a direct cause of PU. Pressure-induced injury (PI) in patients with limited mobility is a healthcare issue worldwide. PU resulted in 29,000 deaths worldwide in 2013, which is up from 14,000 deaths in 1990. The rate of PU in hospital settings is high; the prevalence in European hospitals ranges from 8.3% to 23%, and the prevalence is 26% in Canadian healthcare settings (McInnes et al. 2015). There is a higher rate of bedsores in intensive care units because of immunocompromised individuals, with 8% to 40% of those in the ICU developing bed-sores. The prevalence of PU in intensive care units in the U.S. range from 16.6% to 20.7%. Using the European Pressure Ulcer Advisory Panel (EPUAP) methodology, similar figures are available for PU in acutely sick people. PU prevalence in Europe was high, from 8.3% (Italy) to 22.9% (Sweden) (Tubaishat et al. 2010). A study in Jordan showed a similar figure (Vanderwee et al. 2007). There is some evidence of differences in PU detection among white and black residents in nursing homes (Li et al. 2011). From 2003 to 2008, the prevalence of pressure ulcers among high-risk nursing home residents was higher in black residents that in white residents. This disparity was in part related to the site of nursing home care. The cost associated with PU is enormous and needs serious attention. If PU is acquired in the hospital, the hospital no longer receives reimbursement. Hospitals spend ~$5 billion annually for the treatment of PU. According to Centers for Medicare and Medicaid Services, PU is one of the eight preventable iatrogenic illnesses.

This chapter describes causes, symptoms, risk factors, complications, pathophysiology, stages, prevention, treatment, and the theranostic significance of CP in the TSE-EBPT of PU.

PU occurs due to pressure applied to the soft tissue, resulting in complete or partial obstruction of blood flow. Shear is also a cause, as it can pull blood vessels that nourish the skin. Other factors can also influence the tolerance of skin for pressure and shear, thereby increasing the risk of PU such as protein-calorie malnutrition, microenvironment (skin wetness caused by sweating or incontinence), diseases that reduce blood flow to the skin (arteriosclerosis), or those reduce the sensation in the skin (paralysis or neuropathy). The healing of PU may be slowed as a function of aging, medical conditions (arteriosclerosis, diabetes, or infection), smoking or medications (anti-inflammatory drugs). PU can be difficult to prevent in critically-ill frail elders, and wheelchair users (spinal cord injury, cerebral palsy). People who cannot make even small movements are at increased risk of developing PU.

The primary method of prevention is to redistribute pressure by regularly turning the patient, providing a balanced diet with adequate protein, and keeping the skin free from exposure to sweat, urine, and stool. Some complications of PU include autonomic dysreflexia, bladder distension, bone infection, pyarthroses, sepsis, amyloidosis, anemia, urethral fistula, gangrene, and rarely malignant transformation (Marjolin's ulcer: *secondary carcinomas in chronic wounds*). Sores may recur if those with PU do not follow recommended guidelines or may develop seromas, hematomas, infections, or wound dehiscence. Paralyzed individuals are the most likely to have PU recurrence. In some cases, complications from PU can be life-threatening. The most common causes of fatality stem from kidney failure and amyloidosis. *Serou*s is usually seen in healing ulcer and *purulent* is seen in infected ulcer. Yellow creamy discharge is observed in staphylococcal infection; bloody opalescent discharge in streptococcal infection, while greenish discharge is seen in a pseudomonas ulcer. Bloody discharge (sanguineous) is usually seen in malignant ulcers and in healing ulcers with granulation tissue. Seropurulent, serosanguinous, serous with sulphur granules are seen in actinomycosis while yellowish discharge is seen in tuberculous ulcer. Chronic wounds and ulcers, especially, are caused by poor circulation, either through cardiovascular issues or external pressure from a bed or a wheelchair. Other causes of skin ulcers include bacterial, viral, fungal infections, and cancers. Blood disorders and chronic wounds can result in skin ulcers as well. Venous leg ulcers due to impaired circulation or a blood flow disorder are more common in the elderly. Rare causes of skin ulcers include pyoderma gangranosum, lesions caused by Crohn's disease or ulcerative colitis, granulomatosis with polyangitis, morbus Bchçet, and infections in immunocompromised patients, such as ecthyma gangranosum. Surgical procedures should be avoided on ulcerations caused by Behçet or pyoderma gangranosum as these exhibit pathergy.

Some of the investigations done for ulcer are: study of discharging fluid, culture and sensitivity; edge biopsy (edge contains multiplying cells); radiograph of affected area to evaluate periostitis or osteomyelitis; fine needle aspiration cytology of lymph node; chest X-ray and Mantoux test in suspected tuberculous skin ulcers may take a long time to heal. Treatment involves preventing the ulcer from getting infected, removing excess discharge, maintaining a moist wound environment, controling the edema, and easing pain caused by nerve and tissue damage. Topical antibiotics are used to prevent the ulcer getting infected, and the wound or ulcer is kept clear of dead tissue through surgical debridement. Patients are advised to change their lifestyle and their diet to boost MB and prevent CBMP. Improving the circulation, proper nutrition, moderate exercise, smoking cessation, and lose weight. Healing may be accelerated by replacing or stimulating growth factors implicated in CP regulation. Leg ulcers can be prevented by wearing compression stockings to prevent blood pooling and back flow for at least five years to prevent recurrence. Bedsores are treatable, but, if treatment comes too late, they can lead to fatality.

Causes of PU

According to Johns Hopkins Medicine, a sore can develop if blood supply is cut off for more than 2–3 hrs. PU are usually caused by: (a) *Continuous pressure*: if there is pressure on the skin on one side, and bone on the other, the skin and underlying tissue may not receive an adequate blood supply; (b) *Friction:* For some patients, especially those with thin, frail skin and poor circulation, turning and moving may damage the skin, raising the risk of bedsores; (c) *Shear:* If the skin moves one way while the underlying bone moves in the opposite direction, there is a risk of shearing. Cell walls and minute blood vessels may stretch and tear. This can happen if a patient slides down a bed or a chair, or if the top half of the bed is raised too high. Injured tissue can develop an infection, which can spread, leading to serious illness. There are primarily four mechanisms that contribute to PU development (Grey et al. 2006):

1. **External Pressure** especially over the bony prominences can result in obstruction of the blood capillaries, which deprives tissues of O_2 and nutrients, causing ischemia, hypoxia, edema, inflammation, and, finally, necrosis and ulcer formation due to increased accumulation of toxic CBMP metabolite from the destabilized CS. Ulcers due to external pressure occur over the sacrum and coccyx, followed by the trochanter and the calcaneus.

2. **Friction** is damaging to the superficial blood vessels directly under the skin. It occurs when two surfaces rub against each other. The skin over the elbows can be injured due

to friction. The back can also be injured when patients are pulled or slide over bedsheets while being moved up in bed or transferred onto a stretcher.

3. ***Shearing*** is a separation of the skin from underlying tissues. When a patient is sitting up in bed, their skin may stick to the sheet, making them susceptible to shearing when underlying tissues move downward with the body towards the foot of the bed. This may also be possible on a patient who slides down while sitting in a chair.

4. ***Moisture*** due to sweat, urine, feces, or wound drainage can exacerbate the damage. It may contribute to maceration of surrounding skin thus expanding the deleterious effects of PU.

Risk Factors for PU

There are over 100 risk factors for PU (Lyder 2003). Factors that may place a patient at increased risk include immobility, diabetes mellitus, peripheral vascular disease, malnutrition, cerebral vascular accident, and HTN (Berlowitz and Wilking 1989). Other factors are an age greater than 70 years, current smoking history, xeroderma, low BMI, urinary and fecal incontinence, physical restraints, malignancy, and a history of PU. In old age, the MB is compromised to trigger CBMP involved in the development of PU. It is more common among those who: (i) are immobilized because of injury, illness, or sedation, (ii) have long-term spinal cord injuries or neuropathic conditions, including diabetes, have reduced sensation. They may not feel a bedsore developing, and continue to lie on it, making it worse. Factors that increase the risk include: (i) Older age as skin gets thinner and more vulnerable, (ii) reduced pain perception due to a spinal cord or other injury, as they may not notice the sore, (iii) inadequate blood circulation due to diabetes, vascular diseases, smoking, and compression, (iv) poor diet, lacking proteins, vitamin C, and zinc (as it transcriptionally-regulates MTs implicated in CP regulation and CBMP inhibition by activating genes involved in cell proliferation, development, and differentiation to heal PU), (v) reduced mental awareness, due to a disease, injury, or medication, can reduce the patient's ability to take preventive action, (vi) incontinence of urine or feces can cause areas of moist skin, increasing the risk of skin breakdown and damage, (vii) reduced or high BMI. A person with a low body weight will have less padding around their bones, while those with obesity can develop sores in unusual places. People with a BMI of 30–40 have a 1.5X higher risk of developing PU. Various risk factors for PU and their alleviation by preventing CBMP are presented in Fig. 22.

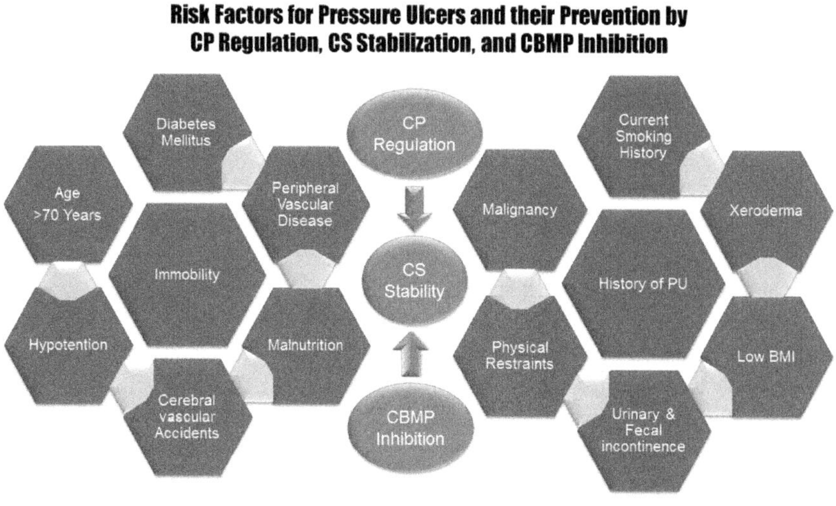

Risk Factors for Pressure Ulcers and their Prevention by CP Regulation, CS Stabilization, and CBMP Inhibition

Figure 22

Complications of PU

Without treatment, PU can lead to serious complications. Cellulitis could be potentially life-threatening. Bacterial infection from the surface to the deepest layer of skin and can result in septicemia, or toxemia. Bone and joint infections can arise if a PU spreads, resulting in damage to cartilage and tissue, and a reduction in limb and joint function. Sepsis, in which bacteria can enter through sores infect the bloodstream, resulting in shock and organ failure, is a life-threatening condition. There is a higher risk of developing cancer in the squamous cells if the patient has bedsores. Stage 2 bedsores can heal within 1–6 weeks, but ulcers that reach stage 3 or 4 may take several months, or they may never heal, especially in people with pre-existing conditions. With the appropriate measures, patients and medical staff can significantly reduce the risk of developing PU.

Pathophysiology of PU

A mild pressure sore may be experienced by healthy individuals while sitting in the same position for extended periods of time: the dull ache experienced is indicative of impeded blood flow to affected areas. Within 2 hrs, ischemia may lead to tissue damage and cell death involving CBMP. The other process of PU development is seen when pressure is high enough to damage the cell membrane of muscle cells. The sore initially starts as a red, painful area. The deep-tissue-injury form of PU begins as purple intact skin.

Stages of PU

The severity of PU develop in four stages: (a) the skin will look red and feel warm to the touch. It may be itchy; (b) There may be a painful open sore or a blister, with discolored skin around it; (c) A crater-like appearance develops, due to tissue damage below the skin's surface; (d) severe damage to skin and tissue with infection. Muscles, bones, and tendons may be visible: (e) an infected sore takes longer to heal and can spread elsewhere in the body; (f) various PUs can be prevented by CP regulation, CS stabilization, and CBMP inhibition by developing novel TSE-EBPT-CPTs. The four PU stages are revised periodically by the National Pressure Ulcer Advisor Panel (NPUAP) in the U.S.A. and in Europe by the European Pressure Ulcer Advisory Panel (EPUAP-2014). They are as follows according to Edsberg (2016):

Stage I   Intact skin with non-blanchable redness of a localized area over a bony prominence. Darkly pigmented skin may not have visible blanching; its color may differ from the surrounding area. The area differs in characteristics such as thickness and temperature as compared to adjacent tissue. This stage may be difficult to detect in individuals with dark skin and may indicate "at risk" persons.

Stage II   Partial thickness loss of dermis as a shallow open ulcer with a red PINK wound bed, without slough. May also present as an intact or open/ruptured serum-filled blister. Presents as a shiny or dry shallow ulcer without slough or bruising. This stage should not be used to describe skin tears, tape burns, perineal dermatitis, maceration, or excoriation.

Stage III   Full thickness tissue loss. s.c. fat may be visible but bone, tendon or muscle are not exposed. Slough may be present but does not obscure the depth of tissue loss. May include undermining and tunneling. The depth of a stage 3 PU varies by anatomical location. The bridge of the nose, ear, occiput, and malleolus do not have (adipose) s.c. tissue and can be shallow. In contrast, areas of significant adiposity can develop extremely deep stage 3 PU. Bone/tendon is not visible or directly palpable.

Stage IV Full thickness tissue loss with exposed bone, tendon or muscle. Slough or eschar may be present on the wound bed. Often include undermining and tunneling. The depth of a stage 4 PU varies by anatomical location. Stage 4 ulcers can extend into muscle and/or supporting structures (e.g. fascia, tendon or joint capsule) making osteomyelitis likely to occur. Exposed bone/tendon is visible or directly palpable. In 2012, the NPUAP stated that PU with exposed cartilage are also classified as a stage 4.

Unstageable Full thickness tissue loss in which actual depth of the ulcer is completely obscured by slough (yellow, tan, gray, green, or brown) and/or eschar (tan, brown, or black) in the wound bed. Until enough slough and/or eschar is removed to expose the base of the wound, the true depth, and therefore stage, cannot be determined. Stable (dry, adherent, intact without erythema or fluctuance) eschar on the heels is normally protective and should not be removed. CBMP in PU progression is presented in Fig. 23.

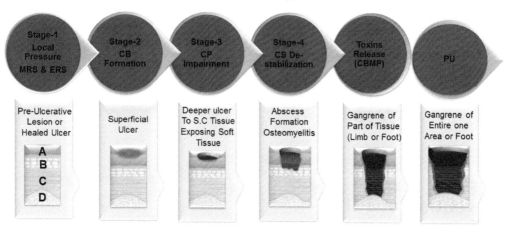

CBMP in Pressure Ulcers Progression
(Wagner's Grading)

A: Skin, B: Adipose Tissue, C: Muscle Tissue, D: Bone

Figure 23

Suspected Deep Tissue Injury

A purple or maroon area of discolored intact skin or blood-filled blister due to damage of underlying soft tissue from PU. The area may be preceded by tissue that is *painful, firm, mushy, boggy, warmer or cooler* as compared to the adjacent tissue. A deep tissue injury may be difficult to detect in individuals with dark skin tones. Evolution may include a thin blister over a dark wound bed. The wound may further evolve and become covered by thin eschar. Evolution may be rapid, exposing additional layers of tissue even with optimal treatment. CBMP-mediated PU complications are presented in Fig. 24.

Biofilm

Biofilm is one of the most common reasons for delayed healing in PU. Biofilm occurs rapidly in wounds and stops healing by keeping the wound inflamed. Frequent debridement and antimicrobial dressings are needed to control the biofilm. Infection prevents healing of PU. Signs of PU infection include slow or delayed healing and pale granulation tissue. Symptoms of systemic infection include fever, pain, redness, swelling, warmth of the area, and purulent discharge. Infected wounds may have a gangrenous smell, be discolored, and eventually produce more pus. It is important to apply antiseptics at once. H_2O_2 is not recommended as it enhances inflammation, dysregulates CP, augments CBMP, and impedes healing. Dressings with cadexomer iodine, silver, or honey can penetrate biofilms. Systemic antibiotics are not recommended in treating local infection in a PU, as it can lead to bacterial resistance. These are recommended if there is evidence of cellulitis, bony infection, or bacteria in the blood.

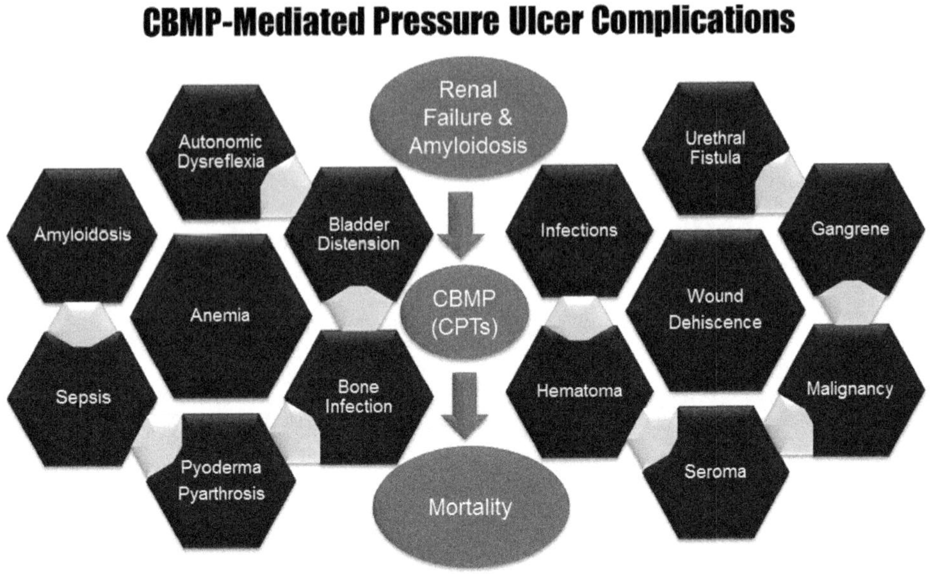

Figure 24

Prevention of PU

Preventing bedsores is easier than treating them, but this can be challenging. Tips to reduce the risk of PU developing include: (a) moving the patient at least every 15 min for wheelchair users and at every 2 hrs for people in bed, (b) daily skin inspections, (c) keeping the skin healthy and dry, (d) maintaining good nutrition to enhance general health and wound healing (e) quitting smoking (f) exercise, even if it is carried out in bed with assistance, as it improves circulation, (g) patients should mention any possible bedsores to their doctor, (h) a physical therapist can advise on the most appropriate positions to avoid PU. In the UK, the Royal College of Nursing has published guidelines in PU risk assessment and prevention to identify people at risk and taking preventative action. The U.S.A. and South Korea automate risk assessment and classification by training machine learning models on electronic health records (Cho et al. 2013, Kaewprag et al. 2017, Cramer et al. 2019). The NPUAP, EPUAP, and Pan Pacific Pressure Injury Alliance (Australia, New Zealand, Singapore and Hong Kong) published EBPT guidelines in 2014 developed by an international team of over 100 specialists and updated the 2009 EPUAP and NPUAP guidelines with recommendations on strategies to prevent PU including: the use of pressure redistributing support surfaces, repositioning, and maintaining appropriate nutritional support. The most important care for a person at risk for PU and those with bedsores is the redistribution of pressure so that no/or minimum pressure is applied to the PU (Reilly et al. 2007). Nursing homes and hospitals set programs to avoid the development of PU in those who are bedridden, such as using a routine timeframe for turning and repositioning the patient to reduce pressure. The frequency of turning and repositioning the patient depends on his or her level of risk (Witteridge and Guttman 2004).

Treatment of PU

Strategies to treat PU, include bed rest, pressure redistributing support surfaces, nutritional support, repositioning, wound care (e.g. debridement, wound dressings) and biophysical agents (e.g. electrical stimulation).

Support Surfaces

A 2015 Cochrane review found that people who lay on high specification or high-density foam mattresses were 60% less likely to develop PU compared to regular foam mattresses. Sheep-skin overlays on top of mattresses could prevent new PU formation. The effectiveness of alternating pressure mattresses remains uncertain. Pressure-redistribution mattresses are used to reduce pressure on prominent or bony areas of the body. Many support surfaces redistribute pressure by immersing and/or enveloping the body into the surface. Some support surfaces, including anti-decubitus mattresses and cushions, contain multiple air chambers that are alternately pumped (Guy et al. 2004). Methods to standardize the products and evaluate the efficacy of these products have only been developed through the work of the S3I within NPUAP (Bain and Ferguson-Pell 2002). For individuals with paralysis, pressure shifting on a regular basis and using a wheelchair cushion equipped with pressure relief components can help prevent PU. Controlling the heat and moisture levels of the skin surface, known as skin microclimate management, also plays a significant role in the prevention and treatment of PU. The following steps should be taken:

(a) **Remove the pressure** from the sore by moving the patient or using foam pads or pillows to prop up parts of the body.

(b) **Clean the wound**: Minor wounds may be gently washed with water and a mild soap. Open sores need to be cleaned with a saline solution each time the dressing is changed.

(c) **Control incontinence** as far as possible.

(d) **Remove dead tissue**: A wound does not heal well if dead or infected tissue is present, so debridement is necessary.

(e) **Apply dressings**: These protect the wound and accelerate healing. Some dressings help prevent infection by dissolving dead tissue.

(f) **Use antibiotic cream or oral antibiotics**: These can help treat an infection.

(g) **Negative pressure wound therapy**: Also known as vacuum-assisted therapy, which involves the attachment of a suction tube to the bedsore. The tube draws moisture from the ulcer, improving the healing time and reducing the risk of infection. Wounds heal within ~6 weeks at half the cost of surgery.

Skin Care

Skin Care is also important because damaged skin cannot tolerate pressure. However, skin that is damaged by exposure to urine or stool is not considered a PU. These skin wounds should be classified as incontinence associated dermatitis.

Nutrition

Bedridden people with higher intakes of vitamin C have a lower frequency of bed sores than those with lower intakes. Maintaining proper nutrition in newborns is also important for preventing PU. If a patient is unable to access proper nutrition through protein and calorie intake, he or she is advised to use supplements to support proper nutrition. For more details please refer to Langer and Fink (2014).

Surgery

Some bedsores may become so severe that surgical intervention is necessary. Surgery aims to clean the sore, treat or prevent infection, reduce fluid loss, aerate the lesion, and lower the risk of further complications. A pad of muscle, skin, or other tissue from the patient's body is used to cover the wound and cushion the affected bone through flap reconstruction employing CT-guided surgery.

Debridement

Necrotic tissue should be removed in most PU. However, healing may not occur in cases when the limb has an inadequate blood supply. Necrotic tissue is a safe haven for bacterial growth, which can compromise wound healing. There are five ways to remove necrotic tissue:

(a) *Autolytic debridement,* is the use of moist dressings to promote autolysis with the body's own enzymes and leukocytes. It is a slow process, but mostly painless, and is effective in individuals with a properly functioning immune system.

(b) *Biological debridement,* or maggot debridement therapy, is the use of medical maggots to feed on necrotic tissue and clean the wound of excess bacteria. Although this fell out of favor for many years, in January 2004, the FDA approved maggots as a live medical device.

(c) *Chemical debridement,* or enzymatic debridement, is the use of prescribed enzymes that promote the removal of necrotic tissue.

(d) *Mechanical debridement,* is the use of debriding dressings, whirlpool, or ultrasound for slough in a stable wound.

(e) *Surgical debridement,* or sharp debridement, is the fastest method, as it allows a surgeon to quickly remove dead tissue. For more details please refer to Moor and Cowman 2013, De Marco (2014), and Sieggreen (2016).

Guidelines for dressing PU are presented in Table 10.

Table 10 Guidelines for Dressing PU (DeMarco 2014)

S.No	Condition	Cover Dressing
1.	None to moderate exudate	Gauge with tape or composite
2.	Moderate to heavy exudate	Foam dressing with tape and composite
3.	Frequent soiling	Hydrocolloid dressing, film, or composite
4.	Fragile skin	Stretch gauze or stretch net

Note: These guidelines suggest that both IMD and ICD by CP regulation as well as extracellular detoxification (ECD) by using proper cover dressing are highly prudent for a better TSE-EBPT of PU. The guidelines for dressing PU are illustrated in Fig. 25.

More research is needed to assess how to support the treatment of PU, for example by repositioning (Langer and Fink 2014, Moore and Cowman 2015, Moore et al. 2016). Also, the benefit of using systemic or topical antibiotics in the management of PU is still uncertain (Norman et al. 2016). A 2017 Cochrane review found that it was unclear whether one topical agent or dressing was better than another for treating PU. Protease-modulating dressings, foam dressings, or collagenase ointment may be better at healing than gauze (Westby et al. 2017). The dressing should be selected based on the wound and condition of the surrounding skin. Some studies indicate that antimicrobial products that stimulate the epithelization may improve the wound healing (Sipponen et al. 2008). However, there is no global consensus on the selection of the dressings for PU. Placing a pillow under the affected area can help to alleviate pressure and symptoms. Less severe PU often heal within a few weeks with proper treatment, but serious wounds may need CT-guided surgery.

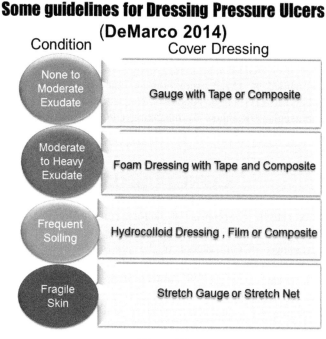

Some guidelines for Dressing Pressure Ulcers (DeMarco 2014)

Condition	Cover Dressing
None to Moderate Exudate	Gauge with Tape or Composite
Moderate to Heavy Exudate	Foam Dressing with Tape and Composite
Frequent Soiling	Hydrocolloid Dressing , Film or Composite
Fragile Skin	Stretch Gauge or Stretch Net

Figure 25

Significance of CP in PU

CP/ATG and Apoptosis in PU

The molecular mechanism that contributes to the pathogenesis of deep PU remains to be elucidated. Teng et al. (2011) tested the hypotheses that: (i) CP/ATG and apoptosis are induced in compression-induced muscle pathology and (ii) CP/ATG and apoptotic changes precede pathological changes in skeletal muscle in response to prolonged compression. Adult SD rats were subjected to pressure-induced deep tissue injury. Static pressure of 100 mm Hg was applied to an area of 1.5 cm^2 over the mid-tibialis region of right limb for one single session of 6-hr compression (1D) or two sessions of 6 compression over two consecutive days with rats sacrificed one day (2D) or immediately after (2D-IM) the compression. Muscle tissues underneath the compression region were collected for analysis. The rounding contour of myofibres and massive nuclei accumulation were demonstrated in muscles of 2D and 2D-IM. These changes were not found in muscle following 1D. Apoptotic DNA fragmentation, TUNEL index, and caspase-3 activity were elevated in compressed muscles of all groups. Caspase-9 activity was increased in compressed muscles of 2D and 2D-IM whereas increase in caspase-8 activity was found in compressed muscle of 1D. FoxO3 and LC3 was reduced whereas Beclin-1 was decreased only in 2D. No differences were noticed in the Akt and phospho-Akt in muscles, demonstrating that the opposing responses of CP/ATG and apoptosis to moderate compression in muscle and that cellular changes in CP/ATG and apoptosis occurred in the early stage. Tam et al. (2018) reported that PU is mediated by intrinsic apoptosis and exacerbated by ATG. Conditional ablation of Bax and Bak activates the Akt-mTOR pathway and Bnip-3-mediated CP and preserves mitochondrial contents in compressed muscle. The Bax and Bak alter the function of CP/ATG in PU, suggesting that manipulating CP/ATG and apoptosis are potential theranostic targets for the treatment and prevention of PU. Recently, Liu et al. (2019) observed degeneration, enhanced ATG, and apoptosis in deep PU muscle tissues. Muscular proteome of deep PU revealed 520 differentially expressed proteins; particularly, JAK2 was downregulated. JAK2 expression in C2C12 myoblasts exposed to O_2-glucose deprivation and re-oxygenation (OGD/R) was also reduced. In transfected C2C12 myoblasts with lentivirus carrying the JAK2 plasmid, myoblasts exhibited a decrease in ATG and apoptosis after OGD/R treatment. p-JAK2, p-Akt, p-mTOR, and p-ERK1/2 levels were elevated, accompanied by JAK2 overexpression but without p-STAT3. Inhibition of the Akt and ERK1/2 enhanced ATG and/or apoptosis, suggesting that JAK2 may play a protective role in PU-induced muscular I/R injury by inhibiting CP/ATG and apoptosis through the Akt and ERK1/2 pathways.

CONCLUSION

This chapter described causes, symptoms, risk factors, complications, pathophysiology, stages, prevention, and treatment for PU including: CT-guided surgical interventions, proper antibiotics, specialized sterile dressings, vacuum suction of the pus from deep abscesses of the ulcerated region, and sanitary precautions, particularly for the management of deep ilio-sacral ulcers of diabetic patients as these can easily get contaminated with urine, feces, and sweat. Abnormally lean or obese subjects are more prone to develop PU during chronic bed-ridden conditions. Hence, PU-specific CB antagonists, CP modulators/regulators, and CS stabilizers are recommended to prevent CBMP and biofilm development implicated in ulcer progression and poor prognosis due to ischemia, CMB, ICT, and release of toxic metabolites from the destabilized CS from the ulcerated tissue. In addition to postural adjustments, debridement, special dressing, antibiotics, vacuum suction of pus from the ulcerated abscess, proper nutrition and vitamins (Ascorbate), zinc and antioxidants as novel TSE-EBPT-CPTs are recommended for chronic bedridden patients, severely injured war-wounded patients, burned patients, organ-transplanted patients, spinal cord injury patients, wheelchair ridden cerebral palsy patients, immobile congenital syndrome patients, astronauts, organ-transplanted, and chronically ill old cancer patients to boost keratinocytes MB, regulate CP ,and prevent or inhibit CBMP to prevent PU development because a PU develops primarily due to CMB, dysregulated CP, and CBMP.

REFERENCES

Bain, D.S. and M. Ferguson-Pell. 2002. Remote monitoring of sitting behavior of people with spinal cord injury. J Rehabil Res Dev 39: 513–520.

Berlowitz, D.R. and S.V.B. Wilking. 1989. Risk factors for pressure sores. A comparison of cross-sectional and cohort-derived data. Journal of the American Geriatrics Society 37: 1043–1050.

Bhat, S.M. 2013. SRB's Manual of Surgery, 4th Ed. Jaypee Brothers Medical Publishers (P) Ltd., New Delhi, India.

Cho, I., I. Park, E. Kim, E. Lee, et al. 2013. Using EHR data to predict hospital-acquired pressure ulcers: A prospective study of a Bayesian Network model. Int J Med Inform 82: 1059–1067.

Cramer, E.M., M.G. Seneviratne, H. Sharifi, A. Ozturk, et al. 2019. Predicting the incidence of pressure ulcers in the intensive care unit using machine learning. eGEMs. 7(1): 49.

DeMarco, S. 2014. Wound and Pressure Ulcer Management. Johns Hopkins Medicine. Johns Hopkins University.

Edsberg, L.E., J.M. Black, M. Goldberg, L. McNichol. 2016. EPUAP – European Pressure Ulcer Advisory Panel.

Grey, J.E., K.G. Harding and S. Enoch. 2006. Pressure ulcers. BMJ 332 (7539): 472–475.

Guy, H. 2004. Preventing pressure ulcers: Choosing a mattress. Professional Nurse 20: 43–46.

International Pressure Ulcer Clinical Practice Guideline.

Kaewprag, P., C. Newton, B. Vermillion, S. Hyun, et al. 2017. Predictive models for pressure ulcers from intensive care unit electronic health records using Bayesian networks. BMC Medical Informatics and Decision Making 17 (Suppl 2): 65.

Kumar, V., N. Fausto and A. Abbas 2004. Robbins and Cotran Pathologic Basis of Disease, 7th Ed. Saunders, US.

Langer, G. and A. Fink. 2014. Nutritional interventions for preventing and treating pressure ulcers. The Cochrane Database of Systematic Reviews (6): CD003216.

Li, Y., J. Yin, X. Cai, J. Temkin-Greener, et al. 2011. Association of race and sites of care with pressure ulcers in high-risk nursing home residents. JAMA 306: 179–186.

Liu, Z., L. Ren, X. Cui, L. Guo, et al. 2019. Muscular proteomic profiling of deep pressure ulcers reveals myoprotective role of JAK2 in ischemia and reperfusion injury. Am J Transl Res 10: 3413–3429.

Lyder, C.H. 2003.Pressure Ulcer Prevention and Management. JAMA. 289: 223–6.

McInnes, E., A. Jammali-Blasi, S.E.M. Bell-Syer, J.C. Dumville, et al. 2015. Support surfaces for pressure ulcer prevention. The Cochrane Database of Systematic Reviews (9): CD001735.

Moore, Z.E. and S. Cowman. 2013. Wound cleansing for pressure ulcers. The Cochrane Database of Systematic Reviews (3): CD004983.

Moore, Z.E. and S. Cowman. 2015. Repositioning for treating pressure ulcers. The Cochrane Database of Systematic Reviews 1: CD006898.

Moore, Z.E., M.T. van Etten and J.C. Dumville. 2016. Bed rest for pressure ulcer healing in wheelchair users. The Cochrane Database of Systematic Reviews 10: CD011999.

Norman, G., J.C. Dumville, Z.E. Moore, J. Tanner, et al. 2016. Antibiotics and antiseptics for pressure ulcers. The Cochrane Database of Systematic Reviews 4: CD011586. Pressure Relief and Wound Care Independent Living (UK).

Reilly, E.F., G.C. Karakousis, S.P. Schrag and S.P. Stawicki. 2007. Pressure ulcers in the intensive care unit: The 'forgotten' enemy. OPUS 12 Scientist 1(2): 17–30.

Sieggreen, M. 2016. Revised national pressure ulcer advisory panel pressure injury staging system. Journal of Wound, Ostomy, and Continence Nursing 43(6): 585–597.

Sipponen, A., J.J. Jokinen, P. Sipponen, A. Papp, et al. 2008. Beneficial effect of resin salve in treatment of severe pressure ulcers: a prospective, randomized and controlled multicentre trial. Br J Dermatol 158: 1055–1062.

Tam, B.T., A.P. Yu, E.W. Tam, D.A. Monks, et al. 2018. Ablation of bax and bak protects skeletal muscle against pressure-induced injury. Sci Rep 8: 3689.

Teng, B.T., X.M. Pei, E.W. Tam, I.F. Benzie, et al. 2011. Opposing responses of apoptosis and ATG to moderate compression in skeletal muscle. Acta Physiol (Oxf) 201: 239–254.

Tubaishat, A., D.M. Anthony and M. Saleh. 2010. Pressure ulcers in Jordan: A point prevalence study. J Tissue Viability 20(1): 14–19.

Vanderwee, K., M. Clark, C. Dealey, L. Gunningberg, et al. 2007. Pressure ulcer prevalence in Europe: a pilot study. Journal of Evaluation in Clinical Practice 13(2): 227–235.

Westby, M.J., J.C. Dumville, M.O. Soares, N. Stubbs, et al. 2017. Dressings and topical agents for treating pressure ulcers. The Cochrane Database of Systematic Reviews 6: CD011947.

Whitteridge, D. and S.L. Guttmann. K. 2004. Luddwig (1899–1980)', rev. Oxford Dictionary of National Biography, Oxford University Press, 2004; online edn, May 2012 Dealing with Pressure Sores

6

Charnolophagy in Toxicology

INTRODUCTION

Many genetic differences leading to mitochondrial diseases affect ~1 person in 4,300, creating a large number of gene-environment interactions in mitochondrial toxicity. Recently, a rapid surge in the toxic effects of drugs and pollutants on mitochondria has been noticed. CP serves as a gold-standard biomarker to monitor environmental safety and toxicity. There are currently several examples of crosstalk between CP/ATG and other modes of cell death following exposure to toxicants. Although, ATG serves as a protective mechanism in a biological system, its persistence may induce cellular demise through defective CP and CBMP in response to toxic agents. Meyer et al. (2018) described the role of drugs and environmental pollutants in ROS signaling, biological processes involved in mitochondrial homeostasis, DNA maintenance and mutagenesis, stress response pathways, fusion and fission, CP/ATG, biogenesis, exocytosis, systemic effects from MTS in specific cell types, immune dysfunction, long-term effects of toxicity, mitochondrial-epigenetics, and mitochondrial toxicity in response to environmental pollutants. They also discussed the hormetic effects of mitochondrial stressors and future areas of research for mitochondrial toxicology, including integration of clinical, laboratory, and epidemiological data, improved understanding of biomarkers, and other factors that can affect mitochondria, such as diet, exercise, age, and DPCI.

This chapter describes the clinical significance of CP for the assessment of environmental safety and toxicity as a sensitive biomarker and in developing novel DSST-TSE-EBPT-CPTs for the management of victims exposed to organic and inorganic environmental toxins.

Tebufenozide Toxicity

The velvet bean caterpillar, Anticarsia gemmatalis Hübner (*Lepidoptera: Noctuidae*), is a soybean pest. Tebufenozide, a novel nonsteroidal ecdysone agonist is used to control this pest. Fiaz et al. (2018a,b) assessed Tebufenozide toxicity and its effects on their midgut. The toxicity, survival, behavior, and respiration rate for their larvae after exposure to Tebufenozide were evaluated. Damage to midgut cells was increased with exposure time. These cells showed a damaged striated border with release of protrusions to the midgut lumen, damaged nuclear membrane, and nucleus with condensed chromatin and increase in ATG vacuoles. Mitochondria were modified into nanotunnels indicating that Tebufenozide induces damage to cells, resulting in cell death. Tebufenozide also caused paralytic movement with change in homeostasis and compromised larval respiration. Thus, sublethal exposure to Tebufenozide disturbed the ultrastructure of the midgut, which might compromise insect fitness, confirming Tebufenozide as pest-controlling insecticide.

Pyrethrins-induced Toxicity

Natural Pyrethrins, a natural neural toxin for insects, are used for the control of pests affecting crops, livestock, and human beings. Yang et al. (2018) investigated whether natural Pyrethrins (0-40 μg/mL) modulate ATG through the AMPK/mTOR signaling pathway. Natural Pyrethrins inhibited the proliferation of HepG2 cells, induced autophagosome, augmented LC3-II formation and translocation, and led to the accumulation of Beclin-1 and the reduction of p62 and thus ATG. Natural Pyrethrins induced the abnormal redox metabolism in these pests, resulting in mPTP opening, ATP depletion, and mitochondria elimination by ATG. The phosphorylation of AMPK was enhanced, and the mTOR and p70s6k phosphorylation were decreased, suggesting that Pyrethrins-induced ATG of HepG2 cells and activation of the AMPK/mTOR signaling might pose a risk to human health.

Perfluoroalkyl Acid Toxicity

PFAAs accumulates primarily in the liver to cause hepatotoxicity. However, it can also deposit in lungs through air-borne particles and cause pulmonary toxicity. Xin et al. (2018) employed lung cancer cells, A549, to investigate the effects of three PFAAs with different carbon chain lengths on ATG. Through immunoblotting on LC3-I/II ratio of cells exposed to non-cytotoxic concentration (200 μM) and cytotoxic concentration (350 μM), they found increased autophagosomes, which was confirmed by TEM and fluorescence imaging. The p62 increased with the PFAAs concentration indicating ATG inhibition. They identified the involvement of CP and ER-phagy in the disruption of mitochondria and ERs, as confirmed by ROS overproduction, ΔΨ collapse, and upregulation of ERS-related proteins, ATF4 and p-IRE1. PFAAs induced MAPK pathways and inhibited the PI3K/Akt pathway, with potencies: PFDA > PFNA > PFOA. NAC treatment did not rescue cells from death, indicating that oxidative stress is not involved in cytotoxicity. Inhibition of ATG by Atg5 siRNA and Chloroquine (CQ) increased the toxicity of PFAAs, suggesting that CP/ATG was induced as the secondary response and played a protective role during cell death.

Acrolein Toxicity

Acrolein, a highly reactive α, β-unsaturated aldehyde, is a toxic component of cigarette smoke. As a lipid peroxidation biomarker, acrolein plays an important role in a wide variety of diseases such as NDDs, AD, diabetes, atherosclerosis, and cancer. Luo et al. (2018) focused on acrolein-induced ATG-dependent apoptosis. Treatment with acrolein increased the number of intracellular GFP-LC3 II puncta and the expression of the autophagosome biomarker LC3-II, with a low dose (25 μM) or at an early stage of treatment (3 hrs). Treatment of EAhy926 cells with acrolein for 6 hrs induced LMP-induced cathepsin B (CB) release. Acrolein also induced ΔΨ collapse, Cyt-C release, caspase-3, and caspase-9, suggesting that it induces apoptosis. ATG inhibitor 3-Methyladenine (3-MA) and CB inhibitor CA-074 attenuated acrolein-induced apoptosis, suggesting that acrolein-induced apoptosis was a CP/ATG-dependent injury to lysosomes and mitochondria in the endothelial cells.

Atrazine Toxicity

A widely used environmental herbicide, Atrazine (ATR) is neurotoxic and may cause global health risks in mammals, birds, and fishes. To assess the molecular mechanisms of ATR-induced cerebral toxicity through oxidative damage, Lin et al. (2018) treated quails with ATR by oral gavage at doses of 0, 50, 250, and 500 mg/kg body weight daily for 45 days. Increases in the swelling of neuronal cells, the percentage of mean damaged mitochondrial malformation, vacuolar degeneration, and decreases in the cristae and volume density indicated CBMP. ATR induced toxicities in the mitochondrial-related genes and oxidative damage, suggesting that ATR exposure can cause neurological disorders and cerebral injury by activating Bcl-2, Bax, and Caspase-3 expression but failed to induce ATG (because LC3B was not cleaved to LC3BI/ II). ATR induced CYP-related metabolic disorders by activating the nuclear xenobiotic receptors response (NXRs including AHR, CAR, and PXR) and increased CYP isoforms (CYP1B1 and C) to enhance mitochondrial dysfunction. ATR induced oxidative stress and mitochondrial dysfunction by activating the NXR response and by interfering in the CYP450s homeostasis to cause cerebral toxicity.

Chlorpyifos Toxicity

The organophosphate (OP) pesticide Chlorpyifos (CPF), used in agriculture, induces developmental and neurological impairments. Singh et al. (2018) hypothesized that STAT1, a transcription factor, causes DAergic cell death via mitochondrial oxidative stress. Exposure of N27 cells to CPF resulted in apoptotic cell death. Similar effects were observed in CPF-treated LUHMES cells, with an increase in mitochondrial dysfunction involving CBMP. CPF (10 μM) induced time-dependent STAT1 activation coincided with the $\Delta\Psi$ collapse, increase in ROS, proteolytic cleavage of PKCδ, reduced O_2 consumption rate (OCR), with reduction in ATP-linked OCR, increase in Bax/Bcl-2 ratio, and CP induction. STAT1 was bound to a regulatory sequence in the NOX1 and Bax promoter regions in response to CPF in N27 cells. Overexpression of non-phosphorylatable STAT1 mutants (STAT1Y701F and STAT1S727A) but not STAT1 WT attenuated the cleavage of PKCδ and cell death in CPF-treated cells. siRNA knockdown demonstrated STAT1 as a critical regulator of CP/ATG and mitochondria-mediated proapoptotic cell signaling. Oral administration of CPF (5 mg/kg) in 27–81 days postnatal rats induced motor deficits and NS-DAergic degeneration with induction of STAT1-dependent proapoptotic cell signaling, whereas co-treatment with Mitoapocynin and CPF rescued motor deficits, and restored neuronal survival via abrogation of STAT1-dependent proapoptotic cell signaling. This study identified a mechanism by which STAT1 regulates mitochondrial oxidative stress, PKCδ activation, and ATG. The phosphorylation of Tyrosine 701 and Serine 727 in STAT1 was essential for PKCδ cleavage. Hence, Mitoapocynin may have theranostic potential to attenuate CPF-induced DAergic toxicity and neurobehavioral deficits.

Spinosad Toxicity

Spinosad is an extensively used bio-pesticide throughout the world. The effects of pesticide in human health are associated with its residue in food or occupational exposure in agriculture. The lung is the direct target of pesticides exposure. Zhang et al. (2019) demonstrated that Spinosad inhibited the proliferation of human lung epithelial A549 cells, induced DNA damage, and enhanced apoptosis. DNA double strand breaks, cleavage of PARP, release of Cyt-C, $\Delta\Psi$ collapse, ROS generation, caspase-3/9 activation, increase in Bax/Bcl-2 ratio, LC3-I to LC3-II conversion, accumulation of Beclin-1, degradation of p62, phosphorylation of AMPK, and mTOR contributed to its toxic effects. The cytotoxicity of Spinosad may be associated with the mitochondrial apoptotic or AMPK/mTOR-mediated CP/ATG pathways. The DNA strand breaks suggested that it has genotoxic effects on lung cells which pose a risk to human health.

1,4-Benzoquinone Toxicity

1,4-Benzoquinone is a *toxic* metabolite in human blood and can be used to track exposure to benzene or aromatic compounds, such as petrol. It interferes with respiration and induces kidney damage in animals. Hemato-toxicity of benzene is derived mainly from its active metabolite, 1,4-Benzoquinone (1,4-BQ), which induces mitochondrial damage and apoptosis. Zhang et al. (2018) investigated whether PINK1/Parkin-mediated MTG is activated in 1,4-BQ-treated HL-60 cells, and its role in 1,4-BQ-induced apoptosis. 1,4-BQ-induced ATG in HL-60 cells was characterized by increased LC3-II/LC3-I ratio, Beclin1 expression, and decreased p62 expression, which was blocked by pretreatment with Cyclosporine A (CsA). 1,4-BQ induced mitochondrial stress through $\Delta\Psi$ collapse, ROS overproduction, and MTG by increased PINK1/Parkin mRNA and protein expression. 1,4-BQ-induced apoptosis with or without CsA, demonstrated that PINK1/Parkin-mediated MTG exerts a protective effect in 1,4-BQ-induced apoptosis in HL-60 cells.

Paraquat Toxicity

Paraquat (PQ) is an herbicide which was once used globally, but is now prohibited due to its toxicity to humans. However, there are still rare cases of the fetal intoxication of PQ, which was purchased prior to its prohibition in Japan. Hirayama et al. (2018) evaluated cell-death pathways, MTS response, and ATG in SH-SY5Y cells exposed to PQ. A decrease in MTS sensitive-Bnip-3 protein, ATG suppression, lack of apoptosis, necroptosis, and ferroptosis were observed, indicating that although the responses of mitochondria and ATG were observed, subsequent cell death occurred via necrosis.

Squamocin Toxicity

Squamocin was found to be a lethal agent for midgut cells of some insects when tested on their larvae. Fiaz et al. (2018) calculated LC_{50} and LC_{90} of Squamocin for *A. gemmatalis* Hübner (*Lepidoptera: Noctuidae*) using probit analysis. Morphological changes in midgut cells of larvae treated with LC_{50} and LC_{90} of Squamocin for 24, 48 and 72 hrs were analyzed under light, fluorescence, and TEM. The maximum damage to midgut cells was found at LC_{90} where it showed digestive cells with an enlarged basal labyrinth, vacuolated cytoplasm, damaged apical surface, cell protrusions, ATG, and cell death. The goblet cells showed disorganized microvilli. Mitochondria exhibited compromised Mitotracker labeling, indicating a decrease in the respiratory rate, which induced epithelial cell damage.

Methylisothiazolinone Toxicity

Methylisothiazolinone (MIT) is a biocide and preservative, used alone or in a 1:3 ratio with methylchloroisothiazolinone (MCIT) under the trade name, Kathons, during the manufacture of household products. Park et al. (2018) explored the toxicity of MIT on human liver epithelial cells. MIT was bound to the plasma membrane and the inner wall of vacuoles, ruptured cell membrane, and nuclear envelope, inducing autophagosome-like vacuoles formation, and mitochondrial damage within 24 hrs of exposure. Cell viability decreased due to increased LDH, NO, IFN-γ, IL-8, IL-10, and apoptosis. Mitochondrial membrane damage and apoptosis-related proteins were enhanced, and ATP levels were reduced. Increased DNA damage and decreased transcriptional activity were observed. No cell death was specifically induced by ATG modulation, suggesting that MIT may induce multiple pathways of cell death and an inflammatory response through DNA damage caused by nuclear envelope perforation.

Gentamicin Ototoxicity

ATG plays a role during early morphogenesis in the mammalian inner ear, as well as in adult cochlear hair cells exposed to ototoxic insults. Setz et al. (2018) searched for molecular biomarkers of MTG within House Ear Institute-Organ of Corti-1 (HEI-OC1) cells as well as in the organ of Corti (OC). They tested the expression of PINK1/Park2 mRNA in 5-days-old C57BL/6 mice's cochleae using RT-PCR to evaluate Gentamicin-induced MTG in HEI-OC1 cells and in the OC. The translocation of fluorescence-tagged LC3 to mitochondria was observed after a 6 hrs of incubation with CCCP. Incubation with Gentamicin generated no mitochondrial translocation of LC3. MTG was observed after CCCP exposure in HEI-OC1 cells by downregulation of COXIV. A downregulation of COXIV was observed in the OC after CCCP. The O_2 consumption rate (OCR) changed in cells treated with CCCP. Gentamicin generated no impact on OCR or mitochondrial morphology. Changes in the expression of Atg12 and LC3 in both the OC and HEI-OC1 cells after CCCP exposure were observed, indicating that Gentamicin had no impact on the activation of MTG-either in the HEI-OC1 cell line or in the OC and that MTG-independent mechanisms may underlie aminoglycoside ototoxicity.

Doxicycline Toxicity

Although anthracyclines, such as Doxicycline (DOX), are potent anti-cancer agents for the treatment of solid tumors and hematological malignancies, their clinical use is hampered by cardiotoxicity. Li et al. (2018) investigated the role of PI3Kγ in DOX-induced cardiotoxicity and the cardio-protective and anti-cancer effects of PI3Kγ inhibitors. Mice expressing a kinase-inactive PI3Kγ or receiving PI3Kγ selective inhibitors were subjected to chronic DOX treatment. Echocardiography and DOX-mediated signaling were assessed in whole hearts as well as in isolated cardiomyocytes, respectively. PI3Kγ KD mice showed preserved cardiac function after chronic low-dose DOX treatment, and were protected in DOX-induced cardiotoxicity. The beneficial effects were linked to enhanced CP/ATG elimination of DOX-induced CBs. Pharmacological or genetic blockade of CP/ATG *in vivo* abrogated the resistance of PI3Kγ KD mice to DOX cardiotoxicity. PI3Kγ was triggered in DOX-treated hearts, downstream of TLR9, by the mtDNA released by injured organelles, and contained in CSs. The CS-PI3Kγ/Akt/mTOR/Ulk1 signaling provided maladaptive feedback inhibition of CP/ATG. PI3Kγ blockade in mammary gland tumors prevented DOX-induced cardiac dysfunction, synergized with the anti-tumor action of DOX, by unleashing anticancer immunity, suggesting that inhibition of PI3Kγ may provide dual theransostic benefit in regard to cancer by preventing anthracyclines cardiotoxicity and reducing tumor growth.

Iodine-Induced Neurotoxicity

Cui et al. (2019) explored whether high iodine intake may impair intelligence and the role of CP/ATG and apoptosis in high iodine-induced neurotoxicity. Iodine reduced the IQ of rats, and caused abnormalities in the hippocampus by increased apoptosis, as confirmed by apoptotic proteins and TUNEL-positive cells. Iodine impaired the mitochondrial ultrastructure and caused the elevation of Bax, Cyt-C and decline in Bcl_2, indicating CBMP. The expression of autophagosomes protein Atg7, Beclin1 and ATG substrate p62 were elevated, suggesting that their accumulation occurs due to enhanced formation and reduced clearance, indicating a crucial role of CP/ATG in iodine-induced neurotoxicity.

CP in Metal Ion Toxicity

Lead-Induced Nephrotoxicity

Lead (Pb) is a nephrotoxicant that causes damage to renal proximal tubular cells. Wang et al. (2019) showed that Pb induces ERS represented by increased phosphorylation of PERK with activation of the eIF2α-ATF4-CHOP in primary rat proximal tubular (rPT) cells, indicating the activation of the PERK-eIF2α-ATF4-CHOP pathway due to excessive ERS. The Pb-induced PERK pathway was inhibited by 4-Phenylbutyric acid and PERK gene silencing, whereas it was upregulated by Tunicamycin (TM) treatment. Pb-induced apoptosis and inhibition of ATG in rPT cells were augmented by co-treatment with TM, respectively. Pharmacological or genetic inhibition of the PERK pathway resulted in the alleviation of apoptosis and restoration of ATG inhibition in Pb-exposed rPT cells, suggesting that the activation of PERK-eIF2α-ATF4-CHOP triggered by excessive ERS in rPT cells leads to Pb-induced ATG inhibition and apoptosis, resulting in nephrotoxicity.

Cadmium (Cd)-Induced Neurotoxicity

Cadmium (Cd) is an environmental and occupational hazard with neurotoxic consequences. Pi et al. (2018) exposed Neuro-2a cells to different concentrations of $CdCl_2$ (12.5, 25 and 50 μM) for 24 hrs. and found that Cd induces LMP with the release of cathepsin B (CTSB) to the cytosol, causing the release of Cyt-C and triggering caspase-dependent apoptosis. Cd decreased Tfe3 expression but induced the nuclear translocation of Tfe3 and Tfe3 target-gene expression, associated with lysosomal stress. Tfe3 overexpression was protected in Cd-induced neurotoxicity because the lysosomal-mitochondrial axis was maintained. The protective effect of Tfe3 was not dependent on the restoration of ATG, suggesting that lysosomal-mitochondrial axis-dependent apoptosis is involved in Cd-induced neurotoxicity and that manipulation of Tfe3 signaling may be a theranostic approach to curb Cd-induced neurotoxicity.

Methylmercury (MeHg) Toxicity

MeHg is a neurotoxin, which causes changes in various structures of the CNS. Ferreira et al. (2018) investigated the effect of MeHg on the ultrastructure of the cells in the spinal cord. Chicken embryos at E3 were treated *in ovo* with 0.1 μg MeHg/50 μL saline solution and analyzed at E10. A significant number of altered mitochondria were observed with external membrane disruptions, crest disorganization, matrix swelling, and vacuole formation between the internal and external membranes involving CBMP. Methylmercury induced dilation in the Golgi complex and ER cisterns and the myelin-like cytoplasmic inclusions. No difference was observed in the mitochondria number between the control and MeHg-treated groups. However, the MeHg-treated embryos showed CBs and decreased mitochondrial fusion involving CBMP. Unusual CBs were observed in MeHg-treated embryos as well as ATG vacuoles with amorphous, homogeneous, and electron-dense contents, indicating MeHg neurotoxicity in the developing spinal cord through changes in the endomembrane system, mitochondrial damage, mitochondrial dynamics, and CP induction.

Copper (Cu) and Arsenic (As) Toxicity

Wang et al. (2018) showed that environmental pollutants, Arsenic (As) and Copper (Cu) are oxidative stress inducers. A 12-week exposure to Cu or/and As caused chickens to display residual elements in the pectoralis muscle. The pro-oxidant nature of Cu and As was indicated by enzyme/non-enzyme antioxidants. CBs induced by oxidative damage were accompanied by overexpressed DRP-1 and decreased mitochondrial fusion-related genes. A time-dependent conversion of light chain 3 (LC3)-I to LC3-II, increases in ATG-related gene, Beclin-1, and inhibition of the PI3K/Akt/mTOR pathway indicated that Cu and/or As induce ATG. Elevated HSPs suggested adaptation and physiological acclimation in chickens. Combined exposure to Cu and As elicited oxidative damage via inhibition of the PI3K/Akt/mTOR pathway, ATG induction, and CBMP. Shao et al. (2019) investigated Cu-induced testicular toxicity, mitochondrial dynamics, apoptosis, and CP/ATG by dividing 36 1-days-old male Hy-line chickens into a control group (C group) and a test group (Cu group). The chickens were exposed to 0 (C group) or 300 mg/kg (Cu group) of $CuSO_4$ for 30, 60, and 90 days as a dietary supplement. The mitochondrial fission-related genes increased, and the fusion-related genes decreased; ATG-related genes (ATG4B, dynein, LC3-II, Atg5, and Beclin-1) were increased, while mTOR and LC3-I were reduced. Cu induced CBMP and apoptosis, indicating that its exposure can influence the CP dynamics and apoptosis. There was a correlation between mitochondrial dynamics, CP/ATG, and apoptosis in Cu-induced toxicity.

Selenium (Se) Protection in Cadmium (Cd) Cytotoxicity

To investigate molecular mechanism(s) of protection by Se (Na_2SeO_3; Se^{4+}) in Cd ($CdCl_2$; Cd^{2+})-induced cytotoxicity, Binte Hossain et al. (2018) exposed PC-12 cells to Se (5, 10, 20 and 40 μM) and Cd (2.5, 5 and 10 μM). Se ($\geq$10 μM) promoted CP/ATG cell death via inhibition of mTOR activation and p62 accumulation due to increased oxidative stress. Co-administration of Se (5 μM) and Cd (5 μM) increased cell viability, glutathione, glutathione peroxidase 1 (GPx1) levels, and decreased DNA fragmentation and LDH activity compared to Cd-treated (5 μM) cells alone. Immunoblot analyses of Cyt-C and ERK1 indicated that Cd-induces apoptotic cell death. However, the co-exposure of Se with Cd decreased the release of Cyt-C into cytosol from mitochondria, and upregulated ERK1 to inhibit Cd-induced apoptosis, indicating that although Se induced cytotoxicity, its co-administration with Cd attenuated Cd-induced apoptosis by inhibiting oxidative stress apoptosis involving CBMP. Environmental toxins and the transcriptional regulation of CS by CP is presented in Fig. 26.

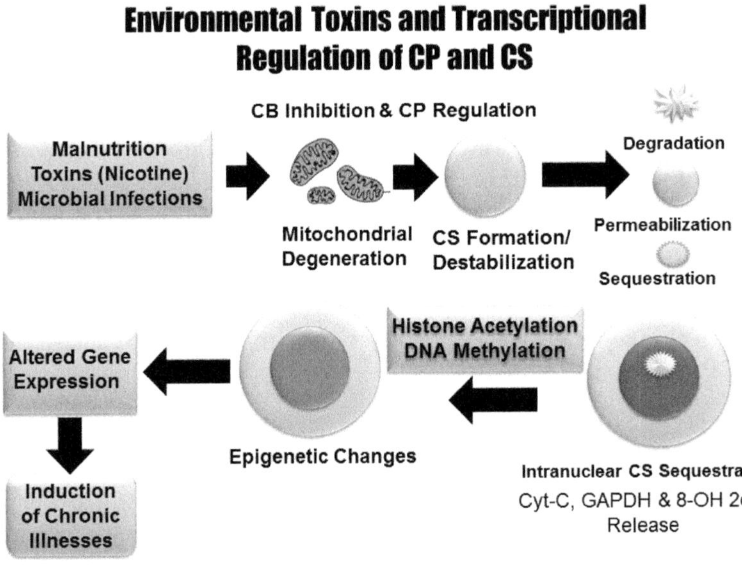

Environmental Toxins and Transcriptional Regulation of CP and CS

Figure 26

CONCLUSION

This chapter described the theranostic potential of CP in evaluating the mitochondrial toxicity of organic and inorganic environmental pollutants. Toxicological effects of Tebufenozide were observed in Anticarsia gemmatalis larvae, while natural Pyrethrins induced ATG of HepG2 cells through the AMPK/mTOR pathway. Perfluoroalkyl acid induced mitochondrial and ER-phagy in lung cells. Acrolein induced ATG-dependent apoptosis via lysosomal-mitochondrial pathway in EAhy926 cells. Atrazine induced mitochondrial dysfunction in quail cerebrum via activating nuclear receptors and the CYP-P450 system. Chlorpyifos impaired STAT1 signaling to induce DAergic toxicity through RONS stress. PINK1/Parkin mediated MTG was induced in 1,4-Benzoquinone-induced apoptosis in HL-60 cells. Necrosis occurred in neuronal cells exposed to Paraquat. Squamocin induced histological changes in the midgut cells of Anticarsia gemmatalis. Methylisothiazolinone induced pro-inflammatory cell death through DNA damage in liver epithelial cells. High dose iodine induced apoptosis and impaired CP/ATG to cause neurotoxicity in SD rats. E3 was protected in Cd-induced apoptosis by the lysosomal-mitochondrial axis in Neuro-2a cells. MeHg caused CP/ATG dysregulation in the chicken spinal cord cells, while Cu and As induced ATG by oxidative stress-related PI3K/Akt/mTOR pathways and mitochondrial-fission/fusion-associated CP/ATG and apoptosis. Inhibitory effects of Se on Cd-induced cytotoxicity in PC12 cells occurred through oxidative stress and apoptosis. MTG and Atg12/LC3 pathways were induced in the HEI-OC1 auditory cell line of the organ of Corti, whereas PI3-kinase-γ inhibition reduced tumor growth and protected from Dox cardiotoxicity. Environmental toxins induce CP during the acute phase as a protective mechanism and CBMP during the chronic exposure. Hence, novel DSST-TSE-EBPT-CPTs can be developed for the clinical management of victims exposed to these toxins.

REFERENCES

Binte Hossain, K.F., M.M. Rahman, M.T. Sikder, T. Saito, et al. 2018. Inhibitory effects of selenium on cadmium-induced cytotoxicity in PC12 cells via regulating oxidative stress and apoptosis. Food Chem Toxicol 114: 180–189.

Cui, Y., Z. Zhang, B. Zhang, L. Zhao, et al. 2018. Excessive apoptosis and disordered ATG flux contribute to the neurotoxicity induced by high iodine in Sprague-Dawley rat. Toxicol Lett 297: 24–33.

Ferreira, F.F., E.M. Nazari and Y.M.R. Müller. 2018. MeHg causes ultrastructural changes in mitochondria and autophagy in the spinal cord cells of chicken embryo. J Toxicol 2018: Article ID 8460490.

Fiaz, M., L.C. Martínez, M.D.S. Costa, J.F.S. Cossolin, et al. 2018a. Squamocin induce histological and ultrastructural changes in the midgut cells of *Anticarsia gemmatalis* (Lepidoptera: Noctuidae). Ecotoxicol Environ Saf 156: 1–8.

Fiaz, M., L.C. Martínez, A. Plata-Rueda, W.G. Gonçalves, et al. 2018b. Toxicological and morphological effects of tebufenozide on *Anticarsia gemmatalis* (Lepidoptera: Noctuidae) larvae. Chemosphere 212: 337–345.

Hirayama, N., T. Aki, T. Funakoshi, K. Noritake, et al. 2018. Necrosis in human neuronal cells exposed to paraquat. J Toxicol Sci 43: 193–202.

Li, M., V. Sala, M.C. De Santis, J. Cimino, et al. 2018. Phosphoinositide 3-kinase gamma inhibition protects from anthracycline cardiotoxicity and reduces tumor growth. Circulation 138: 696–711.

Lin, J., H.S. Zhao, L. Qin, X.N. Li, et al. 2018. Atrazine triggers mitochondrial dysfunction and oxidative stress in quail (*Coturnix C. coturnix*) cerebrum via activating xenobiotic-sensing nuclear receptors and modulating cytochrome P450 systems. J Agric Food Chem 66: 6402–6413.

Luo, S., L. Jiang, Q. Li, X. Sun, et al. 2018. Acrolein-induced ATG-dependent apoptosis via activation of the lysosomal-mitochondrial pathway in EAhy926 cells. Toxicol In Vitro 52: 146–153.

Meyer, J.N., J.H. Hartman and D.F. Mello. 2018. Mitochondrial toxicity. Toxicol Sci 162: 15–23.

Park, E.J., S. Kim and J. Chang. 2018. Methylisothiazolinone may induce cell death and inflammatory response through DNA damage in human liver epithelium cells. Environ Toxicol 33: 156–166.

Pi, H., M. Li, J. Xie, Z. Yang, et al. 2018. Transcription factor E3 protects against cadmium-induced apoptosis by maintaining the lysosomal-mitochondrial axis but not autophagic flux in Neuro-2a cells. Toxicol Lett 295: 335–350.

Setz, C., A.S. Benischke, A.C. Pinho Ferreira Bento, Y. Brand, et al. 2018. Induction of mitophagy in the HEI-OC1 auditory cell line and activation of the Atg12/LC3 pathway in the organ of Corti. Hear Res 361: 52–65.

Shao, Y., H. Zhao, Y. Wang, J. Liu, et al. 2019. Copper-mediated mitochondrial fission/fusion is associated with intrinsic apoptosis and autophagy in the testis tissues of chicken. Biol Trace Elem Res 188: 468–477.

Singh, N., V. Lawana, J. Luo, P. Phong, et al. 2018. Organophosphate pesticide Chlorpyifos impairs STAT1 signaling to induce dopaminergic neurotoxicity: Implications for mitochondria mediated oxidative stress signaling events. Neurobiol Dis 117: 82–113.

Wang, Y., H. Zhao, Y. Shao, J. Liu et al. 2018. Copper or/and arsenic induces autophagy by oxidative stress-related PI3K/Akt/mTOR pathways and cascaded mitochondrial fission in chicken skeletal muscle. J Inorg Biochem 188: 1–8.

Wang, M.G., R.F. Fan, W.H. Li , D. Zhang et al. 2019. Activation of PERK-eIF2α-ATF4-CHOP axis triggered by excessive ER stress contributes to lead-induced nephrotoxicity. Biochim Biophys Acta Mol Cell Res 1866: 713–726.

Xin, Y., B. Wan, Y. Yang, X.J. Cui, et al. 2018. Perfluoroalkyl acid exposure induces protective mitochondrial and endoplasmic reticulum autophagy in lung cells. Arch Toxicol 92: 3131–3147.

Yang, Y., J. Gao, Y. Zhang, W. Xu, et al. 2018. Natural pyrethrins induce autophagy of HepG2 cells through the activation of AMPK/mTOR pathway. Environ Pollut 241: 1091–1097.

Zhang, C., X. Yu, J. Gao, Q. Zhang, et al. 2018. PINK1/Parkin-mediated mitophagy was activated against 1,4-Benzoquinone-induced apoptosis in HL-60 cells. Toxicol In Vitro 50: 217–224.

Zhang, Y., H. Chen, Y. Fan, Y. Yang, et al. 2019. Cytotoxic effects of bio-pesticide spinosad on human lung A549 cells. Chemosphere 230: 182–189.

Part-2

Charnolophagy in Metabolic Disorders

7

Charnolophagy in Congenital Diseases

INTRODUCTION

Congenital defects are defects in an infant at birth, or which develop in the first month of life (Blau et al. 2014). There are two main types of congenital defect. The first is caused by genetic abnormalities; these are hereditary. The second is caused by conditions (such as infectious diseases) which a baby gets from his mother (Stork and Renshaw 2005). The first pathogenic mutation in mtDNA was identified in 1988. Around 275 other disease-causing mutations have been identified (Claiborne et al. 2017). Notable people who suffered from mitochondrial disease include: (a) Mattie Stepanek, a poet, peace advocate, and motivational speaker who suffered from dysautonomic mitochondrial myopathy, who died at age 13; (b) Rocco Baldelli, a coach and former center fielder in Major League Baseball who had to retire at age 29 due to mitochondrial channelopathy; (c) Charlie Gard, a British boy who suffered from mtDNA depletion syndrome; decisions about his care were taken to law courts. About 1 in 4,000 children in the U.S.A. develop mitochondrial disease by the age of 10 years. Up to 4,000 children are born with a mitochondrial disease per year in the U.S.A.

Because mitochondrial disorders contain many variations and subsets, some of these are rare. The average number of births per year among women at risk for transmitting mtDNA disease is estimated to ~150 in the U.K. and 800 in the U.S.A. (Gorman et al. 2015). About 3% of all babies have a major physical anomaly (Finsterer 2007). Birth defects involving the brain are the most common (~10 per 1000 live births), compared to heart problems at 8 per 1000, kidney problems at 4 per 1000, and limbs at 1 per 1000. All other physical anomalies occur in 6 per 1000 live births. Birth defects of the cardiovascular system have the highest risk of death during childhood. They are the cause of 28% of infant mortalities. Chromosomal and respiratory abnormalities each account for 15%, and brain malformations ~12%. Genetic diseases cause ~10% of deaths in children. This is more than the number of deaths caused by infectious diseases (Stork and Renshaw 2005). One baby with birth defects is born every 30 seconds in China (Lax et al. 2009). We can find out that a baby has a congenital disorder before its birth by prenatal screening tests, such as amniocentesis (Pieczenik et al. 2007). Genetic defects occur due to the induction of lethal or damaging genes during embryonic development. Some gene alleles can damage the infant. Conditions like dwarfism are genetic in origin. For instance, achondroplasia happens when a child's bones grow incorrectly. Another type is caused when the pituitary, responsible for releasing growth hormones, does not work properly (Nierenberg et al. 2012). Many genetic disorders are caused by mutations in gene alleles, which can cause abnormal development, or a biochemical deficiency. In chemical deficiency, the problem may be curable. For example, phenylketonuria (PKU) is a cause of mental retardation. If these children are treated and follow a strict diet, they can have BQL and can live long. PKU now causes few cases of mental retardation. Teinert et al. (2018) provided an update on the clinical, imaging, and genetic studies of congenital disorders of CP/ATG and highlighted its importance in childhood-onset neurological diseases. Recently, several single-gene disorders have been discovered to give rise to a group of inborn errors of metabolism (IEM) referred to as congenital disorders of CP/ATG. While these are heterogeneous, they share several clinical and molecular characteristics including involvement of the CNS leading to brain malformations, developmental delay, intellectual disability, epilepsy, movement disorders, and cognitive decline. A brain MRI reveals involvement of the corpus callosum, corticospinal tracts, and cerebellum. A storage disease phenotype is present in some diseases, suggesting both clinical and molecular overlaps to lysosomal storage diseases (LSDs).

CP is a fundamental and highly conserved intracellular process that mediates the degradation of nonfunctional mitochondria and associated macromolecules in lysosomes through CB formation. CP regulation is highly crucial for the normal growth and development of CNS, particularly during the first trimester (gastrulation phase) of pregnancy. A slight physico-chemical perturbation during this critical period can have deleterious consequences on the CNS, the cardiovascular, musculoskeletal, pulmonary, hepatic, renal, integumentary systems, and in many other parts of body possessing maximum mitochondria and high metabolic needs such as gastrointestinal system and endocrine glands. Defective and/or nonfunctional CP is a serious event which occurs due to mtDNA and/or nDNA mutations during the prezygotic or postzygotic phase of intrauterine life. Microcephaly, cleft palate, cleft lip, ectrodactyly, polydactyly, and other musculoskeletal anomalies are observed due to CP dysregulation during congenital life. A genetic disorder is caused by one or more abnormalities in the genome. The earliest known genetic condition in a hominid was in the fossil species *Paranthropus robustus,* with over a third of individuals displaying Amelogenesis imperfecta. Genetic disorders may be hereditary or nonhereditary. However, disorders may be caused by mutations, altered phenotype, or changes in the DNA. In these cases, the defect is only passed down if it occurs in the germline. Genetic disorders can be monogenic, multi-factorial, or chromosomal. Recessive gene disorders confer an advantage when only one copy of the gene is present. DPCI, including viral infections and drugs of abuse, compromise the pluripotency of stem cells to cause microcephaly, cleft palate, cleft lip, arthrogryposis, and musculoskeletal anomalies, posing lifelong consequences and a socioeconomic burden on society.

This chapter describes CP dysregulation in the pluripotent stem cells (PPCs) during intrauterine life as a mechanism of congenital diseases.

Congenital Diseases

Birth defects are also called congenital anomalies. A brief alphabetic list of congenital diseases include: Albinism, Amelia and hemimelia, Amniotic band syndrome, Anencephaly, Angelman syndrome, Aposthia, Arnold–Chiari malformation, Bannayan–Zonana syndrome, Bardet–Biedl syndrome, Barth syndrome, Basal-cell nevus syndrome, Beckwith–Wiedemann syndrome, Benjamin syndrome, Bladder exstrophy, Bloom syndrome, Cat eye syndrome, Caudal regression syndrome, Sotos syndrome, Cerebral Gigantism, CHARGE syndrome, Chromosome 16 abnormalities, Chromosome 18 abnormalities, Chromosome 20 abnormalities, Chromosome

22 abnormalities, Cleft lip/palate, Cleidocranial dysostosis, Club foot, Congenital adrenal hyperplasia (CAH), Congenital central hypoventilation syndrome, Congenital diaphragmatic hernia (CDH), Congenital Disorder of Glycosylation (CDG), Congenital hyperinsulinism, Congenital insensitivity to pain with anhidrosis (CIPA), Congenital pulmonary airway malformation (CPAM), conjoined twins, Costello syndrome, Craniopagus parasiticus, Cri du chat syndrome, Cyclopia, Cystic fibrosis, De Lange syndrome, Diphallia, Distal trisomy 10q, Down syndrome, Ectodermal dysplasia, Ectopia cordis, Ectrodactyly, Encephalocele, Fetal alcohol syndrome, Fetofetal transfusion, First arch syndrome, Freeman–Sheldon syndrome, Gastroschisis, Goldenhar syndrome, Harlequin-type ichthyosis, Heart disorders (Congenital heart defects), Hemifacial microsomia, Holoprosencephaly, Huntington's disease, Hirschsprung's disease (or congenital aganglionic megacolon), Hypoglossia, Hypomelanism or hypomelanosis (albinism), Hypospadias, Haemophilia, Heterochromia, Hemochromatosis, Imperforate anus, Incontinentia pigmenti, Intestinal neuronal dysplasia, Ivemark syndrome, Katz syndrome, Klinefelter syndrome, Kabuki syndrome, Larsen syndrome, Laurence–Moon syndrome, Anencephaly, Lissencephaly, Microcephaly, Schizencephaly, Marfan syndrome, Microtia, Monosomy 9p, Myasthenic syndrome, Myelokathexis, Nager's Syndrome, Nail–patella syndrome, Neonatal jaundice, Neurofibromatosis, Neuronal ceroid lipofuscinosis, Noonan syndrome, Nystagmus, Ochoa syndrome, Oculocerebrorenal syndrome, Pallister–Killian syndrome, Pectus excavatum, Pectus carinatum, Pierre Robin syndrome, Poland syndrome, Polydactyly, Prader–Willi syndrome, Proteus syndrome, Prune belly syndrome, Radial aplasia, Rett syndrome, Robinow syndrome, Rubinstein–Taybi syndrome, Saethre–Chotzen syndrome, Sirenomelia, Situs inversus, Smith–Lemli–Opitz syndrome, Smith–Magenis syndrome, Spina bifida, Strabismus, Sturge–Weber syndrome, Syphilis, congenital, Teratoma, Treacher Collins syndrome, Trichothiodystrophy, Triple-X syndrome, Trisomy 13, Trisomy 9, Turner syndrome, Umbilical hernia, Usher syndrome, Waardenburg syndrome, Werner syndrome, Wolf–Hirschhorn syndrome, and Wolff–Parkinson–White syndrome. The above short list of congenital diseases indicates that extensive studies are still needed to understand the exact molecular basis of CB formation, CP induction, and CS destabilization involving genetically-linked, disease-specific, spatiotemporal CBMP in these congenital disorders during the early prezygotic and postzygotic phase during intrauterine life to accomplish TSE-EBPT of these developmental anomalies. Particularly, the first trimester (gastrulation phase) of early pregnancy is highly vulnerable to DPCI-mediated free radical-induced CBMPs, which trigger developmental chranolopathies primarily due to the loss of pluripotency of iPPCs implicated in impaired organogenesis.

Single-gene Disorders

Most congenital metabolic disorders known as inborn errors of metabolism (IEM) result from single-gene defects. Over 6000 human diseases are caused by single-gene disorders which can be passed on to successive generations in several ways. However, genomic imprinting and uniparental disomy may affect inheritance. The division between recessive and dominant types is not really strict, although autosomal and X-linked types are based on the chromosomal location of the gene. For example, achondroplasia is considered to be a dominant disorder, but children with two genes have a severe skeletal disorder where these victims could be considered as carriers. Sickle-cell anemia is also considered recessive, but heterozygous carriers have increased resistance to malaria in early childhood, which could be considered as dominant (Williams and Obaro 2011). In a couple where one partner or both are sufferers or carriers of a single-gene disorder and wish to have a child, they can do so through *in vitro* fertilization, which facilitates a preimplantation diagnosis to ascertain whether the embryo has the genetic disorder (Kuliev et al. 2005). An approximate prevalence of single-gene disorders is presented in Fig. 27.

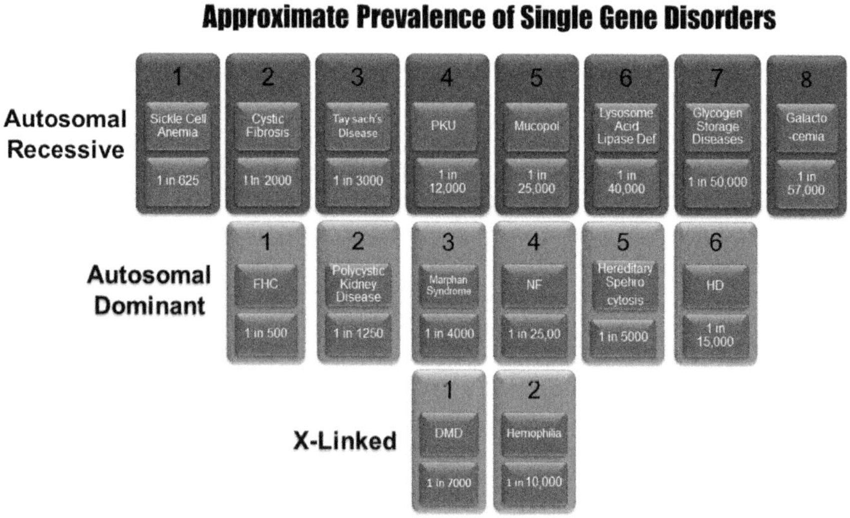

Approximate Prevalence of Single Gene Disorders

	1	2	3	4	5	6	7	8
Autosomal Recessive	Sickle Cell Anemia	Cystic Fibrosis	Tay sach's Disease	PKU	Mucopol	Lysosome Acid Lipase Def	Glycogen Storage Diseases	Galacto -cemia
	1 in 625	1 in 2000	1 in 3000	1 in 12,000	1 in 25,000	1 in 40,000	1 in 50,000	1 in 57,000

	1	2	3	4	5	6
Autosomal Dominant	FHC	Polycystic Kidney Disease	Marfan Syndrome	NF	Hereditary Spehro cytosis	HD
	1 in 500	1 in 1250	1 in 4000	1 in 25,00	1 in 5000	1 in 15,000

	1	2
X-Linked	DMD	Hemophilia
	1 in 7000	1 in 10,000

Figure 27

The most common inborn-movement disorders are presented in Fig. 28.

TSE-EBPT Targets for Most Common Inborn Metabolic Movement Disorders

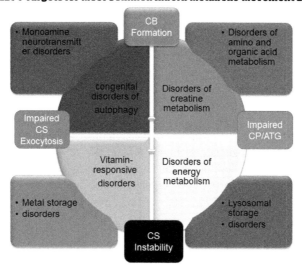

Figure 28

Autosomal Dominant

In this situation, only one mutated copy of the gene will be affected by an autosomal dominant disorder. Each affected person has one affected parent (Griffiths et al. 2012). The probability that a child will inherit the mutated gene is 50%. Sometimes, autosomal dominant conditions have reduced penetrance, which means although only one mutated copy is needed, not all individuals who inherit that mutation will develop the disease as noticed in Huntington's disease, neurofibromatosis type-1 and type-2, Marfan syndrome, hereditary nonpolyposis colorectal cancer, hereditary multiple exostoses, tuberous sclerosis, Von Willebrand disease, and acute intermittent porphyria.

Autosomal Recessive

Here, two copies of the gene need to be mutated to be affected by an autosomal recessive disorder. An affected person has unaffected parents who carry a single copy of the mutated gene. Each carrier parent with a defective gene does not have symptoms. Two unaffected people who each carry one copy of the mutated gene have a 25% risk with each pregnancy of having a child affected by the disorder as observed in albinism, medium-chain acyl-CoA dehydrogenase deficiency, cystic fibrosis, sickle-cell disease, Tay–Sachs disease, Niemann-Pick disease, spinal muscular atrophy, and Roberts syndrome. Other phenotypes, such as wet versus dry earwax, are also determined in an autosomal recessive disorder (Wade et al. 2006, Yoshiura et al. 2006).

X-Linked Dominant

These disorders are caused by mutations in genes in the X chromosome. Only a few disorders have this inheritance pattern; for example X-linked hypophosphatemic rickets. Males and females are both affected, with males being more severely affected than females. Some X-linked dominant conditions, such as Rett syndrome, incontinentia pigmenti type 2, and Alcardi syndrome, are fatal in males either *in utero* or shortly after birth, and are primarily seen in females. Exceptions to this finding are boys with Klinefelter syndrome (47, XXY) who also inherit an X-linked dominant condition and exhibit symptoms similar to those of a female regarding disease severity. The chance of passing on an X-linked dominant disorder differs between men and women. The sons of a man with an X-linked dominant disorder will be unaffected, and daughters will inherit the condition. A woman with an X-linked dominant disorder has a 50% chance of having an affected fetus with each pregnancy, although in incontinentia pigmenti, only female offspring are viable.

X-Linked Recessive

These conditions are caused by mutations in genes in the X chromosome. Males are more frequently affected than females, and the chances of passing on the disorder differs between men and women. The sons of a man with this disorder will not be affected, and his daughters will carry one copy of the mutated gene. A woman who is a carrier of an X-linked recessive disorder ($X^R X^r$) has a 50% chance of having sons who are affected and a 50% chance of having daughters who carry one copy of the mutated gene as carriers. X-linked recessive conditions include diseases such as Hemophilia A, Duchenne muscular dystrophy, and Lesch-Nyhan syndrome, male pattern baldness, and red-green color blindness. X-linked recessive conditions may manifest in females due to skewed X-inactivation or monosomy X (Turner syndrome).

Y-Linked

These disorders are caused by mutations in the Y chromosome and may only be transmitted from the heterogametic sex to offspring of the same sex. This means that Y-linked disorders can only be passed from men to their sons; females are not affected because they do not possess Y-allosomes. Y-linked disorders are rare but may cause infertility. Reproduction in such conditions is possible through the circumvention of infertility by medical intervention. This type of inheritance, also known as maternal inheritance, applies to genes encoded by mtDNA. Because only oocytes contribute mitochondria to the developing embryo, only mothers can pass on mtDNA mutations involving CBMP to their children, as noticed in Leber's hereditary optic neuropathy. The vast majority of mitochondrial diseases is actually caused by a nuclear-gene defect, and often follows autosomal recessive inheritance.

Multifactorial Disorder

Genetic disorders may be complex, multifactorial, or polygenic, and associated with the effects of multiple genes in combination with lifestyle and environmental factors. Multifactorial disorders include CVDs and diabetes. Although complex disorders cluster in families, they do not have a fixed pattern of inheritance, making it difficult to determine a person's risk of inheriting or passing on these disorders. Complex disorders are also difficult to study and treat, because the specific factors that cause these disorders have not yet been established. The genotype-first approach identifies genetic variants within patients and then determines the associated clinical manifestations contrary to the more traditional phenotype-first approach, and may identify causal factors that have been obscured by clinical heterogeneity, penetrance, and expressivity. However, polygenic diseases tend to run among families on pedigree, but the inheritance does not fit simple patterns as with Mendelian diseases. Nevertheless, genes can be identified and there is an environmental component to many of them (HTN).

Chromosomal Disorder

This type of genetic defect is caused by errors in chromosome copying during cell division. Cells divide and copy themselves to produce gametes. Sometimes, errors happen in the way that chromosomes are copied during this process. These errors are copied again and again as cells keep on dividing. Humans have 23 pairs of chromosomes, for a total of 46 chromosomes. These chromosomal pairs are numbered according their size. Chromosome pair-1 is the largest and chromosome pair-23 is the smallest. First 22 pairs of chromosomes are named as autosomes, and the 23rd pair is named as a sex chromosome. In Down's syndrome, chromosome-21 exists as a triplet, hence this syndrome is also named as Trisomy-21 or Mongolism. These children have characteristic moon like face, and mental retardation. Down syndrome causes distinct facial features, intellectual disability, developmental delays, and may be accompanied with thyroid or heart disease. Other clinical features include, decreased or poor muscle tone, short neck, with excess skin at the back of the neck, flattened facial profile and nose, small head,

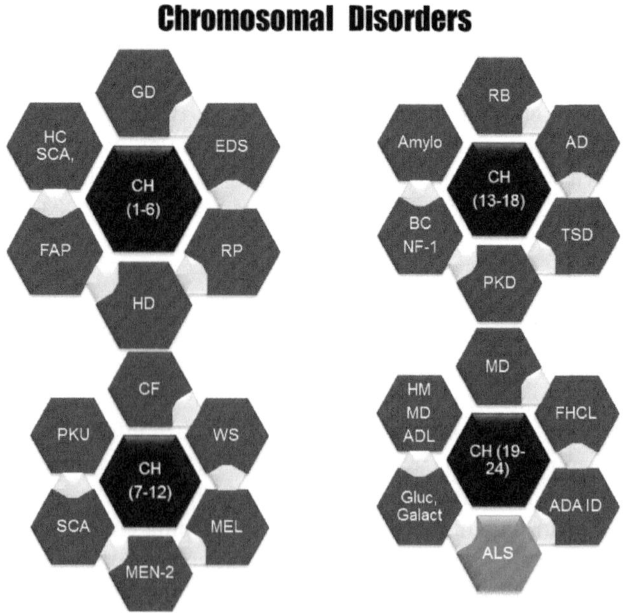

Chromosomal Disorders

Figure 29

ears, and mouth, upward slanting eyes with epicanthal folds. These individuals may develop presenile dementia early in life due to CB formation, CP dysregulation, and CBMP in the hippocampal CA-3 and dentate gyrus regions as observed in Alzheimer's disease (AD) patients. The probability of Down's syndrome increases in a child from a mother over the age of 35. Early intrauterine diagnosis can be made by chorionic villous sampling, amniocentesis, or by cord blood sampling along with ultrasound imaging of the developing fetus. The most common human condition occurs due to aneuploidy. A chromosomal disorder is a missing, extra, or irregular portion of chromosomal DNA. It can be from an atypical number of chromosomes or a structural abnormality in one or more chromosome. An example of these kinds of disorders is Trisomy 21 (Down syndrome: Mongolism), in which there is an extra copy of chromosome 21. The most common chromosomal disorders are illustrated in Fig. 29.

Diagnosis

Most genetic disorders are diagnosed at birth or during early childhood however Huntington's disease can escape detection until the patient enters into adulthood. The basic aspects of a genetic disorder rests on the inheritance of genetic material. With access to family history, it is possible to anticipate possible disorders in children which direct physicians to specific tests depending on the disorder, and allow parents the opportunity to prepare for potential lifestyle changes, anticipate the possibility of stillbirth, or contemplate termination. Prenatal diagnosis can detect the presence of abnormalities in fetal development through ultrasound, or via invasive procedures such as amniocentesis (Milunsky 2004).

Prognosis

Although, not all genetic disorders directly result in death; there are no known cures for genetic disorders. Many genetic disorders affect stages of development, such as Down syndrome, while others result in physical symptoms such as muscular dystrophy. During the active phase of a genetic disorder, patients rely on maintaining or retarding the deterioration of QOL and sustain autonomy. This includes physical therapy, pain management, and alternative medical interventions.

Treatment

Over 1800 gene therapy clinical trials having been completed, are ongoing, or have been approved worldwide. Most treatment options involve treating the symptoms to improve the patient's QOL. Gene therapy refers to treatment where a healthy gene is introduced to a patient, which may alleviate the defect caused by a faulty gene or slow the progression of disease. A major obstacle has been the delivery of genes to the appropriate cell, tissue, and organ affected by the disorder. How one introduces a gene into the potentially trillions of cells which carry the defective copy has been the major challenge in understanding the specific genetic disorder and correcting it (Verma et al. 2013).

Maternal Environment

If a pregnant woman gets toxoplasma, CMV, rubella, or Zika viral infection, her child can have many birth defects as described in author's book *Zika Virus Infection: Prevention and Cure*, Nova Science Publishers, New York, U.S.A. (Sharma 2017) More than 200,000 cases of Zika virus disease were reported and ~8600 infants were born with malformation in Brazil between 2015-2017. As of May 2019 no country has reported active outbreak of Zika virus disease perhaps due to the acquisition of immunity. The prevalence of congenital syphilis was high a century ago; and now we have high prevalence of congenital AIDs. Maternal nutritional defects are much rarer, except in countries where food supply is limited. Sometimes mothers take chemicals which cause damage to the embryo. Any substance that causes birth defects is known as a teratogen (Misiewicz et al. 2019). Drugs taken by the mother may affect development of the embryo. Pregnant women are not allowed to use some drugs. For example, Thalidomide should not be used by a pregnant woman, because it can cause defects in the fetus. If the mother took certain drugs during pregnancy, these can lead to problems with the baby. Common examples are smoking tobacco, or drinking alcohol. If a pregnant woman does not receive enough folic acid, the child can get neural tube defects due to dysregulated CP and CBMP induction in the PPCs (Nunnari and Suomalainen 2012). Pregnancies which do not come to term (miscarriages) have similar causes of birth defects. Most miscarriages (two thirds to three-quarters) occur during the first trimester (Scharfe et al. 2009). Chromosomal abnormalities are found in >50% of embryos miscarried in the first 13 weeks. A pregnancy with a genetic problem has a 95% probability of ending in miscarriage (Petersen et al. 2004). Genetic problems occur more likely to older parents; higher miscarriage rates are observed in older women (Sparks et al. 2005).

Mitochondrial Disorders

Mitochondrial diseases are caused by dysfunctional mitochondria. Ragged red fibers are seen in muscle biopsy with Gomori trichrome stain. Mitochondrial diseases are (~15%) caused by mutations in the mtDNA that affect mitochondrial function (DiMauro and Davidzon 2005). Other mitochondrial diseases are caused by mutations in genes of the nDNA, whose gene products are imported into the mitochondria (mitochondrial proteins) as well as acquired mitochondrial conditions. Mitochondrial diseases exhibit unique characteristics because of the way the diseases are often inherited and because mitochondria are highly crucial to cellular function. A subclass of these diseases that have neuromuscular symptoms are called mitochondrial myopathies. The body is modulated by genome variants; the mutation that in one individual may cause liver disease might in another cause a CNS disorder, or exercise intolerance. These defects affect the mitochondrial function, leading to multisystem disorders (Nunnari and Suomalainen 2012). Mitochondrial diseases are worse when present in the muscles, cerebrum, or nerves because these cells utilize more energy than other cells in the body (Finsterer 2007). Although mitochondrial diseases vary from person to person, several major clinical categories have been defined, based on the most common phenotypic features, symptoms, and signs associated with the mutations. Whether ATP depletion or ROS implicated in CBMP are responsible for the phenotypic consequences is yet to be established. Cerebellar atrophy or hypoplasia is associated with mitochondrial disorders (Lax et al. 2012). The most common congenital disorders of impaired CP/ATG include developmental delay, intellectual disability, epilepsy, motor disorders, cognitive decline, brain malfunctions, and microcephaly.

Causes

Mitochondrial disorders may be caused by mutations (acquired or inherited) in mtDNA, or in nuclear genes that code for mitochondrial proteins. They may also be the result of acquired mitochondrial dysfunction due to the adverse effects of drugs, infections, or other environmental causes. The nDNA has two copies per cell (except for sperm and oocytes), one copy being inherited from the father and the other from the mother. However, the mtDNA is strictly inherited from the mother and each mitochondria contain between 2–10 mtDNA copies. During cell division, the mitochondria segregate randomly and make more copies, generally reaching 500 mitochondria per cell. As mtDNA is copied when mitochondria proliferate, they can also accumulate mutations, a phenomenon called heteroplasmy. If only a few of the mtDNA copies inherited from the mother are defective, mitochondrial division may cause defective copies to end up in just one of the new mitochondria. Mitochondrial disease become clinically significant once the number of affected mitochondria reaches a certain level; this phenomenon is called "threshold expression". mtDNA mutations occur due to the lack of the error checking capability that nDNA has, suggesting that mtDNA disorders may occur spontaneously. Defects in enzymes that control medina (all of which are encoded for by genes in the nDNA) may also cause mtDNA mutations. Human mtDNA encodes 13 proteins of the ETC, while 1,500 mitochondrial proteins are nuclear-encoded. Defects in nuclear-encoded mitochondrial genes are associated with anemia, dementia, hypertension, lymphoma, retinopathy, seizures, and neurodevelopmental disorders (Scharfe et al. 2009). A study explored the role of mitochondria in insulin resistance among the offspring of patients with T2DM (Petersen et al. 2004). Other studies showed that the mechanism may involve the interruption of the mitochondrial-signaling in lipid myocytes. Another study showed that this partially disabled the genes that produce mitochondria (Sparks et al. 2005).

Mechanism

The overall energy for the available body is referred to as the daily glycogen generation capacity, and is used to compare the mitochondrial output of healthy individuals to that of afflicted or chronically glycogen-depleted individuals (Lorini and Ciman 1962, Mitchell 1978, Michelakis 2007). This value is slow to change in a given individual, as it takes between 18 and 24 months to complete a full cycle (Michelakis 2007). The glycogen-generation capacity depends on the capacity of the mitochondria of the human body Stacpoole et al. (1998); however, the relation between the energy generated by the mitochondria and the glycogen capacity is flexible and is mediated by many biochemical pathways (Mitchell 1978). Mitochondrial diseases are diagnosed by analysis of muscle samples because the muscular tissue is highly rich in mitochondria. Southern blotting is performed to detect big deletions or duplications. In addition, polymerase chain reaction (PCR), specific mutation analysis, and gene sequencing can be performed to diagnose mitochondrial diseases.

Treatment

Although, treatment options are currently limited, vitamins are prescribed (Marriage et al. 2003). Pyruvate was proposed as a treatment option (Tanaka et al. 2007). NAC reverses experimental models of mitochondrial dysfunction. In bipolar disorder, NAC, acetyl-L-carnitine (ALCAR), S-adenosylmethionine (SAMe), CoQ_{10}, α-lipoic acid (ALA), Creatine Monohydrate (CM), and melatonin could be potential treatment options (Frantz and Wipf 2010, Nierenberg 2012).

Gene Therapy Prior to Conception

Spindle transfer procedure, where the nDNA is transferred to another healthy oocyte leaving the defective mtDNA behind, is a treatment option that has been carried out in monkeys (Ghosh 2009, Tachibana et al. 2009). Using a similar pronuclear transfer technique, healthy DNA from donor women who were unaffected, was transplanted in the oocyte of recipient woman with mitochondrial disease (Boseley 2010, Craven et al. 2010). Ethical questions were raised regarding biological motherhood, since the child received genes and gene regulatory molecules from two different women. A male baby was born in Mexico in 2016 from a mother with Leigh syndrome using spindle transfer procedure (Hamzelou 2016). In September 2012, a public hearing was launched in the UK to explore the ethical issues (Sample 2012) regarding this topic. Human genetic engineering was used to allow infertile women with genetic defects in their mitochondria to have children. In June 2013, the UK government agreed to develop legislation that would legalize the 'three-person IVF' procedure to eliminate mitochondrial diseases that are passed on from mother to child (Knapton 2014). Embryonic mitochondrial transplant and protofection were proposed for inherited mitochondrial disease, and allotopic expression of mitochondrial proteins as a treatment for mtDNA mutation. In June 2018, the Australian Senate legalized mitochondrial replacement therapy (MRT) in Western Australia. In 2010, the Australian Federal Minister for Mental Health and Aging, appointed a committee to review the two relevant acts: the Prohibition of Human Cloning for Reproduction Act 2002 and the Research Involving Human Embryos Act 2002. The committee's report, released in July 2011, recommended that the existing legislation remain unchanged. Currently, human clinical trials are underway at GenSight Biologics (ClinicalTrials.gov # NCT02064569) at the University of Miami (ClinicalTrials.gov # NCT02161380) to examine the safety and efficacy of mitochondrial gene therapy in Leber's hereditary optic neuropathy.

Congenital Defects and CP (Recent Update)

Cystinosis

Cystinosis is a LSD due to inactivating mutations in CTNS, the cystinosin transporter that exports cystine out of lysosomes. The lysosomal accumulation of cystine leads to dysfunction of the proximal tubule epithelial cells of the kidney, causing defective endocytosis and losses of solutes in the urine. Luciani et al. (2018) reported that lysosomal alterations in cystinosis leads to defective CP and oxidative stress, which destabilizes tight junctions and activates an abnormal YBX3 (Y box binding protein 3) transcription, resulting in loss of differentiation and impaired apical endocytosis in cells. Correction of the primary lysosomal defect, neutralization of oxidative stress, or blockade of tight junction-associated YBX3 signaling, rescue epithelial function and endocytic uptake, suggesting a mechanism that links lysosomal disease, defective CP/ATG, and epithelial dysfunction, providing new perspectives on cystinosis and LSDs.

α1-Antitrypsin Deficiency.

The classical form of α1-antitrypsin deficiency (ATD) is characterized by accumulation of the misfolded variant α1-antitrypsin Z (ATZ) and liver disease. Wang et al. (2019) investigated theranostic agents that would reduce ATZ accumulation in a *C. elegans* model of ATD with genome-wide RNAi screening and computational pharmacological strategies. The RNAi screening was utilized to identify genes that modify the accumulation of ATZ and a novel computational pipeline was developed to make confidence predictions about drugs. This approach identified Glibenclamide (GLB), a sulfonylurea drug, that is used as an oral hypoglycemic agent. GLB promoted CP degradation of misfolded ATZ in cell-line models of ATD. An analog of GLB reduced hepatic ATZ accumulation and fibrosis in a mouse model without affecting blood glucose or insulin levels, providing support for a drug-discovery strategy using simple organisms as human disease models combined with genetic and computational screening. GLB and/or its analogs could be tested to curb the progression of ATD liver disease.

von Gierke's Disease

Glucose-6-phosphatase α (G6Pase) deficiency (*von Gierke's Disease*) or Glycogen storage disease type Ia (GSD Ia), is characterized by the inability of the liver to convert glucose-6-phosphate to glucose leading to glycogen accumulation and hepatosteatosis. Waskowicz et al. (2019) highlighted that long-term complications of GSD Ia, including hepatic adenomas and carcinomas, accompanied with CP/ATG suppression in the liver. The G6pc–/– mouse and canine models for GSD Ia were treated with the pan-PPAR agonist, Bezafibrate, to determine its effect on the liver metabolism. Bezafibrate decreased liver triglyceride and glycogen and ameliorated the CP defect in the GSD Ia models. Changes in medium-chain acyl-CoA dehydrogenase expression and acylcarnintine suggested that fatty acid oxidation was increased and fatty acid synthase associated with lipogenesis was decreased in G6pc–/– mice treated with Bezafibrate, suggesting that it induces CP/ATG while increasing fatty-acid oxidation and decreasing lipogenesis in G6pc–/– mice for glycogen overload and hepatosteatosis associated with GSD Ia, with beneficial effects for NAFLD.

Machado-Joseph Disease (MJD)

Machado-Joseph disease (MJD) is an NDD caused by an abnormal expansion of cytosine-adenine-guanine trinucleotide repeats in the gene, which leads to an abnormal polyglutamine in the protein ataxin-3 (Atx3), resulting in the formation of Atx3 aggregates. Marcelo et al. (2019) reported that reducing the expression of mutant Atx3 led to a mitigation of MJD-related behavior and neuropathological abnormalities. They investigated a pharmacological inhibitor of translation-Cordycepin in preclinical models. Cordycepin reduced (i) the levels of mutant Atx3, (ii) the neuropathological abnormalities in a lentiviral mouse model, (iii) the motor and neuropathological deficits in a transgenic mouse model, and (iv) ubiquitin aggregates in a human neural model, suggesting that its effect is mediated by the increase in phosphorylated AMPK, which is accompanied by a reduction in the translation and by activation of the CP/ATG pathway, suggesting its TSE-EBPT potential for MJD and other poly-glutamine diseases.

SMPD4

Sphingomyelinases synthesize ceramide from sphingomyelin as a second messenger involved in cell proliferation, differentiation, or apoptosis. Magini et al. (2019) presented children from 12 unrelated families with microcephaly, simplified gyral pattern of the cortex, hypo-myelination, cerebellar hypoplasia, arthrogryposis, and fetal/postnatal demise. Genomic analysis revealed biallelic loss-of-function variants in SMPD4, coding for the neutral sphingomyelinase-3 (nSMase-3/SMPD4). Overexpression of human Myc-tagged SMPD4 showed localization in the outer nuclear envelope and the ER and interactions with nuclear pore complex proteins by proteomics analysis. Fibroblasts from affected individuals showed ER cisternae abnormalities, suspected for increased CP/ATG, and were susceptible to apoptosis under stress conditions. Treatment with siSMPD4 caused delayed cell cycle progression, indicating that SMPD4 links homeostasis of membrane sphingolipids to cell fate by regulating the cross-talk between the ER and the outer nuclear envelope, while its loss revealed a pathogenic mechanism in microcephaly.

EPG5 Variants in Vici Syndrome

Congenital disorders of ATG are multisystem disorders with neurological involvement. Ectopic p-granules protein 5 (*EPG5*)-associated Vici syndrome is a congenital disorder of CP/ATG accompanied with the symptoms of agenesis of the corpus callosum, cataracts, cardiomyopathy, immunodeficiency, and oculo-cutaneous hypopigmentation. The majority of *EPG5* variants leading to Vici syndrome are null with only a few missense variants. Kane et al. (2019) reported a 3.5-year-old male with compound heterozygous *EPG5* variants [NM_020964.2: c.772G > T/c.5943-9_5943-5del]. His clinical presentation deviated from classic Vici syndrome with a lack of hypopigmentation, cataracts, immunodeficiency, cardiomyopathy, or failure to thrive. Early-onset developmental delay, hypo-tonia, and microcephaly, seizures, hearing loss, or optic nerve atrophy were absent; however, an MRI demonstrated a thin but fully formed corpus callosum. It was hypothesized that the functional impact of the *EPG5* variants would be milder with a higher amount of residual *EPG5* expression. Analyses of *EPG5* mRNA in the patient and his parents were performed to examine expression and splicing. Aberrant splicing due to the intronic mutation was detected, without loss of expression. A 50% reduction in mRNA expression in Vici-syndrome-patient fibroblasts, suggested a model of disease severity, which correlated with the *EPG5* expression.

Charcot-Marie-Tooth (CMT) Neuropathy Type 2B

Mutation of Rab18 leads to a severe illness known as Warburg-Micro (WARBM) syndrome, characterized by visual impairment, microcephaly, and lower limb spasticity. Dejgaard and Presley (2019) examined the role of Rab18 gene to elucidate its molecular mechanism of action in CMT neuropathy type IIB. Nian et al. (2019) developed Rab18$^{-/-}$ mice which exhibited hind-limb weakness and spasticity as well as signs of axonal degeneration in the spinal cord. Rab18 associated with lysosomes and traffics along neurites in cultured neurons. Rab18$^{-/-}$ neurons exhibited impaired lysosomal transport. Using LC3-II, it was shown that Rab18 dysfunction leads to impaired CP/ATG in the neurons. Accumulation of lipofuscin granules was observed in the dorsal root ganglion of Rab18$^{-/-}$ mice. Rab18 colocalized, cofractionated, and coprecipitated with the lysosomal regulator Rab7, mutations of which induced CMT neuropathy type 2B. Rab7 was upregulated in Rab18-deficient neurons, suggesting a compensatory effect of RAB18 and RAB7 in lysosomes and that CP/ATG may be the mechanism underlying WARBM and CMT pathogenesis in the CNS.

Cardiovascular Ciliopathies

Recently, Chaudhry and Henderson (2019) highlighted that motile cilia provide propulsion, and immotile ones are enriched with receptors to establish left-right identity in the developing embryo and are implicated in human diseases. Abnormalities in ciliary function underlie congenital heart disease (CHD) in individuals with laterality disturbance. Mitochondrial function and cellular energetics, respectively mTOR and ATG, were linked with ciliary function, revealing new mechanisms and candidate genes for syndromic human disease.

Zika Virus Disease

Piontkivska et al. (2019) investigated ZIKV-mediated changes in the expression of adenosine deaminases acting on RNA (ADARs), links between abnormal RNA editing and pathogenesis, and theranostic strategies. Earlier studies on ZIKV pathogenesis have focused primarily on virus-driven pathology and neurotoxicity, as well as host-related changes in cell proliferation, CP/ATG, immunity, and uterine functions. It was hypothesized that ZIKV pathogenesis arises as consequences of the host's innate immunity and a novel strategy of host- immune mechanisms in disease pathogenesis, focusing on dysregulation of post-transcriptional RNA editing as neurodevelopmental defects and clinical symptoms in both infants and adults associated with ZIKV infections.

Ascending Aortopathy

Forte et al. (2019) reported that ATG is currently gaining attention in the pathogenesis of ascending thoracic aortic aneurysm (TAA), a localized or diffused dilatation of the aorta with an abnormal widening >50% of the vessel's normal diameter. TAA is less frequent than abdominal aortic aneurysm (AAA), but is encountered with a higher percentage in patients with congenital heart disease or genetic syndromes. One of the most controversial and important forms of TAA is associated with the congenital bicuspid malformation of the aortic valve (BAV). Dysregulated ATG in response to wall shear stress alterations affect the phenotype of vascular cells, with remodeling and angiogenesis. They summarized the recent findings concerning ATG and its dysregulation, both in general and in different vascular cell types, in TAA progression, with reference to BAV-related aortopathy.

Inclusion Body Myopathy

Disturbances in ATG and stress granule dynamics have been implicated as mechanisms underlying inclusion body myopathy (IBM) and related disorders. Wang et al. (2019) demonstrated that impaired expression of the core ATG proteins (ULK1 and ULK2) in mice causes a vacuolar myopathy with ubiquitin and TDP-43-positive inclusions; similar to that caused by VCP/p97 mutations, the most common cause of familial IBM. ULK1/2 localize to stress granules and phosphorylate VCP, thereby increasing VCP's activity and disassemble stress granules. This suggests that VCP dysregulation and defective stress granule disassembly contribute to IBM-like disease in Ulk1/2-deficient mice. Stress granule disassembly was accelerated by an ULK1/2 agonist, suggesting their role for the regulation of stress granules and theranostic intervention in IBM-related disorders.

Cardiac Laminopathy

Mutations in the human LMNA gene cause a spectrum of diseases known as laminopathies, including myocardial diseases that exhibit age-dependent penetrance of dysrhythmias and heart failure. The LMNA gene encodes A-type lamins and intermediate filaments support nuclear structure and organize the genome. Bhide et al. (2018) modeled human disease-causing mutations in the *Drosophila* Lamin C gene and expressed mutant Lamin C specifically in the heart, resulting in cardiac dysfunction, loss of adipose tissue homeostasis, and a reduced lifespan. Mutant Lamin C aggregated in the cytoplasm, the CncC(Nrf2)/Keap1 redox-sensing pathway was activated, mitochondria exhibited abnormal morphology implicated in CBMP, and the CP/ATG cargo receptor Ref2(P)/p62 was upregulated in the cardiomyocytes. Overexpression of the ATG kinase Atg1 gene and an RNAi against CncC eliminated the protein aggregates, restored cardiac function, and lengthened the lifespan, suggesting that increasing CP/ATG and inhibiting the Nrf2/Keap1 pathway is a potential theranostic strategy for cardiac laminopathies.

mTOR and CREB in zQ175 Model of Huntington's Disease (HD)

Huntington's Disease (HD) is a NDD caused by a genetic abnormality in the huntingtin gene that leads to a polyglutamine repeat expansion of the huntingtin protein. The cleaved polyglutamine expansion of mutant huntingtin (mHTT) form aggregates correlated with HD progression. Abd-Elrahman et al. (2019) showed that the inhibition of mGluR5 using CTEP, a selective negative mGluR5 modulator, can delay disease progression and reduce mHTT aggregates in the zQ175 mouse model of HD, accompanied with enhanced catalytic activity of Unc-51-like kinase 1 (ULK1), which is modulated by mTOR (a key regulator of ATG initiation). CTEP could correct aberrant PI3K/Akt/mTOR signaling in zQ175 mice that may underlie the enhanced ULK1 activity and ATG induction and that CTEP can facilitate CREB-mediated expression of BDNF to foster neuronal survival and reduce apoptosis, providing the evidence for how targeting mGluR5 using a selective NAM can mitigate ATG and apoptosis in NDDs. mTOR-dependent charnolopathogenetic laminopathies are presented in Fig. 30.

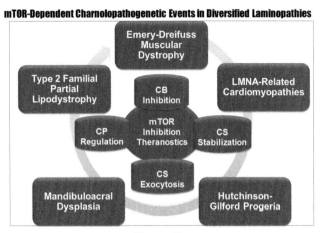

Figure 30

Lattice Corneal Dystrophy

Lattice corneal dystrophy (LCD) is related to the denaturation of TGFBIp. Han et al. (2019) investigated the role of CP/ATG in the degradation of mutant (MU) TGFBIp in macrophages. Corneas from participants were observed by slit-lamp photography and subjected to histopathologic and genetic analysis. Wild-type (WT) and MU TGFBIp were recombined and expressed. Macrophages from MU participants were isolated and co-cultured with the recombinant TGFBIp. Colocalization of the two molecules was observed by immunofluorescent microscopy. Fourteen members from a family of 25 were identified as LCD sufferers. Significant TGFBIp aggregates and macrophage infiltration were found only in the corneas of LCD sufferers. Marker accumulation of TGFBIp was found in macrophages exposed to MU TGFBIp even 5 hrs after MU TGFBIp was withdrawn. High expressions of CD68 and CD36 were found in macrophages exposed to WT TGFBIp, but not to MU TGFBIp. Impaired ATG flux due to defective autophagosome fusion to lysosomes was found in macrophages exposed to MU TGFBIp. ATG inhibition suppressed the expression of CD36 and CD68 in macrophages exposed to WT TGFBIp, similar to those found in macrophages exposed to MU TGFBIp, suggesting that reversion of the defective CP/ATG in macrophages may be a theranostic strategy for patients with LCD.

CEDNIK Syndrome

Homozygous mutations in SNAP29, encoding a SNARE protein involved in membrane fusion, cause cerebral dysgenesis, neuropathy, ichthyosis, and keratoderma (CEDNIK), a rare congenital neuro-cutaneous syndrome with short life expectancy. Mastrodonato et al. (2019) reported the analysis of the first genetic model of CEDNIK in zebrafish. Homozygous snap29 mutant larvae displayed CEDNIK-like features, such as microcephaly and skin defects. Consistent with the Snap29 role in membrane fusion during CP/ATG, they observed the accumulation of p62 and LC3, and formation of multi-lamellar CBs and apoptotic cell death during early development, which might play a role in CEDNIK pathogenesis. Mutant larvae also displayed mouth-opening problems and feeding and swimming difficulties, which correlated with defective trigeminal nerve formation and excess axonal branching. Since Snap25 is known to promote axonal branching, Snap29 might modulate Snap25 activity during neurodevelopment. This vertebrate genetic model of CEDNIK extended the description of the multisystem defects due to the loss of Snap29 and could be used to test compounds that might ameliorate traits of the disease.

Spinocerebellar Ataxia-3 (SCA3)

Mitochondrial dysfunction is implicated in several NDDs including SCA3, which is a poly-glutamine NDD resulting from the misfolding and accumulation of a pathogenic protein, causing cerebellar dysfunction. Duarte-Silva et al. (2018) evaluated whether a creatine-enriched diet would be beneficial for a mouse model of SCA3. Two preclinical trials were performed using the CMVMJD135 mouse with different disease severity, and wild-type mice, to which 2% creatine was provided for 19 or 29 weeks. Motor behavior was evaluated from 5–34 weeks of age. Creatine improved the motoric performance of CMVMJD135 mice in both trials, rescuing motor balance and coordination, restoring brain weight, mitigating astrogliosis, and preserving Calbindin-positive cells in the cerebellum. A reduction in mutant ataxin-3 aggregates occurred despite steady-state levels of the protein and the absence of ATG activation. Creatine also restored the expression of porin and reduced the expression of HO1 and NAD(P)H quinone dehydrogenase 1 (NQO1), suggesting its beneficial effect on oxidative stress. Creatine slowed disease progression and ameliorated neuropathology of the CMVMJD135 animals, highlighting its theranostic potential in SCA3. Liu et al. (2019) assessed the effect of far-infra-red (FIR) therapy on SCA3 by using a mouse model over 28 weeks. Control mice carried a healthy wild-type ATXN3 allele that had a polyglutamine tract with 15 CAG repeats (15Q), whereas SCA3 transgenic mice possessed an allele with a pathological poly-glutamine tract with 84 CAG (84Q) repeats. 84Q SCA3 mice displayed impaired motor coordination, imbalance, and abnormal gait performance, along with a loss of Purkinje neurons in the cerebellum. FIR treatment prevented these defects and improved performance in the maximal contact area and stride length, and support in the forepaws, hind-paws, or both. Its treatment improved the survival of Purkinje neurons and regulated CP/ATG, as reflected by the induction of LC3-II and Beclin-1, concomitant with the reduction of p62 and ataxin-3 as a rescue mechanism, indicating that FIR confers benefit to a SCA3 transgenic animal and has potential for theranostic applications. Harding's classification of SCA based on severity of clinical symptoms and CBMP is presented in Table 11.

Table 11   Harding's Classification of Spinocerebellar Ataxia

ACDA-1	Cerebellar ataxia signs, Additional pyramidal signs, Extrapyramidal signs, Amyotrophy
ACDA-2	Cerebellar ataxia signs, pigmentary retinal degeneration
ACDA-3	Pure cerebellar ataxia symptoms

CONCLUSION

The theranostic significance of CP/ATG was described in genetic and congenital disorders. Impaired CP/ATG and abnormal tight junctions induced epithelial dysfunction in congenital cystinosis. Glibenclamide analog enhanced the CP/ATG of misfolded α1-antitrypsin. Bezafibrate induced CP/ATG to improve hepatic lipid metabolism in GSD Ia. Cordycepin induced CP/ATG through AMPK phosphorylation to minimize abnormalities in Machado-Joseph disease, whereas far-infrared radiation improved motor dysfunction in SCA-3. The neuroprotective role of creatine in the CMVMJD135 mouse model of SCA-3 and the loss of SMPD4-inducing microcephaly and congenital arthrogryposis were described. Enhancing ATG and blocking Nrf2 suppressed laminopathy-induced age-dependent cardiac dysfunction and reduced lifespan. EPG5 variants with a modest functional impact ameliorated neurological phenotype in Vici syndrome. Mitochondrial dysfunction occurred through mTOR and CP/ATG induction in ciliary disorders. Pathogenicity of Zika virus disease was linked to defective CP/ATG in Guillain-Barre' syndrome. Defective CP/ATG was reported in aortic valve malformations. Although ERT cleared Gb3 deposits from a podocyte model of Fabry disease, it could not restore altered cellular signaling. ULK1 and ULK2 regulated stress granule disassembly through phosphorylation of VCP/p97 and modulation of mTOR and CREB. Blockade of mGluR5 improved HD pathology in zQ175 mice. Impaired CP/ATG of TGF-β-induced protein by macrophages caused LCD. A genetic model of CEDNIK syndrome in zebrafish demonstrated Snap29 in neuro-motor and epidermal development. Hence any physiological and/or pharmacological intervention to rectify CP/ATG from the iPPCs during intrauterine life can improve TSE-EBPT of congenital disorders.

REFERENCES

Abd-Elrahman, K.S. and S.S.G. Ferguson. 2019. Modulation of mTOR and CREB pathways following mGluR5 blockade contribute to improved Huntington's pathology in zQ175 mice. Mol Brain 12: 35.

Bhide, S., A.S. Trujillo, M.T. O'Connor, G.H. Young, et al. 2018. Increasing ATG and blocking Nrf2 suppress laminopathy-induced age-dependent cardiac dysfunction and shortened lifespan. Aging Cell 17: e12747.

Blau, N., K.M. Duran, C. Gibson, C. Dionisi-Vici (eds). 2014. Physician's Guide to the Diagnosis, Treatment, and Follow-Up of Inherited Metabolic Diseases. Springer Verlag. Heidelberg, Germany.

Boseley, S. 2010. Scientists Reveal Gene-Swapping Technique to Thwart Inherited Diseases. Guardian, London.

Chaudhry, B. and D.J. Henderson. 2019. Cilia, mitochondria, and cardiac development. J Clin Invest 129: 2666–2668.

Claiborne, M., C. Mark Sokolowski, D. deHaro, K.J. Kines, et al. 2017. Involvement of conserved amino acids in the C-terminal region of LINE-1 ORF2p in retrotransposition. Genetics 205(3): 1139–1149.

Craven, L., H.A. Tuppen, G.D. Greggains, S.J. Harbottle, et al. 2010. Pronuclear transfer in human embryos to prevent transmission of mitochondrial DNA disease. Nature 465: 82–85.

Dejgaard, S.Y. and J.F. Presley. 2019. Rab18: New insights into the function of an essential protein. Cell Mol Life Sci 76: 1935–1945.

Dimauro, S. and G. Davidzon. 2005. Mitochondrial DNA and disease. Ann Med 37: 222–232.

Duarte-Silva, S., A. Neves-Carvalho, C. Soares-Cunha, J.M. Silva, et al. 2018. Neuroprotective effects of creatine in the CMVMJD135 mouse model of spinocerebellar ataxia type 3. Mov Disord 33: 815–826.

Finsterer, J. 2007. Hematological manifestations of primary mitochondrial disorders. Acta Haematologica 118: 88–98.

Forte, A., M. Cipollaro, M. De Feo and A. Della Corte. 2019. Is there a role for autophagy in ascending aortopathy associated with tricuspid or bicuspid aortic valve? Clin Sci (Lond) 133: 805–819.

Frantz, M.C. and P. Wipf. 2010. Mitochondria as a target in treatment. Environ Mol Mutagen 51: 462–475.

Ghosh, P. 2009. Genetic Advance Raises IVF Hopes. BBC News, Science Correspondent, UK.

Gorman, Gráinne, S., J.P. Grady., Y. Ng, A.M. Schaefer, et al. 2015. Mitochondrial donation — How many women could benefit? N Engl J Med 372: 885–887.

Griffiths, A.J.F., S.R. Wessler, S.B. Carroll and J. Doebley. 2012. 2: Single-Gene Inheritance. Introduction to Genetic Analysis, 10th Ed. W.H. Freeman and Company, New York.

Hamzelou, J. 2016. Exclusive: World's first baby born with new "3 parent" technique. New Scientist Updated Sep 27, 2016.

Han, J., M. Zhang, H.Y. Lin, F.Y. Huang, et al. 2019. Impaired autophagic degradation of transforming growth factor-β-induced protein by macrophages in lattice corneal dystrophy. Invest Ophthalmol Vis Sci 60: 978–989.

Kane, M.S., J. Zhao, J. Muskett, A. Diplock, et al. 2019. EPG5 variants with modest functional impact result in an ameliorated and primarily neurological phenotype in a 3.5-year-old patient with vici syndrome. Neuropediatrics 50: 257–261.

Knapton, S. 2014. 'Three-parent babies' could be born in Britain next year. The Daily Telegraph Science News, Retrieved 1 March 2014.

Kuliev, A. and Y. Verlinsky. 2005. Preimplantation diagnosis: A realistic option for assisted reproduction and genetic practice. Curr Opin Obstet Gynecol 17: 179–83.

Lax, N.Z., P.D. Hepplewhite, A.K. Reeve, V. Nesbitt, et al. 2012. Cerebellar ataxia in patients with mitochondrial DNA disease. Journal of Neuropathology & Experimental Neurology 71: 148–161.

Liu, S.W., J.C. Chang, S.F. Chuang, K.H. Liu, et al. 2019. Far-infrared radiation improves motor dysfunction and neuropathology in spinocerebellar ataxia type 3 mice. Cerebellum 18: 22–32.

Lorini, M.M. and M. Ciman. 1962. Hypoglycaemic action of DI*ISO*propylammonium salts in experimental diabetes. Biochemical Pharmacology 11: 823–827.

Luciani, A., B.P. Festa, Z. Chen and O. Devuyst. 2018. Defective autophagy degradation and abnormal tight junction-associated signaling drive epithelial dysfunction in cystinosis. Autophagy 14: 1157–1159.

Magini, P., D.J. Smits, L. Vandervore, R. Schot, et al. 2019. Loss of SMPD4 causes a developmental disorder characterized by microcephaly and congenital arthrogryposis. Am J Hum Genet 105: 689–705.

Marcelo, A., F. Brito, S. Carmo-Silva, C.A. Matos, et al. 2019. Cordycepin activates ATG through AMPK phosphorylation to reduce abnormalities in Machado-Joseph disease models. Hum Mol Genet 28: 51–63.

Marriage, B., M.T. Clandinin and D.M. Glerum. 2003. Nutritional cofactor treatment in mitochondrial disorders. J Am Diet Assoc 103: 1029–1038.

Mastrodonato, V., G. Beznoussenko, A. Mironov, L. Ferrari, et al. 2019. A genetic model of CEDNIK syndrome in zebrafish highlights the role of the SNARE protein Snap29 in neuromotor and epidermal development. Sci Rep 9: 1211.

Michelakis, E. 2007. A mitochondria-K^+ channel axis is suppressed in cancer and its normalization promotes apoptosis and inhibits cancer growth. Cancer Cell 11: 37–51.

Milunsky, A., (ed.) 2004. Genetic Disorders and the Fetus: Diagnosis, Prevention, and Treatment, 5th Ed. Johns Hopkins University Press, Baltimore, Maryland.

Misiewicz, Z., S. Iurato, N. Kulesskaya, L. Salminen, et al. 2019. Multi-omics analysis identifies mitochondrial pathways associated with anxiety-related behavior PLOS Genetics 15(9): e1008358.

Mitchell, P. 1978. Keilin's respiratory chain concept and its chemiosmotic consequences. Sci. 206(4423): 1148–1159.

Nian, F.S., L.L. Li, C.Y. Chen, P.C. Wu, et al. 2019. Rab18 collaborates with Rab7 to modulate lysosomal and autophagy activities in the nervous system: An overlapping mechanism for warburg micro syndrome and charcot-marie-tooth neuropathy type 2B. Mol Neurobiol 56: 6095–6105.

Nierenberg, A., A. Kansky, C. Brennan, P. Brian, et al. 2012. Mitochondrial modulators for bipolar disorder: A pathophysiologically informed paradigm for new drug development. Australian & New Zealand Journal of Psychiatry 47: 26–42.

Nunnari, J. and A. Suomalainen. 2012. Mitochondria: In sickness and in health. Cell 148: 1145–1159.

Petersen, K.F., S. Dufour, D. Befroy, R. Garcia, et al. 2004. Impaired mitochondrial activity in the insulin-resistant offspring of patients with type 2 diabetes. New England Journal of Medicine 350: 664–671.

Pieczenik, S.R. and J. Neustadt. 2007. Mitochondrial dysfunction and molecular pathways of disease. Experimental and Molecular Pathology 83: 84–92.

Piontkivska, H., N.M. Plonski, M.M. Miyamoto and M.L. Wayne. 2019. Explaining pathogenicity of congenital zika and guillain–barré syndromes: does dysregulation of RNA editing play a role? BioEssays 41: e1800239.

Sample, I. 2012. Regulator to consult public over plans for new fertility treatments. The Guardian. London. Retrieved 8 October 2012.

Scharfe, C., H.H. Lu, J.K. Neuenburg, E.A. Allen, et al. 2009. Mapping gene associations in human mitochondria using clinical disease phenotypes. PLoS Comput Biol 5: e1000374.

Sharma, S. 2017. Zika Virus Disease: Prevention and Cure. Nova Science Publishers, New York, U.S.A.

Sparks, L.M., H. Xie, R.A. Koza, R. Mynatt, et al. 2005. A high-fat diet coordinately downregulates genes required for mitochondrial oxidative phosphorylation in skeletal muscle. Diabetes 54: 1926–1933.

Stacpoole, P.W., G.N. Henderson, Z. Yan and M.O. James. 1998. Clinical pharmacology and toxicology of dichloroacetate. Environ. Health Perspect 106(Suppl 4): 989–994. doi:10.1289/ehp.98106s4989

Stork, C. and P.F. Renshaw. 2005. Mitochondrial dysfunction in bipolar disorder: Evidence from magnetic resonance spectroscopy research. Mol Psychiatry 10: 900–919. https: //doi.org/10.1038/sj.mp.4001711.

Tachibana, M., M. Sparman, H. Sritanaudomchai, H. Ma, et al. 2009. Mitochondrial gene replacement in primate offspring and embryonic stem cells. Nature 461: 367–372.

Tanaka, M., Y. Nishigaki, N. Fuku, T. Ibi, et al. 2007. Therapeutic potential of pyruvate therapy for mitochondrial diseases. Mitochondrion 7: 399–401.

Teinert, J., R. Behne, M, Wimmer and D. Ebrahimi-Fakhari. 2018. Novel insights into the clinical and molecular spectrum of congenital disorders of autophagy. Neuropediatrics 49: 018–025. J Inherit Metab Dis 43: 51–62. https://doi.org/10.1002/jimd.12084

Verma, I.M. 2013. Gene therapy that works. Sci 341: 853–855.

Wade., N. 2006. Japanese Scientists Identify Earwax Gene. New York Times.

Wang, B., B.A. Maxwell, J.H. Joo, Y. Gwon, et al. 2019. ULK1 and ULK2 regulate stress granule disassembly through phosphorylation and activation of VCP/p97. Mol Cell 74: 742–757.

Waskowicz, L.R., J. Zhou, D.J. Landau, E.D. Brooks, et al. 2019. Bezafibrate induces autophagy and improves hepatic lipid metabolism in glycogen storage disease type Ia. Hum Mol Genet 28: 143–154.

Williams, T.N. and S.K. Obaro. 2011. Sickle cell disease and malaria morbidity: A tale with two tails. Trends in Parasitology 27: 315–320.

Yoshiura, K., A. Kinoshita, T. Ishida. A. Ninokata, et al. 2006. A SNP in the *ABCC11* gene is the determinant of human earwax type. Nat Genet 38: 324–330.

8

Charnolophagy in Inborn Errors of Metabolism (Recent Update)

INTRODUCTION

The developing embryo is subjected to defect(s) at the cellular, molecular, genetic, and epigenetic level, which cause biochemical and functional impairments in the human body. A metabolic disorder can occur when abnormal chemical reactions in the body alter the normal metabolic process. It can also be defined as inherited single gene anomaly, most of which are autosomal recessive. Numerous mechanisms have been proposed to explain biochemical and clinico-pathological features of inborn errors of metabolism (IEM), including the CP/ATG pathway, representing genetic defects leading to multisystem diseases with predominantly CNS, cardiovascular, and musculoskeletal involvement (Graef et al. 2008). Depending on the type of metabolic disorder, symptoms include lethargy, weight loss, jaundice, and seizures. There are four categories of symptoms: acute symptoms, late-onset acute symptoms, progressive symptoms, and permanent symptoms (Fernandes et al. 2013). Inherited metabolic disorders occur when a defective gene causes an enzyme deficiency. Metabolic diseases can also occur when the liver or pancreas do not function properly. IEM can be present at birth and can be identified by routine screening. Specific blood and DNA tests are performed to diagnose genetic metabolic disorders. The gut microbiota also contribute to metabolism and has a positive function for its host. An abnormal gut microbiome can play a role in metabolic-disorder-related obesity. Metabolic disorder screening can be done in newborns by: (a) blood test, (b) skin test, and (c) hearing test. Metabolic disorders can be treated by nutritional interventions (Acosta 2010). IEMs can be classified in three broad categories: (i) metabolic syndrome, (ii) LSD, and (iii) deficiency disease. Lysosome triggers Ca^{2+} signaling, via the TRPML1/calcineurin/TFEB pathway, which promotes CS exocytosis and clearance of CS in various models of LSDs. Di Paola and Medina (2019) described methods to determine TFEB activation and CS exocytosis, which may represent innovative tools to study lysosomal function and develop novel theranostic strategies to enhance clearance in LSDs.

The transcription factor EB (TFEB) plays a significant role in the regulation of lysosomal biogenesis and CP/ATG. The subcellular localization and activity of TFEB are regulated by mechanistic target of rapamycin (mTOR)-mediated phosphorylation at the lysosomal surface.

This chapter describes the theranostic significance of CP in IEM, congenital neurological CP disorders, and the role of CP/ATG in inherited metabolic and endocrine myopathies. The

TSE-EBPT potential of CP in the clinical management of IEM is highlighted. The chapter also presents a recent update on lysosomal and ER-Ca^{2+} with a focus on ATG defects in LSDs, CP and nucleophagy involving CBMP in congenital muscular dystrophies, defective proteolysis in neuronal ceroid lipofuscinosis, and rectification of ERT with r-Cathepsin-D.

Congenital Disorders of CP/ATG

Recently, clinical, imaging, and genetics of congenital disorders of ATG and its significance in the metabolism and childhood-onset NDDs were described. CP/ATG is particularly important for postmitotic and metabolically active neurons. The complex architecture of neurons and their long axons pose challenges for efficient recycling of cargo. Hence, CP/ATG is required for normal CNS development and function. Several single-gene disorders of the CP/ATG pathway give rise to a novel group of IEM known as congenital disorders of CP/ATG. While these disorders are heterogeneous, they share several clinical and molecular characteristics, including involvement of the CNS leading to brain malformations, developmental delay, intellectual disability, epilepsy, movement disorders, and cognitive impairment. A brain MRI analysis of IEM reveals involvements of corpus callosum. corticospinal tracts, and cerebellum. A storage disease phenotype has been presented in some diseases, emphasizing both clinical and molecular overlaps to LSDs. Major metabolic disorders are presented in Table 12.

Table 12 Major CP/ATG Metabolic Disorders

S.No	Acid-Base Imbalance	Iron Metabolism Disorders	Porphyrines Metabolism Disorders
1.	Metabolic rain disorders, Disorders of Ca^{2+} metabolism, DNA repair deficiency disorder, Glucose metabolism disorder, Hyper-lactemia	Lipid metabolism disorder, Malabsorption syndrome, Metabolic syndrome-X, IEM, Mitochondrial disorders	Porphyrias, Protease deficiency, Metabolic skin disorders, Wasting syndrome, Water & electrolyte imbalance

CAMDs

The last decade saw major advances in understanding the metabolism of CoA thioesters (acyl-CoAs) and IEM (CAMDs). Yang et al. (2019a) highlighted that for diagnosis, Acylcarnitines and organic acids derived from acyl-CoAs are excellent markers of CAMDs. Clinically, each CAMD is unique but three main patterns emerged: (a) systemic decompensations with combinations of acidosis, ketosis, hypoglycemia, hyper-ammonemia, and fatty liver; (b) neurological (particularly acute stroke-like) episodes, involving the basal ganglia, cerebral cortex, brainstem or optic nerves, and (c), long chain fatty acyl-CoA metabolism, lipid myopathy, cardiomyopathy, and arrhythmia. Some patients develop signs from more than one category, which may result from CoA sequestration, toxicity, and redistribution in the mitochondrial matrix. Most CAMDs cause deficiency of CoA, CMB, and abnormal accumulation of acyl-CoAs. Measurements of tissue acyl-CoAs in CAMDs models can be related to clinical features. CAMDs cause changes similar to acyl-CoA degradation. Hence, CoA levels in cells can be influenced pharmacologically. Acylation of intracellular proteins is increased in mammalian tissues of CAMDs.

Neurometabolic Disorders

Many single-gene disorders can be classified as IEM; these are often rare and heterogeneous multisystem diseases with non-neurological and neurological manifestations, with early childhood onset. Movement disorders are among the most common in IEM and contribute to the morbidity with a significant impact on QOL. Ebrahimi-Fakhari et al. (2019) developed a framework for a phenomenology-based approach with regard to movement disorders to identify the "top ten" treatable IEM with movement disorders including monoamine neurotransmitter disorders, disorders of amino and organic acid metabolism, metal storage disorders, LSDs, congenital disorders of ATG, disorders of creatine metabolism, vitamin-responsive disorders, and disorders of energy metabolism. Disease-modifying therapies exist in several IEM, and early recognition and treatment can prevent CNS damage to reduce morbidity and mortality. This approach can facilitate a differential diagnosis and facilitates biochemical, molecular, and imaging evaluation. The complexity of metabolic movement disorders demands an interdisciplinary approach and close collaboration of pediatric neurologists, geneticists, and experts in metabolism. Numerous childhood-onset disorders are caused by mutations that impact the ATG pathway to ataxia, spastic paraplegia, and intellectual disability. Clinically, these disorders affect the CNS at various stages of development, leading to brain malformations, developmental delay, intellectual disability, epilepsy, movement disorders, and neurodegeneration. At a molecular level, mutation in key CP genes led to impairment in membrane and autophagosome maturation, or autophagosome-lysosome fusion. Ebrahimi-Fakhari et al. (2016) discussed CP/ATG' in IEM by using six monogenic diseases: EPG5-related Vici syndrome, β-propeller protein-associated neurodegeneration due to mutations in WDR45, SNX14-associated autosomal-recessive cerebellar ataxia and intellectual disability syndrome, and three forms of hereditary spastic paraplegia SPG11, SPG15, and SPG49 caused by SPG11, ZFYVE26 and TECPR2 mutations, respectively. They also highlighted associations between defective CP/ATG and other IEM such as LSDs and neurodevelopmental disorders associated with the mTOR pathway, and discussed how congenital disorders of CP enhance our understanding of cellular pathway in CNS disorders. Finally, they highlighted modulating CP/ATG as a theranostic strategy and congenital disorders of CP which confer unique possibilities and challenges of pathway-specific CPTs development. Ebrahimi-Fakhari et al. (2018) also provided clinical, imaging, and genetic characteristics of congenital disorders of CP/ATG and significance in childhood-onset neurological diseases. Transcriptionally-regulated CP/ATG is highly crucial for normal CNS development and neuronal function. Several single-gene disorders of the CP/ATG pathway include: EPG5-associated Vici syndrome, WDR45-associated β-propeller protein-associated neurodegeneration, SNX14-associated autosomal-recessive SCA20, Atg5-associated autosomal-recessive ataxia syndrome, SQSTM1/p62-associated childhood-onset neurodegeneration, and hereditary spastic paraplegias characterized by CNS involvement of the white matter tracts and the cerebellum as hallmarks, that include a thinning of the corpus callosum, cerebellar hypoplasia, and atrophy. CP/ATG plays a pivotal role in maintaining cellular homeostasis. Mutations in CP/ATG-related genes are a contributing factor in childhood neurological disorders. Marsh and Dragich (2019) explored the neurodevelopmental aspects of CP/ATG, the process by which cells remove and remodel their structure in a regulated and spatially-restricted manner. These investigators discussed CP/ATG in relation to endosomal sorting to the lysosome, and explored how these mechanisms regulate developmental events. Zhu et al. (2019) summarized single-gene disorders that impair ATG pathways and their roles in childhood neurological diseases. Defective proteins causing such diseases can interfere with CP/ATG flux at different stages of development and may be an important contributor to the pathological features of NDDs with accumulation of aberrant proteins and dysfunctional organelles including CBs, indicating the theranostic significance of CP/ATG restoration in single-gene disorders.

Other Metabolic Disorders

CP/ATG in LSDs

The LSDs encompass a group of >50 inherited diseases characterized by the accumulation of lysosomal substrates. Liu et al. (2019) highlighted that although, two-thirds of Niemann-Pick type C and Gaucher disease patients experience neurological symptoms, the mechanism of neurodegeneration is not well understood. A wide range of LSDs show defects in CP/ATG and Ca^{2+} homeostasis as Ca^{2+} is a key regulator of CP/ATG.

CP/ATG in Wilson Disease

Wilson disease (WD) is an inherited disorder of Cu metabolism that accumulates in the liver and brain causing hepato-lenticular degenerations, with a statue-like appearance. It is caused by mutations in the ATPase Cu-transporting β gene (ATP7B), which encodes a protein that transports Cu from hepatocytes into the bile. Polishchuk et al. (2019) studied ATP7B-deficient cells and animals to decrease Cu toxicity in patients with WD. They used RNA-seq to compare gene expression between wild-type and ATP7B-knockout HepG2 cells exposed to Cu and collected blood and liver tissues from $Atp7b^{-/-}$ and $Atp7b^{+/-}$ (control) rats (LPP) and mice; some mice were given five daily injections of CP inhibitor (Spautin-1) or vehicle. Liver biopsies from two patients with WD and liver tissues from patients without WD (control) were obtained. Cu-exposed ATP7B-knockout cells revealed an increased expression of 103 genes that regulate CP (including MAP1LC3A, known as LC3). EM and confocal microscopy visualized more CS in the cytoplasm of ATP7B-knockout cells than wild-type cells following Cu exposure. Hepatocytes from patients with WD and from $Atp7b^{-/-}$ mice and rats had multiple CSs. In ATP7B-knockout cells, mTOR had decreased activity and was dissociated from lysosomes; resulting in translocation of the mTOR substrate transcription factor EB to the nucleus and activation of CP/ATG-related genes. In wild-type HepG2 cells, exposure to Cu and amino acids induced recruitment of mTOR to lysosomes. Inhibitors of CP/ATG or knockdown of ATG7 and ATG13 accelerated death of ATP7B-knockout HepG2 cells. CP protected ATP7B-knockout cells from Cu-induced toxicity. ATP7B-deficient hepatocytes, as in patients with WD, activated CP to prevent Cu-induced apoptosis, suggesting that CP-inducing agents might attenuate Cu toxicity in WD patients.

Mucopolysaccharidosis

Mucopolysaccharidosis (MPS) is a group of inherited conditions involving metabolic dysfunction. Lysosomal enzyme deficiency causes accumulation of glycosaminoglycan (GAG), resulting in systemic symptoms, and is categorized into seven types caused by deficiency in one of eleven enzymes. Kobayashi (2019) provided a framework for developing novel TSE-EBPT strategies for MPS. The pathophysiological mechanism of these diseases, indicates impaired CP/ATG in neurodegeneration, association of activated microglia and astrocytes with neuro-inflammation, and tauopathy. A new inherited error of metabolism resulting in a multisystem disorder with features of the MPS was also identified. These investigators highlighted the importance of recombinant enzymes that can penetrate the BBB, hematopoietic stem cell transplantation, gene therapy using a viral vector system, gene editing, and substrate reduction therapy for MPS.

Metabolic and Endocrine Cardiomyopathies

The prevalence of cardio-metabolic disease has now reached an exponential rate of rise owing to high fat/high caloric diet intake and satiety lifestyle. Although the presence of dyslipidemia, insulin resistance, hypertension, and obesity contributes to the increased cardio-metabolic diseases, population-based, clinical, and genetic studies have revealed an important role of inherited myopathies and endocrine disorders, such as GSDs and LSDs. An essential role for proteo-toxicity due to CP/ATG dysregulation in the onset of inherited metabolic and endocrine disorders has been demonstrated. Given the key role of CP/ATG in the degradation and removal of proteins and organelles for the maintenance of cellular and organismal homeostasis, Tan et al. (2019) discussed CP/ATG dysregulation in the pathogenesis of inherited myopathies and endocrine disorders, which contribute to increased prevalence of cardio-metabolic disorders.

Muscular Dystrophies

Congenital muscular dystrophies (CMDs) are childhood-onset muscle diseases characterized by weakness, disabilities, and early mortality. CMDs are caused by mutations in the dystrophin-associated transmembrane gene complex. Their primary mechanism is muscle cell injury due to impaired membrane anchorage. Horstick et al. (2013) examined the potential of altering CP as a theranostic strategy to establish the relationship between CMD disease and CBMP and the impact of modulating CP on CMD disease and proposed that aberrant CP is a common feature of CMDs; hence, interventions that regulate CP can reverse CBMP and improve disease prognosis. These investigators studied biopsy material from patients with CMDs and zebrafish models to evaluate impaired CP as compared to other congenital muscle diseases, genetic manipulations, and drugs that modulate CP.

Neuronal Ceroid Lipofuscinosis

Neuronal ceroid lipofuscinosis (NCL) are distinct LSDs with accumulation of protein aggregates and ceroid lipofuscin leading to neurodegeneration and blindness. Marques et al. (2019) demonstrated that recombinant human lysosomal Cathepsin D (rhCTSD) can improve the biochemical phenotype of CTSD-deficient hippocampal slice cultures *in vitro* and retinal cells *in vivo*. Dosing of rhCTSD in the murine CLN10 model resolved lysosomal hypertrophy, and impaired CP/ATG in the CNS and viscera. CTSD is important for the maintenance of cellular proteo-stasis by turning over substrates of endocytosis, phagocytosis, CP, and ATG. CTSD deficiency triggers impairment of the lysosomal-CP/ATG machinery. In mice and humans, CTSD dysfunction underlies the congenital variant (CLN10) of NCL. The approach to treat LSDs is ERT by replacing the defective hydrolase with an exogenously applied recombinant protein. The recombinant human pro-CTSD produced in a mammalian expression can be taken up by a variety of cell models, is targeted to lysosomes and processed in the mature form of the protease. Direct delivery of the recombinant protease to the CNS was required to ameliorate CBMP and longevity. Hence, rhCTSD has potential in the TSE-EBPT of NCL.

Fabry Disease

Fabry disease (FD) is a LSD characterized by impaired α-galactosidase A (α-Gal A) due to mutations in the GLA gene. While virtually all tissues are affected, renal damage is critical for the patient's prognosis. Braun et al. (2019) studied the effects of enzyme replacement therapy (ERT) on a podocyte cell culture model of Fabry disease. They investigated the effect of α-Gal A on podocytes for three days, mimicking ERT. They studied reduction in Gb3 accumulation in podocytes upon α-Gal A treatment. Despite Gb3 clearance, dysregulation of the signaling pathways was not reversed, presenting evidence for Gb3-independent effects. They assumed that alterations observed in FD may have a point of no return after which a reversal of dysregulated cellular signal transduction by α-Gal A treatment was ineffective, despite Gb3 clearance, suggesting further research to determine the appropriate time for initiation of therapy. Yanagisawa et al. (2019) examined the association between methylation and CP/ATG in a female patient with FD, which was caused by mutation of the GLA gene on the X chromosome, and her two sisters, who had few symptoms. They confirmed CP/ATG by LC3 turnover assay using fibroblasts. In the severe female patient, CP/ATG was abnormal while her two sisters with few symptoms had normal CP/ATG, revealing the direct relationship between symptoms and CP/ATG. In the severe patient, lysosomes were enlarged and p62 was accumulated in the CPS. The methylated allele of the GLA gene had a high proportion of wild alleles; whereas, the sisters' methylated allele had a high proportion of mutant alleles. The mRNA expression of the mutant allele by allele-specific PCR was high in the severe patient and low in the siblings with few symptoms. A correlation between the mRNA expression and disease severity was confirmed. There was a correlation between severe symptoms, dysfunction of CP/ATG, and methylation of wild alleles in FD, suggesting that allele-specific PCR may facilitate diagnosis and prognosis of female patients with FD.

mTOR Signaling

The mTOR is a ubiquitous serine/threonine kinase that regulates anabolic and catabolic processes, in response to environmental stimuli. The existence of mTOR in intracellular compartments senses stress, executes growth signals, and regulates CP/ATG. Understanding the mechanism of myeloid differentiation provides insights into the hematopoietic development. By using an ESC-derived myeloid progenitor cell model, Zhang et al. (2019b) found that CSF2/GM-CSF triggered macrophage differentiation and activation of the mTOR signaling. Activation or inhibition of the mTOR signaling enhanced or attenuated macrophage differentiation, respectively. CP/ATG was inhibited with the addition of CSF2. Genetic inhibition and modification of CP/ATG enhanced macrophage differentiation and rescued the inhibitory effect on differentiation caused by mTOR inhibition. The mTOR signaling pathway regulated macrophage differentiation of myeloid progenitors by inhibiting ATG, providing new insights into the mechanisms for myeloid differentiation for theranostic applications of hematopoietic and myeloid progenitor cells. The mTOR signaling deregulation is related to aging and age-related disorders, among which progeroid laminopathies represent clinical entities with well-defined phenotypes. These diseases are caused by LMNA mutations with altered bone turnover, metabolic dysregulation, and mild to severe segmental progeria. Different LMNA mutations cause pathologies in muscles and adipose tissue and neuropathologies in the absence of major systemic involvement. Chiarini et al. (2019) highlighted the recent advances detailing mTOR involvement in progeroid and tissue-specific laminopathies. Hyper-activation of Akt/mTOR signaling was demonstrated in muscular laminopathies, and rescue of mTOR-regulated pathways increased lifespan in animal models of Emery-Dreifuss muscular dystrophy. Rapamycin (mTOR inhibitor) was used to elicit CP/ATG and degradation of mutated lamin A or progerin in progeroid cells. mTOR-dependent charnolopathogenetic events were identified in Emery-Dreifuss muscular dystrophy, LMNA-related cardiomyopathies, Hutchinson-Gilford progeria, mandibuloacral dysplasia, and type 2 familial partial lipodystrophy. LMNA-related laminopathies are presented in Fig. 31.

Tuberous Sclerosis Complex

Tuberous sclerosis complex (TSC) is an autosomal dominant syndrome that causes tumor formation and is caused by mutations in the genes encoding TSC1/2, which are negative regulators of the mTORC1. Downregulation of TSC is associated with GSD. In human and mouse cells with defective or absent TSC2, Pal et al. (2019) demonstrated that the complete loss of TSC2 causes an increase in glycogen synthesis through mTORC1 induction and inhibition of glycogen synthase kinase 3β (GSK3β), a negative regulator of glycogen synthesis. Specific TSC2 pathogenic mutations, however, elevated glycogen levels with no changes in mTORC1 or GSK3β activities. They identified mTORC1-independent lysosomal depletion and CP/ATG impairment underlying GSD in TSC, irrespective of the mutation. The defective CP/ATG degradation of glycogen was associated with abnormal ubiquitination and degradation of essential proteins of the CP/ATG-lysosome pathway, such as LC3 and LAMP1/2, which were restored by mTORC1+ Akt inhibitors, suggesting mTORC1 as the primary theranostic target for TSC pathogenesis. These findings discovered mTORC1-independent dysregulated pathways for the of TSE-EBPT of TSC.

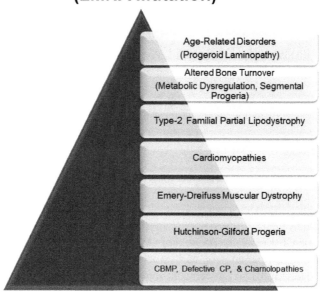

Figure 31

Danon Disease

Danon disease is an X-linked dominant hereditary condition caused by mutations in the gene encoding LAMP2, leading to failure of lysosome binding to CPS, glycogen accumulation in the heart, and abnormal cardiac function. Zhou et al. (2019) described a mutation in LAMP2, c.741+1G>T, in a family with Danon disease by whole exome sequencing. Skeletal muscle biopsy revealed myogenic damage and CP/ATG vacuoles with sarcolemmal features. Numerous vacuoles indicated CP/ATG dysfunction. The mutation did not result in the loss of mRNA exons; rather, a 6-nucleotide (two-codon) insertion, as a stop codon, caused early termination of LAMP2 protein translation. The truncated protein lacked transmembrane domain, which impaired lysosome/CPS fusion and CP, and exhibited clinical manifestations of Danon disease.

Myopathies

Decremental responses in repetitive nerve stimulation are reported in few hereditary myopathies. Elahi et al. (2019) examined the frequency of decrement in myopathy patients. They reviewed myopathy patients who underwent repetitive nerve stimulation by including patients with decrement (>10%) by either a pathological or molecular diagnosis of myopathy. Among 157 patients, four had decrement (2-OHCQ)-associated vacuolar myopathy, one had centro-nuclear myopathy, and one distal myopathy. One OH–CQ-associated vacuolar myopathy patient also had inflammatory myopathy. Pyridostigmine improved weakness in the centro-nuclear myopathy patients, but remained ineffective in distal myopathy patients.

Marinesco-Sjögren Syndrome

Marinesco-Sjögren Syndrome (MSS) is a rare neuromuscular condition caused by recessive mutations in the SIL1 gene, resulting in the absence of functional SIL1 protein, a co-chaperone for the major ER chaperone, BiP. As BiP is required for proper protein processing, loss of SIL1 causes accumulation of misshaped proteins, which destroys cells in vulnerable tissues, leading to cataracts, cerebellar ataxia, vacuolar myopathy, and other MSS phenotypes. To study PNS vulnerability in MSS, Phan et al. (2019) investigated intramuscular nerves fibers from MSS patients and from SIL1-deficient mice (woozy) as well as sciatic nerves and neuromuscular junctions (NMJ) via TEM, immunofluorescence, and proteomic profiling. PNS and NMJ integrity were analyzed via immunofluorescence studies in a MSS-zebrafish model. Morphological changes indicated impaired CP/ATG and CBs in distal axons and in Schwann cells. Changes in the morphology of NMJs as well as in the transcripts encoding proteins for NMJ function were detected in woozy mice, similar to the abnormal structure in SIL1-deficient zebrafish embryos. Proteome profiling of sciatic nerve specimens from woozy mice revealed altered proteins implicated in neuronal maintenance, suggesting the activation of compensatory mechanisms.

Wilms' Tumor

Although, Wilms' tumor treatment has achieved great success in the last decade, some cases still failed to respond to the current multimodality therapy. These cases fall primarily in the unfavorable histology group. CP/ATG regulation affects cancer cell behavior and has emerged as a novel mechanism to improve cancer cell response to theranostics. Guimei et al. (2019) investigated the expression of CP/ATG related markers (ATG4B and Beclin-1) in WT, its association with the clinico-pathological parameters, and impact on patient survival. Twenty-one formalin fixed paraffin embedded (FFPE) WT specimens were stained using ATG-related biomarkers, Beclin-1 and ATG4B. All specimens showed positive expression of both Beclin-1 and ATG4B. The staining score for Beclin-1 varied between 50 and 300, and its expression was associated with favorable histology. ATG4B expression was higher in favorable histology tumors compared to unfavorable histology. A positive correlation between Beclin-1 and ATG4B expression was observed. Disease-free survival in patients with favorable histology was higher compared to those patients with unfavorable histology. Thus, Beclin-1 and ATG4B expression were significant discriminators of survival, suggesting that the expression of CP/ATG-related biomarkers is associated with a favorable histology and could predict better survival in these patients.

Multiple Congenital Anomalies

Data from exome sequencing show that a proportion of individuals in whom a genetic disorder is suspected turn out to have two to four distinct characteristics. Voinea et al. (2019) reported a patient with splenomegaly, pneumopathy, bone changes, and FTD. "Sea-blue histiocytes" in his bone marrow pointed to a LSD. Homozygosity for a pathogenic mutation in the SMPD1 gene confirmed Niemann-Pick disease type B (NPD-B). MCI and abnormal brain FDG-PET were consistent with FTD. They initially tried to fit the skeletal and neurologic phenotype into the NPD-B diagnosis. However, additional studies revealed a mutation in the SQSTM1 gene. Thus, this patient had two distinct diseases; NPD-B, and Paget's disease with FTD. The subsequent finding of a mutation in the SQSTM1 gene explained the combination of a singular "unifying" diagnosis and allowed theranostic decisions. SQSTM1 mutations are associated with FTD, because of defective CP/ATG, suggesting that although for unifying diagnosis remains valid, physicians should consider the possibility of coexisting multiple diagnoses when clinical features are difficult to explain, because an accurate diagnosis can guide genetic counseling and lead to better theranostic management.

Mucolipidosis Type IV

Mucolipidosis type IV (MLIV) is a rare autosomal recessive LSD, causing intellectual disability, motor and speech deficits, retinal degeneration culminating in blindness, and systemic disease leading to a reduced lifespan. MLIV results from mutations in the gene MCOLN1 encoding the transient receptor potential channel mucolipin-1. Research has been focused on understanding the role of mucolipin-1 protein in cell and brain functions and how its absence causes disease. Boudewyn and Walkley (2019) explored current understanding of the mucolipin-1 in relation to neuro-pathogenesis in MLIV and described its role in mTOR and transcription factor EB (TFEB) signaling feedback loops as well as in the endosomal/lysosomal system. These investigators also discussed whether haplo-insufficiency in MCOLN1 heterozygotes was associated with neuronal dysfunction or disease.

Leber's Hereditary Optic Neuropathy

Leber's hereditary optic neuropathy (LHON) is caused by mutations in the mtDNA encoding complex I subunits, resulting in oxidative stress, retinal ganglion cell (RGC) death, and loss of vision. Using cybrid models for LHON, Sharma et al. (2019) reported that CP/ATG is compromised in cells carrying LHON-specific mtDNA mutations, resulting in reduced clearance of CBs and dysregulated CP (which causes CBMP and cell death). CP induction selectively cleared CBs and improved cell survival, suggesting that compromised CP/ATG is the missing link connecting oxidative stress to LHON pathogenesis. CB elimination through ATP-driven lysosomal-dependent CP conferred a protective role by improving LHON mutations and could be utilized as a theranostic target for LHON treatment.

Spinocerebellar Ataxia

Spinocerebellar ataxia (SCA) is a heterogeneous group of neurodegenerative disorders with autosomal-dominant inheritance. Sullivan et al. (2019) provided an update on the clinical and scientific progresses in SCA where numerous genes were identified using the NGS technique. The main disease mechanisms of SCAs included toxic RNA gain-of-function, mitochondrial dysfunction, channelopathies, CP/ATG, and transcriptional dysregulation. Recent studies demonstrated the importance of DNA-repair pathways in modifying SCA with CAG expansions. The latest advances in detecting known and novel repeat expansion in SCA and the roles of antisense oligonucleotides and RNA-based therapy were also emphasized. Machado-Joseph disease (MJD), also known as SCA3, is the most common fatal polyglutamine disease with no disease-modifying treatment. The selective serotonin reuptake inhibitor, Citalopram, was shown in nematode and mouse models to be a candidate for MJD therapeutics (Ashraf et al. 2019). Citalopram decreases ATXN3 aggregation in a mouse model of MJD. Four-week-old YACMJD84.2 mice and non-transgenic littermates were given Citalopram 8 mg/kg in their drinking water for 10 weeks. Brains of Citalopram-treated YACMJD84.2 mice showed ~50% decrease in the cells containing ATXN3-positive inclusions in the substantia nigra and brainstem nuclei compared to the controls. No differences in ATXN3-inclusion load were observed in deep cerebellar nuclei. While lysates from the brainstem and cervical spinal cord of Citalopram-treated mice showed a decrease in soluble forms of ATXN3 and reduction in insoluble ATXN3, no differences in ATXN3 levels were observed between cerebella of Citalopram-treated and vehicle-treated mice. Citalopram altered components of the cellular protein homeostatic machinery that might have enhanced refold and/or degraded mutant ATXN3, suggesting its theranostic potential in this fatal disorder. Matos et al. (2019) analyzed studies dedicated to the MJD/SCA3 pathogenesis and theranostic strategies, focusing on gene therapy and pharmacological approaches based on the molecular and cellular mechanisms of disease.

MJD/SCA3 arises from mutation of the ATXN3 gene, but this monogenic caused contrasts with the complexity of the pathogenic mechanisms that are admitted to underlie neuronal dysfunction and death. The aberrantly expanded ataxin-3, aggregates and generates toxic species that disrupt ATG, proteostasis, transcription, mitochondrial function, and signal transduction. Silencing the pathogenic protein, blocking aggregation, inhibiting proteolytic processing, and counteracting dysfunctions of the cellular systems yielded ameliorating results in cellular and animal models.

Pompe Disease

Pompe disease is caused by mutations in the α-1, 4-glucosidase (GAA) gene. In patients with late onset Pome disease (LOPD), genotype-phenotype correlations are unpredictable. Skeletal muscle pathology includes glycogen accumulation and altered CP of various degrees. A correlation of the muscle morphology with clinical features and the genetic background in GAA may contribute to the understanding of the phenotypic variability. Tarallo et al. (2019) studied microRNAs as biomarkers for Pompe disease. They analyzed microRNA expression by small RNA-seq in tissues from the disease murine model at two different ages (3 and 9 months), and in plasma from Pompe patients. In the mouse model, 211 microRNAs were expressed in the gastrocnemii and 66 in the heart, with a distinct pattern of expression at different ages. In a preliminary analysis in plasma from six patients, 55 microRNAs were differentially expressed. Sixteen of these microRNAs were common to those dysregulated in mouse tissues. These microRNAs modulated the expression of genes involved in Pompe disease pathophysiology (CP/ATG, muscle regeneration, muscle atrophy). MiR-133a, was selected for further qRT-PCR analysis and its levels in 52 Pompe disease patients were higher than those in the controls. This finding correlated with phenotype severity, which was higher in infants compared with late-onset patients. In three infantile patients, miR-133a decreased after initiation of the ERT with evidence of clinical improvement, suggesting that circulating microRNAs as CP modulators may represent biomarkers of the severity and prognosis of Pompe disease severity. Kulessa et al. (2019) took muscle biopsies before the ERT from 53 patients with LOPD. Glycogen accumulation, fibrosis, CP vacuoles, and severity of muscle damage were analyzed and compared with clinical findings. Additional CP markers LC2-IA/LC3-IIA, p62, and Bcl2-associated athanogene 3 were analyzed from 22 LOPD biopsies. The myo-pathology showed a high variability in most patients, with moderate glycogen accumulation and low morphology-scores. High morphology-scores were associated with increased fibrosis and CP, highlighting its role in severe skeletal muscle damage. The morphology-score did not correlate with the patient's age at biopsy, disease duration, residual GAA activity, or creatine-kinase levels. In 37 patients, genetic analysis identified the most frequent mutation, c.-32-13T>G, at 95%, in combination with c.525delT (19%). No significant correlation was found between the different GAA genotypes and muscle morphology which showed a high variability in most cases with moderate pathology. Increased pathology was associated with enhanced fibrosis and CP.

CP in Congenital Diseases

Lipid Droplet Biogenesis in Obesity

Browning induction, transplantation of BAT, or brown/beige adipocytes derived from progenitor or iPSCs can represent a strategy to treat metabolic diseases. Various genetic factors controlling the differentiation of brown adipocytes have been identified, although these studies have been performed using *in vitro* cultured pre-adipocytes. Mayeuf-Louchart et al. (2019) investigated the differentiation of brown adipocytes from adipose progenitors in the mouse embryo and demonstrated the formation of multiple LDs is initiated within clusters of glycogen, which is degraded through glycophagy to provide the metabolic substrates for lipogenesis and LD formation. This indicates the role of glycogen in the generation of LDs as the author discovered in developing UN rat cerebellar Purkinje neurons.

Lipid Droplets in APOL1 Kidney Disease

Two coding variants in the apolipoprotein L1 (APOL1) gene (termed G1 and G2) are associated with increased risk of nondiabetic kidney disease in people of African ancestry. The mechanisms by which the risk variants cause kidney damage involve injury to glomerular podocytes. Chun et al. (2019) demonstrated that APOL1 also localizes to intracellular LDs. While a large fraction of risk variant APOL1 (G1 and G2) localizes to the ER, a significant proportion of wild-type APOL1 (G0) localizes to LDs. APOL1 interacted with ER, mitochondria, and endosomes. The treatment of cells that promote LD formation with oleic acid shifted the localization of G1 and G2 from the ER to LDs, with reduction in CP/ATG and cytotoxicity. Co-expression of G0 APOL1 with risk variant APOL1 enabled recruitment of G1 and G2 from the ER to LDs, accompanied by reduced cell death, suggesting that ability of G0 APOL1 to recruit risk variant APOL1 to LDs may help explain the recessive pattern of kidney disease inheritance and establish APOL1 as a LD-associated protein. Recruitment of risk-variant APOL1 to LDs reduce cell toxicity, CP/ATG, and cell death. Thus, interventions that divert APOL1 risk variants to LDs may be a potential TSE-EBPT strategy to alleviate their cytotoxic effects.

Neuronal Ceroid Lipofuscinoses

The neuronal ceroid lipofuscinoses (NCL) are a group of disorders defined by shared clinicopathological features, including seizures and progressive decline in vision, cognition, motor functioning, and accumulation of autofluorescent lysosomal storage material, or 'ceroid lipofuscin'. Thirteen distinct genetic subtypes were recognized. Most genes causing NCL were identified, emphasizing the need for a shift towards applying genomics to achieve a deeper understanding of the molecular basis of the NCLs and related disorders. Butz et al. (2019) summarized findings of thirteen NCL genes and the proteins they encode, clinical manifestations linked to each of the genes, recent progress leading to a broader understanding of pathways involved in NCL disease pathogenesis, and similarities with other NDDs.

TDP-43 in C9orf72-Associated ALS/FTD

The G4C2 hexanucleotide repeat expansion mutation in the *C9orf72* gene is the most common genetic cause underlying both ALS and FTD. These NDDs are linked by the presence of abnormal phosphorylated TDP-43 neuronal inclusions. Lee et al. (2019a) compared the number of phosphorylated TDP-43 inclusions and their morphology in hippocampi in patients dying with sporadic versus *C9orf72*-related ALS with frontotemporal lobar degeneration with phosphorylated TDP-43 inclusions (the pathological substrate of clinical FTD in patients with ALS). In sporadic cases, there were consolidated phosphorylated TDP-43 inclusions that were variable in size, whereas the inclusions in *C9orf72* ALS/frontotemporal lobar degeneration were smaller. Also, a *C9orf72* ALS /frontotemporal lobar degeneration homogenized brain contained soluble cytoplasmic TDP-43 that was absent in sporadic cases. To better understand these pathological differences, TDP-43 inclusion formation were modulated in fibroblasts derived from sporadic or *C9orf72*-related ALS/FTD. Both sporadic and *C9orf72* ΛLS/FTD patient fibroblasts showed impairment in TDP-43 degradation by the proteasome, which may explain increased TDP-43 protein in both sporadic and *C9orf72* ALS/frontotemporal lobar degeneration in the frontal cortex and hippocampus. Fibroblasts derived from sporadic patients, but not *C9orf72* patients, demonstrated the sequestration of cytoplasmic TDP-43 into aggresomes via microtubule-dependent mechanism. TDP-43 aggresomes *in vitro* and TDP-43 neuronal inclusions were localized with CP/ATG biomarkers and behaved similarly for ATG degradation. The *C9orf72* fibroblasts were unable to form TDP-3 aggresome; whereas TDP-43 protein was soluble in the cytoplasm and formed relatively smaller inclusions in the *C9crf72* brain compared with sporadic disease; suggesting a loss of the protein QC to sequester and degrade TDP-43 in *C9orf72*-related diseases.

TRAPPC11 Variants for Carboxy Terminus

Variants in TRAPPC11 are associated with a broad spectrum of phenotypes but all affected individuals display muscular pathology. TRAPPC11 was identified as a component of the TRAPP III complex that functions in membrane trafficking and ATG. Milev et al. (2019) reported three individuals from families that had bi-allellic TRAPPC11 variants. Subject 1 harbored a compound heterozygous variant (c.1287+5G>A and c.3379_3380insT). The former variant resulted in a partial deletion of the foie gras domain (p.Ala372_Ser429del), while the latter variant resulted in a frame-shift and extension at the C-terminal (p.Asp1127Valfs*47). Subjects 2 and 3 harbored a homozygous missense variant (c.2938G>A; p.Gly980Arg). Fibroblasts from all three subjects displayed membrane trafficking defects manifested as delayed ER-to-Golgi transport and/or protein exit from the Golgi. All three individuals showed a defect in glycosylation of an ER-resident glycoprotein. However, only the compound heterozygous subject displayed impaired ATG. Characterization of these individuals with bi-allelic TRAPPC11 variants highlighted the importance of the C-terminal portion of the protein in muscular pathology.

Hsp70 in Poly-glutamine Diseases

The polyglutamine (polyQ) diseases are a group of nine fatal, adult-onset NDDs characterized by misfolding and aggregation of mutant proteins containing toxic expansions of CAG/polyQ tracts. Davis et al. (2019) reported that the Hsp90/Hsp70 chaperone machinery is a key component of QC, playing a role in the regulation of folding, aggregation, and degradation of polyQ proteins. The ability of Hsp70 to facilitate disaggregation and degradation of misfolded proteins makes it an attractive theranostic target in polyQ diseases. Manipulation of Hsp70 and related co-chaperones can enhance the disaggregation and/or degradation of misfolded proteins in polyQ disease. Therefore, the development of molecules that enhance Hsp70 activity is of great interest. Thus, this research highlighted the multifaceted role of Hsp70 in protein QC and the opportunities and challenges Hsp70 poses as a potential theranostic target in polyQ disease.

Autoinflammation in Familial Mediterranean Fever

Autoinflammatory disorders represent a heterogeneous group of systemic inflammatory diseases caused by genetic or acquired defects in key components of the innate immunity. Familial Mediterranean fever (FMF) is the most common clinical phenotype of the rare hereditary periodic fevers (HPFs) syndromes. Skendros et al. (2019) reported that FMF is associated with mutations in the MEFV gene encoding pyrin and is characterized by recurrent, stress-provoked attacks of fever and serositis, but also by chronic inflammation. FMF is prevalent in Greece and other countries of the eastern Mediterranean region. These investigators focused on FMF during their research on innate immunity and the role of neutrophils. The study of Greek patients with FMF yielded: the epidemiology of the disease, its clinical manifestations and overlaps with other idiopathic inflammatory conditions, its complex genetic background, and the crosstalk between environmental stress and inflammation. During an FMF attack, neutrophils release chromatin structures called neutrophil extracellular traps (NETs), decorated with bioactive IL-1β. REDD1 (regulated in development and DNA damage responses 1), encodes a stress-related mTOR repressors upregulated gene in neutrophils during disease progression. Upon adrenergic stress, REDD1-induced ATG triggers a pyrin-driven IL-1β maturation, and the release of IL-1β-bearing NETs. Consequently, not only the mode of action of IL-1β-targeting therapies was explained, but also new treatment strategies emerged with the evaluation drugs targeting CP/ATG-induced NETosis. Information gained from FMF studies may be applied in more complex inflammatory conditions, such as adult-onset Still's disease, gout, ulcerative colitis, and Behçet's disease.

WDFY3 Variants Cause NDD

Le Duc et al. (2019) presented data on exome and genome sequencing as well as an array analysis of 13 individuals that point to pathogenic, heterozygous, de novo variants in WDFY3 as a monogenic cause of mild and non-specific neurodevelopmental delay. Nine variants were protein-truncating and four missense. The symptoms included neurodevelopmental delay, intellectual disability, macrocephaly, and psychiatric disorders (autism spectrum disorders/ADHD). One pro-band presented with an opposing phenotype of microcephaly and the only missense-variant located in the PH-domain of WDFY3. Pathogenic PH-domain variants could lead to microcephaly via canonical Wnt-pathway upregulation. The ATG scaffolding protein WDFY3 was required for cerebral cortical size regulation in mice, by controlling division of NPCs. These investigators showed that proliferating cortical NPCs of human embryonic brains express high amounts of WDFY3, supporting its role in the regulation of prenatal neurogenesis. They demonstrated wnt-pathway dysregulation in wdfy3-haploinsufficient mice, which displayed microcephaly and deficits in motor coordination and associated learning, similar to human phenotypes, and proposed that WDFY3 loss-of-function variants can lead to microcephaly via downregulation of Wnt pathway. Thus, they presented WDFY3 as a novel gene linked to neurodevelopmental delay and intellectual disability and concluded that variants causing haplo-insufficiency lead to macrocephaly, while an opposing mechanism due to variants in the PH-domain of WDFY3 leads to microcephaly.

Small Molecules Ameliorate Human Fibroblasts

The generation of neural cells is of great interest in medical research because of its promise in the effective treatment of NDDs. Small molecules are used for inducing specific cell types across lineage boundaries. Therefore, to direct neural cell fate, small molecule is a feasible approach for generating clinically-relevant cell types without genetic alterations. Human fibroblasts are induced into neural cells with different combinations of small molecules. Rujanapun et al. (2019) induced human fibroblasts into neural cells by using four small molecules: *WNT activator, DNMT inhibitor, Notch inhibitor, and retinoic acid* within five days. Neural-specific genes, including NESTIN, TUJ1, and SOX2, were upregulated which coincided with the activation of CP/ATG. CP/ATG-related genes, such as LC3, ATG12, and LAMP1, were enhanced upon neural induction. The number of induced-neural cells decreased when ATG was suppressed by CQ. The activation of ATG reduced ROS generation within the induced-neural cells, and the inhibition of ATG by CQ suppressed the expression of antioxidant genes, catalase, SOD, and GPX, suggesting that ATG maintained the optimal level of ROS for neural induction of human fibroblasts. This study presented conditions to induce neural cells from human fibroblasts and revealed the roles of CP/ATG in controlling neural cell induction.

Extracellular Vesicles in LSDs

Extracellular vesicles (EVs) have received attention over the last two decades. Their protein, nucleic acid (miRNA and mRNA), and lipids have signaling functions. Cells release different types of vesicular structures. Many stress conditions, such as hypoxia, senescence, and oncogene activation are associated with the release of higher levels of EVs. CP/ATG-lysosomal pathway abnormalities also affect EV release. In fact, in NDDs characterized by the accumulation of toxic proteins, although it has not become clear to what extent the intracellular storage of undigested material has beneficial/adverse effects, these proteins are released extracellularly via EVs. LSDs are characterized by the accumulation of undigested substrates within the endosomal-lysosomal system, caused either by genetic mutations in lysosomal proteins or due to treatment with pharmacological agents. Tancini et al. (2019) investigated the role of lysosomal and CP/ATG dysfunction on the release of EVs (CS), with a focus on studies exploring the release of EVs in LSD models of both genetic and pharmacological origin. A better knowledge of EV-releasing pathways in lysosomal stress conditions will provide information on their role in both alleviating intracellular storage of undigested materials and spreading the pathology to the neighboring tissue.

RINT1 Bi-Allelic Variations

Pediatric acute liver failure (ALF) is a life-threatening condition with genetic, immunologic, and environmental etiologies. Recurrent ALF (RALF) in infants demonstrates repeated episodes of liver injury with the recovery of hepatic function between crises. Cousin et al. (2019) described bi-allelic RINT1 alterations as the cause of a multisystem disorder including RALF and skeletal abnormalities. Three unrelated individuals with RALF onset ≤3 years of age had splice alterations at the same position (c.1333+1G>A or G>T) in Trans with a missense (p.Ala368Thr or p.Leu370Pro) or in-frame deletion (p.Val618_Lys619del) in RINT1. ALF episodes are concomitant with fever/infection and not all individuals have complete normalization of liver function between episodes. Biopsies revealed nonspecific liver damage including fibrosis, steatosis, or increases in Kupffer cells. Skeletal imaging revealed abnormalities affecting the vertebrae and pelvis. Dermal fibroblasts showed splice-variant mediated skipping of exon 9, leading to an out-of-frame product and nonsense-mediated transcript decay. Fibroblasts also revealed decreased RINT1 protein, abnormal Golgi morphology, and impaired ATG compared to the control. RINT1 interacted with NBAS (implicated in RALF), and UVRAG, to facilitate Golgi-to-ER vesicle transport. During nutrient depletion or infection, Golgi-to-ER transport was suppressed and ATG was promoted through UVRAG regulation by mTOR. Aberrant ATG was associated with the development of similar skeletal abnormalities and with liver disease, suggesting that disruption of RINT1 functions may explain the liver and skeletal findings. Hence, resolving the mechanism underlying this gene-disease relationship may confer theranostic opportunities.

Annexin A7 for Plasma Membrane Repair

By using invasive BC cells, Sønder et al. (2019) showed that the Ca^{2+} – and the phospholipid-binding protein annexin A7 are part of the plasma membrane repair response by enabling assembly of the endosomal sorting complex for transport (ESCRT) III. Following injury to the plasma membrane and Ca^{2+} flux into the cytoplasm, annexin A7 forms a complex with the apoptosis-linked gene-2 (ALG-2) to facilitate recruitment and binding of ALG-2 and the ALG-2-interacting protein X (ALIX) to the damaged membrane. ALG-2 and ALIX assemble the ESCRT III complex, which helps excise and shed the damaged plasma membrane during wound healing, indicating that annexin A7 helps in plasma membrane repair by regulating ESCRT III-mediated shedding of injured plasma membrane.

DTP/MTMR14 in Anoxia and Protein Aggregation

Drosophila egg-derived tyrosine phosphatase (EDTP), a lipid phosphatase that removes 3-position phosphate at the inositol ring, has dual functions in oogenesis and muscle performance in adults.

A mammalian homologous gene MTMR14, which encodes the myotubularin-related protein 14, negatively regulates ATG. Mutation of EDTP/MTMR14, however, causes three deleterious consequences: (1) the lethality in early embryogenesis; (2) a "jumpy" phenotype with impaired motor functions; and (3) an association with a rare genetic centro-nuclear myopathy. The benefit of EDTP/MTMR14 downregulation is masked by the lethality or severe muscle defects due to loss of this gene. Xiao et al. (2019) showed that flies carrying a heterozygous EDTP mutation revealed increased survival to prolonged anoxia; tissue-specific downregulation of EDTP in non-muscle tissues, particularly moto-neurons, extended lifespan, and improved survivorship in $A\beta42$ and poly-glutamine protein aggregates, highlighting the significance of selective downregulation of EDTP for beneficial consequences. MTMR14 expression was evident in the hippocampus and cortex in C57BL/6J and APP/PS1 mice. Compared with C57BL/6J mice, APP/PS1 mice had reduced MTMR14 in the cortex. The hippocampal expression of MTMR14 increased and plateaued at 9–17 months compared with 2–6 months in C57BL/6J mice. MTMR14 was induced by $A\beta42$ in the rat hippocampal neurons and mouse Neuro2a neuroblasts, demonstrating a novel approach to tissue-specific downregulation of the disease-associated gene EDTP/MTMR14 for extended lifespan and improved survival of cellular protein aggregates, which could be extended to mammals.

TLR4-Mediated ATG

Increased orosomucoid-like 3 (ORMDL3) expression, due to SNPs, are associated with inflammatory diseases, including asthma and inflammatory bowel diseases. ORMDL proteins inhibit serine palmitoyltransferase (SPT), the first rate-limiting enzyme in sphingolipid synthesis and alter $[Ca^{2+}]_i$ homeostasis. Both processes are essential for immune response. Kiefer et al. (2019) addressed the ORMDL3 protein involvement in macrophages using an overexpressing knock-in mouse model. Ceramide was different in the bone-marrow-derived macrophages (BMDM) from the transgenic mouse model compared with the wild type (WT) macrophages. Sphinganine production was altered upon BMDM activation in the transgenic mice. Alteration in the ORMDL3 expression did not affect activation or macrophage polarization. These investigators studied phagocytosis and ATG-crucial processes that are dependent on lipid membrane composition. Phagocytosis in transgenic macrophages was not affected by ORMDL3 overexpression, but induced reduction in TLR-4-mediated ATG. Both genetic and functional studies pointed to ATG as an essential pathway which may provide new insights into the functional link between the ORMDL3 expression and inflammatory diseases.

ATG-Related Gene 5 Variants to Aplastic Anemia

Immune-mediated quantitative and qualitative defects of hematopoietic stem/progenitor cells (HSPCs) play a vital role in the pathophysiology of acquired aplastic anemia (AA). ATG is related to T cell pathophysiology and the destiny of HSPCs, in which the ATG-related gene 5 (Atg5) is involved. You et al. (2019) hypothesized that genetic variants of Atg5 might contribute to AA. They studied six Atg5 polymorphisms in a Chinese cohort of 176 patients with AA and compared them with 157 healthy controls. A decreased risk of AA in the recessive models of rs510432 and rs803360 polymorphisms was observed. The decreased risk was more pronounced among AA compared with healthy controls in recessive models. The rs573775 could predict the occurrence of newly onset hematological event in patients with AA, indicating that genetic Atg5 variants contributed to AA; this knowledge may facilitate the understanding of the basic mechanisms of AA and aid in making a patient-tailored medical decision.

Methylomics of CP/ATG in Cystic Fibrosis

CP/ATG is impaired in CF patients and CF mice, as their cells exhibit low expression of essential CP/ATG molecules. The genetic disorder in CF is due to mutations in the CF transmembrane conductance regulator (cftr) gene that encodes for a Cl⁻ channel. CF patients are prone to infection by pathogens that are eliminated by CP/ATG in healthy immune cells including *Burkholderia cenocepacia* (*B. cenocepacia*). Caution et al. (2019) determined the mechanism underlying impaired CP/ATG in CF macrophages and develop DSST-TSE-EBPT-CPTs to resolve it. Using reduced representation bisulfite sequencing (RRBS) to determine the DNA methylation profile, they found that the promoter regions of Atg12 in CF macrophages were more methylated than in the wild-type (WT) immune cells, accompanied by low protein expression. Epigallo-Catechin-3-gallate (EGCG) reduced the methylation of Atg12 promoter, improving its expression. EGCG restricted *B. cenocepacia* replication within CF mice and their macrophages by improving CP/ATG and preventing dissemination. In addition, EGCG improved the function of CFTR protein. Thus, utilizing RRBS revealed a mechanism for reduced CP/ATG in CF.

SQSTM1/p62-Directed Metabolic Reprogramming

Calvo-Garrido et al. (2019) reported that loss-of-function mutations in the ATG adaptor protein SQSTM1/p62 lead to progressive NDDs presenting themselves in childhood. They studied the consequences of loss of p62 in a neuroepithelial stem cell (NESC) model and differentiated neurons derived from reprogrammed p62 patient cells or by CRISPR/Cas9-directed gene-editing in NESCs. Transcriptomic and proteomic analyses suggested that p62 is essential for neuronal differentiation to control the metabolic shift from aerobic glycolysis to O/P required for neuronal maturation, which was blocked by the failure to downregulate LDH expression due to the loss of p62, through Hif-1α downregulation and increased sensitivity to oxidative stress. This indicated the important role of p62 in energy metabolism in the regulation of the shift between glycolysis and O/P for neural differentiation.

Genetics of Spastic Paraplegias

Hereditary spastic paraplegias are a heterogeneous group of neurological disorders. Patients present lower limb weakness and spasticity, complicated with additional neurological symptoms. Boutry et al. (2019) highlighted that the perception of the intricate connections between clinical, genetic, and molecular aspects of NDDs has radically changed owing to the improvements in genetic approaches for hereditary spastic paraplegias, for which >60 genes have been identified, highlighting: (i) the genetic heterogeneity of this group of clinically diverse disorders, (ii) the fuzzy border between recessive and dominant inheritance for several mutations, and (iii) the overlap of these mutations with other neurological conditions. Abnormal intracellular trafficking, changes in ER shaping and defects affecting lipid metabolism, lysosomal physiology, CP/ATG, myelination, and neuronal development have been proposed as mechanisms. Several genes affect these interconnected functions, suggesting a unifying pathogenic model that could be employed for the TSE-EBPT of spastic paraplegias

Hydroxyurea in Down Syndrome

Down syndrome (DS), a genetic disorder caused by partial or complete triplication of chromosome 21, is the most common genetic cause of intellectual disability. DS mouse models and cell lines display defects in cellular adaptive stress responses, including ATG, unfolded protein response, and MB. Brose et al. (2019) tested the ability of Hydroxyurea (HU), an

FDA-approved pharmacological agent that activates adaptive cellular stress response pathways, to improve the cognitive function of Ts65Dn mice. The chronic HU treatment started at a stage when early mild cognitive deficits are present in this model (~3 months of age) and continue until a stage of advanced cognitive deficits in untreated mice (~5–6 months of age). The effects of HU on cognitive performance were analyzed using water maze tasks to detect changes in different types of memory with sensitivity to detect deficits as well as improve spatial memory. The most common characteristic of cognitive deficits at 5–6 months of age was their inability to acquire new information for long-term storage, a feature akin to episodic-memory. HU treatment produced mild benefits in Ts65Dn by improving memory acquisition and short-term retention of spatial information. In control mice, the HU treatment facilitated memory retention in constant as well as time-variant conditions implicating a nootropic effect, indicating that HU has potential for improving memory retention and cognitive flexibility that can be harnessed for the amelioration of cognitive deficits in normal aging and in dementia related to DS and other NDDs.

Parkinsonism and Gluco-cerebrosidase Deficiency

Recently, LSDs appeared as a bridge of knowledge between rare genetic inborn metabolic disorders and NDDs such as PD or FTD. Epidemiological studies have improved our understanding of the link between mutations in the glucocerebrosidase (GBA) gene and PD. Gatto et al. (2019) conducted a review of this link, highlighting the association in GBA mutation carriers and in Gaucher disease type 1 patients (GD type 1). There was a bidirectional interaction between GBA and α-Syn regulatory pathways involving the clearance of aggregated proteins through CP/ATG. The link between GBA deficiency and PD was not restricted to α-Syn aggregates but also involved Parkin and PINK1 mutations. In addition, early and later endosomes and the LAMP-2A involved in the chaperone-mediated CP/ATG can facilitate developing substrate reduction and/or ERT as novel TSE-EBPT strategies in NDDs.

EWSR1 and Aging

Lee et al. (2019b) reviewed the emerging role of EWSR1 genetic mutations and their association with brain diseases, as well as how EWSR1 modulates cellular function via the epigenetic pathway to provide a better understanding of its role in aging and associated brain disorders. They highlighted that Ewing's sarcoma (EWS) is a bone cancer arising primarily in young children. EWSR1 (Ewing Sarcoma breakpoint region 1/EWS RNA binding protein 1) gene is expressed in most cell types, indicating it has diverse roles in various cellular processes and organ development. Missense mutations of EWSR1 genes are associated with ALS and FTD. EWSR1 plays epigenetic roles in gene expression, RNA processing, and signal transduction. EWSR1 controls miRNA levels via Drosha, leading to CP/ATG dysfunction and impaired dermal development. EWSR1 deficiency also leads to premature senescence of RBCs and gamete cells with accelerated apoptosis due to the abnormal meiosis.

T-Cell Antigen 1 in Welander Distal Myopathy

Welander distal myopathy (WDM) is a muscle dystrophy characterized by adult-onset distal muscle weakness, impacting the distal long extensors of the hands and feet. WDM is an autosomal dominant disorder caused by a missense mutation (c.1362G>A; p.E384K) in the TIA1 (T-cell intracellular antigen 1) gene, which encodes an RNA-binding protein required for the post-transcriptional regulation of RNAs. Carrascoso et al. (2018) developed a cell model of WDM to study the molecular and cellular events associated with mutated TIA1 expression by analyzing how this mutation affects three regulatory functions mediated by TIA1: (i) control of alternative SMN2 (survival motor neuron 2) splicing; (ii) formation, assembly, and disassembly of stress granules; and (iii) mitochondrial dynamics and its consequences for CP, ATG, and apoptosis. Whereas WDM-associated TIA1 expression had only a mild effect on SMN2 splicing, it led to suboptimal adaptation to environmental stress, with exacerbated stress granule formation that was accompanied by mitochondrial dysfunction and CP/ATG. This indicatied that the cell phenotype seen in the muscles of patients with WDM can be recapitulated by ectopic expression of WDM-TIA1 in embryonic kidney cells, and highlighted the potential of this model to investigate the pathogenesis of WDM and possible therapeutics.

ATL3 Mutation

Axonopathies are NDDs caused by axonal degeneration, affecting primarily the longest neurons. These axonopathies are caused by genetic defects in proteins involved in the shaping and dynamics of the ER. Given its central and widespread position within a cell, the ER is a pivotal player in inter-organelle communication. Krols et al. (2019) demonstrated that defects in the ER fusion protein ATL3, which were identified in patients suffering from hereditary sensory and autonomic neuropathy, increased the number of ER-mitochondrial contact sites, both in HeLa cells as well as in patient-derived fibroblasts. This increased contact was reflected in higher phospholipid metabolism, upregulated ATG, and augmented Ca^{2+} interaction between both organelles. The mitochondria in these cells displayed reduced motility, and the number of axonal mitochondria in neurons expressing disease-causing mutations in ATL3 decreased, indicating the functional interdependence of subcellular organelles in health and disease.

β-Propeller Protein

Neurodevelopmental/NDD β-Propeller protein-associated neurodegeneration (BPAN) is an X-linked rare dominant disorder of ATG. The role of WDR45 is implicated in BPAN exclusively in females due to male lethality. Characterization of clinical manifestations and complex genetic determinants in rare male patients remain crucial for deciphering BPAN and other X-linked dominant diseases. Akçakaya et al. (2019) performed whole exome sequencing (WES), followed by segregation analysis, and identified a novel mis-sense and mosaic variant in WDR45, namely NM_007075.3:c.873C>G; p. (Tyr291*) in an affected male at the age of 34. His biphasic medical history was compatible with BPAN, characterized by delayed psychomotor development, intellectual disability, and progression into dystonia Parkinsonism in his twenties. The variant had a mosaic pattern in the whole exome and Sanger sequencing findings. To figure out if mosaicism was restricted to this variant or related to a chromosomal-level mosaicism, they used WES data from 129 unrelated individuals to calculate the threshold values of male and female X chromosome heterozygosity (XcHet) in WES data. A Bkg level of heterozygous variants on X chromosome (excluding the pseudo-autosomal loci) was a phenomenon in WES analysis and was used as a QC measure. Utilization of this measure for detection of digital anomalies of the X chromosome in males by observing a higher XcHet value than the threshold value was suggested. This approach revealed a variant level mosaicism in the affected male, which was supported with cytogenetic analyses. Hor and Tang (2019) reported that the BPAN results from heterozygous or hemizygous germline mutations/pathogenic variant of the X chromosome gene WDR45, which encodes WD40 repeat protein to interact with phosphoinostidies 4 (WIPI4). This subtype of the spectrum of neurodegeneration with brain iron accumulation diseases is characterized by a biphasic mode of manifestation and progression. The first phase involves early-onset of epileptic seizures, developmental delay, intellectual disability, and autistic syndrome. Subsequently, Parkinsonism, dystonia, and dementia emerge in adolescence or early adulthood. WIPI4/WDR45 has an essential role in ATG, acting as a PI-3-phosphate binding effector for autophagosome biogenesis and size control. These investigators discussed WIPI4's role in ATG and linked the neuropathological manifestations of BPAN's biphasic infantile onset (epilepsy, autism) and adolescent onset (dystonic, Parkinsonism, dementia) phenotypes to ATG impairment.

Polyrotaxanes

Recently, the application of β-cyclodextrins (β-CDs) has received considerable attention as theranostic agents in Niemann-Pick type C (NPC) disease, a family of LSDs characterized by cholesterol accumulation in the lysosomes. To further improve the theranostic efficacy of β-CDs, the use of β-CD-threaded polyrotaxanes (PRXs) were proposed as a carrier of β-CDs for NPC disease. PRXs are supramolecular polymers composed of many CDs threaded onto a linear polymer chain and capped with bulky stopper molecules. Tamura et al. (2019) described the design of PRXs and their theranostic applications in their research. Recently, Tamura et al (2019) described to achieve the intracellular release of threaded β-CDs from PRXs, stimuli-cleavable linkers were introduced in a polymer of PRXs. The stimuli-labile PRXs could dissociate into their constituent molecules by a cleavage reaction under specific stimuli, such as pH reduction in lysosomes. The release of the threaded β-CDs from acid-labile PRXs in lysosomes resulted in the formation of an inclusion complex with the cholesterol that had accumulated in NPC disease patient-derived fibroblasts, thus promoting the extracellular excretion of the excess cholesterol. The administration of PRXs to a mouse model of NPC disease caused suppression of the tissue cholesterol accumulation, resulting in a prolonged life span in the mouse model. The induction of CP/ATG by the methylated β-CD-threaded PRXs (Me-PRXs) was described. Hence, the stimuli-labile PRXs could be effective carriers of CDs for TSE-EBPT of NPC disease.

PKG1-Modified TSC2 and Cardiac Stress

The mTORC1 coordinates regulation of growth, metabolism, protein synthesis, and CP/ATG. Its hyper-activation contributes to disease in numerous organs, including the heart, although abnormal inhibition of mTORC1 risks interference with its homeostatic roles. Tuberin (TSC2) is a GTPase-activating protein and intrinsic regulator of mTORC1 that acts through modulation of Ras homologue enriched in brain (RHEB). TSC2 inhibits mTORC1; however, this activity is modified by phosphorylation from signaling kinases that inhibits (AMPK and GSK-3β) or stimulates (Akt, ERK, and RSK-1) mTORC1 activity. Each kinase requires engagement of serines, impeding the analysis of their role *in vivo*. Ranek et al. (2019) showed that phosphorylation or gain- or loss-of-function mutations at either of two adjacent serine residues in TSC2 (S1365 and S1366 in mice; S1364 and S1365 in humans) can control mTORC1 activity stimulated by growth factors or hemodynamic stress, and modulate cell growth and CP/ATG. In the heart, or in isolated cardiomyocytes or fibroblasts, PKG1 phosphorylated TSC2 sites. PKG1 is a primary effector of NP and natriuretic peptide signaling, and protected in CVDs. The suppression of hypertrophy and stimulation of CP/ATG in cardiomyocytes by PKG1 required TSC2 phosphorylation. Homozygous knock-in mice that expressed a phosphorylation-silencing mutation in TSC2 (TSC2(S1365A)) developed severe heart disease and had higher mortality following pressure overload of the heart, owing to mTORC1 hyperactivity that could not be rescued by PKG1 stimulation. However, cardiac disease was reduced and the survival of heterozygote Tsc2^{S1365A} knock-in mice subjected to the same stress was improved by PKG1 activation or expression of a phosphorylation-mimicking mutation (TSC2 (S1365E)). Basal mTORC1 activity remained unaltered in either knock-in model. Hence, TSC2 phosphorylation was required for PKG1-mediated cardio-protection in pressure overload. Thus, serine residues conferred a genetic tool for bidirectional regulation of the amplitude of stress-stimulated mTORC1 activity in the heart.

CONCLUSION

An impaired glycogen metabolism induced LD formation during brown adipocyte differentiation. TDP-43 cytoplasmic inclusion was disrupted in C9orf72-associated ALS/FTD. The impaired DNA methylation of the GLA gene was associated with CP/ATG dysfunction. MTOR-mediated charnolo-pathogenetics was detected in laminopathies. Glycogen storage in tuberous sclerosis was associated with impaired mTORC1-mediated signaling. Danon disease caused by a splice mutation in LAMP2 generated a nonfunctional truncated protein. Movement disorders were observed in IEM and neuromuscular transmission defects were observed in myopathies. Deficiency of SIL1 caused degenerative changes in peripheral nerves and neuromuscular junctions. Hepatic tissues from patients with Wilson disease and from ATP7B-deficient animals suggested that CP protects hepatocytes from Cu-induced apoptosis. Impaired CP/ATG was detected in muco-polysaccharidosis and in the SCA model of MJD, and microRNAs were identified as theranostic biomarkers in Pompe disease. Beclin-1 and ATG4B were induced in Wilms' Tumor. Neuropathogenesis of mucolipidosis type IV indicated that CP repairs Leber's hereditary optic neuropathy-associated mitochondrial dysfunction and cardiovascular disorders.

In addition, TSE2 phosphorylation was required for PKG-1-mediated cardioprotection during pressure overload and serine residue provided a genetic tool for the regulation of amplitude of stress-induced mTORC activity in the heart.

REFERENCES

Acosta, P. (ed.) 2010. Nutrition Management of Patients with Inherited Metabolic Disorders. Jones and Bartlett, U.S.A.

Akçakaya, N.H., B. Salman, Z. Görmez, A.Y. Tarkan, et al. 2019. A novel and mosaic WDR45 nonsense variant causes beta-propeller protein-associated neurodegeneration identified through whole exome sequencing and X chromosome heterozygosity analysis. Neuromolecular Med 21: 54–59.

Ashraf, N.S., S. Duarte-Silva, E.D. Shaw, P. Maciel, et al. 2019. citalopram reduces aggregation of ATXN3 in a YAC transgenic mouse model of machado-joseph disease. Mol Neurobiol 56: 3690–3701.

Boudewyn, L.C. and S.U. Walkley. 2019. Current concepts in the neuropathogenesis of mucolipidosis type IV. J Neurochem 148: 669–689.

Boutry, M., S. Morais, G. Stevanin. 2019. Update on the genetics of spastic paraplegias. Curr Neurol Neurosci Rep 19: 18.

Braun, F., L. Blomberg, S. Brodesser, M.C. Liebau, et al. 2019. Enzyme replacement therapy clears Gb3 deposits from a podocyte cell culture model of fabry disease but fails to restore altered cellular signaling. Cell Physiol Biochem 52: 1139–1150.

Brose, R.D., A. Savonenko, B. Devenney, K.D. Smith, et al. 2019. Hydroxyurea improves spatial memory and cognitive plasticity in mice and has a mild effect on these parameters in a down syndrome mouse model. Front Aging Neurosci 11: 96.

Butz, E.S., U. Chandrachud, S.E. Mole and S.L. Cotman. 2019. Moving towards a new era of genomics in the neuronal ceroid lipofuscinoses. Biochim Biophys Acta Mol Basis Dis 30: 165571.

Calvo-Garrido, J., C. Maffezzini, F.A. Schober, P. Clemente, et al. 2019. SQSTM1/p62-directed metabolic reprogramming is essential for normal neurodifferentiation. Stem Cell Reports 12: 696–711.

Carrascoso, I., C. Sánchez-Jiménez, E. Silion, J. Alcalde, et al. 2018. A heterologous cell model for studying the role of T-cell intracellular antigen 1 in welander distal myopathy. Mol Cell Biol 39(1): e00299–18.

Caution, K., A. Pan, K. Krause, A. Badr, et al. 2019. Methylomic correlates of ATG activity in cystic fibrosis. J Cyst Fibros 18: 491–500.

Chiarini, F., C. Evangelisti, V. Cenni, A. Fazio, et al. 2019. The cutting edge: The role of mTOR signaling in laminopathies. Int J Mol Sci 20: 847.

Chun, J., J.Y. Zhang, M.S. Wilkins, B. Subramanian, et al. 2019. Recruitment of APOL1 kidney disease risk variants to lipid droplets attenuates cell toxicity. PNAS 116: 3712–3721.

Cousin, M.A., E. Conboy, J.S. Wang, D. Lenz, et al. 2019. RINT1 Bi-allelic variations cause infantile-onset recurrent acute liver failure and skeletal abnormalities. Am J Hum Genet 105: 108–121.

Davis, A.K., W.B. Pratt, A.P. Lieberman and Y. Osawa. 2019. Targeting Hsp70 facilitated protein quality control for treatment of polyglutamine diseases. Cell Mol Life Sci 77: 977–996.

Di Paola, S. and D.L. Medina. 2019. TRPML1-/TFEB-Dependent regulation of lysosomal exocytosis. Methods Mol Biol 1925: 143–144.

Ebrahimi-Fakhari, D. 2018. Congenital disorders of autophagy: What a pediatric neurologist should know. Neuropediatrics 49: 18–25.

Ebrahimi-Fakhari, D., A. Saffari, L. Wahlster, J. Lu, et al. 2016. Congenital disorders of autophagy: An emerging novel class of inborn errors of neuro-metabolism. Brain 139: 317–337.

Ebrahimi-Fakhari, D., C. Van Karnebeek and A. Münchau. 2019. Movement disorders in treatable inborn errors of metabolism. Mov Disord 34: 598–613.

Elahi, B., R.S. Laughlin, W.J. Litchy, M. Milone, et al. 2019. Neuromuscular transmission defects in myopathies: Rare but worth searching for. Muscle Nerve 59: 475–478.

Fernandes, J., J.M. Saudubray, G. vanden Berghe and J.H. Walter (eds). 2013. Inborn Metabolic Diseases: Diagnosis and Treatment. Springer Medizin, Heidelberg, Germany.

Gatto, E.M., G. Da Prat, J.L. Etcheverry, G. Drelichman, et al. 2019. Parkinsonisms and glucocerebrosidase deficiency: A comprehensive review for molecular and cellular mechanism of glucocerebrosidase deficiency. Brain Sci 9(2): 30.

Graef, J.W., J.I. Wolfsdorf and D.S. Greenes (eds). 2008. Manual of Pediatric Therapeutics. Lippincott Williams & Wilkins, Philadelphia, PA, US.

Guimei, M., M.A. Eladl, A.V. Ranade and S. Manzoor. 2019. Autophagy related markers (Beclin-1 and ATG4B) are strongly expressed in Wilms' tumor and correlate with favorable histology. Histol Histopathol 34: 47–56.

Hor, C.H.H. and B.L. Tang. 2019. Beta-propeller protein-associated neurodegeneration (BPAN) as a genetically simple model of multifaceted neuropathology resulting from defects in autophagy. Rev Neurosci 30: 261–277.

Horstick, E., X. Li, S. Moore and J.J. Dowling. 2013. P.1.13 Autophagy and the pathogenesis of congenital muscular dystrophies. Neuromuscular Disorders 23: 745.

Kiefer, K., J. Casas, R. García-López and R. Vicente. 2019. Ceramide imbalance and impaired TLR4-mediated autophagy in BMDM of an ORMDL3-overexpressing mouse model. Int J Mol Sci 20: 1391.

Kobayashi, H. 2019. Recent trends in mucopolysaccharidosis research. J Hum Genet 64: 127–137.

Krols, M., B. Asselbergh, R. De Rycke, V. De Winter, et al. 2019. Sensory neuropathy-causing mutations in ATL3 affect ER-mitochondria contact sites and impair axonal mitochondrial distribution. Hum Mol Genet 28: 615–627.

Kulessa, M., I. Weyer-Menkhoff, L. Viergutz, C. Kornblum, et al. 2019. An integrative correlation of myopathology, phenotype and genotype in late onset Pompe disease. Neuropathol Appl Neurobiol 46: 359–374.

Le Duc, D., C. Giulivi, S.M. Hiatt, E. Napoli, et al. 2019. Pathogenic WDFY3 variants cause neurodevelopmental disorders and opposing effects on brain size. Brain 142: 2617–2630.

Lee, S.M., S. Asress, C.M. Hales, M. Gearing, et al. 2019a. TDP-43 cytoplasmic inclusion formation is disrupted in C9orf72-associated amyotrophic lateral sclerosis/frontotemporal lobar degeneration. Brain Commun 1(1): fcz014.

Lee, J., P.T. Nguyen, H.S. Shim, S.J. Hyeon, et al. 2019b. EWSR1, a multifunctional protein, regulates cellular function and aging via genetic and epigenetic pathways. Biochim Biophys Acta Mol Basis Dis 1865(7): 1938–1945.

Liu, E.A. and A.P. Lieberman. 2019. The intersection of lysosomal and endoplasmic reticulum calcium with autophagy defects in lysosomal diseases. Neurosci Lett 697: 10–16.

Marques, A.R.A., A. Di Spiezio, N. Thießen, L. Schmidt, et al. 2019. Enzyme replacement therapy with recombinant pro-CTSD (cathepsin D) corrects defective proteolysis and ATG in neuronal ceroid lipofuscinosis. Autophagy 16: 1–15.

Marsh, D and J.M. Dragich. 2019. Autophagy in mammalian neurodevelopment and implications for childhood neurological disorders. Neurosci Lett 697: 29–33.

Matos, C.A., L.P. de Almeida and C. Nóbrega. 2019. Machado–Joseph disease/spinocerebellar ataxia type 3: lessons from disease pathogenesis and clues into therapy. J Neurochem 148: 8–28.

Mayeuf-Louchart, A., S. Lancel, Y. Sebti, B. Pourcet, et al. 2019. Glycogen dynamics drives lipid droplet biogenesis during brown adipocyte differentiation. Cell Rep 29: 1410–1418.

Milev, M.P., D. Stanga, A. Schänzer, A. Nascimento, et al. 2019. Characterization of three TRAPPC11 variants suggests a critical role for the extreme carboxy terminus of the protein. Sci Rep 9: 14036.

Pal, R., Y. Xiong and M. Sardiello. 2019. Abnormal glycogen storage in tuberous sclerosis complex caused by impairment of mTORC1-dependent and -independent signaling pathways. PNAS 116: 2977–2986.

Phan, V., D. Cox, S. Cipriani, S. Spendiff, et al. 2019. SIL1 deficiency causes degenerative changes of peripheral nerves and neuromuscular junctions in fish, mice and human. Neurobiol Dis 124: 218–229.

Polishchuk, E.V., A. Merolla, J. Lichtmannegger, A. Romano, et al. 2019. Activation of autophagy, observed in liver tissues from patients with wilson disease and from ATP7B-deficient animals, protects hepatocytes from copper-induced apoptosis. Gastroenterology 156: 1173–1189.

Ranek, M.J., K.M. Kokkonen-Simon, A. Chen, B.L. Dunkerly-Eyring, et al. 2019. PKG1-modified TSC2 regulates mTORC1 activity to counter adverse cardiac stress. Nature 566: 264–269.

Rujanapun, N., N. Heebkaew, W. Promjantuek and A. Sotthibundhu. 2019. Small molecules re-establish neural cell fate of human fibroblasts via ATG activation. In Vitro Cell Dev Biol Anim 55: 622–632.

Sharma, S. 2019. The Charnoly Body: A Novel Biomarker of Mitochondrial Bioenergetics. CRC Press, Taylor & Francis Group, Boca Raton, FL, U.S.A.

Skendros, P., C. Papagoras, I. Mitroulis and K. Ritis. 2019. Autoinflammation: Lessons from the study of familial Mediterranean fever. J Autoimmun 104: 102305.

Sønder, S.L., T.L. Boye, R. Tölle, J. Dengjel, et al. 2019. Annexin A7 is required for ESCRT III-mediated plasma membrane repair. Sci Rep 9: 6726.

Sullivan, R., W.Y. Yau, E. O'Connor, H. Houlden. 2019. Spinocerebellar ataxia: An update. J Neurol 266: 533–544.

Tamura, A. 2019. Intracellularly degradable polyrotaxanes for therapeutic applications. Yakugaku Zasshi 139: 143–155.

Tan, Y., Y. Gong, M. Dong, Z. Pei, et al. 2019. Role of autophagy in inherited metabolic and endocrine myopathies. Biochim Biophys Acta Mol Basis Dis 1865: 48–55.

Tancini, B., S. Buratta, K. Sagini, E. Costanzi, et al. 2019. Insight into the role of extracellular vesicles in LSDs. Genes (Basel) 10(7): 510.

Tarallo, A., A. Carissimo, F. Gatto, E. Nusco, et al. 2019. microRNAs as biomarkers in Pompe disease. Genet Med 21: 591–600.

Voinea, C., E. Gonzalez Rodriguez, C. Beigelman-Aubry, V. Leroy, et al. 2019. Hepatosplenomegaly, pneumopathy, bone changes and fronto-temporal dementia: Niemann-Pick type B and SQSTM1-associated Paget's disease in the same individual. J Bone Miner Metab 37: 378–383.

Xiao, C., S. Qiu, X. Li, D.J. Luo, et al. 2019. EDTP/MTMR14: A novel target for improved survivorship to prolonged anoxia and cellular protein aggregates. Neurosci Lett 705: 151–158.

Yanagisawa, H., M.A. Hossain, T. Miyajima, K. Nagao, et al. 2019. Dysregulated DNA methylation of GLA gene was associated with dysfunction of ATG. Mol Genet Metab 126: 460–465.

Yang, H., C. Zhao, M.C. Tang, Y. Wang, et al. 2019a. Inborn errors of mitochondrial acyl-coenzyme a metabolism: Acyl-CoA biology meets the clinic. Mol Genet Metab 128: 30–44.

Yang, H., Y. Wen, M. Zhang, Q. Liu, et al. 2019b. MTORC1 coordinates the autophagy and apoptosis signaling in articular chondrocytes in osteoarthritic temporomandibular joint. Autophagy 16: 271–288.

You, Y., J.H. Huo, J. Huang, M. Wang, et al. 2019. Contribution of autophagy-related gene 5 variants to acquired aplastic anemia in Han-Chinese population. J Cell Biochem 120: 11409–11417.

Zhang, M., F. Liu, P. Zhou, Q. Wang, et al. 2019. The MTOR signaling pathway regulates macrophage differentiation from mouse myeloid progenitors by inhibiting ATG. Autophagy 15(7): 1150–1162.

Zhou, N., J. Cui, W. Zhao, Y. Jiang, et al. 2019. A family with Danon disease caused by a splice site mutation in LAMP2 that generates a truncated protein. Mol Genet Genomic Med Mar 7(3): e561.

Zhu, Y., G. Runwal, P. Obrocki and D.C. Rubinsztein. 2019. Autophagy in childhood neurological disorders. Dev Med Child Neurol 61: 639–645.

9

Charnolophagy in Malnutrition

INTRODUCTION

ATG (particularly, CP) is induced in response to changes in nutrients and is the defense mechanism against cellular nutritional stress. When cells face nutritional stress, caused by either nutrient deficiency or nutrient excess, CP/ATG pathways are activated. CS is destabilized and is not efficiently exocytosed during chronic malnutrition due to free radical overproduction, ATP depletion, inadequate lysosomal enzymes, compromised IMD, and ICD accompanied with defective CP and CBMP.

This chapter highlights the theranostic significance of CP dysregulation in malnutrition which represents both overnutrition as well as undernutrition.

Evidence-based Nutrition

Although malnutrition is prevalent in the inpatient setting, particularly in older morbid patients, the medical community has struggled to find an efficient, EBPT approach for its prevention and treatment. Merker et al. (2019) highlighted that from an evolutionary perspective, illness-related low appetite may be seen as a protective response to accelerate recovery from disease by improving CP. Earlier trials in the intensive care units in severely ill patients have demonstrated the undesired effects of overnutrition. Uncertainties regarding the best approach to the malnourished patient in conjunction with a lack of robust clinical data may explain the low level of attention that medical staff have paid to malnutrition in the non-critical care inpatient setting. The effect of early nutritional support on frailty, functional outcomes, and recovery of malnourished inpatients trial (EFFORT) has shown that personalized nutritional support reduces severe complications and improves mortality, with a positive impact on functional outcomes and BQL. These results from a high-quality effectiveness trial in conjunction with other studies, such as the nutrition opportunities to understand reform involving student health (NOURISH), should improve management of malnutrition. A systematic screening for risk of malnutrition in admitted patients, assessment of nutritional status by a multidisciplinary team of dieticians, nurses, and physicians, and the early initiation of personalized nutritional support of at-risk patients is highly crucial to accomplish nutritional goals. Understanding the optimal use of nutritional support in patients with an acute illness is complex because the timing, route of delivery, and the amount and type of nutrients may influence prognosis. Particularly for patients in the medical ward, logistics of catering, staffing to provide food and support (nurses and dieticians), motivation/understanding of the patient to encourage eating in defiance of appetite, the empathic human factor of nutritional care, the quality of meal, the taste of supplements, and unnecessary fasting have a significant influence on the nutritional care of patients. Further research and clinical trials are needed to better understand how we can use clinical nutrition to maximize recovery, improve functional status, and QOL of patients. Such an EBPT strategy will allow us to implement personalized nutrition-driven interventions.

Parenteral Nutrition

In critically-ill children admitted to pediatric intensive care units (PICUs), enteral nutrition (EN) is often interrupted or delayed due to GIT dysfunction. Jacob et al. (2019) provided evidence to suggest that early supplemental parenteral nutrition (PN) in critically-ill children. Since a macronutrient deficit in these patients is associated with adverse outcomes, supplemental PN is advised to meet nutritional requirements. However, uncertainty of timing of initiation, optimal dose, and composition of PN has led to a wide variation in parenteral nutrition. The early versus late PN in the randomized controlled trial showed that withholding PN in the first week in PICUs reduced incidence of new infections and accelerated recovery as compared to providing supplemental PN early (within 24 hrs after PICU admission), irrespective of diagnosis, severity of illness, risk of malnutrition, or age. The early withholding of amino acids in particular (they are suppressors of CP, MD, and ICD) has explained this outcome benefit of parenteral nutrition. Two years after PICU admission, restricting supplemental PN early in PICUs did not negatively affect mortality, growth, or health status, and improved neurocognitive development. These findings have a theranostic impact on PN administration to critically-ill children.

Starvation-Induced α-Syn Degradation

Impaired CP/ATG clearance of aggregated α-Syn is considered as one the key mechanisms of PD (Sharma et al. 2013). The high-mobility group protein B1 (HMGB1) mediates ND by promoting inflammatory and neurotoxic factors. Guan et al. (2018) examined the influence of the overexpression of wild-type (WT) and mutant-type (MT, A53T and A30P) α-Syn on the CP/ATG in SH-SY5Y cells during starvation, and the regulation of endogenous HMGB1 on the α-Syn degradation and on the starvation-induced CP in the α-Syn-overexpressed SH-SY5Y cells. The overexpression of WT or MT α-Syn downregulated the starvation-induced conversion of LC3-I to LC3-II and CP protein (Atg5) expression and inhibited the starvation-downregulated mTOR in SH-SY5Y cells. However, the lentivirus-mediated upregulation of endogenous HMGB1 promoted the degradation of WT or MT α-Syn, CP-dependently, via promoting Atg5, but not mTOR. The Atg5 knockdown downregulated the HMGB1-mediated α-Syn degeneration, indicating that α-Syn inhibits starvation-induced CP in the SH-SY5Y cells by blocking the mTOR/Atg5 signaling pathway. However, endogenous HMGB1 promoted the CP degradation of α-Syn via the Atg5-dependent pathway, indicating the protective role of endogenous HMGB1 during α-Syn accumulation.

Metabolic Nutrients

Guillaume et al. (2019) described methods to quantify CP/ATG using a fluorescent sensor of ATG membranes and to estimate the impact of specific nutrients on CP/ATG, employing fluorescent microscopy. Although, tumorigenesis relies on the ability of cancer cells to obtain nutrients and fulfill energy demands associated with rapid proliferation, owing to increased metabolite consumption and poor vascularization, most cancer cells survive in a nutrient-poor and cellular-stress microenvironment. Cancer cells undergo metabolic reprogramming to evade cell death and ensure proliferation because they utilize the catabolic process of CP/ATG involving CBMP, which creates metabolites by sequestering cytosolic macromolecules in double-membrane vesicles for lysosomal degradation. During environmental and nutritional stress, CP/ATG is upregulated through AMPK and mTOR interactions, in cooperation with Unc-51 like CP/ATG-activating kinase 1 (ULK1). A lack of metabolic nutrients plays a crucial role in inducing CP/ATG, while their metabolites serve as fuel for the starving cell.

Serum and Nutrient Deprivation

The loss of nutrient supply is a contributor to intervertebral disc degeneration. Yurube et al. (2019) investigated the effects of limited nutrients on disc AF cell fate, including ATG. Rabbit disc AF cells were cultured in 5% oxygen in differential media with varying serum concentrations. The cellular responses to changes in serum and nutrient concentrations were determined by measuring their proliferation and metabolic activity. ATG flux in AF cells was monitored using flow cytometry and immunoblotting for LC3, HMGB1, and p62/SQSTM1. Apoptosis (caspase-3 and TUNEL) and cellular senescence (β-galactosidase and p16/INK4A) were measured. The biomarkers of apoptosis and senescence increased, while cell proliferation and metabolic activity decreased during serum and nutrient withdrawal without any change in O_2, confirming cellular stress. Increases in ATG biomarkers, including LC3 puncta, LC3-II expression, and HMGB1, were observed during nutritional stress, while an ATG substrate, p62/SQSTM1, decreased, suggesting an increased ATG flux in disc AF cells under serum and nutrient deprivation. Cellular responses included cell death, quiescence, reduced proliferation, and metabolic activity, and CP/ATG induction during nutritional stress.

mtDNA Mutation and Nutrient-Regulated CP

Mitochondria are highly susceptible to nutrient deficiencies, and nutritional intervention is an essential way to maintain MQC. Cancer, NDDs, and metabolic disorders are associated with mitochondrial dysfunction through multiple molecular mechanisms. Yang et al. (2019) discussed mtDNA mutations and their implications for human diseases. They examined how nutrients may eliminate mtDNA mutations through CP/ATG induction. Recent advances in genetic manipulation and NGS reveal the crucial roles of mtDNA in various pathophysiological conditions. Given the high prevalence of mtDNA mutations in humans and their impact on mitochondrial function, it is important to investigate the CP dynamics that regulate mtDNA mutation.

Starvation-Protective Membrane Domains

The eukaryotic plasma membrane is compartmentalized into domains enriched in specific lipids and proteins. The best-studied domain in yeast is the membrane compartment containing the arginine permease Can1 (MCC) which clusters additional transporters. MCCs correspond to invaginations of the plasma membrane and associate with subcortical "eisosomes" that include upstream regulators of the TORC2 in sensing sphingolipids and membrane stress. Gournas et al. (2018) reported that the clustering of Can1 in MCCs is governed by its conformation, requires proper sphingolipid biosynthesis, and controls its ubiquitin-dependent endocytosis. In the substrate-free outward-open conformation, Can1 accumulated in MCCs depending on sustained biogenesis of complex sphingolipids. An arginine transport-elicited shift to an inward-facing conformation promoted its cell-surface dissipation and made it accessible to the ubiquitylation machinery triggering endocytosis. During starvation, MCCs increased in number and size, depending on the BAR domain containing the Lsp1 eisosome component. This expansion of MCCs provided protection for nutrient transporters from endocytosis occurring concomitantly with ATG upon TORC1 inhibition, suggesting the importance of nutrient-regulated protection from endocytosis for protein partitioning into membrane domains.

Fructose in PER Old Rats

Dardevet et al. (2018) hypothesized that fructose feeding during a catabolic situation corresponding to protein-energy restriction (PER) in older rats would reduce AA utilization for energy purposes, thus slowing down the loss of body weight (BW) and improving body composition. Twenty-two month old male Wistar rats were fed a control ration (13% protein) either at normal (20 g/d), restricted (PER: 10 g/d), or at PER levels supplemented with glucose (3 g/d) or fructose (3 g/d) for 45 days, and subsequently studied in the post-absorptive state. BW, body composition, enzyme activities, and metabolites related to glucose, fructose, and AA metabolism were measured. Both glucose and fructose feeding reduced the PER-induced loss of BW and lean mass (–27% compared with PER), but only fructose reduced the loss of fat mass (–28% compared with PER). Fructose prevented the PER-induced loss of muscle and intestinal mass, reduced circulating branched-chain AA by 50% (compared with PER), and increased those of alanine (+65% compared with PER). A reduction in hepatic enzymes related to AA catabolism was observed during fructose feeding (compared with PER), whereas glycogen was increased in both the intestine (+300%) and muscle (+21%), indicating that in PER older rats, fructose feeding improves body composition and the weight of organs by reducing AA catabolism and utilization for energy production and ATG. This could be advantageous in sparing body proteins during catabolic states related to malnutrition during aging.

Non-Suckling Starvation

During oocyte meiotic arrest, germ cell nest breakdown occurs, and primordial follicle (PF) formation is initiated at the perinatal stage. CP is induced by nutrient starvation. Watanabe and Kimura (2018) investigated how starvation affects PF formation and CP induction during neonatal life. Suckling of neonatal female mice was prevented after birth for 12–36 hrs to induce starvation. The numbers of PFs were counted from serial sections of ovaries and CP-related proteins were evaluated. The number of PFs peaked at 60 hrs after birth in the control group. The numbers for the starvation groups were higher than those for the control groups at 12 and 36 hrs. LC3B was present in the oocyte cytoplasm. At 36 hrs after birth, the starvation group showed a higher rate of LC3-II/LC3-I expression as a marker for CP. The expression of p62 (a CP substrate) was decreased compared to the control group. The expression of caspase-9 (an apoptotic marker) remained lower at 36 hrs. Starvation promoted PF formation with a concomitant CP induction in early neonatal ovaries. Hence, CP induction during follicle assembly might increase the number of PFs.

Amoeba Chaos Cell Survival in Starvation

Cubic membranes (CM) are highly organized, well defined, and reveal a 3-D nano-periodic structure with symmetry in biological systems including CBs. These membrane arrangements are induced in cells under stress, disease conditions, or upon viral infection. Chong et al. (2018) investigated CM formation in the mitochondria of amoeba Chaos and observed a correlation between the organism's ability to generate CM and the cell survival during starvation. Rapamycin was used to pharmacologically induce CP, and CM formation. Inhibition of CP reverted the cubic IMM morphology to tubular structure. In starved Chaos cells, mitochondria and CPS did not co-localize and ATP production was sustained. CM transition in the mitochondria during starvation or upon induction of CP might prevent their sequestration by CPS, thus slowing their rate of degradation. Such mitochondrial activity may allow these cells to survive for a longer period during the organism's starvation, as discovered in developing prenatal and postnatal UN rat Purkinje neurons (Sharma et al 1993).

Vitamin D Deficiency and Crohn's Disease

Recently, White (2018) highlighted vitamin D as a key regulator of innate immune responses to pathogen threat. Vitamin D signals through a nuclear receptor transcription factor and regulates gene transcription. Vitamin D signaling remains active both upstream and downstream of pattern recognition receptors, as vanguards of innate immune responses. Crohn's disease (CD) is a relapsing-recurring IBD that arises from dysregulated intestinal innate immunity. Genetic studies have identified several CD-susceptibility biomarkers linked to innate immune responses to infection. Recent studies have discovered that the pathogenesis of CD contributes to vitamin D deficiency (Li et al. 2019). Clinical trials have shown that vitamin D supplementation may confer benefits to patients with CD.

Glutamine/Glucose Deprivation

To improve our knowledge concerning how cancer cells respond to nutrient withdrawal, Chiodi et al. (2019) studied the effect of glutamine and /or glucose starvation in transformed fibroblasts, characterized at the cellular and molecular level. Concomitant starvation of both nutrients led to loss of cellular adhesion (~16 hrs after starvation), followed by cell death. Deprivation of glucose alone had the same effect, although at a later time (~48 hrs after starvation), suggesting that glucose plays a crucial role in cell attachment. Glutamine deprivation did not induce rapid cell death, but arrested cell proliferation; the cells started dying only 96 hrs after starvation. Before massive cell death occurred, the effects of all the starvation conditions were reversible. CP induction was observed in cells incubated in the absence of glucose for >48 hrs. Apoptotic biomarkers, such as caspase 3, caspase 9, and PARP1 proteolytic fragments, were not observed under any growth condition. Glucose and/or glutamine deprivation induced PARP1 activation, with PARP1 (polyADP) ribosylation. This activation was not due to starvation induced DNA double strand breaks, and appeared at the late stages of deprivation, when most cells die. This indicates the diverse consequences of glucose and glutamine starvation, which may be considered when nutrient availability is used as a target for anticancer therapies.

Hibernating Bears

Although physical inactivity and malnutrition lead to a profound loss of muscle mass as well as metabolic dysfunction in humans, hibernating bears show limited muscle atrophy and can maintain locomotive function. Miyazaki et al. (2019) hypothesized that hibernating bears can alter the regulation of protein and energy metabolism in skeletal muscle which contributes to "muscle atrophy resistance" during physical inactivity. They examined the alteration of signaling pathways governing protein and energy metabolisms in skeletal muscle of the Japanese black bear. Sartorius muscle samples were collected from bear legs during late November (pre-hibernation) and early April (post-hibernation). Protein degradation pathways, through an ubiquitin-proteasome system (murf1 mRNA expression) and CP-dependent system (Atg7, Beclin-1, and map1lc3 mRNAs expression), were induced in skeletal muscle following hibernation. As indicated by an increase in S6K1 phosphorylation, motor induction, which functions as a regulator of protein synthesis, increased in post-hibernation samples, whereas gene expression of myostatin, a negative regulator of skeletal muscle mass, was decreased post-hibernation. The phenotype shifted toward slow-oxidative muscle and MB, suggesting that protein and energy metabolism is altered in hibernating bears to cause a limited loss of muscle mass and efficient energy utilization.

Growth Hormone in Starved Mice

When mice are subjected to 60% calorie restriction (CR) for several days, they lose their body fat. Although the animals lack energy stores, their livers produce enough glucose to maintain blood glucose even after a 23 hrs fast. This adaptation is mediated by an increase in plasma GH, induced by an increase in plasma ghrelin. In the absence of ghrelin, CR mice developed hypoglycemia due to reduced glucose production. To determine the site of GH action, Fang et al. (2019) employed CRISPR/Cas9 and Cre recombinase technology to produce mice that lack GH receptors in liver (*L-Ghr$^{-/-}$* mice) or in adipose tissue (*Fat-Ghr$^{-/-}$* mice). When subjected to CR and then made to fast for 23 hrs, the *L-Ghr$^{-/-}$* mice, but not the *Fat-Ghr$^{-/-}$* mice, developed hypoglycemia. The reduction in blood glucose in *L-Ghr$^{-/-}$* mice was correlated with a depletion in hepatic triglycerides. Hypoglycemia was prevented by the injection of lactate or octanoate to enhance gluconeogenesis. TEM analysis revealed CP induction in livers of CR control mice but not in *L-Ghr$^{-/-}$* mice, suggesting that GH acts through its receptor in the liver to induce CP, preserve triglycerides, enhance gluconeogenesis, and prevent hypoglycemia in CR mice.

Barriers to Cancer Nutrition Therapy

Cancer-associated malnutrition is driven by reduced dietary intake and by metabolic changes (such as inflammation, anabolic resistance, proteolysis, lipolysis, and futile cycling) induced by the tumor and activated immune cells. Cytotoxic and targeted chemotherapies also elicit proteolysis and lipolysis at the tissue level. Schiessel and Baracos (2018) highlighted chemotherapeutic effects that provoke proteolysis in muscle and lipolysis in adipose tissue. They explored whether these catabolic changes can be reversed by nutritional therapy. In skeletal muscle, tumor factors and chemotherapeutics activated intracellular signals to suppress protein synthesis and induce a transcriptional program leading to CP and the degradation of myofibrillar proteins. Cancer nutrition therapy is intended to ensure the adequate provision of energy fuels and a complete repertoire of biosynthetic building blocks. Cancer- and chemotherapy-associated metabolic alterations may be corrected by individual nutrients. The amino acids leucine and arginine supplemented in the diet reverse anabolic suppression in the muscle, while n-3 PUFA inhibit the transcriptional activation of muscle catabolism involving CBMP.

Septin in ATG

Although, >40 ATG proteins and several organelles have been identified as membrane source, the exact cellular and molecular mechanism of autophagosome biogenesis remains uncertain. Barve et al. (2018) discovered that the GTP-binding proteins, called septins, contribute to autophagosome biogenesis. Septins are localized at the bud-neck region and are involved in cytokinesis. During ATG, septins traffic between different cellular compartments such as Golgi, mitochondria, endosomes, plasma membrane, and vacuolar membranes to influence cellular response.

Maternal Quercetin Intake

The maternal restriction of dietary proteins during pregnancy and lactation can induce renal disease in later life. A high fructose diet (HFD) causes metabolic syndrome, resulting in an increased risk of developing CKD. Sato et al. (2019) investigated whether Quercetin intake during lactation affects HFD-induced inflammation and ATG in the kidneys of HFD-fed adult female offspring exposed to maternal normal-protein (NP) or low-protein (LP) diets. Pregnant Wistar rats received diets containing 20% (NP) or 8% (LP) casein, and 0 or 0.2% Quercetin containing NP diets (NP/NP or NP/NPQ) in experiment (Expt.) 1 and 0 or 0.2% Quercetin containing LP diets (LP/LP or LP/LPQ) in Expt. 2 during lactation. At weaning, pups that received a diet of distilled water (Wa) or 10% fructose solution (Fr) were divided into six groups: NP/NP/Wa, NP/NP/Fr, NP/NPQ/Fr in Expt. 1, and LP/LP/Wa, LP/LP/Fr, LP/LPQ/Fr in Expt. 2. At week 12, macrophage infiltration, mRNA of TNF-α and IL-6, and markers of ATG in the kidneys of male offspring were examined. The number of macrophages, TNF-α, and IL-6 mRNA increased in the kidneys of the NP/NP/Fr or LP/LP/Fr, respectively. The macrophage number and IL-6 in the NP/NPQ/Fr or LP/LPQ/Fr decreased. LC3B-II levels were downregulated in the NP/NP/Fr or LP/LP/Fr rats. LC3B-II was upregulated, while p62 was downregulated in the NP/NPQ/Fr and LP/LPQ/Fr rats, indicating that maternal Quercetin intake during lactation may cause long-term alterations in the ATG and inflammation in the kidneys of HFD-fed adult female offspring.

Mucosal Proteome in Anorexia

Anorexia nervosa is an eating disorder associated with intestinal disorders. Nobis et al. (2018) evaluated the colonic proteome during activity-based anorexia. Female C57Bl/6 mice were randomized into three groups: control, limited food access (LFA), and activity-based anorexia (ABA). LFA and ABA mice had a limited access to food but only ABA mice had access to an activity wheel. A 2D PAGE-based comparative proteomic analysis was performed on colonic mucosal protein extracts and differentially-expressed proteins were identified by LC-ESI-MS/MS. Twenty-seven proteins differentially expressed between control, LFA, and ABA groups were identified. The ABA mice exhibited alteration in mitochondrial proteins (such as dihydrolipoyl dehydrogenase and 3-mercaptopyruvate sulfurtransferase) involved in energy metabolism. Downregulation of mTOR pathway was observed leading to the inhibition of protein synthesis (Puromycin was incorporated and mediated by the increased phosphorylation of eukaryotic elongation factor 2), and to the activation of ATG (increase in the marker of ATG, the LC3-phosphatidylethanolamine conjugate/cytosolic form of LC3-II/LC3-I ratio). The colonic mucosal proteome was altered during ABA, suggesting a downregulation of the energy metabolism. An mTOR-mediated decrease in protein synthesis and an activation of ATG were also observed.

BmCalpains in Metamorphosis and Starvation

CP and apoptosis play crucial roles during Bombyx mori metamorphosis and starvation. Recently, calpain, as an intracellular proteases, was involved in CP and apoptosis. BmAtg5 and BmATG6 mediate apoptosis following CP induced by 20-hydroxyecdysone and starvation in *B. mori*. Yi et al. (2018) performed a phylogenetic analysis of calpains from *B. mori*, *Drosophila*, and *Homo sapiens*. Close relationships of BmCalpain-A/B with DmCalpain-A/B, BmCalpain-C with DmCalpain-C, and BmCalpain-7 with HsCalpain-7 were observed. The expression of BmCalpain-A/B, BmCalpain-C and BmCalpain-7 was increased during B. mori metamorphosis and induced in the fat body and midgut of starved larvae, consistent with the expression profiles of BmAtg5, BmAtg6, and BmCaspase-1. The apoptosis-associated cleavage of BmATG6 in Bm-12 cells was enhanced when BmCalpain-A/B and BmCalpain-7 were induced by starvation and was inhibited by the inhibitor of either calpain or caspase, but completely inhibited when both types of inhibitors were applied concomitantly, indicating that BmCalpains may be involved in CP and apoptosis during B. mori metamorphosis and starvation, and contribute to the apoptosis-associated cleavage of BmATG6.

Aldose Reductase Inhibition

Recently, Zhang et al. (2019a) demonstrated that deletion in Aldose reductase (AR) promotes cardiac remodeling via excessive ATG. To determine the role of AR in starvation-induced ATG, WTC57/Bl6 mice were pretreated with the AR inhibitor, Sorbinil, (0.2 g/L for 48 hrs) in drinking water, followed by 24 hrs fasting. Sorbinil pretreatment in fed mice did not affect blood glucose levels, whereas, it decreased the blood glucose levels in fasting mice. In comparison with fed mice, the LC3-II formation and LCII/LCI ratio were increased in the fasted mice hearts and tj\he Sorbinil pretreatment enhanced LC3-II formation and LC3-II/LC3-I ratios. Fasting-induced ATG coincided with AMPK activation in the Sorbinil-pretreated fasting mice hearts. ATG and activation of AMPK was also induced in the gastrocnemius skeletal muscle. Induction of ATG in the cardiac tissues was accompanied by the increased clearance of 4-hydroxytrans-2-nonenal-protein adducts, indicating that the inhibition of AR during fasting activates the ATG response, and increases the clearance of aldehyde-protein adducts to maintain cellular homeostasis during starvation.

mtDNA Copy Number in Starvation

Mitochondria have maintained their own reduced genome, mtDNA, which encodes for a small and highly specialized set of genes. mtDNA exists in tens to thousands of copies packaged in nucleoprotein complexes, termed nucleoids, distributed throughout the mitochondrial network. Medeiros and Graef (2019) summarized their recent findings that Mip1/POLG (mtDNA polymerase-γ) controls the mtDNA copy number by operating in two opposing modes (the synthesis and degradation of mtDNA), when yeast cells face nutrient starvation. The balance of the two modes of Mip1/POLG and thus, the mtDNA copy number depends on the integrity of CP/ATG, which sustains the continuous synthesis and maintenance of mtDNA. In ATG-deficient cells, a combination of nucleotide insufficiency and elevated ROS production impairs mtDNA synthesis and drives its degradation by the $3'$-$5'$-exonuclease activity of Mip1/POLG resulting in mtDNA depletion and irreversible respiratory deficiency.

Sestrin-Like Protein in Starvation

Sestrins are highly conserved, stress-inducible proteins that help maintain metabolic homeostasis and protect cells during stress. Sestrins are upregulated during stress and influence AMPK and mTOR pathways. Rafia et al. (2019) discovered the role of Sestrin from Dictyostelium discoideum (Dd), where starvation initiates multicellular development. The single DdSesn-like gene was expressed and its endogenous functions were characterized. Both, the knockout and constitutively expressing strains, were made and their involvement in starvation-induced ATG was analyzed. Autophagic fluxes and ROS levels were also monitored. Overexpression of DdSesn decreased cell growth and showed a longer lag phase. Upon starvation, both DdSesn and ROS increased. Sesn[OE] showed reduced ROS while sesn⁻ showed increased ROS, suggesting that increased sesn expression may be beneficial in reducing ROS during starvation. Deletion of sesn showed reduced ATG and increased p4EBP1, suggesting that DdSesn promotes ATG in D. discoideum during starvation.

MDR Protein-1 in Glucose Starvation

Glucose starvation induces resistance to Metformin through the elevation of mitochondrial MDR protein-1. Metformin, a drug for T2DM, has shown therapeutic effects for various cancers. However, it had no beneficial effects on the survival rate of human malignant mesothelioma (HMM) patients. Hwang et al. (2019) elucidated the mechanism of Metformin resistance in

HMM cells. Glucose-starved HMM cells were resistant to Metformin, as demonstrated by decreased ATG and apoptosis and increased cell survival. These cells showed abnormalities in mitochondria, such as decreased ATP synthesis, morphological elongation, altered permeability transition pores, and hyperpolarization of $\Delta\Psi$ involving CBMP. Mdr1 was upregulated in mitochondria but not in the cell membrane. The upregulated mitochondrial Mdr1 was reversed by treatment with CCCP, a $\Delta\Psi$ inducer. ATG and apoptosis were increased in the MDR protein-1 knockout HMM cells cultured under glucose starvation with Metformin treatment, suggesting that Mdr1 plays a critical role in the chemoresistance to Metformin in HMM cells, which could be a potential target for improving its theranostic efficacy.

Amino Acid Starvation and Replication of Ibaraki Virus

Ibaraki virus (IBAV) is a strain of epizootic hemorrhagic disease virus 2 that belongs to the genus Orbivirus of the family Reoviridae. IBAV replication is suppressed by the inhibition of ATG, and since mTORC1 is a key regulator of ATG, Onishi et al. (2019) examined if mTORC1 inhibition by amino acid starvation or mTOR inhibitors (Torin 1 and Rapamycin) affects IBAV replication. IBAV replication was enhanced after amino acid starvation, but not after treatment with mTOR inhibitors, during the early stages of viral infection (0–1 hpi). Inhibition of mTORC1 by amino acid starvation was reversible and thus restricted to 0–1 hpi, whereas mTOR inhibitors suppressed mTORC1 even after the 1-hr treatment, suggesting that mTORC1 suppression does not affect IBAV replication. To investigate the mechanism of enhanced IBAV replication by amino acid starvation, they examined the endocytic pathway, since IBAV utilizes acidification of endosomes as a trigger for viral replication. Amino acid starvation, but not mTOR inhibitors, induced acidification of lysosomes and inhibition of acidification by Bafilomycin A1 inhibited IBAV replication, suggesting that the inactivation of mTORC1 by amino acid starvation during the early stages of infection enhances acidification of lysosomes and CSs to augment IBAV replication.

ATG Reduces Mitochondria in Starvation

Starvation alters cellular physiology, and triggers signs of aging. Mitochondria are essential to the regulation of cellular bioenergetics and aging. Hibshman et al. (2018) determined if mitochondria exhibit signs of aging and whether QC mechanisms regulate mitochondrial physiology during starvation. They described the effects of starvation on mitochondria in the first and third larval stages of the nematode *C. elegans*. When starved, the larvae enter developmental arrest. The researchers observed the fragmentation of the mitochondrial network, a reduction in the mtDNA copy number, and DNA damage during starvation-induced developmental arrest involving CBMP. The mitochondrial function was compromised by starvation. The starved worms had lower basal, maximal, and ATP-linked respiration, consistent with reduced MQC and IMD similar to mitochondrial phenotypes during aging. Using pharmacological and genetic approaches, worms deficient of CP/ATG were short-lived during starvation and recovered poorly from starvation, indicating sensitivity to nutrient stress. ATG mutants unc-51/Atg1 and atg-18/Atg18 maintained higher mtDNA content than wild-type worms during starvation, suggesting that CP/ATG promotes mitochondrial degradation involving CBMP during starvation. The unc-51 mutants also had a reduced O_2 consumption rate during starvation, suggesting the contribution of CP/ATG to reduced mitochondrial function. However, mutations in genes involved in mitochondrial fission and fusion as well as CP of damaged mitochondria did not affect mitochondrial content during starvation, indicating the influence of starvation on mitochondrial physiology with organismal consequences, and that these physiological effects were influenced by CP/ATG.

p62-Mediated ATG in 3T3-L1 Pre-adipocytes

Previous studies have shown that an organism's nutritional status changes the protein levels of the insulin receptor substrate 1 (IRS-1) in a tissue-specific manner. Igawa et al. (2019) investigated how IRS-1 protein levels change depending on the nutritional status of 3T3-L1 preadipocytes. 3T3-L1 pre-adipocytes were treated with a glucose-, amino acid- and serum-free medium for starvation. The levels of IRS-1, but not those of the insulin receptor and protein kinase B, decreased when starvation activated ATG. The inhibition of ATG by CQ or ATG-related 7 (Atg7) RNA interference counteracted the starvation-induced decrease in IRS-1. The Atg7 knockdown increased the insulin-stimulated phosphorylation of the protein kinase B. Furthermore, p62 co-localized with IRS-1, and p62 knockdown counteracted the starvation-induced degradation of IRS-1, indicating that ATG through p62 regulates IRS-1 protein levels in response to nutritional deficiency. This suggested that CP/ATG might function as an energy depletion-sensing machinery that modulates insulin signal transduction.

Ribose-Functionalized NAD$^+$ for Poly-ADP-Ribosylation

Nicotinamide adenine dinucleotide (NAD$^+$)-dependent ADP-ribosylation plays an important role in physiology and pathophysiology. Zhang et al. (2019b) studied the synthesis of NAD$^+$ analogs with ribose functionalized by terminal alkyne and azido groups. Azido substitution at 3′-OH of nicotinamide riboside enabled the enzymatic synthesis of an NAD$^+$ analogue with high efficiency and yields. The 3′-azido NAD$^+$ exhibited high activity and specificity for protein PARylation catalyzed by PARP1 and PARP2. The poly-ADP-ribose polymers that were derived showed an increased resistance to poly (ADP-ribose) glycohydrolase-mediated degradation, which led to the enhanced labeling of protein PARylation by 3′-azido NAD$^+$ and facilitated the direct visualization and labeling of the mitochondrial protein PARylation. Thus, 3′-azido NAD$^+$ provided an important tool for studying cellular PARylation.

ATP Hydrolysis by Complex V for Clinical Theranostics

ATP synthase, the mitochondrial complex V, plays a major role in bioenergetics and its defects lead to severe diseases such as muscular hypotonia, hypertrophic cardiomyopathy, psychomotor delay, encephalopathy, peripheral neuropathy, lactic acidosis, 3-methylglutaconic aciduria, and clinical syndromes including neuropathy, ataxia, and retinitis pigmentosa (NARP), and maternally-inherited Leigh's syndrome (MILS). Lack of a consensual protocol for the assay of complex V activity explains the under-representation of a complex V defect among mitochondrial diseases. Haraux and Lambes (2019) elaborated a fast, simple, and reliable method to evaluate complex V capacity in samples relevant to clinical theranostics. Using homogenates from four murine organs, they tested do-decylmaltoside, stability, linearity with protein amount, sensitivity to Oligomycin and to exogenous inhibitory factor 1 (IF1), influence of freezing, and the impact of mitochondrial purification. They obtained similar complex V specific activities from fresh and frozen organs. Similar inhibition by Oligomycin and exogenous IF1 demonstrated the coupling between F1 and F0 domains. A complex V catalytic turnover rate, as measured in preparations solubilized in detergent using immune-titration and activity measurements, was >3X higher in extracts from the brain or muscle than in extracts from the heart or liver, suggesting post-translational modifications. Measurement of respiratory activities showed slightly different complex II/complex V ratio in the four organs. In contrast, the complex I/complex V ratio differed in the brain as compared to other organs because of a high complex I activity in brain. Mitochondrial purification preserved these ratios, except for the brain where selective degradation of complex I occurred. Therefore, mitochondrial purification could introduce a biased enzymatic evaluation, suggesting that a reliable assay of complex V activity is possible with small samples from frozen biopsies.

ATG in Alcohol-Induced Liver Injury

Excessive alcohol consumption induces intestinal dysbiosis of the gut microbiome and reduces epithelial integrity, leading to portal circulation-mediated translocation of gut-derived microbial products, such as LPS, to the liver, where these induce TLR4 and initiate hepatic inflammation to promote alcoholic liver disease (ALD). Liang et al. (2019) used WT and myeloid cell-specific *ATG-related 7* (*Atg7*) knockout (*Atg7*$^{\Delta Mye}$) mice to find that chronic ethanol feeding for six weeks plus an LPS injection enhances the serum ALT and IL-1β levels and augments hepatic C-C motif chemokine ligand 5 (CCL5) and C-X-C motif chemokine ligand 10 (CXCL10) expression in WT mice, a phenotype that was further exacerbated in *Atg7*$^{\Delta Mye}$ mice. *Atg7*$^{\Delta Mye}$ macrophages exhibited defective mitochondrial respiration and elevated ROS and inflammasome activation. Compared with WT cells, *Atg7*$^{\Delta Mye}$ macrophages also had increased abundance and nuclear translocation of interferon regulatory factor 1 (IRF1) after LPS stimulation. LPS induced co-localization of the IRF1 with the ATG adaptor p62 and the autophagosome, resulting in IRF1 degradation. However, upon p62 silencing or Atg7 deletion, IRF1 accumulated in ATG-deficient macrophages and translocated into the nucleus, where it induced CCL5 and CXCL10 expression. This indicated that macrophage ATG protects in ALD by promoting IRF1 degradation and the removal of CBs participating in defective CP and CBMP, thus limiting macrophage activation and inflammation.

Cyanidin and Quercetin

Rafiei et al. (2019) reported that in HepG2 hepatocytes, treatment with Quercetin, Cyanidin, or their phenolic breakdown/digestion products (protocatechuic acid, 2,4,6-trihydroxybenzaldehyde, and caffeic acid), starting 2 hrs prior to oleic acid for 24 hrs, protected against increases in the intracellular lipid and ROS and decreased $\Delta\Psi$. Cyanidin or the phenolic products also protected against decreased mitochondrial content. After pre-incubation for only 1 hr and their removal prior to oleic acid, only the phenolic products protected against decreased mitochondrial content. Without adding oleic acid, only protocatechuic acid and caffeic acid increased mitochondrial content, suggesting that the phenolic breakdown/digestion products of Cyanidin and Quercetin confer cytoprotection.

Methionine Adenosyltransferase α1

Methionine adenosyltransferase α1 (MATα1, encoded by MAT1A) is responsible for hepatic biosynthesis of S-adenosyl methionine, the principal methyl donor. MATα1 also acta as a transcriptional cofactor by interacting and influencing the activity of transcription factors. Mat1a knockout (KO) mice have increased levels of CYP2E1. Murray et al. (2019) identified binding partners of MATα1 and elucidated how MATα1 regulates CYP2E1 expression. They identified binding partners of MATα1 by co-immunoprecipitation (co-IP) and mass spectrometry. The interacting proteins were confirmed by co-immunoprecipitation (co-IP), using recombinant proteins, liver lysates, and mitochondria. ALD samples were used to confirm the relevance of these findings. MATα1 negatively regulated CYP2E1 at mRNA and protein levels, with the latter being the dominant mechanism. MATα1 interacted with many proteins but with a predominance of mitochondrial proteins including CYP2E1. MATα1 was present in the mitochondrial matrix of hepatocytes. Mat1a KO hepatocytes had reduced $\Delta\Psi$ and higher ROS, both of which were normalized when MAT1A was overexpressed. In addition, KO hepatocytes were sensitized to ethanol and TNFα-induced mitochondrial dysfunction. The interaction of MATα1 with CYP2E1 was direct, and facilitated CYP2E1 methylation at R379, leading to its degradation through the proteosomal pathway. Mat1a KO livers had a reduced methylated/total CYP2E1 ratio. MATα1's influence on mitochondrial function was mediated by its effect on CYP2E1 expression. Patients with ALD had reduced MATα1 and a methylated/total CYP2E1 ratio. These findings highlighted the crucial role of MATα1 in regulating mitochondrial function by suppressing CYP2E1 expression.

PI3K/mTOR in HCC Cancer Cells

Sheng et al. (2019) explored the role of mitochondrial-lysosomal crosstalk in the Cisplatin resistance of HCC cells. Huh7 and HepG2 cells were subjected to different treatments. Flow cytometry was conducted to detect ROS, mitochondrial mass, lysosomal function, $\Delta\Psi$, and apoptosis. The O_2 consumption rate was measured to evaluate mitochondrial function. Cisplatin activated CP and lysosomal biogenesis, resulting in crosstalk between mitochondria and lysosomes and Cisplatin resistance in HCC cells. A combination of Cisplatin with the PI3K/mTOR inhibitor PKI-402 induced LMP. This effect changed the role of the lysosome from a protective one to that of a cell-death promoter, destroying the mitochondrial-lysosomal crosstalk and enhancing the sensitivity of HCC cells to Cisplatin.

PI3K Regulates Nuclear Receptor PPARα

Iershov et al. (2019) showed that the liver-specific inactivation of Vps15, the essential regulatory subunit of the class 3 PI3K, elicits mitochondrial depletion and failure to oxidize fatty acids. The transcriptional activity of PPARα, a nuclear receptor orchestrating lipid catabolism, is blunted in Vps15-deficient livers. The PPARα repressors, histone deacetylase 3 (Hdac3), and nuclear receptor co-repressor 1 (NCoR1) accumulated in Vps15-deficient livers due to defective ATG. The activation of PPARα or the inhibition of Hdac3 restored MB and lipid oxidation in Vps15-deficient hepatocytes, suggesting the significance of class 3 PI3K and ATG in the transcriptional regulation of mitochondrial metabolism.

ER-associated Degradation Inhibitor SVIP

The ER of cancer cells adapts to the enhanced proteotoxic stress associated with the accumulation of unfolded, misfolded, and transformation-associated proteins. One way by which tumors thrive in the context of ERS is by promoting ER-associated degradation (ERAD). Llinàs-Arias et al. (2019) showed that the small p97/VCP interacting protein (SVIP), an endogenous inhibitor of ERAD, undergoes DNA hyper-methylation-associated silencing in tumorigenesis to achieve this goal. SVIP exhibited tumor suppressor features and its recovery was associated with increased ERS and growth inhibition. Proteomic and metabolomic analyses showed that cancer cells with the epigenetic loss of SVIP are depleted in mitochondrial enzymes and oxidative respiration activity. This phenotype was reverted upon SVIP restoration. The dependence of SVIP hyper-methylated cancer cells on aerobic glycolysis and glucose was also associated with sensitivity to an inhibitor of the glucose transporter, GLUT1. This could be relevant to the management of tumors carrying SVIP epigenetic loss, because these occur in high-risk patients who manifest poor clinical prognosis. This study provided insights into how epigenetics deal with ERS and SVIP epigenetic loss in cancer which may be amenable to therapies that target glucose transporters.

MAP1B-LC1

In fed cells, syntaxin 17 (Stx17) is associated with microtubules at the ER-mitochondria interface and promotes mitochondrial fission by determining the localization and function of the mitochondrial fission factor Drp-1. Upon starvation, Stx17 dissociates from microtubules and Drp-1, and binds to Atg14L, a subunit of the PI3K complex, to facilitate PI3-phosphate production and thereby, autophagosome (more specifically, CPS) formation. Arasaki et al. (2018) identified MAP1B-LC1 (microtubule-associated protein 1B-light chain 1) as a regulator of Stx17 function. Depletion of MAP1B-LC1 caused Stx17-dependent autophagosome accumulation even under nutrient-rich conditions, whereas its overexpression blocked starvation-induced autophagosome formation. MAP1B-LC1 linked microtubules and Stx17 in fed cells, and starvation caused the de-phosphorylation of MAP1B-LC1 at Thr217, allowing Stx17 to dissociate from MAP1B-LC1 and bind to Atg14L. These results revealed the mechanism by which Stx17 changes its binding partners in response to the organism's nutritional status.

ATG-Deficient NSCLC Cells in Nutrient Deprivation

MacroATG/ATG inhibition under stress conditions is associated with increased cell death. Allavena et al. (2018) found that under nutrient limitation, activation of CASP8/caspase-8 was increased in ATG-deficient lung cancer cells, which precedes mitochondria outer membrane permeabilization (MOMP), CYCS/Cyt-C release, and the activation of CASP9/caspase-9, indicating that the activation of CASP8 is a primary event in that initiates apoptosis and reduces the clonogenic survival of ATG-deficient cells. Starvation leads to the suppression of CFLAR proteo-synthesis and accumulation of CASP8 in SQSTM1 puncta. The overexpression of CFLARs reduced CASP8 activation and apoptosis during starvation, while its silencing promoted the activation of CASP8 and apoptosis in ATG-deficient U1810 lung cancer cells even under nutrient-rich conditions. Similar to starvation, the inhibition of protein translation led to the efficient activation of CASP8 and cell death in ATG-deficient lung cancer cells, indicating that suppressed translation leads to the activation of CASP8-dependent apoptosis in ATG-deficient NSCLC cells during nutrient limitation and that targeting translational machinery can be beneficial for the elimination of ATG-deficient cells via the CASP8-dependent apoptotic pathway.

Nutrient-Driven O-GlcNAc in Proteostasis

Proteostasis is essential in the mammalian brain where post-mitotic cells function for decades to maintain synaptic contacts and memory. The brain is dependent on glucose and other metabolites for proper functioning. Akan et al. (2018) investigated how the nutrient-sensitive nucleocytoplasmic post-translational modification O-linked N-acetylglucosamine (O-GlcNAc) regulates protein homeostasis. The O-GlcNAc modification is abundant in the mammalian brain and has been linked to proteopathies, including NDDs such as AD, PD, and HD. *C. elegans*, *Drosophila*, and mouse models harboring O-GlcNAc transferase- and O-GlcNAcase-knockout alleles have helped define the role O-GlcNAc plays in the development and age-associated NDDs. These enzymes add and remove the single monosaccharide from the protein serine and threonine residues, respectively. Blocking O-GlcNAc cycling is detrimental to brain development and interferes with neurogenesis, neural migration, and proteostasis. Findings in the *C. elegans* and *Drosophila* model indicate that the turnover of O-GlcNAc is critical for maintaining levels of transcriptional regulators for neurodevelopment. In addition, CP/ATG pathways and proteasomal degradation depend on a transcriptional network that is reliant on O-GlcNAc cycling. Like the QC system in the ER which uses a 'mannose timer' to monitor protein folding, the cytoplasmic proteostasis relied on an 'O-GlcNAc timer' to regulate the lifetime fate of nuclear and cytoplasmic proteins. O-GlcNAc-dependent developmental alterations impact metabolism and the growth of the developing mouse embryo and persist into adulthood. Hence, brain-selective knockout mouse models are an important tool for understanding the role of O-GlcNAc in the physiology of the brain and its susceptibility to NDDs.

CONCLUSION

Parenteral nutrition was recommended for critically ill children. Starvation-induced Atg5-dependent CP degradation of α-Syn occurs through HMGB1. Deprivation of serum and nutrients increased ATG in the intervertebral disc annulus fibrosus cells. CP/ATG was modulated by mtDNA mutation, diseases, and nutrients. Fructose feeding during the post-absorptive state altered the body composition and spared nitrogen in protein-energy-restricted old rats while non-suckling starvation of neonatal mice promoted primordial follicular development through ovarian ATG induction. Cubic membrane formation supported the cell survival of the amoeba, Chaos, during starvation whereas vitamin D deficiency ameliorated Crohn's disease. Inhibition of aldose reductase stimulated starvation-induced CP and eliminated aldehyde protein adducts. GH augmented CP in the liver to maintain glucose levels in starved mice. Tumor products and chemotherapy-induced catabolism of muscle and adipose tissues proved barriers to cancer nutrition therapy. Maternal Quercetin intake during lactation attenuated renal inflammation and modulated ATG in high-fructose-fed female rat offspring exposed to maternal malnutrition. Mucosal proteomes revealed reduced energy metabolism and protein synthesis but enhanced ATG during anorexia-induced malnutrition in mice. BmCalpains were involved in CP and apoptosis during metamorphosis and starvation in Bombyx mori. Inhibition of aldose reductase stimulated starvation-induced ATG to eliminate aldehyde protein adducts in *Bombyx mori*. The skeletal muscles of hibernating bears exhibited minimal atrophy and phenotype shifting despite prolonged physical inactivity and starvation in hibernating bears via CP regulation. A sestrin-like protein was detected from Dictyostelium discoideum ATG during nutritional stress. Glucose starvation augmented resistance to Metformin through the elevation of MDR protein-1. Amino acid starvation accelerated the replication of the Ibaraki virus. ATG reduced the mitochondrial content during starvation in *C. elegans*, whereas p62-mediated ATG affected the nutrition-dependent insulin receptor substrate 1 in 3T3-L1 pre-adipocytes. A ribose-functionalized NAD^+ was synthesized to evaluate poly-ADP-ribosylation of proteins implicated in CP/ATG. Suppressed translation was involved in caspase 8-dependent apoptosis in ATG-deficient NSCLC cells during nutritional stress. In addition, nutrient-driven O-GlcNAc was implicated in proteostasis, CP, and neurodegeneration.

REFERENCES

Akan, I., S.O.-V. Stichelen, M.R. Bond and J.A. Hanover. 2018. Nutrient-driven O-GlcNAc in proteostasis and neurodegeneration. J Neurochem 144: 7–34.

Allavena, G., F. Cuomo, G. Baumgartner and T. Bele. 2018. Suppressed translation as a mechanism of initiation of CASP8 (caspase 8)-dependent apoptosis in ATG-deficient NSCLC cells under nutrient limitation. Autophagy. 14: 252–268.

Arasaki, K., H. Nagashima, Y. Kurosawa, H. Kimura, et al. 2018. MAP1B-LC1 prevents autophagosome formation by linking syntaxin 17 to microtubules. EMBO Rep 19(8): e45584.

Barve, G., P. Sanyal and R. Manjithaya. 2018. Septin localization and function during autophagy. Curr Genet 64: 1037–1041.

Chiodi, I., G. Picco, C. Martino and C. Mondello. 2019. Cellular response to glutamine and/or glucose deprivation in in vitro transformed human fibroblasts. Oncol Rep 41: 3555–3564.

Chong, K., Z.A. Almsherqi, H.M. Shen and Y. Deng. 2018. Cubic membrane formation supports cell survival of amoeba Chaos under starvation-induced stress. Protoplasma 255: 517–525.

Dardevet, D., L. Mosoni, J. David and S. Polakof. 2018. Fructose feeding during the postabsorptive state alters body composition and spares nitrogen in protein-energy-restricted old rats. J Nutr 148: 40–48.

Fang, F., X. Shi, M.S. Brown, J.L. Goldstein, et al. 2019. Growth hormone acts on liver to stimulate autophagy, support glucose production, and preserve blood glucose in chronically starved mice. PNAS 116: 7449–7454.

Gournas, C., S. Gkionis, M. Carquin, L. Twyffels, et al. 2018. Conformation-dependent partitioning of yeast nutrient transporters into starvation-protective membrane domains. Proc Natl Acad Sci U S A. 115: E3145–E3154.

Guan, Y., Y. Li, G. Zhao and Y. Li. 2018. HMGB1 promotes the starvation-induced autophagic degradation of α-Syn in SH-SY5Y cells Atg5-dependently. Life Sci 202: 1–10.

Guillaume, J.D., S.L. Celano, K.R. Martin and J.P. MacKeigan. 2019. Determining the impact of metabolic nutrients on autophagy. *In*: S.M. Fendt and S. Lunt (eds), Metabolic Signaling. Methods in Molecular Biology, Vol 1862. Humana Press, New York, NY. pp. 151–162.

Haraux, F. and A. Lombès. 2019. Kinetic analysis of ATP hydrolysis by complex V in four murine tissues: Towards an assay suitable for clinical diagnosis. PLoS One 14: e0221886.

Hibshman, J.D., T.C. Leuthner, C. Shoben, D.F. Mello, et al. 2018. Nonselective autophagy reduces mitochondrial content during starvation in *Caenorhabditis elegans*. Am J Physiol Cell Physiol 315(6): C781–C792.

Hui-Yu, Yi., W.Y. Yang., W.M. Wu and X.X. Li, et al. 2018. BmCalpains are involved in autophagy and apoptosis during metamorphosis and after starvation in *Bombyx mori*. Insect Science 25: 379–388.

Hwang, S.H., M.C. Kim, S. Ji, Y. Yang, et al.. 2019. Glucose starvation induces resistance to Metformin through the elevation of mitochondrial multidrug resistance protein 1. Cancer Sci 110: 1256–1267.

Iershov, A., I. Nemazanyy, C. Alkhoury, M. Girard, et al. 2019. The class 3 PI3K coordinates ATG and mitochondrial lipid catabolism by controlling nuclear receptor PPARα. Nat Commun 10: 1566.

Igawa, H., A. Kikuchi, H. Misu, K.A. Ishii, et al. 2019. p62-mediated ATG affects nutrition-dependent insulin receptor substrate 1 dynamics in 3T3-L1 preadipocytes. J Diabetes Invest 10: 32–42.

Jacobs, A., I. Verlinden, I. Vanhorebeek, G. Van den Berghe. 2019. Early supplemental parenteral nutrition in critically III children: An Update. J Clin Med Jun 8(6): 830.

Li, XX, Y. Liu, J, Luo, Z-D. Huang, et al. 2019. Vitamin D deficiency associated with Crohn's disease and ulcerative colitis: A meta-analysis of 55 observational studies. J Transl Med 17(1): 323.

Liang, S., Z. Zhong, S.Y. Kim, R. Uchiyama, et al. 2019. Murine macrophage autophagy protects against alcohol-induced liver injury by degrading interferon regulatory factor 1 (IRF1) and removing damaged mitochondria. J Biol Chem 294: 12359–12369.

Llinàs-Arias, P., M. Rosselló-Tortella, P. López-Serra, M. Pérez-Salvia, et al. 2019. Epigenetic loss of the endoplasmic reticulum-associated degradation inhibitor SVIP induces cancer cell metabolic reprogramming. JCI Insight 5(8): e125888.

Medeiros, T.C., R.L. Thomas, R. Ghillebert and M. Graef. 2018. Autophagy balances mtDNA synthesis and degradation by DNA polymerase POLG during starvation. J Cell Biol 217: 1601–1611.

Medeiros, T.C. and M. Graef. 2019. Autophagy determines mtDNA copy number dynamics during starvation. Autophagy 15(1): 178–179.

Merker, M., F. Gomes, Z. Stanga and P. Schuetz. 2019. Evidence-based nutrition for the malnourished, hospitalised patient: One bite at a time. Swiss Med Wkly 149: w20112.

Miyazaki, M., M. Shimozuru and T. Tsubota. 2019. Skeletal muscles of hibernating black bears show minimal atrophy and phenotype shifting despite prolonged physical inactivity and starvation. PLoS One 14(4): e0215489.

Murray, B., H. Peng, L. Barbier-Torres, A.E, Robinson, et al. 2019. Methionine adenosyltransferase α1 is targeted to the mitochondrial matrix and interacts with cytochrome P450 2E1 to lower its expression. Hepatology 70: 2018–2034.

Nobis, S., N. Achamrah, A. Goichon, C. L'Huillier, et al. 2018. Colonic mucosal proteome signature reveals reduced energy metabolism and protein synthesis but activated autophagy during anorexia – induced malnutrition in mice. Proteomics 18: e1700395.

Onishi, K., S. Shibutani, N. Goto, Y. Maeda, et al. 2019. Amino acid starvation accelerates replication of Ibaraki virus. Virus Res 260: 94–101.

Rafia, S. and S. Saran. 2019. Sestrin-like protein from Dic*tyostelium discoideum* is involved in autophagy under starvation stress. Microbiol Res 220: 61–71.

Rafiei, H., K. Omidian and B. Bandy. 2019. Phenolic breakdown products of cyanidin and quercetin contribute to protection against mitochondrial impairment and reactive oxygen species generation in an *in vitro* model of hepatocyte steatosis. J Agric Food Chem 67: 6241–6247.

Sato, S., T. Norikura and Y. Mukai. 2019. Maternal quercetin intake during lactation attenuates renal inflammation and modulates autophagy flux in high-fructose-diet-fed female rat offspring exposed to maternal malnutrition. Food Funct 10: 5018–5031.

Schiessel, D.L. and V.E. Baracos. 2018. Barriers to cancer nutrition therapy: Excess catabolism of muscle and adipose tissues induced by tumour products and chemotherapy. Proc Nutr Soc 77: 394–402.

Sharma, S., W. Selvamurthy and K. Dakshinamurti. 1993. Effect of environmental neurotoxins in the developing brain. Biometereology 2: 447-455.

Sharma, S., C. Moon, A. Khogali, A. Haidous, et al. 2013. Biomarkers in Parkinson's disease. Neurochem Int 63(3): 201–229.

Sheng, J., L. Shen, L. Sun, X. Zhang, et al. 2019. Inhibition of PI3K/mTOR increased the sensitivity of hepatocellular carcinoma cells to cisplatin via interference with mitochondrial-lysosomal crosstalk. Cell Prolif 52: e12609.

Watanabe, R. and N. Kimura. 2018. Non-suckling starvation of neonatal mice promotes primordial follicle formation with activation of ovarian autophagy. J Reprod Dev 64: 89–94.

White, J.H. 2018. Vitamin D deficiency and the pathogenesis of Crohn's disease. J Steroid Biochem Mol Biol 175: 23–28.

Yang, X., R. Zhang, K. Nakahira and Z. Gu. 2019. Mitochondrial DNA mutation, diseases, and nutrient-regulated mitophagy. Annu Rev Nutr 39: 201–226.

Yi, H.Y., W.Y. Yang, W.M. Wu, X.X. Li, et al. 2018. BmCalpains are involved in autophagy and apoptosis during metamorphosis and after starvation in *Bombyx mori*. Insect Sci 25(3): 379–388.

Yurube, T., W.J. Buchser, H.J. Moon, R.A. Hartman, et al. 2019. Serum and nutrient deprivation increase autophagic flux in intervertebral disc annulus fibrosus cells: an in vitro experimental study. Eur Spine J 28: 993–1004.

Zhang, D., A. Bhatnagar and S.P. Baba. 2019a. Inhibition of aldol reductase activity stimulates starvation induced autophagy and clears aldehyde protein adducts. Chem. Bio. Interqct. 306: 104–109.

Zhang, X.-N., Q. Chang, J. Chen, A.T. Lam, et al. 2019b. A ribose-functionalized NAD^+ with unexpected high activity and selectivity for protein-ADP-ribosylation. Nat. Commun. 10: 4196.

10

Charnolophagy in Diet Restriction

INTRODUCTION

Traditionally, food deprivation and calorie restriction (CR) have been considered to slow down aging and increase longevity. Fasting on special festivals and auspicious occasions particularly among women is commonly practiced in India. It is regarded as the simple, efficient, and economical way to purify the body, brain, and mind and is common in religious places to accomplish peace, calmness, eternal happiness, and achieve God's blessings. CR has been recognized as one of the most important strategies and plays a crucial role in aiding the anti-aging benefits of CP/ATG. There is now evidence to suggest that dietary restriction (DR) can increase the human lifespan. Recent studies demonstrated the beneficial effects of intermittent fasting due to CP induction. Protein restriction plays a crucial role in the cancer prognosis by modulating CBMP. Since CP inhibition attenuates the anti-aging effects of CR, it plays an important role in CR-mediated longevity.

This chapter highlights that CR augments CP and CS exocytosis as a mechanism of IMD and ICD for MQC and NCF to extend human life-span.

Nutrition and Longevity

Genetic, environmental, and lifestyle factors determine the lifespan of an organism. Nutrition is a key component affecting our health. Rodent models have shown that nutrition has the potential to increase lifespan. Ekmekcioglu (2019) discussed the important nutritional components and diets which have been associated with longevity through mTor, IGF-1, and ATG signaling. CR without malnutrition, methionine restriction, lower protein intake, and Spermidine are life-extending factors in rodent models. Certain healthy foods, which cause an increase in telomere length, and reduction in protein intake with lower IGF-1, are associated with contributing to longer lifespans. A high intake of whole grains, vegetables, fruits, and nuts is associated with a reduced risk of mortality whereas a high intake of processed red meat is related to mortality. Mediterranean and high-quality diets are associated with a reduced risk of mortality.

Intermittent Fasting

Recently, Stockman et al. (2018) reviewed the basic molecular mechanisms and potential benefits of intermittent fasting (IF) in animal models and clinical trials and highlighted that numerous variations of IF exist, and study protocols vary in their interpretations of this weight-loss trend. Most IF studies result in minimal weight loss and marginal improvements in metabolic biomarkers. Animal models have shown that IF reduces oxidative stress, improves cognition, and prolongs the lifespan. IF has anti-inflammatory effects, promotes CP, and benefits the gut microbiome. CR and IF resulted in weight loss and improved insulin sensitivity, suggesting that it may also be a promising weight-loss strategy.

Protein Restriction and Cancer

Protein restriction without malnutrition is currently an effective strategy to prevent diseases and promote health span in organisms ranging from yeast to human. Yin et al. (2018) reported that a low protein diet was associated with lowered incidence and mortality risk of cancers in humans. In murine models, protein restriction inhibited tumor growth via the mTOR signaling pathway. IGF-1, amino acid metabolic programing, FGF21, and CP may also serve as mechanisms of protein-restriction-mediated cancer prevention. Hence, dietary intervention aimed at reducing protein intake can be beneficial and may be widely adopted and effective in preventing and treating cancers because DR causes CBMP in cancer cells to inhibit tumor growth.

AMPK Signaling in Compensatory Growth

Ballester et al. (2018) determined changes in the pig skeletal-muscle transcriptome during the compensatory growth following a feed restriction period. A RNA-Seq experiment was performed on 24 female pigs. Half of the animals received either a restricted (RE) or *ad libitum* (AL) diet during the first fattening period (60–125 days of age). After that, all gilts were fed *ad libitum* for a further ~30 days until the age of ~155 days, when they were sacrificed and gluteus medius muscle samples were harvested to perform RNA-Seq analyses and fat content. During the period following food restriction, RE animals that were fed *ad libitum* again displayed compensatory growth, better feed conversion rate, and more s.c. fat than the AL-fed animals. Animals were sacrificed in the phase of accelerated growth, when RE animals had not completely compensated the performance of the AL group, exhibiting lower live and carcass weights. RE gilts showed a higher content of PUFA during the compensatory growth phase. The comparison of RE and AL expression identified 86 differentially expressed (DE) genes. A functional categorization of DE genes identified AMPK signaling as the canonical pathway. This kinase plays a key role in the maintenance of energy homeostasis and ATG induction. Among the DE genes identified as components of the AMPK-signaling pathway, 5 out of 6 genes were downregulated in RE pigs. Animals fed again after a restriction period exhibited a less oxidative metabolic profile and catabolic processes in the muscles than animals fed ad libitum. The downregulation of ATG observed in the skeletal muscle of pigs undergoing compensatory growth may constitute a mechanism to increase muscle mass thus ensuring an accelerated growth rate, indicating that the downregulation of AMPK signaling plays an important role in compensatory growth in pigs.

Sesamin Extends Lifespan

Sesamin, a polyphenolic compound found in sesame seeds confer health benefits. Nakatani et al. (2018) reported that sesamin increases the lifespan of *C. elegans*. Starting from 3 days of age, *C. elegans* were fed a standard diet alone or supplemented with sesamin. A genome array was used to perform expression analysis. Differentially expressed genes were validated using PCR. Mutant or RNAi-treated animals were fed sesamin, and the lifespan was determined to identify genes involved in the longevity. The microarray analysis revealed that ER unfolded protein-response-related genes, which showed decreased expression in SIR-2.1/Sirtuin 1 (SIRT1) overexpression; these were downregulated in animals supplemented with sesamin. Sesamin failed to extend the lifespan of sir-2.1 knockdown animals and of sir-2.1 loss-of-function mutants. It was also ineffective in bec-1 RNAi-treated animals; a key regulator of CP, and is necessary for longevity induced by sir-2.1 overexpression. The heterozygotic mutation of daf-15, which encodes the TOR-binding partner Raptor, abolished the lifespan extension provided by sesamin. Sesamin did not prolong the lifespan of loss-of-function mutants of aak-2, which encodes the AMPK. Sesamin extended the lifespan of *C. elegans* through dietary restriction-related signaling pathways, involving SIRT1, TOR, and AMPK.

Fesetin as CRM in Aging

Recently, Singh et al. (2018) evaluated the neuroprotective role of Fesetin, a caloric restriction mimetic (CRM), in D-galactose (D-gal)-induced aging models of rats. Fesetin was supplemented (15 mg/kg b.w., orally) to the diet of young, D-gal-induced aged (D-gal 500 mg/kg b.w s.c.) and naturally aged rats for 6 weeks. Standard protocols were employed to measure pro-oxidants, antioxidants, and $\Delta\Psi$ in brain tissues. Gene-expression analysis with RT-PCR was performed to assess the CP, neuronal, aging, as well as inflammatory biomarkers. They also evaluated apoptosis as well as synaptosomal membrane-bound ion transporter activities in brain tissues. Fesetin decreased pro-oxidants and increased antioxidants. Fesetin also ameliorated $\Delta\Psi$, synaptosomal membrane-bound ion transporters, and apoptosis in aging rat brains. Fesetin upregulated the expression of CP genes (Atg-3 and Beclin-1), sirtuin-1 and neuronal markers (NSE and Ngb), and downregulated the expression of inflammatory (IL-1β and TNF-α) and Sirt-2 genes, respectively in the aging brain, suggesting that its supplementation may provide neuroprotection in aging-induced oxidative stress, apoptotic cell death, neuroinflammation, and neurodegeneration by augmenting CP and inhibiting CBMP as a mechanism of IMD, MQC, and ICD.

Calorie Restriction Mimetics (CRMs) as Novel CPTs

The increase in life expectancy has boosted the incidence of age-related pathologies beyond social and economic sustainability. Hence, there is an urgent need for interventions that revert or prevent age-associated deterioration involving CBMP. The permanent or periodic reduction of calorie intake without malnutrition (CR and fasting) may extend health span. However, life-long compliance with these regimens is difficult, which has promoted the emergence of CRMs. Madeo et al. (2019) defined CRMs as compounds that trigger the protective pathways of CR by CP induction, via a reduction in protein acetylation. They described the molecular, cellular, and organismal effects of CRMs and envisaged that CRMs as novel CPTs will become part of the pharmacological intervention in aging and age-related CVDs, NDDs, and MDR malignancies.

Diet and Testicular Development

Energy balance is an important feature for spermatogenesis in the testis. Recently, Pang et al. (2018) highlighted that the AMPK is a sensor of MB, and as a mediator between gonadal function and energy balance. They determined the physiological effects of AMPK on testicular development in feed-energy-restricted and feed-energy-compensated prepubertal rams. Lambs had restricted feeding for two months and compensatory feeding for another three months. Feed levels were 100% (control), 15%, and 30%, for energy restriction (ER) diets, respectively. The lambs fed the 30% ER diet had lower testicular weight and spermatids number in the seminiferous tubules, but there were no differences between control and 15% ER groups. 15% ER and 30% ER diets induced testis CP and apoptosis through activating the AMPK-ULK1(ULK1, Unc-51 like CP-activating kinase) signal pathway with increased Beclin-1 and LC3-II/LC3-I ratio, upregulated the ratio of pro-apoptotic Bcl-2-associated X protein (BAX) and anti-apoptotic Bcl-2, as well as activated AMPK, phosphorylated AMPK(p-AMPK), and ULK1. Furthermore, a compensation of these parameters occurred when the lambs were fed again with normal energy requirements after restriction, suggesting that dietary energy levels influence testicular development through CP and apoptosis mediated by the AMPK-ULK1 signal pathway, and the important role AMPK plays in testicular homeostasis.

Perinatal CR Regulates Hepatic ATG

Intrauterine growth restriction leads to obesity, CVDs, and NAFLD/NASH. Animal models have shown that combined intrauterine and early postnatal CR (IPCR) ameliorates these sequelae in adult life. Recently, Devarajan et al. (2018) hypothesized that IPCR could regulate ATG in the liver of male rat offspring. At birth (d1) and on day 21 (p21) of life, IPCR male rat offspring had decreased hepatic ATG in all three stages of development: *initiation, elongation, and maturation*. However, upon receiving a normal diet ad-lib throughout adulthood, aged IPCR rats (day 450 of life (p450)), had increased hepatic ATG, in direct contrast to what was seen in their early life. The decreased ATG at d21 induced accumulation of ubiquitinated proteins and lipid peroxidative products, whereas the increased ATG in late life had the opposite effect. Oxidized lipids were unchanged at d1 by IPCR indicating that decreased ATG precedes oxidative stress in early life. When cellular signaling pathways regulating ATG were examined, the AMPK, and not ERS pathway, was altered, suggesting that ATG is regulated through the AMPK-signaling pathway in IPCR rats. This study revealed that the perinatal nutritional status establishes a sensitive memory that enhances hepatic ATG in late life, a process that acts as a protective mechanism to limited nutrition.

Stem Cell Rejuvenation by CR

Stem cells being pluripotent in nature can differentiate into a wide array of specific cells and divide to produce new ones; but they may undergo aging by themselves. Recently, Bi et al. (2018) explored the molecular mechanisms on how CR induces appropriate ATG to restore the regenerative ability of aging stem cells. Aging has both quantitative and qualitative effects on stem cells, and could restrain them from replenishing into progenitor cells. ROS accumulated in the aging cells could not only block the cell cycle but also affect ATG by damaging the mitochondria to induce CBMP. ATG could eliminate redundant production of ROS in aging stem cells and maintain the proliferation by restraining the expression of p16^{INK4a}. Improving ATG could restore the regenerative ability of aging stem cells. Hence, it is important to maintain the appropriate ATG. CR retards the stem cell aging by a certain basic level of ATG, suggesting that it is an effective way to extend longevity in mammals because it regulates CP and attenuates CBMP.

Ketogenic Diet in PTZ-Kindled Seizures

The ketogenic diet (KD) ameliorates neuronal loss in seizure models. Wang et al. (2018) determined the role of ATG following seizure under KD. Pentylenetetrazol (PTZ)-kindled rats, which were fed a normal diet (ND) or KD, were pretreated with i.v. infusions of saline, ATG inducer Rapamycin (RAP), or inhibitor 3-MA. KD alleviated seizure severity and decreased the number of Fluoro-jade B (FJB)-positive cells in the hippocampus of kindled rats. These effects were abolished by the 3-MA pretreatment. The RAP pretreatment did not affect seizure severity, but decreased the number of FJB-positive cells in the ND group. KD decreased the percentage of damaged mitochondria implicated in impaired CP in the kindled group. Hippocampal Beclin-1 was increased by KD in the vehicle group. The ATG proteins Atg5 and Beclin-1, and the ratio of LC3-II to LC3-I in kindled KD-fed rats were higher, and the ATG substrate P62 was lower than those in the kindled ND-fed rats, indicating an increase in ATG following KD. Pretreatment with RAP increased LC3-II/LC3-I; and with 3-MA increased P62 in KD-fed rats. The mitochondrial Cyt-C was upregulated, cytosolic Cyt-C and cleaved caspase-3 were downregulated in KD-fed rats, indicating a decrease in mitochondrial apoptosis, and that KD activates ATG pathways and reduces brain injury during PTZ-kindled seizures via reduction in the mitochondrial Cyt-C release.

Aspirin as CRM Augments CP

CRMs are pharmacological agents that recapitulate the biochemical properties of CR, namely a global reduction of protein acetylation and the induction of CP. Generally, the capacity of cells and organisms to sustain, and to eventually adapt to, environmental and genetic insults declines with age. Because CP is regarded as one of the major determinants of cellular fitness *in vitro* and *in vivo*, interventions that aim at promoting CP may slow down aging and promote health span. CR without malnutrition, counteracts aging-associated features. Pietrocola et al. (2018) found that Aspirin and its active metabolite, salicylate, stimulate CP/ATG due to their inhibitory action on acetyltransferase EP300. The inhibition of EP300 resulted from a direct competition between salicylate and acetyl coenzyme A for binding to the catalytic domain of the enzyme. This common mode of action remained conserved across evolution as it accounts for the induction of ATG by Aspirin in mouse models and in the *C. elegans*, suggesting that Aspirin acts as a CRM.

Carbohydrate-restricted Diet

Recently, Wu et al. (2019) used senescence-accelerated prone mice (SAMP8) to examine the effects of a carbohydrate-restricted diet (CRD) on aging and skin senescence, to determine how long-term carbohydrate restriction affects the aging process. Three-week-old male SAMP8 mice were divided into three groups after one week of preliminary feeding: one was given a controlled diet, the other was given a high-fat diet (HFD), and the third was given a CRD. *Ad libitum* feeding was administered until the mice reached 50 weeks of age. Before the end of the test period, a grading test was used to evaluate visible aging in the mice. After the test period, serum and skin samples were obtained and submitted for analysis. There was significant progression of visible aging in the CRD group, as well as a decreased survival rate. The epidermis and dermis in the CRD group had become thinner. An increase in serum IL-6, aggravated skin senescence, inhibition of skin ATG, and activation of skin mTOR, suggests that CRD promotes skin senescence in senescence-accelerated mice.

Hematopoietic Stem Cells and Radiation Exposure

Karabulutoglu et al. (2019) discussed the prominence of dietary and metabolic regulators in maintaining hematopoietic stem cell (HSC) function, long-term self-renewal, and differentiation. Most adult stem cells are preserved in a quiescent, non-motile state *in vivo* which acts as a "protective state" for stem cells to reduce endogenous stress provoked by DNA replication and cellular respiration as well as environmental stress. The balance between quiescence, self-renewal, and differentiation is critical for supporting a functional blood system throughout the life of an organism. Ionizing radiations can trigger HSCs to proliferate and migrate through extramedullary tissues to expand their number and hematopoiesis. Deregulation of this balance plays a role in hematopoietic diseases including leukemia. Understanding the influence of diet, metabolism, and epigenetics on radiation-induced leukemogenesis may lead to the development of theranostic interventions to reduce the risk in the exposed population.

CONCLUSION

Treatment with Sesamin extended the lifespan of the *C. elegans* through DR-related signaling pathways. Fesetin also served as a CRM and as a neuro-protectant in aging. The effect of dietary regimens on sheep testicular development was associated with AMPK/ULK1/CP activation. Protein restriction in MDR malignancies conferred beneficial effects through CP induction, whereas, perinatal CR regulated the CP/ATG in and redox status of the liver, respectively. CR promoted stem cell rejuvenation and age retardation, whereas, a carbohydrate-restricted diet promoted skin senescence. Aspirin augmented CP and served as a CRM. The Ketogenic diet attenuated neuronal injury via CP/ATG induction. CP/ATG was induced in PTZ-kindled seizures in experimental rats whereas, CR improved CS-antioxidant interaction by regulating CP to sustain MQC and ICD for NCF and longevity.

REFERENCES

Ballester, M., M. Amills, O. González-Rodríguez, T.F. Cardoso, et al. 2018. Role of AMPK signalling pathway during compensatory growth in pigs. BMC Genomics 19: Article number 682.

Bi, S., H. Wang and W. Kuang. 2018. Stem cell rejuvenation and the role of autophagy in age retardation by caloric restriction: An update. Mech Ageing Dev 175: 46–54.

Devarajan, A., N.S. Rajasekaran, C. Valburg, E. Ganapathy, et al. 2018. Maternal perinatal calorie restriction temporally regulates the hepatic autophagy and redox status in male rat. Free Radic Biol Med 130: 592–600.

Ekmekcioglu, C. 2019. Nutrition and longevity – From mechanisms to uncertainties. Crit Rev Food Sci Nutr 1–20.

Karabulutoglu, M., R. Finnon, T. Imaoka, A.A. Friedl, et al. 2019. Influence of diet and metabolism on hematopoietic stem cells and leukemia development following ionizing radiation exposure. Int J Radiat Biol 95: 452–479.

Madeo, F., T. Eisenberg, F. Pietrocola and G. Kroemer. 2019. Spermidine in health and disease. Sci 359 (6374): eaan2788.

Nakatani, Y., Y. Yaguchi, T. Komura, M. Nakadai et al. 2018. Sesamin extends lifespan through pathways related to dietary restriction in *Caenorhabditis elegans*. Eur J Nutr 57: 1137–1146.

Pang, J., F. Li, X. Feng, H. Yang, et al. 2018. Influences of different dietary energy level on sheep testicular development associated with AMPK/ULK1/ATG pathway. Theriogenology 108: 362–370.

Pietrocola, F., F. Castoldi, M.C. Maiuri, G. Kroemer. 2018. Aspirin—another caloric-restriction mimetic. Autophagy 14:(7): 1162–1163.

Singh, S., A.K. Singh, G. Garg and S.I. Rizvi. 2018. Fesetin as a caloric restriction mimetic protects rat brain against aging induced oxidative stress, apoptosis and neurodegeneration. Life Sci 193: 171–179.

Stockman, M.C., D. Thomas, J. Burke and C.M Apovian. 2018. Intermittent fasting: Is the wait worth the weight? Curr Obes Rep 7: 172–185.

Wang, B.H., Q. Hou, Y.Q. Lu, M.M. Jia, et al. 2018. Ketogenic diet attenuates neuronal injury via autophagy and mitochondrial pathways in pcntylenetetrazol-kindled seizures. Brain Res 1678: 106–115.

Wu, Q., E.S. Yamamoto and K. Tsuduki. 2019. Carbohydrate-restricted diet promotes skin senescence in senescence-accelerated prone mice. Biogerontology 20: 71–82.

11

Charnolophagy in Gastrointestinal Diseases

INTRODUCTION

GIT disorders include conditions such as constipation, irritable bowel syndrome, hemorrhoids, anal fissures, perianal abscesses, anal fistulas, perianal infections, diverticular diseases, colitis, colon polyps, and cancer. In 2015, annual health care expenditures for GIT diseases reached $135.9 billion in the U.S.A. There were 266,600 new cases of GI cancers and 144,300 cancer deaths. Each year, there were 97,700 deaths from non-malignant GI diseases. In addition, the incidence of acute pancreatitis is increasing globally due to the increased incidence of obesity and cholelithiasis. The reported annual incidence of acute pancreatitis in the U.S.A. ranges from 4.9–35 per 100,000 population. *Helicobacter pylori* (*H. pylori*) causes infections in the stomach and is the primary cause of peptic ulcers; and can also cause gastritis and stomach cancer. About 30–40% of people pick up H. pylori infection, and peptic ulcer disease affects ~4.5 million people annually in the U.S.A. ~10% of the US population has evidence of duodenal ulcer at some time. Of those infected with H pylori, the lifetime prevalence is ~20%.

This chapter emphasizes the TSE-EBPT significance of CP in various GIT disorders including pancreatitis, GIT infections, *H. pylori*-induced ulcers, and colon cancer.

Pancreatitis

Acute pancreatitis (AP) is a potentially lethal inflammatory disease associated with tissue injury and necrosis that lacks specific therapy. The disease can be mild, involving only the pancreas, and resolve within days, or severe, with systemic inflammatory response-associated extra-pancreatic organ failure and even death. Damaged pancreatic acinar cells are the site of AP initiation. The primary function of these cells is the synthesis, storage, and export of digestive enzymes. Beginning in the ER and ending with secretion of proteins stored in zymogen granules, distinct pancreatic organelles use ATP produced by mitochondria to move and modify nascent proteins through vesicular compartments. Compartment-specific accessory proteins concentrate cargo and promote vesicular budding, targeting, and fusion. The ATG-lysosomal-endosomal pathways maintain acinar cell homeostasis by removing damaged/dysfunctional organelles and recycling cell constituents for substrate and energy. Tissues from patients with pancreatitis had biomarkers of mitochondrial damage and impaired ATG. The pathogenesis of AP is associated with abnormal increases in $[Ca^{2+}]_i$, mitochondrial dysfunction, impaired ATG, and ERS. Hence, strategies to restore CP/ATG might be developed for the treatment of AP. Biczo et al. (2018) induced pancreatitis in C57BL/6J mice (control) and mice deficient in peptidyl-prolyl isomerase D (Cyclophilin D, encoded by Ppid) by administrating L-arginine (also in rats), caerulein, bile acid, or an AP-inducing diet. Some mice with AP were given Trehalose to enhance ATG. Mitochondrial dysfunction in pancreas of mice with AP was induced by either mitochondrial Ca^{2+} overload or through a pathway that involved reduced ATP synthase. Both pathways were mediated by Cyclophilin D and led to mitochondrial depolarization and fragmentation. Mitochondrial dysfunction caused pancreatic ERS, impaired ATG, and deregulated lipid metabolism. These pathologic responses were abrogated in Cyclophilin D-knockout mice. Trehalose prevented trypsinogen activation, necrosis, and pancreatic injury in mice with L-arginine AP. Gukovskaya et al. (2019) described studies on experimental and genetic AP models, which demonstrated that acinar cell injury is mediated by distinct mechanisms of organelle dysfunction involved in protein synthesis and trafficking, secretion, energy generation, and ATG. These early events due to impaired $[Ca^{2+}]_i$ in the acinar cell triggered the inflammatory and cell death responses in pancreatitis. Manifestations of acinar cell organelle disorders are also prominent in human pancreatitis, suggesting that targeting specific mediators of organelle dysfunction could reduce disease severity. Habtezion et al. (2019) emphasized that stressors (environmental and genetic) causing AP initially induce injury to organelles of the acinar cell (mitochondria, ER, and endolysosomal-CP/ATG system), and lead to inappropriate intracellular activation of trypsinogen and inflammatory pathways. These investigators suggested the correction of organelle functions in AP for TSE-EBPT of AP.

GIT Infections Theranostics

Recent studies have shown that Schisandrin–C enhances odontoblastic differentiation through ATG and MQC in dental pulp cells. To investigate the role of Schisandrin C in odontoblastic differentiation, and its relations between ATG and MB in dental pulp cells (HPDCs), Takanche et al. (2018) used third molars, and cultured for HDPCs. To understand the mechanism of Schisandrin C, the HDPCs were treated with LPS, ATG, and HO-1 inhibitors: 3-MA and Zinc protoporphyrin IX (ZnPP), respectively. LPS decreased the expression of ATG molecules (Atg5, Beclin-1, and LC3-I/II) and MB molecules (HO-1 and PGC-1α), and disrupted odontoblastic differentiation. The downregulation of ATG and MB with 3-MA and ZnPP inhibited odontoblastic differentiation. However, Schisandrin C restored the expression of all the above molecules, with LPS and inhibitor treatment, suggesting that ATG and MB plays an essential role in odontoblastic differentiation, and Schisandrin C activates these systems to promote odontoblastic differentiation of HDPCs. As Schisandrin C regulates odontoblastic differentiation, it may be recommended for pulp homeostasis. H. pylori (Hp) vacuolating cytotoxin (VacA) enters host cells and induces mitochondrial dysfunction. Kim et al. (2018) reported that VacA perturbations in mitochondria are linked to alterations in cellular amino acid homeostasis, which results in the inhibition of mTORC1 and ATG. mTORC1, which regulates cellular metabolism during nutrient stress, is inhibited during Hp infection by a VacA-dependent mechanism. The VacA-dependent inhibition of mTORC1 signaling is linked to the dissociation of mTORC1 from the lysosomal surface and results in the activation of cellular ATG through the Unc 51-like kinase 1 (Ulk1) complex. VacA intoxication results in reduced cellular amino acids, and bolsters amino acid pools, preventing VacA-mediated mTORC1 inhibition. This strengthens hypothesis that Hp modulates the host cell's metabolism through the action of VacA at mitochondria involving CBMP. Khan (2015) highlighted that the epithelium of GIT organizes many innate defense systems against microbial intruders, such as the integrity of epithelial, rapid eviction of infected cells, quick turnover of epithelial cells, intrinsic immune responses, and ATG. However, entero-pathogenic *E. coli* (EPEC) evades the host defense systems and utilizes the GIT epithelium as a multiplicative site. During multiplication on and within the epithelium, EPEC secrete toxins that weaken, usurp, and use many host cellular systems. The EPEC in colorectal cancer is implicated in the depletion of DNA mismatch repair (MMR) proteins of the host cell in the colon epithelium. The EPEC colonized intracellularly in the mucosa of colorectal carcinoma whereas the extracellular strain was detected in mucosa of normal colon cells. Alteration in MutS, MutL complexes, and MUTYH of cells may be involved in the development of CRC, indicating that MMR of *E. coli* may be potential theranostic targets and biomarkers for CRC. The gut microbiome contributes to IBD, in which bacteria can be present within the epithelium. The epithelial barrier function is decreased in IBD, and dysfunctional epithelial MTS and ERS are associated with IBD. Lopes et al. (2018) hypothesized that the combination of ERS and MRS disrupt epithelial barrier function. They treated human colonic biopsies, epithelial colonoids, and epithelial cells with an uncoupler of O/P, Dinitrophenol (DNP), with or without the ER-stressor Tunicamycin, and assessed the epithelial barrier function by monitoring the internalization and translocation of commensal bacteria. They also examined the barrier function and colitis in mice exposed to Dextran sodium sulfate (DSS) or DNP and co-treated with DAPK6, an inhibitor of death-associated protein kinase 1 (DAPK1). Induction of ERS (that is, the unfolded protein response) prevented decrease in barrier function caused by the disruption of the mitochondrial function. ERS did not prevent DNP-driven uptake of bacteria; rather, the specific mobilization of the ATF6 arm of ERS and recruitment of DAPK1 resulted in enhanced xenophagy of bacteria. Epithelia with a Crohn's disease-susceptibility mutation in the ATG gene ATG16L1 exhibited less xenophagy. Systemic delivery of the DAPK1 inhibitor, DAPK6, increased bacterial translocation in DSS- or DNP-treated mice, indicating that promoting ERS-ATF6-DAPK1 signaling in transporting enterocytes counters the transcellular passage of bacteria evoked by dysfunctional mitochondria involved in CBMP, thereby reducing the potential for metabolic stress to reactivate or perpetuate inflammation.

Inflammatory Bowel Disease (IBD) Theranostics

Inflammatory Bowel Disease (IBD) is a complicated inflammatory colitis disorder (Crohn's disease and ulcerative colitis). Genetic studies have shown the clinical relevance of CP/ATG-related genes in the pathogenesis of IBD. Prevention of IBD relies on tight control of inflammatory, cell death, and ATG mechanisms. ATG is pivotal for intestinal homeostasis maintenance, gut ecology regulation, appropriate intestinal immune responses, and anti-microbial protection. Dysfunctional ATG leads to disrupted intestinal epithelial function, gut dysbiosis, defect in the antimicrobial peptide secretion by Paneth cells, ERS response, and aberrant immune responses to pathogenic bacteria. Conditional knockout mice have led to the understanding of ATGs that affect intestinal inflammation, Paneth cell abnormality, and enteric pathogenic infection during colitis. How alterations in the symbiotic relationship between the genetic composition of the host and the intestinal microbiota, under impact of specific environmental factors, lead to chronic intestinal inflammation, remains uncertain. Despite the availability of new theranostic modalities for IBD, the overall success in treating it remains modest, and full remission is usually accomplished and maintained in ~30% of patients only. The involvement of multiple genetic loci combined with differential environmental exposures suggests that IBD represent a continuum of disorders rather than distinct homogeneous disease entities. This diversity is translated into different disease course patterns, wherein some patients experience a quiescent disease whereas others suffer from a chronic disease. Hence, basic disease pathogenesis sets the stage for differential theranostic responses. Currently, IBD therapy is based on immunosuppression which does not take disease variability into account. Treatments are based on statistical considerations related to the response of the average patient in clinical trials rather than on personal considerations. The prognosis can be improved if physiologic considerations are integrated into the drug selection process. Drugs can be targeted at known patient dysfunctional processes such as in patients carrying ATG-related genetic polymorphisms being treated with Rapamycin (mTOR inhibitor and ATG enhancer) or we can perform high-throughput screening of predictive biomarkers and mechanisms associated with the response to a specific drug therapy. Additional predictive markers for drug safety are needed. IBD is driven by dysfunction between host genetics, the microbiota, and the immune system. Gaps in our knowledge remain regarding how IBD genetic risk loci drive gut microbiota changes. The Crohn's disease risk allele ATG16L1 T300A results in abnormal Paneth cells due to decreased CP, increased cytokine release, and decreased intracellular bacterial clearance. Recently, Kim et al. (2018) discussed various ATGs involved in CP, including ATG16L1, IRGM, LRRK2, ATG7, p62, optineurin, and TFEB in the intestinal homeostasis. Hence, direct targeting of ATGs will facilitate the development of novel TSE-EBPT for IBD. GWAS and functional studies have identified a role for ATG genes in IBD, especially in Crohn's disease. A further understanding of the role of ATG in IBD pathogenesis may provide better classification of IBD phenotypes and novel TSE-EBPT for disease management. To unravel the effects of ATG16L1 T300A on the microbiota and immune system, Lavoie et al. (2019) employed a genotobiotic model using human fecal transfers into ATG16L1 T300A knock-in mice. They observed increases in *Bacteroides ovatus* and Th1 and Th17 cells in ATG16L1 T300A mice. Association of altered Schaedler flora mice with *B. ovatus* specifically increased Th17 cells in ATG16L1 T300A knock-in mice. Changes occurred before the disease onset, suggesting that ATG16L1 T300A contributes to dysbiosis and immune infiltration prior to symptoms. Slowicka et al. (2019) showed that the anti-inflammatory protein A20 and the ATG-mediator, Atg16l1, interact and synergize to regulate the stability of the intestinal epithelial barrier. A proteomic screen using the WD40 domain of ATG16L1 (WDD) identified A20 as a WDD-interacting protein. The loss of A20 and Atg16l1 in the mouse intestinal epithelium induced IBD-like pathology, characterized by severe inflammation and increased intestinal epithelial cell death in both the small and large intestine. The absence of A20 promoted Atg16l1 accumulation, while elimination of Atg16l1 or expression of WDD-deficient Atg16l1 stabilized A20, indicating that A20 and Atg16l1 control intestinal homeostasis by acting at the intersection of inflammatory, ATG, and cell death pathways.

GIT Cancer Theranostics

As the modulation of ATG can be theranostically-beneficial to cancer treatment, the identification of novel ATG enhancers is highly anticipated. However, current ATG-inducing anticancer agents exert undesired side effects owing to their non-specific bio-distribution in off-target tissues. Huang et al. (2018) synthesized mitochondria-targeting near-infrared (NIR) fluorophores to screen and identify their ATG-enhancing activity by using the inhibitors, siRNA, RNA sequencing, and mass spectrometry to screen and identify a new NIR ATG enhancer, IR-58, which exhibited tumor-selective killing effects. IR-58 preferentially accumulated in the mitochondria of CRC cells and xenografts, a process that is glycolysis-dependent and organic-anion-transporter-polypeptide-dependent. IR-58 killed tumor cells and induced apoptosis via ATG induction, through the ROS-Akt-mTOR pathway. RNA sequencing, mass spectrometry, and siRNA interference studies demonstrated that translocase of IMM-44 (TIM44)-SOD2 pathway inhibition was responsible for the ROS overproduction, ATG, and apoptosis. TIM44 expression correlated positively with CRC and poor prognosis in patients. A novel NIR small-molecule ATG enhancer, IR-58, with mitochondria-targeted imaging and therapy was developed for CRC treatment. TIM44 was identified as a potential oncogene, which plays an important role in ATG through the TIM44-SOD2-ROS-mTOR pathway. Yi et al. (2018) synthesized an iridium (III) complex and evaluated its inhibitory effect on the cancer cells' growth. This complex displayed cytotoxic activity in A549 cells with an IC_{50} value of 3.6 ± 0.3 μM and 63.84% tumor growth inhibition compared with the control. The complex also exhibited potencies superior to that of Cisplatin toward A549 cells, enhanced ROS level, decreased ΔΨ, induced ATG, and inhibited cell invasion, indicating that it induced apoptosis in A549 through mitochondria dysfunction and PI3K/Akt/mTOR signaling pathways. In addition, Tang et al. (2018) synthesized a ligand THPDP (THPDP = 11-(6,7,8,9-tetrahydrophenazin-2-yl)dipyrido[3,2-a:2′,3′-c]phenazine) and its iridium(III) complex $[Ir(ppy)_2(THPDP)]PF_6$ (Ir-1), characterized by elemental analysis, IR, ESI-MS, ^1H NMR and ^{13}C NMR. The cytotoxicity of the complex in cancer cells B16, A549, Eca-109, SGC-7901, BEL-7402, and normal NIH 3T3 cell lines was evaluated using MTT. The complex inhibited growth in B16, A549, and Eca-10^9 cells, induced apoptosis, increased ROS, and decreased ΔΨ. The $[Ca^{2+}]_i$ and Cyt-C release were studied under a fluorescent microscope. The complex induced apoptosis through ROS-mediated mitochondrial dysfunction and inhibition of Akt/mTOR pathways, indicating their application as GIT anticancer agents. Almasi et al. (2018) investigated the role of TRPM2 in the survival of gastric cancer cells. TRPM2 knockdown in AGS and MKN-45 cells decreased cell proliferation and enhanced apoptosis. TRPM2 knockdown impaired mitochondrial metabolism, as indicated by a decrease in basal and maximal mitochondrial O_2 consumption and ATP production. The mitochondrial defects coincided with a decrease in ATG and MTG, represented by reduced levels of ATG- and MTG-associated proteins (that is, ATGs, LC3A/B II, and Bnip-3). TRPM2 modulated ATG through a JNK-dependent and mTOR-independent pathway, suggesting that in the absence of TRPM2, downregulation of the JNK signaling pathway impairs ATG, causing CB accumulation and death of gastric cancer cells involving CBMP. By inhibiting cell proliferation and promoting apoptosis, the TRPM2 downregulation enhanced the efficacy of Paclitaxel and Dox in gastric cancer cells, suggesting that TRPM2 inhibition may be utilized for the TSE-EBPT of gastric cancer. DiPrima et al. (2019) reported that phosphotyrosine-dependent Eph receptor signaling sustains colorectal carcinoma cell survival, thereby uncovering a survival pathway active in colorectal carcinoma cells. Genetic and biochemical inhibition of Eph TK activity or depletion of the Eph ligand EphrinB2, induced colorectal carcinoma cell death by CP. Spautin and 3-MA, inhibitors of early steps in the CP pathway, reduced CP-mediated cell death that follows the inhibition of phosphotyrosine-dependent Eph signaling in colorectal cancer cells. A small-molecule inhibitor of the Eph kinase, NVP-BHG712 (or its isomer NVP-Iso), reduced human colorectal cancer cell growth *in vitro* and tumor growth in mice. Colorectal cancers expressed the EphrinB ligand and its Eph receptors at higher levels than other cancer types, supporting Eph signaling inhibition as a novel strategy for the broad treatment of colorectal carcinoma. Liu et al. (2018) reported that GA suppressed colon cancer cell proliferation, migration, invasion, and induced cell death through G0/G1 phase arrest. Apoptosis was induced by GA treatment as confirmed by the release of Cyto-C from the mitochondria into the cytosol. GA-induced CP/ATG was supported by an increase in LC3BII, Atg5, and Beclin-1. Silencing Atg5 reduced the cell viability and enhanced apoptosis in GA-treated colon cancer cells, indicating that GA-induced apoptosis (rather than CP/ATG) contributed to colon cancer cell death. mTORC1 was reduced by GA, as evidenced by the reduction of p-mTOR, p-p70 ribosomal S6 kinase (p70s6k), and p-pras40. GA induced ROS, along with increased H_2O_2 and O_2. However, blocking ROS using its scavenger, NAC recovered GA-induced cells death, represented by an increase in cell viability, and decrease in apoptosis. The expressions of ATG- and cell cycle arrest-related molecules, as well as mTORC1 were reversed by NAC in GA-treated cells.

GA reduced tumor growth without toxicity to animals, suggesting that GA caused G0/G1 phase arrest and triggered apoptosis and ATG modulated by ROS in human colon cancer, and might be considered as a potential TSE-EBPT agent for colon cancer. It has been shown that Tinospora cordifolia (TC) is an ayurvedic herb used in the treatment of diabetes, gonorrhea, secondary syphilis, anemia, rheumatoid arthritis, dermatological diseases, cancer, gout, jaundice, asthma, leprosy, bone fractures, liver and intestinal disorders, blood purification, and confers a new life to the whole body as a rejuvenating herb. Sharma et al. (2018) investigated the anticancer properties of the aqueous alcoholic extract of T. cordifolia using bioassay-guided fractionation. TC-2 was confirmed by X-ray crystallographic analysis. The *in vitro* anti-cancer activity of TC-2 was evaluated by an SRB assay and ATG was investigated by fluorescence microscopy. Annexin-V FITC and PI dual staining was applied for the detection of apoptosis. The studies on $\Delta\Psi$ and ROS production were also conducted. Bioassay-guided fractionation and purification of the aqueous alcoholic extract of TC led to the isolation of clerodane furano diterpene glycoside (TC-2) along with five known compounds, that is, cordifolioside A (β-D-Glucopyranoside,4-(3-hydroxy-1-propenyl)-2,6-dimethoxyphenyl 3-O-D-apio-β-D-furanosyl) (TC-1), β-Sitosterol(TC-3), $2\beta,3\beta$:15,16-Diepoxy-4α, 6β-dihydroxy-13(16),14-clerodadiene-17,12:18,1-diolide (TC-4), ecdysterone(TC-5), and tinosporoside(TC-6). TC-2 emerged as a potential candidate for the treatment of colon cancer. The isolated clerodane furano diterpenoid from TC exhibited anticancer activity via induction of mitochondria-mediated CP/ATG and apoptosis in HCT116 cells for treating colon cancer. In addition, Isovitexin (IV), a glycosylflavonoid, is extracted from rice hulls of Oryza sativa, and has various biological activities. Lv et al. (2018) showed that IV suppressed the growth of liver cancer cells and induced apoptosis by the mitochondrial apoptotic pathway, as evidenced by the increase of Bax, caspase-3 activation, PARP cleavage, and Cyt-C released from mitochondria involving CBMP. IV resulted in ATG in liver cancer cells, as evidenced by the enhancement of LC3-II and ATG-related proteins (Atg) 3, Atg5, and Beclin-1. Suppressing ATG with Bafilomycin A1 (BFA) or siRNA Atg5 reduced apoptotic cells in IV-treated cells, demonstrating that ATG induction regulated apoptosis. IV caused ERS in liver cancer cells, along with the promotion of ERS-related molecules, including inositol-requiring enzyme 1α (IRE1α), X-box-binding protein-1s (XBP-1s), C/EBP homologous protein (CHOP), and glucose-regulated protein (GRP)-78. Inhibition of ERS by its inhibitor, Tauroursodeoxycholate (TUDCA), reversed IV-induced apoptosis and ATG. The IV treatment demonstrated tumor growth inhibition; hence it could be a candidate for liver cancer theranostics.

CONCLUSION

The theranostic significance of CP in acute pancreatitis, GIT infections, IBD (Crohn's disease and ulcerative colitis), and GIT cancer was highlighted. The mitochondrial dysfunction occurred through CP/ATG dysregulation, ERS, and impaired lipid metabolism in experimental pancreatitis. The mitochondrial translocase was targeted by a fluorescently labelled small-molecule enhancer for the colorectal cancer theranostics. Isovitexin-IV induced ATG and apoptosis in HCC through ERS, death-associated protein kinase-1-dependent xenophagy, and ameliorated epithelial barrier dysfunction. The H. pylori infection hijacked host cell metabolism through VacA-dependent inhibition of mTORC1, whereas polymorphism in ATG16L1 T300A genes altered the gut microbiota and enhanced the local Th1/Th17 response to confer cytoprotection in Crohn's disease. CP/ATG-related genes were identified in the pathogenesis of IBD. The potential role of *E. coli* DNA mismatch repair proteins in colon cancer was observed. A polypyridyl complex of Iridium (III) was developed as a potent anticancer agent which induced ATG and apoptosis in B16 cells through inhibition of the Akt/mTOR pathway. Furthermore, regulation of the TRPM2 channel-mediated ATG promoted MQC and gastric cancer cell survival through the JNK signaling pathway. A novel clerodane furano diterpene glycoside from Tinospora cordifolia triggered CP/ATG and apoptosis in HCT-116 colon cancer cells, suggesting its theranostic potential.

REFERENCES

Almasi, S., B.E. Kennedy, M. El-Aghil, A.M. Sterea, et al. 2018. TRPM2 channel-mediated regulation of ATG maintains mitochondrial function and promotes gastric cancer cell survival via the JNK-signaling pathway. J Biol Chem 293: 3637–3650.

Biczo, G., E.T. Vegh, N. Shalbueva, O.A. Mareninova, et al. 2018. Mitochondrial dysfunction, through impaired ATG, leads to endoplasmic reticulum stress, deregulated lipid metabolism, and pancreatitis in animal models. Gastroenterology 154: 689–703.

DiPrima, M., D. Wang, A. Tröster, D. Maric, et al. 2019. Identification of Eph receptor signaling as a regulator of autophagy and a therapeutic target in colorectal carcinoma. Mol Oncol 13: 2441–2459.

Habtezion, A., A.S. Gukovskaya and S.J. Pandol. 2019. Acute pancreatitis: A multifaceted set of organelle and cellular interactions. Gastroenterology 156: 1941–1950.

Huang, Y., J. Zhou, S. Luo, Y. Wang, et al. 2018. Identification of a fluorescent small-molecule enhancer for therapeutic autophagy in colorectal cancer by targeting mitochondrial protein translocase TIM44. Gut 67(2): 307–319.

Khan, S. 2015. Potential role of *Escherichia coli* DNA mismatch repair proteins in colon cancer. Crit Rev Oncol Hematol 96: 475–482.

Kim, I.J., J. Lee, S.J. Oh, M.S. Yoon, et al. 2018. Helicobacter pylori infection modulates host cell metabolism through VacA-dependent inhibition of mTORC1. Cell Host Microbe 23: 583–593.

Lavoie, S., K.L. Conway, K.G. Lassen, H.B. Jijon, et al. 2019. The Crohn's disease polymorphism, *ATG16L1* T300A, alters the gut microbiota and enhances the local Th1/Th17 response. eLife 8: e39982.

Lopes, F., A.V. Keita, A. Saxena, J.L. Reyes, et al. 2018. ER-stress mobilization of death-associated protein kinase-1-dependent xenophagy counteracts mitochondria stress-induced epithelial barrier dysfunction. J Biol Chem 293: 3073–3087.

Lv, S.X. and X. Qiao. 2018. Isovitexin (IV) induces apoptosis and autophagy in liver cancer cells through endoplasmic reticulum stress. Biochem Biophys Res Commun 496: 1047–1054.

Sharma, N., A. Kumar, P.R. Sharma, A. Qayum. 2018. A new clerodane furano diterpene glycoside from *Tinospora cordifolia* triggers autophagy and apoptosis in HCT-116 colon cancer cells. Ethnopharmacol 211: 295–310.

Slowicka, K., I. Serramito-Gómez, E. Boada-Romero, A. Martens, et al. 2019. Physical and functional interaction between A20 and ATG16L1-WD40 domain in the control of intestinal homeostasis. Nat Commun 10: 1834.

Takanche, J.S., J.S. Kim, J.E. Kim, S.H. Han, et al. 2018. Schisandrin C enhances odontoblastic differentiation through autophagy and mitochondrial biogenesis in human dental pulp cells. Arch Oral Biol 88: 60–66.

Tang, B., D. Wan, Y.J. Wang, Q.Y. Yi, et al. 2018. An iridium (III) complex as potent anticancer agent induces apoptosis and ATG in B16 cells through inhibition of the Akt/mTOR pathway. Eur J Med Chem 145: 302–314.

Yi, Q.Y., D. Wan, B. Tang, Y.J. Wang, et al. 2018. Synthesis, characterization and anticancer activity in vitro and in vivo evaluation of an iridium (III) polypyridyl complex. Eur J Med Chem 145: 338–349.

12

Charnolophagy in Liver Diseases

INTRODUCTION

ATG is identified as a molecular mechanism that can be modulated in hepatic diseases to eliminate nonfunctional protein aggregates, damaged organelles, LDs, and regulate inflammatory signaling. Recently, pathophysiology of liver disease, role of P450 enzymes in alcohol liver disease, cell death in drug-induced liver injury, and clinical significance of key proteins in liver regeneration were investigated (Michalopoulos and Bhushan 2020). It was discovered that dietary exacerbation of metabolic stress led to accelerated hepatic carcinogenesis in GSDs. The liver is constantly exposed to pathogens, viruses, chemicals, and toxins, which may cause injury, leading to liver fibrosis, cirrhosis, adenoma, and cancer. Gupta and Venugopal (2018) highlighted the role of the augmenter of liver regeneration (ALR) in normal liver physiology and in liver failure, NAFLD/NASH, viral infections, cirrhosis, and HCC. Under physiological conditions, the liver can regenerate if the loss of cells is less than the proliferation of hepatocytes. If the loss is more than the proliferation, the radical treatment is liver transplantation. Liver regeneration is regulated by several growth factors; one of the key factors is ALR, which is involved in O/P, MB, MQC, regulation of CP/ATG, and cell proliferation. ALR is involved in liver regeneration through its ability to overcome cell cycle inhibition and to maintain the stem cell pool. Thus, it appears to have a role in the maintenance of liver health.

This chapter describes the theranostic significance of CP in various hepatic diseases.

Perinatal CR Regulates Hepatic ATG

Intrauterine growth restriction leads to obesity, CVDs, and NAFLD/NASH. Animal models have shown that combined intrauterine and early postnatal calorie restriction (IPCR) ameliorates these sequelae in adult life. Devarajan et al. (2018) hypothesized that IPCR regulates ATG in the liver of male rat offspring. At birth (d1) and on day 21 (p21) of life, IPCR male rat offsprings had a profound reduction in hepatic ATG in all three stages of development: initiation, elongation, and maturation. However, upon receiving a normal diet ad-lib throughout adulthood, aged IPCR rats (day 450 of life (p450)), had increased hepatic ATG, in direct contrast to what was seen in early life. The decreased ATG at d21 led to the accumulation of ubiquitinated proteins and lipid oxidative products, whereas the increased ATG in late life had an opposite effect. Oxidized lipids were unchanged at d1 by the IPCR treatment, indicating that decreased ATG triggers oxidative stress in early life. When the cellular signaling pathways regulating ATG were examined, the AMPK pathway was altered, suggesting that ATG is regulated through the AMPK signaling pathway in IPCR rats, and that the perinatal nutritional status establishes a nutritionally-sensitive memory that enhances the hepatic ATG in late life, a process which may serve as a protective mechanism to limited nutrition.

Drug-Induced Hepatic Injury

Recently, Iorga and Dara (2019) described apoptosis, necrosis, necroptosis, CP/ATG, pyroptosis, and ferroptosis and their relevance to drug-induced liver injury (DILI) in liver toxicity with varying clinical manifestations, the most severe of which being acute liver failure (ALF). Hepatocyte death as a cause of drug toxicity is a feature of DILI. The mode of cell death in DILI depends on the drug, as it regulates the mechanism and the extent of injury. ATG and its regulated pathways participate in many cellular physiology and pathological processes involving protein aggregates, damaged mitochondria implicated in CB formation and CP induction during the acute phase and CBMP, excessive peroxisomes, ribosomes, and invading pathogens during the chronic phase. Zhou et al. (2018) described the lncRNA-regulated ATG during DILI and its progression to ALF linked to ERS and induced ATG, which protect hepatocytes during DILI. LncRNA influences the regulation of the expression of ATGs to manipulate ATG. The main cell death mechanisms in DILI are apoptosis and necrosis, executed through the mitochondria. For example, Acetaminophen (APAP) can cause direct, dose-dependent toxicity, while the majority of drugs cause idiosyncratic-DILI, which is an unpredictable form of liver injury, occurring in individuals with a genetic predisposition, and presents with variable latency. Cell death in IDILI occurs as a death receptor-mediated apoptosis due to the induction of the innate and adaptive immune system, compounded by genetics, gender, age, and immune tolerance. Alcohol consumption causes liver diseases, named as alcoholic liver disease (ALD). Because alcohol is detoxified by alcohol dehydrogenase (ADH), the development of ALD was initially believed to be due to malnutrition caused by alcohol metabolism in the liver. The discovery of the microsomal ethanol oxidizing system (MEOS) dispelled this myth. CYP2E1 in MEOS is one of the major ROS generators in the liver and contributes to ALD. Lu and Cederbaum (2018) studied the relationship between CYP2E1 and ALD and found that the human CYP2A6 and its mouse analog CYP2A5 are also induced by alcohol. In mice, the alcohol induction of CYP2A5 was CYP2E1-dependent, whereas CYP2E1 and CYP2A5 protected against the development of ALD.

CP and Hepatic Diseases

Hepatic fibrosis increases mortality in humans with NASH, but it remains uncertain how the fibrotic stage and progression affect the NASH pathogenesis. Ipsen et al. (2019) investigated the transcriptional regulation and the impact of the fibrosis stage, the pathways relating to hepatic lipid, and cholesterol homeostasis, inflammation, and fibrosis using RT-qPCR in the guinea pig NASH model. Animals were fed a chow (4% fat), a high-fat (20% fat, 0.35% cholesterol), or high-fat/high-sucrose (20% fat, 15% sucrose, 0.35% cholesterol) diet for 16 or 25 weeks (n = 7/group/time point). The HFD induced NASH where the markers of hepatic lipogenesis were enhanced while markers of mitochondrial, peroxisomal, and cytochrome fatty acid oxidation were reduced. Markers of fatty acid uptake were unaltered or decreased. The expression of cholesterol uptake and synthesis markers were decreased, whereas genes relating to lipid and cholesterol export were unaltered. Inflammatory and chemotactic cytokines were induced along with fibrogenic pathways, including hepatic stellate cell activation and migration, matrix deposition (e.g. MCP1, TNFα, β-PDGF and Col1a1, >3X), and decreased matrix degradation. The fibrosis stage (mild vs. severe) and progression did not affect the expression of afore-mentioned genes, suggesting that liver dysfunction at the transcriptional level is induced early and maintained throughout fibrosis progression, allowing potential treatments to target dysregulated pathways at early disease stages. As the guinea pig NASH model mimics human molecular pathophysiology, these results may be used to augment the understanding of NASH pathology and explore TSE-EBPT strategies. It is known that obesity-related NAFLD is connected with mitochondrial stress and hepatocyte apoptosis. Parkin-related CP sustains mitochondrial homeostasis and hepatocyte viability. Macrophage stimulating 1 (Mst1) is a novel CP regulator, which exacerbates heart and cancer apoptosis by repressing CP.

Zhou et al. (2019) explored whether Mst1 contributes to NAFLD via disrupting Parkin-related CP. A NAFLD model was generated in wild-type (WT) mice and Mst1 knockout (Mst1-KO) mice using HFD. Experiments were conducted via palmitic acid (PA) treatment in the primary hepatocytes. Mst1 was upregulated in HFD-treated livers. The genetic ablation of Mst1 attenuated HFD-mediated hepatic injury and sustained hepatocyte viability. Mst1 knockdown reversed Parkin-related CP and the latter protected mitochondria and hepatocytes against HFD. Mst1 modulated Parkin expression via the AMPK pathway; the blockade of AMPK repressed Parkin-related CP, recalled hepatocytes mitochondrial apoptosis, and helped identify NAFLD's association with the defective Parkin-related CP due to Mst1 upregulation which might provide the TSDE-EBPT of fatty liver disease.

To probe into the mechanism and interventional effects of Silybin-phospholipid complex on Amiodarone-induced steatosis in mice, Sun et al. (2019) divided 8-week-old male C57BL/6 mice into three groups (5 mice in each group): a control group (WT) with a normal diet, a model group with Amiodrone 150 mg/kg/day by oral gavage (AM), and an intervention group on Amiodrone 150 mg/kg/day combined with Silybin-phospholipid complex (AM+SILIPHOS). All mice were fed their diet for one week. Serum AST, ALT, total cholesterol, and HDL were detected in each group. RT-q PCR was used to detect the expression of PPARα and its regulated lipid metabolism genes CPTI, CPTII, Acot1, Acot2, ACOX, Cyp4a10, and Cyp4a14. Intrahepatic steatosis was reduced in intervention group compared to model group with Amiodrone having pyknotic nuclei, mitochondrial swelling, structural damage, and lysosomal degradation whereas the intervention group had hepatic nucleus without pyknosis, reduced mitochondrial swelling, and slight structural damage. The expression of PPARα, CPTI, CPTII, Acot1, Acot2, ACOX, Cyp4a10, and Cyp4a14 were increased in the model group but the expression of CPTI, Cyp4a14, Acot1, and PPARα were decreased in the intervention group, suggesting that the Silybin-phospholipid complex can alleviate Amiodrone-induced steatosis and may protect mitochondrial function and regulate fatty acid metabolism by preventing CBMP. Thus, the Silybin-phospholipid complex may have an ameliorating effect on Amiodrone-induced fatty liver.

Ding et al. (2019) showed that MTG is enhanced with increased apoptosis in hepatic stellate cells during the reversal of hepatic fibrosis. The inhibition of MTG suppressed apoptosis in HSCs and aggravated hepatic fibrosis in mice. In contrast, the activation of MTG induced apoptosis in HSCs. Furthermore, BCL-B, as a regulator, mediates MTG-related apoptosis. The knockdown of BCL-B increased apoptosis and MTG in HSCs, while its overexpression caused the opposite effects. BCL-B inhibited the phosphorylation of Parkin (a key regulator of MTG) and bound phospho-Parkin. Enhanced MTG promoted apoptosis in HSCs during the reversal of hepatic fibrosis. BCL-B suppressed MTG in HSCs by binding and suppressing phospho-Parkin, thereby inhibiting apoptosis. BCL-B-dependent MTG is a new pathway for regulating apoptosis in HSCs during the regression of hepatic fibrosis. The increasing epidemic of fine particulate matter (PM2.5) is a serious threat to human health as it increases the occurrence of liver fibrosis. Qiu et al. (2019) investigated the molecular mechanisms of PM2.5 inducing liver fibrosis. PM2.5 activated LX-2 cells and primary HSCs, inducing liver fibrosis along with the downregulation of the gelatinases MMP-2, and upregulation of myofibroblast markers collagen type I and α-SMA. The levels of RONS, as well as the lipid peroxidation marker MDA were upregulated in LX-2 cells and primary HSCs treated with PM2.5. The antioxidant levels were disturbed by PM2.5, which decreased the MTP, releasing Cyt-C from the mitochondria to the cytosol. The mitochondrial dynamics was regulated by PM2.5 via their fission. The excess ROS induced by PM2.5 triggered CP/ATG by activating the PINK1/Parkin pathway, and by inhibiting CP/ATG induced by PM2.5 which diminished the liver fibrosis, suggesting that PM2.5 may induce MTG via activating the PINK1/Parking pathway by increasing ROS, thereby inducing HSCs and liver fibrosis.

Recently, Ghorbani et al. (2019) reported that NAFLD develops in concert with related metabolic diseases, such as obesity, dyslipidemia, and insulin resistance. Prolonged lipid accumulation and inflammation can progress to NASH. Recent findings revealed the possible regulation of NASH by metabolites of the mevalonate pathway. Mevalonate is converted to the farnesyl-diphosphate (FPP) and geranylgeranyl diphosphate (GGPP). GGPP synthase (GGPPS), the enzyme that converts FPP to GGPP, is dysregulated during NASH. Both FPP and GGPP can be conjugated to proteins through prenylation, modifying protein function and localization. Deletion or knockdown of GGPPS favors FPP prenylation (farnesylation) and augments liver kinase B1, an upstream kinase of AMPK. Despite AMPK activation, livers in Ggpps-deficient mice on a HFD poorly oxidize lipids due to mitochondrial dysfunction. Besides abstinence and nutritional support, there is no clinical treatment for AFLD patients.

Gao et al. (2019) demonstrated the therapeutic effects and mechanism of action of wolfberry-derived zeaxanthin dipalmitate (ZD) on AFLD models. The hepato-protective effects of ZD were evaluated *in vitro* and *in vivo*. The directly interacting receptors of ZD on cell membranes were identified by liver-specific knockdown and biophysical measurements. ZD attenuated hepatocyte and whole-liver injury in ethanol-treated cells (dose: 1 µm) and a chronic binge AFLD rat model (dose: 10 mg kg^{-1}), respectively. ZD targeted receptor P2X7 and adiponectin receptor 1 (adipoR1) on the cell membrane. The signals from P2X7 and adipoR1 modulated the PI3-kinase-Akt and/or AMP-activated protein kinase-Foxo3a pathways, to restore CP/ATG suppressed by ethanol intoxication. In addition, ZD alleviated hepatic inflammation via the inhibition of Nod-like receptor 3 inflammasome, whose activation was a consequence of suppressed CP. Liver-specific inhibition of P2X and adipoR1 receptors or inhibition of CP, impaired the beneficial effects of ZD on AFLD model.

The protein and organelle turnover by ATG is a key component in maintaining cellular homeostasis. Loss of the ATG protein ATG16L1 is associated with reduced bacterial killing and aberrant IL-1β production, perpetuating inflammation, and carcinogenesis. Reuken et al. (2019) hypothesized that the functional p.T300A gene variant in ATG16L1 is associated with an increased risk for HCC in cirrhosis. A case-control study was performed using a prospective derivation cohort (107 patients with HCC and 101 controls) and an independent validation cohort (124 patients with HCC and 108 controls) of patients with cirrhosis. ATG16L1 p.T300A (rs2241880) and PNPLA3 p.I148M (rs738409) variants were determined by PCR. In the derivation cohort and validation cohort, G allele of the ATG16L1 p.T300A varient was more frequent in HCC patients compared to controls (without HCC). In a combined analysis (Reuken et al. 2019), the odd ratios (OR) were 1.76 for G allele positivity and 2.43 for p.T300A G allele homozygosity. This association was independent from the presence of a PNPLA3 variant, which was also associated with HCC, and remained significant after adjustment for male sex, age, and etiology in multivariate analysis, suggesting that the common germ-line ATG16L1 gene variant is a risk factor for HCC in patients with cirrhosis. Hence, personalized strategies employing the genetic risk conferred by ATG16L1 and PNPLA3 may be used for risk-based surveillance in cirrhosis.

Liver endothelial cells are the first liver cell type affected after any kind of liver injury. The loss of their phenotype during injury amplifies the liver damage by orchestrating the response of the liver microenvironment. Ruart et al. (2019) investigated the role of ATG in the regulation of endothelial dysfunction and the impact of its manipulation during liver injury. They analyzed primary LSECs from Atg7^{control} and Atg7^{endo} mice as well as rats after CCl$_4$-induced liver injury. Liver tissue and primary isolated stellate cells were used to analyze liver fibrosis. ATG, microvascular function, NO bioavailability, superoxide, and the antioxidant response were evaluated in endothelial cells. ATG maintains LSEC homeostasis and was upregulated during angiogenesis. Pharmacological and genetic downregulation of endothelial ATG increased oxidative stress *in vitro*. During liver injury, the selective loss of endothelial ATG resulted in cellular dysfunction and reduced NO. The loss of ATG also impaired LSECs' ability to handle oxidative stress and aggravated fibrosis. ATG contributed to maintaining endothelial phenotype and protecting LSECs from oxidative stress during the early phases of liver disease. Selectively potentiating ATG in LSECs during the early stages of liver disease may be an approach to modify the disease course and prevent fibrosis.

Wang et al. (2019) investigated theranostic agents that would reduce ATZ accumulation by employing a *C. elegans* model of α1-antitrypsin deficiency (ATD) with high-content genome-wide RNAi screening and computational systems pharmacology. The RNAi screening was utilized to identify genes that modify the intracellular accumulation of ATZ and a computational pipeline was developed to make high-confidence predictions on drugs. This approach identified Glibenclamide (GLB), a sulfonylurea drug that is used as an oral hypoglycemic agent. GLB promoted CP/ATG elimination of misfolded ATZ in cell line models of ATD. An analog of GLB reduced hepatic ATZ accumulation and fibrosis in a mouse model without affecting blood glucose or insulin levels. Hence GLB and/or its analogs can be tested to inhibit the progression of the human ATD liver disease.

Lee et al. (2019) evaluated the effects of sodium molybdate (SM) on hepatic steatosis and associated disturbances in a mouse model of the metabolic disease. Male C57Bl/6 mice at 10 weeks of age were fed a diet deficient in methionine and choline (MCD) and water containing SM for four weeks. The SM treatment attenuated MCD-induced accumulation of triglycerides in the liver. The lipid catabolic ATG pathways were activated by SM in the MCD-fed mouse livers, as evidenced by a decreased level of p62 expression. MCD-induced oxidative damage, such as lipid and protein oxidation, was alleviated by SM in the liver. However, MCD-induced hepatocellular damage was not affected by SM, suggesting that molybdate can be used for the treatment of hepatic steatosis. Genetic factors are associated with a familial predisposition for developing liver cirrhosis and HCC during a chronic hepatitis B virus (HBV) infection. ATG plays a role in HBV replication and the course of the disease. More than 190 host genes can modify ATG. Tian et al. (2018) recruited chronic hepatitis B (CHB) patients to investigate the expression of ATG-modulating genes in PBMCs. mRNA prepared from PBMCs from members of two families with clustering HBV infection, including 11 CHB patients and nine healthy spouses, was hybridized into high-density oligonucleotide arrays. Of the 192 ATG-modulating genes, 18 were differentially expressed. Of these, 11 displayed decreased expression in CHB patients, while seven displayed increased expression compared to those in healthy controls. These genes are involved in initiation, nucleation, elongation of phagophores, formation of CPS transportation to lysosomes, and degradation. An immunoblot analysis revealed inhibited ATG based on decreased lipidation of LC3-II. A differential-expression profile of ATG-modulating genes, and decreased ATG was associated with chronicity of HBV infection, suggesting a novel TSE-EBPT strategy for chronic HBV infection. Abdel-Mohsen et al. (2018) investigated the interaction between CP/ATG and apoptosis, and the therapeutic role of vitamin-D and its receptors in hepatitis-C viral HCV) infection and in the progression of HCC. The serum levels of LC3, marker of ATG (caspase-3), marker of apoptosis (vitamin D3), and vitamin D receptor (VDR) were measured by ELISA. The liver profile revealed hepatic dysfunctions in HCV patients with or without HCC. A significant reduction in the serum concentration of LC3 and caspase-3 were observed indicating the downregulation of ATG and host-mediated apoptosis in HCV patients with or without HCC. Deficiency of vitamin D and decreased levels of its receptor were observed in HCV and HCV-HCC patients. The perturbation in the vitamin D/VDR axis, which modulates both CP/ATG and apoptosis in HCV infection, suggested its involvement and implication in the pathogenesis of an HCV infection and the development of HCV-related HCC. Hence, supplementation with vitamin D may not be the only solution to restore the biological functions of vitamin D; VDR-targeted therapy may be of great importance in this respect.

Recently, Lei et al. (2018) reported that a liver I/R injury occurs through the induction of oxidative stress and release of DAMPs, including cytosolic DNA released from dysfunctional mitochondria or from the nucleus. cGAMP synthase (cGAS) is a cytosolic DNA sensor (known to trigger stimulation of interferon genes (STING)) and downstream type 1 interferon (IFN-I) pathways are innate immune system responses to pathogen. The researchers subjected C57BL/6 (WT), cGAS knockout (cGAS$^{-/-}$), and STING-deficient (STING$^{gt/gt}$) mice to a warm liver I/R injury and found that cGAS$^{-/-}$ mice had significantly increased liver injuries compared with WT or STING$^{gt/gt}$ mice, suggesting a protective effect of cGAS independent of STING. Liver I/R upregulated cGAS in hepatocytes subjected to anoxia/re-oxygenation (A/R). Hepatocytes did not express STING under normoxic conditions or after A/R. Hepatocytes and liver from cGAS$^{-/-}$ mice had increased cell death and reduced induction of ATG under hypoxic conditions as well as increased apoptosis. Protection could be restored in cGAS$^{-/-}$ hepatocytes by the over-expression of cGAS or by pretreatment of mice with the ATG-inducer Rapamycin, indicating a protective role of cGAS in the regulation of ATG during I/R injury that occurred independently of STING. This study confirmed the role of cGAS in the acute setting of an injury induced by I/R, providing evidence that cGAS protects the liver from I/R injury in a STING-independent manner.

Due to the lack of adequate organs, the number of patients with end-stage liver diseases, acute liver failure, or hepatic malignancies waiting for liver transplantation is increasing. Kan et al. (2018) highlighted that accepting aged liver grafts is one of the strategies to expand the donor pool, easing the discrepancy between the growing demand and the limited supply of donor organs. However, recipients of organs from old donors may show an increased post-transplantation morbidity and mortality due to enhanced I/R injury. Energy metabolism, inflammatory response, and ATG are involved in the aging progress as well as in hepatic I/R injury. Compared with young liver grafts, impairment of energy metabolism in aged liver grafts leads to lower ATP production and ROS overproduction, both aggravating the inflammatory response, which determines the extent of hepatic I/R injury and augments the liver damage. CP induced the attenuation of lipid accumulation by molybdate in the livers of mice fed on methionine and choline-deficient diet, whereas hepatitis C virus induced HCC. cGAS-mediated ATG protected the liver from I/R injury independently of STING. Furthermore, Cu is an essential trace element for the catalysis of several cellular enzymes. Excessive Cu could induce hepatotoxicity in humans and multiple animals. Yang et al. (2018) investigated the effects of ATG on Cu-induced hepatotoxicity. Chicken hepatocytes were cultured in a medium in the absence and presence of $CuSO_4$ (0, 10, 50, and 100 µM) for 0, 6, 12, and 24 hrs, and in a combination of $CuSO_4$ and NAC (1 mM), Rapamycin (10 nM), 3-MA (5 mM) for 24 hrs. Cu increased the number of autophagosomes and LC3 puncta, induced ATG-related genes (Beclin-1, Atg5, LC3 I, LC3 II, mTOR, and Dynein) mRNA expression and protein (BECN1, LC3 II/ LC3) expression. NAC relieved Cu-induced changes of above genes and proteins. Rapamycin attenuated Cu-induced LDH, AST, and ALT, and SOD-1 mRNA expression and decreased cell viability, ROS, H_2O_2, SOD, MDA, CAT, HO-1 mRNA expression, TP levels, mitochondrial mass, and $\Delta\Psi$. But 3-MA had the opposite effects on above factors, indicating that Cu induces ATG by generating excessive ROS in hepatocytes, and ATG might attenuate Cu-induced mitochondrial dysfunction by regulating oxidative stress.

CP/ATG and Signal Transduction in Hepatic Diseases

ATG plays an important role in cell survival, sequestering, and degrading a wide variety of substrates. An increase in autophagosomes is noticed in the livers of sepsis patients and in septic mice; Oami et al. (2018) elucidated on the contribution of liver ATG to the pathophysiology of sepsis in their study. They performed a cecal ligation and puncture on liver-specific ATG-deficient (Alb-Cre/Atg5) mice (6-8-week-old male). The accumulation of p62 in the liver and a greater number of cleaved caspase-3 immuno-reactive hepatocytes were observed in the KO mice. A significant increase in ATG vacuoles in the control mice as compared to the KO mice was observed. In contrast, cell shrinkage and apoptosis were seen in the KO mice. Mitochondrial damage was also prominent in KO mice, associated with an increase of ROS. Serum AST and IL-6 were increased in the KO mice compared with the controls. Deficiency of ATG in the liver decreased survival in the sepsis model, indicating that blocking liver ATG accelerates mortality, and that it plays a protective role in organ failure through the degradation of CBs participating in CBMP, as well as by preventing apoptosis. NAFLD is becoming the most common cause of fatal liver diseases such as cirrhosis, liver cancer, and indications for liver transplantation. Lee et al. (2019) highlighted the involvement of mitochondrial processes in the development of NAFLD and the potential targets for its theranostics. In the pathogenesis of NAFLD, mitochondrial dysfunction arises as a result of changes in ETC complexes, $\Delta\psi$ collapse, and decreased ATP synthesis. Due to their role in energy metabolism and cell death, alterations in mitochondria are critical factors causing NAFLD through CB formation. Reduced β-oxidation, along with increased lipogenesis, result in lipid accumulation in hepatocytes, the production of ROS and hepatocyte injury, thus contributing to hepatic inflammation and fibrosis through the activations of Kupffer cells and hepatic stellate cells. The author proposed liver-specific CB antagonists, CP agonists, and CS stabilizers and CS exocytosis-enhancers for the TSE-EBPT of NAFLD. Hepatic fibrosis increases mortality in humans with NASH. Ipsen et al. (2019) investigated the transcriptional regulation of pathways in hepatic lipid and cholesterol homeostasis, inflammation, and fibrosis using RT-qPCR in the guinea pig NASH model. Animals were fed a chow (4% fat), a high-fat (20% fat, 0.35% cholesterol) or high-fat/high-sucrose (20% fat, 15% sucrose, 0.35% cholesterol) diet for 16 or 25 weeks. In HFD-induced NASH, markers of mitochondrial, peroxisomal, and cytochrome fatty acid oxidation were reduced. Markers of fatty acid uptake were unaltered or decreased. Similarly, the expression of cholesterol uptake and synthesis markers were decreased, whereas genes involved in lipid and cholesterol export remained unaltered. Inflammatory and chemotactic cytokines were enhanced along with fibrogenic pathways, including increased hepatic stellate cell activation and migration, matrix deposition, and decreased matrix degradation. The fibrotic stage (mild vs. severe) and progression did not affect the expression of the investigated pathways, suggesting that liver dysfunction at the transcriptional level is induced early and maintained throughout fibrosis progression, allowing potential treatments to target dysregulated pathways at early disease stages. Zhang et al. (2019) investigated how CP/ATG affects NLRP3 inflammasome activation in hepatic lipotoxicity. Mice were fed a high fat/calorie diet (HFCD) for 24 weeks. Primary rat hepatocytes were treated with palmitic acid (PA) for various periods of time. CP was measured by protein levels of LC3-II and P62. NLRP3, caspase-1, IL-18, and IL-1β at mRNA and protein levels were used as indicators of inflammasome activation. Along with steatotic progression in HFCD-fed mice, the ratio of LC3-II/β-actin was decreased with increased levels of liver P62, NLRP3, caspase-1, IL-1β, IL-18, and serum IL-1β levels in late-stage NASH. The PA treatment resulted in mitochondrial oxidative stress and initiated CP in primary hepatocytes. Cyclosporine A did not change LC3-II/Tomm20 ratios; but P62 levels were increased after an extended duration of PA exposure, indicating defective CP accompanied with the upregulation of the mRNA and protein levels of NLRP3, caspase-1, IL-18, and IL-1β by PA treatment. Pretreatment with MCC950, NAC, or acetyl-L-carnitine attenuated inflammasome activation and a pyroptotic cascade. CP was partially recovered as indicated by an increase in the LC3-II/Tomm20 ratio, parkin, and PINK1 expression, and decreased P62 expression, suggesting that defective CP triggers hepatic NLRP3 inflammasome activation in a murine NASH model and primary hepatocytes. The new insights into inflammasome activation through CP advances our understanding of how fatty acids elicit lipotoxicity through oxidative stress and CP.

The class 3 PI3K is required for lysosomal degradation by ATG and vesicular trafficking, assuring nutrient availability. Mitochondrial lipid metabolism is another energy source. ATG and mitochondrial metabolism are transcriptionally regulated by nutrient-sensing nuclear receptors. Iershov et al. (2019) showed that the liver-specific inactivation of Vps15, the essential regulatory subunit of the class 3 PI3K, elicits mitochondrial depletion and a failure to oxidize fatty acids. The transcriptional activity of PPARα, a nuclear receptor orchestrating lipid catabolism, is blunted in Vps15-deficient livers. The PPARα repressor histone deacetylase 3 (Hdac3) and nuclear receptor co-repressor 1 (NCoR1) accumulated in Vps15-deficient livers due to defective ATG. The activation of PPARα or inhibition of Hdac3 restored MB and lipid oxidation in Vps15-deficient hepatocytes. These findings revealed roles for the class 3 PI3K and ATG in the transcriptional regulation of mitochondrial metabolism.

GSD1a deficient in glucose-6-phosphatase-α (G6Pase-α) is a rare metabolic disease characterized by hypoglycemia, steatosis, excessive glycogen accumulation with glycogen accumulation in hepatocytes, steatosis, and hepatocellular carcinoma (HCC). Mitochondrial dysfunction is implicated in GSD-Ia. Cho et al. (2018) showed that hepatic G6Pase-α deficiency leads to the downregulation of sirtuin 1 (SIRT1) signaling, which underlies defective hepatic ATG in GSD-Ia. SIRT1 is a NAD^+-dependent deacetylase that can deacetylate and activate PGC-1α, a regulator of mitochondrial integrity, biogenesis, and function. These investigators hypothesized that the downregulation of hepatic SIRT1 signaling in G6Pase-α-deficient livers impairs PGC-1α activity, leading to mitochondrial dysfunction. The G6Pase-α-deficient livers displayed defective PGC-1α signaling, reduced functional mitochondria, and impaired O/P. The overexpression of hepatic SIRT1 restored PGC-1α activity, normalized ETC components, and increased mitochondrial complex IV activity. The restoration of hepatic G6Pase-α expression normalized SIRT1 signaling, PGC-1α activity, and mitochondrial function. HCA/HCC lesions found in G6Pase-α-deficient livers contain mitochondrial and oxidative DNA damage, demonstrating that downregulation of hepatic SIRT1/PGC-1α signaling induces mitochondrial dysfunction and that oxidative DNA damage (induced by damaged mitochondria involving CBMP) may contribute to HCA/HCC development in GSD-Ia.

Metabolic syndrome, characterized by central obesity, hypertension, and hyperlipidemia, increases the morbidity and mortality of CVDs, type 2 diabetes, NAFLD, and other metabolic diseases. Hepatic insulin resistance is a risk factor for metabolic syndrome. Fatty acid accumulation can cause hepatic insulin resistance through increased gluconeogenesis, lipogenesis, chronic inflammation, oxidative stress, ERS, and impaired insulin signal pathway. Mitochondria are the major sites of β-oxidation of fatty acids. Mitochondrial dysfunction involving CBMP is involved in the development of fatty-acid-induced hepatic insulin resistance. CP, a catabolic process, degrades damaged mitochondria participating in pleomorphic CB formation to reverse mitochondrial dysfunction and preserve MQC and function. Hence, CP can promote mitochondrial fatty acid oxidation to inhibit fatty acid accumulation and improve hepatic insulin resistance. Ye et al. (2019) highlighted the relationship between CP and hepatic insulin resistance as well as the theranostic significance of CP in the TSE-EBPT of hepatic insulin resistance and metabolic syndrome. Despite the identification of Atg5 involved in CP/ATG induction during a hepatitis B virus (HBV) infection and HCC, the consequences of Atg5 mutation for patients with a chronic HBV infection remains uncertain.

Hepatic encephalopathy (HE) is reported in >40% of patients with cirrhosis in clinical practice. HE induces mitochondrial dysfunction. Bai et al. (2018) evaluated changes in mitochondrial dynamics and ATG of the substantia nigra (SN) and prefrontal cortex (PFC) in HE, which increased CBMP and CP/ATG in the SN (not seen in the PFC), induced Drp-1 transformation from the cytosolic to the mitochondria, and increased mitochondrial fission and the number of mitochondria. The long isoforms of fusion protein OPA1 (L-OPA1) were increased in the SN of HE mice. HE also increased CP/ATG proteins PINK1/Parkin and P62/LC3-B in the SN, which selectively removed CBs and cells, respectively. There were no significant changes in the fission, fusion, or ATG proteins in PFC-purified mitochondrial proteins in HE mice. The number of mitochondria also did not show alterations in the PFC of HE mice, suggesting that mitochondria can protect by changing the dynamics and ATG in the SN of HE mice. Changes in the mitochondrial dynamics and ATG related to HE can help repair damaged mitochondria involved in CBMP and confer further understanding of the mechanisms of HE.

CP in Hepatic Carcinogenesis

Most patients with GSDIa develop hepatocellular adenomas (HCA), which can progress to HCC. Gjorgjieva et al. (2018) characterized metabolic reprogramming and cellular defense alterations during tumorigenesis of hepatocyte-specific-G6pc-deficient (L.G6pc$^{-/-}$) mice, which develop the hepatic hallmarks of GSDIa. Liver metabolism and cellular defenses were assessed at pre-tumoral (4 months) and tumoral (9 months) stages in L.G6pc$^{-/-}$ mice fed a high fat/high sucrose (HF/HS) diet, which accelerated HCC since 85% of the L.G6pc$^{-/-}$ mice developed multiple hepatic tumors within nine months, with 70% classified as HCA and 30% as HCC. Tumor development was associated with the high expression of the malignancy markers of HCC, that is, α-fetoprotein, glypican 3, and β-catenin. In addition, L.G6pc$^{-/-}$ livers exhibited a loss of tumor suppressors. L.G6pc$^{-/-}$ steatosis exhibited a low-inflammatory state and was less pronounced than in wild-type livers. This was associated with an absence of epithelial-mesenchymal transition and fibrosis, while HCA/HCC showed epithelial-mesenchymal transition in the absence of TGF-β1 increase. In HCA/HCC, glycolysis was characterized by the enhanced expression of PK-M2, decreased O/P, and pyruvate entry in the mitochondria, confirming a "Warburg-like" phenotype. These metabolic alterations led to a decrease in antioxidant defenses, and ATG and chronic ERS in L.G6pc$^{-/-}$ livers and tumors. ATG was reactivated in HCA/HCC. The metabolic remodeling in the L.G6pc$^{-/-}$ liver generates a pre-neoplastic status and leads to a loss of cellular defenses and tumor suppressors that facilitates tumor development in GSDI. The GSDIa livers reprogram their metabolism in a similar way to cancer cells, which facilitates tumor formation and progression, in the absence of hepatic fibrosis. Moreover, the hepatic burden due to the overload of glycogen and lipids in the cells leads to a decrease in cellular defenses, such as CP/ATG, which further promote tumorigenesis in GSDI. To construct the recombinant adenoviral containing fructose 1, 6-biphosphatase 1 (FBP1), and to investigate whether FBP1 has an effect on CP and proliferation in HepG2 cells, Pan et al (2019) amplified the FBPI cDNA sequence by PCR and cloned it in adenovirus vector pAdTrack-TO4, and then constructed the recombinant adenovirus plasmid pAdTrack-FBP. The recombinant adenovirus plasmid was transfected into HEK293 cells by Lipofectamine 3000. The high-titer of recombinant adenovirus AdFBP1 was obtained by packaging and amplification. HepG2 cells were infected with the recombinant adenovirus AdFBP1, and the mock and AdGFP group were set at the same time. The level of ATG in the AdFBP1 group was lower than that in AdGFP group. The average number of autophages in AdGFP was 28.33 ± 1.53, whereas it was 12.33 ± 1.53 in the AdFBP1group. The results of the colony formation assay and MTT assay showed that the proliferation of liver cancer cells in the AdFBP1 group was significantly inhibited compared with the AdGFP group. The results of colony formation showed that the cell clones in the AdGFP group was 65.66 ± 2.57 and 34.00 ± 2.00 in the AdFBP1 group. The absorbance of AdGFP group at 96 hrs was 39.13 ± 2.21 and 30.61 ± 3.33 in the AdFBP1 group for the same time period. FBP1 inhibited CP and proliferation in liver cancer cells (HepG2).

Recently, Li et al. (2019) examined the association of Atg5 polymorphisms with HBV-related HCC. Two polymorphisms, Atg5 rs573775 and rs510432, were genotyped by ligase detection reaction-PCR in 403 patients with chronic HBV infection (171 chronic hepatitis, 119 cirrhosis, and 113 HCC) and 196 healthy controls. The rs573775 genotype and allele frequencies showed no differences amongst patients with different clinical conditions. However, HCC patients had a higher frequency of the rs510432 genotype AA than chronic hepatitis patients. In multivariate analyses, rs510432 allele A-containing genotypes (AA+GA) were associated with cirrhosis rather than chronic hepatitis. The rs510432 genotypes AA+GA were also associated with HCC in comparison to chronic hepatitis or chronic HBV infection without HCC, indicating that rs510432 genotypes AA+GA are associated with disease progression and HCC risk in a chronic HBV infection, and highlighting the role of Atg5 in the pathogenesis of HBV-related HCC.

Ionizing Radiation-Induced Hepatic Injury

Lysek-Gladysinska et al. (2018) investigated the long-term effects of radiation on the wild-type C57BL/6J and ApoE$^{-/-}$ male mice which received a single dose (2 or 8 Gy) of X-rays to the heart with simultaneous exposure to low doses (no >30 and 120 mGy, respectively). Livers were collected for analysis 60 weeks after irradiation and used for ultrastructural and biochemical analyses. An increased damage to the mitochondrial ultrastructure and lipid deposition in hepatocytes of irradiated animals was observed. Radiation-related effects were stronger in ApoE$^{-/-}$ mice than wild-type animals. Radiation-related changes in the activity of lysosomal hydrolases, including acid phosphatase, β-glucuronidase, N-acetyl-β-D-hexosaminidase, β-galactosidase, and α-glucosidase, were observed in wild type but not in ApoE-deficient mice, suggesting a higher activity of ATG in ApoE-proficient animals. Irradiation caused a reduction in plasma biomarkers of liver damage in wild-type mice, while an increased hepatic lipase was observed in plasma of ApoE-deficient mice, indicating a higher resistance of hepatocytes from ApoE-proficient animals to radiation-induced damage. Liver dysfunctions were observed as late effects of irradiation, in association with malfunction of the lipid metabolism. In addition, Wieczorek et al. (2018) studied the effect of ionizing radiation on the lysosomes of the mouse liver after *in vivo* exposure. Activities of selected lysosomal enzymes were assessed in 12, 36, and 120 hrs after exposure to the mean dose of 1 Gy. The ATG-related proteins LC3-II and p62 were compared by immunoblotting between untreated and irradiated animals (120 hrs after exposure). An increased number of ATG vacuoles were observed in the hepatocytes from exposed animals. These vacuoles contained degenerated mitochondria implicated in CBMP. The lysosomal hydrolases activity was increased after exposure. However, ATG substrates LC3-II and p62 were barely affected in exposed animals 120 hrs after irradiation. The effects of irradiation included an increased number of autophagosomes and increased activity of lysosomal enzymes. However, putative markers of ATG were not observed, suggesting suppression of the radiation-mediated ATG pathway.

Theranostic Significance of Antioxidants as CP Regulators in Liver Diseases

Resveratrol in Hepatic Steatosis

In the liver, ATG mediates the breakdown of lipid droplets. Milton-Laskibar et al. (2018) compared the involvement of ATG and the oxidative status on the effects of Resveratrol (Res) and energy restriction as theranostic strategy for managing liver steatosis. They fed rats a HF/HS diet for 6 weeks and then divided them into four groups and fed them a standard diet: a control group (C), a Res-treated group (RSV, 30 mg kg^{-1} day^{-1}), an energy- restricted group (R, –15%), and an energy-restricted group treated with Res (RR). Liver triacylglycerols (TGs) were measured by Folch's method. TBARS, GSH, GSSG, GPx, and SOD were assessed using commercial kits. The protein expression of Beclin, Atg5, and p62, as well as ratios of pSer555 ULK1/total ULK1, pSer757 ULK1/total ULK1, and LC3 II/I were determined by immunoblotting. Energy restriction increased Beclin, Atg5, and pSer757 ULK1/total ULK1 and LC3 II/I ratios, and reduced the expression of p62, indicating that it induced ATG. The effects of RR were similar but less marked than the hypocaloric diet. No differences were observed in oxidative stress determinants except for TBARS, which was decreased by energy restriction, suggesting that RR can reverse partially dietary-induced hepatic lipid accumulation, although less efficiently than energy restriction. The dyslipidating effect of energy restriction was mediated by ATG activation; however, its involvement following Res treatment was less clear. The author proposed that antioxidants such as Res exert their beneficial effect by boosting the MB and by augmenting CP for IMD and ICD, as observed during CR (Sharma 2019).

Melatonin in HCC

Mortezaee (2018) highlighted that melatonin (N-acetyl-5-methoxytryptamine) is a multi-tasking hormone that has anti-cancer activity in various human cancers, including HCC. Melatonin inhibits MDR and induces apoptosis in HCC. Melatonin induces ER- and ATG-mediated apoptosis in cancer cells and inhibits cancer cell proliferation, motility, and invasiveness by modulating various transcription factors and related pathways. Melatonin also relieves an immunosuppressive state in HCC cancer cells by controlling tumor-derived exosomes. Both pro-and anti-oxidative functions of melatonin are essential for combating HCC. Combination of melatonin with chemotherapy confers cumulative effects on cancer cells by acting on the MAPK family members.

Betaine in MCD-Induced Fatty Liver Disease

Veskovic et al. (2019) examined the effects of betaine (an endogenous and dietary methyl donor essential for the methionine-homocysteine cycle) on oxidative stress, inflammation, apoptosis, and ATG in methionine-choline deficient diet (MCD)-induced NAFLD. The male C57BL/6 mice received standard chow (control), standard chow and betaine (1.5% w/v in drinking water), MCD, or MCD and betaine. After six weeks, serum and liver samples were collected for analysis. Betaine reduced the MCD-induced increase in liver transaminases and inflammatory infiltration, as well as the hepatosteatosis and serum levels of LDL, while it increased HDL. The MCD-induced production of hepatic RONS was significantly reduced by Betaine, which improved the antioxidant defense by increasing glutathione and SOD, catalase, glutathione peroxidase, and paraoxonase. Betaine reduced the expression of pro-inflammatory cytokines TNF and IL-6, as well as the pro-apoptotic mediator Bax, while increasing anti-inflammatory cytokine IL-10 and anti-apoptotic Bcl-2 in MCD-fed mice. In addition, Betaine increased the expression of ATG-activators Beclin-1, ATG-related (ATG)4 and Atg5, as well as the presence of ATG vesicles and degradation of the ATG target sequestosome 1/p62 in the liver of NAFLD mice. These effects of Betaine coincided with the increase in the phosphorylation of mTOR and its activator Akt, suggesting that the beneficial effect of Betaine in MCD-induced NAFLD is associated with the reduction in liver oxidative stress, inflammation, and apoptosis, and an increase in cytoprotective Akt/mTOR signaling and ATG.

Formononetin in Hepatic Steatosis

Formononetin ameliorates hyperlipidemia and obesity. Lipophagy is a protective mechanism during steatosis that results in the decomposition of LDs through ATG and the prevention of cellular lipid accumulation. Wang et al. (2019) investigated the beneficial role of Formononetin in treating NAFLD and the mechanism of lipophagy in anti-hepatic steatosis effects. Formononetin ameliorated hepatic steatosis in HFD mice and reduced FFAs-stimulated lipid accumulation in HepG2 cells and primary mouse hepatocytes. Steatosis increased LC3B-II, a marker of ATG, but caused the blockade of ATG associated with a lack of lysosomes. Treatment with Formononetin promoted lysosome biogenesis and autophagosome-lysosome fusion, relieving the blockade in ATG and further inducing lipophagy. Formononetin activated AMPK and promoted the nuclear translocation of transcription factor EB (TFEB), a key regulator of lysosome biogenesis. TFEB inhibition abolished Formononetin-induced lysosome biogenesis, autophagosome-lysosome fusion, lipophagy, alleviated lipid accumulation, improved hepatic steatosis via TFEB-mediated lysosome biogenesis, providing evidence of its anti-NAFLD effects.

Kaempferol Lowers Hepatic Triglyceride

The number of people with hyperlipidemia is growing in both developed and developing societies. Kaempferol could be used for theranostic interventions for the treatment of these individuals. Kaempferol is a dietary flavonoid in various plant-based foods, and is used in functional foods, with beneficial properties such as anticancer, antioxidant, and anti-atherosclerotic activities. Kaempferol exerts its TG-lowering effect via Akt inhibition and the activation of PPARα and PPARδ. Hoang et al. (2019) studied the mechanism of the TG-lowering effect of Kaempferol. It showed LXR-agonistic activities without inducing TGs or the expression of lipogenic genes in cultured cells. A luciferase and qPCR analysis showed that Kaempferol induced PPARα, PPARδ, and gene expression associated with fatty acid oxidation and uptake in hepatocytes. Kaempferol inhibited protein kinase B (Akt) activity and suppressed SREBP-1 activation via increasing Insig-2a expression, reducing SREBP-1 phosphorylation, and increasing GSK-3 phosphorylation. These actions inhibited the SREBP-1 activation process. As an Akt/mTOR pathway inhibitor, Kaempferol induced hepatic ATG and decreased LD formation in the mouse liver, suggesting that it exerts a TG-lowering effect via Akt inhibition and the activation of PPARα and PPARδ.

Mst1 Inhibition Attenuates NAFLD

Obesity-related NAFLD is associated with MTS and hepatocyte apoptosis. Parkin-related CP sustains mitochondrial homeostasis and hepatocyte viability. Macrophage stimulating 1 (Mst1) is a novel CP upstream regulator which exacerbates heart and cancer apoptosis via repressing CP. Zhou et al. (2019) explored whether Mst1 contributes to NAFLD via disrupting Parkin-related CP. A NAFLD model was generated in wild-type (WT) mice and Mst1 knockout (Mst1-KO) mice using HFD. Experiments were conducted via PA treatment in the primary hepatocytes. Mst1 was upregulated in HFD-treated livers. The genetic ablation of Mst1 attenuated HFD-mediated hepatic injury and sustained hepatocyte viability. The Mst1 knockdown reversed

Parkin-related CP and protected mitochondria and hepatocytes against HFD challenges. Besides, Mst1 modulated Parkin expression via the AMPK pathway; the blockade of AMPK repressed Parkin-related CP and recalled hepatocytes' mitochondrial apoptosis, suggesting that NAFLD is associated with the defective Parkin-related CP due to Mst1 upregulation, which may pave the way to theranostic modalities for the treatment of fatty liver disease.

Cyanidin and Quercetin in Hepatocyte Steatosis

Rafiei et al. (2019) reported that in HepG2 hepatocytes, treatment with Quercetin, Cyanidin, or their phenolic breakdown/digestion products (protocatechuic acid, 2,4,6-trihydroxybenzaldehyde, and caffeic acid), starting 2 hrs prior to oleic acid for 24 hrs, protected against increases in intracellular lipid, ROS, and $\Delta\Psi$ collapse. Cyanidin and its phenolic products also protected against decreased mitochondrial content. After pre-incubation for only 1 hr and removal prior to oleic acid, only the phenolic products protected against decreased mitochondrial content, without adding oleic acid. Only Protocatechuic acid and Caffeic acid, and less so Cyanidin, increased mitochondrial content, suggesting that phenolic breakdown products of Cyanidin and Quercetin contribute to the protective effects.

MATα1 Interacts with Cytochrome P450 2E1

Methionine adenosyltransferase α1 (MATα1, encoded by MAT1A) is responsible for hepatic biosynthesis of SAM, the principal methyl donor. MATα1 also acts as a transcriptional cofactor by interacting and influencing the activity of several transcription factors. Mat1a knockout (KO) mice have increased levels of CYP2E1. Murray et al. (2019) identified the binding partners of MATα1 and elucidated how MATα1 regulates CYP2E1 expression. They identified the binding partners of MATα1 by co-immunoprecipitation (co-IP) and mass spectrometry. Interacting proteins were confirmed using recombinant proteins, liver lysates, and mitochondria. ALD samples were used to confirm the relevance of these findings. MATα1 negatively regulated CYP2E1 at mRNA and protein levels, with the latter being the dominant mechanism. MATα1 interacted with many proteins but with a predominance of mitochondrial proteins including CYP2E1. MATα1 was present in the mitochondrial matrix of hepatocytes. Mat1a KO hepatocytes had reduced $\Delta\Psi$ and higher ROS, both of which were normalized when MAT1A was overexpressed. In addition, KO hepatocytes were sensitized to ethanol and TNFα-induced mitochondrial dysfunction. Interaction of MATα1 with CYP2E1 was direct, and facilitated CYP2E1 methylation at R379, leading to its degradation through the proteasomal pathway. Mat1a KO livers have a reduced methylated/total CYP2E1 ratio. MATα1's influence on mitochondrial function is mediated by its effect on CYP2E1 expression. Patients with ALD have reduced MATα1 levels and a decrease in the methylated/total CYP2E1 ratio, suggesting the critical role of MATα1 in regulating mitochondrial function by suppressing CYP2E1 expression.

Vinyl Chloride-Induced Steatohepatitis

Vinyl chloride (VC), an environmental contaminant causes steatohepatitis at high levels, but is considered safe at lower (that is, sub-OSHA) levels. Chen et al. (2019) showed that even low concentrations of VC exacerbate NFALD caused by HFD. Mitochondrial oxidative injury and subsequent metabolic dysfunction play key roles in mediating this interaction. Mitochondrial aldehyde dehydrogenase 2 (ALDH2) serves as a key line of defense against endogenous and exogenous reactive aldehydes. Mice were exposed to low VC concentrations (<1 ppm), or room air for 6 hrs/day, 5 days/week for 12 weeks, while on HFD or LFD. Some mice received Alda-1 (20 mg/kg i.p., 3 × /week) for the last 3 weeks of the diet/VC exposure. Indices of liver injury, oxidative stress, and metabolic and mitochondrial function were measured. A low-dose of VC did not cause liver injury in control mice; liver injury caused by HFD was enhanced by VC, which decreased the hepatic ALDH2 activity of mice fed a HFD. Alda-1 attenuated oxidative stress, liver injury, and impaired metabolism in mice exposed to HFD+VC under these conditions. Alterations in the mitochondrial function caused by VC and HFD were diminished by Alda-1. Liver injury caused by HFD was mediated by enhanced CP. Alda-1 suppressed PINK1/Parkin-mediated CP, supporting the hypothesis that ALDH2 is a defense system against mitochondrial injury caused by VC in NAFLD. The ALDH2 activator Alda-1 conferred protection in liver damage by increasing the clearance of aldehydes through CP and preserving mitochondrial O/P.

PPARδ Attenuates Hepatic Steatosis

PPARδ belongs to the nuclear receptor family and is involved in metabolic diseases. Tong et al. (2019) showed that PPARδ is a potent stimulator of hepatic ATG. The expression of PPARδ and ATG-related proteins were decreased in liver tissues from obese and aging mice. Pharmacological and adenovirus-mediated increases in PPARδ expression and activity were achieved in obese transgenic db/db and HFD-fed mice. Using genetic, pharmacological, and metabolic approaches, these investigators demonstrated that PPARδ reduces intrahepatic lipids and stimulates β-oxidation in liver and hepatocytes by an ATG-lysosomal pathway involving AMPK/mTOR signaling, providing novel insight into the lipolytic actions of PPARδ through ATG and its potential beneficial effects during NAFLD.

Catalase Protects Hepatic Cells

CeNPs with a predominantly high Ce +4 oxidation state exhibit biological catalase enzyme-like activity. Catalase is present in mammalian cells and facilitates the protection from ROS, generated due to the decomposition of H_2O_2. The inactivation of catalase causes several diseases such as acatalasemia, T2DM, and vitiligo. Singh and Singh (2019) inhibited the activity of catalase from human liver cells (WRL-68) using 3-Amino-1,2,4-Triazole (3-AT). CeNPs were used for their protective effect against the deleterious effects of cellular H_2O_2. CeNPs (+4) protected hepatic cells from cytotoxicity and damage from the high concentrations of H_2O_2 in the absence of functional catalase enzyme. CeNPs were internalized in WRL-68 cells and scavenge the free radicals generated due to elevated H_2O_2. CeNPs protected cells from undergoing early apoptosis and DNA damage induced due to the 3-AT exposure. CeNPs did not elicit the natural antioxidant defense system of the cells even in the absence of catalase, suggesting that the observed protection was due to the H_2O_2 degradation activity of CeNPs (+4). This study confirmed CeNPs for the treatment of diseases related to a nonfunctional catalase enzyme in the mammalian cells.

Proinflammatory and Profibrotic Events of ALD

Zhong et al. (2018) explored how early mitochondrial adaptations for alcohol metabolism lead to ALD pathogenesis. Ethanol (EtOH) acutely causes a near doubling of hepatic EtOH metabolism and O_2 consumption within 2–3 hrs. This swift increase in alcohol metabolism (SIAM) is an adaptive response to enhance the metabolic elimination of both EtOH and its toxic metabolite, acetaldehyde (AcAld). In association with SIAM, EtOH causes widespread hepatic mitochondrial depolarization (mtDepo), which stimulates O_2 consumption. Parallelly, voltage-dependent anion channels (VDAC) in the OMM close. VDAC closure and respiratory stimulation promote the selective oxidation of EtOH, first to AcAld in the cytosol, and then to nontoxic acetate in mitochondria, since the membrane-permeant AcAld does not require VDAC to enter mitochondria. VDAC closure also inhibits mitochondrial fatty acid oxidation and ATP release, promoting steatosis and a decrease in cytosolic ATP. After acute EtOH, these changes reverted as EtOH is eliminated by just a little hepatocellular lethality. mtDepo also stimulated MTG. After chronic high EtOH exposure, the capacity to process depolarized mitochondria by MTG was compromised, leading to the intra- and extracellular release of damaged mitochondria, mitophagosomes, and/or autolysosomes containing mtDAMP molecules. mtDAMPs caused inflammasome activation and promoted inflammatory and profibrogenic responses, causing hepatitis and fibrosis, suggesting that the persistence of mitochondrial responses to EtOH metabolism links initial adaptive EtOH metabolism to maladaptive changes initiating the onset and progression of ALD due to the induction of CBMP.

Akebia Saponin D Alleviates Hepatic Steatosis

Akebia Saponin D (ASD) is the constituent of the rhizome of the Dipsacus asper Wall. ASD alleviates hepatic steatosis targeted at the modulation of ATG and exerts protective effects through mitochondria. Gong et al. (2018) explored the mechanisms through which ASD alleviates hepatic steatosis. ASD reduced lipid accumulation in BRL cells and increased CP as demonstrated by co-localization between mitochondria and punctate EGFP-LC3. ASD treatment increased the expression of Bnip-3 and phospho-AMPK, as well as prevented oleic-acid (OA)-induced LC3-II and phospho-mTOR expression similar to co-treatment with Rapamycin. However, ASD could not attenuate the expression of Bnip-3 blocked by CQ or the siRNA-mediated knockdown of Bnip-3, suggesting that Akebia saponin D alleviates hepatic steatosis targeted at Bnip-3-mediated CP. Hence, the activation of Bnip-3 via ASD may offer a new strategy for treating NAFLD.

ROS-MTG Signaling in I/R Injury

I/R injury (IRI) is the primary cause of complications following liver transplantation. ROS were thought to be the main regulators of IRI. However recent studies demonstrate that ROS activates the cyto-protective mechanism of ATG, promoting cell survival. Liver IRI initially damages the liver endothelial cells (LEC). Bhogal et al. (2018) isolated primary human LEC from human liver tissue and exposed it to an *in vitro* model of IRI to assess the role of ATG in LEC using a murine model of partial liver IRI. During IRI, ROS activates ATG7, promoting autophagic flux and the formation of LC3B positive puncta around mitochondria in human LEC. The inhibition of ROS reduced autophagic flux in LEC during IRI, inducing necrosis. In addition, the siRNA knockdown of ATG7 sensitized LEC to necrosis during IRI. Uninjured liver lobes indicated that ATG within LEC was reduced following IRI with concomitant reduction in ATG flux and increased cell death, indicating that during IRI, ROS-dependent ATG promotes LEC survival and therapeutic targeting of this signaling pathway may reduce liver IRI following transplantation.

Mitochondrial Stasis Alleviates NAFLD

Yamada et al. (2018) introduced mitochondrial stasis by deleting two dynamin-related GTPases for division (Drp-1) and fusion (Opa1) in livers. Mitochondrial stasis rescued liver damage and hypotrophy caused by the single knockout (KO). At the cellular level, mitochondrial stasis re-established mitochondrial size and rescued CP defects caused by division deficiency. Using Drp-1KO livers, they found that the ATG adaptor protein p62/sequestosome-1-which functions downstream of ubiquitination promotes mitochondrial ubiquitination. The p62 recruits two subunits of a cullin-RING ubiquitin E3 ligase complex, Keap1 and Rbx1, to mitochondria. Diet-induced NAFL resembles Drp-1KO and enlarges mitochondria and accumulate CP intermediates. Opa1KO resembling Drp-1Opa1KO rescues liver damage in this disease model. This study provided the novel concept that mitochondrial stasis leads the spatial dimension of mitochondria to a stationary equilibrium and showcases a new mechanism for mitochondrial ubiquitination in CP.

Tanshinone IIA Reduce Liver I/R Injury

ATG is a highly conserved cell program in eukaryotic cells, which plays an important role in dealing with adverse external stimuli such as I/R. Tanshinone IIA (TanIIA) has a protective effect on myocardial disease and could regulate ATG in different cells. Wang et al. (2018a) detected the role of TanIIA in regulating ATG and the subsequent protective effects on hepatocytes. TanIIA pre-treatment enhanced ATG by the MEK/ERK/mTOR pathway in hepatocytes after liver I/R, which enhanced ATG, and decreased ROS generation by clearing damaged mitochondria implicated in CBMP, providing a protective effect on liver I/R, which was manifested as reduced serum enzyme levels, reduced liver tissue damage, decreased inflammatory cell infiltration, decreased inflammatory cytokines, and reduced hepatocyte apoptosis. Hence, TanIIA might be a potential theranostic approach for liver I/R.

Liver-specific Deletion of Eva1a/Tmem166

Acute liver failure (ALF) is an inflammation-mediated hepatocellular injury associated with cellular ATG. Lin et al. (2018) demonstrated that Eva1a (eva-1 homolog A)/Tmem166 (transmembrane protein 166), an ATG-related gene, can protect mice from ALF induced by D-galactosamine (D-GalN)/lipopolysaccharide (LPS) via ATG. A hepatocyte-specific deletion of Eva1a aggravated hepatic injury in ALF mice, as evidenced by increased ALT and AST, myeloperoxidase (MPO), and inflammatory cytokines (e.g., TNFα and IL-6), which was associated with disordered liver architecture exhibited by Eva1a$^{-/-}$ mouse livers with ALF. The decreased ATG in Eva1a$^{-/-}$ mouse liver resulted in the accumulation of swollen mitochondria in ALF, resulting in a lack of ATP generation, and hepatocyte apoptosis or death involving CBMP. The administration of Adeno-Associated Virus Eva1a (AAV-Eva1a) or ATG-inducer Rapamycin increased the ATG and provided protection against liver injury in Eva1a$^{-/-}$ mice with ALF, suggesting that defective ATG is a mechanism of ALF in mice. Thus, Eva1a-mediated ATG-ameliorated liver injury in mice with ALF by attenuating inflammatory responses and apoptosis, indicating a potential theranostic application for ALF.

NPC2 Regulates Cholesterol Accumulation

Liver fibrosis is the first step towards progression to cirrhosis, portal hypertension, and HCC. A high-cholesterol diet is associated with liver fibrosis via the accumulation of free cholesterol in hepatic stellate cells (HSCs). Niemann-Pick type C2 (NPC2) plays an important role in the regulation of intracellular free cholesterol homeostasis via direct binding with free cholesterol. Wang et al. (2018b) reported that NPC2 was downregulated in liver cirrhosis. The loss of NPC2 enhanced the accumulation of free cholesterol in HSCs and made them more susceptible to TGF-β1. The knockdown of NPC2 resulted in an increase in PDGF-BB-induced HSC proliferation through enhanced ERK, p38, JNK, and protein kinase B (Akt) phosphorylation, whereas, NPC2 overexpression decreased PDGF-BB-induced cell proliferation by inhibiting p38, JNK, and Akt phosphorylation. Although NPC2 expression did not affect caspase-related apoptosis, the ATG marker LC3-β was decreased in NPC2 knockdown, and free cholesterol accumulated in the HSCs. The mitochondrial respiration functions (such as the O_2 consumption rate, ATP production, and maximal respiratory capacity) were decreased in NPC2 knockdown, and free cholesterol accumulated in the HSCs, while NPC2-overexpressed cells remained normal. In addition, NPC2 expression did not affect the susceptibility of HSCs to LPS, and U18666A treatment induced free cholesterol accumulation, which enhanced LPS-induced TLR4, NF-κB (p65) phosphorylation, IL-1 and IL-6 expression, indicating that NPC2-mediated free cholesterol homeostasis controls HSC proliferation and mitochondrial function.

Maternal Physical Activity in Mitochondrial Health

Maternal exercise and physical activity during the gestational period can be protective against maternal HFD-induced hepatic steatosis in older offspring. Cunningham et al. (2018) investigated whether maternal physical activity would attenuate maternal western diet (WD)-induced steatosis in young adult rats. Female Wistar rats (7–8 weeks of age) were randomized into having a WD (42% fat, 27% sucrose) or a normal chow diet (ND), and further randomized into physical activity (RUN) or sedentary (SED) conditions for a total of four groups. The dams returned to ND/SED conditions after parturition. Post-weaning, the offspring were maintained in ND/SED conditions for 18 weeks. Maternal WD-induced increases in male offspring body mass was attenuated in the WD/RUN offspring. Maternal WD feeding increased hepatic steatosis in male (but not female offspring), which was not attenuated by maternal RUN. However, the maternal RUN group had increased hepatic markers of MB and MTG (mitochondrial transcription factor A, PPAR-γ, and nuclear factor E2-related factor 2) in all offspring and the MTG marker, BCL2-interacting protein 3, in WD/RUN offspring. Hepatic markers of *de novo* lipogenesis (fatty acid synthase and acetyl coenzyme A carboxylase), MTG (ATG-related gene 12:5, BCL2-interacting protein 3, p62, and LC3 II/I), and mitochondria biogenesis/content (mitochondrial transcription factor A and OXPHOS-Complex II) were significantly increased in female versus male offspring. Although maternal physical activity did not attenuate WD-induced hepatic steatosis in older adult offspring, it did increase hepatic markers of MB and MTG. Female offspring had elevated hepatic markers of mitochondrial health, providing evidence as to why female rats are protected against maternal WD-induced hepatic steatosis.

Sirtuin 1 and Mitofusin 2 in I/R Hepatic Injury

CP/ATG is energy (ATP)-driven, lysosomal-dependent event which occurs in the most vulnerable hepatocytes in response to DPCI-induced free radical injury. It is not a mutually-exclusive event and is executed sequentially by Akt-ubiquitination of CB for lysosomal recognition, activation and phagocytosis. CP plays a predominant role during the acute phase of ischemic insult, whereas ATG plays a predominant role during reperfusion and the chronic phase of disease progression due to free radical overproduction and compromised ATP synthesis from functionally-impaired mitochondria. Thus, I/R injury contributes to morbidity and mortality during liver resection and transplantation. Livers from elderly patients have a poorer recovery from these surgeries, indicating reduced restorative capacity with aging. Chun et al. (2018) investigated how sirtuin 1 (SIRT1) and mitofusin 2 (Mfn-2) are affected by I/R in aged livers. Young (3 months) and old (23–26 months) male C57/BL6 mice were subjected to hepatic I/R *in vivo*. Primary hepatocytes isolated from each age group were also exposed to *in vitro* I/R. Compared to young mice, old livers showed accelerated liver injury following mild I/R. Reperfusion of old hepatocytes also showed necrosis, defective CP/ATG, onset of the mitochondrial permeability transition and dysfunction, and loss of both SIRT1 and Mfn-2 after I/R involving CBMP. Overexpression of either SIRT1 or Mfn-2 alone in old hepatocytes failed to mitigate I/R injury, while co-overexpression of both proteins promoted ATG and prevented mitochondrial dysfunction and cell death after reperfusion. Genetic approaches with deletion and point mutants revealed that SIRT1 de-acetylated K655 and K662 residues in the C-terminus of Mfn-2, leading to CP/ATG induction. The SIRT1-Mfn-2 axis was pivotal during I/R recovery and may be a theranostic target to reduce I/R injury in aged livers.

Fenofibrate in Acetaminophen (APAP) Hepatotoxicity

An Overdose of APAP induces acute liver injury due to the destruction of mitochondria and oxidative stress involving CBMP. Recently, the fibroblast growth factor 21 (FGF21) has been demonstrated to protect liver from oxidative stress. Zhang et al. (2018) explored the role of FGF21 in the protective effect of Fenofibrate, an agonist of PPARα, in APAP-induced liver injury. Mice and primary cultured hepatocytes were used to test the protective effect of Fenofibrate in APAP-induced hepatotoxicity. FGF21-deficient mice were used to evaluate the role of FGF21 in Fenofibrate in APAP-induced acute liver injury. Treatment with Fenofibrate inhibited APAP-induced hepatotoxicity, as evidenced by decreased serum ALT and AST levels and hepatic necrosis in liver tissue as well as an increased survival rate in response to APAP overdose, which was attenuated in FGF21 KO mice. Fenofibrate increased ATG and alleviated hepatotoxicity in APAP-treated WT mice. However, such an effect was attenuated in APAP-treated FGF21 KO mice, suggesting that Fenofibrate in APAP-induced hepatotoxicity is mediated by upregulating the expression of FGF21, which promotes ATG-mediated protective effects.

Fucoxanthin

Laminaria japonica has been used as a food supplement and drug in traditional medicine. Among the major active constituents responsible for the bioactivities of L. japonica, fucoxanthin (FX) is considered a potential antioxidant. Jang et al. (2018) examined the effects of an L. japonica extract (LJE) or FX in oxidative stress on hepatocytes and elucidated on their cellular mechanisms of action. They constructed an *in vitro* model which was given a treatment of arachidonic acid (AA)+iron in the HepG2 cells to stimulate the oxidative stress. The cells were pre-treated with LJE or FX for 1 hr, and incubated with AA + iron. The effect on oxidative damage and cellular mechanisms of LJE or FX were assessed by a cytological examination and biochemical assays under conditions which did and did not include kinase inhibitors. LJE or FX pretreatment attenuated the pathological changes caused by AA+ iron treatment, such as cell death, altered expression of apoptosis-related proteins such as procaspase-3 and PARP, and caused mitochondria dysfunction. FX induced AMPK activation and the AMPK inhibitor, compound C, reduced the protective effect of FX on mitochondria dysfunction. Consistent with AMPK activation, FX increased the ATG markers (LC3-II and Beclin-1) and the number of Acridine orange-stained cells, decreased the phosphorylation of mTOR, and increased the phosphorylation of ULK1. The inhibition of ATG by 3-MA or Bafilomycin A1 attenuated the protective effect of FX, suggesting that FX confers protection in oxidative damages through the AMPK pathway by regulating CP/ATG.

Fatty Liver Preservation in Cold Ischemia Injury

Institute Goeorges Lopez 1 (IGL-1) and Histidine-Tryptophan-Ketoglutarate (HTK) preservation solutions are used for liver transplantation besides the University of Wisconsin (UW) solution and Celsior. Several clinical trials have been carried out comparing these solutions; however the comparative IGL-1 and HTK appraisals are poor, especially when they deal with the protective mechanisms of the fatty liver graft during cold storage. Panisello-Roselló et al. (2018) conserved fatty livers from male obese Zücker rats for 24 hrs at 4°C in IGL-1 or HTK preservation solutions. After organ recovery and rinsing of fatty liver grafts with the Ringer Lactate solution, they measured the changes in mTOR signaling, liver ATG markers (Beclin-1, Beclin-2, LC3B, and ATG7) and apoptotic markers (caspase 3, caspase 9, and TUNEL). These determinations were correlated with the prevention of liver injury (AST/ALT), and mitochondrial damage (glutamate dehydrogenase). Liver grafts preserved in an IGL-1 solution showed a reduction in p-TOR/mTOR ratio compared to HTK, concomitant with increased protective ATG and prevention of apoptosis, including inflammatory cytokines such as HMGB1. These results revealed that the IGL-1 preservation solution better protected fatty liver grafts from cold ischemia damage than the HTK solution and that this protection was associated with a reduced liver damage, induced CP/ATG, and decreased apoptosis. All these effects would contribute to limit the subsequent extension of I/R injury after graft revascularization in liver transplantation.

CONCLUSION

Sirtuin signaling regulated mitochondrial function in GSD-Ia. CP/ATG was dysregulated in hepatic insulin resistance. The molecular drivers of NASH were sustained in mild-to-late fibrosis in a guinea pig model. The progression from NAFLD to NASH by ethanol was associated with impaired CP-mediated NLRP3 inflammasome activation. LncRNA-regulated ATG and drug-induced hepatic injury in mice. ATG attenuated Cu-induced CBMP by regulating oxidative stress in chicken hepatocytes. Chronic low-dose mouse liver irradiation induced lysosomal changes in hepatocytes depending on the lipid metabolism. Blocking ATG accelerated apoptosis and mitochondrial injury in hepatocytes and mortality in a murine sepsis model. Fructose-1, 6-bisphosphatase inhibited CP and proliferation in liver cancer cells. The theranostic significance of antioxidants as CP regulators in hepatic disease was explored. CP was implicated in the beneficial effects of Res in hepatic steatosis and Melatonin-mediated protection in HCC. Natural and synthetic antioxidants: Betaine, Formononetin, Kaempferol, Cyanidin, Quercetin, Wolfberry-derived zeaxanthin dipalmitate, Cerium oxide-based nanozyme, Akebia aponin D, Tanshinone IIA conferred hepato-protection by CP/ATG induction. Fucoxanthin triggered AMPK-mediated cytoprotection and ATG during oxidative stress. CP/ATG induction attenuated hepatic I/R Injury through the MEK/ERK/mTOR pathway, whereas loss of sirtuin 1 and mitofusin 2 enhanced I/R injury in aged livers. Impaired CP/ATG induced hepatic encephalopathy and deletion of Eva1a/Tmem166 aggravated acute hepatic injury. Neiman-Pick type C2 protein regulated cholesterol accumulation, stellate cell proliferation, and O/P, whereas maternal physical activity influenced the hepatic mitochondrial biomarkers of mouse progeny. Fenofibrate provided FGF21-mediated protection in APAP-induced hepatotoxicity by CP/ATG induction. Furthermore, the IGL-1 preservation solution better protected fatty liver grafts from cold ischemic damage than the HTK solution by inducing CP/ATG and inhibiting apoptosis.

REFERENCES

Abdel-Mohsen, M.A., A.A. El-Braky, A.A.E. Ghazal and M.M. Shamseya. 2018. Autophagy, apoptosis, vitamin D, and vitamin D receptor in hepatocellular carcinoma associated with hepatitis C virus. Medicine (Baltimore) 97: e0172.

Bai, Y., Y. Wang and Y. Yang. 2018. Hepatic encephalopathy changes mitochondrial dynamics and autophagy in the substantia nigra. Metab Brain Dis 33: 1669–1678.

Bhogal, R.H., C.J. Weston, S. Velduis, H.G.D. Leuvenink, et al. 2018. The reactive oxygen species-mitophagy signaling pathway regulates liver endothelial cell survival during ischemia/reperfusion injury. Liver Transpl 24: 1437–1452.

Chen, L., A.L. Lang, G.D. Poff, W.X. Ding, et al. 2019. Vinyl chloride-induced interaction of nonalcoholic and toxicant-associated steatohepatitis: Protection by the ALDH2 activator Alda-1. Redox Biol 24: 101205.

Cho, J.H., G.Y. Kim, B.C. Mansfield and J.Y. Chou. 2018. Sirtuin signaling controls mitochondrial function in glycogen storage disease type Ia. J Inherit Metab Dis 41: 997–1006.

Chun, S.K., S. Lee, J. Flores-Toro, Rebecca Y.U., et al. 2018. Loss of sirtuin 1 and mitofusin 2 contributes to enhanced ischemia/reperfusion injury in aged livers. Aging Cell 17: e12761.

Cunningham, R.P., M.P. Moore, G.M. Meers, G.N. Ruegsegger, et al. 2018. Maternal physical activity and sex impact markers of hepatic mitochondrial health. Med Sci Sports Exerc 50: 2040–2048.

Devarajan, A., N.S. Rajasekaran, C. Valburg, E. Ganapathy, et al. 2018. Maternal perinatal calorie restriction temporally regulates the hepatic ATG and redox status in male rat. Free Radic Biol Med 130: 592–600.

Ding, Q., X.L. Xie, M.M. Wang, J. Yin, et al. 2019. The role of the apoptosis-related protein BCL-B in the regulation of MTG in hepatic stellate cells during the regression of liver fibrosis. Exp Mol Med 51(1): 6.

Gao, H., Y. Lv, Y. Liu, J. Li, et al. 2019. Wolfberry-derived zeaxanthin dipalmitate attenuates ethanol-induced hepatic damage. Mol Nutr Food Res 63: e1801339.

Ghorbani, P., T.R. Smith and M.D. Fullerton. 2019. Does prenylation predict progression in NAFLD? J Pathol 247: 283–286.

Gjorgjieva, M., J. Calderaro, L. Monteillet, M. Silva, et al. 2018. Dietary exacerbation of metabolic stress leads to accelerated hepatic carcinogenesis in glycogen storage disease type Ia. J Hepatol 69: 1074–1087.

Gong, L.L., S. Yang, W. Zhang, F.F. Han, et al. 2018. Akebia saponin D alleviates hepatic steatosis through Bnip-3 induced mitophagy. J Pharmacol Sci 136: 189–195.

Gupta, P. and S.K. Venugopal. 2018. Augmenter of liver regeneration: A key protein in liver regeneration and pathophysiology. Hepatol Res 48: 587–596.

Hoang, M.H., Y. Jia, J.H. Lee, Y. Kim, et al. 2019. Kaempferol reduces hepatic triglyceride accumulation by inhibiting Akt. J Food Biochem 43: e13034.

Iershov, A., I. Nemazanyy, C. Alkhoury, M. Girard, et al. 2019. The class 3 PI3K coordinates autophagy and mitochondrial lipid catabolism by controlling nuclear receptor PPARα. Nat Commun 10: 1566.

Iorga, A.L. and L. Dara. 2019. Cell death in drug-induced liver injury. Adv Pharmacol 85: 31–74.

Ipsen, D.H., J. Skat-Rørdam, M.M. Tsamouri, M. Latta, et al. 2019. Molecular drivers of non-alcoholic steatohepatitis are sustained in mild-to-late fibrosis progression in a guinea pig model. Mol Genet Genomics 294: 649–661.

Jang, E.J., S.C. Kim, J.H. Lee, J.R. Lee, et al. 2018. Fucoxanthin, the constituent of *Laminaria japonica*, triggers AMPK-mediated cytoprotection and autophagy in hepatocytes under oxidative stress. BMC Complement Altern Med 18: 97.

Kan, C., L. Ungelenk, A. Lupp, O. Dirsch, et al. 2018. Ischemia-reperfusion injury in aged livers—the energy metabolism, inflammatory response, and autophagy. Transplantation 102: 368–377.

Lee, J., J.S. Park and Y.S. Roh. 2019. Molecular insights into the role of mitochondria in non-alcoholic fatty liver disease. Arch Pharm Res 42: 935–946.

Lei, Z., M. Deng, Z. Yi, Q. Sun, et al. 2018. cGAS-mediated ATG protects the liver from ischemia-reperfusion injury independently of STING. Am J Physiol Gastrointest Liver Physiol 314: G655–G667.

Li, N., X. Fan, X. Wang, H. Deng, et al. 2019. Autophagy-related 5 gene rs510432 polymorphism is associated with hepatocellular carcinoma in patients with chronic hepatitis b virus infection. Immunol Invest 48: 378–391.

Lin, X., M. Cui, D. Xu, D. Hong, et al. 2018. Liver-specific deletion of Eva1a/Tmem166 aggravates acute liver injury by impairing ATG. Cell Death Dis 9: 768.

Lu, Y. and A.I. Cederbaum. 2018. Cytochrome P450s and alcoholic liver disease. Curr Pharm Des 24: 1502–1517.

Lysek-Gladysinska, M., A. Wieczorek, A. Walaszczyk, K. Jelonek, et al. 2018. Long-term effects of low-dose mouse liver irradiation involve ultrastructural and biochemical changes in hepatocytes that depend on lipid metabolism. Radiat Environ Biophys 57: 123–132.

Michalopoulos, G.K., B. Bhushan. 2020. Liver regeneration: Biological and pathological mechanisms and implications. Nat Rev Gastroenterol Hepatol. https://doi.org/10.1038/s41575-020-0342-4

Milton-Laskibar, I., L. Aguirre, U. Etxeberria, F.I. Milagro, et al. 2018. Involvement of ATG in the beneficial effects of Resveratrol in hepatic steatosis treatment. A comparison with energy restriction. Food Funct 9: 4207–4215.

Mortezaee, K. 2018. Human hepatocellular carcinoma: Protection by melatonin. J Cell Physiol 233: 6486–6508.

Murray, B., H. Peng, L. Barbier-Torres, A.E. Robinson, et al. 2019. Methionine adenosyltransferase α1 is targeted to the mitochondrial matrix and interacts with cytochrome P450 2E1 to lower its expression. Hepatology 70: 2018–2034.

Oami, T., E. Watanabe, M. Hatano, Y. Teratake, et al. 2018. Blocking liver ATG accelerates apoptosis and mitochondrial injury in hepatocytes and reduces time to mortality in a murine sepsis model. Shock 50: 427–434.

Pan, X.M., G.J. Zhang, X.M. Chen, L. Liang, et al. 2019. Fructose-1, 6-bisphosphatase inhibits ATG and proliferation in liver cancer cells. Zhonghua Gan Zang Bing Za Zhi 27: 687–692.

Panisello-Roselló, A., E. Verde, A. Lopez, M. Flores, et al. 2018. Cytoprotective mechanisms in fatty liver preservation against cold ischemia injury: A comparison between IGL-1 and HTK. Int J Mol Sci 19(2): 348.

Qiu, Y.N., G.H. Wang, F. Zhou, J.J. Hao, et al. 2019. PM2.5 induces liver fibrosis via triggering ROS-mediated mitophagy. Ecotoxicol Environ Saf 167: 178–187.

Rafiei, H., K. Omidian and B. Bandy. 2019. Phenolic breakdown products of cyanidin and quercetin contribute to protection against mitochondrial impairment and reactive oxygen species generation in an *in vitro* model of hepatocyte steatosis. J Agric Food Chem 67: 6241–6247.

Reuken, P.A., P. Lutz, M. Casper, E. Al-Herwi, et al. 2019. The *ATG16L1* gene variant rs2241880 (p.T300A) is associated with susceptibility to HCC in patients with cirrhosis. Liver Int 39: 2360–2367.

Ruart, M., L. Chavarria, G. Camprecios, N. Suárez-Herrera. 2019. Impaired endothelial autophagy promotes liver fibrosis by aggravating the oxidative stress response during acute liver injury. J Hepatol 70: 458–469.

Sharma, S. 2019. The Charnoly Body: A Novel Biomarker of Mitochonndrial Bioenergetics. CRC Press, Taylor & Francis Group, Boca Raton, FL, U.S.A.

Singh, R. and S. Singh. 2019. Redox-dependent catalase mimetic cerium oxide-based nanozyme protect human hepatic cells from 3-AT induced acatalasemia. Colloids Surf B Biointerfaces 175: 625–635.

Sun, S.S., Y.X. Wu, M.L. Cheng, C.W. Chen, et al. 2019. Experimental study of silybin-phospholipid complex intervention on amiodarone-induced fatty liver in mice. Zhonghua Gan Zang Bing Za Zhi 27: 45–50.

Tian, B., J. Li, R. Pang, S. Dai, et al. 2018. Gold NPs biosynthesized and functionalized using a hydroxylated tetraterpenoid trigger gene expression changes and apoptosis in cancer cells. ACS Appl Mater Interfaces 10: 37353–37363.

Tong, L., L. Wang, S. Yao, L. Jin, et al. 2019. PPARδ attenuates hepatic steatosis through ATG-mediated fatty acid oxidation. Cell Death Dis 10(3): 197.

Veskovic, M., D. Mladenovic, M. Milenkovic, J. Tosic, et al. 2019. Betaine modulates oxidative stress, inflammation, apoptosis, ATG, and Akt/mTOR signaling in methionine-choline deficiency-induced fatty liver disease. Eur J Pharmacol 848: 39–48.

Wang, Y., Q. Ni, Q. Ye, F. Liu, et al. 2018a. Tanshinone IIA activates autophagy to reduce liver ischemia-reperfusion injury by MEK/ERK/mTOR pathway. Pharmazie 73: 396–401.

Wang, Y.H., Y.C. Twu, C.K. Wang, F.Z. Lin, et al. 2018b. Niemann-pick type C2 protein regulates free cholesterol accumulation and influences hepatic stellate cell proliferation and mitochondrial respiration function. Int J Mol Sci 19(6): 1678.

Wang, Y., H. Zhao, X. Li, Q. Wang, et al. 2019. Formononetin alleviates hepatic steatosis by facilitating TFEB-mediated lysosome biogenesis and lipophagy. J Nutr Biochem 73: 108214.

Wieczorek, A., M. Lysek-Gladysinska, A. Walaszczyk, K. Jelonek, et al. 2018. Changes in activity and structure of lysosomes from liver of mouse irradiated in vivo. Int J Radiat Biol 94: 443–453.

Yamada, T., D. Murata, Y. Adachi, K. Itoh, et al. 2018. Mitochondrial stasis reveals p62-mediated ubiquitination in Parkin-independent MTG and mitigates nonalcoholic fatty liver disease. Cell Metab 28: 588–604.

Yang, F., J. Liao, R. Pei, W. Yu, et al. 2018. ATG attenuates Cu-induced mitochondrial dysfunction by regulating oxidative stress in chicken hepatocytes. Chemosphere 204: 36–43.

Ye, J., X. Hu, T. Wu, Y. Wu, et al. 2019. Insulin resistance exhibits varied metabolic abnormalities in nonalcoholic fatty liver disease, chronic hepatitis B and the combination of the two: a cross-sectional study. Diabetol Metab Syndr 11: 45.

Zhang, Y., Y. Pan, R. Xiong, J. Zheng, et al. 2018. FGF21 mediates the protective effect of Fenofibrate against acetaminophen-induced hepatotoxicity via activating ATG in mice. Biochem Biophys Res Commun 503: 474–481.

Zhang, N.P, X.I. Liu, L. Xie, X.Z. Shen, et al. 2019. Impaired mitophagy triggers NLRP3 inflammasome activation during the progression from nonalcoholic fatty liver to nonalcoholic steatohepatitis. Lab Invest 99: 749–763.

Zhong, Z. and J.J. Lemasters. 2018. A unifying hypothesis linking hepatic adaptations for ethanol metabolism to the proinflammatory and profibrotic events of alcoholic liver disease. Alcohol Clin Exp Res 42: 2072–2089.

Zhou, J., Y. Li, X. Liu, Y. Long, et al. 2018. LncRNA-regulated autophagy and its potential role in drug-induced liver injury. Ann Hepatol 17: 355–363.

Zhou, T., L. Chang, Y. Luo, Y. Zhou, et al. 2019. Mst1 inhibition attenuates non-alcoholic fatty liver disease via reversing Parkin-related mitophagy. Redox Biol 21: 101120.

13

Charnolophagy in Diabetes

INTRODUCTION

Prevalence of Type 2 Diabetes Mellitus (T2DM) has reached pandemic levels in Western societies. ATG is an important regulatory signaling pathway for insulin-resistant T2DM and is induced by cellular stress that could affect many tissues, glucose, and lipid metabolism as well as the secretion of insulin. Hence, understanding the interaction between ATG and the important protein kinase (AMPK) might serve as a potential theranostic strategy. Both T2M and obesity are characterized by hyperlipidemia and LD accumulation in adipose tissue. To investigate whether LDs also accumulate in β-cells of T2D patients, Ji et al. (2019) assessed the expression of PLIN2, a LD-associated protein, in non-diabetic (ND) and T2D pancreas. They observed an upregulation of PLIN2 mRNA and protein in β-cells of T2D patients, along with significant changes in the lipid metabolism, apoptosis, and oxidative-stress genes. The increased LD buildup in T2D β-cells was accompanied by the inhibition in nuclear translocation of TFEB, a master regulator of ATG, and by downregulation of the lysosomal biomarker LAMP2. To investigate whether LD accumulation and ATG are influenced by diabetic conditions, they used INS-1 cells to evaluate the effects of hyperglycemia and hyperlipidemia on ATG and metabolic gene expression. Both LD formation and PLIN2 expression were enhanced in INS-1 cells in hyperglycemia, whereas TFEB activation and ATG gene expression were reduced, suggesting that lipid clearance and mitochondrial homeostasis is disrupted in β-cells during hyperglycemia due to CP dysregulation and CBMP induction. Hence interventions ameliorating lipid clearance could be beneficial in reducing functional impairments in β-cells caused by glucolipotoxicity.

This chapter describes the theranostic significance of CP/ATG in diabetes, with a primary focus on the TSE-EBPT of T2DM.

ATG in DE

Maternal diabetes induces neural tube defects and stimulates the activity of the Foxo3a gene in the embryonic neuro-epithelium. Xu et al. (2019) demonstrated that deleting the Foxo3a gene ameliorates maternal diabetes-induced neural tube defects. Rescuing ATG suppressed by maternal diabetes in the developing neuro-epithelium inhibited the neural tube defect in diabetic pregnancies, suggesting a possible link between Foxo3a and impaired ATG in diabetic embryopathy (DE), which can be more specifically described as diabetic charnolopathy (DC). They determined whether maternal diabetes suppresses ATG through Foxo3a, and if its transcriptional activity is required for the induction of DE by employing the STZ–induced mouse model of T1DM embryopathy. To determine if Foxo3a mediates the inhibitory effect of maternal diabetes on ATG in the developing neuro-epithelium, they induced DE in the Foxo3a gene knockout mice and Foxo3a dominant negative transgenic mice as well. Embryos were harvested at day 8.5 to determine Foxo3a and ATG and at day 10.5 for the presence of neural tube defects. They also examined ATG-related genes. Neural stem cells (C17.2) were used for examining the effects of Foxo3a on ATG *in vitro*. Deletion of the Foxo3a gene restored the ATG markers, lipidation of microtubule-associated protein 1A/1B-LC3-I to light chain 3II, in neurulation-stage embryos. Maternal diabetes decreased LC3-I-positive puncta in the neuro-epithelium, which was restored by deleting Foxo3a. Maternal diabetes also decreased the expression of positive regulators of ATG-related gene 5 and the negative regulators of ATG, and protein p62. Foxo3a gene ablation abrogated the dysregulation of ATG genes. The active form of Foxo3a mimicked high glucose in repressing ATG. In cells cultured under high-glucose conditions, overexpression of the dominant negative Foxo3a mutant blocked ATG impairment. Dominant negative Foxo3a overexpression in the developing neuro-epithelium restored ATG and reduced maternal diabetes-induced apoptosis and neural tube defects, indicating that diabetes-induced Foxo3a activation inhibited ATG in the embryonic neuro-epithelium and that Foxo3a transcriptional activity mediated the teratogenic effect of maternal diabetes. This is because dominant negative Foxo3a prevented maternal diabetes-induced ATG impairment and neural tube defects, suggesting that ATG inducers could be developed for the TSE-EBPT of maternal diabetes-induced neural tube defects.

Pancreatic β-Cell CP/ATG Dysfunction

Lee et al. (2019) summarized results from studies about the role of CP/ATG and its dysregulation in the physiology, metabolism, and pathogenesis of diabetes, with an emphasis on pancreatic β-cell CP/ATG. They discussed generalized ATG and the significance of selective CP/ATG of pancreatic β-cells. Novel findings regarding ATG types other than macroATG were also covered, since several types of ATGs or lysosomal degradation pathways other than macroATG may coexist in pancreatic β-cells. Impaired CP/ATG due to aging, obesity, or genetic predisposition could be a factor in the development of β-cell dysfunction and diabetes associated with lipid overload or islet amyloid deposition. Modulation of CP/ATG of pancreatic β-cells would be valuable in the treatment of diabetes associated with lipid overload or the accumulation of islet amyloid. Hoshino and Matoba (2018) described a protocol to monitor Parkin-mediated MTG in pancreatic MIN6 β-cells using flow cytometry and a pH-sensitive fluorophore, mKeima. In pancreatic islet β-cells, mitochondria play a pivotal role in glucose-stimulated insulin secretion through ATP production from glucose oxidation. Impaired ATGs and the subsequent CBMPs contribute to β-cell dysfunction and glucose intolerance.

Atp6ap2 Deletion Consumes Pancreatic β-Cells Insulin

Pancreatic β-cells store insulin within secretory granules which undergo exocytosis upon the elevation of blood glucose. Crinophagy and ATG deliver damaged or old granules to lysosomes for degradation. However, excessive elimination of insulin granules can impair β-cell function and cause diabetes. Atp6ap2 is an accessory component of the vacuolar ATPase required for lysosomal degradation and ATG. Binger et al. (2019) showed that Cre recombinase-mediated conditional deletion of Atp6ap2 in mouse β-cells causes accumulation of large, multi-granular vacuoles in the cytoplasm, with a reduction in insulin and compromised glucose homeostasis. Loss of insulin stores and gigantic vacuoles were also observed in cultured insulinoma INS-1 cells upon CRISPR/Cas9-mediated removal of Atp6ap2. These phenotypic alterations could not be attributed to a deficiency in ATG or acidification of lysosomes, indicating that Atp6ap2 is critical for regulating the insulin pool and that a balanced regulation of granule turnover is key to maintaining β-cell function and diabetes prevention.

p53 in Diabetes

Itahana and Itahana (2018) discussed the roles of the p53 family in glycolysis, gluconeogenesis, aerobic respiration, and ATG. They also discussed how the dysregulation of the p53 family leads to diseases such as cancer and diabetes. Elucidating the complexities of the p53 family members in glucose homeostasis will improve our understanding of these diseases. Glucose is the key source of energy, as well as the metabolites which generate building blocks in cells. The deregulation of glucose homeostasis occurs in enhanced aerobic glycolysis that is observed in cancers, and insulin-resistant diabetes. Although p53 suppresses tumorigenesis by inducing cell cycle arrest, apoptosis, and senescence in response to stress, other functions of p53 in cellular energy homeostasis and metabolism are also emerging as critical factors for tumor suppression. p53 plays a significant role in regulating glucose homeostasis. The p53 family members p63 and p73, as well as gain-of-function p53 mutants, are also involved in glucose metabolism.

Skeletal Muscle Insulin Resistance Triggers Diabetes

T2DM begins with the development of peripheral insulin resistance which may originate within the skeletal muscle. A number of mechanisms including classical glucose handling, cellular derangements (mitochondrial degeneration), alterations in muscle protein turnover, and microRNAs dysregulation have been proposed for the development of muscle insulin resistance. Greene et al. (2018) examined the recent findings on mitochondrial maintenance, protein turnover and miRNA dysregulation along with implications for these derangements in the development of T2DM. They highlighted the evidence detailing the degeneration of mitochondria and compromised MQC involving CBMP. They examined the current findings of the alterations in muscle protein synthesis and ATG protein degradation as well as the feedback of these systems to insulin signaling in T2DM. The dysregulation of miRNAs is involved in muscle insulin resistance. Several miRNAs are altered by the insulin resistance which regulate insulin signaling and the other processes. Considering that T2DM may be initiated with muscle insulin resistance, improved understanding of the dysregulation of these metabolic parameters of skeletal muscle in the pathogenesis of T2DM may be key to developing TSE-EBPT of T2DM. Skeletal muscle ATG is suppressed by insulin, but it remains uncertain if such suppression is altered with insulin resistance. Ehrlicher et al. (2018) investigated the possibility of the inhibitory action of insulin on ATG remaining intact despite insulin resistance to glucose metabolism. The C57BL/6J mice consumed either a low-fat (10% fat) diet as control or high-fat (60% fat) diet for 12 weeks to induce insulin resistance. Following a 5 hrs fast, mice underwent either hyperinsulinemic-euglycemic, hyperinsulinemic-hyperglycemic, or saline infusion to test the effect of insulin on ATG markers in the quadriceps muscle. Despite the high-fat group having lower insulin-stimulated glucose uptake, both low-fat and high-fat groups had similar autophagosomes during hyperinsulinemic conditions. The lipidation of LC3-II/LC3-I was decreased in hyperinsulinemia versus saline control conditions in low-fat and high-fat groups, demonstrating similar suppression of ATG in the diet groups. Mitochondrial-associated LC3-II was greater in the high-fat group as compared to the low-fat group across clamp conditions, suggesting a greater localization of autophagosomes with mitochondria. L6 myotubes were treated with insulin and Rapamycin to determine the role of mTORC1 in insulin-mediated suppression of ATG. Inhibition of mTORC1 blunted the decline of LC3-II/LC3-I with insulin, suggesting that mTORC1 mediates the insulin action to suppress ATG, which remained responsive to the suppressive effects of insulin in insulin-resistant obese mice.

Recently, Monaco et al. (2018) highlighted that we have achieved a limited theranostic success particularly in the management of chronic MDR diseases. Sometimes it is the intricate MB of microbes (bacteria, virus, fungus, amoeba) and sometimes these are our own mitochondria which play an intricate role in the progression and/or regression of chronic diseases, such as NDDs, CVDs, infectious diseases, and cancer. Why is it that highly toxic substances released from degenerating mitochondria cannot suppress the growth and proliferation of cancer cells, whereas Cyt-C, acetaldehyde, H_2O_2, GAPDH, ammonia, and 8-OG, 2dG are highly toxic to the normal CNS and cardiovascular system and induce chronic NDDs and CVDs? A study was aimed to assess skeletal muscle mitochondrial phenotype in young adults with type 1 diabetes. Physically active, young adults (men and women) with type 1 diabetes (HbA_{1c} 63.0 ± 16.0 mmol/mol [$7.9\% \pm 1.5\%$]) and without type 1 diabetes (control), matched for sex, age, BMI, and level of physical activity, were recruited (n = 12/group) to undergo vastus lateralis muscle microbiopsies. Mitochondrial respiration (high-resolution respirometry), site-specific mitochondrial H_2O_2 emission, and Ca^{2+} retention capacity (CRC) were assessed using permeabilized myofiber bundles. The mitochondrial oxidative capacity was lower in participants with type 1 diabetes versus the control group, at Complex II of the ETC, without differences in mitochondrial content between the groups. The muscles of those with type 1 diabetes also exhibited increased H_2O_2 emission at Complex III and decreased CRC relative to control individuals. TEM revealed an increase in the size and number of ATG remnants in the muscles of participants with type 1 diabetes. Despite this, the levels of the ATG regulatory protein, p-AMPKα^{Thr172}, and its downstream targets, phosphorylated Unc-51 like ATG-activating kinase 1 (p-ULK1^{Ser555}) and p62, were similar across the groups. No differences in muscle capillary density or platelet aggregation were observed between the groups. Alterations in the mitochondrial ultrastructure and bioenergetics implicated in CBMP were evident within the skeletal muscle of active young adults with type 1 diabetes. Whether more rigorous exercise may help to prevent skeletal muscle metabolic deficiencies in both active and inactive individuals with type 1 diabetes remains uncertain.

MSCs from Metabolic Syndrome and T2DM

The unique features of mesenchymal stem cells (MSC), including self-renewal, pluripotency, and immunomodulatory properties have drawn the global attention of researchers and physicians with respect to their disease-specific theranostic applications. Although, MSCs have become a promising tool for theranostic interventions, their source of origin and quality are highly important. Hence, the microenvironment (niche) from which these are isolated may determine their theranostic potential. MSCs are involved in disease and aging. Kornicka et al. (2018) highlighted how T2DM and metabolic syndrome (MS) may affect MSC properties, and thus limit their theranostic potential. They focused primarily on ATG and apoptosis and mitochondrial deterioration processes involving CBMP that affect MSC fate and suggested that special attention should be paid when considering autologous MSC therapy in T2D or MSC treatments, as their theranostic potential may be compromised.

MSCs with PPAR-γ Agonist or Exendin-4

Therapy targeting mitochondria may provide novel ways to treat diabetes and its complications. Wassef et al. (2018) reported that bone marrow-derived MSCs, the PPAR-γ agonists, and exendin-4 (an analog of glucagon-like peptide-1) have shown protective properties in many cardiac injuries. Hence, these researchers evaluated their effects in diabetic cardiomyopathy (DCM) in relation to mitochondrial dysfunction implicated in CBMP. This work included seven groups of adult male albino rats: the control group, the non-treated diabetic group, and the treated diabetic groups: one group was treated with MSCs only, the second with Pioglitazone only, the third with MSCs and Pioglitazone, the forth with exendin-4 only, and the fifth with MSCs and exendin-4. All treatments were initiated after six weeks from the induction of diabetes and continued for the next four weeks. Their blood samples were collected for the assessment of glucose, insulin, and cardiac enzymes. Their hearts were removed to study gene expression of myocyte enhancer factor-2 (*Mef2*), *PGC1α*, *NF-κB* and ATG markers: *LC3* and Beclin by PCR. The mitochondrial levels of Cardiolipin and UCP2 were assessed by ELISA and immunoblotting, respectively. The treated groups showed improvement in left ventricular function associated with amelioration in the cardiac injury and myopathic markers. *NF-κB* was downregulated while Cardiolipin, *PGC1α*, *LC.3,* and Beclin were upregulated in treated groups, suggesting the protective effects of MSCs, exendin-4, or Pioglitazone, based on their ability to improve mitochondrial functions by inhibiting CBMP through targeting inflammatory and ATG signaling. The co-administration of Pioglitazone or exendin-4 with MSCs resulted in superior improvement compared with MSCs alone.

Suppression of CP in T2DM

Diabetes is a devastating disease with severe complications in the cardiovascular system. A multidisciplinary, integrative, and translational approach to validate that defective CP-dependent CB clearance is critical in diabetic cardiomyopathy. To demonstrate the specific modulation of CP by stimulating the Sirtuin 1-FoxO1 signaling pathway is a novel approach to preventing heart failure in T2DM patients. Mitochondria are essential for ATP synthesis, but if damaged, they become a source of ROS and pro-apoptotic factors involving CBMP and cellular demise. Hence, the selective removal of dysfunctional mitochondria participating in CB formation via CP/ATG is an important mechanism to maintain IMD, ICD, and MQC and thus preserve cell viability. CP eliminates only a limited number of degenerated mitochondria in response to immature pleomorphic CB formation during the acute phase, whereas massive degeneration of mitochondria triggers the formation of mature, condensed, multi-lamellar CB during the chronic phase of disease progression, which persists as an intracellular nonfunctional inclusion and is only partially phagocytosed by lysosomes due to CMB in diabetes, AD, and aging. Zhonglin and Ming-Hui (2011) suggested that ATG is suppressed and CBs are accumulated in the diabetic heart, both of which contribute to cardiomyocyte apoptosis and cardiac dysfunction in T2DM hearts. Reduced Sirtuin 1 activity-mediated deacetylation of FoxO1 in T2DM hearts suppresses CP of mature CB, leading to cardiomyopathy by accentuating cardiomyocyte apoptosis through p62-dependent activation of caspase-8 and ROS. These investigators evaluated the possibility of defective ATG-dependent mitochondrial clearance causing cardiac structural and functional damage during diabetes. They delineated the mechanism of action to test the hypothesis that defective CP causes cardiomyopathy by potentiating apoptosis through p62-dependent activation of caspase-8 and/or mitochondrial ROS in T2DM. They also elucidated how CP is impaired in the diabetic heart by determining whether diabetes-inhibited Sirtuin 1 signaling results in CP suppression through down-egulation of PINK1 and Beclin-1, which may provide new insights into how diabetes induces cardiomyopathy and the modulation of CP via stimulation of SIRT1-FoxO1 signaling. This could be a potential theranostic target to prevent or delay cardiomyopathy in diabetic patients.

Low-Protein Diet for Diabetic Kidney Disease

Kitada et al. (2018) reported that a low-protein diet (LPD) can retard renal functional decline in advanced stages of CKD, including diabetic kidney disease (DKD), and is recommended in a clinical setting. LPD exerts reno-protection through improvement of glomerular hyper-filtration/hypertension due to the reduction of intra-glomerular pressure. However, LPD, particularly a very-LPD (VLPD), improved tubulo-interstitial damage, inflammation, and fibrosis through the restoration of ATG via the reduction in mTORC1 activity in T2DM in the animal model of obesity. Based on animal studies, a VLPD may have a beneficial effect in advanced DKD. VLPD slows the progression of renal dysfunction in patients with chronic glomerulonephritis. The patients with CKD, including DKD, are at high-risk malnutrition, manifesting as protein-energy wasting (PEW), sarcopenia, and frailty. Therefore, an LPD, including a VLPD, should be prescribed to patients when the benefits of LPD outweigh the risk, depending on the patient's age and nutritional status. Hence, VLPD replacement therapy without malnutrition may be beneficial for reno-protection in the advanced stages of DKD, through the regulation of mTORC1 and CP.

p62-Mediated CP in 3T3-L1 Pre-adipocytes

Previous studies have shown that an organism's nutritional status changes the protein levels of IRS-1 in a tissue-specific manner. Igawa et al. (2019) investigated how IRS-1 protein levels change depending on the nutritional status of 3T3-L1 pre-adipocytes. Starvation in 3T3-L1 pre-adipocytes was induced by culturing them in glucose, amino acid, and a serum free medium. The effect of CP and p62 on the IRS-1 protein during starvation was examined. The levels of IRS-1, but not those of the insulin receptor and protein kinase B, decreased when starvation induced CP. The inhibition of CP by CQ or CP-related 7 (ATG7) RNA interference counteracted the starvation-induced decrease in IRS-1. The ATG7 knockdown increased insulin-stimulated phosphorylation of protein kinase B during starvation. Furthermore, p62 co-localized with IRS-1 during starvation, and the p62 knockdown counteracted the starvation-induced degradation of IRS-1, suggesting that CP regulates IRS-1 protein levels through p62 in response to nutritional deficiency and that it might function as an energy depletion-sensing machinery that regulates insulin signal transduction.

CP in Hepatic Insulin Resistance

Hepatic insulin resistance is a risk factor for metabolic syndrome, characterized by central obesity, hypertension, and hyperlipidemia (hypercholesterolemia, hypertriglyceridemia). It increases the morbidity and mortality of CVDs, T2DM, NAFLD, and other metabolic diseases. Su et al. (2019) highlighted the significance of MTG in the treatment of hepatic insulin resistance and metabolic syndrome. Hepatic fatty acid accumulation can cause insulin resistance through increased gluconeogenesis, lipogenesis, chronic inflammation, oxidative stress and ERS, and an impaired insulin signal pathway. Mitochondria are the sites for β-oxidation of fatty acids, which is the major degradation mechanism of fatty acids. Mitochondrial dysfunction is involved in the development of hepatic fatty-acid-induced hepatic insulin resistance. CP, a catabolic process, selectively eliminates CBs to reverse mitochondrial dysfunction and preserve mitochondrial dynamics and function to promote mitochondrial fatty acid oxidation, inhibit hepatic fatty acid accumulation, and improve hepatic insulin resistance.

Autophagosome in Pancreatic β-Cells

Dysfunctional mitochondria participating in CB formation are observed in β-cells of diabetic patients; these are removed by CP/ATG. VAMP7, a vesicular SNARE protein, regulates autophagosome formation to maintain MQC and control insulin secretion in pancreatic β-cells. Aoyagi et al. (2018) investigated the molecular mechanism of VAMP7-dependent autophagosome formation using VAMP7-deficient β-cells and β-cell-derived Min6 cells. VAMP7 localized in ATG9a-resident vesicles of recycling endosomes (REs), which contributed to autophagosome formation, and interacted with Hrb, Syntaxin16, and SNAP-47. Hrb recruited VAMP7 and ATG9a from the plasma membrane to REs. Syntaxin18 and SNAP-47 mediated autophagosome formation occurred at a step later than the proper localization of VAMP7 to Atg9a-resident vesicles. The knockdown of Hrb, Syntaxin16, and SNAP-47 resulted in defective autophagosome formation, accumulation of CBs, and the impairment of glucose-stimulated insulin secretion, indicating that VAMP7 and ATG9a are initially recruited to REs to organize VAMP7 and ATG9a-resident vesicles in a Hrb-dependent manner. In addition, VAMP7 forms a SNARE complex with Syntaxin16 and SNAP-47, which may cause fusions of ATG9a-resident vesicles during autophagosome formation. Thus, VAMP7 participates in autophagosome formation by supporting ATG9a that maintains MQC.

Pancreatic β-Cells Overexpressing hIAPP

Human islet amyloid polypeptide (hIAPP), or amylin, has the tendency to aggregate into insoluble amyloid fibrils, a typical feature of islets from T2DM patients. Hernández et al. (2018) investigated the impact of hIAPP on key pathways involved in pancreatic β-cell survival. INS1E-hIAPP cells present a hyper-activation of MTORC1 and an inhibition of CP/ATG signaling, with the cells showing an increase in cell size. Resveratrol, a MTORC1 inhibitor, can reverse TSC2 degradation that occurs in INS1E-hIAPP cells and diminish MTORC1 hyper-activation with concomitant ATG stimulation. Simultaneously, a blockade in CP was found in INS1E-hIAPP cells, as compared with control or INS1E-rIAPP cells. Human amylin overexpression increased nitrotyrosine and poly-ubiquitinated aggregates. Failure of the protein degradation machinery induced the accumulation of damaged and fissioned mitochondria participating in CB formation, ROS production, and increased susceptibility to ERS-induced apoptosis. hIAPP overexpression in INS1E cells induced MTORC1 activation and CP inhibition, favoring a pro-fission scenario of CBMP. Hence, these cells are more susceptible to the ERS-stress-induced apoptosis and malfunction.

Neuro-2a Cell Damage

Song et al. (2018) highlighted that chronic cerebral hypoperfusion (CCH) plays an insidious role in the development of cognitive impairment. DM as a vascular risk factor may exacerbate CCH and is related to cognitive decline. Dysregulation of CP followed by ATG is associated with the pathogenesis of NDDs such as AD. To elucidate the role of CP/ATG in CCH- and/or DM-related pathogenesis, mouse Neuro-2a cells were exposed to hypoxia and/or high glucose for 48 hrs, mimicking CCH complicated with DM pathologies. Chronic hypoxia reduced cell proliferation and increased cleaved caspase-3, whereas high glucose had no synergistic toxic effects. The accumulation of CP/ATG vacuoles under hypoxia may be due to both ATG impairment and induction, with the former accounting for Neuro-2a cell death. The aberrant accumulation of mitochondria in Neuro-2a cells may be attributed to insufficient Bnip-3-mediated MTG due to the poor interaction between Bnip-3 and LC3-II implicated in CBMP. These data indicate that impaired CP/ATG and inefficient Bnip-3-mediated MTG may constitute neuronal cell damage during chronic hypoxia.

Theranostic Significance of Antioxidants as CP Regulators in Diabetes

Ginsenoside Rb1

Panax ginseng and Panax notoginseng, two well-known medical plants have a long history of use for managing various diseases in Asian countries. Clinical and experimental evidence suggests that Notoginsenosides and Ginsenosides have beneficial effects on metabolic, vascular, and CNS diseases. Considerable attention has been focused on Ginsenoside Rb1 as an anti-diabetic agent that can attenuate insulin resistance and other complications. Ginsenoside Rb1 exerts pharmacological effects by attenuating glycemia, hypertension, and hyperlipidemia, depending on the modulation of oxidative stress, inflammatory response, CP/ATG, and anti-apoptosis. Regulation of these pathophysiological mechanisms can improve blood glucose, insulin resistance, and protect micro/macrovascular complications. Zhou et al. (2019) summarized the pharmacological effects and mechanisms of the action of Ginsenoside Rb1 in the management of diabetes or diabetic complications. Ginsenoside Rb1 exerted significant anti-obesity, anti-hyperglycemic, and anti-diabetic effects by regulating glycolipid metabolism and improving insulin and leptin sensitivities, suggesting that it exerts protective effects in diabetes and diabetic complications by regulating MB, and thus, improving insulin resistance. Hence, it may be considered as a potential anti-obesity, anti-hyperglycemic, and anti-diabetic agent.

Vildagliptin

In HFD-fed rats, neuronal insulin resistance and brain mitochondrial dysfunction were evident, along with impaired learning and memory (Pintana et al. 2013). Vildagliptin prevented insulin resistance by restoring long-term depression and neuronal insulin receptor (IR), insulin receptor substrate (IRS)-1, Akt/protein kinase B-serine phosphorylation, MB, and cognitive performance. Vildagliptin also restored neuronal IR function, increased glucagon-like-peptide 1 levels, and attenuated the impaired cognitive function caused by the HFD, suggesting the clinical significance of MB, which is compromised during nutritional and environmental toxic stress and alleviated by nutritional rehabilitation, physiological zinc supplementation, and MTs as potent CB inhibitors. The natural abundance and genetic susceptibility of mtDNA qualify CB, CP, and CS as a universal biomarkers of cell injury and apoptosis to evaluate the theranostic potential of Vildagliptin in HFD-induced insulin resistance.

Carnosic Acid

Hu et al. (2019) provided evidence that Carnosic acid (CA) attenuates the I/R injury of diabetic myocardium via CP/ATG induction. Hence, increased understanding of the target molecule in CA-enhanced CP/ATG is necessary for the development of potential chemotherapy for I/R injury in diabetic myocardium.

Ubiquitin-Dependent CP

Pancreatic islet β-cells, which release insulin in response to circulating blood glucose levels, are susceptible to mitochondrial dysfunction due to their high metabolic activity and energy requirements for insulin processing, maturation, and secretion. Dysregulated CP has drawn interest in the etiology of β-cell failure in diabetes. Pearson and Soleimanpour (2018) demonstrated that the β-cell CP regulator, CLEC16A, is an E3 ligase that forms ubiquitin-dependent tripartite complex with RNF41/NRDP1 and USP8. Maintenance of the CLEC16A-RNF41-USP8 CP complex is necessary for cellular respiration and insulin secretion. Diabetogenic metabolic stressors, including elevated glucose and fatty acids, destabilized the CLEC16A-RNF41-USP8 complex and induced β-cell apoptosis, suggesting, that the β-cell CP pathway requires ubiquitin signals to stabilize the CLEC16A-RNF41-USP8 complex and maintain MQC.

IL-6 Reduces β-Cell Oxidative Stress

Production of RONS is a key instigator of β-cell dysfunction in diabetes. The cytokine IL-6 has been linked to β-cell ATG but has not been studied in the context of β-cell antioxidant response. Marasco et al. (2018) used a combination of animal models of diabetes and cultured human islets and rodent β-cells to study how IL-6 influences the antioxidant response. IL-6 coupled CP/ATG to the antioxidant response and reduced ROS in β-cells and human islets. The β-Cell-specific loss of IL-6 signaling rendered mice more susceptible to oxidative damage and cell death through the selective β-cell toxins Streptozotocin and Alloxan. IL-6-driven ROS reduction was associated with an increase in the antioxidant factor NRF2, which translocated to the mitochondria to decrease mitochondrial activity and stimulate MTG. IL-6 also initiated a transient decrease in cAMP, contributing to the stimulation of MTG to mitigate ROS, suggesting that coupling ATG to antioxidant response in β-cells leads to stress adaptation that can reduce apoptosis. These findings have implications for β-cell survival under diabetogenic conditions and confer novel TSE-EBPT interventions.

Melatonin

Diabetic retinopathy (DR), a microvascular complication of DM, remains a major cause of blindness worldwide. Dehdashtian et al. (2018) highlighted the effects of Melatonin on DR, focusing on its ability to regulate ATG. The release of pro-inflammatory cytokines and the adhesion of leukocytes to retinal capillaries are primary events in DR development. Inflammation, ERS, oxidative stress, and CP/ATG are involved in the pathogenesis of DR. Diabetes associated hyperglycemia leads to mitochondrial ETC dysfunction culminating in a rise in ROS overproduction. Since mitochondria are the major source of ROS production, oxidative stress induced by CBs also contribute to the development of DR. CP/ATG increases in the retina of diabetic patients and is regulated by ERS, oxidative stress, and inflammation-related pathways. Under mild stress, CP/ATG can lead to cell survival while during severe stress, dysregulated CP/ATG results in massive cell death and may participate in the initiation and exacerbation of DR. Melatonin and its metabolites confer protective roles during inflammation, ERS, and oxidative stress due to their direct free radical scavenging activities and indirect antioxidant activity via the antioxidant enzymes glutathione reductase, glutathione peroxidase, SOD, and catalase by regulating CP and attenuating CBMP. Melatonin also serves as a cell survival agent by modulating CP/ATG in various cell types through the amelioration of oxidative stress, ERS, and inflammation.

CONCLUSION

The skeletal muscle CP/ATG remained responsive to hyperinsulinemia and hyperglycemia even at higher plasma insulin concentrations in insulin-resistant mice. The p62-mediated CP/ATG influenced nutrition-dependent insulin receptor substrate-1 in 3T3-L1 pre-adipocytes. CP/ATG was impaired in hepatic insulin resistance and VAMP7 regulated CPS formation by augmenting ATG9a in pancreatic β-cells from male mice, whereas, cells overexpressing hIAPP impaired CP and induced CBMP. The MQC was compromised in the skeletal muscle of adults with type 1 diabetes. Impaired CP/ATG and MTG were implicated in Neuro-2a cell damage under hypoxic and/or high-glucose conditions. HFD-induced insulin resistance, brain CBs, and cognitive impairments were ameliorated by Ginsenoside Rb1 and Vildagliptin. Carnosic acid protected from I/R injury in T2DM by CP/ATG induction, whereas ubiquitin-dependent CP/ATG sustained MQC and insulin secretion, and IL-6 reduced pancreatic β-cell oxidative stress by CP/ATG induction to attenuate DR. Furthermore, inflammation and oxidative stress in DR were ameliorated by melatonin, suggesting the theranostic potential of antioxidants in DR via CP/ATG regulation.

REFERENCES

Aoyagi, K., M. Itakura, T. Fukutomi, C. Nishiwaki, et al. 2018. VAMP7 regulates autophagosome formation by supporting Atg9a functions in pancreatic β-cells from male mice. Endocrinology 159: 3674–3688.

Binger, K.J., M. Neukam, S.G. Tattikota, F. Qadri, et al. 2019. *Atp6ap2* deletion causes extensive vacuolation that consumes the insulin content of pancreatic β cells. PNAS 116: 19983–19988.

Dehdashtian, E., S. Mehrzadi, B. Yousefi, A. Hosseinzadeh, et al. 2018. Diabetic retinopathy pathogenesis and the ameliorating effects of melatonin; involvement of ATG, inflammation and oxidative stress. Life Sci 193: 20–33.

Ehrlicher, S.E., H.D. Stierwalt, S.A. Newsom and M.M. Robinson. 2018. Skeletal muscle autophagy remains responsive to hyperinsulinemia and hyperglycemia at higher plasma insulin concentrations in insulin-resistant mice. Physiol Rep 6(14): e13810.

Greene, N.P., J.L. Brown, M.E. Rosa-Caldwell, D.E. Lee, et al. 2018. Skeletal muscle insulin resistance as a precursor to diabetes: Beyond glucoregulation. Curr Diabetes Rev 14: 113–128.

Hernández, M.G., A.G. Aguilar, J. Burillo, R.G. Oca, et al. 2018. Pancreatic β-cells overexpressing hIAPP impaired mitophagy and unbalanced mitochondrial dynamics. Cell Death Dis 9: 481.

Hoshino, A. and S. Matoba. 2018. Observation of Parkin-mediated mitophagy in pancreatic β-Cells. Methods Mol Biol 1759: 41–46.

Hu, M., T. Li, Z. Bo and F. Xiang. 2019. The protective role of carnosic acid in ischemic/reperfusion injury through regulation of autophagy under T2DM. Exp Biol Med (Maywood) 244: 602–611.

Igawa, H., A. Kikuchi, H. Misu, K.A. Ishii, et al. 2019. p62-mediated ATG affects nutrition-dependent insulin receptor substrate 1 dynamics in 3T3-L1 preadipocytes. J Diabetes Investig 10: 32–42.

Itahana, Y. and K. Itahana. 2018. Emerging roles of p53 family members in glucose metabolism. Int J Mol Sci Mar 8;19(3).

Ji. Jeff., M. Petropavlovskaia, A. Khatchadourian, J. Patapas., et al. (2019) Type 2 diabetes is associated with suppression of autophagy and lipid accumulation in β-Cells. J Cellular & Molecular Medicine 23: 2890–2900.

Kitada, M., Y. Ogura, I. Monno and D. Koya. 2018. A low-protein diet for diabetic kidney disease: Its effect and molecular mechanism, an approach from animal studies. Nutrients 10(5): 544.

Kornicka, K., J. Houston and K. Marycz. 2018. Dysfunction of mesenchymal stem cells isolated from metabolic syndrome and type 2 diabetic patients as result of oxidative stress and ATG may limit their potential therapeutic use. Stem Cell Rev 14: 337–345.

Lee, Y.H., J. Kim, K. Park and M.S. Lee. 2019. β-cell autophagy: Mechanism and role in β-cell dysfunction. Mol Metab 27: S92–S103.

Marasco, M.R., A.M. Conteh and C.A. Reissaus. 2018. Interleukin-6 reduces β-cell oxidative stress by linking autophagy with the antioxidant response. Diabetes 67: 1576–1588.

Monaco, C.M.F., M.C. Hughes, S.V. Ramos, N.E. Varah, et al. 2018. Altered mitochondrial bioenergetics and ultrastructure in the skeletal muscle of young adults with type 1 diabetes. Diabetologia 61: 1411–1423.

Pearson, G. and S.A. Soleimanpour. 2018. A ubiquitin-dependent mitophagy complex maintains mitochondrial function and insulin secretion in beta cells. Autophagy 14: 1160–1161.

Pintana, H., N. Apaijai, N. Chattipakorn and S.C. Chattipakorn. 2013. DPP-4 inhibitors improve cognition and brain mitochondrial function of insulin-resistant rats. J Endocrinol 218: 1–11.

Song, Y., Y. Du, W. Zou, Y. Luo, et al. 2018. Involvement of impaired autophagy and mitophagy in Neuro-2a cell damage under hypoxic and/or high-glucose conditions. Sci Rep 8: Article number 3301.

Su, Z., Y. Nie, Z. Huang, Y. Zhu, et al. 2019. Mitophagy in hepatic insulin resistance: Therapeutic potential and concerns. Front Pharmacol 10: 1193. doi: 10.3389/fphar.2019.01193.

Wassef, M.A.E., O.M. Tork, L.A. Rashed, W. Ibrahim, et al. 2018. Mitochondrial dysfunction in diabetic cardiomyopathy: Effect of mesenchymal stem cell with PPAR-γ agonist or exendin-4.. Exp Clin Endocrinol Diabetes 126: 27–38.

Xu, C., X. Chen, E.A. Reece, W. Lu, et al. 2019. The increased activity of a transcription factor inhibits autophagy in diabetic embryopathy. Am J Obstet Gynecol 220(1): 108.e1–108.e12. doi.org/10.1016/j.ajog.2018.10.001

Zhonglin, X. and Z. Ming-Hui. 2011. Suppression of autophagy-dependent clearance of mitochondria in type-2 diabetes. Autophagy 10: 1522–1534.—Please recheck given description.

Zhou, T., L. Chang, Y. Luo, Y. Zhou, et al. 2019. Mst1 inhibition attenuates non-alcoholic fatty liver disease via reversing Parkin-related mitophagy. Redox Biol 21: 101120. doi: 10.1016/j.redox.2019.101120

14

Charnolophagy in Obesity

INTRODUCTION

Obesity is a complex disease characterized by the accumulation of excess body fat, which is caused by an adipocyte hypertrophy and/or hyperplasia due to excessive accumulation of triacylglycerol in white adipose tissue (WAT). Various mechanisms allowing the regulation of triacylglycerol storage and mobilization by LD-associated proteins and lipolytic enzymes have been identified in obesity. Recent studies have associated obesity with the dysfunction of mitochondria and ER in variety of cells, resulting in oxidative stress, accumulation of residual damaged cell organelles (mitochondria) involving CB formation, and ERS leading to unfolded protein responses (UPRs) accumulation in the cytoplasm. Obesity is also associated with compromised CP/ATG. Recently, Wu et al. (2018) investigated latest development in mitochondria-based targets for therapies. They highlighted that we need to know how drugs initiate mitochondrial dysfunction, the exact role of nuclear messages in mtDNA regulation, and mitochondrial communication between and with other cells. We also need to learn how mitochondria control immune response, CP/MTG/ATG, genome activation, and inter- and intracellular communication. How the transcription is triggered and terminated, how the proteins and other organelles interact, and how mtDNA, miRNA, and mtmiRNA regulate respiratory complexes is yet to be established for the theranostic management of obesity. Pan et al. (2018) determined the effects of maternal low-protein (LP) diet on s. c fat deposition of weaning piglets. Sows were fed either a standard protein (SP), 15 and 18% crude protein or a LP diet (50% protein levels of SP) throughout pregnancy and lactation. s.c. fat and blood from male piglets at 28 days of age were analyzed. Body weight, back fat thickness, triglycerides in s.c. fat tissue, and serum, and FFA were significantly reduced in LP piglets when compared with SP piglets. mRNA and the protein expression of acetyl-CoA carboxylase and fatty acid synthase (enzymes of lipogenesis) were reduced in LP piglets, while mRNA expression and the lipolytic enzymes activities of lipolysis genes, triglyceride lipase, and hormone-sensitive lipase, were increased in the same piglets. The expression of ATG-related gene 7 and ATG marker gene LC3 as well as the conversion of LC3-I to LC3-II were elevated, along with the expression of activating transcription factor-4 and eukaryotic translation initiation factor-2a, indicating that amino acid starvation-induced CP is involved in reduced s.c. fat deposition in maternal LP weaning piglets, demonstrating links between maternal protein restriction and offspring fat deposition.

This chapter highlights the pivotal role of CP to accomplish TSE-EBPT of obesity in light of the emerging literature in this clinically-significant area of global interest. The chapter also highlights the unique role of mitochondria in cellular toxicity as a potential drug target in obesity.

Browning of WAT

The browning of WAT holds great promise for the treatment of obesity and metabolic syndrome. DJ-1 is evolutionarily conserved across species, and its mutations were identified in PD. Higher levels of DJ-1 are associated with obesity as well. Silvester et al. (2018) used DJ-1 knockout (KO) mouse models and wild-type littermates maintained on a normal diet or HFD as well as in *in vitro* cell models to show the direct effects of DJ-1 depletion on adipocyte phenotype, thermogenic capacity, fat metabolism, and microenvironment profile. Global DJ-1 KO mice showed increased sympathetic input to WAT and intracellular β3-adrenergic receptor signaling, leading to high mitochondrial content, reduced lipid accumulation, and adequate vascularization and attenuated ATG. DJ-1 KO mice had normal body weight, energy balance, and adiposity, associated with protective effects on healthy WAT expansion by hyperplasia. Browning of inguinal WAT occurred in DJ-1 KO mice that did not show increased predisposition to obesity, suggesting that such a mechanism may overcome the adverse metabolic consequences of obesity independent of an effect on body weight. Hence, targeting DJ-1 in adipocyte may offer a unique strategy for the TSE-EBPT of obesity. The thyroid hormone T_3 activates thermogenesis by uncoupling ETC from ATP synthesis in BAT mitochondria. These investigators examined the effects of T_3 on mitochondrial activity, ATG, and metabolism in primary brown adipocytes and BAT and found that T_3 increased fatty acid oxidation and mitochondrial respiration as well as CP, ATG, MTG, and MB. There was no significant induction of ROS despite high mitochondrial respiration and UCP1 induction by T_3. However, when cells were treated with Atg5 siRNA to block ATG, induction of mitochondrial respiration by T_3 decreased, and was accompanied by ROS accumulation, indicating the critical role of CP/ATG turnover in body fat regulation. They generated an Atg5 conditional knockout mouse model (Atg5 cKO) by injecting Ucp1 promoter-driven Cre-expressing adenovirus into $Atg5^{Flox/Flox}$ mice to determine the effects of BAT-specific ATG on thermogenesis *in vivo*. Hyperthyroid Atg5 cKO mice exhibited a lower body temperature than hyperthyroid or euthyroid control mice. T_3 increased short and long chain acyl-carnitines in BAT, consistent with increased β-oxidation. T_3 also decreased amino acid levels, and in conjunction with SIRT1 activation, decreased mTOR activity to stimulate ATG, suggesting that it has direct effects on CP and turnover in BAT for thermogenesis. Hence, stimulation of BAT by thyroid hormone or its analogs may represent a potential theranostic strategy for obesity and metabolic diseases.

Obesity and Late Gestation Diet

Intrauterine growth restriction in late pregnancy can contribute to adverse long-term metabolic health effects in the offspring. Saroha et al. (2018) used a sheep model to monitor maternal dietary manipulation in late pregnancy, combined with exposure of the offspring to a low-activity, obesogenic environment after weaning, to characterize the effects on glucose homeostasis. Dizygotic twin-pregnant sheep were either fed 60% of requirements (nutrient restriction (R)) or fed *ad libitum* (~140% of requirements (A)) from 110 days gestation until term (~147 days). After weaning (~3 months of age), the offspring were kept in either a standard or low-activity, obesogenic environment. R mothers gained less weight and produced smaller offspring. As adults, obese offspring were heavier and more obese with reduced glucose tolerance, regardless of maternal diet. Molecular markers of stress and CP in liver and adipose tissue were increased with obesity, with gene expression of hepatic Grp78 and omental activation transcription factor 6 (Atf6), Grp78m, and ERS degradation enhancer molecule 1 (Edem1) increased only in R offspring, suggesting that the adverse effect of juvenile-onset obesity on insulin-responsive tissues can be amplified by previous exposure to a suboptimal nutritional environment *in utero*, thereby contributing to an earlier onset of insulin resistance.

HG-Dependent MSCs Adipogenesis

Although, the major source of adipocytes comes from mesenchymal stem cells (MSCs), their exact role in obesity remains uncertain. An understanding of the mechanisms, regulation, and outcomes of adipogenesis is crucial for the development of novel EBPT of obesity-related diseases. Recently, an unexpected role of the tumor suppressor promyelocytic leukemia protein (PML) in hematopoietic stem cell biology and metabolic regulation has emerged. Morganti et al. (2019) investigated the molecular pathway underlying the role of PML in the control of adipogenic MSC differentiation. Muscle-derived stem cells (MDSCs) and adipose-derived stem cells (ADSCs) obtained from mice and voluntary patients were cultured in the presence of high glucose (HG), a nutrient stress condition known to promote MSCs differentiation in mature adipocytes and the adipogenic potential of PML was assessed. PML is essential for a correct HG-dependent adipogenic differentiation, and the enhanced PML levels is fundamental during adipogenesis. Increased PML expression upregulated PKCβ, which, by regulating CP/ATG permitted an increase in PPARγ that led to the adipogenic differentiation. Genetic and pharmacological depletion of PML prevented PKCβ expression, and by increasing CP/ATG, impaired the MSCs adipogenic differentiation. Human ADSCs isolated from overweight patients displayed increased PML and PKCβ compared to normal weight individuals, indicating that the PML-PKCβ pathway enhanced adipogenesis and human metabolism. The new link found among PML, PKCβ, and ATG opened a novel EBPT avenue for diseases characterized by an imbalance in the MSCs differentiation process, such as metabolic syndromes and cancer.

CB/ATG in Obesity

While, overnutrition and a sedentary lifestyle are the driving forces behind the development of metabolic diseases; CR and exercise are the most effective strategies in combating metabolic diseases of aging by augmenting CP and preventing CBMP. Interestingly, exercise and CR share a common feature: both represent a mechanism of upregulating CP, which can be induced by CR, and inactivated by amino acids as well as growth factors (for example, insulin). Recently, van Niekerk et al. (2018) provided evidence that CP is attenuated in metabolic tissue such as liver, muscle, and adipose tissue in obesity. They also highlighted the mechanism by which defective CP may contribute to metabolic diseases, including a compromised IMD, ICD, and MQC, since CP plays a crucial role in the elimination of defective mitochondria involved in CB formation and CBMP. CP plays an indispensable role in the clearance of protein aggregates and redundant large protein aggregates such as inflammasomes, apoptosome, and necro-apoptosome. CP also plays a pivotal role in the metabolism of endotoxins, suggesting its importance in the pathogenesis of metabolic endotoxemia and obesity-induced metabolic derangements.

Arsenic (As) and High Fat Diet (HFD) Exposure

Arsenic (As) is a toxic and hazardous metalloid. Its presence in drinking water, together with an impaired nutritional status, is associated with metabolic disorders in young people. Degradation of mitochondria represented by functionally-impaired CP and CBMP is an important landmark leading to apoptosis during lipo-toxicity. Recently, Zeinvand-Lorestani et al. (2018) reported that lipotoxicity and cellular toxicity due to As can induce changes in CP and apoptosis. The protein derived from SQSTM1 gene, also called p62, plays an important role in energy homeostasis in the liver, and can contribute to the regulation of ATG by influencing mTOR, MAPK, and NF-KB signaling. Hence, changes in Sqstm1, CP (Bnip-3), and apoptotic (caspase 3) genes in the livers of NMRI mice were examined by real-time RT-PCR Array followed by exposure to As (50 ppm) in drinking water while being fed with a HFD or LFD for 20 weeks (LFD-As and HFD-As groups). While LFD-As and HFD groups showed a decrease in Bnip-3 expression, a significant increase was observed in the HFD-As group. P62 gene was downregulated in LFD-As and HFD groups, and upregulated in the HFD-As group. Caspase 3 showed increased expression as apoptotic liver cell death in the three groups, with the highest value in HFD-As group. The changes observed in the expression of Sqstm1, Bnip-3, and caspase 3 were related to the extent of liver damage caused by exposure to AS, HFD, and Bnip-3 pro-apoptotic protein, which led to an increased incidence of cell death.

CP in Adipogenesis

Obesity is related to the abnormal differentiation of adipocytes, those are subjected to high plasma levels of FFAs. As the most abundant FFA in the bloodstream, oleic acid (OA) induces adipogenic differentiation in human adipose-derived stromal cells (hADSCs). Recently, p62, an ATG mediator, was shown to play an important role in obesity and adipose tissue metabolism. Therefore, Zeng et al. (2018) investigated the roles of ATG and mitochondrial function at different stages of OA (in combination with insulin and Dexamethasone)-induced adipogenesis in hADSCs. The hADSCs were incubated with OA, insulin, and Dexamethasone after pretreatment with ATG inhibitors or knockdown of p62 with shRNA. Treatment with 80 μM OA (substituted for Isobutylmethylxantine; IBMX) for 10 days induced hADSCs in adipocytes. During OA-induced adipogenesis, ATG was induced, with an increased LC3-II/I ratio on day 3 and a decreased protein level of p62 on and after day 3. Inhibition of ATG with 3MA at the early stage (day 0 to day 3) of differentiation, but not at the middle or late stage, decreased OA-induced adipogenesis; while knockdown of p62 with shRNA promoted adipogenesis in hADSCs. The copy number of mtDNA (the ND1 gene) and TOM20, a mitochondrial membrane protein, were increased following OA treatment; this was related to the mitochondrial stability. Knockdown of p62 increased the mito-LC3-II/I and cyto-LC3-II/I ratios by 110.1% and 73.3%, respectively. The increase in the ratio of mito-LC3-II/I was higher than that of cyto-LC3-II/I. Furthermore, p62 knockdown-enhanced adipogenesis in hADSCs was abolished by inhibiting CP with Cyclosporine A, suggesting that p62 plays a protective role in adipogenesis of hADSCs through CP regulation.

CP Controls Beige Adipocytes

Beige adipocytes are an inducible form of mitochondria-enriched thermogenic adipocytes that emerge in response to external stimuli, such as chronic cold exposure. Lu et al. (2018) showed that after the withdrawal of external stimuli, beige adipocytes acquired a white-fat-like phenotype through CP/ATG-mediated mitochondrial degradation. They investigated the upstream pathway that mediates mitochondrial clearance and reported that Parkin-mediated MTG plays a key role in the beige-to-white adipocyte transition. Mice genetically deficient in *Park2* showed reduced mitochondrial degradation and retained thermogenic beige adipocytes even after the withdrawal of external stimuli. NE signaling through the PKA pathway inhibited the recruitment of Parkin protein to mitochondria in beige adipocytes. However, mitochondrial proton uncoupling by UCP-1 was dispensable for Parkin recruitment and beige adipocyte maintenance, suggesting a physiological mechanism by which external cues control mitochondrial homeostasis in thermogenic fat cells through CP.

PINK1-Parkin and Obesity-Induced Metabolic Stress

Several studies have shown that MTG mediated by PINK1 and Parkin may play a critical role in clearing the damaged mitochondria participating in CB formation and maintaining MQC. PINK1 and Parkin were overexpressed in adipose tissue in obese subjects. Cui et al. (2018) created a HFD-induced obese mouse model and examined the expression of PINK1 and Parkin in adipose tissue. There was significant difference between regular-chow-fed mice and HFD-induced obese mice in the expression of PINK1 and Parkin *in vivo*; the expression of PINK1 and Parkin in 3T3-L1 pre-adipocytes *in vitro* was tested by treating cells with palmitic acid (PA) to induce metabolic stress. To better understand the role of PINK1 and Parkin in metabolic stress, 3T3-L1 pre-adipocytes were transfected with siRNA of PINK1 and Parkin followed by PA treatment. At lower concentrations of PA, PINK1 and Parkin could be activated and played a protective role in resisting the harmful effects of PA, including the mitochondrial function and cell-death resistance, while at higher concentrations of PA, the expression of PINK1 and Parkin was inhibited, suggesting that PINK1-Parkin protect mitochondrial function in metabolic stress induced by obesity or PA.

Roux-en-Y Gastric Bypass in Obesity

Bariatric surgery provides improvement in glycemic control and hepatic steatosis. Recently, alterations in mitochondrial morphology have shown a direct link to nutrient adaptations in obesity. Sacks et al. (2018) evaluated the effects of Roux-en-Y gastric bypass (RYGB) surgery on biomarkers of liver mitochondrial dynamics in a diet-induced obese rat model. Livers were harvested from adult male rats, 90 days after either Sham or RYGB surgery or continuous high-fat feeding. They assessed the expression of mitochondrial proteins involved in fusion, fission, CP/ATG, and biogenesis, as well as differences in citrate synthase and biomarkers of oxidative stress. The expression for mitochondrial fusion genes, mitofusin 1 (Mfn-1), mitofusin-2 (Mfn-2; and optic atrophy 1 (OPA1) increased following RYGB surgery. Biogenesis regulators, PGC1α, and Nrf1, also increased in the RYGB group, as well as the MTG marker, Bnip-3. Protein expression for Mfn-1, PGC1α, Bnip-3, and mitochondrial complexes I-V was also increased by RYGB, and Mfn-1 expression negatively correlated with body weight, insulin resistance, and fasting plasma insulin. In the RYGB group, citrate synthase was increased and ROS was decreased. The total antioxidant capacity remained unchanged between groups, demonstrating an association between RYGB surgery and improved markers of liver mitochondrial dynamics. These improvements may be related to weight loss and reduced energetic demand in the liver, which could facilitate normalization of glucose homeostasis and protect against hepatic steatosis.

B1a B Cells Require ATG

Specific metabolic programs are activated by immune cells to fulfill their functional roles, which include adaptations to their microenvironment. B1 B cells are tissue-resident, innate-like B cells. They have many distinct properties, such as the capacity to self-renew and the ability to respond to a limited repertoire of epitopes. Clarke et al. (2018) showed that B1 B cells are metabolically more active than B2 B cells, with higher rates of glycolysis and O/P, and depend on glycolysis. They acquire exogenous fatty acids and store lipids in droplet form. ATG is differentially activated in B1a B cells, and deletion of the ATG gene, ATG7, leads to a selective loss of B1a B cells caused by a failure in self-renewal. ATG-deficient B1a B cells downregulated metabolic genes and accumulated CBs involved in functionally-impaired CP and CBMP. B1 B cells, therefore, have evolved a distinct metabolism adapted to their specific functional properties.

Carnitine as a CP/ATG Modulator

CP/ATG is suppressed in skeletal muscle and the liver with insulin resistance induced by HFD as it is essential for maintaining mitochondrial function, and dysfunctional mitochondria are associated with insulin resistance involving CBMP. As Carnitine treatment is known to improve insulin resistance by promoting mitochondrial function, Choi et al. (2018) investigated if it affects CP/ATG in the skeletal muscle of HFD-induced rodent model of obesity. After six weeks on HFD (48 kcal% fat), mice developed glucose intolerance, and the gastrocnemius muscle showed a decrease in insulin signaling and mitochondrial function, which was reversed by Carnitine (100 mg/kg/day) treatment by oral gavage for two weeks. Swollen mitochondria with destroyed cristae implicated in CB formation were observed in the skeletal muscle of HFD-fed mice; however, the same were not observed after the Carnitine treatment. After the Carnitine treatment, HFD decreased LC3B-II (a marker of autophagosome formation) while increased sequestosome 1 (SQSTM1) expression was reversed. In C2C12 myotubes, prolonged treatment with palmitate suppressed ATG, which was relieved by the Carnitine treatment. However, the induction of CP/ATG by Carnitine in C2C12 myotubes was not observed after knockdown of an ATG-regulator, PPARγ, indicating that the elimination of dysfunctional mitochondria involved in CBMP by ATG induction through PPARγ may be a novel mechanism by which Carnitine improves insulin resistance and MB in obesity.

HSL/ATGL in 3T3-L1 Adipocytes

Increasing energy expenditure by inducing a mild uncoupling of mitochondria in adipocytes might represent an anti-obesity strategy as it reduces the adipose tissue triacylglycerol content (limiting alterations caused by cell hypertrophy) by stimulating lipolysis, limiting the adverse effects of adipocyte hypertrophy. Demine et al. (2018) characterized the molecular mechanisms involved in lipolysis induced by uncoupling of mitochondria in white 3T3-L1 adipocytes. Mitochondrial uncoupling-induced lipolysis was independent from pathways that involve lipolytic enzymes such as HSL and ATGL. Enhanced lipolysis of LDs in response to mitochondrial uncoupling relied on CP, because these are captured by endocysosomal vesicles.

Chemerin

Adipocyte endocrine function is affected by altered ATG in individuals with obesity. Genetic variants in the ATG-related gene 7 (ATG7), correlated with the serum Chemerin's (RARRES2) concentrations. A study investigated a functional interplay between Chemerin and ATG7, how it may relate to ATG-mediated adipocyte dysfunction in obesity, and the relevance of genetic ATG7 variants in Chemerin physiology. Adipose ATG7 mRNA expression and adiposity measures were available in two human study cohorts. The effect of a high-calorie diet on adipose Rarres2 and ATG7 gene expression was investigated in mice. In 3T3-L1 adipocytes, the effect of ATG7 knockdown on Chemerin expression and secretion was studied. The influence of SNP on ATG7 transcription and Chemerin physiology was investigated using a luciferase reporter assay. Heinitz et al. (2019) investigated vitro studies, mouse models, and clinical trials on Native American (n = 83) and white (n = 100) cohorts. In mice fed a high-calorie diet, adipose ATG7 mRNA expression and Rarres2 mRNA expression did not show a parallel increase. ATG7 mRNA expression in s.c. adipose tissue correlated with BMI, fat mass, and adipocyte cell size. ATG7 knockdown in 3T3-L1 adipocytes decreased Chemerin secretion by 22%. Rs2606729 may alter ATG7 transcription and induce higher luciferase activity *in vitro*. Human adipose ATG7 mRNA expression related to measures of adiposity. ATG7 knockdown reduced Chemerin secretion from adipocytes *in vitro*, indicating a functional relationship between ATG7 and Chemerin in CP/ATG-mediated adipocyte dysfunction.

CONCLUSION

Nutritional excess compromised CP/ATG in obese mice. Chronic exposure to As and HFD induced dysregulation of Sqstm1, CP/ATG, and apoptotic genes. Loss of DJ-1 promoted browning of WAT in diet-induced obese mice, and T_3 stimulated BAT through mTOR-mediated CP/ATG induction. The p62 gene was linked to CP/ATG in oleic acid-induced abiogenesis in adipose-derived stromal cells. CP controlled beige adipocytes through a Parkin-dependent and UCP1-independent mechanism. PINK1-Parkin alleviated metabolic stress in adipose tissue and in 3T3-L1 pre-adipocytes. The hepatic mitochondrial dynamics was altered by the Roux-en-Y gastric bypass in a rat model of obesity, whereas, B1a cells required CP/ATG for intracellular homeostasis and self-renewal. Treatment with Carnitine induced CP/ATG and ameliorated HFD-induced CBMP in obesity. Mitochondrial uncoupling induced HSL/ATGL-independent lipolysis by CP/ATG in 3T3-L1 adipocytes, whereas, ATG7 knockdown reduced Chemerin secretion in murine adipocytes to modulate obesity.

REFERENCES

Choi, J.W., J.H. Ohn, H.S. Jung, Y.J. Park, et al. 2018. Carnitine induces autophagy and restores high-fat diet-induced mitochondrial dysfunction. Metabolism 78: 43–51.

Clarke, A.J., T. Riffelmacher, D. Braas, R.J. Cornall, et al. 2018. B1a B cells require autophagy for metabolic homeostasis and self-renewal. J Exp Med 215: 399–413.

Cui, C., S. Chen, J. Qiao, L. Qing, et al. 2018. PINK1-Parkin alleviates metabolic stress induced by obesity in adipose tissue and in 3T3-L1 preadipocytes. Biochem Biophys Res Commun 498: 445–452.

Demine, S., S. Tejerina, B. Bihin, M. Thiry, et al. 2018. Mild mitochondrial uncoupling induces HSL/ATGL-independent lipolysis relying on a form of ATG in 3T3-L1 adipocytes. J Cell Physiol 233: 1247–1265.

Heinitz, S., C. Gebhardt, P. Piaggi, J. Krüger, et al. 2019. ATG7 knockdown reduces chemerin secretion in murine adipocytes. J Clin Endocrinol Metab 104: 5715–5728.

Lu, X., S. Altshuler-Keylin, Q. Wang, Y. Chen, et al. 2018. Mitophagy controls beige adipocyte maintenance through a Parkin-dependent and UCP1-independent mechanism. Sci Signal 11(527): eaap8526.

Morganti, C., S. Missiroli, M. Lebiedzinska-Arciszewska, L. Ferroni, et al. 2019. Regulation of PKCβ levels and autophagy by PML is essential for high-glucose-dependent mesenchymal stem cell adipogenesis. Int J Obes 43: 963–973.

Pan, S., Y. Jia, X. Yang, D. Cai, et al. 2018. Amino acid starvation-induced ATG is involved in reduced subcutaneous fat deposition in weaning piglets derived from sows fed low-protein diet during gestation and lactation: ATG is involved in reduced fat deposition in maternal low-protein piglets. Eur J Nutr 57: 991–1001.

Sacks, J., A. Mulya, C.E. Fealy, H. Huang, et al. 2018. Effect of Roux-en-Y gastric bypass on liver mitochondrial dynamics in a rat model of obesity. Physiol Rep 6(4): e13600.

Saroha, V., N.S. Dellschaft, D.H. Keisler, D.S. Gardner, et al. 2018. Tissue cell stress response to obesity and its interaction with late gestation diet. Reprod Fertil Dev 30: 430–441.

Silvester, A.J., K.R. Aseer, H.J. Jang, R. Ryu, et al. 2018. Loss of DJ-1 promotes browning of white adipose tissue in diet-induced obese mice. J Nutr Biochem 61: 56–67.

van Niekerk, G., A. du Toit, B. Loos and A.M. Engelbrecht. 2018. Nutrient excess and autophagic deficiency: Explaining metabolic diseases in obesity Metabolism 82: 14–21.

Wu, D., X. Wang and H. Sun. 2018. The role of mitochondria in cellular toxicity as a potential drug target. Cell Biol Toxicol 34: 87–91.

Zeinvand-Lorestani, M., H. Kalantari, M.J. Khodayar, A. Teimoori, et al. 2018. Dysregulation of Sqstm1, mitophagy, and apoptotic genes in chronic exposure to arsenic and high-fat diet (HFD). Environ Sci Pollut Res Int 25: 34351–34359.

Zeng, R., Y. Fang, Y. Zhang, S. Bai. 2018. p62 is linked to mitophagy in oleic acid-induced adipogenesis in human adipose-derived stromal cells. Lipids Health Dis 17: 133.

15

Charnolophagy in Hyperlipidemia

INTRODUCTION

Although, it remains uncertain whether hypercholesterolemia impairs CP/ATG or the mTOR pathways, the efficiency of ischemic conditioning is significantly diminished in hypercholesterolemia. Disturbed metabolism of cholesterol and trigylceroles (TGs) carries an increase risk of coronary artery calcification (CAC). Under normal physiological conditions and concentrations, cholesterol and triglyceroles are useful for our body. Djekic et al. (2019) identified disturbances in lipid profiles in the calcification process and proposed potential biomarker candidates for hypercholesterolemia. They investigated the lipidome of 70 patients at intermediate risk for CAD who had undergone CAC assessment using CT and Agatston coronary artery calcium score (CACS). Patients were divided into three groups: those with no CAC (NCC; CACS: 0; n = 26), those with mild coronary calcification (MCC; CACS: 1-250; n = 27), and those with severe CAC (SCC; CACS: >250; n = 17). Serum samples from each group were analyzed using LC-MASS to determine the lipidomic profile. As many as 103 lipids were identified within the glycerolipid, glycerophospholipid, sphingolipid, and sterol lipid classes. Increased Phosphatidylcholine (PC)(16:0/20:4), and reduced PC(18:2/18:2), PC(36:3), and phosphatidylethanolamine (20:0/18:2) correlated with the severity of SCC. No significant differences were observed in individual TGs between the three groups; however, clustering the lipid profiles revealed a trend for higher levels of saturated and monounsaturated TGs in SCC compared to NCC. There was also a trend for lower TG(49:2), TG(51:1), TG(54:5), and TG(56:8) levels in SCC compared to MCC, suggesting that the CAC is associated with CP/ATG dysfunction.

The lipidomic biomarker profile in this study may aid in better assessment of patients with sub-clinical CAD.

This chapter highlights the TSE-EBPT significance of CP/ATG in hyperlipidemia.

Hyperlipidemia is the underlying cause of both myocardial infarction and stroke. Dietary management and CR are beneficial in reducing the complications of diabetes-mediated obesity. Elevated glucose and saturated fatty acids induce metabolic, oxidative, and mitochondrial stress, accompanied with inflammation that may lead to chronic complications in diabetes. Alnahdi et al. (2019) used HepG2 cells to investigate the effects of high glucose (25 mM and palmitic acid (up to 0.3 mM) on metabolic, inflammatory, and redox stress. Increased lipid, protein, and DNA damage, caspase-dependent apoptosis, and mitochondrial dysfunction were observed. Increased ROS production and redox stress altered $\Delta\Psi$ and MB, suggesting that cytochrome P450s-dependent drug metabolism and antioxidant adaptation in HepG2 cells treated with palmitic acid were augmented with high glucose. Altered NF-kB/AMPK/mTOR-dependent cell signaling and inflammatory (IL6/TNF-α) responses were also observed. The high-energy metabolites enhanced apoptosis while suppressing CP/ATG by inflammatory and oxidative-stress-induced alterations in cell signaling and metabolism. Recently, Liu et al. (2019) described the interaction between RAS and AMPK to highlight AMPK as a dynamic balance between physiological and pathological roles of the RAS. The RAS is the most critical regulator of arterial BP, fluid volume, as well as renal function and is implicated in the development of obesity, diabetes, hyperlipidemia, other diseases, and in the regulation of cell proliferation, apoptosis, CP/ATG, and insulin resistance. AMPK, an essential energy sensor is also involved in these diseases, indicating a link between the RAS and AMPK. Although it is well-established that diet, hormones, gene transcription, and post-translational modifications control the hepatic metabolism of FAs, metabolic dysregulation causing CVDs warrants further evaluation of FA, triacylglycerol (TAG) synthesis, and degradation. Long-chain FA metabolism begins with the formation of an acyl-CoA by a member of the acyl-CoA synthase (ACSL) family. TAG synthesis begins with acyl-CoA esterification to glycerol-3-phosphate by a member of the glycerol-3-phosphate acyltransferase (GPAT) family. Studies conducted by Coleman (2019) on the isoforms ACSL1 and GPAT1 suggested that these proteins are members of large *interactomes.* The ER-targeted ACSL1 interacts with peroxisomal LD and tethering proteins. PPARα upregulates ACSL1, interacts with proteins, and tethers LDs to the OM, whereas, GPAT1 is upregulated by carbohydrate and insulin from saturated FA via lipogenesis to FA esterification by GPAT1 through the TAG biosynthesis pathway. This suggests that enzymes form a protein *interactome* to enhance esterification and other lipid-metabolic pathways.

PLIN2 in Atherosclerosis

Hyperglycemia and hyperlipidemia are the hallmarks of diabetes and obesity and major risk factors for CVDs and atherosclerosis. The Pro251 variant of perilipin-2 reduces plasma triglycerides and may be beneficial in reducing atherosclerosis development. Saliba-Gustafsson et al. (2019) determined the beneficial effects of the Pro251 variant of perlipin-2 on atherosclerosis and its mechanism of action. Whole blood from individuals recruited, based on perilipin-2 genotype, was used to prepare primary monocytes-derived macrophages from buffy coats. The Pro251 variant of perilipin-2 was associated with decreased intima-media thickness at baseline and >30 months of follow-up. Using human primary monocyte-derived macrophages from carriers of the Pro251 variant, it was shown that this variant increased ATG activity, cholesterol efflux, and the inflammatory response. An increase in ATG was accompanied with an increase in liver-X-receptor (LXR) activity, and LXR and ATG activated each other in a feed-forward loop, regulated by CYP27A1 and 27OH-cholesterol. This study showed that perilipin-2 affects susceptibility to human atherosclerosis through the activation of ATG and the stimulation of cholesterol efflux. It also showed that perilipin-2 modulates levels of the LXR ligand 27OH-cholesterol and initiates a feed-forward loop where LXR and ATG activate each other; the mechanism by which perilipin-2 exerts its beneficial effects in atherosclerosis.

Indole-3-Carbinol in Hyperlipidemia

Indole-3-carbinol (I3C) is extracted from cruciferous vegetables and is known for its anti-cancer, antioxidant, and anti-inflammatory properties. Jiang et al. (2019) investigated the protective effect of I3C in hyper-lipidemic zebrafish larvae and early stage toxicity of I3C on zebrafish embryos and their larvae. Zebrafish larvae were fed with a 4% high-cholesterol diet (HCD) and treated with I3C 2.5 µmol/L and 5 µmol/L for two weeks. Confocal image analysis and oil Red O staining were used to analyze vascular lipid accumulation, while immunoblotting was used to evaluate possible mechanics. In addition, the zebrafish embryos were treated with I3C for 96 hrs to assess cardiotoxicity. The lipid deposition on vasculature had decreased in the I3C treated groups as compared with the control group (47%, 23%). I3C inhibited lipid deposition by inducing CP/ATG, as identified by the enhancement of LC3-II, Beclin-1, hVps34, and m-cathepsin D, as well as by the reduction of P62, Bcl-2, Akt, p- Akt, mTOR, and p-mTOR in HCD-fed zebrafish larvae. This indicated that I3C has a protective effect on hyper-lipidemic zebrafish larvae and may be a promising drug in the prevention and treatment of atherosclerosis.

Chemokine (C-C motif) Ligand 2 Gene Ablation

The risk of non-alcohol fatty liver disease (NAFLD) increases with obesity. Vulnerability to oxidative stress and/or inflammation represents a crucial step in NAFLD progression through abnormal metabolic responses. Luciano-Mateo et al. (2019) investigated the role of CCL2 gene ablation in mice that were double deficient in lDL receptor and paraoxonase-1. Mass spectrometry was used to assess the liver metabolic response in mice fed either regular chow or a HFD. The dietary fat caused liver steatosis, oxidative stress, and the accumulation of proinflammatory macrophages in the livers of the double deficient mice. Alterations in the energy metabolism-related pathways and in metabolites associated with the methionine cycle and the glutathione reduction pathway were observed. This metabolic response was associated with impaired ATG. In mice with CCL2 deficiency, histologic features of fatty liver disease were abrogated, hepatic liver oxidative stress decreased, and anti-inflammatory macrophage marker expression levels increased. These changes were associated with the normalization of metabolic disturbances and increased LAMP2 expression, suggesting enhanced chaperone-mediated ATG. This study demonstrated that CCL2 (a key molecule for metabolic and histological alterations in the mouse liver) is sensitive to the development of hyperlipidemia and hepatic steatosis, which could be used to identify novel theranostic targets in liver diseases.

Cholesterol and CoQ$_{10}$ Deficiency in FH

Familial Hypercholesterolemia (FH) is an autosomal co-dominant genetic disorder characterized by elevated LDL cholesterol, and an increased risk of premature CVDs. Suárez-Rivero et al. (2018) examined FH pathophysiology in skin fibroblasts derived from FH patients harboring heterozygous mutations in the LDL-receptor. These fibroblasts showed a reduced LDL-uptake associated with increased intracellular cholesterol and CoQ$_{10}$ deficiency, suggesting dysregulation of the mevalonate pathway. Reduced CoQ$_{10}$ and mitochondrial dysfunction may play an important role in the pathophysiology of early atherosclerosis in FH. A secondary CoQ$_{10}$ deficiency was associated with mitochondrial depolarization and CP induction in FH fibroblasts. Persistent CP altered ATG flux and induced inflammasome to enhance cytokine production by mutant cells. All the pathological alterations in FH fibroblasts were also reproduced in a human endothelial cell line by LDL-receptor gene silencing. Both, increased intracellular cholesterol and mitochondrial dysfunction in FH fibroblasts, were restored by CoQ$_{10}$ supplementation. The dysregulated mevalonate pathway in FH, including the increased expression of cholesterol synthesizing enzymes and decreased expression of CoQ$_{10}$ biosynthetic enzymes, was corrected by the CoQ$_{10}$ treatment. Hence, the diagnosis of CoQ$_{10}$ deficiency and mitochondrial impairment in FH patients may be important to establish an early treatment with CoQ$_{10}$.

ApoE Mimetic Peptide AEM-2

CVDs, specifically atherosclerosis, is exacerbated by hypercholesterolemia. Current therapies that target lipid lowering, however, are not effective in all patients. apoE plays an important role in mediating the clearance of plasma cholesterol and also exerts protective responses. Giordano-Mooga et al. (2018) synthesized novel therapeutics that mimic the ability of apoE to decrease plasma cholesterol. The apoE mimetic peptide, AEM-2, is a dual-domain peptide composed of an amphipathic helical region that binds phospholipids, and a positively-charged region that mediates the hepatic clearance of lipoproteins. The administration of AEM-2 to apoE null mice reduced their plasma cholesterol concentration by 80% one hr post-administration. Since apoE also exerts anti-inflammatory effects that are independent of its ability to lower cholesterol, these investigators tested the effects of AEM-2 on LPS-induced responses in human THP-1 macrophages. The pre-treatment of THP-1 cells with AEM-2 reduced the LPS-induced secretion of IL-6 and TNFα. Since LPS administration is associated with an increase in mitochondrial injury, they monitored the effects of AEM-2 on mitochondrial function. AEM-2 reduced mitochondrial superoxide formation, prevented the LPS-induced $\Delta\Psi$ collapse, and attenuated mitochondrial Cyt-C release. AEM-2 also inhibited the activities of initiator caspases 8 and 9 and effector caspase 3. The attenuation of apoptosis in AEM-2 treated cells was associated with an increase in CP/ATG, suggesting that AEM-2 attenuates cellular injury in LPS-treated THP-1 macrophages and facilitates the removal of cellular debris and damaged organelles via CP/ATG induction.

Neuronal Dysfunction and Cholesterol Deregulation

Cholesterol metabolism is crucial for cells. It's important to note that its biosynthesis in the CNS occurs *in situ*, and its dysregulation involves morphological changes that cause functional variations and trigger apoptosis. The pathogenesis of rare diseases, such as mevalonate kinase deficiency or Smith-Lemli-Opitz syndrome, arises due to enzymatic defects in the cholesterol metabolic pathways, resulting in a shortage of downstream products. The most severe clinical manifestations of these diseases appear as neurological defects. Deregulation of the cholesterol pathway induces mitochondrial dysfunction as a result of respiratory chain damage. Marcuzzi et al. (2018) determined whether mitochondrial damage may be prevented by using protective mitochondrial-targeted compounds, such as MitoQ, in a neuronal cell line treated with a statin to induce a biochemical block of the cholesterol pathway. Mitochondria play a crucial role in the apoptotic mechanism involving CBMP, secondary to blocking the cholesterol pathway. This study showed that MitoQ, administered as a preventive agent, could counteract the cell damage induced by statins in the early stages, but its protective effect fades over time.

CONCLUSION

Fatty acid and triacylglycerol metabolism were investigated via protein *interactome* analysis. Palmitic acid induced glucotoxicity, oxidative stress, mitochondrial dysfunction, and apoptosis, whereas AMPK regulated the RAS gene in HepG2 cells. Atherosclerosis was modulated by PLIN2 through a loop between LXR and ATG. Indole-3-carbinol inhibited lipid deposition and promoted ATG in hyper-lipidemic zebrafish larvae. The Chemokine (C-C motif) ligand 2 gene ablation protected from liver injury, oxidative stress, and inflammation in LDL and paraoxonase-1 double deficient mice. Concomitant CoQ_{10} deficiency and intracellular cholesterol accumulation occurred in FH. The ApoE mimetic peptide AEM-2 attenuated CBMP in human

THP-1 macrophages. Furthermore, neuronal dysfunction was associated with cholesterol dysregulation due to the induction of CBMP, whereas MitoQ alleviated statins-induced neuronal dysfunction and cholesterol deregulation in FH; although, its protective effect was attenuated as a function of time.

REFERENCES

Alnahdi, A., A. John and H. Raza. 2019. Augmentation of glucotoxicity, oxidative stress, apoptosis and mitochondrial dysfunction in HepG2 cells by palmitic acid. Nutrients 11(9): 1979.

Coleman, R.A. 2019. It takes a village: Channeling fatty acid metabolism and triacylglycerol formation via protein interactomes. J Lipid Res 60: 490–497.

Djekic, D., R. Pinto, D. Repsilber, T. Hyotylainen, et al. 2019. Serum untargeted lipidomic profiling reveals dysfunction of phospholipid metabolism in subclinical coronary artery disease. Vasc Health Risk Manag 15: 123–135.

Giordano-Mooga, S., G. Datta, P. Wolkowicz, D.W. Garber, et al. 2018. The apolipoprotein E mimetic peptide AEM-2 attenuates mitochondrial injury and apoptosis in human THP-1 macrophages. Curr Top Pept Protein Res 19: 15–25.

Jiang, Y., G. Yang, Q. Liao, Y. Zou, et al. 2019. Indole-3-carbinol inhibits lipid deposition and promotes autophagy in hyperlipidemia zebrafish larvae. Environ Toxicol Pharmacol 70: 103205.

Liu, J., X. Li, Q. Lu, D. Ren, et al. 2019. AMPK: A balancer of the renin–angiotensin system. Biosci Rep 339(9): BSR20181994.

Luciano-Mateo, F., N. Cabré, S. Fernández-Arroyo, G. Baiges-Gaya, et al. 2019. Chemokine (C–C motif) ligand 2 gene ablation protects low-density lipoprotein and paraoxonase-1 double deficient mice from liver injury, oxidative stress and inflammation. Biochim Biophys Acta Mol Basis Dis 1865: 1555–1566.

Marcuzzi, A., C. Loganes, E. Valencic, E. Piscianz, et al. 2018. Neuronal dysfunction associated with cholesterol deregulation. Int J Mol Sci 19(5): 1523.

Saliba-Gustafsson, P., M. Pedrelli, K. Gertow, O. Werngren, et al. 2019. Subclinical atherosclerosis and its progression are modulated by *PLIN2* through a feed-forward loop between LXR and autophagy. J Intern Med 286: 660–675.

Suárez-Rivero, J.M., M. de la Mata, A.D. Pavón, M. Villanueva-Paz, et al. 2018. Intracellular cholesterol accumulation and coenzyme Q_{10} deficiency in Familial Hypercholesterolemia. Biochim Biophys Acta Mol Basis Dis 1864: 3697–3713.

Part-3

Charnolophagy in Systemic Disorders

16

Charnolophagy in Skin and Hair Diseases

INTRODUCTION

Skin is the largest organ of human body, with a surface area of around two square meter. It is the first line of defense against numerous environmental insults, including UV radiation, microbial infections, mechanical stresses, and toxic chemicals. CP/ATG is an important mediator of cell fate and has effects on inflammation, pathogen clearance, and antigen presentation. CP/ATG is a vital process for endogenous defenses against environmental derangements. In the adult mammalian skin, cells are constantly renewing, differentiating, and moving upward, to finally die. Wang et al. (2019) provided an overview of CP/ATG machinery in keratinocytes, skin fibroblasts, and melanocytes related to skin diseases and strategies for theranostic modulation, for the treatment of these diseases.

Recent studies documented that CP/ATG is intricately related to skin and hair diseases. CP/ATG plays a pivotal role in maintaining intracellular homeostasis under physiological and pathophysiological conditions and its upregulation may serve as an adaptive process to provide nutrients and energy during stress. Lysosomes support the degradation, signaling, and mitochondrial metabolism for epidermal differentiation, which is impaired in skin and hair diseases. Keratinocytes undergo structural remodeling during epidermal differentiation, including transformation of the proteome coupled with a reduction in cellular biomass, suggesting that intracellular digestion of proteins and organelles is necessary for keratinocyte differentiation. Monteleon et al. (2018) used both genetic and pharmacologic approaches to demonstrate that transcriptionally regulated ATG and lysosomal functions are required for keratinocyte differentiation in organotypic human skin. Lysosomal activity was required for mTOR signaling and mitochondrial oxidative metabolism, whereas, ROS are necessary for keratinocyte differentiation. Treatment with exogenous ROS rescued the differentiation defect in lysosome-inhibited keratinocytes, indicating a reciprocal relationship between lysosomes and mitochondria, in which lysosomes support mitochondrial metabolism and ROS production. The ROS released to the cytoplasm in keratinocytes triggers CP/ATG and lysosome-mediated degradation for epidermal differentiation. As defective lysosome-dependent CP/ATG is associated with common skin diseases including psoriasis and atopic dermatitis, a better understanding of the role of lysosomes in epidermal homeostasis may confer TSE-EBPT strategies for skin diseases. Guo et al. (2019) provided a brief synopsis of CP/ATG, to elucidate its role in various skin disorders and the need for further research on skin and hair diseases. CP/ATG plays an important role in maintaining cellular homeostasis under pathophysiological conditions and its upregulation may serve as an adaptive response to provide nutrients and energy during physicochemical stress to skin or hair.

This chapter describes the pivotal role of CP/ATG in malnutrition-associated dermatosis, molecular genetics of skin disorders such as acne, psoriasis, pemphigus vulgaris, SAPHO, eczema and vitiligo, and UVB-irradiated keratinocytes damage, and proposes to discover DSST-CP regulators for the TSE-EBPT of chronic skin and hair disorders.

CP/ATG in Malnutrition-associated Dermatoses and Hair Loss

Malnutrition-associated dermatoses and hair loss including necrolytic migratory erythema (NME) and pellagra share common clinico-pathological features; particularly, necrolytic changes in the epidermis. Hirai et al. (2019) reported the involvement of ATG in the development of necrolysis in three patients with malnutrition-associated dermatoses. They examined an ATG-specific molecule, LC3, using a monoclonal antibody. LC3 was expressed in the granular layers of the active border, and less intensely in the perilesional areas. Faint LC3 staining or only background levels were observed in control skin diseases including atopic dermatitis, psoriasis vulgaris, basal cell carcinoma with amyloid deposits, and squamous cell carcinoma. Autophagosome-like structures were observed near in the necrolytic areas. No apoptotic signals were observed in the necrolytic lesion as determined by TUNEL method. Epidermal Langerhans cells determined by the anti-CD1a antibody were decreased, suggesting that malnutrition-associated necrolysis, NME, and pellagra, may be induced by dysregulated CP/ATG. Garg and Sagwan (2019) established dysregulated ATG of skin and hair in a low dietary protein scenario by determining the facial profile, clinical presentation, and histopathological correlates deficient protein intake and missing of meals in a tertiary care aesthetic skin institute. A total of 98 patients of skin- and hair-related complaints were enrolled and a histopathological correlation was established by skin and scalp biopsies in high and low protein groups. A significant number of subjects were taking less than half of the recommended daily allowance of proteins and faced problems like hair fall, acne, pigmentation, vitiligo, hirsutism, melasma, and premature aging. Subjects missing breakfast suffered from hypothyroidism, diffuse hair fall, and autoimmune disorders like vitiligo, lichen planus, and alopecia areata. Histopathological images from the submental area showed loose and fragmented collagen in the high carbohydrate group in comparison to the high protein group where thick, uniformly stained collagen bundles were found in the dermis. The histopathology of the scalp tissue showed chronic perifollicular inflammatory infiltrates and fibrosis in the high carbohydrate group, which were absent in the histopathology specimen of the high protein group. Patients eating an early and nutrient-rich breakfast had higher mean protein intakes and less severe skin and hair problems, suggesting that circadian rhythm, dietary protein adequacy and eating an early breakfast all had significant influence in preventing the self-destruction or dysregulated CP/ATG in trichology, cosmetic dermatology, and various autoimmune, inflammatory, and metabolic diseases.

CP/ATG in Molecular Genetics of Skin and Hair Diseases

PNPLA1 Mutations in Ichthyosis

Autosomal recessive congenital ichthyosis (ARCI) is a group of epidermal keratinization disorders. One of the disease-associated proteins, patatin-like phospholipase domain-containing protein-1 (PNPLA1), plays a crucial role in the epidermal omega-O-acylceramide synthesis and localizes on the surface of LDs. Earlier clinical tests showed abnormal LD accumulation in blood smear samples of ARCI patients with PNPLA1 mutations. To investigate the abnormal accumulation of LDs, Onal et al. (2019) analyzed the primary fibroblasts of ARCI patients with PNPLA1 mutations (p.Y245del and p.D172N). They hypothesized that PNPLA1 mutations might affect the lipophagy-mediated regulation of LDs and cause intracellular lipid accumulation in ARCI patients. LD accumulation was analyzed by fluorescence staining with BODIPY®493/503 in the fibroblasts of patient cells and PNPLA1-siRNA-transfected control fibroblasts. The expression of PNPLA1 and its effects on the lipophagy-mediated degradation of LDs were analyzed by immunocytochemistry and immunoblotting. Mutant or downregulated PNPLA1 protein caused abnormal intracellular LD accumulation. PNPLA1 mutations affected neither the cellular localization nor the protein expression in the fibroblasts. When they analyzed the lipophagic degradation process, LC3 expression and the number of CPS were decreased in fibroblasts of these patients. In addition, the co-localization of LDs with CPS and lysosomes was reduced. Thus, PNPLA1 mutations caused disturbances in both CPS-formation and its fusion lysosomes, indicating a possible role for PNPLA1 protein in LD regulation via lipophagy-mediated degradation. Although LD is a highly-specialized form of CB and occurs primarily in skin and hair disorders, it may be detected in various NDDs, CVDs, musculoskeletal diseases, autoimmune and inflammatory diseases, and in MDR malignancies. Similarly, lipophagy is a highly specialized form of CP, which particularly eliminates LDs from the biological system as a mechanism of ICD for NCF. Nevertheless, both CP as well as lipophagy require Akt-ubiquitination, lysosomal activation, and MB to synthesize sufficient ATP for their execution.

MDA-7/IL-24 Protein in Skin Diseases

Mda-7/IL-24 is implicated in many pathological conditions involving inflammation and may play a role in IBD, psoriasis, CVDs, rheumatoid arthritis, tuberculosis, and viral infection. Menezes et al. (2018) provided a recent update on the multifunctional gene mda-7/IL-24 for the treatment of not only cancer, but also other pathological conditions. These investigators identified gene displaying differential expression by subtraction hybridization method. Metastatic human melanoma cells were terminally-differentiated and lost their tumorigenic properties by treatment with recombinant fibroblast interferon and Mezerein. This approach permitted cloning of multiple genes displaying enhanced expression when melanoma cells terminally differentiated, called melanoma differentiation associated (mda) genes. One mda gene, mda-7, has emerged based on its relevance to cancer, inflammation, and other pathological states, which based on the presence of a secretory sequence, chromosomal location, and IL-10 signature motif has been named IL-24 (mda-7/IL-24). Mda-7/IL-24 is a potent cancer suppressor gene capable of inducing cancer cell death through ATG and apoptosis in preclinical animal models. Mda-7/IL-24 demonstrated profound anticancer activity in a Phase I/II clinical trial following a direct injection with an adenovirus (Ad.mda-7; INGN-241) in tumors in patients with advanced cancers.

SAPHO and Propionibacterium Acnes

Recently, Berthelot et al. (2018) reported that many patients with SAPHO syndrome may lack overt infection by Propionibacterium acnes, which is a dominant member of cutaneous microbiota, and antibiotics have only a transient and incomplete effect, either in SAPHO syndrome or acne. As several auto-inflammatory bone disorders sharing overproduction of IL-1β can mimic SAPHO; this syndrome depends on genetically encoded overproduction of IL-1β. However, cyclic intracellular infections by P. acnes can contribute to the enhanced IL-1β release by skin cells and bone cells. P. acnes is a powerful trigger of NLRP3-inflammasome activation and IL-1β, leading to osteitis and enhanced mesenchymal cells differentiation in osteoblasts. The first steps of this disorder are not driven by P. acnes, but by a relative deficiency of FoxO1 within the nucleus of sebaceous cells. A similar defect of FoXO1 in bone cells should also be sought in SAPHO, since repression of the FoxO1 gene is found in psoriasis skin, and is associated with an increased number of osteoblasts and high bone mass in mice. FoxO1 promotes IL-1β production, so that its downregulation could help P. acnes escape innate immunity and persist in a latent state in bone cells, including mesenchymal stem cells. However, P. acnes itself contributes to FoxO1 downregulation, like a H. pylori infection which induces nuclear inactivation of FoxO1 in gastric cells to slow down CP/ATG clearance. Bisphosphonates, which often improve SAPHO syndromes and enhance CP/ATG may be worth testing to see whether their combination with antibiotics confers synergistic benefit in SAPHO syndromes. SAPHO and acnes treatment protocol is presented in Fig. 32.

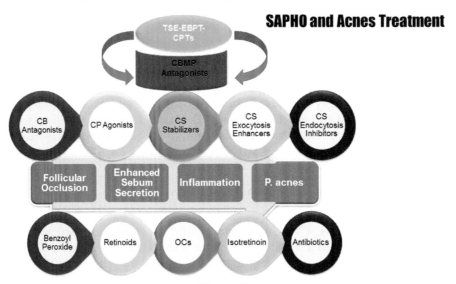

Figure 32

Propionibacterium acnes in Keratinocytes

Megyeri et al. (2018) evaluated the effects of different P. acnes strains and propionic acid on ATG in keratinocytes. P. acnes strain 889 altered the architecture of the mitochondrial network, elevated LC-3B-II, Beclin-1, and AMPKα, stimulated ATG, facilitated the intracellular redistribution of LC-3B-II, increased the number of autophagosomes per cell, and enhanced the development of acidic vesicular organelles in the HPV-KER cell line. Propionic acid increased AMPKα, enhanced lipidation of LC-3B-II, stimulated ATG, and facilitated the translocation of LC-3B-II into autophagosomes in HPV-KER cells. P. acnes strains 889 and 6609 and heat-killed strain 889 also stimulated autophagosome formation in primary keratinocytes, indicating that the cell wall components and secreted propionic acid metabolite of P. acnes evoke mitochondrial damage, thereby triggering AMPKAα-associated activation of CP/ATG, which facilitates the removal of dysfunctional mitochondria implicated in CP dysregulation and CBMP. It also promotes keratinocytes' survival, suggesting that low-level colonization of hair follicles with noninvasive P. acnes strains, by triggering a local increase in CP/ATG, might exert a profound effect on physiological processes for the maintenance of skin tissue homeostasis. A Schematic algorithm of TSE-EBPT of Acne and SAPHO syndrome and its treatment based on mild, moderate, and severe symptoms is presented in Fig. 33.

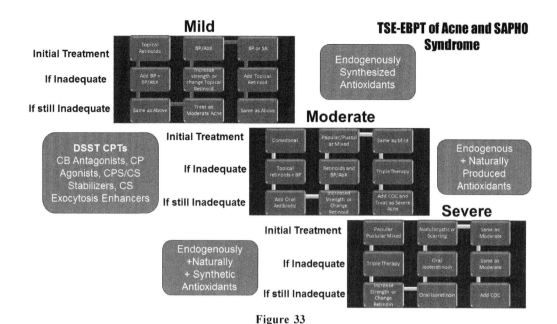

Figure 33

CP/ATG in Skin Diseases

Koenig et al. (2019) provided evidence that CP/ATG has a dual role in the skin. In addition to its known protective role as an evolutionary conserved upstream regulator of lysosomal degradation, ATG-induced cell death (CDA) occurred in epithelial lineage-derived organs, such as the inter-follicular epidermis, the sebaceous gland, and the Harderian gland. By utilizing GFP-LC3 transgenic and ATG7-deficient mice, these investigators showed that CDA is initiated during terminal differentiation when the cells become highly resistant to apoptosis. In these transitional cells, the Golgi compartment expanded, which accounted for the formation of primary lysosomes, and the nucleus started to condense. During CDA, a burst of autophagosome formation was observed; first the ER was phagocytosed, followed by ATG of the nucleus. By this selective form of cell death, most of the cytoplasmic organelles were degraded, but structural proteins remained intact. In the absence of ATG, parts of the ER, ribosomes, and chromatin remained. A burst of CP/ATG was observed in single cells of the epidermis and in larger areas of ductal cells, suggesting induction and an integral role of CP/ATG in the death of keratinocyte lineage cells as well as participation of these cells in terminal cell fate.

MCM7 Silencing

Cutaneous melanoma (CM) has become a major public health concern. Recent studies illustrate that mini-chromosome maintenance protein 7 (MCM7) participates in various diseases including skin disease. Yang et al. (2020) studied the effects of MCM7 silencing on CM cell ATG and apoptosis by modulating the Akt threonine kinase 1 (Akt1)/mTOR kinase signaling pathway. Initially, a microarray analysis was used to screen the CM-related gene expression data as well as differentially expressed genes. Subsequently, MCM7 expression vector and lentivirus RNA used for MCM7 silencing (LV-shRNA-MCM7) were constructed, and these vectors, dimethyl sulfoxide (DMSO) and Akt-activator SC79, were then introduced into CM cell line SK-MEL-2 to validate the role of MCM7 in ATG, viability, apoptosis, cell cycle, migration, and invasion. To further investigate the regulatory mechanisms of MCM7 in CM, the expression of MCM7, Akt1, mTOR, cyclin D1, as well as CP/ATG and apoptosis relative factors, such as LC3B, SOD2,

DJ-1, p62, Bcl-2, Bax, and caspase-3 in melanoma cells were determined. MCM7 mediated the Akt1/mTOR signaling to influence the progress of melanoma. MCM7 silencing contributed to the increased expression of Bax, capase-3, and CP/ATG-related genes (LC3B, SOD2, and DJ-1), but decreased the expression of Bcl-2, suggesting that MCM7 silencing promoted CP/ATG and apoptosis. MCM7 silencing also attenuated cell viability, invasion, and migration, and reduced the cyclin D1 expression and protein levels of p-Akt1 and p-mTOR. Thus, MCM7-silencing inhibited CM via the inactivation of the Akt1/mTOR signaling pathway.

CP/ATG in Alopecia

Alopecia areata (AA) is a highly prevalent autoimmune disease that attacks the hair follicle and leads to hair loss that can range from small patches to the complete loss of scalp and body hair. Previous linkages and GWAS generated evidence for etiological contributions from inherited genetic variants at different population frequencies, including both rare mutations and common polymorphisms. Petukhova et al. (2019) conducted gene expression (GE) studies on scalp biopsies of 96 patients and controls to establish signatures of the active disease. They performed an integrative analysis on these two datasets to test the hypothesis that rare CNVs in patients with AA could be leveraged to identify the drivers of disease in the AA GE signatures. Copy number variants (CNVs) in a case-control cohort of 673 patients with AA and 16 311 control independent of these case-control cohort of 96 participants were used in the GE study. Using an integrative computational analysis, 14 genes were identified whose expression was altered by CNVs, corresponding to gene expression changes in the lesioned skin of patients. Four of these genes were affected by CNVs in three or more unrelated patients with AA, including ATG4B and SMARCA2, involved in ATG and chromatin remodeling, respectively. These findings identified new classes of genes with contributions to AA pathogenesis.

Small Extracellular Vesicles and Cutaneous Wound Healing

A diabetic foot ulcer is a life-threatening clinical problem in diabetic patients. Endothelial cell-derived small extracellular vesicles (sEVs) are important mediators of intercellular communication in the pathogenesis of several diseases. Zeng et al. (2019) isolated sEVs from human umbilical vein endothelial cells (HUVECs) pretreated with or without advanced glycation end products (AGEs). The roles of HUVEC-derived sEVs on the biological characteristics of skin fibroblasts were investigated both *in vitro* and *in vivo*. sEVs derived from AGEs-pretreated HUVECs (AGEs-sEVs) inhibited collagen synthesis by activating ATG of human skin fibroblasts. Treatment with AGEs-sEVs delayed the wound healing in SD rats. miR-106b-5p was upregulated in AGEs-sEVs and in exudate-derived sEVs from patients with diabetic foot ulcers. Consequently, the sEV-mediated uptake of miR-106b-5p in recipient fibroblasts reduced the expression of ERK1/2, resulting in fibroblasts' ATG activation and subsequent collagen degradation, demonstrating that miR-106b-5p could be enriched in AGEs-sEVs. It then decreases collagen synthesis and delays cutaneous wound healing by triggering fibroblasts' ATG by reducing ERK1/2 expression.

Melanin Processing by Keratinocytes

Moreiras et al. (2019) identified a parallelism between melanin processing within keratinocytes and the host-pathogen interaction with plasmodium, opening new avenues to understand the molecular mechanisms that ensure skin pigmentation and photo-protection. In contrast with melanin biogenesis and transport within melanocytes, little is known about how melanin is transferred and processed within keratinocytes. Several models have been proposed, with evidence supporting coupled exo/endocytosis. Upon internalization, melanin is stored within keratinocytes in an arrested compartment, allowing the pigment to persist for long periods.

Psoriasis

Psoriasis is an immune-mediated inflammatory disease of the skin and IL-17A plays a crucial role in its pathogenesis. Cytokines like TNFα and IL-23 are also important in mediating the disease and CP/ATG serves as a novel mechanism by which cytokines controls the immune response. Varshney and Saini (2018) investigated the effect of IL-17A on ATG and revealed crosstalk between ATG and cholesterol signaling in keratinocytes, suggesting that IL-17A stimulated keratinocytes activated PI3K/Akt/mTOR signaling and inhibited CP/ATG by inhibiting autophagosome formation and enhancing CP/ATG. Immunoblotting was utilized to detect the expression of ATG biomarkers (LC3 and p62), PI3K, mTOR, and Akt. Induction of CP/ATG by the mTOR inhibitor, Rapamycin, and/or starvation also inhibited IL-17A, secreted IL-8, CCL20, and S100A7 in keratinocytes. The inhibition of ATG by IL-17A was accompanied by enhanced cholesterol levels which regulated the ATG. To investigate the interaction between CP/ATG and cellular cholesterol, methyl-β-cyclodextrin (MβCD) was used, which disrupted detergent-insoluble microdomains (DIMs) by depleting cells of cholesterol and checked CP/ATG. The decreased expression of LC3-II in psoriatic lesional skin compared to non-lesional skin and induction of CP/ATG by the anti-psoriatic drug Methotrexate in keratinocytes confirmed the role of CP/ATG in psoriasis, suggesting that modulators of CP/ATG and/or cholesterol may be developed as novel TSE-EBPTs for psoriasis. Progranulin (PGRN), a secreted glycoprotein, has been investigated in many skin diseases. It plays an important role in the inflammatory response and ATG, mediated through the Wnt/β-catenin pathway. Farag et al. (2019) investigated the role of progranulin in psoriasis pathogenesis by evaluating its immune-histochemical expression in lesional and perilesional skin to gather information on the role of β-catenin. They performed this study on 37 patients presented with variable degrees of psoriasis vulgaris severity vs 37 age and sex-matched healthy volunteers. Psoriasis area and severity index (PASI) score were used to evaluate the severity of psoriasis. From all cases (lesional and perilesional) and controls, skin biopsies were taken for histopathological and immune-histochemical evaluation of PGRN and β-catenin. There was a significant upregulation of PGRN from the samples taken from the controls to the ones taken from those with perilesional and lesional psoriatic skin. The PGRN expression was then correlated with psoriasis severity. β-Catenin showed downregulation from control to peri-lesional and lesional psoriatic skin. There was a negative correlation between PGRN and β-catenin expression in psoriatic skin, indicating that it has a pro-inflammatory effect in the psoriasis pathogenesis, which could be mediated through a decreased β-catenin expression. Hence, PGRN may be used as a target for immunotherapy in psoriasis.

Transcriptome-Wide Expression of cEDS Skin Fibroblasts

Classical Ehlers-Danlos syndrome (cEDS) is a dominant inherited connective tissue disorder caused by mutations in the COL5A1 and COL5A2 genes encoding type V collagen (COLLV), which is a fibrillar COLL in connective tissues. cEDS patients suffer from skin hyper-extensibility, abnormal wound healing/atrophic scars, and joint hypermobility. Most of the causative variants result in a non-functional COL5A1 allele and COLLV haplo-insufficiency, whilst COL5A2 mutations affect its structural integrity. Chiarelli et al. (2019) performed gene expression profiling in skin fibroblasts from four patients harboring haplo-insufficient and structural mutations in both disease genes. Transcriptome profiling revealed changes in the expression of the extracellular matrix (ECM)-related genes, such as SPP1, POSTN, EDIL3, IGFBP2, and C3, which encode both matri-cellular and soluble proteins involved in cell proliferation and migration, and cutaneous wound healing. These gene expression changes were consistent with previous protein findings on *in vitro* fibroblasts from other cEDS patients, which exhibited reduced migration and poor wound repair owing to COLLV disorganization, altered deposition of fibronectin into ECM, and an abnormal integrin pattern. A microarray analysis also indicated the decreased expression of

DNAJB7, VIPAS39, CCPG1, ATG10, and SVIP, which encode molecular chaperones facilitating protein folding, enzymes regulating post-Golgi COLLs processing, and proteins acting as cargo receptors required for ER proteostasis and implicated in the ATG. Patients' cells also showed altered mRNA of many cell-cycle-regulating genes including CCNE2, KIF4A, MKI67, DTL, and DDIAS. Protein studies showed that aberrant COLLV expression caused the disassembly of itself and many structural ECM constituents including COLLI, COLLIII, fibronectin, and fibrillins. These findings provided the evidence of significant gene expression changes in cEDS skin fibroblasts, emphasizing that defective ECM remodeling, ER homeostasis, and CP/ATG might play a crucial role in the pathogenesis of cEDS.

IL-17 in Vitiligo

Mitochondrial dysfunction, which can induce the excessive production of ROS, is emerging as a mechanism that underlies various inflammatory and autoimmune diseases, including vitiligo. This is a de-pigmentary disorder that develops as a result of the progressive disappearance of epidermal melanocytes. Stress can precipitate or exacerbate skin disease through psychosomatic mechanisms. Stress induces vitiligo-like symptoms in mice, as cellular damage to melanocytes causes synthetic pigment loss. Stress also increases IL-17, IL-1β, and anti-melanocyte IgG in mouse serum. Upregulation of the IL-1β transcript in patients suggests its role in the autoimmune pathogenesis of vitiligo. Zhou et al. (2018) demonstrated that IL-17 promoted IL-1β secretion from keratinocytes. They demonstrated that IL-17 inhibits melano-genesis of zebrafish, normal human epidermal melanocytes, and B16F10 cells. IL-17 increased mitochondrial dysfunction, and ROS accumulation was related to CP/ATG induction, which is needed for the apoptosis of B16F10 cells. To inhibit ROS generation, B16F10 cells were pretreated with NAC, which inhibited ATG. 3-MA also had an inhibitory effect on ATG. NAC or 3-MA pretreatments inhibited IL-17-mediated cell apoptosis, suggesting that IL-17 induces a cellular stress microenvironment in melanocytes to promote ATG cell apoptosis in vitiligo.

Nucleophagy in Skin Diseases

Nucleophagy is a selective ATG, which removes damaged or non-essential nuclear material from a cell. Fu et al. (2018) elucidated on the signal pathways of nucleophagy as well as its role in human diseases. Nucleophagy is crucial for promoting cell longevity and ensures normal body function and may play a crucial role in degenerative disorders, tumorigenesis, malnutrition, metabolic disorders, parakeratosis, and psoriasis. Nucleophagy can improve degenerative disorders by delaying premature cell senescence, prevent malnutrition and metabolic disorder by maintaining nuclear structure and releasing nutrients for energy production, and alleviate parakeratosis and psoriasis. Some studies indicated that overexpression of the lamin B1 delays cell senescence. Appropriate nucleophagy can drive RAS-induced cell senescence and DNA damage-induced cell senescence to restrain cell proliferation, and degrade excessive DNA in polyploid tumor cells. Hence, selective nucleophagy may protect cells from tumorigenesis and maintain cell and tissue integrity. However, uncontrolled nucleophagy can attack normal cells and lead to cytotoxicity. Hence, nucleophagy may be a potential theranostic target in human diseases, including skin and hair disorders.

CP/ATG in UVB-Irradiated Keratinocytes

UV-B radiation is a major environmental risk factor for the development and progression of skin cancers. CP/ATG is an important process for maintaining intracellular homeostasis, which is downregulated in UVB-irradiated keratinocytes. Raffinose is a natural oligosaccharide that serves as a novel activator of ATG and as a balancing agent to regulate the diversity of environmental stress. Lin et al. (2019) found that Raffinose treatment inhibited the LDH release and Trypan blue staining in UVB-challenged human keratinocytes cell line HaCaT but did not affect the cleavage of caspase-3 and PARP, as well as their translocation into the nucleus of other cell death markers, endonuclease G and AIF. The Raffinose treatment enhanced CP/ATG flux in an mTOR-independent manner. Decreased LC3-II turnover in UVB-irradiated keratinocytes could be rescued by Raffinose treatment, indicating that its treatment increased CP/ATG in UVB-irradiated HaCaT cells. Raffinose's effect on cell death was inhibited when CP/TG was suppressed with either a siRNA targeting Atg5 (siAtg5) or CP/ATG inhibitor Wortmannin, suggesting that Raffinose increases mTOR-independent ATG and reduces cell death in UVB-irradiated keratinocytes, indicating its theranostic potential in attenuating photo-damage to the skin. Apigenin, a bioflavonoid inhibit UVB-induced skin cancer. Li et al. (2019) performed LDH release assay to determine that Apigenin increased cell death in the primary human epidermal keratinocytes (HEKs) and the cutaneous squamous cell carcinoma cell line COLO-16. Apigenin reduced LC3-II turnover, Acridine orange staining, and GFP-LC3 puncta in both cell types, suggesting ATG inhibition. However, Apigenin restored the inhibition of ATG in UVB-challenged HEKs. Apigenin restored the UVB-induced downregulation of ataxia-telangiectasia mutated (ATM), ataxia-telangiectasia, Rad3-related (ATR) and the UPR regulatory proteins, BiP, IRE1α and PERK in HEKs. Apigenin also inhibited UVB-induced apoptosis and cell death in HEKs. ATG inhibition by the ATG-related gene, (ATG) 5 RNA interference, interrupted the Apigenin-induced restoration of ATR, ATM, and BiP, which were downregulated in HEKs, indicating that Apigenin exhibits a protective effect in keratinocytes with UVB damage, suggesting its potential application as a photo-protective agent. Sun or therapy-related UVB irradiation induce diversified cell death modalities such as apoptosis, necrosis/necroptosis, and CP/ATG. An understanding of the mechanisms implicated in the regulation and execution of the cell death program is imperative for the prevention and treatment of skin diseases. An essential component of death-inducing complex is Fas-associated protein with death domain (FADD), involved in the conduction of death signals of different death modalities. Antunovic et al. (2019) investigated the role of FADD in the selection of the cell death mode after narrow-band UVB (NB-UVB) irradiation using specific cell death inhibitors (carbobenzoxy-valyl-alanyl-aspartyl-[O-methyl]-fluoromethylketone (zVAD-fmk), Necrostatin-1, and 3-MA) and FADD-deficient (FADD$^{-/-}$) mouse embryonic fibroblasts (MEFs) and their wild type (WT) counterparts. A lack of FADD sensitized MEFs to the induction of receptor-interacting protein 1 (RIPK1)-dependent apoptosis by the ROS generation, but without the activation of p53, Bax, and Bcl-2, as well as without the enrolment of calpain-2. ATG was established as a contributing factor to NB-UVB-induced death execution. By contrast, WT cells triggered an intrinsic apoptotic pathway that was resistant to the inhibition by zVAD-fmk and Necrostatin-1, indicating a mechanism overcoming the cell survival and supporting the role of FADD in the prevention of CP/ATG-dependent apoptosis.

CONCLUSION

CP/ATG and nucleophagy play pivotal role in preventing skin and hair diseases. A CP/ATG defect was observed in malnutrition-associated dermatoses and hair loss. Dietary protein deficiency dysregulated CP/ATG to cause skin disorders, alopecia, and early aging. Impaired lipophagy due to PNPLA1 mutations induced LD accumulation in the primary fibroblasts of ichthyosis patients. Impaired mda-7/IL-24 was observed in human skin and other diseases. Lysosomes induced degradation, signaling, and mitochondrial metabolism for epidermal differentiation, whereas PI3K/Akt/mTOR activation and CP inhibition increased cholesterol accumulation in the IL-17A-mediated inflammatory response of psoriasis patients. Progranulin and β-Catenin expression were also impaired in psoriasis. A functional association between SAPHO, CP/ATG, IL-1, FoxO1, and Propionibacterium acnes was observed. Propionibacterium acnes induces ATG in keratinocytes through multiple mechanisms. Cell death induced CP/ATG in terminal differentiation of keratinocytes. Raffinose increased CP/ATG and reduced cell death in UVB-irradiated keratinocytes. MCM7 silencing promoted cutaneous melanoma cell CP/ATG and apoptosis by inactivating Akt1/mTOR signaling. An etiological role of CP/ATG was observed in alopecia. An analysis of rare copy number variants and gene expression in alopecia was involved in the CP/ATG pathogenesis. Endothelial cell-derived extracellular vesicles suppressed cutaneous wound healing by dysregulating fibroblasts' CP/ATG. Melanin processing by keratinocytes was recognized as a non-microbial type of host-pathogen interaction in the skin. Apigenin restored impaired CP/ATG and downregulated UPR regulatory proteins in keratinocytes exposed to UV-B radiation. FADD-deficient mice embryonic fibroblasts were highly vulnerable to RIPK1-dependent CP/ATG and apoptosis following UV irradiation. The pathogenesis of cEDS was explored from the transcriptome-wide expression of patients' skin fibroblasts. IL-17 induced a cellular stress microenvironment of melanocytes to impair CP/ATG, and induced apoptosis in vitiligo.

REFERENCES

Antunovic, M., I. Matic, B. Nagy, K. Caput Mihalic, et al. 2019. FADD-deficient mouse embryonic fibroblasts undergo RIPK1-dependent apoptosis and ATG after NB-UVB irradiation. J Photochem Photobiol B 194: 32–45.

Berthelot, J.M., S. Corvec and G. Hayem. 2018. SAPHO, ATG, IL-1, FoxO1, and Propionibacterium (Cutibacterium) acnes. Joint Bone Spine 85: 171–176.

Chiarelli, N., G. Carini, N. Zoppi, M. Ritelli, et al. 2019. Molecular insights in the pathogenesis of classical Ehlers-Danlos syndrome from transcriptome-wide expression profiling of patients' skin fibroblasts. PLoS One 14: e0211647.

Farag, A.G.A., M.A. Shoaib, R.M. Samaka, A.G. Abdou, et al. 2019. Progranulin and beta-catenin in psoriasis: An immunohistochemical study. J Cosmet Dermatol 18: 2019–2026.

Fu, N., X. Yang and L. Chen. 2018. Nucleophagy plays a major role in human diseases. Curr Drug Targets 19: 1767–1773.

Garg, S. and A. Sangwan. 2019. Dietary protein deficit and deregulated autophagy: A new clinico-diagnostic perspective in pathogenesis of early aging, skin, and hair disorders. Indian Dermatol Online J 10(2): 115–124.

Guo, Y., X. Zhang, T. Wu, X. Hu, et al. 2019. ATG in skin diseases. Dermatology 235: 380–389.

Hirai, Y., T. Miyake, T. Hamada, Q. Yamasaki, et al. 2019. ATG in malnutrition-associated dermatoses. J Dermatol 46: 43–47.

Koenig, U., H. Robenek, C. Barresi, M. Brandstetter, et al. 2019. Cell death induced ATG contributes to terminal differentiation of skin and skin appendages. Autophagy 4: 1–14.

Li, L., M. Li, S. Xu, H. Chen, et al. 2019. Apigenin restores impairment of ATG and downregulation of unfolded protein response regulatory proteins in keratinocytes exposed to ultraviolet B radiation. J Photochem Photobiol B 94: 84–95.

Lin, S., L. Li, M. Li, H. Gu, et al. 2019. Raffinose increases ATG and reduces cell death in UVB-irradiated keratinocytes. J Photochem Photobiol B 201: 111653.

Megyeri, K., L. Orosz, S. Bolla, L. Erdei, et al. 2018. Propionibacterium acnes induces ATG in keratinocytes: Involvement of multiple mechanisms. J Invest Dermatol 138: 750–759.

Menezes, M.E., P. Bhoopathi, A.K. Pradhan, L. Emdad, et al. 2018. Role of MDA-7/IL-24 a multifunction protein in human diseases. Adv Cancer Res 38: 143–182.

Monteleon, C.L., T. Agnihotri, A. Dahal, M. Liu, et al. 2018. Lysosomes support the degradation, signaling, and mitochondrial metabolism necessary for human epidermal differentiation. J Invest Dermatol 138: 1945–1954.

Moreiras, H., M. Lopes-da-Silva, M.C. Seabra and D.C. Barral. 2019. Melanin processing by keratinocytes: A non-microbial type of host-pathogen interaction? Traffic 20: 301–304.

Onal, G., O. Kutlu, E. Ozer, D. Gozuacik, et al. 2019. Impairment of lipophagy by PNPLA1 mutations causes lipid droplet accumulation in primary fibroblasts of autosomal recessive congenital ichthyosis patients. J Dermatol Sci 93: 50–57.

Petukhova, L., A.V. Patel, R.K. Rigo, L. Bian, et al. 2019. Integrative analysis of rare copy number variants and gene expression data in alopecia areata implicates an aetiological role for autophagy. Exp Dermatol 29: 243–253.

Varshney, P. and N. Saini. 2018. PI3K/Akt/mTOR activation and ATG inhibition plays a key role in increased cholesterol during IL-17A mediated inflammatory response in psoriasis. Biochim Biophys Acta Mol Basis Dis 1864: 1795–1803.

Wang, Y., X. Wen, D. Hao, M. Zhou, et al. 2019. Insights into ATG machinery in cells related to skin diseases and strategies for therapeutic modulation. Biomed Pharmacother 113: 108775.

Yang, Y., S. Ma, Z. Ye and X. Zhou. 2020. MCM7 silencing promotes cutaneous melanoma cell ATG and apoptosis by inactivating the Akt1/mTOR signaling pathway. J Cell Biochem 121: 1283–1294.

Zeng, T., X. Wang, W. Wang, Q. Feng, et al. 2019. Endothelial cell-derived small extracellular vesicles suppress cutaneous wound healing through regulating fibroblasts autophagy. Clin Sci 133(9): CS20190008. doi: https://doi.org/10.1042/CS20190008.

Zhou, J., X. An, J. Dong, Y. Wang, et al. 2018. IL-17 induces cellular stress microenvironment of melanocytes to promote autophagic cell apoptosis in vitiligo. FASEB J 32: 4899–4916.

17

Charnolophagy in Musculoskeletal Diseases

INTRODUCTION

Osteoarthritis (OA) is the most prevalent musculoskeletal disorder in the world and aging is the main risk factor, causing chronic disability. Recent studies have shown that ATG serves as a protective mechanism in normal cartilage, and its aging-related loss is linked to cell death in OA. Lysosomes are ubiquitous intracellular organelles that have an acidic pH because these are highly rich in acid phsophatases and play a crucial role in cellular clearance through ATP-driven CP and ATG, which is involved in bone homeostasis and the onset of osteoporosis. Artesunate protected against surgery-induced knee arthro-fibrosis by activating Beclin-1-mediated ATG through the inhibition of mTOR signaling. The intake of alcohol induced impaired CP and caused muscle protein imbalance. Recently, mitochondrial breakdown in skeletal muscle and the role of lysosomes in this process was investigated. It was shown that effects of 17β-estradiol on ATG in the murine MC3T3-E1 osteoblast cell line is mediated via the G-protein-coupled estrogen receptor and the ERK1/2 signaling. Yin et al. (2019) introduced ATG, summarized its relevance in bone physiology, and discussed its role in the onset of osteoporosis and its theranostic potential. Multiple proteins involved in ATG are critical to the survival, differentiation, and functioning of bone cells, including osteoblasts, osteocytes, and osteoclasts. Dysregulated ATG disturbs the balance between bone formation and bone resorption and mediates the onset and progression of multiple bone diseases, including osteoporosis. Oxidative stress (OS) is involved in the pathogenesis of OA and defective ATG accompanies age-related OA. ATG induction could serve as the theranostic mean, as it alleviates several symptoms in OA animal models. However, over-activation of ATG may cause cell death and may also contribute to the development of OA. Goutas et al. (2018) analyzed the ATG response in the acute exogenous oxidative insult of chondrocytes from healthy individuals (control) and OA patients (OA). Cells were treated with sub-lethal concentrations of H_2O_2 and then allowed to recover. The mRNA levels of ATG-related genes (Atg5, Beclin-1, and LC3) were reduced in OA chondrocytes as compared to the control chondrocytes. Following exposure to OS, in control cells, the mRNA and proteins of these genes initially increased and restored back to their basal levels 6–24 hrs. In OA chondrocytes, however, ATG-related genes remained high even after 24 hrs of treatment, indicating their inability to attenuate ATG. The higher number of impaired mitochondria as well as increased APS in OA cells suggested that a deregulation of ATG response and oxidative stress were responsible for the progression of OA.

Muscle mitochondrial networks changes from a longitudinal, parallel orientation to a perpendicular configuration during postnatal development. Mitochondrial dynamics, CP, and

Ca^{2+} uptake proteins are abundant during early postnatal development. MB and O/P proteins are upregulated throughout muscle development. Postnatal muscle mitochondrial network formation is accompanied by a change in the protein expression profile from mitochondria designed for co-ordinated cellular assembly to mitochondria specialized for cellular energy metabolism. Striated muscle mitochondria form networks for rapid cellular energy distribution. However, the mitochondrial reticulum is not formed at birth. Kim et al. (2019) established the network formation time course and protein expression profile during the postnatal development of the murine muscle mitochondrial reticulum. Two-photon microscopy was used to observe mitochondrial network orientation in the tibialis anterior (TA) muscles of live mice at postnatal days (P) 1, 7, 14, 21, and 42, respectively. All muscle fibers maintained a longitudinal, fiber parallel mitochondrial network orientation early in development (P1-7). Mixed networks were most common at P14 but, by P21, almost all fibers had developed the perpendicular mitochondrial orientation in mature glycolytic fibers. Tandem mass tag proteomics were applied to examine changes in 6869 protein abundances in developing TA muscles. Mitochondrial proteins increased by 32% from P1 to P42. In addition, both nuclear- and mtDNA encoded O/P components had increased during development, whereas O/P assembly factors had decreased. Although mitochondrial dynamics and CP were induced at P1-7, MB was enhanced after P14. Ca^{2+} signaling proteins and the mitochondrial Ca^{2+} uniporter had the highest expression early on in postnatal development, suggesting that mitochondrial networks transform from a parallel to perpendicular orientation during the second and third weeks after birth in murine glycolytic skeletal muscle. This structural transition was accompanied by a change in the protein expression profile from mitochondria designed for coordinated cellular assembly to mitochondria specialized for cellular energy metabolism. Recently, Li et al. (2018a) reported that high intensity interval training (HIIT) is more effective for improving exercise performance than continuous moderate intensity (MIST) training and this improvement is related to mitochondrial function and basal CP/ATG adaptation in the cardiac muscle.

This chapter emphasizes the protective role of CP in various musculoskeletal disorders. It also describes the TSE-EBPT significance of CP in musculoskeletal disorders.

CP/ATG in Young and Aged Skeletal Muscle

A healthy mitochondrial pool relies on the removal of dysfunctional organelles via CP. Chronic contractile activity (CCA) is an exercise model that can elicit mitochondrial adaptations in both young and aged muscle, albeit to a lesser extent in the older age groups. The assessment of CP revealed the enhanced targeting of mitochondria for degradation in aged muscle. CP was reduced as an adaptation to CCA, suggesting that an improvement in organelle quality reduces the need for mitochondrial turnover. CCA enhances lysosomal capacity and may ameliorate lysosomal dysfunction in aged muscle. Skeletal muscle exhibits deficits in MQC with age. Carter et al. (2018) assessed CP using Colchicine following CCA of muscle in young and aged rats. CCA evoked MB in young muscle, with an attenuated response in aged muscle. CP was higher in aged muscle and was correlated with the enhanced expression of CP receptors and transcriptional regulators. CCA decreased CP in both age groups, suggesting an improvement in organelle quality. CCA also reduced the enhanced expression of TFEB in aged muscle, which promoted the age-induced increase in lysosomal markers. Thus, aged muscle possesses an elevated drive for CP/ATG which may contribute to the decline in organelle content observed with age, but which may serve to maintain MQC. CCA improves organelle integrity and reduces CP, illustrating that chronic exercise improves muscle quality in aged populations.

Mitochondrial Breakdown in Skeletal Muscle

Triolo and Hood (2019) summarized how CP and lysosomal biogenesis are regulated in exercising skeletal muscle, with potential theranostic implications. Skeletal muscle mitochondria are essential in providing the energy required for locomotion. In response to contractile activity, the mitochondrial production is upregulated to meet the energy demands on muscle cells. Exercise also promotes the breakdown of dysfunctional mitochondria via CP induction characterized by the selection of poorly functioning organelles, engulfment in CPS and transport to lysosomes for degradation. Exercise also enhances lysosomal biogenesis. This increase in CP targeting and lysosomal biogenesis enhances the capacity for CPS degradation to sustain MQC. Lysosomal dysfunction, as observed in LSDs, negatively impacts mitochondrial function through CP suppression. Since exercise activates CP and lysosomal biogenesis, physical activity could be an effective therapy for LSDs as well.

Muscle Wasting During Cachexia

Skeletal muscle atrophy is a pathological condition characterized by the loss of muscular mass and the contractile capacity of the skeletal muscle as a consequence of muscular weakness and decreased force generation. Oxidative stress is the most common mechanism of cachexia. It results in increased ROS levels, increased oxidation-dependent protein modification, and decreased antioxidant functions. Ábrigo et al. (2018) described the importance of oxidative stress in skeletal muscles, its sources, and how it can regulate protein synthesis/degradation imbalance, ATG deregulation, increase myo-nuclear apoptosis, and mitochondrial dysfunction in cachexia (a pathological condition secondary to illness characterized by the progressive loss of muscle mass with or without loss of fat and with diminution of muscle strength). The molecular mechanisms involved in cachexia include oxidative stress, protein synthesis/degradation imbalance, CP/ATG dysregulation, increased myo-nuclear apoptosis, and mitochondrial dysfunction implicated in CBMP.

Alcohol-Induced Muscle Protein Imbalance

Both the acute and chronic ingestion of alcohol impact the metabolic phenotype of skeletal and cardiac muscle, independent of overt PCM, resulting in the loss of skeletal muscle strength and cardiac contractility. Alcohol-induced changes are mediated by a decrease in protein synthesis due to impaired mTOR activity. Kimball and Lang (2018) summarized the recent advances in understanding mTOR signaling, similarities and differences between the effects of alcohol on this metabolic controller in skeletal muscle and in the heart, and the effects of acute versus chronic alcohol intake. Alcohol-induced alterations in proteolysis via activation of the ubiquitin-proteasome pathway suggested that alcohol impairs ATG in muscle. Hence, further studies are needed to define the role of these changes in protein synthesis and ATG (particularly CP) in the etiology of alcoholic myopathy in the skeletal muscle and the heart.

RINT1 Variations in Liver Failure and Skeletal Abnormalities

Pediatric acute liver failure (ALF) is life-threatening with genetic, immunologic, and environmental etiologies. Recurrent ALF (RALF) in infants represents repeated episodes of severe liver injury with intermittent recovery of the hepatic function. Cousin et al. (2019) posited bi-allelic RINT1 alterations as the cause of RALF and skeletal abnormalities. Three unrelated individuals with RALF onset ≤3 years of age had splice alterations at the same position (c.1333 + 1G>A or G>T) in trans with a missense (p.Ala368Thr or p.Leu370Pro) or in-frame deletion (p.Val618_Lys619del) in RINT1. ALF episodes were concomitant with fever/infection and not all individuals had full normalization of liver function between episodes. Liver biopsies revealed nonspecific damage including fibrosis, steatosis, or mild increases in Kupffer cells. Skeletal imaging revealed abnormalities affecting the vertebrae and pelvis. Dermal fibroblasts showed splice-variant-mediated skipping of exon 9, leading to an out-of-frame product and nonsense-mediated transcript decay. Fibroblasts also revealed decreased RINT1 protein, abnormal Golgi morphology, and impaired ATG. RINT1 interacts with NBAS (implicated in RALF) and UVRAG, to facilitate Golgi-to-ER retrograde vesicle transport. During the nutrient depletion or infection, the Golgi-to-ER transport was suppressed and ATG was promoted through UVRAG regulation by mTOR. Aberrant ATG was associated with the development of similar skeletal abnormalities and liver disease, suggesting that disruption of RINT1 functions may explain the liver and skeletal findings. Hence, learning the mechanism underlying this gene-disease relationship may confer unique theranostic strategies to deal with this disease.

Neuromuscular Transmission in Myopathies

Elahi et al. (2019) reviewed all patients referred for myopathy who had undergone repetitive nerve stimulation. They included patients with decrement (>10%) and either a pathological or molecular diagnosis of myopathy. Among 157 patients, four had decrement (2-OH-CQ-associated vacuolar myopathy, 1 centro-nuclear myopathy, and 1 distal myopathy) myopathy. One 2-OH-CQ-associated vacuolar myopathy patient also had inflammatory myopathy. Pyridostigmine improved weakness in the centro-nuclear myopathy patient, but not in the distal myopathy patient. No patient with an acquired myopathy received Pyridostigmine. Despite the rare occurrence of decrement in myopathy, its presence may encourage pharmacological intervention.

p53 in Skeletal Muscle

Beyfuss et al. (2018) investigated the role of p53 in regulating mitochondria both basally, and under the influence of exercise, by subjecting C57Bl/6J whole-body (WB) and muscle-specific p53 knockout (mKO) mice to a six-week training program. p53 was important in regulating mitochondrial content and function, as well as proteins within the ATG and apoptotic pathways. Despite an increased proportion of phosphorylated p53 (Ser^{15}) in the mitochondria, p53 was not required for the training-induced adaptations in the exercise capacity or in mitochondrial content and function. Similar directional alterations were observed in basal and exercise-induced signaling in WB and mKO mice; however the magnitude of change was less pronounced in the mKO mice, suggesting that p53 is required for MQC in skeletal muscle, but is not required for the adaptive responses to exercise training.

IP$_3$ Receptor Blockade in Skeletal Muscle

Duchenne muscular dystrophy (DMD) is characterized by a progressive destruction of muscle fibers associated with altered Ca^{2+} homeostasis. Valladares et al. (2018) showed that the IP$_3$ receptor (IP$_3$R) plays a crucial role in increasing $[Ca^{2+}]_i$ and that the pharmacological blockade of IP$_3$R restores muscle function. The IP$_3$R pathway negatively regulates ATG by controlling $[Ca^{2+}]_m$ levels. The elevated basal ATG and induced ATG were normalized when IP$_3$R was downregulated in mdx fibers. The blockade of IP$_3$R in mdx fibers restored both increased $[Ca^{2+}]_m$ levels as well as $\Delta\Psi$. The mdx mitochondria changed from a fission to an elongated state after IP$_3$R knockdown, and the elevated CP in mdx fibers were normalized. This study associated IP$_3$R1 activity with changes in ATG, $[Ca^{2+}]_m$, $\Delta\Psi$, and CP dynamics, suggesting that increased IP$_3$R in mdx fibers plays an important role in the pathophysiology of DMD. Hence, specific IP$_3$R blockers can be developed as novel TSE-EBPT-CPTs for DMD.

ATG Suppression in Skeletal Muscle Cells

Parousis et al. (2018) showed that chronic contractile activity (CCA) in muscle cells induced MB and enhanced the expression of the transcription factor EB (TFEB) and PPARGC1A/PGC-1α, as regulators of lysosome and MB, respectively. CCA also enhanced the expression of PINK1 and the lysosomal protease CTSD (cathepsin D). The ATG blockade with Bafilomycin A_1 (BafA) reduced state 3 and 4 respiration, increased ROS production, and enhanced the accumulation of MAP1LC3B-II/LC3-II and SQSTM1/p62. CCA ameliorated mitochondrial dysfunction during defective ATG, increased PPARGC1A, normalized LC3-II levels, and reversed SQSTM1 toward control levels. NAC emulated the LC3-II reductions induced by contractile activity, suggesting that a decrease in oxidative stress could represent a mechanism of ATG normalization by CCA, which enhances MB and lysosomal activity, and normalizes ATG during ATG suppression, via ROS-dependent mechanism(s). Thus, contractile activity represents a potential theranostic intervention for diseases in which CP/ATG is inhibited (such as vacuolar myopathies in skeletal muscle), by establishing the equilibrium of anabolic and catabolic pathways.

VCP Lysosomal Homeostasis and TFEB in Skeletal Muscle

Differentiated tissue is vulnerable to alterations in protein and organelle homeostasis. The essential protein VCP, mutated in hereditary inclusion body myopathy, ALS and FTD, is critical for efficient clearance of misfolded proteins and damaged organelles in dividing cells. To understand the relevance of VCP in differentiated tissue, Arhzaouy et al. (2019) inactivated it in the skeletal muscle of adult mice. The knockout muscle demonstrated a necrotic myopathy with increased CP/ATG proteins and damaged lysosomes. This was not only due to a defect in ATG degradation; age-matched mice with muscle inactivation of the ATG essential protein, Atg5, did not demonstrate myopathy either. Myofiber necrosis was preceded by upregulation of LGALS3/Galectin-3, a marker of damaged lysosomes, and TFEB activation, suggesting defects in the lysosomal system. The myofiber necrosis was recapitulated by the chemical induction of LMP in skeletal muscle. TFEB was activated after LMP, but its activation and nuclear localization occurred upon VCP inactivation or disease mutant expression. These data identified VCP as the central mediator of both lysosomal clearance and biogenesis in skeletal muscle.

Parthenolide Regulates CP

Parthenolide (PTL), a sesquiterpene lactone found in the leaves of feverfew, possesses anti-inflammatory, anti-migraine, and anticancer properties. PTL alleviated cancer cachexia and improves skeletal muscle characteristics in a cancer cachexia model. Ren et al. (2019) reported that PTL attenuated H_2O_2-induced growth inhibition and morphological changes. PTL exhibited ROS scavenging activity, protected C2C12 cells from apoptosis in response to H_2O_2, and attenuated $\Delta\Psi$ collapse, thereby normalizing H_2O_2-induced CP and ATG; this is correlated with its inhibiting degradation of mitochondrial marker protein TIM23, the increase in LC3-II expression, and the reduction of mtDNA. PTL also prevented H_2O_2-induced lysosomal damage in C2C12 cells. The phosphorylation of p53, cathepsin B, and Bax/Bcl-2, and the translocation of Bax from the cytosol to mitochondria by H_2O_2 was reduced by PTL, suggesting that it modulates oxidative stress-induced CP and protects C2C12 myoblasts during apoptosis in oxidative stress-associated skeletal muscle diseases.

Skeletal Muscle mTORC1 Regulates NMJ Stability

Skeletal muscle is a plastic tissue that can adapt to different stimuli. mTORC1 signaling is a key modulator in mediating increases in skeletal muscle mass and function. Baraldo et al. (2019) generated inducible, muscle-specific Raptor and mTOR$_{ko}$ mice. Muscles at 1 and 7 months after deletion were analyzed to assess muscle histology and muscle force. No change in muscle size or contractile properties was observed 1 month after deletion. Prolonging deletion of Raptor to seven months, however, lead to a phenotype characterized by weakness, muscle regeneration, mitochondrial dysfunction implicated in CBMP, and CP/ATG impairment. Reduced mTOR signaling was accompanied by the appearance of markers of fiber denervation, like the increased expression of the neural cell adhesion molecule (NCAM). Muscle-specific deletion of mTOR, Raptor, and Rapamycin induced 3-8% NCAM-positive fibers, muscle fibrillation, and NMJ fragmentation in 24% of fibers. Reactivation of ATG with Tat-Beclin-1 prevented mitochondrial dysfunction and the appearance of NCAM-positive fibers in Raptor k.o. muscles by inhibiting CBMP, indicating that mTOR signaling is critical for maintaining $[Ca^{2+}]_m$ innervation, thus preserving the NMJ structure in both the muscle fibers and the moto-neurons. The beneficial effects of exercise in most pathologies affect the NMJ, through the activation of mTORC1.

Lipin 1-Mediated PAP Activity

Lipin 1 regulates glycerolipid homeostasis by acting as a phosphatidic acid phosphohydrolase (PAP) in the triglyceride-synthesis pathway and by regulating transcription factor activity. Schweitzer et al. (2018) reported that mutations in lipin 1 are a common cause of rhabdomyolysis in children. Mice with lipin 1 deficiency were used to examine mechanisms connecting lipin 1 deficiency to myocyte injury. However, the mouse model was confounded by lipodystrophy not pheno-copied in people. Two muscle-specific mouse models were studied: 1) Lpin1 exon 3 and 4 deletion, resulting in a hypomorphic protein without PAP activity, but a preserved transcriptional coregulatory function; and 2) Lpin1 exon 7 deletion, resulting in total protein loss. In both models, skeletal muscles exhibited myopathy with muscle fiber necrosis, regeneration, and the accumulation of phosphatidic acid and diacylglycerol. Lipin 1-deficient mice had abnormal mitochondrial abundance because of impaired ATG and exhibited an increase in plasma creatine kinase following exhaustive exercise when unfed. This suggested that mice lacking lipin-1-mediated PAP in their skeletal muscle may be used for determining the mechanisms by which lipin 1 deficiency leads to myocyte injury, and for testing potential theranostic agents.

Myosin VI-Dependent Actin Cages

MQC is essential to maintaining cellular homeostasis and is achieved by removing damaged, ubiquitinated mitochondria via Parkin-mediated MTG. Kruppa et al. (2018) demonstrate that MYO6 (myosin VI), which moves toward the minus end of actin filaments, forms a complex with Parkin and is selectively recruited to CBs via its ubiquitin-binding domain. This myosin motor initiates the assembly of F-actin cages to encapsulate CBs by forming a physical barrier that prevents re-fusion with neighboring populations. The loss of MYO6 results in an accumulation of CPS and an increase in mitochondrial mass. In addition, mitochondrial dysfunction manifesting as reduced respiratory capacity and decreased ability to rely on O/P for energy production was observed. These findings demonstrated a crucial step in MQC: the formation of MYO6-dependent actin cages that ensure isolation of CBs from the network.

Skeletal Muscle of Fasted, Castrated Mice

Androgen deficiency promotes muscle atrophy by increasing ATG-mediated muscle protein breakdown during the fasted state, but factors contributing to this remain undefined. Rossetti et al. (2018) subjected mice to sham or castration surgery. Seven-weeks later, mice were fasted overnight, refed for 30 min, and fasted another 4.5 hrs before sacrifice. The Bnip-3-mediated turnover of mitochondria was increased within the atrophied tibialis anterior (TA) of castrated mice and related to the magnitude of muscle atrophy and ATG activation (decreased p62), thus linking the turnover of CBs to ATG-mediated atrophy. ATG induction was facilitated by AMPK activation as a stress survival mechanism since phosphorylation of AMPK (Thr172), as well as the pro-survival kinases Akt (Thr308) and (ERK1/2 the Thr202/Tyr204), were increased by castration, indicating a relationship between mitochondrial turnover in the fasted state with ATG induction and muscle atrophy following androgen depletion.

mTORC1 and PKB/Akt

The loss of innervation of skeletal muscle is detrimental in several muscle diseases. Castets et al. (2019) demonstrated that PKB/Akt and mTORC1 play crucial roles in regulating muscle homeostasis and maintaining neuromuscular endplates after nerve injury. To allow dynamic changes in ATG, mTORC1 activation must be balanced following denervation. Acutely activating or inhibiting mTORC1 impaired ATG regulation and altered homeostasis in denervated muscle. PKB/Akt inhibition, conferred by sustained mTORC1 activation, abrogated denervation-induced synaptic remodeling and induced neuromuscular endplate degeneration. PKB/Akt activation promoted the nuclear import of HDAC4 and was required for epigenetic changes and synaptic gene upregulation upon denervation. This study revealed the functions of PKB/Akt-mTORC1 signaling in the muscle response to nerve injury, with implications for neuromuscular integrity in various pathological conditions.

Artesunate in Surgery-induced Knee Arthro-fibrosis

Wan et al. (2019) reported that intraarticular fibrosis following knee surgery remains a challenging problem. Artesunate (ART), a classical anti-malarial drug extracted from the Chinese medicinal herb Artemisia annua L, has been associated with fibrosis-related diseases. ART induced cellular ATG flux and inhibited cell proliferation in fibroblasts. The genetic depletion of Beclin-1 abolished ART-induced ATG and attenuated the inhibitory effect of ART on fibroblasts' proliferation. ART-induced ATG was associated with the inhibition of mTOR signaling through PI3K/Akt/mTOR and AMPK/mTOR pathways. ART triggered ATG and alleviated surgery-induced knee arthro-fibrosis, indicating that it has anti-proliferative efficacy in fibroblasts and alleviates the severity of knee arthro-fibrosis by inducing Beclin-1-mediated CP/ATG via the inhibition of mTOR signaling. It was also suggested that ART might be a potential theranostic agent for preventing the progression of surgery-induced intraarticular fibrosis of knee.

17β-Estradiol on MTG in the MC3T3-E1 Osteoblasts

Osteoporosis is associated with 17β-estradiol deficiency. The G-protein-coupled receptor 30 (GPR30) is an estrogen-responsive receptor. Sun et al. (2018) evaluated the effects of 17β-estradiol, GPR30, and its signaling pathway, on MTG in the murine MC3T3-E1 osteoblast cell line. These cells were treated, either with 17β-estradiol, or G15, a selective GPR30 antagonist, or U0126, a MAP kinase (ERK1/2) inhibitor, or with vehicle as control. The optimum concentration of 17β-estradiol that resulted in GPR30 expression in MC3T3-E1 cells was 10^{-7} M, which led to the accumulation of mitochondrial APSs and increased the protein phosphorylation of Hsp60, Tom20, and LC3. In cells pretreated with G15 or U0126, the 17β-estradiol treatment did not increase MTG in MC3T3-E1 cells. In murine osteoblasts cultured *in vitro*, treatment with 17β-estradiol enhanced MTG through the GPR30 and ERK1/2 signaling pathway.

Transnasal Sphenopalatine Ganglion Blockade

Long-term physical inactivity can cause the atrophy of skeletal muscle. Zanella et al. (2018) explored the underlying mechanisms of physical inactivity-induced atrophy of skeletal muscle. 14 SD male rats were divided into two groups, comprising the normal control (NC) and hind-limb suspension (HS) groups. After two weeks of HS stimulation, the ratio between skeletal muscle weight and body weight, and the cross-sectional area (CSA) of skeletal muscle fibers, were measured. The rats subjected to a two-week HS treatment presented atrophy of the skeletal muscle with a reduced ratio between skeletal muscle weight and body weight, and smaller cross-sectional area (CSA) of skeletal muscle fibers when compared with control rats. HS stimulation induced mitochondrial damage, the increased expression of MuRF1 and Atrogin-1/MAFbx, and enhanced apoptosis, as well as dysfunctional ATG. HS-induced skeletal muscle atrophy involved the activation of the AMPK/FoxO3 signal pathway, evidenced as AMPK phosphorylation, FoxO3 activation, and Atrogin-1 and MuRF1 upregulation, suggesting that FoxO3-mediated ATG plays an important role in HS-induced skeletal muscle atrophy.

27-Deoxyactein in MC3T3-E1 Osteoblastic Cells

2,3,7,8-Tetrachlorodibenzo-p-dioxin (TCDD) is an environmental contaminant that exerts its toxicity through a variety of signaling mechanisms. Suh et al. (2018) evaluated the effects of 27-Deoxyactein, one of the major constituents isolated from Cimicifuga racemosa, on TCDD-induced toxicity in osteoblastic MC3T3-E1 cells. TCDD reduced cell survival, increased apoptosis, and enhanced ATG. However, pre-treatment with 27-Deoxyactein attenuated all TCDD-induced effects and decreased $[Ca^{2+}]_i$ concentrations, the $\Delta\Psi$ collapse, ROS overproduction, and Cardiolipin peroxidation compared to the TCDD-treated controls. TCDD-induced increases in the aryl hydrocarbon receptor (AhR), CYP1A1, and ERK were inhibited by 27-Deoxyactein. The mRNA levels of SOD, ERK1, and NF-κB were also restored by pretreatment with 27-Deoxyactein. Furthermore, 27-Deoxyactein increased the expressions of genes associated with osteoblast differentiation, including ALP, osteocalcin, bone sialoprotein (BSP), and osterix, indicating the preventive effect of 27-Deoxyactein on TCDD-induced damage in osteoblasts.

ERS in EMS Horses

In horses, reduced physical activity combined with carbohydrate and sugar overload may result in the development of equine metabolic syndrome (EMS), characterized by insulin resistance, hyperinsulinemia, elevated blood triglyceride concentrations, and obesity. Marycz et al. (2018) analyzed insulin-sensitive tissues (that is, muscles, liver, and adipose tissue) to evaluate insulin resistance and apoptosis. They assessed mitochondrial dynamics and MTG in those tissues, because mitochondrial dysfunction is linked to the development of the metabolic syndrome and established the expression of genes related to insulin resistance, ERS, and mitochondria clearance by MTG. Adipose tissue and the liver of EMS horses were characterized by increased mitochondrial damage and MTG, followed by apoptosis as MTG could not restore cellular homeostasis. However, in muscles, apoptosis was reduced, suggesting the existence of a protective mechanism to maintain homeostasis.

TOMM22 Phosphorylation

In yeast, Tom22, the central component of the translocase of the outer mitochondrial membrane (TOMM) receptor complex, is responsible for the recognition and translocation of synthesized mitochondrial precursor proteins, and its protein kinase CK2-dependent phosphorylation, for TOMM-complex biogenesis and proper mitochondrial protein import. Kravic et al. (2018) used a skeletal muscle-specific Csnk2b/Ck2β-conditional knockout (cKO) mouse model. The skeletal muscle of Csnk2b cKO mice showed reduced muscle strength and abnormal metabolic activity of oxidative muscle fibers, due to mitochondrial dysfunction. Active muscle lysates from skeletal muscle Csnk2b cKO mice phosphorylate murine TOMM22, the mammalian ortholog of yeast Tom22, to a lower extent than lysates prepared from controls. The CSNK2-mediated phosphorylation of TOMM22 changes its binding affinity for mitochondrial precursor proteins. However, in contrast to yeast, mitochondrial protein import was not affected using mitochondria isolated from the skeletal muscle of the Csnk2b cKO mice. PINK1, a mitochondrial health sensor that undergoes constitutive import under physiological conditions, accumulates within skeletal muscle Csnk2b cKO fibers and labels abnormal mitochondria for removal by MTG. as demonstrated by mitochondria-containing APSs through EM. MTG can be normalized by either the introduction of a phosphomimetic TOMM22 mutant in cultured myotubes, or by the electroporation of phosphomimetic Tomm22 into muscles of mice. Transfection of the phosphomimetic Tomm22 mutant in muscle cells with ablated Csnk2b restored their O_2 consumption rate comparable to wild-type levels, suggesting that CSNK2-dependent phosphorylation of TOMM22 is a critical switch for MTG and reveal CSNK2-dependent physiological implications on metabolism, muscle integrity, and behavior.

Apobec2 Deficiency

Recently, Sato et al. (2018) reported that Apobec2 is a member of the activation-induced deaminase/apolipoprotein B mRNA editing. Apobec2 deficiency causes mitochondrial defects and MTG in the skeletal muscle enzyme catalytic polypeptide cytidine deaminase expressed in differentiated skeletal and cardiac muscle. Apobec2 deficiency in mice leads to a shift in muscle fiber type, myopathy, and diminished muscle mass. Although Apobec2 localized to the sarcomeric Z-lines in mouse tissue and cultured myotubes, the sarcomeric structure was not affected in Apobec2-deficient muscle. Enlarged mitochondria and mitochondria engulfed by ATG vacuoles suggested that Apobec2 deficiency causes mitochondrial defects leading to increased MTG in skeletal muscle. Apobec2 deficiency induced ROS generation and depolarized mitochondria, leading to MTG as a defensive response. The exercise capacity of Apobec2$^{-/-}$ mice was impaired, implying Apobec2 deficiency resulted in muscle dysfunction. The presence of rimmed vacuoles in myofibers from 10-month-old mice suggested that chronic muscle damage impairs normal ATG and that Apobec2 deficiency causes mitochondrial defects that induce muscle MTG, leading to myopathy and atrophy. It also suggested that Apobec2 is required for IMD, ICD, and MQC to maintain normal skeletal muscle function.

Parkin Clearance of Human Chondrocytes

Mitochondrial dysfunction, oxidative stress, and chondrocyte death are important contributors to the development and pathogenesis of OA. Ansari et al. (2018) determined the expression and role of Parkin in the clearance of damaged/dysfunctional mitochondria, regulation of ROS levels, and chondrocyte survival under pathological conditions. Human chondrocytes were taken from the unaffected area of knee OA cartilage and were stimulated with IL-1β to mimic pathological conditions. IL-1β-stimulated OA chondrocytes showed high levels of ROS generation, mitochondrial membrane damage, accumulation of damaged mitochondria, and a higher incidence of apoptosis. The IL-1β stimulation of chondrocytes with depleted Parkin expression resulted in high levels of ROS, accumulation of damaged/dysfunctional mitochondria implicated in CBMP, and enhanced apoptosis. Parkin translocation to depolarized/damaged mitochondria and the recruitment of p62/SQSTM1 was required for the elimination of CBs in IL-1β-stimulated OA chondrocytes. Parkin elimination of CBs required Parkin ubiquitin ligase activity and reduced ROS and apoptosis in OA chondrocytes under pathological conditions, indicating that Parkin functions to eliminate CBs is necessary for MQC, regulation of ROS levels, and chondrocyte survival under pathological conditions.

mTORC1 in OA Temporomandibular Joint

A switch from CP to ATG to apoptosis is implicated in chondrocytes during the OA progression. Yang et al. (2020) utilized a flow fluid shear stress (FFSS) model in cultured chondrocytes and a unilateral anterior cross-bite (UAC) animal model. Both FFSS and UAC induced ERS in the temporomandibular joints (TMJ) chondrocytes, as demonstrated by increases in expression of HSPA5, p-EIF2AK3, p-ERN1, and ATF6. Both FFSS and UAC activated pro-death p-EIF2AK3-mediated ERS-apoptosis programs and pro-survival p-ERN1-mediated ATG in chondrocytes. mTORC1, a downstream of p-ERN1, suppressed ATG but promoted p-EIF2AK3 mediated ERS-apoptosis. At the early stage, both the p-ERN1 and p-EIF2AK3 were activated, and mTORC1 was inhibited in TMJ chondrocytes. mTORC1-p-EIF2AK3-mediated ERS apoptosis was predominant, while p-ERN1 and ATG were inhibited. The inhibition of mTORC1 by a TMJ local injection of Rapamycin in rats or the induced ablation of mTORC1 expression in chondrocytes promoted ATG and suppressed apoptosis, and reduced TMJ cartilage loss induced by UAC in mice. mTORC1 activation by the TMJ local administration of mTORC1 activation of TMG chondrocytes, local administration of MHY1485, or genetic deletion of Tsc1 (an upstream mTORC1 suppressor) resulted in opposite effects. Aberrant mechanical loading caused cartilage degeneration by activating mTORC1 signaling, which modulated ATG and apoptosis in TMJ chondrocytes. Thus, the inhibition of mTORC1 provides a novel TSE-EBPT strategy for the prevention and treatment of OA.

CRISPR/Cas9 Correction of DNM2 Mutation

Genome editing with the CRISPR/Cas9 technology has emerged recently as a theranostic strategy for dealing with genetic diseases. For dominant mutations linked to gain-of-function effects, allele-specific correction may be the most suitable approach. Rabai et al. (2019) tested the allele-specific inactivation or correction of a heterozygous mutation in the Dynamin 2 (DNM2) gene that causes the autosomal dominant form of centro-nuclear myopathies (CNMs), a rare muscle disorder belonging to the large group of congenital myopathies. Truncated single-guide RNAs specifically targeting the mutated allele were tested on cells derived from a mouse model and patients. The mutated allele was targeted in patient fibroblasts and $Dnm2^{R465W/+}$ mouse myoblasts, and clones were obtained with precise genome correction or inactivation. $Dnm2^{R465W/+}$ myoblasts showed an alteration in transferrin uptake and ATG. Specific inactivation or correction of the mutated allele rescued these phenotypes, indicating the potential of CRISPR/Cas9 to target and correct in an allele-specific heterozygous-point mutations leading to a gain-of-function effect, and to rescue autosomal dominant CNM-related phenotypes. This strategy may be suitable for a large number of diseases caused by germline or somatic mutations resulting in a gain-of-function mechanism.

Zidovudine-Mediated CP/ATG Inhibition

NRTI, such as the thymidine analogue Zidovudine (AZT), are used in HIV-1 therapy and are used for the prevention of mother-to-child transmission. Prolonged thymidine analogue exposure causes mitochondrial toxicities to the heart, liver, and skeletal muscle. Lin et al. (2018) hypothesized that AZT might interfere with CP/ATG in myocytes, implicated in the regulation of mitochondrial recycling, cell survival, and the pathogenesis of NDDs. The impact of AZT and Lamivudine (3TC) on the C2C12 myocyte ATG was studied using LC3-green fluorescent protein overexpression or LC3 staining in combination with immunoblotting, flow cytometry, confocal, and TEM. Lysosomal and mitochondrial functions were studied using specific staining for lysosomal mass, acidity, cathepsins, as well as mitochondrial mass and $\Delta\Psi$ in combination with flow cytometry and confocal microscopy. AZT, but not 3TC, exerted an inhibitory effect on the late stages of APS maturation, which was reversible upon mTOR inhibition. The inhibition of late ATG at therapeutic drug concentrations led to dysfunctional mitochondrial accumulation with membrane hyperpolarization and increased ROS and compromised cell viability triggering CBMP. These AZT effects could be replicated by pharmacological and the genetic inhibition of myocyte CP/ATG and rescued by the stimulation of autophagolysosomal biogenesis, indicating that AZT inhibits CP/ATG in myocytes, which leads to the accumulation of CBs with increased ROS generation involving CBMP and compromised cell viability. This novel mechanism could contribute to our understanding of the long-term side effects of antiviral agents.

Fis1 Deficiencies in Skeletal Muscle

Mitochondrial dynamics and CP are important aspects of MQC, and are linked to NDDs and muscular diseases. Fis1, a protein on the OMM, mediates mitochondrial fission. However, Fis1 null worms and mammalian cells only display mild fission defects but show aberrant CP. To assess Fis1 function *in vivo*, Zhang et al. (2019) generated conditional knock-out Fis1 mice to allow for specific Fis1 deletion in adult skeletal muscle. In the absence of Fis1 in Type I muscle, mitochondrial hyper-fusion, respiratory chain deficiency, and increased CP were found. Abnormal ATG was aggravated by endurance exhaustive exercise stress (EEE), suggesting that Fis1 is involved in maintaining normal CP in mitochondria-rich Type I muscle during exercise. The loss of Fis1 induced a delayed onset change in Type I muscle and inflammation in response to acute exhaustive exercise (EE). Thus, a new role of Fis1 in maintaining normal mitochondrial structure and function at rest and under exercise stress was established.

TAK1 Regulates Skeletal Muscle Mitochondrial Function

Skeletal muscle mass is regulated by a complex array of signaling pathways. TGF-β-activated kinase 1 (TAK1) is a signaling protein, which regulates context-dependent activation of multiple intracellular pathways. Hindi et al. (2018) reported that inducible inactivation of TAK1 causes muscle wasting, leading to kyphosis, in both young and adult mice. The inactivation of TAK1 inhibits protein synthesis and induces proteolysis, through upregulating the ubiquitin-proteasome system and ATG. Phosphorylation and enzymatic activity of AMPK are increased, whereas phosphorylated mTOR and p38 MAPK are diminished upon inactivation of TAK1 in skeletal muscle. In addition, targeted inactivation of TAK1 leads to the accumulation of CBs and oxidative stress in the skeletal muscle of adult mice. Inhibition of TAK1 does not attenuate denervation-induced muscle wasting in adult mice. Finally, TAK1 activity is upregulated during overload-induced skeletal muscle growth, and inactivation of TAK1 prevents myofiber hypertrophy in response to functional overload. This study demonstrated that TAK1 is a key regulator of skeletal muscle mass and oxidative metabolism.

Rapamycin Rescues Mitochondrial Myopathy

The mTOR inhibitor Rapamycin ameliorates the clinical and biochemical phenotype of mouse, worm, and cellular models of mitochondrial disease. Civiletto et al. (2018) demonstrated that prolonged Rapamycin treatment improves motor endurance, corrects morphological abnormalities of muscle, and increases the cytochrome c oxidase (COX) activity of a muscle-specific Cox15 knockout mouse (Cox15$^{sm/sm}$). Rapamycin restored CP/ATG, which was impaired in naïve Cox15$^{sm/sm}$ muscle, and reduced CBs accumulated in untreated Cox15$^{sm/sm}$ mice. Rilmenidine, an mTORC1-independent CP/ATG inducer, was ineffective on the myopathic features of Cox15$^{sm/sm}$ animals, confirming that inhibition of mTORC1 by Rapamycin plays a key role in the improvement of the mitochondrial function in Cox15$^{sm/sm}$ muscle. In contrast to Rilmenidine, Rapamycin also activated lysosomal biogenesis in muscle, associated with increased nuclear localization of TFEB, a major regulator of lysosomal biogenesis, and was inhibited by mTORCl-dependent phosphorylation, suggesting that the regulated induction of CP/ATG and lysosomal biogenesis contribute to the CB clearance through CP by Rapamycin.

The Theranostic Significance of Antioxidants as CP Agonists in Musculoskeletal Disorders

Placental Hydrolysate

Sarcopenia, which refers to the muscle loss that accompanies aging, is a complex neuromuscular disorder with a high prevalence and mortality. Despite many efforts to protect against muscle weakness and muscle atrophy, the incidence of sarcopenia and its related permanent disabilities continue to increase. Bak et al. (2018) found that treatment of this disease with human placental hydrolysate (hPH) increased the viability (~15%) of H_2O_2-stimulated C2C12 cells. While H_2O_2-stimulated cells revealed irregular morphology, hPH restored their morphology to that of cells cultured under normal conditions. hPH inhibited H_2O_2-induced cell death. ROS generation and Mstn expression induced by oxidative stress were associated with muscular dysfunction followed by atrophy. Exposure of C2C12 cells to H_2O_2 induced ROS, mitochondrial superoxide, and mitochondrial dysfunction as well as myostatin expression via NF-κB signaling; these effects were attenuated by hPH, which decreased mitochondria-fission-related gene expression (Drp-1 and Bnip-3) and increased mitochondria biogenesis via the Sirtl/AMPK/PGC-1α pathway and CP/ATG regulation. hPH-mediated prevention of atrophy was achieved through regulation of myostatin and PGC-1α expression and CP/ATG, indicating that it is protective in muscle atrophy and oxidative cell death.

Resveratrol and 5-Azacytydine in Equine Metabolic Syndrome (EMS)

EMS is characterized by insulin resistance, hyper-leptinemia, hyperinsulinemia, inflammation, and pathological obesity. When there is an increased inflammatory response in the adipose tissue, physiological properties of adipose derived stem cells (ASC) get impaired, which limits their theranostic potential. Excessive accumulation of ROS, mitochondrial deterioration implicated in CBMP, and accelerated aging of those cells affect their pluripotency and restrict the effectiveness of the differentiation process. Marycz et al. (2018) treated ASC isolated from EMS individuals with a combination of 5-Azacytydine (AZA) and RES to reverse their aged phenotype and enhance osteogenic differentiation. AZA/RES enhanced early osteogenesis of ASC derived from EMS animals. Increased matrix mineralization, RUNX-2, collagen type I, and osteopontin were noted. AZA/RES exerted its beneficial effects by modulating CP/ATG and mitochondrial dynamics through Parkin and RUNX-2 activity.

Lipin-1 Regulates Bnip-3-Mediated CP/ATG

CP is essential for maintaining muscle mass and healthy skeletal muscle. Patients with heritable phosphatidic acid phosphatase lipin-1-null mutations present with rhabdomyolysis and muscle atrophy in glycolytic muscle fibers, accompanied with mitochondrial aggregates participating in CB formation, defective CP, reduced Cyt-C oxidase activity, and CBMP. Alshudukhi et al. (2018) found that lipin-1 deficiency in mice is associated with CB accumulation and CP/ATG vacuoles involved in CBMP in glycolytic muscle fibers. Studies using lipin-1-deficient myoblasts suggested that lipin-1 participates in BCl-2 adenovirus E1B 19 kDa Bnip-3-regulated CP by interacting with a microtubule-associated protein 1A/1B-light chain (LC)3, which is an important step in the recruitment of mitochondria to CPS. The requirement of lipin-1 for Bnip-3-mediated CP was verified *in vivo* in lipin-1$^{-/-}$-GFP-LC3 mice. A lipin-1 deficiency in mice resulted in defective CB adaptation to starvation-induced metabolic stress and impaired contractile muscle force in glycolytic muscle fibers, suggesting that dysregulated CP originating from lipin-1 deficiency is associated with impaired muscle function and rhabdomyolysis.

ATG-Related Factors in Contusion Repair

To explore the molecular mechanism of skeletal muscle contusion repair through changes in the expression of ATG-related genes and proteins in SD rats with acute skeletal muscle contusion, Luo et al. (2018) selected six rats as the control group from 30 male SD rats. The acute skeletal muscle contusion model was established in the remaining 24 rats with a self-made hitter. The model rats were divided into four groups (3 days, 5 days, 7 days, 14 days groups, $n = 6$). On the 3rd, 5th, 7th and 14th days after injury, the injured gastrocnemius of each group was harvested. The inflammation reached its peak on the 5th days after injury, while new muscle fibers were observed in the 7 days group. Oncotic mitochondria were seen in the 3 days, 5 days, 7 days groups. Also, the Z line changed from disappearing to drift thickening, and SR dilatation gradually improved, without any difference between the 14 days group and the control group, suggesting that the damage has healed. The expressions of LC3-II and p62 were increased at first and then decreased. The LC3-II expression was up-regulated in the 3 days, 5 days, 7 days groups compared with the control group and the 14 days group. The expression of p62 reached its peak on the 3rd days after injury, and returned to the normal level on the 14th days. The expression of ATG10 mRNA in the natural recovery group of 3 days, 5 days, 7 days, 14 days was initially decreased and then increased, the ATG10 mRNA was downregulated in the 3 days, 5 days, 7 days groups and the 14 days group. The expression of ATG7, ATG12, ATG16L1 mRNA was increased initially and then decreased. It was upregulated in the 3 days, 5 days, 7 days groups, and the 14 days group, indicating that ATG was involved in the repair of skeletal muscle injury through its own mediators following contusion. Hence, the rate of damage repair may be related to the level of ATG.

Heat Stress in Sus scrofa

Prolonged environment-induced hyperthermia causes morbidities, mortality, and organ-specific injury and dysfunction in humans and animals. It represents a threat to human health and agricultural products. Ganesan et al. (2018a) determined the extent to which prolonged environment-induced hyperthermia altered ATG in oxidative skeletal muscle in an animal model, serving the dual purpose of accurately modeling human physiology as well as agricultural production. Pigs were treated as follows: thermoneutral (20°C), heat stress (35°C), or were held under thermoneutral conditions but pair-fed to the heat stress group for seven days. Upon euthanasia, the red portion of the semitendinosus was collected. Prolonged hyperthermia increased oxidative stress without a corresponding change in antioxidant enzyme activities. Hyperthermia prevented initiation of ATG despite increased markers of nucleation, elongation and autophagosome (APS) formation. However, p62-relative protein abundance, which was inversely correlated with ATG degradation, was increased suggesting the reduced degradation of APS. Markers of CP and mitochondrial abundance were similar between groups, indicating that defective CP plays a key role in hyperthermic muscle dysfunction. Furthermore, Ganesan et al. (2018b) determined ATG dysfunction and apoptotic signaling in oxidative skeletal muscle following prolonged hyperthermia. Pigs were assigned to four groups ($n = 8$/group) and exposed to environmental heat stress (37°C) for 0, 2, 4, or 6 hrs. Markers of apoptotic signaling were increased following 2 hrs of heating but returned to baseline thereafter, while caspase 3 activity remained elevated 2–3X throughout the hyperthermic period. Heat stress increased markers of ATG, nucleation, as well as APS formation and degradation throughout the heating intervention. In addition, 6 hrs of hyperthermia increased markers of MTG, suggesting that apoptotic signaling precedes increased ATG during acute heat stress in oxidative skeletal muscle.

Ketogenic Diet

Li et al. (2018b) reported that a diet with ketogenic amino acids rich replacement (KAAR) ameliorated HFD-induced hepato-steatosis via activation of the ATG system. KAAR ameliorated the mitochondrial morphological alterations and associated mitochondrial dysfunction involving CBMP induced by an HFD through induction of the Akt/4EBP1 and ATG signaling in both fast and slow muscles. The mice were fed with a standard HFD (30% fat in food) or an HFD with KAAR (HFD^{KAAR}). In both the gastrocnemius and the soleus, HFD^{KAAR} ameliorated HFD-impaired mitochondrial morphology and function, characterized by decreased mitofusin 2, optic atrophy 1, PPARγ coactivator-1α, and PPARα, and increased DRP-1 implicated in CBMP. The decreased levels of phosphorylated Akt and 4EBP1 in the gastrocnemius and soleus of the HFD-fed mice were remediated by HFD^{KAAR}. The HFD^{KAAR} ameliorated the HFD-induced CP/ATG defects, suggesting that KAAR may be a novel strategy to combat obesity-induced CBMP, through the induction of the Akt/4EBP1 and CP/ATG pathways in skeletal muscle.

Nor-1 in Exercise-Induced Adaptations

Exercise induces physical and metabolic changes in skeletal muscle that reprograms to physiological and environmental demands. Underlying these changes are modifications to gene expression. Pearen and Muscat (2018) postulated that the nuclear hormone receptor, Nor-1, is induced after exercise, and this transcription factor modifies gene expression to drive the molecular and cellular adaptations associated with contractile reorganization. The mitochondrial network in muscle is controlled by the opposing processes of MB and MTG. The PGC-1α regulates biogenesis, while the transcription of MTG-related genes is controlled by TFEB. PGC-1α activation is induced by exercise; however, the effect of exercise on TFEB is not fully known. Erlich et al. (2018) investigated the interaction between PGC-1α and TFEB on mitochondria in response to acute contractile activity in C_2C_{12} myotubes and following exercise in wild-type and PGC-1α knockout mice. TFEB nuclear localization increased 1.6-fold following 2 hrs of acute myotube contractile activity in culture, while TFEB transcription also increased twofold to threefold. Viral overexpression of TFEB in myotubes increased PGC-1α and cytochrome-c oxidase-IV gene expression. In wild-type mice, TFEB translocation to the nucleus increased 2.4X in response to acute exercise, while TFEB transcription, assessed through the electroporation of a TFEB promoter construct, was elevated fourfold. These exercise effects were dependent on the presence of PGC-1α, indicating that acute exercise provokes TFEB expression and activation in a PGC-1α-dependent manner and suggested that TFEB, along with PGC-1α, is an important regulator of MB in muscle as a result of exercise.

Magnesium as a Ca^{2+} Antagonist

Mg^{2+}, as a Ca^{2+} antagonist, plays a vital role in bone metabolism and the balance between Mg^{2+} and Ca^{2+} is crucial in bone physiology. Li et al. (2018c) demonstrated that matrix mineralization in human bone marrow-derived mesenchymal stem cells (hBMSCs) can be suppressed by high Mg^{2+}. As mitochondrial calcium phosphate granules depletion manifests concurrently with the appearance of matrix vesicles (MVs), and ATG is associated with matrix mineralization, these researchers studied the effect of high extracellular Mg^{2+} on these pathways. High Mg^{2+}

had inhibitory effect on the extracellular mineral aggregates and the expression of collagen 1 along with the growth of the mineral crystals. A relatively less amount of MVs were observed inside hBMSCs treated with high Mg^{2+}; high Mg^{2+} inhibited the release of MVs. High Mg^{2+} suppressed mitochondrial Ca^{2+} accumulation. ATG was induced in response to osteogenesis of hBMSCs. High Mg^{2+} inhibited ATG upon osteogenesis and 3-MA suppressed mineralization. ATP reversed the inhibitory effect of high Mg^{2+} by augmenting ATG, indicating that high Mg^{2+} may modulate MVs-mediated mineralization via suppressing $[Ca^{2+}]_m$; it also regulates ATG of hBMSCs upon osteogenesis, resulting in decreased extracellular mineral deposition, and thus indicating the significant role of Mg^{2+} homeostasis in osteoporosis and the design of Mg^{2+} alloys.

AMP-Induced Protein Kinase

AMPK is a highly crucial enzyme in cellular energy deficit such as exercise, hypoxia, or nutritional stress as it regulates protein degradation through a FOXO-related axis. Sanchez et al. (2018) investigated AMPK activation in FOXO3 expression and stability in skeletal muscle primary myotubes. A Cycloheximide treatment demonstrated that AICAR infusion extends FOXO3 half-life, suggesting that AICAR or nutrient depletion increases FOXO3 expression and the mitochondrial E3 ligase Mul1 is involved in mitochondrial turnover in primary myotubes. In AMPK KO cells, nutrient depletion failed to alter the level of FOXO3-dependent atrophic genes, including LC3B, Bnip-3, and the mitochondrial E3 ligase Mul1, but not the expression of other genes (that is, FOXO1, Gabarapl1, MAFbx, MuRF1), highlighting that AMPK stabilizes FOXO3 as an initial step of CBMP in myocytes.

CONCLUSION

Transmission defects were observed in myopathies and p53 determined mitochondrial adaptations to endurance training in SMCs. The IP_3-receptor blockade restored CP/ATG and MQC in dystrophic mice. The CP/TG response to oxidative stress was dysregulated in OA chondrocytes. Contractile activity attenuated ATG inhibition and reversed mitochondrial defects in SMC. CP/ATG were investigated in young and aged SMC following chronic contractile activity. The loss of lipin 1-mediated phosphatidic acid phosphohydrolase caused skeletal myopathy in mice. Myosin VI-dependent actin encapsulated Parkin-positive CBs were implicated in CBMP. A transnasal sphenopalatine ganglion blockade was used to alleviate acute facial pain. 27-Deoxyactein prevented 2,3,7,8-tetrachlorodibenzo-p-dioxin-induced damage in MC3T3-E1 osteoblastic cells. Oxidative stress regulated muscle wasting during cachexia. Excessive ERS correlated with impaired mitochondrial dynamics, MTG, and apoptosis in liver and adipose tissue but not in muscles in EMS horses. The phosphorylation of TOMM22 in skeletal muscle by protein kinase CSNK2/CK2 regulated MTG. An Apobec2 deficiency caused CP/ATG defect in skeletal muscle. The Parkin clearance of CBs regulated ROS and increased the survival of chondrocytes in the OA cartilage. MTORC1 regulated ATG and apoptosis in articular chondrocytes in the OA temporomandibular joint. An allele-specific CRISPR/Cas9 correction of a heterozygous DNM2 mutation rescued centro-nuclear myopathy, whereas Zidovudine-induced CP/ATG inhibition enhanced CBMP in CMCs. Human placental hydrolysate demonstrated an antioxidant effect during oxidative stress in muscular atrophy. A combination of Res and 5-Azacytidine improved the osteogenesis of metabolic syndrome mesenchymal stem cells. Lipin-1 regulated Bnip-3-mediated CP in glycolytic muscle. Changes in expression of CP/ATG-related factors were observed during the acute contusion repair of skeletal muscle. Short-term heat stress increased CP/ATG and apoptosis in skeletal muscle, whereas prolonged hyperthermia altered CP/ATG in the skeletal muscles of wild pigs. A ketogenic diet improved mitochondrial homeostasis by modifying Akt/4EBP1 and CP/ATG signaling in the gastrocnemius and soleus muscle. The nuclear receptor Nor-1 was the pleiotropic regulator of exercise-induced adaptation. Exercise induced TFEB expression in SMC in a PGC-1α-dependent manner. High Mg^{2+} prevented matrix vesicle-mediated mineralization in bone marrow-derived mesenchymal stem cells through CP/ATG, whereas AMP-induced protein kinase stabilized FOXO3 in primary myotubes to confer protection.

REFERENCES

Ábrigo, J., A.A. Elorza, C.A. Riedel and C. Vilos. 2018. Role of oxidative stress as key regulator of muscle wasting during cachexia. Oxid Med Cell Longev 2018: 2063179.

Alshudukhi, A.A., J. Zhu, D. Huang, A. Jama, et al. 2018. Lipin-1 regulates Bnip3-mediated MTG in glycolytic muscle. FASEB J 32(12): 6796–6807.

Ansari, M.Y., N.M. Khan, I. Ahmad and T.M. Haqqi. 2018. Parkin clearance of dysfunctional mitochondria regulates ROS levels and increases survival of human chondrocytes. Osteoarthr. Cartil. 26: 1087–1097.

Arhzaouy, K., C. Papadopoulos, N. Schulze, S.K. Pittman, et al. 2019. VCP maintains lysosomal homeostasis and TFEB activity in differentiated skeletal muscle. Autophagy 15: 1082–1099.

Bak, D.H., J. Na, S.I. Im, C.T. Oh, et al. 2018. Antioxidant effect of human placenta hydrolysate against oxidative stress on muscle atrophy. J Cell Physiol 234(2): 1643–1658

Baraldo, M., A. Geremia, M. Pirazzini, L. Nogara, et al. 2019. Skeletal muscle mTORC1 regulates neuromuscular junction stability. J Cachexia Sarcopenia Muscle 11: 208–225.

Beyfuss, K., A.T. Erlich, M. Triolo, D.A. Hood. 2018. The role of p53 in determining mitochondrial adaptations to endurance training in skeletal muscle. Sci Rep 8: 14710.

Carter, H.N., Y. Kim, A.T. Erlich, D. Zarrin-Khat, et al. 2018. ATG and MTGflux in young and aged skeletal muscle following chronic contractile activity. J Physiol 596: 3567–3584.

Castets, P., N. Rion, M. Théodore, D. Falcetta, et al. 2019. mTORC1 and PKB/Akt control the muscle response to denervation by regulating ATG and HDAC4. Nat Commun 10: 3187.

Civiletto, G., S.A. Dogan, R. Cerutti, G. Fagiolari, et al. 2018. Rapamycin rescues mitochondrial myopathy via coordinated activation of ATG and lysosomal biogenesis. EMBO Mol Med 10: e8799.

Cousin, M.A., E. Conboy, J.S. Wang, D. Lenz, et al. 2019. RINT1 Bi-allelic variations cause infantile-onset recurrent acute liver failure and skeletal abnormalities. Am J Hum Genet 105: 108–121.

Elahi, B., R.S. Laughlin, W.J. Litchy, M. Milone, et al. 2019. Neuromuscular transmission defects in myopathies: Rare but worth searching for. Muscle Nerve 59: 475–478.

Erlich, A.T., D.M. Brownlee, K. Beyfuss, D.A. Hood. 2018. Exercise induces TFEB expression and activity in skeletal muscle in a PGC-1α-dependent manner. Am J Physiol Cell Physiol 314: C62–C72.

Ganesan, S., A.J. Brownstein, S.C. Pearce, M.B. Hudson, et al. 2018a. Prolonged environment-induced hyperthermia alters ATG in oxidative skeletal muscle in Sus scrofa. J Therm Biol 74: 160–169.

Ganesan, S., S.C. Pearce, N.K. Gabler and L.H. Baumgard. 2018b. Short-term heat stress results in increased apoptotic signaling and ATG in oxidative skeletal muscle in Sus scrofa. J Therm Biol 72: 73–80.

Goutas, A., C. Syrrou, I. Papathanasiou, A. Tsezou, et al. 2018. The autophagic response to oxidative stress in osteoarthritic chondrocytes is deregulated. Free Radic Biol Med 126: 122–132.

Hindi, S.M., S. Sato, G. Xiong, K.R. Bohnert, et al. 2018. TAK1 regulates skeletal muscle mass and mitochondrial function. JCI Insight 3(3): e98441. https://doi.org/10.1172/jci.insight.98441.

Kim, Y., D.S. Yang, P. Katti and B. Glancy. 2019. Protein composition of the muscle mitochondrial reticulum during postnatal development. J. Physiol. 597: 2707–2727.

Kimball, S.R. and C.H. Lang. 2018. Mechanisms underlying muscle protein imbalance induced by alcohol. Annu Rev Nutr 28: 197–217.

Kravic, B., A.B. Harbauer, V. Romanello, L. Simeone, et al. 2018. In mammalian skeletal muscle, phosphorylation of TOMM22 by protein kinase CSNK2/CK2 controls mitophagy. Autophagy 14(2): 311–335.

Kruppa, A.J., C. Kishi-Itakura, T.A. Masters, J.E. Rorbach, et al. 2018. Myosin VI-dependent actin cages encapsulate Parkin-positive damaged mitochondria. Dev Cell 44: 484–499.

Li, F.H., T. Li, Y.M. Su and J.Y. Ai. 2018a. Cardiac basal autophagic activity and increased exercise capacity. J Physiol Sci 68: 729–742.

Li, J., M. Kanasaki, L. Xu, M. Kitada, et al. 2018b. A ketogenic amino acid rich diet benefits mitochondrial homeostasis by altering the Akt/4EBP1 and ATG signaling pathways in the gastrocnemius and soleus. Biochim Biophys Acta 1862: 1547–1555.

Li, Y., J. Wang, J. Yue, Y. Wang, et al. 2018c. High magnesium prevents matrix vesicle-mediated mineralization in human bone marrow-derived mesenchymal stem cells via mitochondrial pathway and ATG. Cell Biol Int 42: 205–215.

Lin, H., M.V. Stankov, J. Hegermann, R. Budida, et al. 2018. Zidovudine-mediated autophagy inhibition enhances mitochondrial toxicity in muscle cells. Antimicrob. Agents Chemother 63(1): e01443-18.

Luo, A., C.L. Tang, S.Q. Huang, D.D. Zhao, et al. 2018. Changes in expression of autophagy-related factors during acute contusion repair of skeletal muscle. Zhongguo Ying Yong Sheng li xue za zhi = Zhongguo Yingyong Shenglixue Zazhi = Chinese Journal of Applied Physiology 34(2): 97–101. DOI: 10.12047/j.cjap.5647.2018.024.

Marycz, K., K. Kornicka, J. Szlapka-Kosarzewska and C. Weiss. 2018. Excessive endoplasmic reticulum stress correlates with impaired mitochondrial dynamics, MTG and apoptosis, in liver and adipose tissue, but not in muscles in EMS horses. Int J Mol Sci 19(1): E165.

Parousis, A., H.N. Carter, C. Tran, A.T. Erlich, et al. 2018. Contractile activity attenuates ATG suppression and reverses mitochondrial defects in skeletal muscle cells. Autophagy 14: 1886–1897.

Pearen, M.A and G.E.O. Muscat. 2018. The nuclear receptor Nor-1 is a pleiotropic regulator of exercise-induced adaptations. Exerc Sport Sci Rev 46(2): 97–104.

Rabai, A., L. Reisser, B. Reina-San-Martin and K. Mamchaoui. 2019. Allele-Specific CRISPR/Cas9 correction of a heterozygous DNM2 mutation rescues centronuclear myopathy cell phenotypes. Mol Ther Nucleic Acids 16: 246–256.

Ren, Y., Y. Li, J. Lv, X. Guo, et al. 2019. Parthenolide regulates oxidative stress-induced MTG and suppresses apoptosis through p53 signaling pathway in C2C12 myoblasts. J Cell Biochem 120: 15695–15708.

Rossetti, M.L., J.L. Steiner and B.S. Gordon. 2018. Increased mitochondrial turnover in the skeletal muscle of fasted, castrated mice is related to the magnitude of autophagy activation and muscle atrophy. Mol Cell Endocrinol 473: 178–185.

Sanchez, A.M.J., R. Candau and H. Bernardi. 2018. AMP-activated protein kinase stabilizes FOXO3 in primary myotubes. Biochem Biophys Res Commun 499: 493–498.

Sato, Y., H. Ohtsubo, N. Nihei, T. Kaneko, et al. 2018. Apobec2 deficiency causes mitochondrial defects and MTG in skeletal muscle. FASEB J 32: 1428–1439.

Schweitzer, G.G., S.L. Collier, Z. Chen, K.S. McCommis, et al. 2018. Loss of lipin 1-mediated phosphatidic acid phosphohydrolase activity in muscle leads to skeletal myopathy in mice. FASEB J 33(1): 652–667.

Suh, K.S., E.M. Choi, W.W. Jung, S.Y. Park, et al. 2018. 27-Deoxyactein prevents 2,3,7,8-tetrachlorodibenzo-p-dioxin-induced cellular damage in MC3T3-E1 osteoblastic cells. J Environ Sci Health A Tox Hazard Subst Environ Eng 53: 561–570.

Sun, X., X. Yang, Y. Zhao, Y. Li, et al. 2018. Effects of 17β-Estradiol on MTGin the Murine MC3T3-E1 osteoblast cell line is mediated via G protein-coupled estrogen receptor and the ERK1/2 signaling pathway. Med Sci Monit 24: 903–911.

Triolo, M. and D.A. Hood. 2019. Mitochondrial breakdown in skeletal muscle and the emerging role of the lysosomes. Arch Biochem Biophys 661: 66–73.

Valladares, D., Y. Utreras-Mendoza, C. Campos, C. Morales, et al. 2018. IP3 receptor blockade restores ATG and mitochondrial function in skeletal muscle fibers of dystrophic mice. Biochim Biophys Acta Mol Basis Dis 1864: 3685–3695.

Wan, Q., H. Chen, G. Xiong, R. Jiao, et al. 2019. Artesunate protects against surgery-induced knee arthrofibrosis by activating Beclin-1-mediated ATG via inhibition of mTOR signaling. Eur J Pharmacol 854: 149–158.

Yang, H, Y. Wen, M. Zhang, Q. Liu, H. Zhang, et al. 2020. MTORC1 coordinates the autophagy and apoptosis signaling in articular chondrocytes in osteoarthritic temporomandibular joint. Autophagy 16(2): 271–288.

Yin, J., X. Lu, Z. Qian, W. Xu, et al. 2019. New insights into the pathogenesis and treatment of sarcopenia in chronic heart failure. Theranostics 9(14): 4019–4029.

Zanella, S., F. Buccelletti, F. Franceschi, A. Vassiliadis, et al. 2018. Transnasal sphenopalatine ganglion blockade for acute facial pain: A prospective randomized case-control study. Eur Rev Med Pharmacol Sci 22: 210–216.

Zhang, S., Z. Song, L. An, X. Liu, et al. 2019. WD40 repeat and FYVE domain containing 3 is essential for cardiac development. Cardiovasc Res 115: 1320–1331.

18

Charnolophagy in Pulmonary Diseases

INTRODUCTION

CP/ATG prevents or promotes the progression of pulmonary diseases by exerting its diverse functions, including regulation of cell proliferation, cell death, cell survival, and innate and adaptive immune responses. Dysregulated CP is implicated in viral infections (including COVID-19-induced fever, fatigue, dry cough, rhinorrhea, nostrilitis, bronchitis, pharyngitis, fatal pneumonia, in addition to nausea, vomiting, and diarrhea). When CP/ATG is dysregulated by cigarette smoking, environmental insults, microbial infection, or aging, it can lead to the formation of CS-bodies and ROS overproduction due to CS destabilization, which contribute to the pathogenesis of COPD as the author described in his book, *Nicotinism and Emerging Role of Electronic Smoking* by Nova Science Publishers, New York. U.S.A. Vol. 1–4 (Sharma 2018). COPD is a lung disease characterized by irreversible airflow limitation. Multiple regulatory pathways are involved in COPD pathogenesis. CP/ATG—a highly conserved catabolic process mediated under various cellular stress conditions—plays a crucial role in the pathogenesis and prognosis of COPD. Mitochondria contain numerous copies of their genomic (mtDNA), creating a genetic redundancy for buffering mutations to sustain cellular function. Medeiros et al. (2018) found that DNA synthesis and the degradation by mtDNA polymerase γ (POLG)-controlled mtDNA copy number in starving yeast cells depends on metabolic homeostasis through CP/ATG. The mtDNA synthesis by POLG in starving wild-type cells was inhibited by nucleotide insufficiency and elevated ROS during CP/ATG dysfunction. After prolonged starvation, $3'$–$5'$ exonuclease-dependent mtDNA degradation by POLG adjusted the increasing mtDNA copy number in wild-type cells, but caused mtDNA instability and respiratory dysfunction in CP/ATG-deficient cells owing to nucleotide limitations, suggesting that mitochondria rely on the homeostatic functions of CP/ATG to balance synthetic and degradative modes of POLG, which control the copy number and stability of the mtDNA. Recently, Hara et al. (2018) outlined the role of MQC systems in the pathogenesis of age-associated lung diseases, COPD, and idiopathic pulmonary fibrosis (IPF). Mitochondrial dynamics and CP are two main QC mechanisms in cells. Mitochondria fuse to increase energy production in response to stress, and the damaged ones are segregated by fission and eliminated by CP. Once these systems are disrupted, CBs with decreased ATP production and increased ROS impact cell fate. The compromised MQC is pathogenic in several age-related diseases. Jiang et al. (2019)

determined the functional consequences of ATG and highlighted CP as highly crucial in cellular energy homeostasis. Tan et al. (2019) aimed to decipher the pathogenic process of ATG that is dysregulated by various risk factors of COPD, leading to either cell death or senescence. In a yeast model, Timón-Gómez et al. (2018) investigated how different protein complexes of the ETC are subject to degradation upon increased respiration load and organelle damage. The turnover of subunits of the ETC-I equivalent and complex III was stimulated upon high respiration rates. Particular mitochondrial proteases, but not MTG, were involved in this degradation. Further mitochondrial damage by Valinomycin triggered MTG removal of the same respiratory complexes which were dependent on the mitochondrial fusion and fission and the ATG adaptor protein ATG11, but not on the MTG receptor ATG32 in the yeast. The loss of autophagosomal protein function induced Valinomycin sensitivity and ROS overproduction upon mitochondrial damage. A specific event in this turnover of ETC complexes was due to the association of ATG11 with the mitochondrial network, which could be achieved by overexpression of the ATG11 protein in the absence of ATG32. The interaction of various ATG11 molecules via the C-terminal coil domain was stimulated upon mitochondrial damage and could be an early trigger of MTG in response to the organelle dysfunction, indicating that CP/ATG QC operates in a MTG-selective manner upon mitochondrial damage. Recently, Suliman and Nozik-Grayck (2019) highlighted that pulmonary hypertension (PH) is a progressive disease, characterized by vascular remodeling and lung vasculo-pathy. The disease causes dyspnea, pulmonary artery uncoupling, and right ventricular (RV) dysfunction. Metabolic impairment contributes to the pathophysiology of PH with mitochondrial dysfunction due to impaired CP and CBMP. Hence, antioxidants as CP regulators and apoptosis inhibitors can be developed for the TSE-EBPT of PH. The eradication of pathogenic microbes by CP/ATG, including M. tuberculosis (Mtb), is an effective host immune process that protects hosts from developing diseases associated with intracellular pathogens. Cheng et al. (2019) investigated the association between the SNPs of the ATG-related genes VAMP8 and VTI1B, and their susceptibility to pulmonary tuberculosis (PTB). Two SNPs, rs1010 from the VAMP8 gene and rs15493 from the *VTI1B* gene, were examined in 202 PTB patients and 216 healthy controls using melt-PCR. The rs1010 SNP genotypes AG and GG were associated with increased susceptibility to PTB. The VTI1B rs15493 SNP had no impact on the susceptibility to PTB, demonstrating that the rs1010 SNP of the VAMP8 gene was associated with the susceptibility to PTB. Hence, rs1010 genotyping could be used as theranostic biomarker to predict the risk of Mtb infection and/or PTB disease development after Mtb infection.

This chapter highlights the TSE-BPT significance of CP in various pulmonary diseases.

CP Theranostics in Lung Inflammation

Mechanical ventilation (MV) is used to maintain life in patients with sepsis and sepsis-related acute lung injury (ALI), which may cause diaphragm weakness due to muscle injury and atrophy resulting in the development of ventilator-induced diaphragm dysfunction (VIDD). Prolonged MV activates CP/ATG in the diaphragm due to ROS overproduction, causing fatality in COVID-19 victims. Pulmonary-macrophage-mediated CP/ATG is compromised and genes involved in the pluripotency of stem cells are downregulated to enhance IS activation and the induction of pro-inflammatory cytokines and fatal pneumonia. Smuder et al. (2018) tested the hypothesis that accelerated ATG is a key contributor to VIDD; and that oxidative stress is required to increase the expression of ATG genes in the diaphragm. The targeted inhibition of ATG in the rat diaphragm prevented MV-induced muscle atrophy and contractile dysfunction. The attenuation of VIDD occurred as a result of the increased concentration of catalase and reduced ROS production, corresponding to reductions in the calpain and caspase-3 activity. Increased

ROS production was required for the upregulation of ATG biomarkers. The mitochondrial-targeted peptide SS-31-administered rats revealed ROS overproduction during MV for the enhanced expression of key CP/ATG genes (LC3, ATG7, ATG12, Beclin-1 and p62) and increased activity of cathepsin L, indicating that CP/ATG is required for VIDD, and that its inhibition reduces MV-induced ROS production and prevents a positive feedback loop whereby CP/ATG is stimulated by oxidative stress. The NLR family pyrin domain containing 3 (NLRP3) inflammasome (IS) is a vital component of innate immunity and is related to ventilator-induced lung injury (VILI). Furthermore, Lyu et al. (2019) transfected mouse lung epithelial (MLE-12) cells with NLRP3 siRNA or sc siRNA and subjected them to 20% cyclic stretch (CS). The wild-type C57BL/6 mice were injected with a complex of NLRP3 siRNA/sc siRNA-Lipofectamine 2000 through the fundus venous plexus before MV. CS activated the NLRP3 IS by activating NIMA-related kinase 7 (NEK7). NLRP3 depletion inhibited NLRP3 IS activation, alleviated the degradation of cell junction proteins (including p120-catenin (p120) and occludin), ameliorated the colocalization of p120 and E-cadherin, and mitigated the decrease in $\Delta\Psi$ caused by mechanical stretch. Furthermore, after NLRP3 depletion, VILI was attenuated by decreasing IL-1β secretion and pulmonary edema. Inhibiting NLRP3 IS activation ameliorated VILI, suggesting a potential target for the TSE-EBPT of VILI. TLR4 and NF-κB signaling may elicit sepsis-related acute inflammatory responses and muscle protein degradation and mediate the pathogenic mechanisms of VIDD. Li et al. (2018) hypothesized that mechanical stretch with or without endotoxin treatment would augment diaphragmatic structural damage, the production of free radicals, muscle proteolysis, mitochondrial dysfunction, and ATG of the diaphragm via the TLR4/NF-κB pathway. Male C57BL/6 mice, either wild-type or TLR4-deficient, aged between 6 and 8 weeks were exposed to MV (6 mL/kg or 10 mL/kg) with or without endotoxemia for 8 hrs. MV with endotoxemia aggravated VIDD, as demonstrated by the increases in the expression levels of TLR4, caspase-3, atrogin-1, muscle ring finger-1, and LC3-II. Increased NF-κB phosphorylation and oxidative loads, disorganized myofibrils, disrupted mitochondria, ATG, and myo-nuclear apoptosis were also observed. MV with endotoxemia reduced p62 levels and diaphragm muscle fiber size. Endotoxin-exacerbated VIDD was attenuated at NF-κB inhibitor in TLR4-deficient mice, indicating that endotoxin-augmented MV-induced diaphragmatic injury occurs through the activation of the TLR4/NF-κB signaling. Mesenchymal stem cells (MSC) and MSC-derived exosomes (EXO) confer a theranostic benefit in animal models of inflammation and injury.

Maremanda et al. (2019) studied the role of MSC and EXO in CS-induced lung inflammation with focus on mitochondrial dysfunction. They characterized EXO by immunoblotting for exosomal markers and tunable resistive pulse sensing by qNano and TEM. Mt-Keima and mito-QC mice were exposed to air or CS for 10 days. mt-Keima mice were treated with MSC or EXO or MSC and EXO (MSC + EXO) i.p. for 10 days. CS exposure increased the inflammatory cellular infiltrations in the lungs of the mt-Keima mice. MSC + EXO treatment showed protection compared to individual treatments (MSC or EXO). There were no changes in the MTG proteins like PINK1 and Parkin, which was also found in the mitoQC mice. CS exposure increased the amount of the mitochondrial fission protein Drp-1 and other DAMPs pathway mediators like S100A4 and S100A8, HMGB1, RAGE and AGE. MSC + EXO increased the gene expression of (fusion genes) like Mfn-1, Mfn-2, and opa1. The rhot1 gene expression was increased in the MSC + EXO treatment group compared to the Air- and CS-exposed groups. BEAS2B-MSC co-cultures showed a protective response against the CSE-altered mitochondrial respiration parameters, confirming the beneficial effect of MSC towards human bronchial lung epithelial cells. CS affects some of the early mitochondrial genes involved in the fission/fusion, enhancing the damage response along with altering cytokine levels. The combined treatment of MSC + EXO showed both their protective effects; hence, this combination may protect against early events caused by CS exposure owing to its anti-inflammatory and other mitochondrial-transfer mechanisms. The incidence of cancer, diabetes, and autoimmune diseases has been increasing and there are more and more patients with solid organ transplants. The survival rate of these immunocompromised individuals is significantly reduced when they are smokers and severely affected. Lyu et al. (2018) established a cardiac arrest-CPR model in SCID mice, analyzed the activation of CP and NLRP3 IS/caspase-1, and explored mitochondrial repair and inflammatory injury in immunodeficiency during systemic I/R injury. A KCl-induced cardiac arrest model was established in C57BL/6 and non-obese diabetic/SCID (NOD/SCID) mice. One hundred male C57BL/6 mice and 100 male NOD/SCID mice were divided into five groups (control, 2 hrs post-CPR, 12 hrs post-CPR, 24 hrs post-CPR, and 48 hrs post-CPR). A temporal dynamic view of alveolar epithelial cells, macrophages, and neutrophils from the broncho-alveolar lavage fluid (BALF) was obtained using Giemsa staining. (1) In NOD/SCID mice, macrophages were disintegrated in BALF, and the alveolar epithelial cells were shed at 48 hrs after resuscitation. Compared with C57BL/6 mice, the ratio of macrophages/total cells peaked at 12 hrs and was higher in NOD/SCID mice. After 24 hrs, macrophages were disintegrated in the BALF. (2) Mitochondrial ATG was present in both C57BL/6 and NOD/SCID mice after CPR, but it began late in the NOD/SCID mice. Compared with C57BL/6 mice, phos-ULK1 (Ser^{327}) expression was lower at 2 hrs and 12 hrs after CPR. (3) NLRP3 IS/caspase-1 activation occurred early and for only a short time in C57BL/6 mice, but was sustained in NOD/SCID mice. The expression of the NLRP3 IS increased in the C57 mice, but this increase was higher in the NOD/SCID mice than in the C57BL/6 mice, especially at 12, 24, 48 hrs after CPR. The expression of caspase-1-20 followed the same pattern as the NLRP3 IS. There was a regulatory relationship between the NLRP3 IS and mitochondrial ATG after CPR in the healthy mice, which was disturbed in the NOD/SCID mice because the signals for CP occurred late, and NLRP3 IS- and caspase-1-dependent cell injury was sustained.

CP/ATG Theranostics in Cigarette Smoking

Cigarette smoke (CS)-induced airway epithelial cell MTG is involved in the pathogenesis of COPD. Mitochondrial protein Nix (also known as BNIP3L) is a selective ATG receptor and participates in several human diseases. Zhang et al. (2019) investigated the effects of Nix on MTG and mitochondrial function in airway epithelial cells exposed to CSE, which increased Nix expression and induced MTG in airway epithelial cells. Nix siRNA inhibited MTG and attenuated mitochondrial dysfunction and cell injury when airway epithelial cells were stimulated with 7.5% CSE, while Nix overexpression enhanced MTG and aggravated mitochondrial dysfunction and cell injury when airway epithelial cells were incubated with 7.5% CSE, suggesting that Nix-dependent MTG promotes airway epithelial cell and mitochondrial injury induced by CS, and may be involved in the pathogenesis of COPD and other CS-associated diseases. Considering that CSC is primarily absorbed through the alveoli in the lungs, Park et al. (2018) used a mouse alveolar macrophage cell line (MH-S cells). After 24 hrs, CSC decreased cell viability with increased ROS and NO level. CSC damaged mitochondria, ER, and lysosomes and enhanced the expression of proteins related to apoptosis, ERS, and DNA damage accompanying elevated annexin V-bound cells. The expression of proteins related to mitochondrial dynamics (OPA1 and Drp-1) and ATG (Atg5) did not show change in cells exposed to CSC. The level of IFN-γ and MIP-1α was elevated in CSC-exposed cells, whereas the MCP-1α level decreased. The expression of chemokine receptors (CD195 and CXCR2) and an adhesion molecule (CD54) were increased by the CSC treatment; the expression of antigen- presentation-related proteins (MHC class II, CD40, and CD80) were also enhanced. The expression of CD86, a co-stimulatory molecule for antigen presentation decreased, suggesting that CSC may induce apoptotic cell death and disturbance in host defense mechanisms by impairing the function of cellular components. CS causes mitochondrial dysfunction leading to cellular senescence in lung cells due to the induction of CBMP.

Sundar et al. (2019) determined the mechanism of mitochondrial dysfunction by CS in lung epithelial cells. CSE affected mitochondrial function, such as $\Delta\Psi$, ROS, and mitochondrial mass, and were associated with altered O/P protein levels (Complexes I–IV) in primary lung epithelial cells (SAEC and NHBE), and (complexes I and II) in BEAS2B cells. There were changes in mitochondrial respiration (O_2 consumption, that is, maximal respiration, ATP production, and spare capacity) in the control versus the CSE-treated BEAS2B and NHBE/DHBE cells. The EM analysis revealed perinuclear CB clustering. CS mediated an increase in Drp-1 and decrease in Mfn-2 levels, which were involved in mitochondrial fission/fusion. CSE reduced Miro1 and PINK1 abundance; these play a crucial role in the intercellular transfer mechanism and CP, indicating the role of Miro1 in CS-induced mitochondrial dysfunction in lung epithelial cells that may contribute to the pathogenesis of inflammatory lung diseases.

To determine the involvement of PRKN-regulated CP in COPD pathogenesis, Araya et al. (2019) used prkn knockout (KO) mouse models. To illuminate how PINK1 and PRKN regulate CP in relation to the CS-induced mitochondrial damage and cellular senescence, overexpression, and knockdown experiments performed in airway epithelial cells (AEC). In comparison to wild-type mice, prkn KO mice demonstrated enhanced airway wall thickening with emphysematous changes following CS exposure. AEC in CS-exposed prkn KO mice showed the accumulation of damaged mitochondria and increased oxidative modifications, accompanied by accelerated cellular senescence implicated in CBMP. PRKN overexpression induced MTG during CSE exposure (even during reduced PINK1 protein levels), resulting in the attenuation of ROS production and cellular senescence. PINK1 overexpression could not recover the impaired MTG caused by PRKN knockdown, indicating that it can be the rate-limiting factor in PINK1-PRKN-mediated MTG during CSE exposure, that PRKN levels may play a pivotal role in COPD pathogenesis by regulating MTG, and that PRKN induction could mitigate COPD progression. The mechanisms by which lung structural cells survive toxic exposures to CS are not well defined but may involve the disposal of damaged mitochondria by CP that may be influenced by ceramide (Cer), or its precursor dihydroceramide (DHC). Mizumura et al. (2018) demonstrated that lung epithelial and endothelial cells exposed to CS-exhibited mitochondrial damage, signaled by PINK1 phosphorylation, ATG, and necroptosis. Although cells responded to CS by the rapid inhibition of DHC desaturase, which elevated DHC levels, palmitoyl (C16)-Cer also increased in CS-exposed cells. Whereas DHC augmentation triggered ATG without cell death, the exogenous administration of C16-Cer triggered necroptosis. The inhibition of Cer-generating acid sphingomyelinase reduced both CS-induced PINK1 phosphorylation and necroptosis. When exposed to CS, PINK1$^{-/-}$ mice, which are protected from airspace enlargement compared with wild-type littermates, had blunted C16-Cer elevations and less lung necroptosis. CS-exposed PINK1$^{-/-}$ mice also exhibited increased lignoceroyl (C24)-DHC, along with increased expression of Cer synthase 2 (CerS2), suggesting that a combination of high C24-DHC and low C16-Cer levels might protect in CS-induced necroptosis. CerS2$^{-/-}$ mice, which lack C24-DHC at the expense of increased C16-Cer, were more susceptible to CS, developing airspace enlargement within one month of exposure. These results implicated DHCs, in particular, C24-DHC, as protective against CS toxicity by enhancing CP/ATG, whereas C16-Cer accumulation contributed to mitochondrial damage and PINK1-mediated necroptosis, which may be amplified by the inhibition of C24-DHC-producing CerS2.

CP in Lung Injury and Pulmonary Fibrosis

Hyperoxia-Induced CB Formation

Recently, Ma et al. (2018) explored mechanisms that alter mitochondrial structure and function in pulmonary endothelial cells (PEC) function after hyperoxia. The mitochondrial structures of PECs exposed to hyperoxia or normoxia were visualized and mitochondrial fragmentation implicated in CB formation were quantified. The expression of pro-fission or fusion proteins or ATG-related proteins were assessed by immunoblotting. The mitochondrial oxidative state was determined using mito-roGFP. Tetramethylrhodamine methyl ester estimated mitochondrial polarization in treatment groups. The role of ROS in mitochondrial fragmentation with mito-TEMPOL was investigated. The mtDNA damage was studied using ENDO III (mt-tat-endonuclease III), a protein that repairs mDNA damage. Drp-1 was overexpressed or silenced to determine the role of this protein in cell survival and trans-well resistance. Hyperoxia induced CB formation in PEC by enhanced phosphorylation of Drp-1 (serine 616), decreased mitofusion protein 1 (Mfn-1), increased optic atrophy 1 (OPA-1), pro-ATG proteins (p62), LC3 adapter-binding protein SQSTM1/p62 (LC-3), PINK-1, and LC3B within 48 hrs. Returning cells to normoxia for 24 hrs reversed the increased CB formation and changes in the expression of pro-fission proteins. Hyperoxia-induced CBMP was mitigated by antioxidants mito-TEMPOL, Drp-1 silencing, or inhibition or protection by the mitochondrial endonuclease ENDO III. Hyperoxia induced oxidation and mitochondrial depolarization and impaired trans-well resistance. The decrease in resistance was mitigated by mito-TEMPOL or ENDO III and reproduced by overexpression of Drp-1. Because hyperoxia evoked mt-fragmentation, cell survival and trans-well resistance were prevented by ENDO III and mito-TEMPOL and Drp-1 silencing, and these data linked hyperoxia-induced mt-DNA damage, Drp-1 expression, mt-fragmentation, and PEC dysfunction implicated in CBMP.

Critically ill patients are treated with high levels of O_2, hyperoxia, for prolonged periods of time which can exacerbate respiratory failure and lead to a high mortality rate. Mitochondrial A-kinase anchoring protein (Akap) regulates mitochondrial function. Under hypoxic conditions, Akap121 undergoes proteolytic degradation and promotes cardiac injury. To understand the role of Akap1 in hyperoxia-induced acute lung injury (ALI), Narala et al. (2018) exposed wild-type (WT) and Akap1$^{-/-}$ mice to 100% O_2 for 48 hrs, a time point associated with lung damage in the murine model of ALI. Under hyperoxia, Akap1$^{-/-}$ mice displayed induced pro-inflammatory cytokines, immune cell infiltration, and protein leakage in lungs, as well as increased alveolar capillary permeability. Akap1 deletion enhanced lung NF-κB p65 activity as assessed by immunoblotting, aDNA-binding assay, and mitochondrial ATG-related markers, PINK1 and Parkin. Akap1 deletion was associated with CBs in type II alveolar epithelial cells, indicating that Akap1 genetic deletion increases the severity of hyperoxia-induced acute lung injury in mice. Li et al. (2019) determined whether PD activates Parkin-dependent MTG to provide protection in LPS-induced mitochondria-dependent apoptosis and lung injury. C57BL/6 mice were injected i.t. with LPS (5 mg/kg) *in vivo* and Beas-2B cells were exposed to 0.5 mM LPS *in vitro* to prepare experimental model of ARDS. PD facilitated Parkin translocation to mitochondria and promoted MTG in ARDS-challenged mice and LPS-treated Beas-2B cells. However, PD-induced MTG was suppressed in Parkin$^{-/-}$ mice and Parkin siRNA transfected cells, indicating that PD activates Parkin-dependent MTG. The protective effects of PD in LPS-induced mitochondria-dependent apoptosis and lung injury were suppressed when Parkin was depleted both *in vivo* and *in vitro*. The inhibition of MTG with MTG inhibitor, mitochondrial division inhibitor-1, *in vivo* and the silencing of the ATG-related gene 7 *in vitro* also attenuated the protective effects mediated by PD, suggesting that Parkin-dependent MTG induced by PD confers protection in mitochondria-dependent apoptosis in ARDS.

Corrole is a new photosensitizer (PS) in cancer photodynamic therapy (PDT). Zhang et al. (2019) prepared water-soluble cationic sulfonated Corrole (1) and its metal complexes (1-Fe, 1-Mn, and 1-Cu), and investigated anti-cancer activity in various tumor cells. The 1's phototoxicity induced ROS overproduction, causing $\Delta\Psi$ collapse and apoptosis via ROS-mediated mitochondrial caspase activation, in which SIRT1 protein degradation played a key role. PTD activity *in vivo* shown in 1 reduced the growth of A549 xeno-grafted tumor, without loss of body weight. Thus, cationic sulfonated Corrole was a candidate for PS. The photo-toxicity of 1 induced A549 cell apoptosis by ROS overproduction to enhance the mitochondrial apoptosis involving CBMP, suggesting that SIRT1 protein is a target in this process. Bueno et al. (2019) showed that ERS represses the PINK1 in lung type II alveolar epithelial cells (AECII) reducing CP and increasing the susceptibility to lung fibrosis. ERS and PINK1 deficiency in AECII led to MTS with oxidative damage to mtDNA and subsequent extracellular release. Extracellular mtDNA was recognized by TLR9 in AECII by an endocytic-dependent pathway. PINK1 deficiency-dependent mtDNA release enhanced the activation of TLR9 and triggered the secretion of the pro-fibrotic factor, TGF-β, which was attenuated by PINK1 overexpression. Enhanced mtDNA oxidation and damage were found in aging and IPF human lungs and circulating mtDNA were elevated in plasma and broncho-alveolar lavage from patients with IPF. Free mtDNA was elevated in other ILDs with low expression of PINK1, including hypersensitivity pneumonitis and autoimmune interstitial lung diseases, suggesting the role of PINK1 mediated CP/ATG in the attenuation of DAMP release and control of TGF-β mediated pro-fibrotic responses.

CP/ATG in Lung Cancer Theranostics

Lei et al. (2018) focused on the mechanisms of metastasis-associated lung adenocarcinoma transcript 1 (MALAT1) expression in various physiological and pathological processes. MALAT1 is a long noncoding RNA whose transcript is ~8 kb in length and can be expressed differentially under stress conditions, such as hypoxia, high glucose, H_2O_2, UV irradiation, microbial infection, and chemical stimulation. MALAT1 is involved in regulating proliferation, apoptosis, differentiation, migration, epithelial-mesenchymal transition, ATG, and morphological maintenance. MALAT1 plays critical roles in embryo implantation, angiogenesis, tissue inflammation, tumor progression, liver fibrosis, cardiovascular remodeling, and diabetes by regulating gene transcription, forming RNA-protein complexes with proteins, regulating protein activity, assisting protein localization, mediating epigenetic changes, and by acting as a competing RNA. Furthermore, MALAT1 can affect the sensitivity of chemotherapy and radiotherapy; hence it could be used as a drug target for chemotherapy and radiotherapy. MALAT1 is overexpressed in most tumor tissues or sera, and its expression affects the tumor size, stage, lymph node metastasis, and distant invasion; hence, it can be used as a biomarker for early diagnosis, severity assessment, and prognosis in cancer.

Non-small cell lung cancer (NSCLC) survival rates are dismal and high βIII-tubulin expression is associated with MDR and tumor aggressiveness in this disease. βIII-tubulin promotes cell survival in the harsh tumor microenvironment, which is characterized by poor nutrient supply. Parker et al. (2016) investigated the role of βIII-tubulin in glucose stress response and the survival and proliferation of NSCLC cells. βIII-tubulin regulated cellular metabolism and glucose stress-response signaling in NSCLC cells to promote cell survival and proliferation in glucose starvation. BIII-Tubulin decreased the reliance of cells on glycolytic metabolism, priming them to cope with variable nutrient supply within the tumor microenvironment. BIII-Tubulin protected cells from ERS and reduced both basal and glucose starvation-induced ATG to maintain cell survival and proliferation. βIII-Tubulin enabled rapid Akt activation in response to glucose starvation and co-immunoprecipitated with the master regulator of the ERS response GRP78. Suppression of βIII-tubulin delayed the association of GRP78 with Akt in response to glucose starvation with the potential to influence Akt activation and ER homeostasis under these conditions. These results highlighted that βIII-tubulin regulates glucose metabolism and alters glucose starvation stress to promote cell proliferation and survival in NSCLC cells, elucidating the role of this microtubule protein and insight into correlations between high βIII-tubulin expression and poor patient outcome in this disease.

The expression of TRAP1, a member of the HSP90 chaperone family, has been implicated in tumor protective effects, based on its mitochondrial localization and function. Barbosa et al. (2018) provided new insights into the pathways involved in TRAP1-mediated protection on NSCLC. TRAP1-depleted A549 human NSCLC cells and MRC-5 normal lung fibroblasts were produced using a siRNA approach and the main cellular QC mechanisms (IMD, ICD, and MQC) were investigated. TRAP1-depleted A549 cells displayed decreased cell viability due to impaired mitochondrial function, including decreased ATP/AMP ratio, O_2 consumption and $\Delta\Psi$ collapse, and increased apoptotic indicators. The negative impact of TRAP1 depletion on mitochondrial function was not observed in normal MRC-5 lung cells, which might be due to the differential intracellular localization of the chaperone in tumor versus normal cells. A549 TRAP1-depleted cells showed increased ATG. ATG inhibition decreased cell viability in both TRAP1-expressing and TRAP1-depleted tumor cells with minor effects on MRC-5 cells, whereas, ATG stimulation decreased cell viability of both A549 and MRC-5 TRAP1-expressing cells. In A549, TRAP1-depleted cells increased ATG augmented viability, indicating that even though TRAP1 depletion affects both normal MRC-5 and tumor A549 cell proliferation, inhibition of ATG decreased in tumor cell mass, while having a reduced effect on the normal cell line. The strategy of targeting TRAP1 in NSCLC revealed theranostic applications. Betula platyphylla (BP) is used in the treatment of various human diseases, including cancers. Jung et al. (2019) observed that BP extracts and 1,7-bis(4-hydroxyphenyl)-4-hepten-3-one (BE1), one of the components of BP, decreased the cell viability of several lung cancer cell lines. BE1-treated cells exhibited apoptosis and cell cycle arrest at the G2/M phase. The BE1 treatment resulted in the suppression of CP, as evidenced by increased LC3 II and p62/SQSTM1 expression. The induction of CP with Rapamycin reduced the BE1-induced apoptosis, indicating that apoptosis induced by BE1 was associated with CP inhibition, suggesting that BE1 exposure activated the p38 pathway to regulate pro-apoptotic activity, and that BE1 is a potential anticancer agent for human lung cancer, which exerts its effect by enhancing apoptosis via regulating CP and the p38 pathway. PARK2, which encodes Parkin, is a disease-causing gene for both NDDs and cancer. Parkin as a neuroprotective protein plays a crucial role in the regulation of MTG, and germline mutations in PARK2 are associated with PD. Parkin serves as a tumor suppressor under normal physiological conditions. However, when it is mutated or becomes nonfunctional, it may induce Parkinson's disease or tumor progression depending on its tissue localization, inducers and microenvironment. Somatic and germline mutations in PARK2 are associated with cancers, including lung cancer. Zhang et al. (2019) showed that wild-type (WT) Parkin can translocate onto mitochondria following mitochondrial damage and that Parkin promotes CP in lung cancer cells. However, lung cancer-linked mutations inhibit the mitochondrial translocation and ubiquitin-associated activity of Parkin. A46T Parkin failed to translocate onto mitochondria and recruit downstream CP regulators, including optineurin (OPTN) and TFEB, whereas N254S and R275W Parkin displayed slower mitochondrial translocation than WT Parkin. Deferiprone (DFP), an iron chelator that can induce CP, increased the death of A46T Parkin-expressing lung cancer cells, suggesting that lung cancer-linked mutations in PARK2 are associated with impaired CP, and that DFP, a novel theranostic agent for PARK2-linked lung cancer and other types of cancers, is driven by CP dysregulation.

The Theranostic Significance of Antioxidants as CB Regulators in Respiratory Diseases

CO is an endogenously-produced gas which is a biological signal transduction effector with properties similar, but not identical, to that of NO. CO, which binds primarily to heme iron, may activate the hemoprotein guanylate cyclase, although with lower potency than NO. Recently,

Ryter et al. (2018) highlighted that CO can modulate the activities of signaling molecules such as p38 MAPK, ERK1/2, JNK, Akt, NF-κB, and others. Mitochondria represent a key target of CO action in eukaryotes. The dose-dependent modulation of mitochondrial function by CO can result in alteration of ΔΨ, ROS production, release of pro-apoptotic and pro-inflammatory mediators, as well as the inhibition of respiration at a high concentration. CO, through modulation of signaling pathways, can impact key biological processes including CP, ATG, MB, apoptosis, cellular proliferation, inflammation, and innate immune responses. Inhaled CO is hazardous due to its rapid complexation with hemoglobin, resulting in impaired O_2 delivery to tissues and hypoxemia. Despite systemic and cellular toxicity at high concentrations, CO has demonstrated cyto- and tissue-protective effects at low concentration in animal models of organ injury and disease. These include models of acute lung injury (hyperoxia, hypoxia, I/R, mechanical ventilation, Bleomycin) and sepsis. The success of CO as a therapeutic in preclinical models suggests its potential clinical application in inflammatory and proliferative disorders. Recent studies demonstrated that the MTG mediates pulmonary epithelial cell death in response to CSE exposure, and contributes to emphysema. Son et al. (2018) investigated the role of MTG in regulating apoptosis in CSE-exposed human lung bronchial epithelial cells. They investigated the potential of the poly-methoxylated flavone antioxidant Quercetogetin (QUE) to inhibit CSE-induced MTG-dependent apoptosis. CSE induced MTG in epithelial cells via mitochondrial dysfunction, and caused the increased expression of the MTG-regulator protein, PINK1, and the mitochondrial fission protein, DRP-1. CSE induced epithelial cell death and increased the expression of the cleaved caspase-3, -8, and -9. Caspase-3 was increased in Beas-2B cells exposed to CSE, and decreased by the siRNA-dependent knockdown of DRP-1. The treatment of epithelial cells with QUE inhibited CSE-induced mitochondrial dysfunction and MTG by inhibiting phospho (p)-DRP-1 and PINK1 expression. QUE suppressed MTG-dependent apoptosis by inhibiting the expression of cleaved caspase-3, -8, and -9 and downregulating caspase activity in human bronchial epithelial cells, suggesting that QUE may serve as a potential therapeutic in CS-induced pulmonary diseases. Recent studies show that MTG, the ATG-dependent turnover of mitochondria, mediates pulmonary epithelial cell death in response to CSE and contributes to the development of emphysema *in vivo* during chronic CS exposure. Kyung et al. (2018) investigated the role of MTG in the regulation of CSE-exposed lung bronchial epithelial cell (Beas-2B) death. They also investigated the role of a phosphodiesterase 4 inhibitor, Roflumilast, in CSE-induced CP-dependent cell death. CSE induced CP in Beas-2B cells through mitochondrial dysfunction and increased the expression of the CP regulator protein, PINK1, and Drp-1. CSE-induced epithelial cell death was increased in Beas-2B cells but was decreased by the siRNA-dependent knockdown of Drp-1. Treatment with Roflumilast in Beas-2B cells inhibited CSE-induced mitochondrial dysfunction and CP by inhibiting the expression of phospho-Drp-1 and -PINK1. Roflumilast increased cell viability in Beas-2B cells exposed to CSE, suggesting that it plays a protective role in CS-induced CP-dependent cell death. Pulmonary fibrosis (PF) is an irreversible lung disorder with decline in lung function leading to respiratory insufficiency. Idiopathic pulmonary fibrosis is a disease in older adults, leading to progressive dyspnea and reduced exercise capacity, and resulting in death within 3–5 years of diagnosis. Winters et al. (2019) highlighted that underlying genetic susceptibility combined with environmental insults is to trigger a chronic wound repair response, leading to activation of the fibrotic cascade. Perturbations in several molecular pathways mediate vulnerability of the alveolar epithelium to injurious agents, including the unfolded protein response, ATG, CP, and cellular senescence. These cellular responses link genetic susceptibility to the progressive fibrotic phenotype. Pirfenidone and Nintedanib are the only two US FDA-approved drugs to treat PF. Prashanth et al. (2019) investigated the role of Nimbolide, an active constituent of Neem in TGF-β1 induced *in vitro* and Bleomycin induced *in vivo* model of PF, with emphasis on the regulation of fibrosis-related CP. The reduction in mesenchymal and fibrotic markers, and a substantial upregulation of epithelial markers upon treatment with Nimbolide, which regulated CP signaling by dampening LC-3 and p62 expression and increasing Beclin-1 expression, suggesting Nimbolide as a potent anti-fibrotic agent and its ability to regulate PF-associated CP. Recently, NOD-like receptor family pyrin domain containing 3 (NLRP3) IS, which is activated by ROS and repressed by ATG, has been identified as a novel agent of PF. AngII, the bioactive pro-oxidant in the RAS, aggravates lung fibrosis. Meng et al. (2018) investigated the link between AngII-induced ATG in the regulation of the NLRP3 IS/IL-1β axis in PF. *In vivo*, ATG and the NLRP3 IS were activated in fibrotic patients and correlated with oxidation. Treatment with Rapamycin promoted ATG but inhibited oxidation, NLRP3 IS, and PF after Bleomycin infusion. The ATG inhibitor 3-MA reduced BLM-induced PF and facilitated NLRP3 IS activation and oxidation in fibroblasts. *In vitro*, AngII promoted ROS, H_2O_2, and NADPH oxidase 4 (NOX4) levels and reduced glutathione, resulting in NLRP3 IS activation and consequent collagen synthesis. Ang-II induced CP/ATG, while VAS2870, NOX4, siRNA, and compound C eliminated AngII-induced LC3B augmentation. Moreover, blocking ATG with Bafilomycin A1 or LC3B siRNA resulted in oxidant accumulation, NLRP3 IS activation, and collagen deposition. AngII induced P62/SQSTM1, targeting ubiquitinated apoptosis-associated speck-like protein containing a CARD for degradation, thereby contributing to NLRP3 IS inactivation. CP/ATG attenuated PF by regulating NLRP3 IS activation induced by AngII-mediated ROS via redox balance.

CONCLUSION

The dual role of CP/ATG was demonstrated in COPD. Lamin B1 and PRKN regulated CP and cellular senescence during COPD pathogenesis. The ventilation-induced diaphragm dysfunction was attenuated through TLR4 and NF-κB in a murine endotoxemia model. Hyperoxia caused CB formation in pulmonary endothelial cells by increasing the expression of pro-fission proteins. The genetic deletion of Akap1 increased hyperoxia-induced acute lung injury in mice. Ventilator-induced lung injury was alleviated by inhibiting NLRP3 IS activation. The association of VAMP8 rs1010 polymorphism with host susceptibility to PTB was demonstrated. The metastasis-associated lung adenocarcinoma transcript, Nix/BNIP3L-dependent MTG was responsible for airway epithelial cell injury (Zhang et al. 2019a). Pulmonary HTN was driven by mitochondrial dysfunction. TRAP1 regulated ATG in lung cancer cell. 1,7-Bis(4-hydroxyphenyl)-4-hepten-3-one from Betula-platyphylla-induced apoptosis by regulating CP and p38 pathway in lung cancer cells. The stress induced the degeneration of mitochondrial respiratory complexes in yeast. Crosstalk between ATG and oxidative stress regulated proteolysis in the diaphragm during mechanical ventilation. The Sphingolipid metabolism was impaired, whereas Quercetogetin protected in CSE-induced apoptosis in LECs by inhibiting MTG and necroptosis. The phosphodiesterase 4 inhibitor, Roflumilast, provided protection in CSE-induced MTG-dependent cell death in LECs. LEC injury and dysfunction were involved in the pathogenesis of idiopathic PF. ATG attenuated Ang-II-induced PF by inhibiting redox imbalance-mediated NOD-like receptor family pyrin domain in IS activation. Polydatin mediated Parkin-dependent CP and prevented CBMP in ARDS. The photocytotoxic effect of cationic sulfonated Corrole was also studied in lung cancer cells (Zhang et al 2019b).

REFERENCES

Araya, J., K. Tsubouchi, N. Sato, S. Ito, et al. 2019. PRKN-regulated mitophagy and cellular senescence during COPD pathogenesis. Autophagy 15: 510–526.

Barbosa, I.A., I. Vega-Naredo, R. Loureiro, A.F. Branco, et al. 2018. TRAP1 regulates autophagy in lung cancer cells. Eur J Clin Invest 48(4): e12900.

Bueno, M., D. Zank, I. Buendia-Roldán, K. Fiedler, et al. 2019. PINK1 attenuates mtDNA release in alveolar epithelial cells and TLR9 mediated profibrotic responses. PLoS One 14: e0218003.

Cheng, S., C. Sun, W, Lao and H. Kang. 2019. Association of VAMP8 rs1010 polymorphism with host susceptibility to pulmonary tuberculosis in a chinese han population. Genet Test Mol Biomarkers 23: 299–303.

Hara, H., K. Kuwano and J. Araya. 2018. Mitochondrial quality control in COPD and IPF. Cells 7(8): 86.

Jiang, S., J. Sun, N. Mohammadtursun, Z. Hu, et al. 2019. Dual role of ATG/MTG in chronic obstructive pulmonary disease. Pulm Pharmacol Ther 56: 116–125.

Jung, H.J., K.S. Song, Y.K. Son, J.K. Seong, et al. 2019. 1,7-Bis(4-hydroxyphenyl)-4-hepten-3-one from *Betula platyphylla* induces apoptosis by suppressing autophagy flux and activating the p38 pathway in lung cancer cells. Phytother Res 34: 126–138.

Kyung, S.Y., Y.J. Kim, E.S. Son, S.H. Jeong, et al. 2018. The phosphodiesterase 4 inhibitor roflumilast protects against cigarette smoke extract-induced mitophagy-dependent cell death in epithelial cells. Tuberc Respir Dis (Seoul) 81: 138–147.

Lei, L., J. Chen, J. Huang, J. Lu, et al. 2018. Functions and regulatory 7(8), 86 mechanisms of metastasis-associated lung adenocarcinoma transcript 1. J Cell Physiol 234: 134–151.

Li, L.F., Y.Y. Liu, N.H. Chen, Y.H. Chen, et al. 2018. Attenuation of ventilation-induced diaphragm dysfunction through toll-like receptor 4 and nuclear factor-κB in a murine endotoxemia model. Lab Invest 98: 1170–1183.

Li, T., Y. Liu, W. Xu, X. Dai, et al. 2019. Polydatin mediates Parkin-dependent MTG and protects against mitochondria-dependent apoptosis in acute respiratory distress syndrome. Lab Invest 99: 819–829.

Lyu, J.J., J.L. Mehta, Y. Li, L. Ye, et al. 2018. Mitochondrial ATG and NLRP3 IS in pulmonary tissues from severe combined immunodeficient mice after cardiac arrest and cardiopulmonary resuscitation. Chin Med J (Eng) 131: 1174–1184.

Ma, C., A.M. Beyer, M. Durand, A.V. Clough, et al. 2018. Hyperoxia causes mitochondrial fragmentation in pulmonary endothelial cells by increasing expression of pro-fission proteins. Arterioscler Thromb Vasc Biol 38: 622–635.

Maremanda, K.P., I.K. Sundar and I. Rahman. 2019. Protective role of mesenchymal stem cells and mesenchymal stem cell-derived exosomes in cigarette smoke-induced mitochondrial dysfunction in mice. Toxicol Appl Pharmacol 385: 114788.

Medeiros, T.C., R.L. Thomas, R. Ghillebert and M. Graef. 2018. ATG balances mtDNA synthesis and degradation by DNA polymerase POLG during starvation. J Cell Biol 217: 1601–1611.

Meng, Y., M. Pan, B. Zheng, Y. Chen, et al. 2018. Autophagy attenuates angiotensin II-induced pulmonary fibrosis by inhibiting redox imbalance-mediated NOD-like receptor family pyrin domain containing 3 inflammasome activation. Antioxid Redox Signal 30(4): 520–541.

Mizumura, K., M.J. Justice, K.S. Schweitzer and S. Krishnan. 2018. Sphingolipid regulation of lung epithelial cell MTG and necroptosis during cigarette smoke exposure. FASEB J 32: 1880–1890.

Narala, V.R., J. Fukumoto, H. Hernández-Cuervo, S.S, Patil, et al. 2018. Akap1 genetic deletion increases the severity of hyperoxia–induced acute lung injury in mice. Am J Physiol Lung Cell Mol Physiol 314: L860–L870.

Park, E.J., H.S. Lee, S.J. Lee, Y.J. Park, et al. 2018. Cigarette smoke condensate may disturb immune function with apoptotic cell death by impairing function of organelles in alveolar macrophages. Toxicol in Vitro 52: 351–364.

Parker, A.L., N. Turner, J.A. McCarroll and M. Kavallaris. 2016. βIII-Tubulin alters glucose metabolism and stress response signaling to promote cell survival and proliferation in glucose-starved non-small cell lung cancer cells. Carcinogenesis 37(8): 787–798.

Prashanth, G.M., S. Bale, G. Pulivendala and C. Godugu. 2019. Therapeutic effects of Nimbolide, an ATG regulator, in ameliorating pulmonary fibrosis through attenuation of TGF-β1 driven epithelial-to-mesenchymal transition. Int Immunopharmacol 75: 105755.

Ryter, S.W., K.C. Ma and A.M.K. Choi. 2018. Carbon monoxide in lung cell physiology and disease. Am J Physiol Cell Physiol 314: C211–C227.

Sharma, S. 2018. Nicotinism and Emerging Role of eCigarettes (with special reference to adolescents), Vol. 1–4. Nova Science Publishers, New York, U.S.A.

Smuder, A.J., K.J. Sollanek, W.B. Nelson, K. Min, et al. 2018. Crosstalk between ATG and oxidative stress regulates proteolysis in the diaphragm during mechanical ventilation. Free Radic Biol Med 115: 179–190.

Son, E.S., S.H. Kim, S.W. Ryter, E.J. Yeo, et al. 2018. Quercetogetin protects against cigarette smoke extract-induced apoptosis in epithelial cells by inhibiting mitophagy. Toxicol in Vitro 48: 170–178.

Suliman, H.B. and E. Nozik-Grayck. 2019. Mitochondrial dysfunction: Metabolic drivers of pulmonary hypertension. Antioxid Redox Signal 31: 843–857.

Sundar, I.K., K.P. Maremanda and I. Rahman. 2019. Mitochondrial dysfunction is associated with Miro1 reduction in lung epithelial cells by cigarette smoke. Toxicol Lett 317: 92–101.

Tan, W.S.D., H.M. Shen and W.S.E. Wong. 2019. Dysregulated ATG in COPD: A pathogenic process to be deciphered. Pharmacol Res 144: 1–7.

Timón-Gómez, A., D. Sanfeliu-Redondo, A. Pascual-Ahuir and M. Proft. 2018. Regulation of the stress-activated degradation of mitochondrial respiratory complexes in yeast. Front Microbiol 9: 106.

Winters, N.I., A. Burman, J.A. Kropski, T.S. Blackwell. 2019. Epithelial injury and dysfunction in the pathogenesis of idiopathic pulmonary fibrosis. Am J Med Sci 357: 374–378.

Zhang, M., R. Shi, Y. Zhang, H. Shan, et al. 2019a. Nix/BNIP3L-dependent MTGaccounts for airway epithelial cell injury induced by cigarette smoke. J Cell Physiol 234: 14210–14220.

Zhang, Z., H.J. Yu, H. Huang, B. Wan, et al. 2019b. The photocytotoxicity effect of cationic sulfonated corrole towards lung cancer cells: *In vitro* and *in vivo* study. Lasers Med Sci 34: 1353–1363.

19

Charnolophagy in Cardiovascular Diseases

INTRODUCTION

Cardiac mitochondria are heavy duty organelles and are frequently destroyed; hence, they need continuous repair, replacement, and remodeling for normal cardiovascular functioning. The heart needs sufficient energy (ATP) to supply blood against gravity to meet the requirement of glucose, oxygen, and other trophic factors in the brain and other organs of our body. Therefore, >40% of the cardiac tissue is composed of exclusively mitochondria, arranged like a compact battery in the myocardium. Degenerated, undesired, and nonfunctional mitochondria are involved in CB formation and CP induction as an immediate and early response to eradicate CBs to prevent free radical-induced CBMP in HTN, atherosclerosis, coronary artery disease (CAD), cardiac arrhythmia, angina pectoris, myocardial ischemia, myocardial infarction, cardiovascular remodeling due to volume and pressure overload, ventricular thinning, plaque rupture, and congestive heart failure (CHF), if left untreated. Characteristic features of the cardiovascular system (contractility, rhythmicity, automaticity, and elasticity) are compromised depending on the severity of CVD due to CMB, dysregulated CP, and CBMP. The primary goal of treating cardiovascular diseases is to improve blood supply in the affected organ to restore MB. Pharmacological interventions (nitro-vasodilators, β-blocker, calcium channel blocker, ACE inhibitors, and ARBs) balloon angioplasty, drug-eluting stents, cardiac pacemakers, defibrillators, coronary bypass surgery, and eventually heart transplantation are performed to improve blood supply to all parts of our body for survival. Recently, Moyzis and Gustafsson (2018) highlighted that cardiomyocytes require tremendous energy to sustain contraction. Mitochondria generate most of the energy for the heart via O/P. To ensure a healthy population of mitochondria which can efficiently generate ATP, myocytes eliminate unhealthy, nonfunctional, or unwanted mitochondria via ATP-driven, lysosomal-dependent CP. This selectively eliminates damaged, undesired, nonfunctional, or aged mitochondria since these can become a constant source of ROS and release pro-death proteins through CS destabilization. Sato and Sadoshima (2015) discussed the current understanding of mitochondrial ATG in mammals with reference to yeast. They emphasized on the roles of CP, ATG, and MTG in the heart. MQC is a crucial determinant of cell viability. MTG plays a pivotal role in this control mechanism.

Recently, the role of microRNAs has been investigated in CVDs. An intimate link between ATG and cardiac disorders, including myocardial infarction, cardiac hypertrophy, cardiomyopathy, cardiac fibrosis, and heart failure, has been demonstrated. MiRNAs are small non-coding RNAs with a length of ~21‾22 nucleotides (NT), and are distributed widely in viruses, plants, protists, and animals. They function in regulating the post-transcriptional gene silencing and cardiac CP/ATG by suppressing the expression of genes involved in the pathogenesis of heart diseases in a targeted manner. Sun et al. (2018a) highlighted the role of microRNAs in cardiac CP/ATG and related cardiac disorders and focused on regulatory pathways consisting of miRNAs and their targeted genes. CP and ATG contribute to the cardiac homeostasis in physiological conditions. However, impaired or excessive ATG is implicated in a variety of CVDs. Although Doxycycline (Dox) is effective as an antineoplastic drug, it causes severe cardiotoxicity. Song et al. (2018) determined the role of histone deacetylase 6 (HDAC6) in Dox-induced cardiomyopathy. Dox increased the HDAC6 protein level and activity and decreased α-tubulin acetylation. HDAC6 knockout (HDAC6$^{-/-}$) mice revealed anti-Dox cardiotoxicity by conserved cardiac function monitored by ECoG and the protection was reversed by Nocodazole, a drug-lowering α-tubulin acetylation. Improvement of mitochondrial function and ATG were inhibited by Nocodazole and Colchicine, which lowers α-tubulin acetylation in neonatal rat cardiac myocytes. Tubastatin A, a HDAC6-selective inhibitor, protected in Dox-induced acute cardiomyopathy without influencing the effect of Dox on inhibiting MDA-MB-231 tumorigenesis, suggesting a novel theranostic strategy for cancer with Dox by combining it with HDAC6 inhibitors. PTEN plays an important role in tumor suppression, and PTEN family members are involved in biological processes. Li et al. (2018) reported that PTENα regulates CP by promoting PARK2 recruitment to damaged mitochondria. PTENα-deficient mice exhibited cardiac mitochondria with structural and functional abnormalities, and PTENα-deficient mouse hearts were highly susceptible to injury induced by I/R and Isoprenaline. Mitochondrial clearance by CP is impaired in PTENα-deficient cardiomyocytes. PTENα interacted with the E3 ubiquitin ligase PRKN, which is an important mediator of CP and binds PRKN through the membrane binding helix in its N-terminus, and promotes PRKN mitochondrial translocation through enhancing PRKN self-association in a phosphatase-independent manner. Loss of PTENα compromised the mitochondrial translocation of PRKN and CP following mitochondrial depolarization, suggesting its functions as a MQC mechanism to sustain normal cardiovascular function.

This chapter describes the basic molecular mechanisms of CP/ATG in the heart and its significance in CVDs. The TSE-EBPT significance of antioxidants as CP regulators/modulators in various CVDs is also highlighted.

CP in Cardiovascular Development

WD40 repeat and FYVE domain-3 have been implicated in cardiac development. WD40 repeat and FYVE domain containing 3 (WDFY3) is an adaptor protein involved in selective degradation of protein aggregates by CP/ATG. Wdfy3 is critical in the regulation of brain development and osteoclastogenesis *in vivo*. Zhang et al. (2018) explored the role of Wdfy3 in cardiac morphogenesis using Wdfy3-deficient mice. Wdfy3 was expressed in the developing heart in mice and peaked at embryonic day 12.5 (E12.5). The loss of Wdfy3 in mice led to embryonic and neonatal lethality. Wdfy3-deficient mice displayed congenital heart defects including membranous ventricular septal defect (VSD), aortic overriding (AO), double outlet right ventricle (DORV), thinning of ventricular wall, ventricular dilation, and disorganized ventricular trabeculation at E14.5. Cell proliferation was reduced in the hearts of Wdfy3-deficient mice at E12.5 and E14.5, which was associated with enhanced p21 expression. Cardiomyocyte differentiation was diminished as demonstrated by reduced Myh6 and MLC2v in Wdfy3-deficient mice at E14.5. Two cardiac transcription factors regulating cardiomyocyte differentiation, Nkx2-5 and Mef2c, were decreased in Wdfy3-deficient mice at E14.5. Apoptotic cell death remained unaltered, suggesting that reduced cell proliferation and cardiomyocyte differentiation contribute to cardiac defects in Wdfy3-deficient mice. The loss of Wdfy3 led to a reduction in Notch1 intracellular domain and its downstream targets Hes1 and Hey1, which was accompanied with enhanced full-length Notch1 protein levels. An *in vitro* luciferase assay showed that Wdfy3 deficiency induced p21 promoter, while diminished Hes1 promoter activity through modulation of Notch1 signaling. Wdfy3 was co-localized with Notch1 in primary embryonic cardiomyocytes. Endogenous Wdfy3 interacted with full-length Notch1 in the developing heart, suggesting that Notch1 signaling is perturbed in the hearts of the Wdfy3-deficient mice. No alteration in CP/ATG was detected in the Wdfy3-deficient mice, suggesting that it plays an essential role in cardiac development, mediated by modulating Notch1 signaling.

CP in Atherosclerosis

Platelets circulate in the bloodstream for a finite period: upon vessel injury, they are activated to participate in hemostasis; upon senescence, unused platelets are cleared by CP/ATG. Thrombocytopenia leads to bleeding, whereas, platelet activation leads to occlusive events that trigger strokes and heart attacks. Banerjee et al. (2019) showed that ATG occurs in platelets to facilitate their production and normal functions including hemostasis and thrombosis. Due to the unique properties of platelets, such as their lack of nuclei and propensity for activation, methods for studying platelet ATG must be specifically tailored. ATG becomes dysfunctional during the progression of atherosclerosis, regardless of whether there are many CP/ATG-stimulating factors (for example, ROS, oxidized lipids, and cytokines) within the atherosclerotic plaque. Grootaert et al. (2018) highlighted recent insights into the defective CP/ATG in atherosclerosis, with a special focus on their role in macrophage plaques, vascular smooth muscle cells (VSMCs), and endothelial cells (ECs). Although, defective CP/ATG promotes apoptosis in macrophages, it accelerates premature senescence in VSMCs. In the ECs, defective CP promotes both apoptosis and senescence. There is discrepancy between the three cell types in their response to ATG deficiency and the cell type-dependent role of ATG, which may have implications for the ATG-targeted treatments of atherosclerosis. Cholesteryl esters accumulation in macrophage foam cells drives the development of atherosclerosis. ATG plays a key role in the degradation of intracellular LDs via autolysosome, and in the release of lipids via cholesterol efflux. Ma et al. (2019) identified that a mitochondria-targeted antioxidant, Mito-Tempol, has protective effects on cholesteryl esters accumulation by activating ATG as it ameliorates the lipid burden of atherosclerosis. In the *in vitro* foam cell formation system using oxidized LDL (ox-LDL)-loaded THP-1 macrophages, Mito-Tempol prevented oxidative stress and attenuated lipid accumulation and rescued ox-LDL-impaired ATG, thereby facilitating lipid degradation in THP-1 macrophages and increasing the efflux of cholesterol via ATG-dependent ABCA1 and ABCG1 upregulation. This leads to the recommendation of the ATG pathway of mTOR for the ATG restoration of Mito-Tempol, and that CVDs may benefit from the treatment of Mito-Tempol on reversing atherosclerosis via CP/ATG. Docherty et al (2018) assessed defects in mitochondrial respiration in atherosclerotic plaques and identified the appropriate markers that may reflect a switch in VSMC energy metabolism. Human plaque tissue and cells were assessed for composition and DNA damage, repair potential, and mitochondrial dysfunction implicated in CBMP. Plaque tissue was evaluated using high resolution O_2 respirometry to assess oxidative metabolism. Recruitment and processing of the mitochondrial regulator of ATG PINK1 kinase was investigated in combination with transcriptional and protein markers associated with a switch to a more glycolytic metabolism. Human VSMC had increased nDNA and mtDNA damage and reduced repair potential. A subset of VSMCs within plaque had decreased O/P and the expression of PINK1 kinase. Plaque cells demonstrated increased glycolysis in response to a loss of mitochondrial function. A compensatory glycolytic program may act as energetic switch via

AMPK and hexokinase 2. They identified a subset of VSMCs required for plaque stability that had increased mitochondrial dysfunction and decreased O/P implicated in CBMP.

CP and CVDs

MQC in Cardiac Cells

Mitochondria play an important role in maintaining cardiac homeostasis by supplying the energy required for cardiac excitation-contraction coupling as well as controlling the key intracellular survival and death pathways. Tahrir et al. (2018) assessed the impact of the Tat gene on mitochondrial function and MB pathways in a primary cell culture of neonatal rat ventricular cardiomyocytes (NRVCs). The presence of Tat in cardiomyocytes was associated with decreases in O/P, ATP depletion, and ROS accumulation. Tat impaired $[Ca^{2+}]_m$-uptake electrophysiological activity, protein clearance, and ATG in cardiomyocytes under stress due to I/R. A reduction in ubiquitin along with impaired degradation of ATG proteins including SQSTM1/p62 and a reduction of LC3 II were detected in cardiomyocytes harboring Tat, suggesting that, by targeting mitochondria and PQC, Tat impacts bioenergetics and ATG, resulting in the dysregulation of cardiomyocyte homeostasis. Furthermore, Tahrir et al. (2019) demonstrated the effects of MQC dysregulation in the development of CVDs. Mitochondrial injury during myocardial infarction (MI) impairs O/P and results in the excessive production of ROS, CMB, and contributes to the development of CVDs. Therefore, MB along with proper MQC machinery (which removes CBs) is pivotal for MQC and cardiac health. Upon damage to the mitochondrial network, MQC components are recruited to segregate the CBs and target aberrant mitochondrial proteins for degradation and elimination through CP. Impaired MQC and accumulation of abnormal mitochondria are involved in the CBMP of various cardiac disorders and heart failure.

Septic Cardiomyopathy

Pan et al. (2018a) provided an overview of the recent insights into the factors contributing to septic cardiomyopathy, which is one of the most serious complications of sepsis or septic shock. As the heart is highly dependent on adequate ATP to maintain its contraction and diastolic function, impaired mitochondrial function is detrimental to the heart. Mitochondria play an important role in organ damage during sepsis. The mitochondria-related mechanisms in septic cardiomyopathy have been discussed in terms of restoring mitochondrial function. Mitochondrial uncoupling proteins located in the IMM promotes proton leakage across it, which is the regulator of ΔΨ, ROS, and ATP. Other mechanisms involved in septic cardiomyopathy include ROS production and oxidative stress, mitochondria Ca^{2+} mishandling, mtDNA impairment, mitochondrial fission and fusion, MB, mitochondrial gene and CP dysregulation, and CBMP.

TLR3, Persistent ATG, and Heart Failure

TLRs are immune-receptors involved in host defense against invading microbes. Certain TLRs activate immunological ATG to eliminate microbes. Gao et al. (2018) demonstrated that activation of TLR3 in cultured cardiomyocytes increased LC3-II, a specific marker for ATG induction, and p62/SQSTM1, an ATG receptor degraded in the final step of ATG. The results of transfection with a tandem mRFP-GFP-LC3 adenovirus and use of the ATG-inhibitor CQ suggested that TLR3 in cardiomyocytes promotes ATG without affecting ATG flux. Gene-knockdown experiments showed that the TRIF-dependent pathway mediates the autophagic effect of TLR3. In the mouse model of chronic MI, persistent ATG was observed, concomitant with upregulated TLR3 expression and increased TLR3-Trif signaling. Germline knockout (KO) of TLR3 inhibited ATG, reduced infarct size, attenuated heart failure, and improved survival, which were abolished by the ATG inducer, Rapamycin. TLR3-KO did not prevent ATG in the mouse heart. This study failed to detect inflammation in TLR3-KO-derived protection, as wild-type and TLR3-KO hearts were comparable in inflammatory activity, suggesting that upregulated TLR3 expression contributes to persistent ATG following MI, which promotes heart failure and lethality.

STIM1 Inhibitor ML9 Impairs ATG

Stromal-interaction molecule 1 (STIM1)-mediated store-operated Ca^{2+} entry (SOCE) plays a key role in mediating cardiomyocyte hypertrophy. SOCE is implicated in the Ca^{2+} overload associated with I/R injury. Shaikh et al. (2018) proposed STIM1 inhibition for controlling hypertrophy and I/R-induced Ca^{2+} overload to evaluate the effect of ML9, a STIM1 inhibitor, on cardiomyocyte survival. ML9 induced cell death in cultured neonatal rat cardiomyocytes. Caspase-3 activation, apoptotic index, and release of the necrosis marker LDH in the extracellular medium were evaluated. ML9-induced cardiomyocyte death was not associated with increased ROS or decreased ATP levels. Treatment with ML9 increased the ATG marker LC3-II, without altering Beclin-1 or p62 proteins. Treatment with ML9 followed by Bafilomycin-A1 did not produce further increases in LC3-II content. Treatment with ML9 decreased *LysoTracker®* Green staining, suggesting that cardiomyocyte death is triggered by a ML9-dependent impaired CP/ATG due to lysosomal dysfunction.

PINK1/Parkin-Mediated MTG

Recently, Kang et al. (2018) reported that Duchenne muscular dystrophy (DMD) is an inherited muscle disease with severe and often lethal cardiac complications. The evolution of the pathology in DMD is accompanied by the accumulation of mitochondria with a defective structure and function involving CBMP. Extensive structural damage of mitochondria and a significant decrease in ATP in the hearts of mdx animals led to the development of cardiomyopathy. Enhanced ATG and suppressed MTG were observed. Significantly decreased proteins involved in the PINK1/Parkin MTG pathway and insignificant Parkin protein phosphorylation at the S65 residue upon MTG induction, suggested defective MTG in dystrophic hearts due to the impaired PINK1/Parkin pathway.

Stress Response in CHF

Cardiac malfunction can occur as a result of an imbalance in proteostasis, the homeostatic balance between protein removal and regeneration during the remodeling process involving ER and UPR. Badreddin et al. (2018) discussed the importance of this with respect to an imbalance between muscle breakdown and repair in a stressful environment, especially as a result of RONS overproduction. The normal repair is a remodeling, but under this circumstance, the cell undergoes CP/ATG, or even necrosis instead of apoptosis. There exists an intimate relationship between the UPR pathway and CHF. The importance of mitochondria is not only limited to high energy dependence on ETC, but it also has a signaling role between the mitochondria and the ER under stress. Proteins made in the ER are folded by -SH and the electrostatic force of attraction and repulsion in the tertiary structure.

Small-vessel Vasculopathy in LAMP-2 Deficiency

LAMP2 is physiologically implicated in ATG. A genetic LAMP2 defect causes Danon disease, with myopathy and cardiomyopathy. Arterio-pathy may manifest on rare occasions. Nguyen et al.

(2018) investigated two Danon families that developed small-vessel vasculo-pathy in the coronary or cerebral arteries. They characterized the biological features of LAMP-2-deficient mice and cultured cells. LAMP-2-deficient mice at 9–24 months of age showed medial thickening with luminal stenosis due to the proliferation of VSMC in muscular arteries. Various ATG vacuoles were scattered throughout the cytoplasm, suggesting impaired ATG of long-lived metabolites and degraded mitochondria implicated in CBMP. The VSMC in LAMP2 null mice expressed more vimentin but less α-smooth muscle actin (α-SMA), indicating a switch from contractile to synthetic phenotype. Silencing of LAMP2 in cultured human brain VSMC showed the same phenotypic transition with mitochondrial fragmentation, enhanced mitochondrial respiration, and ROS overproduction, indicating that LAMP-2 deficiency leads to arterial medial hypertrophy with the phenotypic conversion of VSMC, resulting from the age-dependent accumulation of cellular waste generated by impaired CP/ATG.

Umbilical Vein Endothelial Cell Proteomics

The disorders of hemostasis and coagulation are the main contributors to the pathogenesis of pulmonary thromboembolism (PTE). Platelets regulate hemostasis and coagulation, and play important roles in thrombosis. Yue et al. (2019) investigated the proteome of human umbilical vein endothelial cells (HUVECs) with platelet endothelial aggregation receptor-1 (PEAR1) knockdown, using the isobaric tags for the relative and absolute quantitation (iTRAQ) method and analyzed the role of differential abundance proteins (DAPs) in the regulation of platelet aggregation. The conditioned media-culturing HUVECs with PEAR1 knockdown suppressed ADP-induced platelet aggregation. The proteomics analysis was performed by using the iTRAQ technique, and a total of 215 DAPs (124 proteins were upregulated and 91 proteins were downregulated) were identified. The gene ontology enrichment (GOE) analysis showed that proteins related to platelet α granule, ATP metabolism, and endocytosis were significantly enriched. The KEGG pathway analysis also helped identify the enrichment of endocytosis-related pathways. The RT-PCR analysis confirmed that the expression of $P2Y_{12}$, mitochondrial carrier 2, NADH dehydrogenase (ubiquinone) iron-sulfur protein 3, and ubiquinol-Cyt-C reductase hinge protein were downregulated in the HUVECs with PEAR1 knockdown, indicating that the DAPs induced by PEAR1 knockdown contribute to the platelet aggregation. Proteomic studies using GO enrichment and KEGG analysis suggested that the effects of DAPs on platelet aggregation may be linked to the balance of ADP synthesis or degradation in mitochondria.

Cardiac Fibrosis

Proteinopathy in the heart, which manifests excessive misfolded/aggregated proteins in cardiac myocytes, can result in severe fibrosis and heart failure. Chen et al. (2018) developed a mouse model, which express tetrameric DsRed, a red fluorescent protein (RFP), to mimic the pathological mechanisms of cardiac fibrosis. Whilst DsRed is expressed and forms aggregation in most mouse organs, certain pathological defects are recapitulated in cardiac muscle cells including mitochondria damage, aggresome-like residual bodies, ubiquitinated proteins, and the induction of ATG. The proteinopathy and cellular injuries caused by DsRed aggregates may be due to an impaired ubiquitin-proteasome system and ATG-lysosome systems. DsRed was ubiquitinated and associated with MuRF1, a muscle-specific E3 ligase. The concomitant activation of NF-κB signaling and TIMP1 induction were noted, suggesting that RFP-induced fibrosis was augmented by a skewed balance between TIMP1 and MMPs, highlighting the consequences of uncontrolled protein aggregation leading to CHF, and novel insights into fibrosis that can be targeted for improved therapy.

Cardiovascular Calcification

Cardiovascular calcification is a disorder with increasing prevalence and high morbidity and mortality. It is an active process, which provides an opportunity for effective theranostic targeting. The only available therapeutic options for calcific vascular and valvular heart disease are invasive trans-catheter procedures or surgeries that do not fully address the wide spectrum of these conditions; hence, an urgent need exists for novel theranostic interventions. Numerous biological processes are involved in calcific diseases, including matrix remodeling, transcriptional regulation, mitochondrial dysfunction, oxidative stress, Ca^{2+} and phosphate signaling, ERS, lipid and mineral metabolism, ATG, inflammation, apoptosis, loss of mineralization inhibition, impaired mineral resorption, cellular senescence, and extracellular vesicles that act as precursors of cardiovascular micro-calcification. Rogers and Aikawa (2019) discussed calcification processes in the cardiovascular system, based on patient data and imaging methods, experimental models, and omics data. They highlighted the potential and challenges of artificial intelligence, machine learning, and deep learning to integrate imaging and mechanistic data for novel drug discovery.

MQC in the Heart in Chronic Hypoxia

Mitochondrial bioenergetics (MB) is a regulatory mechanism in the heart under chronic hypoxia. The precise quantity and MQC is critical for the survival and function of cardiomyocytes. Zhang et al. (2018) investigated the role of AMPK in MTG regulation in cardiomyocytes under chronic hypoxia. H9c2 cells were cultured under hypoxic conditions (1% O_2) for different time periods. MB was confirmed and hypoxia induced $\Delta\Psi$ collapse and increased the number of dysfunctional mitochondria involved in CBMP. MTG was increased in cardiomyocytes exposed to hypoxic conditions for 48 hrs. AMPK was activated under hypoxia. When the activation of AMPK was enhanced by the AMPK agonist AICAR, MTG was also increased. However, when AMPK activation was blocked, MTG was decreased and cardiomyocyte apoptosis was increased. Hence, hypoxia-induced MTG induction played a crucial role in cardio-protection under chronic hypoxia. AMPK was involved in MTG regulation, thereby providing a potential theranostic target for CVDs associated with chronic hypoxia.

miR-27a-5p Attenuates Cardiomyocyte Injury

Acute myocardial infarction (AMI) is an ischemic heart disease with high mortality. AMI triggers a hypoxic microenvironment and induces myocardial injury, including ATG and apoptosis. The post-transcriptional regulators, miRNAs, are involved in the development of ischemic heart diseases. Zhang et al. (2018) reported that hypoxia alters the miRNA transcriptome in rat cardiomyoblast cells (H9c2), including miR-27a-5p. They investigated the role of miR-27a-5p in the cardiomyocyte response to hypoxia, and showed that its expression was downregulated in the H9c2 cells during hypoxia in the myocardium of AMI rat. MiR-27a-5p attenuated hypoxia-induced cardiomyocyte injury by regulating ATG and apoptosis via ATG7, indicating it has a cardio-protective effect on hypoxia-induced H9c2 cell injury, and is significant for the TSE-EBPT of hypoxia-related heart diseases.

Mst1 Knockout Enhances Cardiomyocyte ATG

AngII plays a central role in the pathogenesis of RAAS-induced heart failure. Mst1 exerts its function in cardiomyocytes subjected to pathological stimuli via inhibiting ATG and aggravating apoptosis. Cheng et al. (2018) determined whether cardiomyocyte-specific Mst1 knockout can alleviate AngII-induced cardiac injury by improving cardiomyocyte ATG and whether these functions depend on AngII receptors. Mst1 knockout alleviated AngII-induced heart failure, without affecting BP and compensatory hypertrophy. Mst1-specific knockout improved the effects of AngII on cardiomyocyte ATG, as evidenced by enhanced LC3-II expression and decreased P62 expression. The more typical APS, accompanied by less damaged mitochondria, were also detected in AngII-treated Mst1$^{\Delta/\Delta}$ mice. *In vitro*, Mst1 knockdown promoted cardiomyocyte ATG, as demonstrated by GFP-mRFP-LC3 puncta per cell. Increased LC3-II and decreased P62 expression in the presence and absence of CQ were observed in Mst1 knockdown cardiomyocytes administered with AngII. Treatment with 3-MA, an inhibitor of ATG, abolished the beneficial effects of Mst1 knockout against AngII-induced cardiac dysfunction. The compensatory effects of AngII on upregulated ATG were associated with Mst1 inhibition. The knockdown or AT$_1$R antagonists inhibited ATG, which may compromise cardiac function. Mst1 knockout enhanced cardiomyocyte ATG following the knockdown or blocking of AT$_1$R and AT$_2$R, indicating that cardiomyocyte-specific Mst1 knockout alleviates AngII-induced cardiac injury by enhancing ATG. Mst1 inhibition may counteract the undesirable effects of blockage of the AngII receptors on ATG and represent a complementary TSE-EBPT strategy in AngII-induced cardiac injury.

ERK-Drp-1 Signaling During Heart Failure

Mitochondrial dysfunction is a major contributor to myocyte loss and the development of heart failure. Myocytes have QC mechanisms to retain functional mitochondria by removing damaged mitochondria via specialized ATG, that is, CP. Huang et al. (2018) demonstrated the effect and potential mechanisms of mitochondrial functional defects associated with abnormal mitochondrial dynamics in heart failure. IGF-IIR signaling produced changes in mitochondrial morphology and function, associated with the altered expression and distribution of Drp-1 and Mfn-2. IGF-IIR signaled ERK activation to promote Drp-1 phosphorylation and translocation to mitochondria to induce CBMP. IGF-IIR signaling triggered Rab9-dependent CS formation by the JNK-mediated phosphorylation of Bcl-2 at serine 87 and promoted ULK1/Beclin-1-dependent CP/ATG membrane formation. Excessive mitochondrial fission by Drp-1 enhanced the Rab9-dependent CS recognition and engulfing of CBs and decreased cardiomyocyte viability, suggesting the connection between Rab9-dependent CS and mitochondrial fission in cardiac myocytes, which provides a potential TSE-EBPT strategy for treating heart disease.

Function and Regulation of Mitofusin 2

Yu et al. (2018) summarized the structural and functional properties of Mfn-2, with focus on recent advances in its regulatory role in the cardiovascular system. Mfn-2 is a dynamin-related protein whose activity promotes mitochondrial fusion and maintains the homeostasis of mitochondrial dynamics. Mfn-2 is a multifunctional protein with signaling roles beyond fusion. Mfn-2 is involved in various biological processes under both physical and pathological conditions, including mitochondrial transport and the interaction between ER/SER and mitochondria, as well as cell metabolism, apoptosis, and CP/ATG.

Age-Dependent Cardiac Function in Sepsis

Age represents a major risk factor for multiple organ failure, including cardiac dysfunction, in patients with sepsis. AMPK is a key regulator of energy homeostasis that controls MB by activation of the PPAR-γ coactivator-1α and disposal of defective organelles by ATG. Inata et al. (2018) investigated whether AMPK dysregulation contributes to age-dependent cardiac injury in young (2–3 mo) and mature adult (11–13 mo) male mice subjected to sepsis by cecal ligation and puncture and whether AMPK activation by 5-amino-4-imidazole carboxamide riboside conferred cardio-protection. Plasma pro-inflammatory cytokines and myokine follistatin were elevated in vehicle-treated young and mature adult mice at 18 hrs after sepsis. However, despite equivalent troponin I and T levels compared with similarly treated young mice, vehicle-treated mature adult mice exhibited more severe cardiac damage with intercellular edema, inflammatory cell infiltration, and mitochondrial derangement involving CBMP. ECoG revealed that vehicle-treated young mice exhibited left ventricular dysfunction after sepsis, whereas mature adult mice exhibited a reduction in stroke volume without changes in load-dependent indexes of cardiac function. Phosphorylation of the catalytic subunits AMPK-α_1/α_2 was associated with nuclear translocation of PPAR-γ coactivator-1α in vehicle-treated young but not mature adult mice. Treatment with 5-amino-4-imidazole carboxamide riboside ameliorated cardiac architecture derangement in mice of both ages. The protective effects were associated with attenuation of the systemic inflammation and amelioration of cardiac dysfunction in young mice but not in the mature adult animals, suggesting that sepsis-induced cardiac dysfunction manifests with age-dependent characteristics, associated with the regulation of AMPK-dependent metabolic pathways. Hence, age-related deterioration and pharmacological activation of AMPK may influence protective effects.

α7nACh Receptor Activation in Myocardial I/R Injury

Hou et al. (2018) investigated the role of ATG in α7nAChR-mediated cardio-protection. Activating α7nAChR with PNU-282987 at the initiation of reperfusion reduced infarct size in I/R rats. PNU-282987 treatment also inhibited I/R-induced ATG dysfunction as evidenced by the reduction of LC3-II/LC3-I ratio, Beclin-1 and p62 abundance. In addition, PNU-282987 treatment reduced H/R-induced cardiomyocyte injury *in vitro*, accompanied with the inhibition of Beclin-1-associated ATG and the restoration of ATG. Inhibiting ATG attenuated α7nAChR-afforded improvement of mitochondrial function as well as inhibition of apoptosis *in vitro*. Co-administration of PNU-282987 with LY294002 (a PI3K inhibitor), AG490 (a JAK2 inhibitor), or Bcl-2 siRNA, but not compound C (an AMPK inhibitor), reduced Bcl-2 and prevented PNU-282987-mediated ATG modulation in H/R cardiomyocytes, suggesting that α7nAChR activation inhibits Beclin-1-associated CP/ATG dysfunction via the JAK2/Bcl-2 and PI3K/Bcl-2 cascades, leading to cardio-protection in I/R injury.

PINK1 Alleviates Ang-II-induced Cardiac Injury

PINK1 is efficiently degraded in normal mitochondria but accumulates in damaged mitochondria participating in CB formation, triggering CP/ATG to protect cells. Xiong et al. (2018) investigated the function of PINK1 in an AngII stimulation model and its regulation of AngII-induced CP. They studied the function of PINK1 in MQC in AngII-stimulated cardiomyocytes via siRNA-mediated knockdown and adenovirus-mediated over-expression of the PINK1 protein. $\Delta\Psi$, ROS production, ATP, apoptosis rates, and cardiomyocyte hypertrophy were measured, in addition to the expression of LC3B, Beclin-1, and p62. Endogenous PINK1, phosphorylated PINK1, mito-PINK1, total Parkin, cyto-Parkin, mito-Parkin and increased Parkin protein phosphorylation. Cardiomyocytes untreated by AngII had very low levels of total and phosphorylated PINK1. However, in the AngII stimulation model, the $\Delta\Psi$ was decreased, and the total and phosphorylated PINK1 were increased. Knocking down PINK-1 inhibited mitochondrial Parkin translocation. Phosphorylated Parkin was reduced, and ATG markers were downregulated. ATP and $\Delta\Psi$ were further reduced, ROS production and the apoptotic rate were increased, and myocardial hypertrophy was aggravated compared with those in the AngII group. However, PINK1 overexpression promoted Parkin translocation and phosphorylation, ATG markers were upregulated, and myocardial injury was reduced. The effects of PINK1 overexpression were reversed by ATG inhibitors. Decreased $\Delta\Psi$ induced by AngII maintained the stability of PINK1, causing PINK1 auto-phosphorylation. PINK1 activation promoted Parkin translocation and phosphorylation and increased CP to eliminate CBs. Thus, PINK1/Parkin-mediated CP conferred a compensatory, protective role in Ang-II-induced cytotoxicity.

ATG Modulation to Treat CVDs

Madrigal-Matute et al. (2018) highlighted that ATG evolved to acquire far more diverse functions than the original response to nutrient depletion. ATG, a process in which almost every cellular compartment, including organelles, are transported to lysosomes for recycling, is essential for MQC and ICD. Three main types of ATG exist: macroautophagy, chaperone-mediated ATG (CMA), and microATG. Nonetheless, almost all research in the cardiovascular system has focused on macroATG, in which double-membrane vesicles, called APS, transport molecules and organelles to lysosomes to be degraded and recycled. MacroATG is also a regulator in the vasculature, preventing progression of atherosclerosis via efferocytosis. CMA is another highly selective type of ATG in which chaperones bind to recognition motifs in specific proteins and transport them to lysosomes for recycling. CMA plays a regulatory role in glucose and lipid metabolism. MacroATG and CMA are differentially modulated by various stresses in a context-dependent manner, and any failure in this regulation can contribute to the pathogenesis of CVDs. It was hypothesized that: (i) autosis, a novel form of cell death by ATG is important in the pathogenesis of ischemic injury, heart failure, and atherosclerosis; (ii) CMA and cardiovascular metabolism reciprocally modulate each other's functions; (iii) MTG and mitochondria reciprocally modulate each other's functions; and (iv) specific modulators of macroATG, CMA, and autosis can provide novel therapies for CVD. To address these hypotheses, we need to: (i) determine the contribution of autosis, as well as other forms of ATG-related cell death, to the pathogenesis of CVD; (ii) delineate the roles of macroATG and CMA as mediators of the metabolic derangements in CVD and the dysregulation of ATG by alterations in the cardiovascular metabolism; (iii) identify molecular mechanisms mediating MTG and its contribution to the pathogenesis of CVD; and (iv) determine whether manipulation of macroATG, CMA, and autosis can provide novel theranostics to CVD. Disruption of the regulatory complex formed by Beclin-1 and BCL2 promotes extended lifespan and improved health span, reducing cardiac alterations in aging mice with increased ATG. Aspirin has recently been shown to recapitulate the effects of CRM. Another CRM, Trehalose, reduces MI-induced cardiac remodeling through ATG induction. Trehalose improved both systolic and diastolic left ventricular functioning by reducing cardiac hypertrophy, apoptosis, and fibrosis. Particularly, the exact theranostic significance impaired CP-driven apoptosis (also named charnoptosis), involving CBMP in various CVDs and other chronic diseases needs further investigations.

Theranostic Significance of Antioxidants, Physiological, and Drug-induced CP Regulation in CVDs

H_2S-mediated Regulation of Cell Death

The cardiomyocytes demise is a precursor for the cascade of hypertrophic and fibrotic remodeling that leads to cardiomyopathy. In diabetes mellitus (DM), hyperglycemia, hyperlipidemia, and oxidative stress causes cardiomyocyte demise, leading to diabetic cardiomyopathy (DMCM). Understanding the roles of the cell death signaling pathways involved in the development of cardiomyopathies is crucial to the discovery of novel biomarkers and TSE-EBPT of DMCM. H_2S, an endogenous gaseous molecule, has cardio-protective effects. Kar ct al. (2019) focused on H_2S in the signaling of apoptotic, ATG, necroptotic, and pyroptotic cell death in DMCM and other cardiomyopathies, abnormalities in H_2S synthesis in DM, and potential H_2S-based theranostic strategies to mitigate myocardial cell death to ameliorate DMCM.

Melatonin Normalizes LPS-induced Cardiomyopathy

To explore the mechanism of mitochondrial UCP2 mediating the protective effect of melatonin in septic cardiomyopathy, Pan et al. (2018b) used UCP2 knocked out mice and cardiomyocytes to study the effect of melatonin in response to LPS. Indicators of myocardial and mitochondrial injury, including $\Delta\Psi$, mitochondrial permeability transition pore, Ca^{2+} loading, ROS, and ATP were estimated. In addition, cell viability and apoptosis and ATG-associated proteins were evaluated. Melatonin protected heart function from LPS, which was attenuated in the UCP2-knockout mice. Genipin, a pharmacologic inhibitor of UCP2, augmented LPS-induced damage of AC16 cells. Melatonin upregulated UCP2 expression and protected the cells from the changes in morphology, $\Delta\Psi$ collapse, $[Ca^{2+}]_m$ overload, the opening of mPTP, increased ROS generation, and ATP depletion. ATG proteins (Beclin-1 and LC-3β) were increased while apoptosis-associated proteins (Cyt-C and caspase-3) were decreased when UCP2 was upregulated, indicating that UCP2 may play a protective role in LPS septicemia by regulating ATG and apoptosis in cardiomyocytes, and may contribute to homeostasis of cardiac function and cardio-myocytes activity by modulating UCP2.

Ginsenoside Rb1 Alleviates Vascular Endothelium Senescence

Oxidative LDL (ox-LDL) induces endothelium senescence and promotes atherosclerosis. Ginsenoside Rb1 (gRb1) protects HUVECs. Shi et al. (2019) explored SIRT1/Beclin-1/ATG axis in gRb1-mediated protection of endothelium in Ox-LDL-induced senescence. Hyperlipidemia in SD rats was induced by HFD and gRb1 was injected in the i.p. Ox-LDL-induced senescence model of HUVECs. gRb1 alleviated hyperlipidemia-induced endothelial senescence, Ox-LDL-induced HUVECs' senescence, and restored SIRT1 and ATG, which were involved in the senescence retardation. Beclin-1 acetylation was reduced, and the correlation between SIRT1 and Beclin-1 was increased, suggesting the anti-senescence function of gRb1 in the endothelium and hyperlipidemia through the SIRT1/Beclin-1/ATG pathway.

Cardio-protective Effects of Sirt1

Sirtuin 1 (Sirt1) exerts its protective effects on various CVDs via multiple cellular pathways. Luo et al. (2019) investigated the Sirt1-mediated regulation of ATG and apoptosis in hypoxic H9C2 cardiomyocytes and in the hypoxic mouse model. Right ventricular outflow tract biopsies were obtained from patients with cyanotic or acyanotic congenital heart diseases. Adenovirus AdSirt1 was used to activate Sirt1 and AdShSirt1 was used to inhibit Sirt1 expression in H9C2 cells to investigate the effect of Sirt1 on ATG and apoptosis. SRT1720, a pharmacological activator of Sirt1 and EX527, a Sirt1 antagonist, were administered to mice to explore their roles in creating hypoxic cardiomyocytes *in vivo*. Heart tissue samples from cyanotic patients exhibited increased ATG and apoptosis, as well as elevated Sirt1 levels. Sirt1 promoted ATG flux and reduced apoptosis in hypoxic H9C2 cells. In addition, Sirt1 activated AMPK, and the AMPK inhibitor, Compound C, abolished the effect of Sirt1 on ATG induction. Sirt1 protected hypoxic cardiomyocytes from apoptosis through inositol requiring kinase enzyme 1α (IRE1α). Treatment with the Sirt1 activator SRT1720 activated AMPK, inhibited IRE1α, enhanced ATG, and decreased apoptosis in the heart tissues of normoxic mice compared with the hypoxia control group. Opposite changes were observed in hypoxic mice treated with the Sirt1 inhibitor EX527, suggesting that Sirt1 promoted ATG via AMPK activation and reduced hypoxia-induced apoptosis via the IRE1α pathway, to protect cardiomyocytes from hypoxic stress.

Gastrodin Alleviates Myocardial I/R Injury

It has been proposed that Gastrodin (GAS), a monomeric component extracted from the herb Gastrodia elata Bl, may have cardio-protective effects in myocardial I/R injury. Fu et al. (2018) investigated male C57BL/6 mice which were subjected to reversible left coronary artery ligation and cultured neonatal rat cardiomyocytes (NRCs) exposed to hypoxia and were preconditioned with GAS prior to ischemia or hypoxia, following reperfusion for 2 hrs or re-oxygenation for 3 hrs, respectively. The GAS pretreatment increased ATG and reduced apoptosis during I/R; this effect was attenuated by co-treatment with the ATG inhibitor, CQ. Compared to mice subjected solely to I/R, GAS-pretreated mice had smaller infarct size and elevated cardiac function. In GAS-pretreated NRCs, ATG was promoted (expression of p62 was inhibited and LC3-II was increased). Tandem fluorescent mRFP-GFP-LC3 assays revealed that APS were degraded due to an increase in ATG flux. The co-administration of CQ blocked ARG. The GAS pretreatment increased $\Delta\Psi$ of NRCs subjected to H/R and increased the cardiomyocyte survival rate which were reversed with CQ. Besides, the GAS-induced ATG may be correlated with activating AMPK phosphorylation and reducing mTOR phosphorylation, which were abrogated by Compound C (AMPK-specific *inhibitor*), to establish that GAS pretreatment attenuates I/R injury by increasing ATG by eliminating CBs to protect penumbral mitochondria and cardiomyocytes.

Beclin-1-Dependent CP/ATG Protects the Heart During Sepsis

Cardiac dysfunction is a major component of sepsis-induced multi-organ failure in critical care units. Sun et al. (2018b) reported that Beclin-1-dependent ATG in the heart during sepsis and the therapeutic benefit of targeting this pathway were investigated in a mouse model of LPS-induced sepsis. LPS induced increase in CP/ATG at low doses, followed by a decline that was in conjunction with mTOR activation at high doses. The cardiac-specific overexpression of Beclin-1 promoted ATG, suppressed mTOR signaling, improved cardiac function, and alleviated inflammation and fibrosis following the LPS challenge. Haplo-sufficiency for Beclin-1 resulted in opposite effects including cardiac-specific suppression of Beclin-1, ATG inhibition, impaired cardiovascular function, enhanced inflammation, and fibrosis following LPS challenge. Beclin-1 also protected mitochondria, reduced the release of DAMPs, and promoted MTG via PINK1-Parkin but not adaptor proteins in response to LPS. The injection of a cell-permeable Tat-Beclin-1 peptide to induce ATG improved cardiac function, attenuated inflammation, and rescued the phenotypes caused by Beclin-1 deficiency in LPS-challenged mice, suggesting that Beclin-1 protects the heart during sepsis and that the targeted induction of Beclin-1 may have TSE-EBPT potential in sepsis-induced multi-organ failure.

Mitochondria and Sex-specific Cardiac Function

Mitochondrial disorders are affected by mutations in either nuclear or mitochondrial genes involved in the synthesis of respiratory chain subunits or in their post-translational control. Vona et al. (2018) presented evidence for the involvement of mitochondria in the sex specificity of CVDs, which can be due to mutations of the mtDNA transmitted by the mother or mutations in the nDNA. Because natural selection on mitochondria operates only in females, mutations may have more deleterious effects in males than in females. As mitochondrial mutations can affect all tissues, they are responsible for a large panel of pathologies including neuromuscular disorders, encephalopathies, metabolic disorders, cardiomyopathies, neuropathies, renal, and reproductive dysfunction, etc. Many of these pathologies present sex/gender specificity. Thus, alleviating or preventing mitochondrial dysfunction will mitigate the severity or progression in the development of diseases.

Estrogen Inhibits Bnip-3-induced Apoptosis

The ATG in the cardiomyocytes maintains homeostasis during cellular stress such as hypoxia by removing aggregated proteins and damaged organelles and thereby protects the heart during starvation and ischemia. However, ATG can lead to cell death under certain circumstances. BCL2/ adenovirus E1B 19 kDa protein-interacting protein 3 (Bnip-3), a hypoxia-induced biomarker induces both CP/ATG and apoptosis. A Bnip-3-docked organelle, for example, mitochondria, also determines whether ATG or apoptosis will take place. Estrogen (E2) and estrogen receptor (ER) α (E2 & ERα) protect the heart in mitochondria-dependent apoptosis. Chen et al. (2018) investigated the mechanisms by which ER&α; regulates Bnip-3-induced apoptosis and ATG, which were associated with hypoxic injury, in cardio-myoblasts. An *in vitro* model to mimic hypoxic injury in the heart by engineering H9c2 cardio-myoblasts to overexpress Bnip-3 was established. Further, the effects of E2 and ER&α; in Bnip-3-induced apoptosis and ATG were determined in Bnip-3-expressing H9c2 cells. ER&α;/E2 suppressed Bnip-3-induced apoptosis and ATG. ER&α/E2 decreased caspase 3 (apoptotic marker), Atg5, and LC3-II (ATG markers). Co-immunoprecipitation of Bnip-3 and immunoblotting of Bcl-2 and Rheb showed that ER&α; reduced the interaction between Bnip-3 and Bcl-2 or Rheb, confirming that ER&α; binds to Bnip-3, causing a reduction in Bnip-3 and thereby inhibiting ATG and apoptosis. In addition, ER&α attenuated Bnip-3 promoter activity by binding to SP-1 or NF&$\kappa\beta$ sites.

p53 Inhibition Attenuates Myocardial I/R Injury

p53 is well known as a regulator of apoptosis and ATG and is a modulator of the opening of the mPTP, a trigger for necrosis. Yano et al. (2018) determined the role of p53 in acute myocardial I/R injury in perfused mouse hearts. In male C57BL6 mice between 12 and 15 weeks of age, two types of p53 inhibitors were used to suppress p53 function during I/R: Pifithrin-α, an inhibitor of transcriptional functions of p53, and Pifithrin-μ, an inhibitor of p53 translocation from the cytosol to mitochondria. Neither infusion of these inhibitors before ischemia nor for the first 30 min period of reperfusion reduced infarct size after 20 min ischemia/ 120 min reperfusion. Infarct sizes were similar in p53 heterozygous knockout mice (p53$^{+/-}$) and wild-type mice (WT), but recovery of the rate pressure product (RRP) 120 min after reperfusion was higher in p53$^{+/-}$ than in WT. The protein expression of p53 in WT was negligible under baseline conditions, during ischemia, and at 10 min after initiating reperfusion, but it became detectable at 120 min after reperfusion, indicating that upregulation of p53 during the late phase of reperfusion plays a significant role in contractile dysfunction after reperfusion. However, p53 was not involved in cardiomyocyte necrosis during ischemia or in the early phase of reperfusion.

Parkin-mediated MTG in Cardio-protection

Late exercise preconditioning (LEP) has a protective effect on acute cardiovascular stress. LEP may involve MTG mediated by the receptors PARK2 gene-encoded E3 ubiquitin ligase (Parkin) and BCL2/adenovirus E1B 19 kDa protein-interacting protein 3 (Bnip-3) to scavenge CBs. Yuan et al. (2018) prepared an EP protocol which involved four 10 min periods of running, separated by 10 min recovery intervals, plus a period of exhaustive running at 24 hrs after EP. They assessed this late protective effect by injection of the ATG inhibitor Wortmannin by using TEM, laser scanning confocal microscopy, and other molecular biotechnology methods to detect related biomarkers, specific relationships between MTG proteins, and mitochondrial translocation. Exhaustive exercise (EE) caused serious injuries to cardio-myofibrils, inducing hypoxic-ischemia and changing their ultrastructure. EE failed to clear CBs' accompanied with LC3 accumulation. LEP suppressed EE-induced injuries, as confirmed by reduced mitochondrial-localized proteins COX4/1 and TOM20. LEP exhaustion caused mitochondrial degradation by increasing LC3-OMM translocation in a Parkin-dependent manner, where activated protein kinase and TOM70 may play key roles. However, MTG was not associated with Bnip-3-mediated LEP-induced cardio-protection. Hence, Bnip-3 may play a role in inducing mitochondrial LC3-II increase. Wortmannin had no effect on LC3 translocation; instead, it influenced LC3-I to convert to LC3-II. Thus, suppressing MTG caused attenuation of EP-induced cardio-protection.

Rab9 Protects the Heart in Ischemia

Saito et al. (2019) showed that CP during myocardial ischemia is mediated through ATG characterized by Rab9-associated autophagosome (APS), rather than the well-characterized form of ATG that is dependent on the ATG-related 7 (ATG) conjugation system and LC3. This form of ATG played a role in protecting the heart in ischemia and was mediated by a complex consisting of unc-51 like kinase 1 (Ulk1), Rab9, receptor-interacting serine/thronine protein kinase 1 (Rip1), and Drp-1, which allowed the recruitment of trans-Golgi membranes associated with Rab9 to damaged mitochondria through the S179 phosphorylation of Rab9 by Ulk1 and S616 phosphorylation of Drp-1 by Rip1. Knockin of Rab9 (S179A) abolished CP and exacerbated the injury in response to myocardial ischemia, without affecting general ATG. CP mediated through the Ulk1/Rab9/Rip1/Drp-1 pathway protected the heart in ischemia by maintaining MQC.

Humanin Activates Chaperone-mediated ATG

Chaperone-mediated ATG (CMA) serves as a QC mechanism during stress through selective degradation of cytosolic proteins in lysosomes. Humanin (HN) as a mitochondria-associated peptide offers cyto-protective, cardio-protective, and neuro-protective effects *in vivo* and *in vitro*. Gong et al. (2018) demonstrated that HN activates CMA by increasing substrate binding and translocation into lysosomes. The potent HN analogue HNG protects from stressor-induced cell death in fibroblasts, cardiomyoblasts, neuronal cells, and primary cardiomyocytes. The protective effects were lost in CMA-deficient cells, suggesting that they are mediated through the activation of CMA. A fraction of endogenous HN was present at the cytosolic side of the lysosomal membrane, where it interacted with HSP-90 and stabilized binding of this chaperone to membrane-bound CMA substrates. Inhibition of HSP-90 blocked the effect of HNG on substrate translocation and abolished the cyto-protective effects, suggesting a novel mechanism by which HN exerts its cardioprotective and neuroprotective effects.

DUSP1 Alleviates Cardiac I/R Injury

Mitochondrial fission and MTG form an axis of MQC that plays a critical role in the development of cardiac IR injury. Dual-specificity protein phosphatase1 (DUSP1) regulates cardiac metabolism. Jin et al. (2018) demonstrated that cardiac DUSP1 was downregulated following acute cardiac IR injury. DUSP1 transgenic mice (DUSP1^{TG} mice) demonstrated a smaller infarcted area and improved myocardial function. The IR-induced DUSP1 deficiency promoted the activation of JNK which upregulated the expression of the mitochondrial fission factor (Mff). Increased Mff expression was associated with elevated mitochondrial fission and apoptosis. The loss of DUSP1 also amplified the Bnip-3 phosphorylated activation via JNK, leading to the activation of MTG. Increased MTG consumed mitochondrial mass, resulting in mitochondrial metabolism disorder. However, the reintroduction of DUSP1 blunted Mff/Bnip-3 activation and alleviated the fatal mitochondrial fission/MTG by inactivating the JNK pathway, providing a survival advantage to myocardial tissue following IR stress, suggesting that DUSP1 and JNK pathway are theranostic targets for protection in IR injury by repressing Mff-mediated mitochondrial fission and Bnip-3-mediated MTG.

FKBP8 Protects Heart

PQC in cardiomyocytes is crucial for maintaining cellular homeostasis. The accumulation of damaged organelles, such as mitochondria and misfolded proteins, in the heart is associated with heart failure. During identification of MTG receptors, Misaka et al. (2018) found the FK506-binding protein 8 (FKBP8), also known as FKBP38, shares similar structural characteristics with a yeast MTG receptor, ATG-related 32 protein. However, knockdown of FKBP8 had no effect on MTG in HEK293 cells or H9c2 myocytes. They determined the role of FKBP8 in the heart. These investigators generated mice with the Fkbp8$^{-/-}$ allele and crossed them with mice expressing α-myosin heavy chain promoter-driven Cre recombinase transgenic mice (αMHC-Cre) to obtain cardiac-specific FKBP8-deficient mice. Fkbp8$^{-/-}$ mice showed no cardiac phenotypes under baseline conditions. The Fkbp8$^{-/-}$ and control wild type littermates (Fkbp8$^{+/+}$) mice were subjected to pressure overload by means of transverse aortic constriction (TAC). Fkbp8$^{-/-}$ mice showed left ventricular dysfunction and chamber dilatation with lung congestion one week after TAC. The number of apoptotic cardiomyocytes was elevated in TAC-operated Fkbp8$^{-/-}$ hearts, accompanied with an increase in cleaved caspase-12 and ERS markers. Caspase-12 inhibition resulted in the attenuation of H_2O_2-induced apoptotic cell death in FKBP8 knockdown H9c2 myocytes. FKBP8 is localized to the ER and mitochondria in the isolated cardiomyocytes, where it interacts with HSP-90. Furthermore, there was accumulation of misfolded protein aggregates in FKBP8 knockdown H9c2 myocytes and electron-dense deposits in the perinuclear region in TAC-operated Fkbp8$^{-/-}$ hearts, suggesting that FKBP8 plays a protective role in hemodynamic stress mediated via inhibition of the accumulation of misfolded proteins and ER-associated apoptosis.

Irisin Alleviates Cardiac Hypertrophy

In hypertrophic hearts, ATG flux insufficiency is a key pathology leading to maladaptive cardiac remodeling and heart failure. Li et al. (2018) investigated the protective role of a new myokine and adipokine, Irisin, in cardiac hypertrophy and remodeling. Adult male wild-type mouse, FNDC5 (Irisin-precursor)-knockout, and FNDC5 transgenic mice received four weeks of transverse aortic constriction (TAC), alone or in combination with CP inhibitor, Chloroquine (CQ) i.p. Endogenous FNDC5 ablation aggravated and exogenous FNDC5 overexpression attenuated the TAC-induced hypertrophic damage, which was comparable to the protection of Irisin against cardiomyocyte hypertrophy induced by AngII or Phenylephrine (PE). Accumulated autophagosome and impaired ATG occurred in the TAC-treated myocardium and AngII- or PE-insulted cardiomyocytes. Irisin deficiency caused reduced ATG and aggravated ATG flux failure, whereas, Irisin overexpression or supplementation-induced protective and improved ATG, were reversed by ATG inhibitors, Atg5 siRNA, 3-MA, and CQ. Irisin induced AMPK but not Akt and MAPK family members in hypertrophic hearts and cultured cardiomyocytes and further activated ULK1 at Ser555 but not Ser757 and did not affect the mTOR-S6K axis. Blockage of AMPK and ULK1 with compound C and SBI-0206965, respectively, abrogated Irisin's protection in cardiomyocyte hypertrophic injury and reversed CP/ATG, suggesting that Irisin protects in pressure overload-induced cardiac hypertrophy by inducing protective CP/ATG via activating AMPK-ULK1 signaling.

Empagliflozin in Diabetic Hearts

To explore mechanisms by which SGLT2 inhibitors protect diabetic hearts from heart failure, Mizuno et al. (2018) examined the effect of Empagliflozin (Empa) on the ultrastructure of cardiomyocytes in the non-infarcted region of the diabetic heart after MI. OLETF, a rat model of T2DM, and its nondiabetic control, LETO, received a sham operation or left coronary artery ligation 12 hrs before tissue sampling. Tissues were sampled from the posterior ventricle (that is, the remote non-infarcted region in rats with MI). The number of mitochondria was larger and small mitochondria were more prevalent in OLETF than in LETO. The Fis1 expression level was higher in OLETF than in LETO, while phospho-Ser637-Drp-1, total Drp-1, Mfn-1/2, and OPA1 levels were comparable. MI further reduced the mitochondrial size with increased Drp-1-Ser616 phosphorylation in OLETF. The number of ATG vacuoles was unchanged after MI in LETO but was decreased in OLETF. LDs in cardiomyocytes and tissue triglycerides were increased in OLETF. Empa (10 mg/kg per day) reduced blood glucose and triglycerides and increased LDs in cardiomyocytes in OLETF. Empa suppressed Fis1 upregulation, increased Bnip-3 expression, and prevented reduction in both mitochondrial size and ATG after MI in OLETF, indicating that along with upregulation of SOD2 and catalase by Empa, Empa normalizes the size and number of mitochondria in diabetic hearts and diabetes-induced reduction in mitochondrial size after MI was prevented by it via suppression of ROS and CP/ATG restoration.

Thymoquinone in Cardiac Damage

Sepsis is a major health complication causing mortality due to cardiac dysfunction and increased healthcare costs. Thymoquinone (TQ) offers protection during hyperlipidemia and Dox-induced cardiac damage. Liu et al. (2019) investigated these protective effects of TQ during cardiac damage in septic BALB/c mice. Eight-week-old male BALB/c mice were divided into four groups: control, TQ, cecal ligation and puncture (CLP), and TQ+CLP. CLP was performed after a two-week TQ gavage. After 48 hrs, they measured the histopathological alterations of the cardiac tissue and the plasma troponin-T (cTnT) and ATP. ATG (p62 and Beclin-1), pyroptosis (NLRP3, caspase-1, IL-1β, and IL-18) at the gene and protein levels and IL-6 and TNF-α at the gene level were evaluated. TQ reduced intestinal histological alterations, inhibited plasma cTnT levels, improved ATP, inhibited p62, NLRP3, caspase-1, IL-1β, IL-18, IL-6, TNF-α, and MCP-1expressions, and increased Beclin-1 and IL-10 level. The PI3-kinase was significantly decreased in the TQ+CLP group versus the CLP group, suggesting that TQ modulates ATG, pyroptosis, and pro-inflammatory response, suggesting its clinical significance in the treatment of sepsis-induced cardiac damage.

Pitavastatin Attenuates AGEs-Induced MTG

Zha et al. (2018) investigated whether Pitavastatin protected in advanced glycation end products (AGEs)-induced injury in neonatal rat cardiomyocytes. Cardiomyocytes of neonatal rats were incubated for 48 hrs with AGEs (100 µg/mL),), an antibody called the receptor for advanced glycation end products (RAGE) (1 µg/mL), and Pitavastatin (600 ng/mL). In the AGEs group, Beclin-1 expression was increased, while p62 expression was decreased. AGEs also decreased $\Delta\Psi$ and increased ROS. Following treatment with either the RAGE antibody or Pitavastatin, Beclin-1 was decreased compared with the AGEs group, but p62 was increased. In the AGEs+ RAGE antibody group and AGEs+ Pitavastatin group, $\Delta\Psi$ was increased and ROS was decreased compared with the AGEs group, indicating that AGEs-RAGE may induce ATG by ROS generation and Pitavastatin could protect in AGEs-induced injury in cardiomyocytes.

Cardioprotection by Exercise Preconditioning

Early exercise preconditioning (EEP) imparts a protective effect on acute cardiovascular stress. EEP may involve mitochondrial protection, which interacts with H_2O_2 oxidative stress. Yuan et al. (2018) used EEP protocol involving four periods of 10 min running with 10 min recovery intervals. A period of exhaustive running and a pretreatment using PI3K/ATG inhibitor Wortmannin was added to test this protective effect. Exhaustive exercise was associated with elevated myocardial injuries, oxidative stress, hypoxia-ischemia, and abnormal mitochondrial ultrastructure. However, exhaustion induced limited mitochondrial protection in a H_2O_2-independent manner to inhibit voltage-dependent anion channel isoform 1 (VDAC1) instead of CP. EEP was safe for the heart and provided suppression of exhaustive exercise (EE) injuries by translocating Bnip-3 to the mitochondria by recruiting the autophagosome protein LC3 to induce CP, which was triggered by H_2O_2 and influenced Beclin-1-dependent ATG. Pretreatment with the Wortmannin attenuated these effects and resulted in the expression of pro-apoptotic phenotypes such as oxidative injury, elevated Beclin-1/Bcl-2 ratio, Cyt-C leakage, Drp-1 expression, and VDAC1 dephosphorylation, suggesting that H_2O_2 regulates mitochondrial protection in EEP-induced cardioprotection.

Cardiac ATG and Increased Exercise Capacity

To investigate whether high-intensity interval training (HIIT) and continuous moderate-intensity training (CMT) have differential impacts on exercise performance and cardiac function and to determine the influence of these interventions on modulating basal ATG in the cardiac muscle, Li et al. (2018) used three groups of rats: sedentary control (SC), CMT, and HIIT. The total exercise volume and mean intensity were matched between the two protocols. After a 10 week training program, rats were evaluated for exercise performance, including exercise tolerance and grip strength. Blood lactate levels were measured after an incremental exercise test. Cardiac function and morphology were assessed by ECoG. The time to exhaustion and grip strength increased significantly in the HIIT group compared with the SC and CMT groups. Both training interventions increased time to exhaustion, reduced blood lactate (after an incremental exercise test), and induced adaptive changes in cardiac morphology, but without altering cardiac systolic function. The greater improvements in exercise performance with the HIIT than with the CMT protocol were related to improvement in basal ATG adaptation and mitochondria function in cardiac muscle. Mitochondrial biomarkers were positively correlated with ATG biomarkers, suggesting that HIIT is more effective in improving exercise performance than CMT and is related to mitochondrial function and basal CP/ATG adaptation in cardiac muscle.

Treatment of Sarcopenia in CHF

Sarcopenia is an age-related geriatric syndrome characterized by a loss of muscle mass, strength, and function. CHF, the final stage of various CVDs, may be correlated to sarcopenia. Sarcopenia and CHF are mutually interacting clinical syndromes. Patients with these two syndromes endure a double burden, with no effective way to halt their progression. Yin et al. (2019) highlighted the latest development in the pathogenesis and treatment of sarcopenia in patients with CHF which promotes sarcopenia through multiple pathophysiological mechanisms, including malnutrition, inflammation, hormonal changes, oxidative stress, dysregulated CP, and apoptosis. CHF can aggravate the adverse outcomes associated with sarcopenia, including falls, osteoporosis, frailty, cachexia, hospitalization, and mortality. However, physical exercise, nutritional supplements, and drug therapy may counteract the development of these maladies.

Theranostic Potential of Antioxidants and other Agents in Congential Syndromes with CVDs

Resveratrol in Marfan Syndrome

Marfan syndrome (MFS) patients are at risk for CVDs. In particular, for aortic aneurysms, resulting in a life-threatening aortic dissection or rupture. The biologically potent polyphenol,

Resveratrol (RES), is found in nuts, plants, and grapes skin, and has a positive effect on aortic repair in rodent aneurysm models (van Adel et al. 2019). RES seemed to affect aortic integrity and dilatation. The beneficial processes relevant for MFS included the improvement of endothelial dysfunction, extracellular matrix degradation, and smooth muscle cell death. Evidence was found for the following pathways: alleviating oxidative stress (change in eNOS/iNOS balance and decrease in NOX4), reducing protease activity to preserve the extracellular matrix (decrease in MMP2), and improving smooth muscle cell survival, and thus affecting aortic aging (changing the miR21/miR29 balance). MFS patients may also suffer from mitral valve prolapse and left ventricular impairment, where evidence from rodent models shows that RES may aid in promoting cardiomyocyte survival directly (by SIRT1 activation or by reducing oxidative stress by increasing SOD) and increasing AMPK activation. These investigators discussed recent RES studies in animal models of aortic aneurysm and heart failure, where advantageous effects were reported that may improve the aortic and cardiac pathology in patients with MFS. The theranostic potential of Resveratrol in Marfan syndrome with CVDs is presented in Fig. 34.

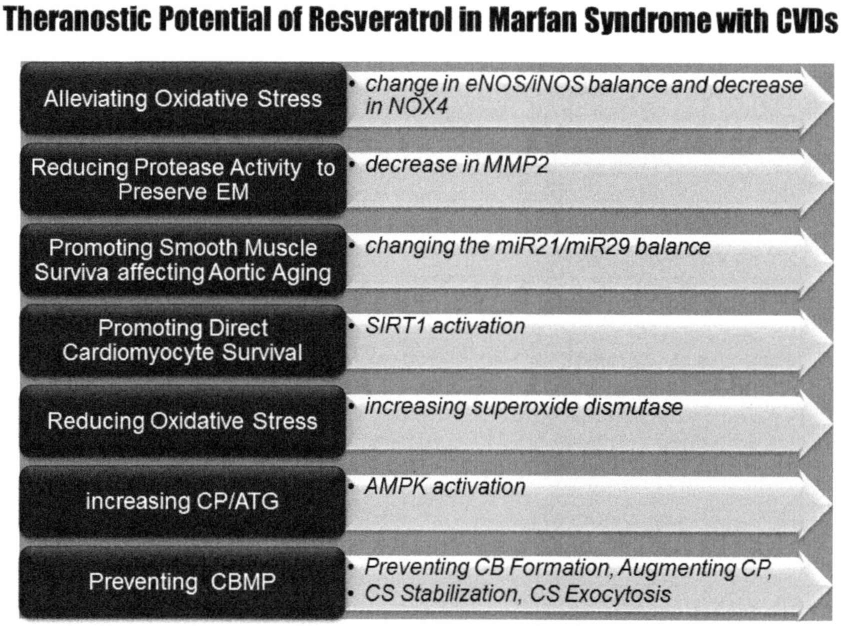

Theranostic Potential of Resveratrol in Marfan Syndrome with CVDs

Alleviating Oxidative Stress	• *change in eNOS/iNOS balance and decrease in NOX4*
Reducing Protease Activity to Preserve EM	• *decrease in MMP2*
Promoting Smooth Muscle Surviva affecting Aortic Aging	• *changing the miR21/miR29 balance*
Promoting Direct Cardiomyocyte Survival	• *SIRT1 activation*
Reducing Oxidative Stress	• *increasing superoxide dismutase*
increasing CP/ATG	• *AMPK activation*
Preventing CBMP	• *Preventing CB Formation, Augmenting CP, CS Stabilization, CS Exocytosis*

Figure 34

Table 13 Beneficial Effect of Resverarol on Cardiovascular Complications in Marfan Syndrome.

S. No	Physiological and Pharmacological Effect	Pharmacodynamics
1.	Alleviating oxidative stress	Changes in eNOS/iNOS balance and decrease in NOX-14
2.	Reducing protease activity to preserve ECM	Decrease in MMP2
3.	Improving smooth muscle cell survival and thus affecting aortic aging	Changing the mir21/mir29 balance
4.	Promoting cardiomyocyte survival directly	SIRT1 activation
5.	Reducing oxidative stress	Increasing SOD activity
6.	Increasing ATG	AMPK activation
7.	Mitochondrial quality control (MQC)	Preventing CBMP: CB inhibition, CP regulation, CS stabilization, CS exocytosis, promoting IMD and ICD

Cardiolipin in Congenital CVDs

Mitochondrial membranes are unique in the cell as they contain the phospholipid Cardiolipin. The protective role of Cardiolipin in cardiovascular health is highlighted by several cardiac diseases, in which it plays a fundamental role. Barth syndrome, Sengers syndrome, and dilated cardiomyopathy with ataxia (DCMA) are genetic disorders, which affect Cardiolipin biosynthesis. Other CVDs, including ischemia/reperfusion injury and heart failure, are also associated with changes in the Cardiolipin pool. Dudek et al. (2019) summarized the molecular functions of Cardiolipin in MB and MTG. I have highlighted the role of Cardiolipin in the respiratory chain, metabolite carriers, mitochondrial metabolism, and its links to apoptosis and mitochondria-specific CP with potential implications in CVDs. The TSE-EBPT significance of Cardiolipin in health and disease is presented in Fig. 35.

TSE-EBPT Significance of Cardiolipin in Health & Disease

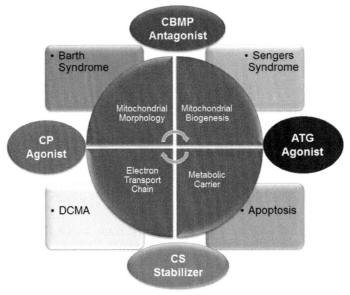

Figure 35

CONCLUSION

Cardiovascular calcification, artificial intelligence, and omics data are accelerating novel discovery of TSE-EBPT-CPTs. TLR3 contributed to persistent CP/ATG and heart failure in mice after MI. A defective ATG in atherosclerosis and CB formation was explored in cardiomyopathy. Impaired mitochondrial respiration in atherosclerotic plaques occurred due to PINK1 in vascular smooth muscle cells and small-vessel vasculopathy due to aberrant ATG in LAMP-2 deficient mice. The iTRAQ-based proteomic analysis of umbilical vein endothelial cells with platelet endothelial aggregation receptor-1 knockdown was investigated. The STIM1 inhibitor, ML9, impaired CP/ATG in cardiomyocytes by decreasing lysosomes. A deficit in PINK1/Parkin-mediated CP/ATG occurred in dystrophic cardiomyopathy. HIV-1 Tat induced dysregulation of MQC in cardiomyocytes. Thymoquinone conferred protection in cardiac damage caused by sepsis in BALB/c mice. FKBP8 protected the heart from hemodynamic stress by preventing the accumulation of misfolded proteins and ERS-associated apoptosis in mice. AMPK activation in MQC occurred via modulating MTG in the heart during chronic hypoxia. H_2S-mediated cell death signaling ameliorated remodeling in diabetic cardiomyopathy. Ginsenoside Rb1 alleviated Ox-LDL-induced vascular endothelium senescence via the SIRT1/ Beclin-1/ATG pathway and miR-27a-5p attenuated hypoxia-induced rat cardiomyocyte injury by inhibiting ATG7. Sirt1 promoted ATG and inhibited apoptosis to protect from hypoxic stress, whereas, Mst1 knockout enhanced ATG to attenuate Ang-II-induced cardiac injury. Modulation of CP/ATG was proposed for the treatment of sarcopenia in chronic heart failure. Inhibition of ERK-Drp-1 and CB formation alleviated IGF-IIR-induced mitochondria dysfunction during heart failure. Irisin alleviated pressure overload-induced cardiac hypertrophy by inducing protective CP/ATG through mTOR-independent activation of the AMPK-ULK1 pathway. The role of mitochondria in sex-specific cardiac function was explored in addition to regulation of Mfn 2 in cardiovascular pathophysiology by modulating CP/ATG to treat CVDs. Age-dependent cardiac function was investigated during sepsis; the effect of AMPK induction by AICAR. $\alpha 7$ nAch receptor activation conferred protection in myocardial I/R through CP/ATG modulation. Gastrodin and inhibition of p53 also alleviated I/R injury by regulating CP/ATG. In addition, Empagliflozin normalized the size and number of mitochondria and prevented reduction in mitochondrial size after MI in diabetic hearts. PINK1 alleviated Ang-II-induced cardiac injury by ameliorating mitochondrial dysfunction, whereas Beclin-1-dependent ATG protected the heart during sepsis. Estrogen and estrogen receptor α inhibited Bnip-3-induced apoptosis and ATG in H9c2 cardiomyoblasts. Melatonin balanced the CP/ATG and apoptosis by regulating UCP2 in the LPS-induced cardiomyopathy. H_2O_2 signaling triggered PI3K-mediated mitochondrial protection to confer cardio-protection in exercise preconditioning. Parkin-mediated MTG conferred cardio-protection by exercise preconditioning. TAK1 regulated skeletal muscle mass and mitochondrial function and Humanin induced chaperone-mediated CP/ATG. DUSP1 alleviated cardiac I/R injury by suppressing the Mff-mediated CBMP and Bnip-3-related MTG via the JNK signaling. In addition, Pitavastatin attenuated AGEs-induced MTG by inhibiting ROS, while cardiac basal CP/ATG could be modulated by exercise.

REFERENCES

Badreddin, A., Y. Fady, H. Attia, M. Hafez, et al. 2018. What role does the stress response have in congestive heart failure? J Cell Physiol 233: 2863–2870.

Banerjee, M., Y. Huang, M.M. Ouseph, S. Joshi, et al. 2019. Autophagy in platelets. Methods Mol Biol 1880: 511–528.

Chen, B.C., Y.J. Weng, M.A. Shibu, C.-K. Han, et al. 2018. Estrogen and/or estrogen receptor α inhibits Bnip-3-induced apoptosis and autophagy in H9c2 cardiomyoblast cells. Int J Mol Sci 19(5): 1298. https://doi.org/10.3390/ijms19051298.

Cheng, Z., M. Zhang, J. Hu, J. Lin, et al. 2018. Mst1 knockout enhances cardiomyocyte autophagic flux to alleviate angiotensin II-induced cardiac injury independent of angiotensin II receptors. J Mol Cell Cardiol 125: 117–128.

Docherty, C.K., A. Carswell, E. Friel and J.R. Mercer. 2018. Impaired mitochondrial respiration in human carotid plaque atherosclerosis: A potential role for PINK1 in vascular smooth muscle cell energetics. Atherosclerosis 268: 1–11.

Dudek, J., M. Hartmann and P. Rehling. 2019. The role of mitochondrial cardiolipin in heart function and its implication in cardiac disease. Biochim Biophys Acta Mol Basis Dis 1865(4): 810–821.

Fu, S., L. Chen, Y. Wu, Y. Tang, et al. 2018. Gastrodin pretreatment alleviates myocardial ischemia/ reperfusion injury through promoting autophagic flux. Biochem Biophys Res Commun 503: 2421–2428.

Gao, T., S.P. Zhang, J.F. Wang, L. Liu, et al. 2018. TLR3 contributes to persistent ATG and heart failure in mice after myocardial infarction. J Cell Mol Med 22: 395–408.

Gong, Z., I. Tasset, A. Diaz, J. Anguiano, et al. 2018. Humanin is an endogenous activator of chaperone-mediated ATG. J Cell Biol 217: 635–647.

Grootaert, M.O.J., L. Roth, D.M. Schrijvers, G.R.Y. De Meyer, et al. 2018. Defective ATG in atherosclerosis: To die or to senesce? Oxid Med Cell Longev 2018: 7687083.

Hou, Z., Y. Zhou, H. Yang, Y. Liu, et al. 2018. Alpha7 nicotinic acetylcholine receptor activation protects against myocardial reperfusion injury through modulation of ATG. Biochem Biophys Res Commun 500: 357–364.

Huang, C.Y., C.H. Lai, C.H. Kuo, S.F. Chiang, et al. 2018. Inhibition of ERK-Drp-1 signaling and mitochondria fragmentation alleviates IGF-IIR-induced mitochondria dysfunction during heart failure. J Mol Cell Cardiol 122: 58–68.

Inata, Y., G. Piraino, P.W. Hake, M. O'Connor, et al. 2018. Age-dependent cardiac function during experimental sepsis: Effect of pharmacological activation of AMP-activated protein kinase by AICAR. Am J Physiol Heart Circ Physiol 315: H826–H837.

Jin, Q., R. Li, N. Hu, T. Xin, et al. 2018. DUSP1 alleviates cardiac ischemia/reperfusion injury by suppressing the Mff-required mitochondrial fission and Bnip-3-related mitophagy via the JNK pathways. Redox Biol 14: 576–587.

Kang, C., M.A. Badr, V. Kyrychenko, E.L. Eskelinen, et al. 2018. Deficit in PINK1/Parkin-mediated mitochondrial ATG at late stages of dystrophic cardiomyopathy. Cardiovasc Res 114: 90–102.

Kar, S., T.N. Kambis and P.K. Mishra. 2019. Hydrogen sulfide-mediated regulation of cell death signaling ameliorates adverse cardiac remodeling and diabetic cardiomyopathy. Am J Physiol Heart Circ Physiol 316: H1237–H1252.

Li, R.L., S.S. Wu, Y. Wu, X.X. Wang, et al. 2018. Irisin alleviates pressure overload-induced cardiac hypertrophy by inducing protective ATG via mTOR-independent activation of the AMPK-ULK1 pathway. J Mol Cell Cardiol 121: 242–255.

Liu, H., Y. Sun, Y. Zhang, G. Yang, et al. 2019. Role of thymoquinone in cardiac damage caused by sepsis from BALB/c mice. Inflammation 42: 516–525.

Luo, G., Z. Jian, Y. Zhu, Y. Zhu, et al. 2019. Sirt1 promotes ATG and inhibits apoptosis to protect cardiomyocytes from hypoxic stress. Int J Mol Med 43: 2033–2043.

Ma, Q., Z. Zhang, J.K. Shim, T.N. Venkatraman, et al. 2019. Annexin A1 bioactive peptide promotes resolution of neuroinflammation in a rat model of exsanguinating cardiac arrest treated by emergency preservation and resuscitation. Front Neurosci 13: 608. doi: 10.3389/fnins.2019.00608.

Madrigal-Matute, J., L. Scorrano and J. Sadoshima. 2018. Leducq Network: Modulating autophagy to treat cardiovascular disease. Circ Res 123: 323–325.

Misaka, T., T. Murakawa, K. Nishida, Y. Omori, et al. 2018. FKBP8 protects the heart from hemodynamic stress by preventing the accumulation of misfolded proteins and endoplasmic reticulum-associated apoptosis in mice. J Mol Cell Cardiol 114: 93–104.

Mizuno, M., A. Kuno, T. Yano, T. Miki, et al. 2018. Empagliflozin normalizes the size and number of mitochondria and prevents reduction in mitochondrial size after myocardial infarction in diabetic hearts. Physiol Rep 6(12): e13741.

Moyzis, A. and A.B. Gustafsson. 2018. Multiple recycling routes: Canonical vs. non-canonical mitophagy in the heart. Biochim Biophys Acta Mol. Basis Dis 1865(4): 797–809.

Nguyen. H.T., S. Noguchi, K, Sugie, Y. Matsuo, et al. 2018. Small-vessel vasculopathy due to aberrant autophagy in LAMP-2 deficiency. Sci Rep 8(1): 3326.

Pan, P., X. Wang and D. Liu. 2018a. The potential mechanism of mitochondrial dysfunction in septic cardiomyopathy. J Int Med Res 46: 2157–2169.

Pan, P., H. Zhang, L. Su, X. Wang, et al. 2018b. Melatonin balance the autophagy and apoptosis by regulating UCP2 in the LPS-induced cardiomyopathy. Molecules 23(3): 675. https://doi.org/10.3390/molecules23030675.

Rogers, M.A. and E. Aikawa. 2019. Cardiovascular calcification: Artificial intelligence and big data accelerate mechanistic discovery. Nat Rev Cardiol 16: 261–274.

Saito, N., J. Araya, S. Ito, K. Tsubouchi, et al. 2019. Involvement of lamin B1 reduction in accelerated cellular senescence during chronic obstructive pulmonary disease pathogenesis. J Immunol 202: 1428–1440.

Sato, T. and J. Sadoshima. 2015. Molecular mechanisms of mitochondrial ATG/MTG in the heart. Circ Res 116: 1477–1490.

Shaikh, S., R. Troncoso, D. Mondaca-Ruff, V. Para, et al. 2018. The STIM1 inhibitor ML9 disrupts basal ATG in cardiomyocytes by decreasing lysosome content. Toxicol in Vitro 48: 121–127.

Shi, G., D. Liu, B. Zhou, Y. Liu, B. Hao, et al. 2019. Ginsenoside Rb1 alleviates oxidative low-density lipoprotein–induced vascular endothelium senescence via the SIRT1/Beclin-1/autophagy axis. J Cardiovasc Pharmacol 75(2): 155–167.

Song, R., Y. Yang, H. Lei, G. Wang, et al. 2018. HDAC6 inhibition protects cardiomyocytes against Dox-induced acute damage by improving α-tubulin acetylation. J Mol Cell Cardiol 124: 58–69.

Sun, T., M.Y. Li, P.F. Li and J.M. Cao. 2018a. MicroRNAs in cardiac autophagy: Small molecules and big role. Cells 7(8): 104.

Sun, Y., X. Yao, Q.-J. Zhang, M. Zhu, et al. 2018b. Beclin-1-dependent autophagy protects the heart during sepsis. Circulation 138: 2247–2262.

Tahrir, F.G., S. Shanmughapriya, T.M. Ahooyi, T. Knezevic, et al. 2018. Dysregulation of mitochondrial bioenergetics and quality control by HIV-1 Tat in cardiomyocytes. J Cell Physiol 233: 748–758.

Tahrir, F.G., D. Langford, S. Amini, T.M. Ahooyi, et al. 2019. Mitochondrial quality control in cardiac cells: Mechanisms and role in cardiac cell injury and disease. J Cell Physiol 234: 8122–8133.

van Andel, M.M., M. Groenink, A.H. Zwinderman, B.J.M. Mulder, et al. 2019. The potential beneficial effects of resveratrol on cardiovascular complications in marfan syndrome patients–insights from rodent-based animal studies. Int J Mol Sci 20(5): 1122.

Vona, R., B. Ascione, W. Malorni, E. Straface. 2018. Mitochondria and sex-specific cardiac function. Adv Exp Med Biol 1065: 241–256.

Xiong, W., J. Hua, Z. Liu, W. Cai, et al. 2018. PTEN induced putative kinase 1 (PINK1) alleviates angiotensin II-induced cardiac injury by ameliorating mitochondrial dysfunction. Int J Cardiol 266: 198–205.

Yano, T., K. Abe, M. Tanno, T. Miki, et al. 2018. Does p53 inhibition suppress myocardial ischemia-reperfusion injury? J Cardiovasc Pharmacol Ther 23: 350–357.

Yin, J., X. Lu, Z. Qian, W. Xu, et al. 2019. New insights into the pathogenesis and treatment of sarcopenia in chronic heart failure. Theranostics 9(14): 4019–4029.

Yu, F., T. Xu, M. Wang, W. Chang, et al. 2018. Function and regulation of mitofusin 2 in cardiovascular physiology and pathology. Eur J Cell Biol 97: 474–482.

Yuan, Y. and S.S. Pan. 2018. Parkin mediates MTG to participate in cardioprotection induced by late exercise preconditioning but Bnip-3 does not. J Cardiovasc Pharmacol 71: 303–316.

Yuan, Y., S.S. Pan, D.F. Wan, J. Lu, et al. 2018. H_2O_2 Signaling-triggered PI3K mediates mitochondrial protection to participate in early cardioprotection by exercise preconditioning. Oxid Med Cell Longev Article ID 1916841. 16 p.

Yue, Y., S. Liu, X. Han, M. Wang, et al. 2019. iTRAQ-based proteomic analysis of human umbilical vein endothelial cells with platelet endothelial aggregation receptor-1 knockdown. J Cell Biochem 120: 12300–12310.

Zha, Z.M., J.H. Wang, S.L. Li and Y. Guo. 2018. Pitavastatin attenuates AGEs-induced MTG via inhibition of ROS generation in the mitochondria of cardiomyocytes. J Biomed Res 32: 281–287.

Zhang, H., B. Liu, T. Li, Y. Zhu, et al. 2018 AMPK activation serves a critical role in mitochondria quality control via modulating MTG in the heart under chronic hypoxia. Int J Mol Med 41: 69–76.

20

Charnolophagy in Renal Diseases

INTRODUCTION

Recent studies have shown that the dysregulation of ATG is implicated in the pathogenesis of various renal disorders. Chronic kidney disease (CKD) patients have elevated oxidative stress and increased ROS production in the mitochondria in addition to altered body homeostasis, protein aggregation, and inflammation. CP is highly crucial in maintaining the cellular homeostasis and protein recycling and its induction is also implicated in IS activation and severity of inflammatory responses. Choi (2019) highlighted ATG as an important modulator of human disease. MacroATG, aggrephagy, and selective ATG (for example, CP, MTG) can influence cellular processes, including inflammation, and immune responses, and cell death, thereby exerting both adaptive and maladaptive roles in disease pathogenesis. CP/ATG is implicated in acute kidney injury, which can arise in response to nephrotoxins, sepsis, I/R, and CKD. The latter includes comorbidities of diabetes and COPD-associated kidney injury. ATG is a cellular recycling process (CRP) which involves auto-elimination and reconstruction of damaged organelles and proteins; whereas CP involves energy (ATP)-driven, lysosomal-dependent elimination of inclusion bodies (known as CBs). CP is a mitochondrially-derived inclusionophagy which serves as a primary event of IMD and ICD. Oxidative stress, inflammation, mitochondrial dysfunction, and CBMP are involved in many renal diseases, CP/ATG induction/inhibition, and ICT due to functionally-impaired CRP. Similar to CP, ATG is involved in normal kidney function and intracellular homeostasis. Clinical studies have suggested ATG induction and inhibition in acute kidney injuries, chronic kidneys diseases, diabetic nephropathies, and polycystic kidney diseases. Recently, Lin et al (2019) reported that abnormal ATG function can cause loss of podocytes, damage proximal tubular cells, and glomerulosclerosis. Following acute renal injuries, ATG protects tubular cells from apoptosis and improves cellular regeneration. Patients with chronic kidney diseases have impaired CP/ATG that cannot be reversed by hemodialysis. Various nephrotoxins and medications also modify CP/ATG signaling pathways, which can be followed to elucidate the exact molecular mechanism(s) of drugs action and their nephrotoxicity to establish their theranostic potential in renal diseases. These researchers highlighted emerging concepts of ATG and its molecular mechanisms in renal pathophysiology and discussed the role of ATG in acute kidney injury, chronic kidney disease, drug toxicity, and aging. In addition, they suggested the theranostic potential of targeting ATG system in renal diseases. However, exact functional relationship between CP and ATG and clinical significance in spatiotemporal induction and inhibition in chronic kidneys diseases is yet to be established. Hence, targeting the ATG pathway will have theranostic potential in the treatment of CKD.

This chapter describes CP as the most suitable biomarker to accomplish TSE-EBPT of CKD.

CP in Iodinated Contrast-induced Renal Injury

Contrast induced-acute kidney injury (CI-AKI) is one of the most common causes of acute kidney injury (AKI) in hospitalized patients. CP, the selective elimination of CB via ATG, is an important mechanism of MQC in physiological and pathological conditions. Lei et al (2018) determined the effects of Iohexol and Iodixanol on mitochondrial ROS production, CP/ATG induction, and their role in cultured CI-AKI cell models. Cell viability was measured by cell counting kit-8. Apoptosis, mitochondrial ROS, and $\Delta\Psi$ were detected by immunoblot, MitoSOX fluorescence, and TMRE staining, respectively. CP was detected by the co-localization of LC3-FITC with MitoTracker Red, immunoblot, and TEM. CP was induced in human renal tubular cells (HK-2 cells) under different concentrations of iodinated contrast media. Mitochondrial ROS were elevated after the treatment. Rapamycin enhanced CP and alleviated contrast media induced HK-2 cells injury. In contrast, the CP/ATG inhibitor 3-MA downregulated CP and aggravated cell injury, indicating that Iohexol and Iodixanol contribute to the generation of ROS and CP, which protect the kidney from iodinated contrast (iohexol)-induced renal tubular epithelial cell injury.

Cisplatin-Mediated Nephrotoxicity

Acute kidney injury is the most critical dose-limiting factor in cancer patients treated with Cisplatin. Mitochondrial dysfunction and resultant cell damage by RONS released from damaged mitochondria are involved in the kidney injury. Ichinomiya et al. (2018) demonstrated mitochondrial damage and CP clearance in Cisplatin-mediated nephrotoxicity. Three groups of rats received a single injection of Cisplatin at 20 mg/kg i.p. and were sacrificed at 24, 48, and 72 hrs after the treatment. A time-dependent increase in the number of damaged renal tubules and the serum BUN, creatinine, and mitochondrial AST were observed in rats after the treatment. The increased numbers of swollen and fragmented mitochondria (implicated in CBMP) and of cytochrome c oxidase IV- and 8-nitroguanosine-positive cytoplasmic granules were observed in the degenerated renal tubules. CP induction was indicated in the degenerated renal epithelial cells, based on the detection of LC3, a CP/ATG marker, and LAMP-1, and swollen and fragmented mitochondria in CPS, suggesting that CB formation and CP induction occurs in response to Cisplatin-mediated nephrotoxicity.

Rapamycin in Renal Tubular Apoptosis

Recently, Yang et al. (2018) reported that ROS overproduction and renal tubular epithelial cell (TEC) apoptosis are key mechanisms of contrast-induced acute kidney injury (CI-AKI). The characteristics of CP and the effects of Rapamycin on contrast-induced abnormalities in oxidative stress, mitochondrial injury and CP, TEC apoptosis, and renal function were investigated in the CI-AKI rat model. Rats were divided into the control group, CI-AKI group, and pretreatment groups (Rapamycin: 2 or 5 mg/kg). CI-AKI was induced by i.p. injection of Iohexol (12.25 g iodine/kg). MDA and CAT were measured as oxidative markers. LC3, P62, Beclin-1, PINK1, and Cyt-C expression were also measured. The co-localization of LC3-labeled CPS with TOMM20-labeled mitochondria or LAMP2-labeled lysosomes was observed. Significantly increased serum creatinine, MDA and CAT, mitochondrial injury (including increase in cytosolic Cyt-C, $\Delta\Psi$ collapse), and apoptosis were induced, resulting in an increased expression of LC3-II/I,

Beclin-1, and PINK1 and a decreased expression of P62. The Rapamycin pretreatment induced the overexpression of LC3 II / I and Beclin-1. LC3-labeled CPS overlapped with TOMM20-labeled mitochondria and LAMP2-labeled lysosomes in CI-AKI, which was enhanced by Rapamycin. Contrast-induced Scr increase, oxidative stress, mitochondrial injury, TEC apoptosis, and necrosis were attenuated by Rapamycin pretreatment, suggesting that it confers reno-protection by attenuating mitochondrial injury and oxidative stress associated with CP dysregulation.

Optineurin-Mediated MTG

The premature senescence of renal tubular epithelial cells (RTEC) in diabetic nephropathy (DN) may result from the accumulation of damaged mitochondria. Premature senescence is a key process in the progression of DN. MTG eliminates damaged mitochondria through the PINK1-mediated recruitment of optineurin (OPTN) to mitochondria. Chen et al. (2018) examined the involvement of OPTN in the MTG regulation of cellular senescence in RTEC in the context of DN. The expression of senescence markers P16, P21, DcR2, SA-β-gal, SAHF, and insufficient MTG-degradation marker (p62) in mouse RTECs increased in culture in response to a 30 mM high-glucose (HG) exposure for 48 hrs. Mitochondrial fission/MTG inhibitor Mdivi-1 enhanced RTEC senescence under HG conditions, whereas ATG/MTG agonist Torin1 inhibited cell senescence. *MitoTempo* inhibited HG-induced ROS and cell senescence with or without Mdivi-1. The expression of PINK1 and OPTN, two regulatory factors for mitophagosome (MPS) formation, decreased after HG stimulation. The overexpression of PINK1 did not enhance MPS formation under HG conditions. OPTN silencing inhibited HG-induced MPS formation, and overexpression of OPTN relieved cellular senescence through promoting MTG. In clinical specimens, renal OPTN expression was decreased with increased tubulointerstitial injury scores. OPTN-positive renal tubular cells did not express the senescence marker P16. OPTN expression also negatively correlated with serum creatinine levels, and positively correlated with eGFR. Thus, OPTN-mediated MTG plays a regulatory role in HG-induced RTEC senescence in DN. Hence, OPTN may be a potential anti-senescence factor in DN.

Podocyte Injury and Repair

Recently, Cellesi et al. (2015) highlighted that podocytes are the main gatekeeper of protein filtration in the glomerulus. These are key cells in the glomerulus, and their damage leads to proteinuria and glomerular dysfunction.

When podocytes work inefficiently, this translates to proteins in the urine, a condition that, if not promptly treated, leads to the progression of glomerular damage and renal failure. Novel gene mutations have been identified in patients with nephrotic syndrome combined with a better definition of the role of podocin mutations. Numerous potential therapeutic targets have been identified and the data support the possibility of boosting podocyte regeneration. However, translation of experimental results into the clinic would depend on the avoidance of undesired side-effects; nanomedicine could provide the means to target conventional and novel drugs specifically to the podocytes.

Albumin Overload and PINK1/Parkin in Renal TECs

As a major urinary protein component, albumin is a risk factor for CKD progression. Mitochondrial dysfunction is one of the main causes of albumin-induced proximal tubule cell injury. Proteinuria (albuminuria) is an important cause of aggravating tubulointerstitial injury. Tan et al. (2018a) determined whether albumin overload-induced mitochondrial dysfunction can activate PINK1/Parkin-mediated MTG in renal tubular epithelial cells (TECs). They also explored the role of PINK1/Parkin signaling in albumin-induced MTG by inhibiting MTG by knockdown of PARK2 (Parkin). The expression level of LC3-II increased, and the maximum increase was observed after 8 hrs of albumin treatment. Albumin overload induced mitochondrial injury and the quantity of autophagosomes increased. The expression of INK1 and cytosolic Cyt-C increased and mitochondria Cyt-C decreased in the albumin group. The co-localization of acidic lysosomes and mitochondria demonstrated that the number of albumin-overload-induced MTG-positive dots increased. The transfection of PARK2 siRNA suggested that knockdown of the expression level of PARK2 can inhibit MTG induced by albumin. Thus, mitochondrial dysfunction activated the PINK1/Parkin signaling and MTG in renal tubular epithelial cells under the albumin-overload condition. Furthermore, Tan et al. (2018b) investigated the role of the clearance of damaged mitochondria. The albumin overload induced an increase in turnover of LC3-II and decrease in the p62 protein in renal proximal tubular (HK-2) cells *in vitro*. The albumin overload also induced an increase in mitochondrial damage. ALC, a mitochondrial torpent, alleviated albumin-induced mitochondrial damage and decreased ATG, while mitochondrial-damage revulsant, CCCP, further increased ATG. Pretreatment of HK-2 cells with Rapamycin reduced the number of CBs and apoptosis induced by albumin overload. In contrast, blocking ATG with CQ exerted the opposite effect, indicating that CP/ATG induction promotes the removal of CBs and protects in renal tubular injury caused by albumin overload.

PINK1-PRKN/PARK2 Pathway in Renal I/R Injury

Damaged or dysfunctional mitochondria participating in CBMP are toxic to the cell by producing RONS and releasing cell death factors. Hence, the timely removal of CBs is critical to cellular homeostasis and viability. MTG is the mechanism of selective degradation of mitochondria via CP/ATG. Tang et al. (2018) showed that MTG is induced in renal proximal tubular cells in both *in vitro* and *in vivo* models of ischemic AKI. MTG in AKI is abrogated by PINK1 and Park2 deficiency, supporting a critical role of the PINK1-PARK2 pathway in tubular cell MTG. Moreover, ischemic AKI is aggravated in PINK1 and Park2 single- as well as double-knockout mice. PINK1 and Park2 deficiency enhanced CB formation, ROS production, and inflammatory response, suggesting that PINK1-PARK2-mediated MTG plays a pivotal role in MQC, tubular cell survival, and renal function during AKI.

Renal I/R-Induced CP

Li et al. (2018) observed CPS and engulfed mitochondria after renal IRI by TEM. The increase of LC3-II and decrease of mitochondrial proteins were detected by immunoblotting, suggesting the presence of CP. Drp-1 translocated to the mitochondria and was phosphorylated at S616 in response to IRI. Inhibiting Drp-1 phosphorylation with mdivi-1 suppressed IRI-induced CP without affecting the general ATG. The downregulation of CP exacerbated apoptosis and kidney dysfunction, indicating that CP is induced via the Drp-1-dependent pathway as a mechanism to protect cells from IRI-induced apoptosis.

LSDs and Epithelial Dysfunction

The endolysosomal system sustains the re-absorptive activity of specialized epithelial cells. LSDs such as nephropathic cystinosis cause a major dysfunction of epithelial cells lining the kidney tubule, resulting in losses of vital solutes in the urine. Festa et al. (2018) demonstrated that by combining genetic and pharmacologic approaches, lysosomal dysfunction in cystinosis results in defective CP/ATG-mediated clearance of damaged mitochondria. This promotes the generation of oxidative stress that stimulates the $G\alpha 12$/Src-mediated phosphorylation of tight junction ZO-1 and triggers a signaling cascade involving ZO-1-associated Y-box factor ZONAB, resulting in cell proliferation and transport defects. The correction of the primary lysosomal defect, neutralization of mitochondrial oxidative stress, and blockage of tight junction-associated ZONAB signaling rescued the epithelial function, suggesting a link between defective lysosome-CP/ATG degradation and epithelial dysfunction, thus, providing new theranostic perspectives for LSDs.

CONCLUSION

Ischemia/reperfusion (I/R)-induced CP prevented renal dysfunction via the Drp-1-dependent-pathway. Iodinated contrast-induced RTEC injury was protected by CP/ATG regulation. Albumin overload and PINK1/Parkin signaling-related MTG was involved in RTEC necrosis. Optineurin-mediated MTG protected RTECs and prevented accelerated senescence in DN. CP/ATG induction promoted the elimination of CBs and albumin-induced RTEC injury implicated in CBMP whereas PINK1-PRKN/PARK2 pathway ameliorated renal I/R injury. Podocyte injury and repair involved CP/ATG modulation, while its dysregulation combined LSD and epithelial dysfunction in renal diseases.

REFERENCES

Cellesi, F., M. Li and M.L. Rastaldi. 2015. Podocyte injury and repair mechanisms. Curr Opin Nephrol Hypertens 24: 239–44.

Chen, K., H. Dai, J. Yuan, J. Chen, et al. 2018. Optineurin-mediated mitophagy protects renal tubular epithelial cells against accelerated senescence in diabetic nephropathy. Cell Death Dis 9: 105. https://doi.org/10.1038/s41419-017-0127-z.

Choi, M.E. 2019. Autophagy in kidney disease. Annu Rev Physiol 82: 297–322.

Festa, B.P., Z. Chen, M. Berquez, H. Debaix, et al. 2018. Impaired autophagy bridges lysosomal storage disease and epithelial dysfunction in the kidney. Nat Commun 9(1): 161.

Ichinomiya, M., A. Shimada, N. Ohta, E. Inouchi, et al. 2018. Demonstration of mitochondrial damage and mitophagy in cisplatin-mediated nephrotoxicity. Tohoku J Exp Med 246(1): 1–8.

Lei, R., F. Zhao, C.Y. Tang, M. Luo. et al. 2018. Mitophagy plays a protective role in iodinated contrast-induced acute renal tubular epithelial cells injury. Cell Physiol Biochem 46: 975–985.

Li, N., H. Wang, C. Jiang, M. Zhang. 2018. Renal ischemia/reperfusion-induced mitophagy protects against renal dysfunction via Drp-1-dependent-pathway. Exp Cell Res 369(1): 27–33.

Lin, T.A., V.C.C. Wu, C.Y. Wang. 2019. Autophagy in chronic kidney diseases. Cell 8: 61.

Tan, J., Q, Xie, S. Song, Y. Miao, et al. 2018a. Albumin overload and PINK/Parkin signaling-related mitophagy in renal tubular epithelial cells. Med. Sci. Monit. 24: 1258–1267.

Tan, J., M. Wang, S. Song, Y. Miao, et al. 2018b. Autophagy activation promotes removal of damaged mitochondria and protects against renal tubular injury induced by albumin overload. Histol Histopathol 33: 681–690.

Tang, C., H. Han, M. Yan, S. Zhu, et al. 2018. PINK1-PRKN/PARK2 pathway of mitophagy is activated to protect against renal ischemia reperfusion injury. Autophagy. 14: 880–897.

Yang, X., X. Yan, D. Yang, J. Zhou, et al. 2018. Rapamycin attenuates mitochondrial injury and renal tubular cell apoptosis in experimental contrast-induced acute kidney injury in rats. Biosci Rep 38(6): BSR20180876.

21

Charnolophagy in Reproductive Diseases

INTRODUCTION

Reproduction involves a series of biological activities, such as cell proliferation, differentiation, and apoptosis. ATG promotes cell survival, intercellular interactions, and guides cell function by eliminating excess proteins and organelles during the reproductive process. CP/ATG is a lysosomal degradation and recycling process for maintaining an intracellular balance for NCF and plays a pro-survival role in spermatocytes and promotes successful fertilization as described in author's books: *Fetal Alcohol Spectrum Disorders* (Sharma 2017a) and *Zika Virus Disease, Prevention and Cure* by Nova Science Publishers, New York, U.S.A. (Sharma 2017b). CP is involved in diversified diseases of the male and female reproductive system. Miscarriage is a common complication during pregnancy. A reduced expression of Mfn-2 was associated with miscarriage due to CP dysregulation in the trophoblasts. Recently molecular biomarkers involved in ATG and apoptosis between the spermatozoa of infertile men with varicocele and fertile individuals were evaluated in addition to the role of ATG in patients with endometriosis of different stages. Mitofusin-2 (Mfn-2) deficiency in trophoblasts, which regulates CP, is an important cause of early miscarriage. Cai et al. (2018) investigated the role of Mfn-2 and CP in miscarriage. Immunohistochemistry and immunoblotting were used to detect the Mfn-2 expression in villous tissues from women who had an early miscarriage, and to detect the expression of CP/ATG-related proteins (Atg5, Beclin-1, and LC3), MMP-2, MMP-9, and integrin $\beta1$. Immunofluorescence was used to detect the expression of APS after transfection with GFP-LC3. JC-1 was used to measure $\Delta\psi$ and TEM to observe the ultrastructure of mitochondria. B-hCG and progesterone in the trophoblast were determined by chemiluminescence. Mfn-2 in the villous tissues of women with an early miscarriage was lower compared to women with a normal pregnancy. Transfection with Mfn-2-siRNA decreased Mfn-2, whereas LC3, Atg5, and Beclin-1 were increased. Abnormal mitochondrial function and increased APS were observed. β-hCG, progesterone, MMP-2, MMP-9, and integrin $\beta1$ were reduced in the Mfn-2-siRNA group. The low expression of Mfn-2 induced CBMP and trophoblast cell dysfunction to cause early miscarriage.

This chapter describes (a) the crucial role of CP during prezygotic, fertilization, postzygotic, and adult life; (b) the function of CP in menstruation, miscarriage, embryogenesis, fetal development, eclepmpsia, and in genitourinary tract infections to discover the TSE-BPT of congenital diseases including microcephaly, cryptorchidism, hypospadias, arthrogryposis, infertility, and acquired (smoking and alcohol-induced) reproductive disorders; and (c) theranostic significance of antioxidants such as CP regulators and CBMP antagonists in various male and female diseases of the reproductive system. The chapter is divided systematically in two parts: (a) CP in male reproductive diseases and (ii) CP in female reproductive diseases.

CP in Male Reproductive Diseases

Cryptorchidism

It is a common male urogenital defect of childhood which impairs fertility during adult life and is characterized by the presence of one unilateral (one) or bilateral (both) undescended testes, which can lead to male infertility, testicular cancer, and psychological issues in the inflicted individual. Zeng et al. (2019) prepared a surgery-induced cryptorchid (SIC) mouse model to investigate the condition's effects on spermatogonia and seminiferous epithelial cycles. SIC led to a reduced testicular weight, aberrant seminiferous epithelial cycles, and spermatogenesis characterized by degenerating spermatogonia and multinucleated giant cells. SIC induced CP/ATG and apoptosis of spermatogonia, suggesting its role in promoting germ cell degeneration. These results provided novel insights into the development of male contraceptive strategies as well as treatment options for male infertility caused by cryptorchidism. Wei et al. (2018a) constructed two rat models to investigate the roles of CP/ATG and apoptosis in cryptorchidism. Pregnant rats were divided into three groups. Group I: non-treated rats were used as controls. Group II: the rats were injected with Flutamide (Flu) 25 mg/kg/bw/day from gestation day (GD) 11–19. Group III: daily intra-gastric administration of 750 mg/kg/bw/day Di-2-ethylhexylphosphate (DEHP) from GD 7–19. The cubs were fed normally and the testes were excised on postnatal day 30. The cryptorchidism models revealed severe testicular damage, increased sperm abnormality, decreased fertility, sperm count, and testosterone. The apoptotic markers FAS, Cyt-C, and caspase-3 were increased in Flu and DEHP-induced groups. DEHP treatment increased CPS and CP/ATG markers (LC3-II and p62). A significant decrease of CP gene (LC3-II and p62) expression was observed in flu-treated rat testes. Thus, impaired CP/ATG was involved in the impaired spermatogenesis of cryptorchidism.

CP in Spermatozoa

Abnormal dilatation and tortuosity of the pampiniform plexus within the spermatic cord are termed varicocele which leads to impaired spermatogenesis due to heat-induced oxidative stress and cell death. Both apoptosis and ATG pathways were activated by heat in the germ cells of mouse *in vivo* and *in vitro*. Foroozan-Broojeni et al. (2018) accessed sperm apoptotic markers (active caspases 3/7 and DNA fragmentation), ATG markers (Atg7 and LC3 proteins), and also sperm parameters and protamine deficiency as secondary outcomes from 23 infertile men with varicocele and 16 fertile individuals. The sperm parameters were assessed according to the WHO-2010 protocol. Apoptotic markers (active caspases 3/7 and DNA fragmentation), ATG markers (Atg7 and LC3 proteins), and protamine deficiency were evaluated by flow cytometry, fluorescence microscope, and immunoblotting. ATG flux, apoptotic markers, and protamine deficiency were increased in infertile men with varicocele compared to fertile individuals, but ATG and apoptosis markers did not correlate with each other, indicating that both ATG and apoptosis are independently active in the spermatozoa of infertile men with varicocele. A cell-free system using oocyte extracts is a valuable tool to study early events of fertilization and protein-protein interactions. Song and Sutovsky (2019) described the protocol to study the interaction of oocyte-derived CP factors with paternal sperm mitochondria from porcine permeabilized spermatozoa co-incubated with cell extracts from oocytes. The post-fertilization sperm CP revealed the timely elimination of paternal, sperm-contributed mitochondria carrying potentially defective mtDNA. The investigation of cell-free systems would be advantageous for studying post-fertilization sperm CP as large amounts of oocyte extracts can be incubated with spermatozoa in a single trial, while only one spermatozoon per zygote can be examined employing whole-cell approaches. Since sperm CP is species-specific, the frog oocyte extracts used for cell-free systems can be replaced with difficult to obtain iso-specific mammalian oocyte extracts.

Hedgehog and Insulin Signaling

Egg production declines with age in many species, a process linked with stem cell depletion. Diet-dependent signaling is critical for stem cell maintenance during aging. Follicle stem cells (FSCs) in the *Drosophila* ovary are responsive to diet-induced signals including Hedgehog (Hh) and insulin-IGF signaling (IIS), entering quiescence in the absence of nutrients and initiating proliferation upon feeding. Although highly proliferative FSCs exhibit an extended lifespan, Singh et al. (2018) found that Hh signaling drives FSC loss and premature sterility despite high proliferative rates. This occurs due to the Hh-mediated induction of ATG in FSCs via a Ptc-dependent and Smo-independent mechanism. Hh-dependent ATG increased during aging, triggering FSC loss and reproductive arrest. IIS was necessary to suppress Hh-induced ATG, promoting a stable proliferative state, suggesting that opposing action of diet-responsive IIS and Hh signals determine reproductive lifespan by modulating the proliferation-ATG balance in FSCs during aging.

CP in Sertoli Cells

Sertoli cells (SCs) maintain spermatogenesis via paracrine interactions with germ cells and other somatic cells in the testis. Eid et al. (2018) provided a methods to detect MTG in SCs in animal models of ethanol toxicity using a single i.p injection (5 g/kg) of ethanol in rats. A proper understanding of MTG and mechanisms in SCs may have theranostic implications for infertility associated with alcoholism and other diseases characterized by mitochondrial dysfunction involving CBMP. In addition, Eid and Kondo (2018) induced MTG in SCs of adult male rats using a single injection of ethanol (5 g/kg) and observed MTG via TEM 24 hrs later. They discussed the possible clinical implications of enhanced ATG and MTG in stressed SCs in their model and in other models of acute stress (for example, heat and transplantation stress). Further studies are needed to fully understand the molecular mechanisms controlling CP/ATG in stressed SCs which may have theranostic implications for infertility treatment. Recently, the author described CB formation and delayed CP during prezygotic phase and CP dysregulation and CS destabilization in the neural progenitor cell during postzygotic phase and their implication in microcephaly in his book, *Fetal Alcohol Spectrum Disorders*, published by Nova Science Publishers, New York, U.S.A. (Sharma 2017a). Sertoli cell death contributes to impaired spermatogenesis, associated with male infertility. Testicular I/R injury induces the cell death of germ cells and Sertoli cells, whereas the inhibition of cell death ameliorates acute testicular I/R damage. Li et al. (2018a) investigated the mechanism of I/R stress-induced cell death in TM4 cells. O_2 glucose deprivation and re-oxygenation (OGD/R) induced I/R injury and cell death in TM4 cells was blocked by the ROS inhibitor, NAC, lipid peroxidation inhibitor, Liproxstatin1, and iron chelator, Deferoxamine. However, the inhibitors of apoptosis, necrosis, or ATG had no effect. Iron and ROS were elevated in I/R injury, mitochondrial size was decreased, and membrane density was increased (indicative of ferroptosis). The ROS overproduction suggested iron accumulation and GSH depletion. The expression of ferroportin (Fpn) and its mRNA was decreased in TM4 cells. Overexpression of Fpn inhibited ferroptosis, ROS production and iron accumulation. GSH dependent peroxidase 4 (GPX4) was inactivated via GSH depletion following I/R injury, whereas GPX4 activation blocked I/R induced ferroptosis by reducing ROS production. I/R induced ferroptosis was blocked by inhibiting p38 MAPK activation, indicating that it is induced by OGD/R injury in Sertoli cells which may provide a novel strategy for the cyto-protection in testicular I/R induced cell loss.

Sexual Development in *C. elegans*

Basal levels of ATG are required to remove aggregate prone proteins, paternal mitochondria, and spermatid-specific membranous organelles. Studies on *C. elegans* have provided valuable insights into the physiological relevance of ATG during metazoan development. Palmisano and Meléndez (2018) discussed the developmental contexts where ATG has been shown to be important. ATG has a role in many biological processes during the development of the nematode *C. elegans*. During larval development, ATG is required for the remodeling that occurs during dauer development, and ATG can selectively degrade and modulate components of the miRNA-induced silencing complex. Basal levels of ATG are important in synapse formation and in the germ line to promote the proliferation of stem cells and for the efficient removal of apoptotic cell corpses by promoting phagosome maturation, in lipid homeostasis, and in the aging process.

PM2.5 Exposure

The blood-testis barrier (BTB), composed of tight junctions (TJs), adherens junctions, and gap junctions, is important for spermatogenesis. PM2.5 impairs testicular functions and reproduction. To investigate the roles of ATG in PM2.5-induced BTB toxicity, Wei et al. (2018b) exposed rats to normal saline (NS) or PM2.5 with the doses of 9 mg/kg b.w. and 24 mg/kg b.w. via i.t. for seven weeks. These investigators determined the success rate of mating, sperm quality, testicular morphology, and expression of BTB junction proteins and ATG-related proteins. Developmental PM2.5 exposure induced decreased fertility, reduced sperm count, increased sperm abnormality, and testicular degeneration. The expressions of TJ (ZO-1 and occludin) and gap junction (connexin43) were downregulated after the PM2.5 treatment. PM2.5 increased the number of CPS and CP markers LC3-II and p62, suggesting that CPS accumulation results from impaired CP. The expressions of HO-1 increased and those of Gpx and SOD were decreased after PM2.5 exposure. Vitamins E and C alleviated the PM2.5-induced oxidative stress, reversed the CP defect, and restored BTB impairment, suggesting that PM2.5 exposure destroys BTB integrity through ROS-mediated CP. These finding could contribute to a better understanding of PM2.5-induced male reproductive toxicity.

Diabetic Testicular Dysfunction

Abnormal ATG play a significant role in accelerating diabetic reproductive injury. Testicular dysfunction is one of the serious secondary complications in diabetes. Lycium barbarum polysaccharide (LBP) possessed beneficial properties such as antiaging, anticancer, and reproduction-enhancing. Shi et al. (2018) investigated the protective effects of LBP on diabetic testicular dysfunction. The protective effects of LBP (40 mg/kg) on testicular function was assessed by evaluating sperm parameters and testosterone levels. Beclin-1 and LC3-I decreased in the LBP 40 mg/kg group. LBP downregulated Beclin-1 and LC3-I protein expressions upregulated p-PI3K and p-Akt protein expressions and decreased Beclin-1 and LC3-I mRNA expressions in treated as compared with untreated diabetic mice, indicating that the inhibition of PI3K/Akt-pathway-mediated testicular ATG may be a novel theranostic target with regard to the protective effects of LBP on diabetic testicular dysfunction.

Heat Stress and Testicular Injury

Wang et al. (2019) investigated the global protein expression in response to acute heat stress in the testes of a broiler-type strain of Taiwan country chickens (TCCs). Twelve 45-week-old roosters were allocated to the control group maintained at 25°C, and three groups subjected to acute heat stress at 38°C for 4 hrs, with 0, 2, and 6 hrs of recovery, respectively. As many as 101 protein spots differed from the control following exposure to acute heat stress. The proteins that were differentially expressed participated in protein metabolism and other metabolic processes, responses to stimuli, apoptosis, cellular organization, and spermatogenesis. Proteins that negatively regulate apoptosis were downregulated and proteins involved in ATG and HSPs (HSP90α, HSPA5, and HSPA8) were upregulated, suggesting that acute heat stress causes a change in protein expression to impair cell morphology, spermatogenesis, and apoptosis. The expression of HSPs increased to attenuate the testicular injury induced by acute heat stress.

CP in Female Reproductive Diseases

LC3 Abundance

Recently, Kang et al. (2018) explored the relationship between cell death and ATG by examining granulosa cell layers that control oocyte quality for successful fertilization. These layers were collected from infertile women and divided into four types, viz., mature (MCCs), immature (ICCs), dysmature cumulus cells (DCCs), and mural granulosa cells (MGCs). LC3, which is involved in APS formation, was over-expressed in DCCs and MGCs, and their chromosomal DNA was fragmented. However, ATG initiation was limited to MGCs, as indicated by the expression of membrane-bound LC3-II and ATG7, an enzyme that converts LC3-I to LC3-II. Although pro-LC3 was accumulated, ATG was disabled in DCCs, resulting in cell death, suggesting the possibility that ATG-independent accumulation of pro-LC3 proteins leads to the death of granulosa cells surrounding the oocytes, reducing oocyte quality and female fertility.

Endometriosis

Endometriosis (EMs) is a disease in which endometrium-like tissues abnormally grow outside the uterus and possesses the characteristics of tumor because of its malignant behavior. CP/ATG may play a role in the Ems' proliferative-phase. Li et al. (2018b) explored ATG between the normal endometrium and EMs during the different phases of the menstrual cycle and EMs. The endometrial samples from 73 women were selected, including 30 healthy individuals and 43 patients with EMs. The participants were divided into two groups according to the menstrual cycle, namely the proliferative-phase group and the secretive-*phase* group. Among the patients with EMs, 22 individuals in the proliferative phase and the other 21 individuals in the secretory phase were further classified into the groups of Stage I–II and Stage III–IV according to the revised-American Fertility Society(r-AFS). Two ATG-related proteins, LC3B-II and sequestosome protein (P62), as markers of ATG were explored in this study. The expression of LC3B-II decreased and that of P62 increased in the secretory phase of the healthy group. The expression of LC3B-II in the ectopic endometrium group was lower than that of its eutopic endometrium group. Compared to the Stage I–II EMs group, the expression of LC3B-II was lower and P62 was higher in Stage III–IV EMs during the secretory phase. The periodicity-losing in EMs and the decreased ATG in ectopic endometrium may exert a potential role in the pathogenesis of EMs. Hence, the downregulated ATG of ectopic endometrium during the secretory phase may be related to the progression of EMs. Homeobox A10 (HOXA10) is a transcription factor necessary for embryonic and adult uterine development, and studies indicate that its expression decreases in endometriosis. Homeobox A10 may negatively regulate ATG in endometriosis. Zheng et al. (2018) measured the expression of autophagic biomarkers (Beclin-1 and LC3-II) and HOXA10 proteins by immunoblotting and mRNA by quantitative real-time PCR. They evaluated the serum cancer antigen 125 (CA-125) levels by immunoassay. The most tested ATG biomarker proteins and mRNAs were upregulated, whereas the HOXA10 protein and mRNA were decreased in ovarian endometriomas compared with the eutopic endometria of women with endometriosis and normal endometria. Compared with normal endometrium, only the protein expression of ATG biomarkers were increased in the eutopic endometrium of women with endometriosis. HOXA10 had a negative correlation with ATG. Serum CA125 was at a high level in endometriosis and increased with elevated revised American Fertility Society staging (I–IV). There was a positive correlation between serum CA125 and LC3-II protein and/or LC3-II/ LC3-I ratio and a negative correlation between serum CA125 and HOXA10-gene expression, suggesting that the deficiency of HOXA10 may induce ATG in endometriosis. Hence, the relationship among CA125, ATG, and HOXA10 in endometriosis requires further investigation.

Polycystic Ovary Syndrome (PCOS)

PCOS is the most common endocrinopathy in women of reproductive age and also an important metabolic disorder associated with insulin resistance (IR). Hyperandrogenism is a key feature of PCOS. Whether hyperandrogenism can cause IR in PCOS remains unknown. The mTORC1 and its regulated ATG are associated with IR. Song et al. (2018) investigated the role of mTORC1-ATG pathway in skeletal muscle IR in a dehydroepiandrosterone (DHEA)-induced PCOS mouse model. DHEA-treated mice exhibited whole-body and skeletal muscle IR, along with the activated mTORC1, repressed ATG, impaired mitochondria, and reduced plasma-membrane GLUT4 expression in the skeletal muscle of the mice. In cultured C2C12 myo-tubes, treatment with a high dose testosterone activated mTORC1, reduced ATG, impaired mitochondria, decreased insulin-stimulated glucose uptake, and induced IR. The inhibition of mTORC1 or induction of ATG restored mitochondrial function, upregulated insulin-stimulated glucose uptake, and increased insulin sensitivity, whereas, inhibition of ATG exacerbated testosterone-induced impairment, suggesting that the mTORC1-ATG pathway might contribute to androgen excess-induced skeletal muscle IR in pre-pubertal female mice by impairing mitochondrial function and reducing insulin-stimulated glucose uptake. This may help in understanding the role of hyper-androgenism and the underlying mechanism in the pathogenesis of skeletal muscle IR in PCOS.

Preeclampsia

The contribution of mitochondrial dynamics to preeclampsia, a hypertensive disorder of pregnancy characterized by placental cell ATG and death, remains unknown. Ausman et al. (2018) showed that the mitochondrial dynamic balance in pre-eclamptic placentae is tilted toward fission (increased Drp-1 expression/activation and decreased OPA1 expression). Increased phosphorylation of Drp-1 (p-DRP1) in mitochondrial isolates from pre-eclamptic placentae and TEM corroborated augmented mitochondrial fragmentation in the cytotrophoblast cells of PE placentae. Increased fission was accompanied by ceramides (CERs) build-up in mitochondria from pre-eclamptic placentae. The treatment of human choriocarcinoma JEG3 cells and primary isolated cytrophoblast cells with CER 16:0 enhanced mitochondrial fission. Bcl-2 member BOK, whose expression is increased by CER, regulated p-DRP1/Drp-1 and Mfn-2 expression, and localized mitochondrial fission in the ER/MAM compartments to participate in CBMP. The BH3 and transmembrane domains of BOK were vital for BOK regulation of fission. PINK1 and Parkin were elevated in mitochondria from PE placentae, indicating that CP degrades excess mitochondrial fragments produced from CER/BOK-induced fission in preeclampsia. This study revealed a novel CER/BOK-induced regulation of mitochondrial fission and its functional consequences for heightened trophoblast cell ATG involving functionally-impaired CP and CBMP in preeclampsia.

NRTI- Induced Oocyte Dysfunction

Low fertility is one of the most common side effects caused by nucleoside reverse transcriptase inhibitors (NRTIs). Recently, Tang et al. (2017) investigated whether ATG plays a role in NRTIs-induced oocyte dysfunction and low fertility in female rats. Both *in vivo* and *in vitro* experiments were conducted. For the *in vivo* experiment, female adult SD rats were subjected to Zidovudine (AZT) and Lamivudine (3TC) intra-gastric treatment for 3, 6, 9, and 12 weeks. Oocytes were collected for evaluating maturation, *in vitro* fertilization, mitochondrial function, apoptosis, and CP/ATG. For the *in vitro* experiment, the oocytes were collected and assigned to the control, 3-MA (an ATG inhibitor), AZT, AZT+3-MA, 3TC, and 3TC+3-MA groups. The oocytes were cultured with these drugs for 24, 48, and 72 hrs and then, subjected to the same assays as in the *in vivo* study. A significant decrease in oocyte maturation-related markers, oocyte cleavage, blastocyst formation, mtDNA copy number, ATP, apoptosis, and RONS overproduction was seen. These changes were attenuated by 3-MA, indicating that NRTIs can cause oocyte dysfunction and reduced CP/ATG-mediated fertility.

Tsetse Reproduction

Tsetse flies are vectors of human and animal trypanosomiasis. The ability to reduce tsetse populations is an effective means of disease control. Lactation is an essential component of tsetse's viviparous reproductive physiology and requires a dramatic increase in the synthesis of milk proteins by the milk gland to nurture larval growth. In between each gonotrophic cycle, the tsetse ceases milk production and its milk gland tubules undergo involution. Benoit et al. (2018) examined the role of ATG during tsetse fly milk gland involution and reproductive output. ATG genes showed enhanced expression in tissues associated with lactation, immediately before or within 2 hrs post-parturition, and a decline in the 24–48 hrs post-parturition. This expression pattern was inversely correlated with that of the milk gland proteins (lactation-specific protein-coding genes) and the ATG inhibitor, fk506-bp1. The increased expression of the *Drosophila* inhibitor of apoptosis 1, diap1, was also observed during involution, when it prevented the apoptosis of milk gland cells. The RNAi-mediated knockdown of the ATG-related gene 8a (ATG8a) prevented milk gland ATG during involution, prolonging gestation, and reducing fecundity in the subsequent gono-trophic cycle. The inhibition of ATG reduced the recovery of stored lipids during the non-lactating periods by 15–20%. Ecdysone application induced ATG and increased milk gland involution even before abortion as observed immediately before birth, suggesting that the ecdysteroid peak preceding parturition triggers milk gland ATG in tsetse fly. Population modeling revealed that a delay in involution would yield a negative population growth rate. Milk gland CP/ATG during involution is critical to restore nutrient reserves and efficient transition between pregnancy cycles. Hence, targeting post-birth phases of reproduction could be utilized to suppress the tsetse populations and reduce trypanosomiasis.

Lhx8 Ablation

Following the proliferation of oogonia in mammals, numerous germ cells are discarded, primarily by apoptosis, while the remainder form primordial follicles (the ovarian reserve) that determine fertility and reproductive lifespan. Massive, rapid, and essentially total loss of oocytes, however, occurs when the transcription factor Lhx8 is ablated—though the germ cell loss from the

Lhx8$^{-/-}$ ovaries remain unknown. D'Ignazio et al. (2018) found that Lhx8$^{-/-}$ ovaries maintain the same number of germ cells throughout embryonic development; a rapid decrease in the pool of oocytes starts shortly before birth. The loss results from the activation of ATG becomes overwhelming within the first postnatal week, with extracellular matrix proteins filling the space previously occupied by follicles to produce a fibrotic ovary. As early as a few days before birth, Lhx8$^{-/-}$ oocytes failed to repair DNA damage, which normally occurs when meiosis is initiated during embryonic development, and DNA damage repair genes are downregulated throughout the oocyte short lifespan. Based on gene expression and morphological analyses, these investigators proposed a model in which the lineage-restricted failure of DNA repair triggers germ cell ATG, causing premature depletion of the ovarian reserve in Lhx8$^{-/-}$ mice.

Ovarian Germ Cell Depletion

Yadav et al. (2018) highlighted that an ovary contains millions of germ cells during embryonic life but only few of them are culminated into oocytes that achieve meiotic competency just prior to ovulation. The majority of germ cells are depleted from the ovary through several pathways. Follicular atresia is one of the major events that eliminate germ cells from the ovary by engaging apoptotic as well as non-apoptotic pathways. Although necro-apoptosis has been implicated in germ cell depletion, CP/ATG seems to play an active role in the life and death decisions of ovarian follicles. CP/ATG is characterized by the intracellular reorganization of membranes and increased number of vesicles that engulf bulk cytoplasm as well as organelles. CP/ATG begins with the encapsulation of cytoplasmic constituents in APS. The CP/ATG vesicles are then destroyed by the lysosomal hydrolases, resulting in follicular atresia. CP/ATG as well as apoptosis play active roles in germ cells depletion from the ovary. Hence, it is important to prevent these two pathways from retaining the germ cells in the ovary of several biological species that are either threatened or on the verge of extinction.

Di (2-Ethylhexyl) Phthalate

The female reproductive lifespan is primarily determined by the size of the primordial follicle pool, which is established early in life. Zhang et al. (2018) reported that Di (2-ethylhexyl) phthalate (DEHP), an environmental endocrine disruptor and a widely-spreading plasticizer, impairs primordial folliculogenesis (FG). DEHP altered the number and sex ratio of the offspring of neonatal-exposed mice. DEHP activated ATG in the ovary, with increased ATG-related gene expression and APS, while inhibition of ATG by 3-MA attenuated the adverse impact of DEHP on primordial FG. The key components of AMPK-SKP2-CARM1 signaling were upregulated by DEHP in the ovary, and the AMPK inhibitor, Compound C, reduced ATG-related gene expression and recovered primordial follicle assembly, indicating that DEHP induces ATG by activating AMPK-SKP2-CARM1 signaling in mice perinatal ovaries, resulting in disrupted primordial FG and reduced female fertility.

Trifolium Pratens L.

Glioblastoma multiforme (GBM) is the most malignant form of brain tumors. Trifolium pratense L. has been suggested for cancer treatment in traditional medicine. Khazaei et al. (2018) investigated the effects of a T. pratense extract on the GBM cell line (U87MG). They investigated the effect of the T. pratense extract on cell viability. Treatment with the T. pratense extract reduced the cell viability. ATG and apoptosis were increased. the T. pratense extract decreased NO production in U87MG cells. The combination of TMZ and T. pratense extract had a synergistic cytotoxic effect. T. pratense also showed anti-cancer properties via induction of ATG and apoptotic cell death.

The Theranostic Significance of Antioxidants as CP Regulators in Reproductive Diseases

Lycium Barbarum Polysaccharide

Lycium barbarum polysaccharide (LBP) contributes to the recovery of male hypogonadism and infertility. Yang et al. (2018) investigated the underlying mechanisms of LBP on male infertility. ERS-induced apoptosis was distinguished from that induced by death reporters and mitochondrial pathways. The death reporters and mitochondrial pathways can independently induce apoptosis. LBP protected Leydig MLTC-1 cells in Cisplatin (DDP) by regulating the ERS-mediated signal pathway, which was evidenced by the downregulation of phosphorylation PERK, phosphorylation of eukaryotic translation-initiation factor 2α, and activation of the transcription factor 4. LBP decreased DDP-induced MLTC-1 cell apoptosis via reducing ERS apoptosis-relative proteins caspase 3, caspase 7, and caspase 12. The result of mono-dansyl-cadaverine staining indicated that LBP inhibited DDP-induced autophagosome formation in MLTC-1 cells. LBP reversed DDP-induced LC3-II and Atg5 upregulation in MLTC-1 cells. In addition, LBP recovered MLTC-1 cells' testosterone level even in the presence of DDP, suggesting that LBP protected MLTC-1 cells against DDP via regulation of ERS-mediated apoptosis and ATG.

Morusin

Epithelial ovarian cancer (EOC) is the leading cause of death among all gynecological cancers. Morusin, a prenylated flavonoid extracted from the root bark of Morus australis, exhibits anti-tumor activity in various human cancers except EOC. Xue et al. (2018) explored the anti-cancer activity of Morusin in EOC. Morusin inhibited EOC cell proliferation and survival *in vitro* and suppressed tumor growth *in vivo*. Treatment of EOC cells with Morusin induced paraptosis-like cell death, a novel mode of non-apoptotic cell death that is characterized by extensive cytoplasmic vacuolation due to the dilation of the ER and mitochondria and a lack of apoptotic hallmarks. Morusin induced an increase in mitochondrial Ca^{2+}, accumulation of ERS markers, generation of ROS, and $\Delta\psi$ loss in EOC cells. Pretreatment with 4, 4′-diisothiocyanostilbene-2, 2′-disulfonic acid (DIDS), an inhibitor of the voltage-dependent anion channel (VDAC) on the OMM, inhibited mitochondrial Ca^{2+} influx, cytoplasmic vacuolation, and cell death induced by Morusin. DIDS pretreatment also suppressed the Morusin-induced accumulation of ERS markers, ROS production, and $\Delta\psi$ loss. Tumor xenograft assays showed that co-treatment with DIDS reversed the inhibitory effects of Morusin on tumor growth *in vivo* and inhibited the increased levels of ERS markers induced by Morusin in tumor tissues, suggesting that VDAC-mediated Ca^{2+} influx into mitochondria. The subsequent mitochondrial Ca^{2+} overload contributed to mitochondrial swelling and dysfunction, leading to a Morusin-induced paraptosis-like cell death in EOC. This study may provide alternative theranostic strategies for EOC exhibiting resistance to apoptosis.

Melatonin

In previous studies, oxidative stress damage was considered to be the mechanism of ovarian aging, and several antioxidants were used to delay ovarian aging. But recently, more reports have found that ERS, ATG, sirtuins, mitochondrial dysfunction, telomere length, gene mutation, premature ovarian failure, and polycystic ovary syndrome are all related to ovarian aging, and all these factors interact with oxidative stress. Yang et al. (2018) highlighted these novel insights on ovarian aging. As a pleiotropic molecule, melatonin was identified as an important antioxidant, which regulates not only oxidative stress, but also various molecules, and normal and pathological processes involved in ovarian functions and aging. They described the intricate role of melatonin in delaying ovarian aging.

Anti-Müllerian Hormone

The follicular ovarian reserve, constituted by primordial follicles (PMF), is established early in life, then keeps declining regularly along reproductive life. The maintenance of a normal female reproductive function implies the presence of a vast amount of dormant PMF. This process involves the continuous repression of PMF activation in the early growing follicle through balancing factors activating the initiation of follicular growth, mainly actors of the PI3K signaling pathway, and inhibiting factors such as anti-Müllerian hormone (AMH). Any disruption of this balance may induce follicle depletion and subsequent infertility. Cyclophosphamide (Cy), an alkylating agent used for treating BC, triggers PMF activation, leading to premature ovarian insufficiency. Preventing chemotherapy-induced ovarian dysfunction is highly crucial for preserving chances of natural or medically-assisted conceptions after healing. Sonigo et al. (2019) evaluated in a model of Cy-treated pubertal mice, whether AMH administration might restrain PMF depletion. Recombinant AMH prevented Cy-induced PMF loss. Activation of the PI3K signaling pathway was noticed after Cy administration. After AMH injection, Foxo3a phosphorylation was decreased, suggesting a protective role of AMH during Cy-induced follicular loss. Evidence for a possible role of CP/ATG in the preservation of follicular pool reserve was also provided. Therefore, concomitant rAMH administration during chemotherapy might be an option for preserving young patient's fertility.

Vitrification

Ovarian cryopreservation by vitrification and transplantation are useful methods to recover female fertility after radiotherapy and chemotherapy. CP/ATG plays important roles in ovarian follicle development, ovarian follicle atresia, and anti-stress injury. Xian et al. (2018) investigated the potential role of ATG in ovarian vitrification. Mouse ovaries were cryopreserved by vitrification, and ATG was treated, after which the ovarian histology was checked, and ovarian follicles were counted. ATG was significantly increased in the vitrified ovary as compared to fresh ovary. The number of primordial follicles was decreased through inhibiting or over-activating the ATG by the ATG inhibitor or activator. However, the number of primary follicles, antral follicles, and atretic follicles was not significantly different between the vitrified/warm ovaries and the fresh ovaries. The apoptotic rate was significantly increased in the vitrified/warmed, ATG-inhibiting and over-activating groups compared with the fresh group. Thus, ATG was activated in the ovarian cryopreservation by vitrification and played a crucial role in the natural adaptive response to cold stress in ovarian cryopreservation by vitrification.

Fucoxanthin

Moskalev et al. (2018) showed that the carotenoid Fucoxanthin can increase the lifespan in *Drosophila* and *C. elegans*. They studied the effects of Fucoxanthin on the *Drosophila* aging process. Fucoxanthin increased the median lifespan and had a positive effect on fecundity, fertility, intestinal barrier function, and night-time sleep. The transcriptome analysis revealed 57 differentially expressed genes involved in 17 KEGG pathways. A significant molecular pathway induced by Fucoxanthin was shown to be related to longevity, including MAPK, mTOR, Wnt, Notch, and Hippo-signaling pathways, ATG, translation, glycolysis, O/P, apoptosis, immune response, neurogenesis, sleep, and response to DNA damage. The life-extending effects of Fucoxanthin were associated with the differential expression of longevity-associated genes.

Torin1

ATG is a highly conserved mechanism for cellular repair that is downregulated during normal aging. Hence, manipulations that regulate ATG could increase lifespan. Previous reports show that manipulations of the ATG pathway can result in longevity in yeast, flies, worms, and mammals. Under standard nutrition, ATG is inhibited by the nutrient-sensing kinase TOR. Therefore, manipulations of TOR that increase ATG may offer a mechanism for extending lifespans. Such manipulations should be specific and minimize off-target effects, and it is important to discover additional methods for lifespan extension. Mason et al. (2018) reported the effect of upregulating ATG on lifespan and fertility in *Drosophila* by the dietary addition of Torin1. The activation of ATG using this selective TOR inhibitor was associated with increased lifespans in both sexes. Torin1 also induced an increase in the lifespan in once-mated females. Torin1-fed females exhibited elevated fecundity as well as egg fertility, and showed no net change in overall fertility, supporting the hypothesis that lifespan can be extended without trade-offs in fertility and that Torin1 may be a useful molecule to pursue fertility, fecundity, and anti-aging research.

CONCLUSION

CP in sperms and SCs was studied in a porcine cell-free system. Ferroptosis occurred with OGD/re-oxygenation-induced cell death. Ethanol-induced MTG in rat SCs compromised fertility. Surgery-induced cryptorchidism induced CP/ATG and apoptosis in mice spermatogonia. Flutamide and DEHP-induced cryptorchid rat models was characterized by defective ATG and enhanced apoptosis. Acute heat stress altered protein expression in the chicken testes. Lycium barbarum polysaccharide attenuated diabetic testicular dysfunction via inhibition of the PI3K/Akt-mediated abnormal ATG in male mice. Hedgehog and insulin signaling balanced proliferation and ATG to determine the follicle stem cell lifespan. ATG disrupted LC3-induced death of supporting cells of oocytes. Palmisano and Melendez (2019) highlighted that ATG has a pivotal role in multiple biological processes during the development of the *C. elegans*. Basal levels of ATG are required to remove aggregate prone proteins, paternal mitochondria (which exist in the form of undesired, nonfunctional inclusion bodies, also identified as CBs), and spermatid-specific membranous organelles as I have described in my book "Fetal Alcohol Spectrum Disorders: Concepts, Mechanisms, and Cure, Nova Science Publishers, New York, U.S.A. (Sharma 2017a). During larval development, ATG is required for the remodeling that occurs during dauer development, which can selectively eliminate components of the miRNA-induced silencing complex, and modulate miRNA-mediated silencing. Basal levels of ATG are important in synaptogenesis and stem cell proliferation in these nematodes. ATG is required for the efficient removal of apoptotic cell corpses by promoting phagosome maturation and is implicated in lipid homeostasis and in the aging process. These authors described the molecular complexes involved in the process of ATG, its regulation, and mechanisms for cargo recognition and the developmental contexts where ATG is extremely important and suggested that studies in *C. elegans* may provide valuable insights into its physiological relevance during metazoan development. Dehydroepiandrosterone-induced activation of mTORC1 and inhibition of ATG caused skeletal muscle insulin resistance in a mouse model of POCS. Ceramide-induced BOK promoted mitochondrial fission in preeclampsia. NRTI-induced oocyte dysfunction and low fertility in mice was mediated by ATG. ATG induced regression of the milk gland during involution in the viviparous reproduction of the tsetse fly. Lhx8 ablation-induced ATG caused DNA damage in the mouse oocyte. Germ cell depletion in the ovary involved CP, ATG, and apoptosis. Fetal-neonatal exposure of di (2-Ethylhexyl) phthalate disrupted ovarian development in mice via ATG induction. The decreased expression of HOXA10 induced ATG in endometriosis. Morusin induced paraptosis-like cell death via $[Ca^{2+}]_m$ overload in ovarian carcinoma. PM2.5 exposure compromised BTB integrity through ROS-mediated ATG. Melatonin was a potential target for delaying ovarian aging. AMH prevented primordial ovarian follicle loss and infertility in Cyclophosphamide-treated mice. CP/ATG was induced during ovarian cryopreservation by vitrification. Transcriptome analysis revealed the protective effects of Fucoxanthin and an ATG inducer, Torin1, increased the lifespan of *Drosophila* without loss of fertility and fecundity.

REFERENCES

Ausman, J., J. Abbade, L. Ermini, A. Farrell, et al. 2018. Ceramide-induced BOK promotes mitochondrial fission in preeclampsia. Cell Death Dis 9: 298. https://doi.org/10.1038/s41419-018-0360-0.

Benoit, J.B., V. Michalkova, E.M. Didion, Y. 2018. Rapid autophagic regression of the milk gland during involution is critical for maximizing tsetse viviparous reproductive output. PLoS Negl Trop Dis 12(1): e0006204.

Cai, H., L. Chen, M. Zhang, W. Xiang, et al. 2018. Low expression of Mfn-2 is associated with early unexplained miscarriage by regulating ATG of trophoblast cells. Placenta 70: 34–40.

D'Ignazio, L., M. Michel, M. Beyer, K. Thompson, et al. 2018. Lhx8 ablation leads to massive ATG of mouse oocytes associated with DNA damage. Biol Reprod 98: 532–542.

Eid, N., Y. Ito, A. Horibe, H. Hamaoka, et al. 2018. A method for in vivo induction and ultrastructural detection of mitophagy in sertoli cells. *In*: M. Alves and P. Oliveira (eds), Sertoli Cells. Meth. Mole. Bio., Vol 1748. Humana Press, New York, NY, pp. 103–112.

Eid, N. and Y. Kondo. 2018. Ethanol-induced mitophagy in rat Sertoli cells: Implications for male fertility. Andrologia 50(1): e12820.

Foroozan-Broojeni, S., M. Tavalaee, R.A. Lockshin, Z. Zakeri, et el. 2018. Comparison of main molecular markers involved in autophagy and apoptosis pathways between spermatozoa of infertile men with varicocele and fertile individuals. Andrologia 51(2): e13177.

Kang, W., E. Ishida, K. Yamatoya, A. Nakamura, et al. 2018. ATG-disrupted LC3 abundance leads to death of supporting cells of human oocytes. Biochem Biophys Rep 15: 107–114.

Khazaei, M., M. Pazhouhi and S. Khazaei. 2018. Evaluation of hydro-alcoholic extract of Trifolium pratens L. for its anti-cancer potential on U87MG cell line. Cell J 20: 412–421.

Li, L., Y. Hao, Y. Zhao, H. Wang, et al. 2018a. Ferroptosis is associated with oxygen-glucose deprivation/reoxygenation-induced Sertoli cell death. Int J Mol Med 41: 3051–3062.

Li, M., M.S. Lu, M.L. Liu, S. Deng et al. 2018b. An observation on the role of ATG in patients with endometriosis of different stages during secretory phase and proliferative phase. Curr Gene Ther 18: 286–295.

Mason, J.S., T. Wileman and T. Chapman. 2018. Lifespan extension without fertility reduction following dietary addition of the autophagy activator Torin1 in *Drosophila melanogaster*. PLoS ONE 13(1): e0190105.

Moskalev, A., M. Shaposhnikov, N. Zemskaya, A. Belyi, et al. 2018. Transcriptome analysis reveals mechanisms of geroprotective effects of fucoxanthin in *Drosophila*. BMC Genomics 19(Suppl 3): 77.

Palmisano, N.J. and A. Meléndez. 2019. Autophagy in *C. elegans* development. Dev Biol 447: 103–125.

Sharma S. 2017a. Fetal Alcohol Spectrum Disorders: Concepts, Mechanisms, and Cure. Series: Neurology–Laboratory and Clinical Research Developments. Nova Sciences Publishers, New York, U.S.A.

Sharma, S. 2017b. Zika Virus Disease: Prevention and Cure. Nova Science Publishers, New York, U.S.A.

Shi, G.J., J. Zheng, X.X. Han, Y.P. Jiang, et al. 2018. *Lycium barbarum* polysaccharide attenuates diabetic testicular dysfunction via inhibition of the PI3K/Akt pathway-mediated abnormal autophagy in male mice. Cell Tissue Res 374: 653–666.

Singh, T., E.H. Lee, T.R. Hartman, D.M. Ruiz-Whalen, et el. 2018. Opposing action of hedgehog and insulin signaling balances proliferation and autophagy to determine follicle stem cell lifespan. Dev Cell 46: 720–734.e6.

Song, X., Q. Shen, L. Fan, Q. Yu, et al. 2018. Dehydroepiandrosterone-induced activation of mTORC1 and inhibition of ATG contribute to skeletal muscle insulin resistance in a mouse model of polycystic ovary syndrome. Oncotarget 9: 11905–11921.

Wei, Y., Y. Zhou, X.L. Tang XL, B. Liu, et al. 2018a. Testicular developmental impairment caused by flutamide-induced and DEHP-induced cryptorchid rat models is mediated by excessive apoptosis and deficient ATG. Toxicol Mech Methods 28: 507–519.

Wei, Y., X.N. Cao, X.L. Tang, L.J. Shen, et al. 2018b. Urban fine particulate matter (PM2.5) exposure destroys blood-testis barrier (BTB) integrity through excessive ROS-mediated ATG. Toxicol Mech Methods 28: 302–319.

Xian, Y., B. Li, P. Pan, Y. Wang et al. 2018. Role of ATG in Ovarian Cryopreservation by Vitrification. Cryo Letters 39: 201–210.

Xue, J., R. Li, X. Zhao. C. Ma, et al. 2018. Morusin induces paraptosis-like cell death through mitochondrial calcium overload and dysfunction in epithelial ovarian cancer. Chem Biol Interact 283: 59–74.

Yadav, P.K., M. Tiwari, A. Gupta, A. Sharma, et al. 2018. Germ cell depletion from mammalian ovary: possible involvement of apoptosis and ATG. J Biomed Sci 25(1): 36.

Yang, Y., H.H. Cheung, C. Zhang, J. Wu, et al. 2018. Melatonin as potential targets for delaying ovarian aging. Curr Drug Targets 20: 16–28.

Zhang, Y., X. Mu, R. Gao, Y. Geng et al. 2018. Foetal-neonatal exposure of Di (2-ethylhexyl) phthalate disrupts ovarian development in mice by inducing ATG. J Hazard Mater 358: 101–112.

Zheng, J., X. Luo, J. Bao, X. Huang, Y. Jin, et al. 2018. Decreased Expression of HOXA10 May Activate the Autophagic Process in Ovarian Endometriosis. Reprod Sci 25: 1446–1454.

Zheng, Y., P. Zhang, C. Zhang and W. Zeng. 2019. Surgery-induced cryptorchidism induces apoptosis and ATG of spermatogenic cells in mice. Zygote 27: 101–110.

22

Charnolophagy in Ophthalmic Diseases

INTRODUCTION

Age-related macular degeneration (AMD) is a multi-factorial disease that is the leading cause of irreversible and severe vision loss. AMD is caused by the decrease in macular function, due to the degeneration of RPE cells. The aged retina is characterized by increased ROS, impaired CP/ATG, and DNA damage that are linked to AMD pathogenesis. The abundance of ROS, DNA damage, and the excessive energy consumption in the aging retina contribute to the degeneration of RPE cells and their mitochondria. Hyttinen et al. (2018) discussed the role of MTG in the RPE and emphasized that its impairment plays a role in AMD pathogenesis. Hence, MTG can be used as a potential theranostic target in AMD and other degenerative diseases of the eye. Impaired CP has been related to various eye diseases such as glaucoma, cataracts, and age-related macular degeneration (AMD). Generally, ATG plays a dual role in these eye diseases. In some cases, increased ATG can reduce oxidative stress to maintain intracellular homeostasis, while in others, its upregulation results in cell death. ATG plays a critical role in lens fiber cell maturation and the development of glaucoma (obstruction of the flow of the lacrimal fluid due to inflammation and blocking of the Schlem's canal). The regulatory role of ATG has been proposed in ocular diseases and its theranostic potential in the TSE-EBPT of retinal pigment epithelial (RPE) and ganglion cell repair and degeneration. CP/ATG maintains mitochondrial quality control (MQC) by eliminating persistent CBs in the degenerating RPE and ganglion cells during AMD. Central to visual health is mitochondrial homeostasis, and the selective ATG turnover of mitochondria through CP plays a crucial role in this. McWilliams et al. (2019) utilized the *mito*-QC mouse and a related general macroATG reporter model to profile basal CP and macroATG in the adult and developing eye. Ocular macroATG was widespread, but CP did not always followed the same pattern. Low levels of CP were noticed in the lens and ciliary body of the developing eye, in contrast to the high levels of general MAP1LC3-dependent macroATG. There was a significant reversal of this process in the adult retina, where CP accounted for macroATG in the photoreceptor neurons of the outer nuclear layer. CP in the adult mouse retina was reversed during the later stages of development.

This chapter highlights the significance of CP and antioxidants as CP regulators/modulators for the TSE-EBPT in ophthalmic diseases.

Cone-rod Dystrophy by DRAM2 Mutations

Cone-rod dystrophies (CRD) are a group of inherited retinal dystrophies (IRD) characterized by the involvement of photoreceptors, resulting in the degeneration of the central retina, or macula. Although there are >55 CRD genes, a considerable percentage of cases remain unsolved. Abad-Morales et al. (2019) characterized the phenotype and the genetic cause of 3 CRD families from a cohort of IRD cases. Clinical evaluation in each patient was supported by an ophthalmological examination, including visual acuity measurement, fundus retinography, auto-fluorescence imaging, optical coherence tomography, and full-field electroretinography. Molecular diagnoses were performed by the whole exome sequencing analyzing of a group of 279 IRD genes, and co-segregation of the identified pathogenic variants, which was confirmed by Sanger sequencing. Three homozygous mutations in the ATG gene DRAM2 were identified as the molecular targets of disease in the three families: c.518–1G>A, c.628_629insAG, and c.693+2T>A. These patients presented a shared CRD phenotype with adult-onset macular involvement and later peripheral degeneration, although the age of onset, evolution, and severity were variable. Alterations in the DRAM2 transcription, including alternative splicing forms and lower levels of mRNA correlated with the phenotypic variability between patients. Frameshift mutations were related to a less severe phenotype, with mid-peripheral involvement, and lower levels of mRNA, suggesting an activation of the nonsense-mediated decay (NMD) pathway; while a more severe retinal degeneration was associated with the in-frame alternative splicing variant due to a malfunctioning or toxicity of the resulting protein. The DRAM2 expression was assessed in several human tissues by qRT-PCR and two isoforms were detected; however, both had a single tissue-specific pattern in retina and brain. Although the retinal phenotype did not correlate with the ubiquitous expression, the retinal-specific expression and the role of ATG in the photoreceptor survival could explain the DRAM2 phenotype.

Retinal Dystrophy in Danon Disease

LAMP2 plays an important role in ATG and lysosomal function and its mutation is responsible for the pathogenesis of Danon disease, which can cause retinopathy. Fukushima et al. (2019) reported a case of Danon disease retinopathy, where they explained how LAMP2 dysfunction contributes to the pathogenesis of retinopathy. This case underwent slit-lamp exam, fundus imaging, visual field testing, and electroretinogram. In molecular biological study, mRNA expression of three splice variants of Lamp2 or LAMP2 in wild-type mouse retina and RPE, human RPE cell line, and adult RPE-19 were quantified. LAMP2 was knocked down by siRNA in adult RPE-19 and its effect on LC3, an ATG marker, was assessed by immunoblotting. The intracellular localization of LAMP2 and LC3 in untreated and LAMP2-knocked-down adult RPE-19 was analyzed by confocal microscopy. Cone dystrophy was manifested in both eyes. The Lamp2a and Lamp2b expression was higher in RPE than that in neural retina. The expression of Lamp2a and Lamp2b were higher than that of Lamp2c in mouse RPE. Adult RPE-19 cells showed a similar LAMP2 expression to mouse RPE. LAMP2 knockdown in adult RPE-19 reduced LC3-II and the number and size of APS, indicating that LAMP2 plays an important role in its formation in RPE.

Prolactin and PIP in PANDO

Ali and Paulsen (2019) hypothesized the role of Prolactin and Prolactin-inducible protein (PIP) in the pathogenesis of primary acquired nasolacrimal duct obstruction (PANDO). Primary acquired nasolacrimal duct obstruction (PANDO) is a syndrome of unknown etiology, affecting post-menopausal females, characterized by inflammation, fibrosis, and obstruction of the nasolacrimal duct. Numerous factors have been proposed as possible etiologic factors and include anatomical configuration, ocular and nasal infections, peri-lacrimal vascular disorders, hormonal influence, lacrimal drainage lymphoid tissue, GERD, topical medications, swimming-pool exposure, smoking, genetic factors, and autonomic and lysosomal dysregulation.

NRF-2 and PGC-1α Genes

The pathogenesis of dry AMD involves impaired protein degradation in RPE. RPE cells are constantly exposed to oxidative stress that may lead to the accumulation of damaged cellular proteins, DNA, and lipids, resulting in tissue deterioration during aging. The ubiquitin-proteasome pathway and the lysosomal/autophagosomal pathway are the two major proteolytic systems in eukaryotic cells. NRF-2 and PGC-1α are the main transcription factors in the regulation of cellular detoxification. Felszeghy et al. (2019) investigated the role of NRF-2 and PGC-1α in the regulation of the RPE cell structure and function by using double knockout (dKO) mice. The NRF-2/PGC-1α dKO mice exhibited age-dependent RPE degeneration, accumulation of the oxidative stress marker, 4-HNE (4-hydroxynonenal), the ERS marker, glucose-regulated protein 78 (GRP78), activating transcription factor 4 (ATF4), and damaged mitochondria implicated in CBMP. The levels of protein ubiquitination and ATG markers p62/SQSTM1 (sequestosome 1), Beclin-1, and LC3B were increased together with the ionized Ca^{2+} binding adaptor molecule 1 (Iba-1), phagocyte marker, and an enlargement of RPE size. These changes in RPE were accompanied by photoreceptor dys-morphology and vision loss as revealed by electroretinography, suggesting that the NRF-2/PGC-1α dKO mouse can be used for investigating the role of proteasomal and CP/ATG clearance in the RPE and dry AMD.

Pyroptosis in Retinopathy

Retinal neovascularization (RNV) is a principal cause of visual impairment and blindness. Wang et al. (2019) investigated oxidative stress, CP/ATG, and pyroptosis in RNV. The O_2-induced retinopathy (OIR) model was established in C57BL/6J mice by exposing them to a high concentration of O_2. RNV was visible in the fundus images and was analyzed by counting the number of neovascular endothelial cell nuclei on the postnatal day 17. The expression of VEGF-A and HIF-1α at the protein level were measured. Oxidative stress was evaluated using dihydroethidium (DHE) staining, and NADPH oxidase (NOX) 1 and 4 in the retinas were detected using qRT-PCR. Immunostaining of LC3 was performed and the expression levels of the LC3, p62, CP/ATG proteins (Atg5, ATG7, ATG12, Beclin-1), NOD-like receptor family pyrin domain-containing 3 (NLRP3), caspase-1, IL-1β, pro-caspase-1 and pro-IL-1β proteins were determined by immunoblotting to detect pyroptosis and CP/ATG. APS were also detected using TEM. VEGF-A and HIF-1α protein expression levels, the DHE-positive area, and NOX1 and NOX4 mRNA expression, were increased in the OIR mice. Increased NLRP3, caspase-1, IL-1β, pro-caspase-1 and pro-IL-1β proteins demonstrated that pyroptosis was induced. However, an accumulation of p62 and a reduction in the levels of LC3-II/I and APS indicated that CP/ATG induction was compromised. Hence, elevated ROS and pyroptosis along with compromised CP/ATG were demonstrated in the OIR mice. The combination of oxidative stress, pyroptosis, and impaired CP/ATG may be implicated in the pathophysiology of RNV and may serve as a potential theranostic strategy to prevent RNV.

Blue Light-induced Retinal Degeneration

Xia et al. (2018) explored the role of ATG in response to blue light damage in aged mice and in hRPE cells. Blue light damage to the retina was induced in 10-month-old (10 mo) C57 mice and hRPE cells. Flash electroretinography was used to assess retinal function. On day 1, after light damage to the 10 mo mice, their retinal function changed. The latent periods of a-wave and b-wave were delayed, and amplitude was reduced. Mitochondrial damage in the RPE and a disorganized photoreceptor outer segment (OS) was observed. PERK, LC3, and Beclin-1 were upregulated, whereas P62 was not. On day 5 after the blue light damage, restoration of electroretinography and OS was observed. PERK, LC3, and Beclin-1 were downregulated, whereas P62 was not. Protein changes *in vitro* were consistent with the changes *in vivo*. This study provided structural and functional evidence that ATG plays an important role in response to blue light-induced retinal damage.

miR-204 Influences RPE

The RPE is important for maintaining the health and integrity of the retinal photoreceptors. miR-204 is expressed in pulmonary, renal, mammary, and eye tissue, and its reduction can result in multiple diseases, including cancer. Zhang et al. (2019) developed miR-204–/– mice to study the impact of miR-204 loss on retinal and RPE structure and function. miR-204–/– eyes evidenced areas of hyper-autofluorescence and defective photoreceptor digestion, along with increased microglia migration to the RPE. Migratory Iba1+ microglial cells were localized to the RPE apical surface where they participated in the phagocytosis of photoreceptor outer segments (POS) and contributed to a persistent buildup of rhodopsin. These structural, molecular, and cellular outcomes were accompanied by decreased light-evoked electrical responses from the retina and RPE. In parallel experiments, these investigators suppressed miR-204 expression in primary cultures of human RPE using anti-miR-204. The *in vitro* suppression of miR-204 in human RPE showed abnormal ROS clearance and the altered expression of CP-related proteins and Rab22a, a regulator of endosome maturation, suggesting that high levels of miR-204 in RPE can mitigate disease onset by preventing generation of oxidative stress and inflammation originating from the intracellular accumulation of undigested photoreactive POS lipids implicated in the RPE miR-204-mediated regulation of CP and endo-lysosomal interaction as a determinant of normal RPE/retinal structure and function.

Retinal Degeneration in SCA-7

Spino-cerebellar ataxia type 7 (SCA7) is a polyglutamine (polyQ) disorder characterized by neurodegeneration of the brain, cerebellum, and retina caused by a polyglutamine expansion in ataxin7. The presence of an expanded polyQ tract in a mutant protein induces protein aggregation, cellular stress, toxicity, and finally, cell death. Lebon et al. (2019) demonstrated that in a retinal SCA7 mouse model, polyQ ataxin7 induces stress within the retina and activates Muller cells. An unfolded protein response and CP/ATG are activated in SCA7 photoreceptors. The photoreceptor death did not involve a caspase-dependent apoptosis but involved AIF and the leukocyte elastase inhibitor (LEI/L-DNase II). When these two cell death effectors were downregulated by their siRNA, a significant reduction in photoreceptor death was observed, indicating polyQ protein expression in the retina and the role of caspase-independent pathways in the photoreceptor cell death. In a retinal SCA7 mouse model, polyQ ataxin7 induced stress within the retina and activated Muller cells. Moreover, UPR and ATG were activated in SCA7 photoreceptors. The photoreceptor cell death was caspase-3-independent. However, AIF and leucocyte elastase inhibitor (LEI/L-DNase II) were involved in the photoreceptor cell death. When these two cell death effectors were downregulated by their siRNA, a significant reduction in photoreceptor death was observed, highlighting the consequences of polyQ protein expression in the retina and the role of caspase-independent pathways in photoreceptor cell death. Retinal degeneration in the poly-glutamine disorder involving CBMP is presented in Fig. 36.

Retinal Degeneration in Spinocerebellar Ataxia 7
(A Polyglutamine (PolyQ) Disorder involving CBMP)

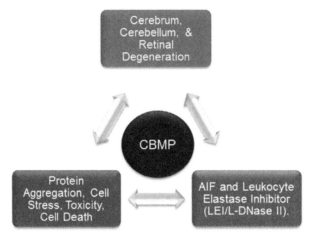

Figure 36

FECD and Mitochondria

Miyai (2018) reported that Fuchs endothelial corneal dystrophy (FECD) is a bilateral progressive corneal endothelial disease characterized by guttae, which presents as a partial descemet membrane thickening, inducing corneal edema at the final stage. Oxidative stress plays an important role in the pathogenesis of FECD. The ETC and O/P system in mitochondria are the main sources of oxidative stress, arising from superoxide generation through premature electron leakage to O_2. In FECD, corneal endothelial cells have altered mitochondria with mtDNA damage, decreased O/P proteins, and lower $\Delta\Psi$. Mitochondrial dynamics and MTG comprise the organelle-level MQC. Mitochondrial dynamics include fusion and fission processes. When mitochondria are severely damaged, fission becomes the dominant process to remove damaged mitochondria through CP. In FECD, corneal endothelial mitochondria have a fission-dominant morphology and low density through MTG upregulation because of QC mechanisms against altered mitochondria implicated in CBMP and, apoptosis implicated in FECD.

Blepharoptosis

To observe the pathological features of levator aponeurosis with involutional ptosis, Zhang et al. (2018a) enrolled 29 patients with involutional blepharoptosis who underwent levator aponeurosis advancement surgery for blepharoptosis correction. Specimens of the levator aponeurosis were obtained during surgery. Twelve normal specimens of fresh levator aponeurosis were obtained from the eye bank as the control group. As many as 14 cases were diagnosed with moderate ptosis and 15 cases with severe ptosis; nine cases involved with both eyes, nine cases with right eyes, and 11 cases with left eyes. Fascicle disruption, scarcity of cross-striations, collagen fibers hyperplasia, fatty infiltration, and a decrease of myoglobin expression were observed in levator aponeurosis. Collagen fiber hyperplasia and cellular degeneration including mitochondrial swelling and hyperplasia, vacuoles, LDs, nucleus pycnosis, chromosome condensation, disintegrated organelles, myeloid body, and ATG were observed. Muscle fiber degeneration, collagen fiber hyperplasia, and cellular degeneration were noticed in patients with involutional blepharoptosis. PRPF8 (pre-mRNA processing factor 8), a core component of the spliceosome, was identified as an essential mediator in hypoxia-induced MTG from an RNAi screen based on a fluorescent MTG reporter mt-Keima analysis. Knockdown of PRPF8 impaired MPS formation and CB clearance through the aberrant mRNA splicing of ULK1, which triggered CP induction (Xu et al 2018a). Autosomal dominant retinitis pigmentosa (adRP)-associated PRPF8 mutant, R2310K, was defective in regulating MTG. Knockdown of other adRP-associated splicing factors, including PRPF6, PRPF31, and SNRNP200, also led to ULK1 mRNA mis-splicing and MTG defects, demonstrating that PRPF8 is essential for MTG and that dysregulation of spliceosome-mediated MTG may contribute to pathogenesis of retinitis pigmentosa.

Ganglion Cells

Retinal explants and mixed primary cultures are currently used to investigate retinal ganglion cells (RGCs) pathophysiology and pharmacology. Zaninello and Scorrano (2018) compared two methods of purification of mouse primary RGCs and showed that mitochondrial and ATG parameters can be measured in RGCs, which were purified from P0 mouse eyes based on the surface antigen Thy1. In a two-step immunopanning purification, a subtraction plate bound macrophage antiserum removed contaminant macrophages and endothelial cells; unbound RGCs were then affinity selected using a plate-bound antiThy1 antibody. In an immunopanning-magnetic separation, macrophage-antiserum bound cells were subtracted and then RGCs were selected using an antiThy1 antibody bound to a magnetic column. The two-steps immunopanning yielded low amounts of 90% pure RGCs, whereas immunopanning-magnetic separation method provided 6X more RGCs from a representative sample of 30% cells. RGCs purified with both methods could be micro-electroporated to image-expressed mitochondria and APS fluorescent probes and to show that expression of the pathogenic optic atrophy mutants caused CB formation implicated in CBMP.

NaIO$_3$

Lin et al. (2018) examined whether NaIO$_3$ treatment disrupted the mitochondrial-lysosomal axis in cultured RPE. The human RPE cell line, ARPE-19, was treated with low concentrations ($\leq$500 µM) of NaIO$_3$. Intracellular acidic compartments and lipofuscinogenesis were evaluated by acridine orange staining and autofluorescence, respectively. Mitochondrial mass, $\Delta\Psi$, and function were quantified by *MitoTracker* Green staining, tetramethylrhodamine methyl ester staining, and the MTT assay, respectively. Treatment with low concentrations of NaIO$_3$ decreased cellular acidity, blocked ATG flux, and increased lipofuscinogenesis in ARPE-19 cells. Despite increases in Sirtuin 1 and PGC-1α, mitochondrial function was compromised, and this decrease was attributed to disrupted $\Delta\Psi$. POS phagocytic activities decreased by 60% in NaIO$_3$-treated cells, and the degradation of ingested POS was also impaired. Pre-treatment and co-treatment with Rapamycin rescued NaIO$_3$-induced RPE dysfunction. Low concentrations of NaIO$_3$ disrupted the mitochondrial-lysosomal axis in RPE and impaired CP/ATG.

Pgc-1α Repression and HFD Induce AMD

AMD is the major cause of blindness in the elderly and its prevalence is increasing with the aging population. AMD initially affects the RPE and gradually leads to secondary photoreceptor degeneration. Zhang et al. (2018b) observed mitochondrial and CP/ATG dysfunction and repressed PGC-1α; (also known as Ppargc1a) in native RPE from AMD donor eyes and induced pluripotent stem cell-derived RPE. They established a mouse model by feeding Pgc-1$\alpha^{+/-}$ mice with a HFD and investigated RPE and retinal health. When mice expressing lower levels of Pgc-1α were exposed to a HFD, they presented AMD-like abnormalities in RPE and retinal morphology and function, including basal laminar deposits, thickening of Bruch's membrane with Drusen marker-containing deposits, RPE and photoreceptor degeneration, decreased mitochondrial activity, ROS overproduction, decreased CP/ATG, and increased inflammatory response in the RPE and retina, confirming that Pgc-1α is important in retina biology and that Pgc-1$\alpha^{+/-}$ mice fed with a HFD provide a promising model to study AMD and discover novel TSE-EBPT-CPTs for it.

Lens Anterior Capsule in Cataract

To observe the ultrastructure of lens epithelial cells in cataract associated uveitis, Yang et al. (2018) conducted a study on seven patients (seven eyes) who received phaco-emulsification due to complicated cataract associated with uveitis [two males and five females, with an average age of (49 ± 20) years] and three patients suffering from age-related cataract (three eyes, females, aged 54, 71, 74 years) were enrolled. Anterior capsules were collected during surgery. Spindle-shaped epithelial cells were observed in cataract associated with uveitis (100%), while 28%, 16.67%, and 16.67% of spindle-shaped epithelial cells were observed in age-related cataract. Mitochondrial swelling and damage to the tight cell junction in cataract were associated with uveitis. The tight junction between two cells was damaged to different degrees, only 8.33% (0–16.67%) of the cell nuclei appeared normal, and increased chromatin density (47.07% ± 22.28%), nuclear pyknosis (38.02% ± 19.61%), and nuclear fragmentation (9.96% ± 8.10%) were observed in cataract secondary to uveitis. The apoptosis was (48.16% ± 26.66%) in cataract associated with uveitis and correlated to the duration of intraocular inflammation. While the apoptosis were 0, 8.33%, and 0 in age-related cataract patients, no APS was observed in cataract associated with uveitis. The increased rate of apoptosis and inhibition of ATG could be the possible mechanisms of cataract formation in uveitic eyes.

d-Galactose Induces Premature Senescence

Cataract is the leading cause of blindness with an estimated 16 million people affected worldwide. d-galactose (d-gal) is a reducing sugar that is widely distributed in foodstuffs, which could promote cataract formation by damaging natural lens epithelial cells (LECs). Xu et al. (2018b) demonstrated that d-gal resulted in premature senescence of LECs. This was confirmed by determining the β-galactosidase activity, cell proliferative potential, and cell cycle distribution, though apoptosis of LECs was not observed. d-gal induced the impairment of ATG flux by measuring the expression of LC3-II and P62. d-gal induced CBMP of LECs through increasing ROS, reducing ATP synthesis and $\Delta\Psi$, and enhancing the concentration of cytoplasm $[Ca^{2+}]_i$ and mPTP opening. Metformin, as a potential anti-aging agent, suppressed the senescence of LECs by restoring ATG flux and mitochondrial function. Although, the antioxidant NAC scavenged ROS significantly but it was inefficient in preventing LECs from premature senescence, suggesting that restoring CP/ATG and improving mitochondrial functions may be a potential strategy for the prevention of LECs senescence-related cataract.

Vitamin D-mediated Protection

Studies on dietary supplementation and AMD occurrence and progression have produced conflicting results. In its advanced stage, AMD may be associated with apoptosis, pyroptosis, or necroptosis of retinal cells. Dietary vitamin D plays an important role in maintaining proper vision by modulating each of these pathways. Vitamin D is a modulator of the immune system and acts synergistically with two members of the regulators of complement activation family H and I, whose specific variants are genetic factors for AMD pathogenesis. Angiogenesis is an essential component of the neovascular form of AMD, whereas, vitamin D possesses anti-angiogenic properties. Cellular DNA damage response is weakened in AMD patients. Several pathways of vitamin D metabolism and AMD pathogenesis overlap, suggesting that vitamin D could modulate the course of AMD by CP/ATG regulation.

MicroRNA-24 Protects Retina

Lian et al. (2019) demonstrated that miR-24 plays an important role in maintaining the retinal structure and visual function of rats by targeting chitinase-3-like protein 1 (CHI3L1). In the RPE cells of the Royal College of Surgeons (RCS) rats, an animal model of genetic retinal degeneration (RD), miR-24, was found lower and the CHI3L1 level was higher compared to those found in SD rats. RCS rats revealed activated Akt/mTOR and ERK pathways and abnormal CP/ATG in the RPE cells. These roles of miR-24 and CHI3L1 were confirmed in RCS rats by a sub-retinal injection of agomiR-24, which decreased the CHI3L1 level and preserved retinal structure and function. NF-κB was identified as the regulator of miR-24 in the RPE cells of these rats. The intraocular treatment of antagomiR-24 in SD rats induced pathological changes similar to those in RCS rats. These investigators proposed the protective role of miR-24 in RPE cells and a mechanism of RD in RCS rats: extracellular stress stimuli first activate the NF-κB signaling pathway, which lowers miR-24 expression to enhance CHI3L1 expression, which results in aberrant CP/ATG and RPE dysfunction by activating the Akt/mTOR and ERK pathways, indicating that miR-24 protects retina by targeting CHI3L1. Hence, miR-24 and CHI3L1 can be utilized for developing the TSE-EBPT of degenerative retinal diseases like AMD.

CONCLUSION

DRAM2 mutations induced a retinal phenotype with cone-rod dystrophy. LAMP-2 mutation caused RPE degeneration in Danon syndrome. Retinal degeneration occurred in a mouse model of SCA7. Prolactin and prolactin-inducible protein induced PANDO pathogenesis. Loss of NRF-2 and PGC-1α genes and implementation of HFD induced RPE degeneration resembling AMD. Oxidative stress, ATG, and pyroptosis were observed in the O_2-induced retinopathy. Fuchs endothelial corneal dystrophy involved CMB. Pathological features of levator aponeurosis were observed in patients with involutional blepharoptosis. Sodium iodate disrupted the mitochondrial-lysosomal axis in cultured RPE cells. Pivotal roles of CP/ATG and CMB were identified in AMD. The d-Galactose induced premature senescence of lens epithelial cells by CMB and CP/ATG, whereas vitamin D ameliorated AMD. Regulation of APS by miR-204 influenced RPE, retinal structure, and function. In addition, microRNA-24 prevented RD by inhibiting chitinase-3-like protein 1 implicated in CP/ATG in rats.

REFERENCES

Abad-Morales, V., A. Burés-Jelstrup, R. Navarro, S. Ruiz-Nogales, et al. 2019. Characterization of the cone-rod dystrophy retinal phenotype caused by novel homozygous DRAM2 mutations. Exp Eye Res 187: 107752.

Ali, M.J. and F. Paulsen. 2019. Prolactin and Prolactin-inducible protein (PIP) in the pathogenesis of primary acquired nasolacrimal duct obstruction (PANDO). Med Hypotheses 125: 137–138.

Felszeghy, S., J. Viiri, J.J. Paterno, J.M.T. Hyttinen, et al. 2019. Loss of NRF-2 and PGC-1α genes leads to retinal pigment epithelium damage resembling dry age-related macular degeneration. Redox Biol 20: 1–12.

Fukushima, M., T. Inoue, T. Miyai and R. Obata. 2019. Retinal dystrophy associated with Danon disease and pathogenic mechanism through LAMP2-mutated retinal pigment epithelium. Eur J Ophthalmol 5: 1120672119832183.

Hyttinen, J.M.T., J. Viiri, K. Kaarniranta and J. Błasiak. 2018. Mitochondrial quality control in AMD: Does MTG play a pivotal role? Cell Mol Life Sci 75: 2991–3008.

Lebon, C., F. Behar-Cohen and A. Torriglia. 2019. Cell death mechanisms in a mouse model of retinal degeneration in spinocerebellar ataxia 7. Neuroscience 400: 72–84.

Lian, C., H. Lou, J. Zha, et al. 2019. MicroRNA-24 protects retina from degeneration in rats by down-regulating chitinase-3-like protein 1. Exp Eye Res 188: 107791.

Lin, Y.C., L.Y. Horng, H.C. Sung and R.T. Wu. 2018. Sodium iodate disrupted the mitochondrial-lysosomal axis in cultured retinal pigment epithelial cells. J Ocul Pharmacol Ther 34: 500–511.

McWilliams, T.G., A.R. Prescott, B. Villarejo-Zori, G. Ball, et al. 2019. A comparative map of macroautophagy and mitophagy in the vertebrate eye. Autophagy 15: 1296–1308.

Miyai, T. 2018. Fuchs endothelial corneal dystrophy and mitochondria. Cornea 37: S74–S77.

Sharma, L.K., M. Tiwari, N.K. Rai and Y. Bai. 2018. Mitophagy activation repairs Leber's hereditary optic neuropathy-associated mitochondrial dysfunction and improves cell survival. Hum Mol Genet 28(3): 422–433.

Wang, S., L.Y. Ji, L. Li, J.M. Li. 2019. Oxidative stress, autophagy and pyroptosis in the neovascularization of oxygen-induced retinopathy in mice. Mol. Med. Rep. 19: 927–934.

Xia, H., Q. Hu, L. Li. et al. 2019. Protective effects of autophagy against blue light-induced retinal degeneration in aged mice. Sci China Life Sci 62: 244–256.

Xu, G., T. Li, J. Chen, C. Li, et al. 2018a. Autosomal dominant retinitis pigmentosa-associated gene PRPF8 is essential for hypoxia-induced MTG through regulating ULK1 mRNA splicing. Autophagy 14: 1818–1830.

Xu, Y., Y. Li, L. Ma, G. Xin, et al. 2018b. D-galactose induces premature senescence of lens epithelial cells by disturbing autophagy flux and mitochondrial functions. Toxicol Lett 289: 99–106.

Yang, M.L. and L. Yang. 2018. Ultrastructure of the lens anterior capsule in secondary cataract associated with uveitis under an electron microscope. Chin J Ophthalmol 54: 357–362.

Zaninello, M. and L. Scorrano. 2018. Rapidly purified ganglion cells from neonatal mouse retinas allow studies of mitochondrial morphology and ATG. Pharmacol Res 138: 16–24.

Zhang, L., B. Li, L. Li, Y. Li, et al. 2018a. Pathological features of levator aponeurosis in patients with involutional blepharoptosis. Zhonghua Yan Ke Za Zhi 54: 671–677.

Zhang, M., Y. Chu, J. Mowery, B. Konkel, et al. 2018b. Pgc-1α repression and high-fat diet induce age-related macular degeneration-like phenotypes in mice. Dis Model Mech 11(9): dmm032698.

Zhang, C., K.J. Miyagishima, L. Dong, A. Rising, et al. 2019. Regulation of phagolysosomal activity by miR-204 critically influences retinal pigment epithelium/retinal structure and function. Hum Mol Genet 28: 3355–3368.

23

Charnolophagy in Neurodegenerative Diseases
(Part-1)

INTRODUCTION

With the global increase in life expectancy, NDDs affect an ever-increasing number of individuals throughout the world. NDDs place an enormous burden on patients and caregivers globally. Over 6 million people in the U.S.A. alone suffer from NDDs, all of which are chronic, incurable, and with unknown causes. Identifying a common molecular mechanism emphasizing NDDs pathology is needed to aid in the design of effective therapies to ease suffering, reduce economic costs, and improve the QOL. New theranostic strategies for NDDs are required given the lack of current therapeutic modalities. Maiese (2018) examined novel strategies for NDDs that included circadian clock genes, ncRNAs, and the mammalian FoxOs, which offer exciting prospects to limit or eliminate morbidity and mortality associated with NDDs. Each of these pathways has a relationship with CP/ATG and apoptosis and share a common link to silent mating type information regulation 2 homolog 1 (S. cerevisiae) (SIRT1) and mTOR. Circadian clock genes modulate CP/ATG, limit cognitive loss, and prevent neuronal injury. ncRNAs control neuronal stem cell development and differentiation and offer protection against vascular diseases such as atherosclerosis. FoxOs activates ATG pathways to remove toxic accumulations and prevent apoptosis implicated in NDDs. Further studies on these genes are promising for the development of novel theranostic strategies for NDDs. Chen et al. (2019) summarized the clinical presentation, molecular pathogenesis, imaging, and genetics of Pantothenate kinase-associated NDD, characterized by iron deposition in specific parts of the brain. It is an autosomal recessive disorder characterized by a variant in the PANK2 gene. Pathogenesis involves mitochondrial dysfunction, oxidative stress, lipid metabolism, and CP/ATG disorders. The phenotypic spectrum includes classic and atypical PKAN. The clinical presentation may range from speech disorder to severe dystonia, dysphagia, mental retardation, and retinal degeneration.

This chapter presents the TSE-EBPT potential of CP in the clinical management of various NDDs.

Original Discoveries

Impaired lysosomal function or CPS/lysosome fusion is observed in most NDDs. CP is the major intracellular event involved in the elimination of abnormal organelles and protein aggregate, the root cause of PD, PDD, MSA, AD, ALS, FTD, HD, Fredrick ataxia, SCA-7, and Cruzfeldt-Jackob disease (a prion disease). The author discovered pleomorphic CB in the developing UN rat cerebellar Purkinje neurons, as well as in the hippocampal CA-3 and dentate gyrus neurons of the intrauterine domoic acid-exposed mice progeny. This original discovery led him to elucidate the CB life cycle involving CP induction, CS stabilization/destabilization, CS exocytosis/CS endocytosis, and eventually, CBMP implicated in diversified congenital and adult neuropathies, encephalopathies and synopathies; collectively classified as *neurodegenerative charnolopathies* (NDCs). Thus, free-radical-induced mitochondrial and lysosomal dysfunction resulting in CBMP participates in the etiopathogenesis of various NDCs.

Basic Molecular Mechanisms of NDDs and CP

Neurodegeneration is characterized by mitochondrial malfunction and protein aggregates due to intracellular redox imbalance. Although therapies that aim at dissolving aggregates remained unsuccessful, the promises of suppressing the expression of ND-associated pathogenic proteins or the deployment of engineered iPSCs are emerging, and these aggregates through CP/ATG-related mechanisms hold the potential for a possible cure for NDDs.

There are primarily three major mechanisms by which mitochondria are targeted for CP: *(a) transmembrane receptor-mediated, (b) ubiquitin-mediated, and (c) Cardiolipin-mediated.* A proteostasis view of ND identifies protein aggregation as the primary cause for degeneration at the cellular, molecular, genetic, epigenetic, and organ levels. The ATG that deals with identification, capture, and degradation of protein aggregates is called aggrephagy. Suresh et al. (2018) described aggrephagy and its selectivity towards aggregates. The diverse cellular adaptors that bridge the aggregates with the core ATG machinery by APS formation were highlighted. In ND, protein QC mechanisms fail as the components also find themselves trapped in these aggregates. Thus, while aggrephagy has the potential to be upregulated, its dysfunction aggravates the pathogenesis. This phenomenon when combined with neurons those can neither dilute the aggregates by cell division nor allow the dead neurons to be replaced due to reduced neurogenesis, makes aggrephagy as a potential theranostic option.

Recently, Audano et al. (2018) provided an update about mitochondria and lysosomal interaction in pathophysiology, focusing on the molecular mechanism that regulates their interdependence. Mitochondria and lysosome are mutually functional, and both maintain proper ICD and cell homeostasis. Restelli et al. (2018) showed that the *in vivo* ablation of the neuron-specific, inducible mitochondrial fission protein Drp-1 causes ERS, resulting in the activation of the stress response to culminate in the neuronal expression of the cytokine Fgf21. Neuron-derived Fgf21 induction occurs also in murine models of tauopathies and prion diseases, suggesting the potential of this cytokine as an early biomarker for latent NDDs. The nuclear-encoded glycyl-tRNA synthetase gene (GARS) is essential for protein translation in both cytoplasm and mitochondria. In contrast, different genes encode the mitochondrial and cytosolic forms of other tRNA synthetases. Dominant GARS mutations were described in inherited neuropathies, while it was shown that recessive mutations cause severe childhood-onset disorders affecting the skeletal muscle and heart. Boczonadi et al. (2018) investigated the mitochondrial function of GARS in human cell lines and in the GarsC210R mouse model. iNPCs carrying dominant and recessive GARS mutations showed alterations of mitochondrial proteins, which were prominent in iNPCs with dominant, neuropathy-causing mutations. Although the comparative proteomic analysis of iNPCs showed changes in the mitochondrial respiratory chain complex subunits, assembly genes, Krebs cycle enzymes, and transport proteins (in both recessive and dominant mutations), proteins involved in the β oxidation of fatty acid were altered only by recessive mutations causing mitochondrial cardiomyopathy. In contrast, significant alterations in the vesicle-associated membrane protein-associated protein B (VAPB) and mitochondrial Ca^{2+} uptake and ATG were detected in GARS mutations. The role of VAPB was supported by similar results in the GarsC210R mice, suggesting that altered mitochondria-associated ER membranes may be disease mechanisms leading to neuropathy.

Chu et al. (2018) summarized key features of the major cargo recognition pathways for selective CP/ATG, highlighting their potential impact in the pathogenesis or amelioration of NDDs. Protein aggregates and damaged mitochondria represent key pathological hallmarks shared by most NDDs. The p62/SQSTM1 as the mammalian selective ATG receptor defined a new family of ATG-related proteins that target protein aggregates, mitochondria, intracellular pathogens, and other cargo to the CP/ATG machinery via the LC3-interacting region (LIR)-motif. Mutations in the LIR-motif proteins p62 (SQSTM1) and optineurin (OPTN) contribute to familial forms of FTD and ALS. Moreover, a subset of LIR-motif proteins participate in CBMP through two recessive familial genes in PD pathogenesis. PINK1 activates the E3 ubiquitin ligase Parkin (PARK2) to mark depolarized mitochondria for CBMP. Liu et al. (2018) reported that reduction in Tom40 expression, a key subunit of the translocase of the OMM complex, led to accumulation of ubiquitin (Ub)-positive protein aggregates engulfed by ATG8a-positive membranes. Other macroATG markers were also accumulated. ATG was induced but the majority of APS failed to fuse with lysosomes when Tom40 was downregulated. In Tom40 RNAi tissues, APS-like (AL) structures were 10X larger than starvation-induced APSs. Atg5 downregulation abolished Tom40 RNAi- induced AL structure formation, but the Ub-positive aggregates remained, whereas knock down of Syx17, a gene required for APS-lysosome fusion, led to the disappearance of giant AL structures and accumulation of small APSs and phagophores near the Ub-positive aggregates.

The protein aggregates contained mitochondrial pre-proteins, cytosolic proteins, and proteosome subunits. Proteasome activity and ATP were reduced and the ROS were increased in Tom40 RNAi tissues. The simultaneous inhibition of proteasome activity, reduction in ATP production, and increase in ROS (but none of these conditions alone) could mimic the imbalanced proteostasis phenotypes observed in Tom40 RNAi cells. Knockdown of ref(2)P or ectopic expression of PINK1 and park reduced the aggregate formation in Tom40 RNAi tissues. Reduction in Tom40 activity lead to aggregate formation and neurodegeneration. Overexpression of PINK1 enhanced NDC phenotypes suggesting that defects in the mitochondrial protein import may be the key to linking imbalanced proteostasis and mitochondrial defects. The translation of mRNAs is constantly regulated and surveyed for errors. Aberrant translation can trigger co-translational protein and RNA-QC, impairments of which cause NDDs. Wu et al. (2018) showed that the QC of translation of OMM-localized mRNA intersects with the turnover of damaged mitochondria participating in CBMP, both orchestrated by the mitochondrial kinase PINK1. CB formation causes stalled translation of complex-I 30 kDa subunit (C-I30) mRNA on OMM, triggering the recruitment of co-translational QC factors Pelo, ABCE1, and NOT4 to the ribosome/mRNA-RNP complex. Damage-induced ubiquitination of ABCE1 by NOT4 generates poly-ubiquitin signals that attract CP/ATG receptors to OMM to trigger CP. In the *Drosophila* PINK1 model, these factors act synergistically to restore CP and neuromuscular tissue integrity. Thus, ribosome-associated co-translational QC generates an early signal to trigger CP. PINK1-catalyzed phosphorylation of ubiquitin (Ub) plays a critical role in the onset of Parkin-mediated CP. PTEN-L is a newly identified isoform of PTEN, with the addition of 173 amino acids to its N-terminus. These findings have theranostic implications for the TSE-EBPT of NDDs. DPCI-induced CB formation and CP dysregulation triggers progressive NDCs as illustrated in Fig. 37.

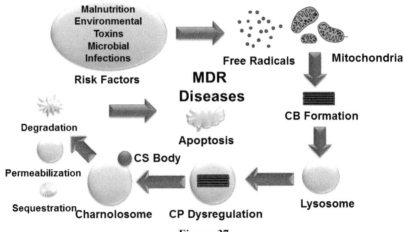

Figure 37

CB prevention, CP induction, and CS stabilization confers neuroprotection by preventing CBMP as illustrated in Fig. 38.

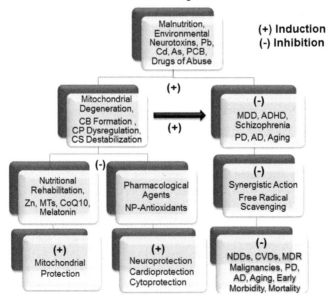

Figure 38

CP Theranostics in NDDs

The onset of progressive NDDs (PD, AD, LSDs, and ALS) is primarily linked to mutations in mitochondrial and lysosomal regulators. The mitochondrial dysfunction leads to lysosomal impairment and buildup of ATG by-products (including CBs), whereas lysosomal imperfections trigger mitochondrial defects to impair CP, implicated in LSDs. Stress adaptation is essential for neuronal health. Neuronal mitochondrial dysfunction triggers the stress response to induce fibroblast growth factor 21 in progressive NDDs. Mutations in glycyl-tRNA synthetase impairs mitochondrial metabolism in neurons to induce CP/ATG in ALS and FTD. A pivotal role of survival motor neuron protein (SMN) has been proposed in protein homeostasis, which is impaired in ALS and FTD. Intracellular homeostasis depends on the spatiotemporal elimination of damaged cellular organelles and proteins via CP, MTG, and ATG. Recent genetic and biochemical evidence has improved our understanding of the mechanisms that lead to ALS and FTD, two devastating NDDs with overlapping symptoms and causes. ALS is a motor neuron disease with connections to other NDDs such as FTD. Impaired RNA metabolism, enhanced aggregation of protein-RNA complexes, aberrant formation of RNP granules, and dysfunctional protein clearance via ATG are emerging as crucial events in ALS/FTD pathogenesis which interact and converge on a common pathogenic cascade. Mandrioli et al. (2019) summarized the key principles underlying ALS and FTD, and discussed how mutations in genes involved in RNA metabolism, protein QC, and protein degradation merge to impair the dynamics of RNP granules, and how this leads to cellular toxicity and death.

Although various signaling pathways become dysfunctional in ALS/FTD due to altered RNP granule dynamics, stress granule-independent mechanisms could also be promising targets for theranostic interventions. Nguyen et al. (2019) discussed ATG that links to the different genetic forms of ALS. Age-dependent NDDs are associated with a decline in protein QC systems, including CP/ATG. There is a recurring theme of protein misfolding as in other NDDs, but there is a distinct common thread among ALS genes that connects them to the cascade of CP/ATG. However, the roles of CP/ATG in ALS remain enigmatic and it is still uncertain whether its activation or inhibition would be reliable to ameliorate the disease. Ever since the loss of SMN protein was discovered as the direct cause of the childhood-inherited NDD, spinal muscular atrophy, significant efforts have been made to reveal the molecular functions of this ubiquitously expressed protein. Chaytow et al. (2018) summarized the diverse functions of SMN, confirming its central role in maintaining the homeostatic environment of the cell. SMN plays pivotal roles in cellular homeostatic pathways, including assembly of the spliceosome and biogenesis of RNPs, mRNA trafficking, local translation, cytoskeletal dynamics, endocytosis, CP, and ATG. SMN influences MB pathways as well as regulates the functioning of the ubiquitin-proteasome system. The diversified functions of SMN protein are presented in Table 14.

Table 14 Diversified Functions of the SMN Protein

S.No	SMN Protein Functions
1.	NCF
2.	Mitochondrial bioenergetics
3.	Skeletal dynamics
4.	Regional translation
5.	CP Regulation and CS stability
6.	IMD and ICD
7.	Endocytosis CP/MTG/ATG
8.	mRNA trafficking
9.	Ubiquinone proteasome system
10.	Spliceosome activity
11.	RNP biogenesis
12.	CBMP inhibition
13.	MQC

A table illustrating the diversified functions of the SMN protein.

Various ALS-causing gene mutations (for example, in FUS, TDP-43, or C9ORF72) have been linked to defects in neuronal trafficking. Burk and Pasterkamp (2019) discussed how endosomal and receptor trafficking are affected in ALS due to dysregulated CP/ATG and/or ER/Golgi trafficking. Changes in axonal transport and nucleocytoplasmic transport suggested that further insight into intracellular trafficking defects will elucidate our understanding of the ALS pathogenesis and will provide novel avenues for theranostic interventions. Mutant Cu/Zn-SOD1 causes mitochondrial alterations that contribute to motor neuron demise in ALS. When mitochondria are damaged, cells activate MQC mechanisms leading to CP. Palomo et al. (2018) showed that in the spinal cord of SOD1-G93A mice, the ATG receptor p62 is recruited to mitochondria and CP is induced. Furthermore, the mitochondrial ubiquitin ligase Parkin and mitochondrial dynamics proteins, such as Miro1 and Mfn-2, are ubiquitinated by Parkin, and the MB regulator PGC1α is depleted.

Parkin genetic ablation delayed disease progression and prolonged survival in SOD1-G93A mice, as it slowed down motoneuron loss and muscle denervation and attenuated the depletion of mitochondrial dynamics proteins and PGC1α, indicating that Parkin is a disease modifier in ALS. This is because chronic Parkin-mediated MQC activation depleted mitochondrial dynamics-related proteins, inhibited MB, and abrogated mitochondrial dysfunction. Wang et al. (2018) reported that PTEN-L is a negative regulator of CP via its protein phosphatase activity against phosphorylated ubiquitin. PTEN-L localizes at the OMM and its overexpression inhibits CP induction by various CB-inducing agents, whereas its deletion promotes it. PTEN-L prevented Parkin mitochondrial translocation, reduced Parkin phosphorylation, maintained its inactive conformation, and inhibited its E3 ligase activity. PTEN-L reduced the level of phosphorylated ubiquitin (pSer65-Ub) in a phosphatase assay, confirming that PTEN-L dephosphorylates pSer65-Ub via its protein phosphatase activity, independently of its lipid phosphatase function. This suggests a novel function of PTEN-L as a protein phosphatase for ubiquitin, which counteracts PINK1-mediated ubiquitin phosphorylation, and leads to the blockage of the feedforward mechanisms in CB induction and CP suppression. Thus, understanding the exact function of PTEN-L will resolve the molecular puzzle involved in CP regulation, which is compromised in various NDDs, including PD, AD, and ALS. Kumar et al. (2018a) reviewed the involvement of mitochondrial CP/ATG dysfunction in AD, PD, and HD. Mitochondria and CP play a pivotal role in cellular health, and failure of these pathways can have deleterious consequences on health and well-being. Neuronal cells are highly vulnerable to CMB since most of their functions depend on ATP derived from mitochondrial metabolism. The NDDs are associated with mitochondrial dysfunction and compromised CP, leading to the accumulation of protein aggregates which culminate in NDDs. Thus, mitochondria and CP/ATG-related proteins and enzymes in NDDs may open the avenues for potential theranostic targets to discover safe and effective therapies. Mutations in the human VPS13 genes are responsible for neurodevelopmental and NDDs including chorea acanthocytosis (VPS13A) and PD (VPS13C). Genetic studies in yeast indicated that Vps13 may have a role in the lipid exchange between organelles. Furthermore, Kumar et al. (2018b) showed that the N-terminal portion of VPS13 is tubular, with a hydrophobic cavity that can solubilize and transport glycerolipids between membranes. Human VPS13A and VPS13C bind to the ER, tethering it to mitochondria (VPS13A), to late endosome/lysosomes (VPS13C), and to LDs (both VPS13A and VPS13C). These findings identified VPS13 as a lipid transporter between the ER and other organelles, involved in defective membrane lipid homeostasis in NDDs due to their mutations. The similarity of the sequence and secondary structure between the N-terminal portions of Vps13 and ATG2 suggested that these proteins have lipid-transport roles as well.

Thioacetamide-induced HE

Hepatic encephalopathy (HE) is a neuropsychiatric syndrome resulting from chronic or acute liver failure. In HE, ROS, inflammatory factors, ammonia poisoning, and amino acids alteration lead to changes in mitochondria. The selective elimination of CB is essential for maintaining the morphology and function of mitochondria and cells. Bai et al. (2018) analyzed mitochondrial morphology in the substantia nigra (SN) and anterior cerebral cortex (ACC) of the HE mice. The Drp-1, Mfn-1, and Mfn-2 increased in mRNA level of SN, which indicated the changes in mitochondrial morphology. The Drp-1 and Mfn-2 genes were upregulated, and Opa1 exhibited no significant change in the ACC. In the HE mice, the CP-related genes, PINK1 and Parkin increased in the SN, while the Parkin reduced in the ACC. The ucp2 increased in the mRNA level of the SN and ACC, and the ucp4 had no change or reduced in the SN and ACC, respectively, suggesting that the mitochondrial dynamics are different in the SN and ACC of HE mice. This indicated that mitochondrial dynamics may confer potential theranostic strategies for HE through the fission, fusion, and CP/ATG of genes.

Lafora Disease

Lafora disease (LD) is a fatal NDD caused by mutations in laforin and malin genes. LD is characterized by accumulation of a poorly branched glycogen in the neurons and other cells. Lahuerta et al. (2018) reported dysfunctional mitochondria in LD models. By using mitochondrial un-couplers and respiratory chain inhibitors, they used fibroblasts to investigate a possible alteration in the selective degradation of CBs. By flow cytometry of *MitoTracker*-labelled cells and measuring the levels of mitochondrial proteins using immunoblot, they found a partial impairment in the increased mitochondrial degradation implicated in CBMP in LD fibroblasts. Co-localization of mitochondrial and lysosomal markers decreased in LD fibroblasts. These results were consistent with a partial impairment in the CP/ATG degradation of CB in LD fibroblasts. However, recruitment of Parkin to the mitochondria under these conditions remained unaffected in LD fibroblasts and in malin and laforin overexpressed SH-SY5Y cells. Neither mitochondrial localization nor protein levels of Bcl-2-like protein 13 (another component of the CP machinery that operates under these conditions) were affected in LD fibroblasts. Although these treatments raised CP/ATG in both control and LD fibroblasts, it was lower in the latter cells. Therefore, the CP/ATG degradation of CBs was impaired in LD, due to a defect in the CP response and not in the MTG signaling pathways.

Spinal Cord Injury

Spinal cord injury (SCI) causes autonomic dysfunction, altered neurohumoral control, hemodynamic changes, and an increased risk of heart disease. Poormasjedi-Meibod et al. (2019) investigated the consequences of chronic SCI in rats by combining *in vivo* MRI and left-ventricular [LV] pressure-volume catheterization with histological and molecular assessments. Twelve weeks post-SCI, MRI-derived structural indices and *in vivo* LV catheterization-derived functional indices indicated the presence of LV atrophy, reduced ventricular volumes, and contractile dysfunction. Cardiac atrophy and contractile dysfunction in SCI were accompanied by reduced BP and circulatory NE, and increased Ang-II. They found reduced cardiomyocyte size, increased expression of AT-II type 1 receptors and TGF-β receptor 1 and 2 post-SCI, and >2X increase in muscle ring finger-1 and Beclin-1 protein following SCI, indicating the upregulation of the UPS and ATG-lysosomal machinery. This provided evidence of SCI-induced cardiomyocyte atrophy and systolic cardiac dysfunction accompanied by an upregulation of proteolytic pathways, the activation of which was due to the loss of trophic support from the sympathetic nervous system, neuro-mechanical unloading, and altered neuro-humoral pathways. ATG and MTG occur in SCI. Bnip-3 and its homolog, NIX, have been implicated in the regulation of MTG. Yu et al. (2018) characterized the mechanisms and role of Bnip-3 in SCI-associated MTG. Bnip-3, targeted to mitochondria, interacted with LC3, which was targeted to APSs, thus forming a mitochondria-Bnip-3-LC3-APS complex resulting in MTG. The downregulation of

Bnip-3 by RNA interference supported the mitochondrial function and decreased cell death in spinal cord neurons under hypoxia. Particularly, the Bnip-3 knockdown improved neurological recovery and the number of neuronal nuclei-positive cells post-SCI, indicating that Bnip-3 interacts with LC3 to induce MTG, while its inhibition conferred protective neuronal effects on SCI rat models.

Autism-Linked Wdfy3 in Brain MTG

WD repeat and FYVE domain-containing 3 (WDFY3; also known as ATG-Linked FYVE or Alfy) is an intellectual disability, developmental delay, and autism risk gene. This gene encodes for a scaffolding protein that is expressed in both the developing and adult CNS and is required for ATG and aggrephagy with as yet unexplored roles in CP. Given that mitochondrial trafficking, dynamics, and remodeling have key roles in synaptic plasticity, Napoli et al. (2018) tested the role of Wdfy3 on brain bioenergetics by using Wdfy3$^{+/lacZ}$ mice, the Wdfy3 mutant animal model with overt neurodevelopmental anomalies that survive to adulthood. Wdfy3 was required for sustaining MB and morphology via CP. The decreased MQC by conventional CP was compensated by the increased formation of mitochondria-derived vesicles (MDV) targeted to lysosomal degradation. The proteomic analysis of mitochondria-enriched cortical fractions showed significant enrichment for pathways associated with CP, mitochondrial transport, and axonal guidance via semaphorin, Robo, L1cam, and Eph-ephrin signaling, suggesting a critical role of Wdfy3 in mitochondrial homeostasis with implications for neuronal differentiation, neurodevelopment, and age-dependent NDDs.

CONCLUSION

Thioacetamide-induced HE revealed mitochondrial changes in the ACC and SN of rats. Lafora disease was characterized by ATG-induced elimination of CBs via CP. Parkin served as a disease modifier in the mutant SOD1 mouse model of ALS. Bcl-2/E1B-19KD-interacting protein 3/LC3 induced MTG in SCI and VPS13A, and VPS13C served as lipid transport proteins at ER contact sites in the rats. Parkin levels were elevated in the CBs implicated in CBMP. Mitochondrial protein import regulated cytosolic protein homeostasis and neuronal integrity. Furthermore, ubiquitination of ABCE1 was induced by NOT4 gene down-regulation in response to mitochondrial degeneration due to compromised MQC and induction of PINK1-directed CP/ATG and MTG. A novel role of autism-linked Wdfy3 gene in the brain MTG was proposed. PTEN-L as a protein phosphatase was required for ubiquitin de-phosphorylation to inhibit PINK1-Parkin-mediated CP, MTG, and ATG.

REFERENCES

Audano, M., A. Schneider and N. Mitro. 2018. Mitochondria, lysosomes, and dysfunction: Their meaning in neurodegeneration. J Neurochem 147: 291–309.

Bai, Y., S. Wang, F. Wu, X. Xie, et al. 2018. The changes of mitochondria in substantia nigra and anterior cerebral cortex of hepatic encephalopathy induced by thioacetamide. Anat Rec (Hoboken) 302: 1169–1177.

Boczonadi, V., K. Meyer, H. Gonczarowska-Jorge, H. Griffin, et al. 2018. Mutations in glycyl-tRNA synthetase impair mitochondrial metabolism in neurons. Hum Mol Genet 27: 2187–2204.

Burk, K. and R.J. Pasterkamp. 2019. Disrupted neuronal trafficking in amyotrophic lateral sclerosis. Acta Neuropathol 137: 859–877.

Chaytow, H., Y.T. Huang, T.H. Gillingwater, K.M.E. Faller, et al. 2018. The role of survival motor neuron protein (SMN) in protein homeostasis. Cell Mol Life Sci 75: 3877–3894.

Chen, X., T. Yu and R. Luo. 2019. Clinical characteristics and molecular pathogenesis of pantothenate kinase-associated neurodegenerative disease. Zhonghua Yi Xue Yi Chuan Xue Za Zhi 36: 175–178.

Chu, C.T. 2018. Mechanisms of selective ATG and mitophagy: Implications for neurodegenerative diseases. Neurobiol Dis 122: 23–34.

Kumar, A., A. Dhawan, A. Kadam and A. Shinde. 2018a. ATG and Mitochondria: Targets in neurodegenerative disorders. CNS Neurol Disord Drug Targets 17: 696–705.

Kumar, N., M. Leonzino, W. Hancock-Cerutti, F.A. Horenkamp, et al. 2018b. VPS13A and VPS13C are lipid transport proteins differentially localized at ER contact sites. J Cell Biol 217: 3625–3639.

Lahuerta, M., C. Aguado, P. Sánchez-Martín, P. Sanz, et al. 2018. Degradation of altered mitochondria by ATG is impaired in Lafora disease. FEBS J 285: 2071–2090.

Liu, W., X. Duan, X. Fang, W. Shang, et al. 2018. Mitochondrial protein import regulates cytosolic protein homeostasis and neuronal integrity. Autophagy 14: 1293–1309.

Maiese, K. 2018. Novel treatment strategies for the nervous system: Circadian clock genes, non-coding RNAs, and forkhead transcription factors. Curr Neurovasc Res 15: 81–91.

Mandrioli, J., L. Mediani, S. Alberti, S. Carra. 2019. ALS and FTD: Where RNA metabolism meets protein quality control. Semin. Cell Dev Biol 99: 183–192.

Napoli, E., P. Song, A. Panoutsopoulos, M.A. Riyadh, et al. 2018. Beyond ATG: A novel role for autism-linked Wdfy3 in brain mitophagy. Sci Rep 8: 11348.

Nguyen, D.K.H., R. Thombre and J. Wang. 2019. ATG as a common pathway in amyotrophic lateral sclerosis. Neurosci Lett 697: 34–48.

Palomo, G.M., V. Granatiero, H. Kawamata, C. Konrad, et al. 2018. Parkin is a disease modifier in the mutant SOD1 mouse model of ALS. EMBO Mol Med 10: e8888.

Poormasjedi-Meibod, M.S., M. Mansouri, M. Fossey, J.W. Squair, et al. 2019. Experimental spinal cord injury causes left-ventricular atrophy and is associated with an upregulation of proteolytic pathways. J Neurotrauma 36: 950–961.

Restelli, L.M., B. Oettinghaus, M. Halliday, C. Agca, et al. 2018. Neuronal mitochondrial dysfunction activates the integrated stress response to induce fibroblast growth factor 21. Cell Rep 24: 1407–1414.

Suresh, S.N., V. Verma, S. Sateesh, J.P. Clement, et al. 2018. Neurodegenerative diseases: Model organisms, pathology and ATG. J Genet 97: 679–701.

Wang, L., Y.L. Cho, Y. Tang, J. Wang, et al. 2018. PTEN-L is a novel protein phosphatase for ubiquitin dephosphorylation to inhibit PINK1-Parkin-mediated mitophagy. Cell Res 28: 787–802.

Wu, Z., Y. Wang, J. Lim, B. Liu, et al. 2018. Ubiquitination of ABCE1 by NOT4 in response to mitochondrial damage links co-translational quality control to PINK1-directed mitophagy. Cell Metab 28: 130–144.e7.

Yu, D., M. Li, P. Nie, B. Ni, et al. 2018. Bcl-2/E1B-19KD-interacting protein 3/light chain 3 interaction induces mitophagy in spinal cord injury in rats both *in vivo* and *in vitro*. J Neurotrauma 35: 2183–2194.

24

Charnolophagy in Neurodegenerative Diseases
(Part-2)

INTRODUCTION

Although the development of neurodegeneration may vary between NDDs, they have common cellular hallmarks, including defects in the ubiquitin-proteasome system involving CP/MTG/ATG dysfunction, CP dysregulation, CS destabilization, and CBMP. CP/ATG dysfunction has been described in many NDDs. It can occur at several steps of the CP/ATG machinery and contribute to tissue repair or degeneration, depending on the intensity and frequency of free radicals generated in response to DPCI and the microenvironment. The author discovered that the structural and functional stability of CS membranes is highly essential following CP for an efficient exocytosis of toxic mitochondrial metabolites to sustain ICD and IMD for NCF to remain healthy. Structural and functional destabilization of CS membranes occurs in response to DPCI-induced oxidative and nitrative stress of free radicals (primarily OH and NO) which triggers CBMP in progressive neurodegenerative disorders including PD, AD, HD, and ALS as highly complex neuropathologies; characterized by chronic pain, agony, physical incapacitation, cognitive (learning, intelligence, memory, and behavior) impairments, and early mortality. Rodolfo et al. (2018) focused on the role played by ATG in the progression of NDDs, and on theranostic approaches involving CP/MTG/ATG modulation. Genetic studies indicate that deficits in the CP/MTG/ATG pathways are implicated in NDDs, including PD, AD, and ALS. Evans and Holzbaur (2019) reviewed the current understanding of the pathways that regulate MQC and compared these mechanisms to those regulating the turnover of the ER and the clearance of protein aggregates. There are multiple mechanisms regulating the degradation of specific cargos, such as dysfunctional organelles and protein aggregates for neuronal health. Neurons are highly vulnerable to impairment in organelle QC pathways due to their morphology, size, polarity, and terminally differentiated post-mitotic nature. Crosstalk in the pathophysiological processes emphasizing metabolic diseases and NDDs have been the subject of extensive investigation, in which insulin signaling and ATG impairment are common factors. Pharmacological and genetic strategies that regulate these pathways may be a promising approach for aggregated protein clearance and delaying the onset or progression of the disease. However, as the response due to this modulation seems to be time-dependent, finding the exact spatiotemporal regulation of ATG may be a potential target for drug development. The role of insulin signaling/resistance and ATG in some NDDs, and pharmacological and non-pharmacological interventions has been highlighted. As neurons are highly specialized cells with minimum or no mitotic potential to regenerate in response to injury, infection, and/or toxic exposure, the only plausible mechanism of elimination of undesirable, nonfunctional, or damaged organelles or macromolecules is through CB formation, CP induction, and CS exocytosis as a mechanism of ICD for NCF. When these sequential events become defective or delayed, the damaged organelles and macromolecules start aggregating to form pleomorphic CBs, as a mechanism of ICD to restrict and nullify the deleterious effect of free radicals and toxic metabolites. Their selective and efficient elimination is highly crucial for the NCF to remain healthy. Thus, CB formation involves MR during DPCI-induced RONS stress to sustain MQC during the acute phase; CP becomes ATP-driven, lysosomal-dependent ATG to sustain ICD during the chronic phase of disease progression.

This chapter highlights the theranostic potential of natural and synthetic antioxidants in the TSE-EBPT of chronic NDDs with currently limited treatment options.

NO and Mitochondria in NDDs

The mitochondrial activity can be modulated by NO, which mediates its function primarily through the activation of the cyclic guanylyl cyclase (cGC) signaling pathway and S-nitrosylation of proteins involved in cellular functioning and mitochondrial dynamics. Excess NO or the formation of RONS, for example, $ONOO^-$, impair mitochondrial function and this, in conjunction with nuclear events, affects neuronal metabolism and survival, contributing to the pathogenesis of NDDs. Ghasemi et al. (2018) highlighted the possible mechanisms underlying the noxious effects of excess NO and RONS on mitochondrial function, including (i) deleterious effects on ETC; (ii) $ONOO^-$-mediated alteration in mitochondrial permeability transition; (iii) enhanced mitochondrial fragmentation and CP/ATG through the S-nitrosylation of DRP-1 and Parkin/PINK1 complex; (iv) alterations in the mitochondrial metabolic pathways, including the Krebs cycle, glycolysis, fatty acid metabolism, and the urea cycle; and eventually (v) mitochondrial $ONOO^-$-induced nuclear toxicity and release of AIF, caspase-3 activation, PARP cleavage, causing apoptotic cell death. These mechanisms highlight the multi-dimensional nature of NO and its signaling in the mitochondrial function. Hence, understanding the mechanisms by which NO mediates mitochondrial function can provide new insights into the TSE-EBPT of NDDs as the author has described in his several publications.

Forward Genetic Screening

Genetic and environmental factors contribute to demise of neurons, leading to diverse cognitive and motor disorders, including PD, AD, and ALS. *Drosophila*, has been used to elucidate the cellular, molecular, and genetic mechanisms of NDDs. Extensive tools and sophisticated technologies allow *Drosophila* geneticists to identify evolutionarily-conserved genes essential for neuronal maintenance. Deal et al. (2019) focused on a large-scale mosaic forward genetic screen on the *Drosophila* X-chromosome that led to the identification of genes that exhibit ND phenotypes when mutated. The electrophysiological and ultrastructural characterization of mutant tissue related to the *Drosophila* visual system, followed by experiments to understand the mechanism of ND in each mutant led to the discovery of molecular pathways for neuronal integrity. Defects in mitochondrial function, lipid and iron metabolism, protein trafficking, and ATG are recurrent themes; hence, DPCI that lead to ND may converge on various cellular processes. Insights from these studies have contributed to our understanding of known NDDs such as Leigh syndrome, Friedreich's ataxia, and identification of new human diseases. By discovering new genes required for neural maintenance in *Drosophila* and working with health professionals to identify patients with deleterious variants in the orthologous human genes, geneticists can play an important role in discovering the TSE-EBPT of NDDs and other chronic MDR diseases.

Ataxia Telangiectasia Mutated (ATM) Gene

Stagni et al. (2018) reported that ATM plays a central role in the DNA damage response (DDR) and mutations in its gene causes a rare autosomal genetic disorder, ataxia telangiectasia (A-T), characterized by ND, premature aging, defects in the immune response, and higher incidence of lymphoma. The ability of ATM to control genome stability indicates that ATM is a tumor-suppressor gene. ATM also has a significant role, in addition to its control on DDR, as the principal modulator of oxidative stress response and MQC, as well as in its regulation of ATG, hypoxia, and cancer stem cell survival. ATM is characterized by aberrant oxidative stress, and an inability to remove damaged organelles such as mitochondria participating in dysregulated CP and CBMP. These findings raise the question of whether ATM may contribute to a general hijack of signaling networks in cancer, therefore, playing a dual role in this context. An unexpected role of ATM in tumorigenesis has been demonstrated. Genetic inactivation of Beclin-1, a CP/ATG regulator, reversed mitochondrial abnormalities and tumor development in ATM-null mice, independently of DDR. Furthermore, ATM sustains cancer stem cell survival by promoting the CP/ATG as ATM kinase activity is enhanced in HER2-dependent tumors.

NGF in Energy Homeostasis and Mitochondrial Remodeling

Neuronal differentiation involves modification of biochemical and morphological properties to meet novel functional requirements. Reorganization of the mitochondrial network to match the higher energy demand plays a pivotal role in this process. Martorana et al. (2018) showed that NGF-induced differentiation requires the activation of ATG mediated by ATG9b and Ambra1, as it is disrupted by their genetic knockdown and by ATG blockers. NGF differentiation involved the induction of P-AMPK and P-CaMK, and is prevented by their pharmacological inhibition. These molecular events correlated with modifications of energy and redox homeostasis, as determined by ATP and NADPH changes, a higher O_2 consumption ratio (OCR), and ROS production, indicating that CP eliminates exhausted mitochondria involved in CB formation, as determined by the enhanced localization of p62 and Lysotracker-red to the mitochondria. NGF differentiation was accompanied by increased MR involving enhanced fission (P-Drp1) and fusion (Opa1 and Mfn-2) proteins, as well as the induction of Sirt3 and the transcription factors mtTFA and PPARγ, which regulate metabolism to sustain increased mitochondrial mass, $\Delta\Psi$, and MB, indicating a NGF-dependent mechanism involving CP and MR, which plays a key role in both neurogenesis as well as regeneration.

Genetic Enhancement of CP

Most of the NDDs that afflict humans manifest with the intra-neuronal accumulation of toxic proteins that are aggregate-prone. Such proteins, like mutant huntingtin or α-Syn, are substrates of CP/ATG. Furthermore, ATG-inducing compounds lower the levels of such proteins and ameliorate their toxicity in animal models of NDDs. However, most of these compounds also have CP/ATG-independent effects and it is important to understand if similar benefits are seen with genetic strategies that upregulate CP/ATG. Ejlerskov et al. (2019) reviewed studies in vertebrate models using genetic manipulations of ATG genes and described how these improve pathology and neurodegeneration, supporting the validity of CP/ATG upregulation as a target for several NDDs.

SCI Endogenous RNA Network

Spinal cord injury (SCI) results from trauma and mostly affects the young male population. SCI imposes major and permanent life changes, and is associated with high mortality and disability rates. lncRNAs serve a critical role in biological processes in various diseases, including SCI. Wang et al. (2019) identified differentially-expressed lncRNAs in SCI based on the competing endogenous RNA (ceRNA) hypothesis by mining data from the Gene Expression Omnibus database of the National Center for Biotechnology Information to unveil their functions. A network consisting of 13 lncRNA, 93 messenger RNA, and 9 microRNA nodes, with a total of 202 edges was established. Three node lncRNAs were identified based on the degree of distribution of the nodes, and their subnetworks were constructed. Based on these subnetworks, the biological pathways and interactions of these three lncRNAs were described using FunRich software. The three lncRNA enrichment analyses revealed that they were associated with ATG, extracellular communication, and transcription factor networks, respectively. The PI3K/PKB/mTOR signaling pathway of XR_350851 was the classic CP/ATG pathway, indicating that it may regulate CP/ATG in SCI; hence, it can be used as a novel biomarker of theranostic significance in SCI.

Epigenetics of miR-34b/c

The exposure to extremely low-frequency magnetic fields (ELF-MFs) has been associated with an increased risk of NDDs. Since epigenetic modulation has been encountered among the key events leading to NDDs, Consales et al. (2018) aimed at investigathing if the control of gene expression mediated by miRs-34 has any role in driving neuronal cell response to a 50-Hz (1 mT) magnetic field *in vitro*. ELF-MFs induced an early reduction of the expression level of miR-34b and miR-34c in SH-SY5Y cells and in mouse primary cortical neurons, by affecting the transcription of the common pri-miR-34. This modulation was p53-independent, but attributed to the hyper-methylation of the CpG island mapping within the miR-34b/c promoter. Incubation with NAC or glutathione ethyl-ester failed to restore miR-34b/c expression, suggesting that these are not responsive to ELF-MF-induced oxidative stress. miRs-34 controlled ROS production and affected mitochondrial oxidative stress triggered by ELF-MFs by modulating its targets identified by an *in silico* analysis. ELF-MFs altered the expression of the α-Syn, which was stimulated upon ELF-MFs exposure via both direct miR-34 targeting and oxidative stress, indicating the potential of the ELF-MFs to regulate redox homeostasis, epigenetic control of gene expression, and the mechanism(s) predisposing neurons to degeneration through CBMP.

MTG in Refractory TLE

Su et al. (2019) determined an association between MTG and refractory temporal lobe epilepsy (rTLE) with hippocampal sclerosis (HS). During epilepsy surgery, they collected tissue samples from the hippocampi and temporal lobe cortexes of rTLE patients with HS. To probe for MTG, they used fluorescent immunolabeling to determine the co-localization of mitochondrial and APS markers. Early APSs were present and mitochondria were differentially impaired in the hippocampi. Co-localization of the APS marker LC3B with the mitochondrial marker TOMM20 in the hippocampi and temporal lobe cortexes indicated the presence of MTG. The mitochondrial and APS marker co-localization was lower in the hippocampus than in the temporal lobe cortex. Accumulation of APSs and MTG activation were implicated in rTLE with hippocampal sclerosis. Aberrant accumulation of damaged mitochondria involving CB formation, especially in the hippocampus, can be attributed to defects in CP/ATG, which may participate in epileptogenesis as the author discovered in IUD Domoic-acid-exposed mouse progeny (Sharma 2019).

Mouse Model of HSPB-8

Mutations in the small heat shock protein B8 gene (HSPB-8/HSP22) have been associated with distal hereditary motor neuropathy, Charcot-Marie-Tooth disease, and distal myopathy. A role of HSPB-8 in chaperone-associated ATG is determinant for the clearance of poly-glutamine aggregates in NDDs and for the maintenance of skeletal muscle myofibrils. Bouhy et al. (2018) generated a new transgenic mouse model leading to the expression of the mutant protein (knock-in lines) or the loss-of-function (functional knock-out lines) of the endogenous protein HSPB-8. While the homozygous knock-in mice developed motor deficits associated with the degeneration of peripheral nerves and severe muscle atrophy corroborating patient data, homozygous knock-out mice had locomotor performances equivalent to those of wild-type animals. The distal skeletal muscles of the post-symptomatic homozygous knock-in displayed Z-disk disorganization and granulofilamentous material accumulation along with HSPB-8, αB-crystallin (HSPB5/CRYAB), and desmin aggregates. The presence of the aggregates correlated with reduced biomarkers of ATG. The sciatic nerve of the homozygous knock-in mice was characterized by a low ATG potential in pre-symptomatic and HSPB-8 aggregates in post-symptomatic animals and presented a normal morphology. Their distal muscle displayed the accumulation of abnormal mitochondria, but had intact myofiber and Z-line organization, suggesting that toxic gain-of-function of mutant HSPB-8 aggregates is a major contributor to peripheral neuropathy and myopathy. In addition, mutant HSPB-8 induces impairments in CP/ATG that may aggravate the phenotype.

BNIP-3L/NIX-Dependent MTG

Esteban-Martínez and Boya (2018) showed that during retinal development, tissue hypoxia triggers HIF1A/HIF-1 stabilization, resulting in increased expression of the MTG receptor BNIP-3L/NIX. BNIP3L-dependent MTG results in a metabolic shift toward glycolysis for RGC neurogenesis. BNIP3L-dependent MTG also regulates the polarization of pro-inflammatory/M1 macrophages, which undergo glycolysis-dependent differentiation during the inflammatory response. These results revealed a new link between hypoxia, MTG, and metabolic reprogramming in the differentiation of several cell types and may have implications for NDDs, metabolic, and other diseases in which mitochondrial dysfunction and metabolic alterations play a pivotal role.

Ca^{2+} Signaling in the Developing Cochlea

Mammano and Bortolozzi (2018) described the intricate interplay between Ca^{2+} signaling, connexin expression and function, and apoptosis. ATG is the crucial step that leads to hearing acquisition. Ca^{2+} signaling plays fundamental roles both in the sensory hair cells and in the matrix of non-sensory, epithelial, and supporting cells, which embed them and are interconnected by a dense network of gap junctions formed by connexin 26 (Cx26) and connexin 30 (Cx30) protein subunits.

Chronic Sleep Fragmentation

Insufficient sleep results in cognitive impairment and emotional changes. Sleep eliminates metabolic wastes in the brain by enhancing CP and CS exocytosis as a mechanism of ICD in the neurons. Xie et al. (2019) proposed that chronic sleep insufficiency in young adult wild-type mice is linked to the dysfunction of intracellular protein degradation pathways and microglia-mediated neuro-inflammation mechanisms involved in the initiation of neurodegeneration involving CBMP. They applied the chronic sleep fragmentation (CSF) model to induce chronic sleep insufficiency in wild-type mice. After 2 months of CSF, cognitive function, amyloid-β accumulation, dysfunction of the endosome-APS-lysosome pathway, and microglia activation were evaluated.

Impairment of spatial learning and memory, and aggravated anxiety-like behavior in mice were identified by behavioral experiments. Increased intracellular amyloid-β accumulation was observed in the cortex and hippocampus due to free radical-induced CMB, dysregulated CP, and CS destabilization. Rab5 (early endosome marker) and Rab7 (late endosome marker) were enhanced in the CSF and LC3B (APS marker), and in the ATG-positive regulatory factors in the brain. The activation of microglia was evident by the enhanced CD68, CD16/32, and CD206 levels. CSF triggered pathogenetic processes similar to the early stage of neurodegeneration, including dysfunction of the endosome-APS-lysosome pathway and microglia-mediated neuro-inflammation, confirming the link between chronic sleep insufficiency and the initiation of neurodegeneration due to induction of CBMP.

CP in Ataxia-Telangiectasia

Ataxia-telangiectasia (A-T) is characterized by neurodegeneration, cancer, diabetes, immune deficiency, and increased sensitivity to ionizing radiation. Desai et al. (2018) introduced MTG and ubiquitin pathways and provided the current understanding of the regulation of MTG by the ubiquitin pathway. They reviewed evidence supporting MTG defects in NDDs and highlighted that the elevated expression of the ubiquitin-like protein interferon-stimulated gene 15 (ISG15), an antagonist of the ubiquitin pathway, was a cause of defective MTG in NDDs. They also summarized the current understanding of the regulation of MTG by the ubiquitin pathway and the targeting of MTG and ubiquitin pathways for the TSE-EBPT of NDDs.

The MQC mechanism is defective in neurons of patients with various NDDs such as A-T, AD, PD, and ALS. Accumulation of defective mitochondria and the production of ROS due to defective MTG have been identified as causes underlying NDDs involving dysregulated CP and CBMP (Sharma and Ebadi 2013). Like MTG, defects in the ubiquitin/26S proteasome pathway is linked to NDDs, resulting in the protein aggregates in neurons. Choy and Watters (2018) examined the roles of ATM in cellular homeostasis and related these functions to the complex A-T phenotype. A-T is attributed to the deficiency of the protein kinase coded by the ATM gene. ATM is a sensor of DNA double-strand breaks (DSBs) and sends signals to cell cycle checkpoints and the DNA repair machinery. ATM phosphorylates numerous substrates and activates many cell-signaling pathways. In proliferating cells, ATM is localized primarily in the nucleus; however, in post-mitotic cells such as neurons, ATM is mostly cytoplasmic. Recent studies reveal diversified roles for ATM in the cytoplasm, including activation by oxidative stress. ATM associates with organelles, including mitochondria and peroxisomes, both sources of RONS which have been implicated in NDDs and aging. ATM is also associated with synaptic vesicles and has a role in regulating cellular homeostasis and CP/ATG. The cytoplasmic roles of ATM provide a new perspective on the neurodegenerative process in A-T. ATM kinase controls the cell cycle G2/M checkpoint and apoptosis in proliferating neuroprogenitor cells. ATM can signal cell cycle arrest, DNA repair, or apoptosis and is required for DNA damage–induced apoptosis in both non – cycling and proliferative cells. However, its exact role in CP/ATG induction or inhibition remains unknown.

CP in ALS and Frontotemporal Lobe Degeneration (FTLD)

ALS is a multifactorial fatal motoneuron disease without an effective cure. Ten percent of ALS cases can be pointed to a clear genetic cause, while the remaining 90% are classified as sporadic. ALS and FTLD are the progressive delocalization and cytosolic accumulation of

TDP-43 inclusions in the CNS. The decrease in the efficiency of the clearance systems in aging, as well as the presence of genetic mutations of proteins associated with cellular proteostasis in the familial forms of proteinopathies, suggest that a failure of these protein degradation systems is a key factor in the etiology of TAR DNA-Binding Protein-43 (TDP-43) associated disorders. The internalization of human pre-formed TDP-43 aggregates in the murine neuroblastoma N2a cells resulted in their ubiquitination and hyper-phosphorylation by endogenous machineries, mimicking the post-translational modifications in patients. Moreover, mitochondria were identified as the main sites for the alteration of Ca^{2+} homeostasis induced by TDP-43 aggregates, which stimulate ROS overproduction and, finally, caspase activation. The inhibition of TDP-43 proteostasis in the presence of selective inhibitors against the proteasome and macroATG systems revealed that these two systems are involved in TDP-43 accumulation and have a robust influence on each other in NDDs associated with TDP. Microsatellite repeat expansion disease loci can exhibit pleiotropic clinical and biological effects depending on repeat length. Large expansions in C9orf72 (100s-1000s of units) are the most common genetic cause of ALS and FTD.

Several studies identified intermediate repeats in PD patients, but the association was not found in autopsy-confirmed cases. Cali et al. (2019) hypothesized that intermediate C9orf72 repeats are a genetic risk factor for cortico-basal degeneration (CBD), a NDD that may be clinically similar to PD but has a distinct tau protein pathology. Intermediate C9orf72 repeats were enriched in autopsy-proven CBD. While large C9orf72 repeat expansions decrease C9orf72 expression, intermediate C9orf72 repeats result in increased C9orf72 expression in human brain tissue and CRISPR/cas9 knockin iPSC-derived neural progenitor cells. In contrast to cases of FTD/ALS with large C9orf72 expansions, CBD with intermediate C9orf72 repeats was not associated with pathologic RNA foci or dipeptide repeat protein aggregates. Knock-in cells with intermediate repeats exhibit numerous changes in gene-expression pathways relating to vesicle trafficking and ATG. Overexpression of C9orf72 without the repeat expansion leads to defects in ATG under nutrient starvation conditions, indicating that theranostic strategies to reduce C9orf72 expression may be beneficial for the treatment of CBD. Coding or non-coding mutation in "fused-in-sarcoma (FUS) gene" causes ALS and FTD. Used in sarcoma (FUS) is a DNA/RNA binding protein containing 526 amino acids. The FUS gene was initially identified as a fusion oncogene on chromosome 16 in human liposarcoma, the translocation and fusion of which to transcription factors results in strong transcriptional activation of the proteins

Ho et al. (2019) reported that in addition to familial ALS, abnormal aggregates of FUS are present in a portion of FTD and other NDDs, independent of their mutations. Broad expression within the CNS of either wild-type or two ALS-linked human FUS mutants produces progressive motor phenotypes accompanied by ALS-like pathology. FUS levels are auto-regulated to maintain an optimal steady-state level. Increasing FUS expression by saturating its auto-regulatory mechanism results in progressive neurological phenotypes and lethality. GWAS revealed genetic dysregulations distinct from those via FUS reduction. Among these are increased expression of lysosomal proteins, suggesting disruption in protein homeostasis as a gain-of-toxicity mechanism. Increased expression of wild-type FUS or ALS-linked mutant forms of FUS inhibit macroATG/ATG. Thus, mice expressing FUS (1) develop progressive motor deficits, (2) increased FUS expression by an overriding of the auto-regulatory mechanism which accelerates neurodegeneration, providing a basis for FUS involvement without mutation, and (3) disruption in both protein homeostasis and RNA processing, which contribute to FUS-mediated toxicity.

Beltran et al. (2019) discovered new connections within the ALS network through a bio-informatics approach: They identified C13orf18, recently named Pacer, as a new component of the ATG machinery, involved in ALS pathogenesis. Initially, they identified Pacer using a network-based bio-informatics. Expression of Pacer was then investigated using spinal cord tissue from two ALS mouse models ($SOD1^{G93A}$ and $TDP43^{A315T}$) and sporadic ALS patients.

Mechanistic studies were performed in cell culture using the mouse moto-neuron cell line NSC34. The loss of function of Pacer was achieved by knockdown using short-hairpin constructs. The effect of Pacer repression was investigated in the context of ATG, SOD1 aggregation, and neuronal death. Using an unbiased network-based approach, they integrated all available ALS data to identify new functional interactions involved in ALS pathogenesis and found that Pacer associates to an ALS-specific subnetwork composed of components of the ATG pathway, one of the main cellular processes affected in the disease. Pacer levels are significantly reduced in spinal cord tissue from sporadic ALS patients and in tissue from ALS mouse models. *In vitro*, a Pacer deficiency lead to impaired ATG and the accumulation of protein aggregates, which correlated with the induction of cell death. This study identified Pacer as a regulator of Proteostasis associated with ALS pathology. In addition, Progranulin (PGL) regulates neuron and immune functions and is implicated in aging. The loss of one functional allele causes haplo-insufficiency and leads to FTLD, the second leading cause of dementia. PGL gene polymorphisms are linked to AD and the loss of function causes neuronal ceroid lipofuscinosis. Despite the critical role of PGL levels in NDDs risk, little is known about their regulation. Deficient PGL levels cause neurological syndromes: haplo-insufficiency leads to FTLD and nullizygosity produces adult-onset neuronal ceroid lipofuscinosis. Elia et al. (2019) performed a genome-wide RNAi screen using ELISA to discover genes that regulate PGL levels in neurons. They identified 830 genes that raise or lower PGL levels by at least 1.5-fold in Neuro2a cells. When inhibited by siRNA or by small-molecule inhibitors, 33 genes of the druggable genome increased PGL levels in mouse primary cortical neurons; several of these also raised PGL levels in FTLD mouse model neurons. "Hit" genes regulated PGL by transcriptional or post-transcriptional mechanisms. A pathway analysis revealed enrichment of hit genes from the CP/ATG-lysosome pathway (ALP), suggesting its key role in regulating PGL levels. PGL also regulated lysosome function and its deficiency increased CP/ATG and caused abnormally enlarged lysosomes. Enhancing PGL levels restored CP/ATG and lysosomal size to control levels. These findings linked the ALP to neuronal PGL. PGL levels were regulated by CP/ATG and, in turn, regulated the ALP. Restoring PGL levels by targeting genetic modifiers reversed FTLD functional deficits, conferring opportunities for theranostic development. An unbiased screen was performed to identify specific pathways controlling PGL levels in neurons. The modulation of these pathways restored levels in PGL-deficient neurons and reversed FTLD phenotypes. These findings provided a new understanding of the genetic regulation of PGL and potential thernoatic strategies to treat FTLD and other NDDs, including AD.

CONCLUSION

Mitochondrial-generated free radicals (OH and NO) play a crucial role in NDDs. NGF differentiation involved energy homeostasis, MR, and CB formation. CP as well as MTG were regulated by the Parkin and Akt-ubiquitin pathways in NDDs. Genetic enhancement of CP occurred in vertebrate models of NDDs due to MR involving CBMP. Molecular mechanism of SCI was accomplished through RNA network analysis. A 50-Hz magnetic field affected the epigenetics of miR-34b/c in neurons, which influenced CBMP implicated in NDDs. A defective MTG was identified in rTLE with sclerosis as the author discovered in the hippocampal CA-3 and dentate gyrus neurons of intra-uterine domoic-acid-exposed mice progeny without any overt clinical seizures. A knock-in/knock-out mouse model of HSPB-8-associated distal hereditary motor neuropathy and myopathy revealed the toxic gain-of-function of mutant HSPB-8. Insulin and BNIP3L/NIX-dependent CP, MTG, and ATG regulated cell differentiation via metabolic reprogramming in NDDs. Neurodegeneration in A-T involved the multiple roles of ATM kinase in cellular homeostasis. Chronic sleep fragmentation shared similar pathogenesis with

NDDs, characterized by a failure of proteostasis counteracting TDP-43 aggregation due to CS destabilization and impaired exocytosis, as a mechanism of ICD. C9orf72 intermediate repeats were associated with CBD, increased C9orf72 expression, and CP downregulation. Elevated FUS levels developed gain-of-toxicity that impaired protein and RNA homeostasis in progressive NDDs by overriding autoregulation. A network approach discovered a Pacer as an ATG protein in ALS pathogenesis. The regulation of neuronal PGL regulated the CP/ATG-lysosomal pathway as mechanism of ICD. Molecular mechanisms of NDDs were further explored through a forward genetic screening in *Drosophila*. ATM kinase was involved in the transcriptional regulation of mitochondrial oxidative stress and CP/ATG in NDDs.

REFERENCES

Beltran, S., M. Nassif, E. Vicencio, J. Arcos, et al. 2019. Network approach identifies Pacer as an autophagy protein involved in ALS pathogenesis. Mol Neurodegener 14, Article number 14.

Bouhy, D., M. Juneja, I. Katona, A. Holmgren, et al. 2018. A knock-in/knock-out mouse model of HSPB-8-associated distal hereditary motor neuropathy and myopathy reveals toxic gain-of-function of mutant HSPB-8. Acta Neuropathol 135: 131–148.

Cali, C.P., M. Patino, Y.K. Tai, W.K. Ho. et al. 2019. C9orf72 intermediate repeats are associated with corticobasal degeneration, increased C9orf72 expression and disruption of ATG. Acta Neuropathol 138: 795–811.

Choy, K.R. and D.J. Watters. 2018. Neurodegeneration in ataxia-telangiectasia: Multiple roles of ATM kinase in cellular homeostasis. Dev Dyn 247: 33–46.

Consales, C., C. Cirotti, G. Filomeni and M. Panatta. 2018. Fifty-hertz magnetic field affects the epigenetic modulation of the miR-34b/c in neuronal cells. Mol Neurobiol 55: 5698–5714.

Deal, S.L. and S. Yamamoto. 2019. Unraveling novel mechanisms of neurodegeneration through a large-scale forward genetic screen in *Drosophila*. Front Genet 9: 700.

Desai, S., M. Juncker and C. Kim. 2018. Regulation of MTG by the ubiquitin pathway in neurodegenerative diseases. Exp Biol Med (Maywood) 243: 554–562.

Ejlerskov, P., A. Ashkenazi and D.C. Rubinsztein. 2019. Genetic enhancement of macroATG in vertebrate models of neurodegenerative diseases. Neurobiol Dis 122: 3–8.

Elia, L.P., A.R. Mason, A. Alijagic and S. Finkbeiner. 2019. Genetic regulation of neuronal progranulin reveals a critical role for the autophagy-lysosome pathway J Neurosci 39(17): 3332–3344.

Esteban-Martínez, L. and P. Boya. 2018. BNIP3L/NIX-dependent mitophagy regulates cell differentiation via metabolic reprogramming. Autophagy 14(5): 915–917.

Evans, C.S. and E.L.F. Holzbaur. 2019. Quality control in neurons: Mitophagy and other selective autophagy mechanisms. J Mol Biol 432: 240–260.

Ghasemi, M., Y. Mayasi, A. Hannoun, S.M. Eslami, et al. 2018. Nitric oxide and mitochondrial function in neurological diseases. Neuroscience 376: 48–71.

Ho, W.Y. and S.C. Ling. 2019. Elevated FUS levels by overriding its autoregulation produce gain-of-toxicity properties that disrupt protein and RNA homeostasis. Autophagy 15: 1665–1667.

Mammano, F. and M. Bortolozzi. 2018. Ca^2+ signaling, apoptosis and ATG in the developing cochlea: Milestones to hearing acquisition. Cell Calcium 70: 117–126.

Martorana, F., D. Gaglio, M.R. Bianco, F. Aprea, et al. 2018. Differentiation by nerve growth factor (NGF) involves mechanisms of crosstalk between energy homeostasis and mitochondrial remodeling. Cell Death Dis 9: 391.

Rodolfo, C., S. Campello and F. Cecconi. 2018. Mitophagy in neurodegenerative diseases. Neurochem Int 117: 156–166.

Sharma, S. 2019. The Charnoly Body: A Novel Biomarker of Mitochondrial Bioenergetics. CRC Press, Taylor & Francis Group, Boca Raton, FL, U.S.A.

Stagni, V., C. Cirotti and D. Barilà. 2018. Ataxia-telangiectasia mutated kinase in the control of oxidative stress, mitochondria, and ATG in cancer: A maestro with a large orchestra. Front Oncol 8: 73.

Su, Z., Y. Nie, Z. Huang, Y. Zhu, et al. 2019. Mitophagy in hepatic insulin resistance: Therapeutic potential and concerns. Front Pharmacol 10: 1193. doi: 10.3389/fphar.2019.01193.

Wang, L., B. Wang, J. Liu and Z. Quan. 2019. Construction and analysis of a spinal cord injury competitive endogenous RNA network based on the expression data of long noncoding, micro- and messenger RNAs. Mol Med Rep 19: 3021–3034.

Xie, Y., L. Ba, M. Wang, S.Y. Deng, et al. 2019. Chronic sleep fragmentation shares similar pathogenesis with neurodegenerative diseases: Endosome-autophagosome-lysosome pathway dysfunction and microglia-mediated neuroinflammation. CNS Neurosci Ther 26(2): 215–227.

25

Charnolophagy in Parkinson's Disease

INTRODUCTION

PD is the most common NDD of movement disorders and affects ~1% of the population worldwide. In PD patients, 70–80% of DAergic cells gradually degenerate, resulting in reduced DA (which controls movement and balance). PD is a progressive, selective, and age-related loss of the NS-DA-ergic system, resulting in bradykinesia, rigidity, and body tremor. The dysregulation of the CP/ATG-lysosomal pathway is involved in the pathogenesis of PD. The author described the theranostic significance of CB, CP, and CS in undernutrition, drug addiction, fetal alcohol spectrum disorder, PD, AD, ALS (also classified as neurodegenerative charnolopathies: NCPs) and the theranostic potential of antioxidants for the TSE-EBPT of these disorders. The importance of lysosomal-based degradative pathways have been highlighted in maintaining the homeostasis of post-mitotic cells, and the contribution of a functional ATG in longevity. In contrast, defects in the clearance of organelles and aberrant protein aggregates are linked to accelerated neuronal loss and NDDs. Balke et al. (2019) evaluated the effects of ATG inhibition in the MPTP mouse model of PD *in vivo*. Adeno-associated viral vector (AAV)-mediated overexpression of a dominant-negative form of the unc-51-like ATG-initiating kinase (ULK1.DN) in the SN was induced three weeks before the MPTP treatment. A significant improvement in the ULK1.DN-expressing mice was observed following the MPTP treatment. DAergic neurons and NS projections revealed that protection from MPTP-induced neurotoxicity after ULK1.DN expression was due to activation of mTOR signaling, indicating that its expression attenuates MPTP-induced axonal degeneration. Hence, ULK1 could be a promising target in the treatment of PD.

LRRK2 is involved in the regulation of intracellular vesicle traffic, CP, and lysosomal activation in PD. Recent studies provided evidence of lysosomal dysfunction in PD. ER-mitochondria signaling is also impaired in PD. Brain mitochondrial aging, loss of the functional mitochondrial network, reduced APS recruitment, DJ-1 mutations, Parkin induction, and compromised MQC are implicated in the etiopathogenesis of PD. In addition, basal MTG occurred independently of PINK1 in mouse tissues of high metabolic demand. Significant oxidative, reductive, metabolic, and proteotoxic alterations were observed in PD postmortem brains. Hence, the alterations of mitochondrial function resulting in CMB needs to be further explored to develop theranostic and prognostic biomarkers for PD. The impact of ATG is context dependent and can have both beneficial and detrimental effects. A significant proportion of genes associated with PD encode proteins involved in the ATG-lysosomal pathway. Zhang et al. (2018) highlighted the evidence for targeting mitochondria by proteotoxic, redox, and metabolic stress, and the role of ATG surveillance in MQC. They summarized the role of α-Syn, LRRK2, and tau in modulating mitochondrial function and CP/ATG. Among the stressors that can overwhelm the MQC mechanisms, they discussed 4-hydroxynonenal and NO. They highlighted the potential of targeting mitochondria and CP/ATG as a theranostic strategy and the contribution of the microbiome to PD susceptibility. Furthermore, Prajapati et al. (2018) identified the miRNA expression in 6-OHDA-induced PD in SH-SY5Y cells. The targets of 5 miRNAs were analyzed by using StarBase. They found that the pathways of miRNAs include neurotrophin signaling, neuronal processes, mTOR, and cell death; miR-5701 was downregulated in the presence of 6-OHDA; and that putative targets of miR-5701 miRNA included genes involved in lysosomal biogenesis and MQC. They also found that transfection of miR-5701 mimic decreased the transcript level of VCP, LAPTM4A, and ATP6V0D1. The expression of miR-5701 mimic induced mitochondrial dysfunction, defect in ATG, and SH-SY5Y cells exposed to 6-OHDA-induced cell death, indicating that the dysregulation of specific miRNAs in PD stress and miR-5701 are regulators of mitochondrial and lysosomal function in PD pathogenesis.

This chapter, describes TSE-EBPT significance of CP and antioxidants in the clinical management of PD.

Mitochondrial Dysfunction in PD

Mitochondrial dysfunction is considered a critical mechanism in PD pathogenesis. Wu et al. (2018a) exposed *C. elegans* to 0.5–10.0 µM Rotenone (RO) or 0.2–1.6 mM Paraquat (PQ) for three days. Both RO and PQ induced Parkinsonism including motor deficits and DAergic degeneration. RO/PQ caused mitochondrial damages characterized by an increase in vacuole areas and ATG vesicles as well as decreased cristae. RO/PQ-impacted mitochondrial function was also demonstrated by the decrease in ATP and $\Delta\Psi$ collapse. The attachment or ER encapsulation of degenerated mitochondria indicated changes in mitochondrial-associated membranes (MAMs). The expression of tomm-7 and complex I, II, and III genes was reduced, whereas the PINK1 expression was increased. To determine MAMs in PD toxicity, they investigated the mutants of hop-1 and PINK1, encoding pre-senilin and PINK1 in MAMs, respectively. The mutation of both hop-1 and PINK1 reduced the vulnerability of lethal, behavioral, and mitochondrial toxicity induced by RO/PQ. These findings suggested that pre-senilin and PINK1 play important roles in RO/PQ-induced neurotoxicity through the MAMs.

It is known that mutations in FOXO genes are implicated in age-dependent NDDs, such as PD. Hence, Tas et al. (2018) investigated the involvement of FOXO in the death of DAergic neurons in *Drosophila*. dFOXO null mutants exhibited a selective loss of DAergic neurons crucial for locomotion, the proto-cerebral anterior medial (PAM) cluster, during development as well as in adulthood. PAM neuron-targeted adult-restricted knockdown demonstrated that dFOXO in adult PAM neurons tissue promoted neuronal survival during aging. dFOXO and the bHLH-TF 48-related-2 (FER2) protected PAM neurons from different forms of cellular stress. However, dFOXO and FER2 shared common processes leading to the regulation of CP/ATG and mitochondrial morphology by inhibiting CBMP. Thus, overexpression of one could rescue the loss of function of the other, indicating a role of dFOXO in neuroprotection and that genetic and environmental factors interacted to increase the risk of DA-ergic degeneration and the development of PD. Parkin and PINK1, gene products mutated in familial PD, play crucial roles in MTG through ubiquitination of mitochondria. Cargo ubiquitination by E3 ubiquitin ligase Parkin is important to trigger CP. Yamano et al. (2018) demonstrated that RABGEF1, the upstream factor of the endosomal Rab GTPase cascade, is recruited to damaged mitochondria participating in CBMP via ubiquitin binding downstream of Parkin in cultured cells. RABGEF1 directs the downstream Rab proteins, RAB5 and RAB7A, to damaged mitochondria, whose associations were regulated by mitochondrial Rab-GAPs. Furthermore, depletion of RAB7A inhibited ATG9A vesicle assembly and the subsequent encapsulation of the mitochondria by autophagic membranes, suggesting that endosomal Rab cycles on damaged mitochondria are crucial regulators of CP/MTG through ATG9A vesicles.

CBMP in PD Pathogenesis

Mitochondrial degeneration triggers MQC pathways, which act to ensure the health of the mitochondrial network. The elimination of damaged mitochondria by CP is initiated by the PD-linked genes, PRKN and PINK1. McLelland and Fon (2018) investigated the role that inter-organellar contact sites between the ER and the OMM. They showed that the ER-OMM tether, Mfn-2, acts as a suppressor of CP by linking the OMM to the ER, limiting the accessibility of other ubiquitination substrates to PINK1 and PRKN. PINK1, PRKN, and the AAA-ATPase VCP disrupt contact between mitochondria and the ER via Mfn-2 ubiquitination, retro-translocation and turnover from the mitochondrial membrane, providing insight into the role of OMM remodeling in CP induction. The pathogenesis of PD involves the impairment of lysosomal CP/ATG, which also contributes to LSDs. Rudenok et al. (2019) analyzed the expression of genes related to lysosomal ATG (Hspa8, Lamp2, Tfam, Slc18a2, and Vps35), in the brain tissues of mice with the earliest stage of MPTP-induced PD. The decrease in Hspa8 and Lamp2 mRNA suggested that dysfunction of lysosomal CP/ATG and CBMP may be involved in the earliest stages of PD. A decrease in the rate of lysosomal CP/ATG may affect the accumulation of CBs, denatured proteins, and the formation of Lewy bodies in PD. Genes related to the lysosome function may be involved in development of both LSD and PD at the earliest stages of these pathophysiological processes. Under physiological conditions, Spermine and Spermidine enhance longevity via CP/ATG induction in aging. Saiki et al. (2019) evaluated polyamine metabolite to act as an age-related, diagnostic, and severity-associated PD biomarker. A metabolome analysis of plasma was performed in Cohort A (controls, n = 45; PD, n = 145), followed by an analysis of seven polyamine metabolites in Cohort B (controls, n = 49; PD, n = 186; progressive supra-nuclear palsy, n = 19; AD, n = 23). Furthermore, 20 patients with PD who were examined within Cohort B were studied using DTI. The association of each polyamine metabolite with disease severity was assessed according to Hoehn and Yahr stage (H&Y) and Unified PD Rating Scale motor section (UPDRS-III). The CP/ATG induction ability of each polyamine metabolite was examined in various cell lines. In Cohort A, N8-Acetylspermidine and N-Acetylputrescine were increased in PD. In Cohort B, Spermine levels and the Spermine/Spermidine ratio were reduced in PD, concomitant with hyper-acetylation. Furthermore, N1, N8-Diacetylspermidine levels had the highest theranostic value, and correlated with H&Y, UPDRS-III, and axonal degeneration quantified by DTI. The Spermine/Spermidine ratio declined with age, but was significantly suppressed in PD. Among polyamine metabolites, Spermine was the strongest CP/ATG inducer in SH-SY5Y cells. No significant genetic variations in five genes encoding enzymes associated with Spermine/Spermidine metabolism were detected. Hence, Spermine synthesis and N1, N8-Diacetylspermidine may be useful theranostic and prognostic biomarkers of PD.

Several genetic mutations have been implicated in PD, including the loss of function of PINK1 and Parkin, which result in the accumulation of damaged mitochondria in the form of CBs and protein aggregates (α-Syn)–leading to neuronal demise (Valente et al. 2004). Mitochondrial dysfunction involving CBMP is implicated in PD progression. In aging-related PD, the disease is caused by dysfunctional mitochondria, oxidative stress, CP/ATG dysregulation and the aggregation of proteins, leading to mitochondrial swelling and depolarization. It is important to eliminate nonfunctional yet highly toxic CBs, because these traits can induce cell death (Esteves et al. 2011). Hence, we need to have efficient CP system to sustain IMD, MQC, and ICD. CMB can cause cellular degeneration, as seen in the SN (Arduíno 2011). PD comprises a spectrum of disorders with differing subtypes, the vast majority of which share LBs as a pathological hallmark. Hence, α-Syn pathology and mitochondrial dysfunction have been implicated in PD pathogenesis. Surmeier (2018) demonstrated that SNc DAergic neurons have an anatomical, physiological, and biochemical phenotype that predisposes them to CBMP and DCPs. α-Syn is a major component of LB and SNCA gene missense mutations or duplications/triplications, which cause hereditary forms of PD. Wang et al. (2016) summarized that the ATG pathway, consists of CP, macroATG, microATG, and chaperone-mediated ATG. They discussed mitochondrial dysfunction, PD-related genes, ATG, and the theranostic significance of functional pathways in PD pathogenesis. ATG and mitochondrial homeostasis are important in the pathogenesis of PD. A better understanding of these pathways can shed light on the novel therapeutic methods for PD prevention and amelioration. As sporadic PD is associated with LB pathology, a factor of major importance is the study of the α-syn protein and its pathology. However, α-Syn pathology is also evident in MSA and LBD and there is an overlap of these synopathies with other protein misfolding diseases, making it non-specific for PD. α-Syn, phosphorylated tau protein (pτ), Aβ, and other proteins show synergistic effects in the pathogenic mechanisms. Multiple cell death mechanisms can induce pathological protein-cascades, but this can also be a reverse process. This holds true for the early phases of the PD progression. Although rare SNCA gene mutations are causal for a minority of familial PD patients, in sporadic PD (where common SNCA polymorphisms are the most consistent genetic risk factor accounting for 95% of PD patients), α-Syn pathology is an important feature of PD progression.

The cellular reprogramming of somatic cells to iPSC represents an efficient tool for the *in vitro* modeling of human brain diseases and identification of novel theranostics. Torrent et al. (2015) explored the PD iPSC-based models, highlighting their role in the discovery of new drugs, as well as discussing the limitations of iPSC-models. Patient-specific iPSC can be differentiated into disease-relevant cell types, including neurons, which carry the genetic Bkg of the donor and enabling the *de novo* generation of human models of genetically complex disorders. Recently, the generation of disease-specific iPSC from patients suffering from PD has unveiled a recapitulation of disease-related cell phenotypes, such as abnormal α-Syn accumulation and alterations in ATG machinery. The use of patient-specific iPSC has a remarkable potential to uncover novel insights of the disease pathogenesis, which will open new avenues for clinical intervention. Our understanding of the mechanisms underlying PD increased with the identification of α-Syn and LRRK2 pathogenic mutations. While α-Syn composes the aggregates that can spread through much of the brain during a disease, LRRK2 encodes a multi-domain dual-enzyme distinct from any other protein linked to ND. Cresto et al. (2019) discussed multiple model systems that suggested these unlikely partners do interact in important ways in a disease, both within cells that express LRRK2 and α-Syn as well as through indirect pathways that might involve neuro-inflammation. Although the link between LRRK2 and disease can be understood through LRRK2 kinase activity (phosphotransferase activity), α-Syn toxicity is multilayered and interacts with LRRK2 kinase activity. These investigators discussed protein interactors like 14-3-3s that may regulate α-Syn and LRRK2 and examined cellular pathways and outcomes to both mutant α-Syn and LRRK2 activity and points of intersection. Understanding the interaction between these two partners may provide novel theranostic opportunities for PD. Mutations in the LRRK2 gene account for the most common causes of familial and sporadic PD and are one of the strongest genetic risk factors in sporadic PD.

Mitochondrial impairment has been observed in fibroblasts and iPSC-derived neural cells from PD patients with LRRK2 mutations localized to mitochondria. Singh et al. (2018) discussed recent discoveries relating to LRRK2 mutations and mitochondrial dysfunction in PD. Pathways implicated in LRRK2-dependent neurodegeneration included cytoskeletal dynamics, vesicular trafficking, ATG, mitochondria, and $[Ca^{2+}]_i$ homeostasis. In PD, LRRK2 is involved in the regulation of intracellular vesicle traffic, CP, and lysosomal function. The current understanding of the mechanisms by which LRRK2 regulates lysosomal-based degradative pathways in neuronal and non-neuronal cells and the impact of PD mutations in contributing to lysosomal dyshomeostasis have been highlighted. Mutations in the genes for PINK1 and Parkin triggers PD. PINK1 and Parkin cooperate in CB elimination through CP in cultured cells. Cornelissen et al. (2018) generated a *Drosophila* model expressing the MTG probe mt-Keima. Using mt-Keima imaging and correlative light and EM, it was shown that MTG occurs in myocytes and DAergic neurons *in vivo*, even in the absence of exogenous mitochondrial toxins. CP increased with aging, which was abrogated by PINK1 or Parkin deficiency. The knockdown of the *Drosophila* homologues of the deubiquitinases USP15 and USP30, rescued CP in the Parkin-deficient flies, suggesting a crucial role for Parkin and PINK1 in age-dependent CP in *Drosophila*.

CP/ATG and MQC in PD

MQC is important in NDDs, but in genetic PD caused by mutations in PINK and Parkin CB elimination through CP, it is crucial. Reductions in CP/ATG are implicated in aging, age-related diseases, and PD. The Parkin null (PK-KO) mice show only a subtle phenotype, apparent with age or with stressors. Gaudioso et al. (2019) studied the changes in the lipidomics of the mitochondrial membranes isolated from the brains of young and old PK-KO mice and compared them to wild type mice to determine the potential implications for PD pathogenesis. They observed an increase in the levels of phosphatidylethanolamine in the young PK-KO mice that is lost in the old and correlated to changes in the phosphatidylserine decarboxylase. PK-KO old mice mitochondria showed lower phosphatidylglycerol and phosphatidylinositol and increased hydroxylated ceramides. Cardiolipins changed in the degree of saturation with age. When mitochondrial homeostasis is compromised, it can lead to ROS formation to further accelerate the accumulation of CBs, resulting in a vicious circle deleterious to the neuron. PINK1 and Parkin, linked to PD, play vital roles in CP in maintaining MQC. Peng et al. (2018) explored MB, CP, and fission/fusion in Rotenone-induced DA toxicity. They focused on interactions between the PINK1/Parkin pathway and PGC-1α in the impaired mitochondrial homeostasis. Both CP and ATG increased significantly and were accompanied by altered levels of PINK1/Parkin proteins in Rotenone-induced neurotoxicity. PINK1 influenced MB by inhibiting PGC-1α and mtTFA expression as well as the mtDNA copy number. PGC-1α inhibited PINK1/Parkin expression and the CP levels, and PINK1 influenced mitochondrial fission/fusion by regulating Mfn-2 and phosphorylating Drp-1. Thus, mutual antagonism of the PINK1/Parkin pathway and PGC-1α formed a balance that regulated MB, fission/fusion, and CP for the maintenance of mitochondrial homeostasis in Rotenone-induced neurotoxicity.

Mitochondria form physical contacts with a specialized domain of the ER, known as the MAM, which constitutes a key signaling hub to regulate several fundamental cellular processes. Gómez-Suaga et al. (2018) highlighted ER-mitochondrial signaling and the evidence concerning damage to this signaling in PD. Alterations in ER-mitochondria signaling have pleiotropic effects on a variety of intracellular events, resulting in mitochondrial damage, Ca^{2+} dyshomeostasis, ERS, and defects in lipid metabolism and ATG through CB formation. Many of these cellular processes are perturbed in NDDs. Thus, functionally impaired ER-mitochondrial signaling contributes to PD. Lee et al. (2019) reported that the mitochondrial matrix protein MsrB2 plays an important role in switching on MTG by reducing Parkin methionine oxidation (MetO), and transducing MTG through ubiquitination by Parkin and interacting with LC3. This signaling occurs only in damaged mitochondria where MsrB2 is released from the mitochondrial matrix to induce CBMP. MsrB2 platelet-specific knockout and *in vivo* peptide inhibition of the MsrB2/LC3 interaction lead to reduced MTG and increased platelet apoptosis. Increased MsrB2 expression in diabetes mellitus and PD induced platelet MTG, whereas, reduced MsrB2 expression inhibited platelet MTG. Parkin mutations at Met192 are associated with PD, highlighting the sensitivity of the Met192 position. The release of the enzyme MsrB2 represented a novel regulatory mechanism for oxidative stress-induced MTG. Dysregulated MTG has been linked to PD due to the role of PINK1 in mediating depolarization-induced MTG *in vitro* (Lee et al. 2019). Mouse reporters have revealed the pervasive nature of basal MTG *in vivo*. Using mito-QC, McWilliams et al. (2018) investigated the contribution of PINK1 to MTG in metabolically active tissues. They observed increased MTG in neural cells, including PD-relevant mesencephalic DAergic neurons and microglia. In all tissues apart from pancreatic islets, loss of PINK1 did not influence basal MTG, despite disrupting depolarization-induced Parkin activation, indicating that PINK1 is detectable at basal levels and that basal MTG occurs independently of PINK1, suggesting multiple pathways orchestrating mitochondrial integrity in a context-dependent fashion, which has profound implications for affecting our understanding of vertebrate MTG. The PINK1 and the E3 ubiquitin ligase Parkin (encoded by the PARK2 gene) act together to mark depolarized mitochondria for degradation. There are multiple pathways of cargo specification for MTG. CP-independent functions of PINK1 and Parkin are also emerging. Chu et al. (2019) summarized key features of three major CP cargo recognition systems: they are (i) receptor-mediated, (ii) ubiquitin-mediated, and (iii) Cardiolipin-mediated. New animal models may be useful for tracking the delivery of mitochondria into lysosomes in different neuronal populations. Combining these research tools with methods to selectively disrupt specific CP pathways may lead to a better understanding of the role of CP in modulating neuronal vulnerability in the PD spectrum (PD/PDD/DLB) and other NDDs.

The deglycase and chaperone protein DJ-1 is pivotal for cellular oxidative stress responses and MQC. Mutations in PARK7, encoding DJ-1, are associated with early-onset familial PD and lead to pathological oxidative stress and/or disrupted protein degradation by the proteasome. Strobbe et al. (2018) investigated the pathogenic mechanisms of selected DJ-1 missense mutations, by characterizing protein-protein interactions, core parameters of mitochondrial function, QC regulation via ATG, and cellular death following DA accumulation. DJ-1[M26I] mutation influenced DJ-1 interactions with SUMO-1, enhancing the removal of dysfunctional mitochondria involved in CBMP and conferring increased cellular susceptibility to DA toxicity. However, the DJ-1[D149A] mutant did not influence CP, but impaired Ca^{2+} dynamics and free radical homeostasis by disrupting DJ-1 interactions with a mitochondrial accessory protein known as DJ-1-binding protein (DJBP/EFCAB6), suggesting that individual DJ-1 mutations have differential effects on mitochondrial function and QC, and thus, implying mutation-specific pathogenesis on impaired mitochondrial homeostasis.

Rango and Bresolin (2018) highlighted the role of mitochondria in aging and in PD. Alterations in mitochondrial activity are typical of aging. Aging is characterized by decreased O/P, and proteasome activity, altered CP/ATG, and mitochondrial dysfunction. Beyond declined O/P, mitochondrial dysfunction consists of a decline of β-oxidation as well as of the Krebs cycle. mtDNA mutations are acquired over time and parallel the decrease in O/P. Many of these mitochondrial alterations are also found in the PD brain, specifically in the SN. mtDNA deletions and development of respiratory chain deficiency in SN neurons of aged individuals as well as of individuals with PD converge towards a shared pathway, which leads to neuronal dysfunction and death due to the induction of CBMP. Several nuclear genes that are mutated in hereditary PD are implicated in mitochondrial impairment triggering CBMP, indicating a tight link between mitochondria and aging. An Autosomal Recessive-Juvenile Parkinsonism (AR-JP) *Drosophila* model exhibits DAergic degeneration as well as aberrant mitochondrial dynamics and their functions. Disruptions in MTG have been observed in Parkin loss-of-function models, and changes in mitochondrial respiration have been reported in patient fibroblasts. More specifically, Park et al. (2006) generated loss-of-function mutants of *Drosophila* PTEN-induced putative kinase 1 (PINK1), a novel AR-JP-linked gene and demonstrated that PINK1 mutants exhibit indirect flight muscle and DAergic degeneration accompanied by locomotive defects. TEM analysis and a rescue experiment with *Drosophila* Bcl-2 demonstrated that mitochondrial dysfunction accounts for the degenerative changes in all phenotypes of PINK1 mutants. PINK1 mutants shared phenotypic similarities with Parkin mutants, whereas transgenic expression of Parkin ameliorated PINK1 loss-of-function phenotypes, but not vice versa, suggesting that Parkin functions downstream of PINK1. This study established that Parkin and PINK1 act in a common pathway in maintaining the structural and functional integrity of mitochondria in both muscles and DAergic neurons. Cackovic et al. (2018) used fluorescent constructs expressed in Drosophila DA neurons that are homologous to those of the mammalian SN. Degenerating DA neurons in Parkin loss-of-function mutant flies had advanced mitochondrial aging, and their networks were fragmented and contained swollen organelles. MTG initiation is decreased in Park (*Drosophila* Parkin/PARK2 ortholog) homozygous mutants, but APS formation was unaffected, and the mitochondrial network volume was decreased. As the fly aged, APS recruitment became similar to control, while mitochondria revealed signs of damage, and climbing deficits. Aberrant mitochondrial morphology, aging, and MTG were not observed in DA neurons that did not degenerate, suggesting that Parkin is important for mitochondrial homeostasis in DA neurons, and that the loss of Parkin-mediated MTG may play a role in the degeneration of DA neurons or motor deficits in this model.

Weil et al. (2018) highlighted recent discoveries about the role of Optn in CP and provided insight into its link with NDDs. They discussed Optn in other pathologies in which CP dysfunctions are involved, including cancer. Optineurin (Optn) is a 577 aa protein encoded by the *Optn* gene. Mutations in *Optn* are associated with glaucoma, ALS, Paget's disease, and Crohn's disease. Optn is involved in NF-κB regulation, membrane trafficking, exocytosis, vesicle transport, reorganization of actin and microtubules, cell cycle control, and ATG. Besides its role in xenophagy and ATG of aggregates, Optn serves as an ATG receptor, among the five adaptors that translocate to mitochondria during CP. One of the important surveillance pathways of mitochondrial health is the signal transduction pathway involving the mitochondrial PINK1 protein and the RING-between-RING ubiquitin ligase Parkin. Mutated forms have been identified in certain types of PD. By targeting ubiquitinated mitochondria to CPS through its association with ATG-related proteins, Optn is responsible for a critical step in CP induction because it targets ubiquinated mitochondria to CPS through its association with ATG-related proteins. Wallings et al. (2019) examined the crucial role of lysosome dysfunction in FTD/ALS and the recent evidence for converging mechanisms. There is evidence from genetic studies, human tissue, iPSCs, and animal models that lysosomal failure is a primary mechanism of disease, rather than merely associated with protein aggregate end-points. STE-EBPT targets lysosomes in therapeutics for both PD and FTD/ALS. Rudenok et al. (2019) analyzed the expression of genes related to lysosomal ATG: Hspa8, Lamp2, Tfam, Slc18a2, and Vps35, in the brain tissues of mice with the earliest stage of MPTP-induced PD. The downregulation in Hspa8 and Lamp2 mRNA suggested that dysfunction of lysosomal ATG may be involved in the earliest stages of PD pathogenesis. A decrease in the rate of lysosomal ATG may affect the accumulation of damaged proteins and the formation of protein inclusions in PD. Thus, genes related to the lysosomal function may be involved in the development of both LSD and PD at the earliest stages of pathogenesis.

Parkin, an E3 ubiquitin ligase and a PD-related gene, translocates to impaired mitochondria and drives their elimination via ATG, a process known as MTG. Mitochondrial pro-fusion protein mitofusins (Mfn-1 and Mfn-2) were targets for Parkin-mediated ubiquitination. Mfns are transmembrane GTPase embedded in the OMM, required on adjacent mitochondria to mediate fusion. Mfn-2 also forms complexes that are capable of tethering mitochondria to ER, a structural feature essential for mitochondrial energy metabolism, Ca^{2+} transfer between the organelles, and Ca^{2+}-dependent cell death. Ubiquitination is a powerful tool to modulate protein function, via regulation of protein subcellular localization and interaction with other proteins. Ubiquitination is also a reversible mechanism, which can be controlled by opposing ubiquitination-deubiquitination events. In Parkin-deficient cells and Parkin mutant human fibroblasts, the tether between ER and mitochondria is decreased. Basso et al. (2018) identified the site of Parkin-dependent ubiquitination and showed that the non-ubiquitinatable Mfn-2 mutant fails to restore ER-mitochondrial interaction. Manipulation of ER-mitochondria tethering by expressing an ER-mitochondria synthetic linker rescues the locomotor deficit associated with an *in vivo Drosophila* model of PD. Recent studies revealed that the ubiquitin-proteasome complex and mitochondrial membrane rupture are key steps preceding CP, in combination with the ubiquitination of specific OMM proteins. The deubiquitinating enzyme ubiquitin-specific peptidase 14 (USP14) modulates both proteasome activity and ATG. Chakraborty et al. (2018) reported that the genetic and pharmacological inhibition of USP14 promotes CP, which occurs in the absence of PINK1 and Parkin. Critical to USP14-induced CP is the exposure of the LC3 receptor Prohibitin 2 by mitochondrial fragmentation and mitochondrial membrane rupture. The genetic or pharmacological inhibition of USP14 *in vivo* corrected the mitochondrial dysfunction and locomotor behavior of the PINK1/Parkin mutant *Drosophila* model of PD, an age-related progressive NDD that is correlated with diminished MQC. This study identified a novel therapeutic target that ameliorates mitochondrial dysfunction and *in vivo* PD-related symptoms. Heterozygous mutations in GBA, the gene encoding the lysosomal enzyme, glucosylceramidase beta/β-glucocerebrosidase, comprise the most common genetic risk factor for PD. Li et al. (2018) showed that in $Gba^{L444P/WT}$ knockin mice, the L444P heterozygous Gba mutation triggers mitochondrial dysfunction by inhibiting ATG and mitochondrial priming, two steps critical for the selective removal of dysfunctional mitochondria by CP/ATG. In SHSY-5Y cells, the overexpression of L444P GBA impeded mitochondrial priming and ATG induction when endogenous lysosomal GBA activity remained intact. Genetic depletion of GBA inhibited the lysosomal clearance of ATG cargo. The link between heterozygous GBA mutations and impaired CP was corroborated in postmortem brain tissue from PD patients carrying heterozygous GBA mutations, where increased mitochondrial content, mitochondria oxidative stress, and impaired CP/ATG, suggested an association of mitochondrial dysfunction with GBA heterozygous mutations (Li et al. 2019).

Monoamine Oxidase and PD

Monoamine oxidase inhibitors (MAOs) are located on the OMM and are drug targets for the treatment of NDDs. MAOs control the levels of neurotransmitters via oxidative deamination and contribute to ROS generation through their catalytic by-product, H_2O_2. Increased ROS may modulate mitochondrial function and is implicated in various disorders. Ugun-Klusek et al. (2019) used MAO-A overexpressing neuroblastoma cells, to demonstrate that higher levels of MAO-A protein/activity result in increased ROS levels with an accompanying increase in protein oxidation. Increased MAO-A results in increased lysine-63 linked ubiquitination of mitochondrial proteins and promoted CP/ATG through Bcl-2 phosphorylation. Furthermore, ROS generated locally on the OMM by MAO-A promoted phosphorylation of the DRP-1 protein, leading to mitochondrial fragmentation and clearance without complete $\Delta\Psi$ collapse. Cellular ATP levels were maintained following MAO-A overexpression and complex IV activity/protein levels increased, revealing a relationship between MAO-A and mitochondrial function. The downstream effects of increased MAO-A are dependent on the availability of amine substrates;

in the presence of an exogenous substrate, cell viability is reduced. This study showed that MAO-A generated ROS is involved in QC, and an increase in MAO-A leads to a protective cellular response to facilitate removal of damaged macromolecules/organelles, but substrate availability may determine cell fate. The latter is important in PD, where a DA precursor (L-DOPA) is used to treat disease symptoms and the fate of MAO-A containing DAergic neurons may depend on both MAO-A and catecholamine substrate availability. Martinez et al. (2018) investigated the effect of α-Syn on mitochondrial dynamics and CP/MTG/ATG in SH-SY5Y cells. Overexpression of wild type α-Syn induced moderated toxicity, ROS generation, and mitochondrial dysfunction. In addition, α-Syn induced Drp-1-dependent mitochondrial fragmentation to trigger CBMP. Overexpression of the fusion protein Opa-1 prevented CBMP. On the other hand, cells expressing α-Syn exhibited activated CP/MTG followed by generalized ATG. CP/ATG was triggered to protect cells from α-Syn-induced cell death. These findings clarified the role of Opa-1 and Drp-1 in mitochondrial dynamics and cell survival, indicating the relevance of mitochondrial homeostasis and CP/ATG in the pathogenesis of PD. Better understanding of the molecular interaction between CP/ATG and α-Syn could confer the TSE-EBPT of PD. An *in vitro* exposure of MPP$^+$ (as cellular model of PD) increased, whereas pretreatment with a specific MAO-B inhibitor, Selegiline, inhibited the α-Syn index (Nitrated α-Syn/Native α-Syn) to provide DA-ergic neuroprotection (Sharma et al. 2003).

α-Syn and CP in PD

PD is associated with intracellular α-Syn accumulation and ventral midbrain DAergic neuronal death in the SN of patients. The abnormal accumulation of α-Syn and mitochondrial dysfunction are involved in the pathogenesis of PD. CP is a crucial component of the network controlling the MQC. Overexpression and/or abnormal accumulation and aggregation of α-Syn can trigger neuronal death. This role of α-Syn in PD pathogenesis is supported by the fact that duplication, triplication, and mutations of α-Syn gene cause familial forms of PD. Ganguly et al. (2018) searched PubMed and Google Scholar for articles describing the pathogenic role of α-Syn and the theranostic implications of targeting pathways related to this protein. These researchers found that the overexpression and accumulation of α-Syn within neurons may involve both transcriptional and post-transcriptional mechanisms including a decreased degradation of the protein through proteasomal or ATG processes. The mechanisms of monomeric α-Syn aggregating to oligomers and fibrils have been investigated, but it remains uncertain which form of this unfolded protein is responsible for toxicity. Mitochondrial dysfunction, ERS, and altered ER-Golgi transport may play crucial roles in DAergic degeneration (Esteves et al. 2011). The ability of α-Syn to form pores in membranes or to interact with specific proteins of the cell organelles and the cytosol could be determining factors in the toxicity of this protein. α-Syn may be a target for the development of neuroprotective drugs in PD. Many potential drugs which prevent the expression, accumulation, and aggregation of α-Syn or its interactions with mitochondria or ER and thereby abolish α-Syn-mediated toxicity have been explored in experimental models. The exposure of cultured primary neurons to preformed α-Syn fibrils (PFFs) leads to the recruitment of endogenous α-Syn and its templated conversion into fibrillar phosphorylated α-Syn (pα-synF) aggregates resembling those involved in PD pathogenesis. It was described as inclusions similar to Lewy bodies and Lewy neurites in PD patients. Grassi et al. (2018) discovered the existence of a conformationally distinct, nonfibrillar, phosphorylated α-Syn species that was named "pα-syn*". They described the existence of pα-syn* in PFF-seeded primary neurons, mice brains, and PD patients' brains. pα-syn* results from the incomplete autophagic degradation of pα-synF. Pα-synF was decorated with ATG markers, but pα-syn* was not. pα-syn* was N- and C-terminally trimmed, resulting in a 12.5 kDa fragment and a SDS-resistant dimer. After lysosomal release, pα-syn* aggregates associated with mitochondria, inducing mitochondrial membrane depolarization, Cyt-C release, and mitochondrial fragmentation involving CB formation visualized by confocal and stimulated emission depletion nanoscopy. Pα-syn* recruited phosphorylated acetyl-CoA carboxylase 1 (ACC1) with which it co-localized. ACC1 phosphorylation indicated low ATP levels, AMPK activation, and oxidative stress and induced mitochondrial fragmentation via reduced lipoylation. Pα-syn* also co-localized with BiP, a master regulator of the unfolded protein response and a resident protein of mitochondria-associated ER membranes that are sites of mitochondrial fission and CP. Pα-syn* aggregates were found in Parkin-positive CP vacuoles and imaged by EM, indicating that pα-syn* induces mitochondrial toxicity and fission, energetic stress, and CP, implicating pα-syn* as a key neurotoxic α-syn species for the TSE-EBPT of PD.

Recently, toxic α-Syn oligomer, which can mediate cell-to-cell propagation is suggested to cause sporadic PD. α-Syn interacts with membrane lipids especially PUFA to stabilize its 3-D structure, whereas peroxidation of PUFA may reduce their affinity to α-Syn and peroxidation byproducts might modify α-Syn. 4-Hydroxy-2-nonenal derived from *n*-6 PUFA modify α-Syn and produce a toxic oligomer. Shamoto-Nagai et al. (2018) found that the accumulation of 4-hydroxy-2-nonenal, induced oligomeriztion of α-Syn in PD brains. Docosahexaenoic acid (DHA), an *n*-3 PUFA abundant in the neuronal membrane, also enhanced α-Syn oligomerization. Propanoylated lysine, a specific indicator of DHA oxidation, was increased in α-Syn overexpressing SH-SY5Y cells. α-Syn is modified by the peroxidation products and degraded by the ATG-lysosome system. In the cells overexpressing α-Syn, the mitochondrial ETC was inhibited. Accumulation of abnormal α-Syn modified by lipid radicals derived from PUFA may be not only an indicator of brain oxidative stress but also causative of PD by impairing mitochondrial function involving CBMP. The Rho GTPase pathway, linking surface receptors to the organization of the actin and microtubule cytoskeletons, participate in PD pathogenesis. To unveil the participation of the Rho GTPase family in the molecular pathogenesis of PD, Kim et al. (2019) used *C. elegans* to demonstrate the role of the small GTPase RAC1 (ced-10 in the worm) in maintaining DAergic function and survival in the presence of α-Syn. In addition, ced-10 mutant worms determined an increase of α-Syn inclusions in comparison to control worms as well as an increase in autophagic vesicles. They used M17 cells over-expressing α-Syn and found that the RAC1 function decreased the amount of amyloidogenic α-Syn. By using DAergic neurons derived from patients of familial LRRK2-PD, they reported that human RAC1 activity is essential in regulating DAergic cell death, α-Syn accumulation, neurite arborization, and ATG modulation. These investigators determined that RAC1/ced-10 participates in PD pathogenesis and established it as a new candidate for further investigation of PD, mainly DAergic function and survival in α-Syn-induced toxicity. Furthermore, Chen et al. (2018) showed that mutant A53T α-Syn accumulation impaired mitochondrial function and Parkin-mediated MTG in α-SynA53T model. α-Syn-A53T overexpression caused p38 MAPK activation. Subsequently, p38 MAPK directly phosphorylated Parkin at serine 131 to disrupt the Parkin's protective function. The p38 MAPK inhibition reduced apoptosis, restored $\Delta\Psi$, as well as increased synaptic density both in SN4741 cells and primary midbrain neurons, indicating that the p38 MAPK-Parkin signaling pathway regulates MQC and NDD, which may form a potential theranostic strategy of PD via enhancing mitochondrial turn-over and maintenance.

Impaired protein degradation and increased α-Syn may trigger its pathological aggregation *in vitro* and *in vivo*. The chaperone-mediated ATG (CMA) pathway is involved in the α-Syn degradation. Dysfunction of the CMA pathway impairs α-Syn degradation and causes cytotoxicity. Wu et al. (2019) investigated the effects on the CMA pathway and α-Syn aggregation using bioactive ingredients (Dihydromyricetin (DHM) and Salvianolic acid B (Sal B)) extracted from natural medicinal plants. In both cell-free and cellular models of α-Syn aggregation, after administration of DHM and Sal B, inhibition of α-Syn accumulation and aggregation was observed. Cells were co-transfected with a C-terminal modified α-Syn (SynT) and Synphilin-1, and treated with DHM (10 μM) and Sal B (50 μM) 16 hrs after transfection; α-Syn aggregation decreased (68% for DHM and 75% for Sal B). Increased LAMP-1 (a marker of lysosomal homeostasis) and LAMP-2A (a key marker of CMA) were observed. Increased colocalization between LAMP-1 and LAMP-2A with α-Syn inclusions was observed after treatment with DHM and Sal B. Increased LAMP-1 and LAMP-2A, along with decreased α-Syn were observed. DHM and Sal B exhibited anti-inflammatory activities, preventing astroglia- and microglia-mediated inflammation in BAC-α-Syn-GFP transgenic mice, indicating that DHM and Sal B modulate α-Syn accumulation, aggregation, and augmenting activation of CMA, holding potential for the PD theranostics.

MUL1 and Parkin in *Drosophila* Model of PD

Sleep disturbance occurs in PD, which may be the result of a disturbed circadian clock. Doktór et al. (2019) highlighted that the ROS level was higher, while the antioxidant enzyme SOD1 level was lower in mull^{A6} and Park^1 mutants than in the white mutant controls. Mutations of both ligases affected circadian rhythms and the clock. The expression of clock genes per time and clock and the level of PER protein were changed in the mutants. The expression of Atg5, an ATG protein also involved in circadian rhythm regulation, was decreased in the brain and in PDF-immunoreactive large ventral lateral clock neurons, resulting in a longer period of locomotor activity, increased total activity, and shorter sleep at night. The lack of both ligases led to decreased longevity and climbing ability. These changes in the brains of the *Drosophila* models of PD, in which mitochondrial ligases MUL1 and Parkin remain nonfunctional, may elucidate the molecular mechanisms of neurological and behavioral symptoms of PD.

LRRK2-associated CP in PD

The LRRK2 is a primarily cytosolic multi-domain protein contributing to the regulation of CP/ATG, mitochondrial function, vesicle transport, nuclear architecture, and cell morphology. Recent advances in cell reprogramming enabled the assessment of disease-related cellular traits in patient-derived somatic cells, providing a platform for disease modeling and drug development. Given the limited access to vital human brain cells, this technology is especially relevant for PD to decipher underlying pathogenesis. Progress in genome-editing technologies analyzed isogenic iPSC pairs that differ only in a single genetic change, thus allowing the assessment of the molecular and cellular phenotypes that result from monogenetic risk factors. Weykopf et al. (2019) summarized the current state of iPSC-based modeling of PD with a focus on LRRK2, one of the most prominent monogenetic risk factors for PD, linked to both familial and idiopathic forms. They summarized iPSC-based studies that contributed to improved understanding of the function of LRRK2 and its variants in PD etiopathology. These data emphasized the multifaceted role of LRRK2 in regulating cellular homeostasis on proteostasis, mitochondrial dynamics, and regulation of the cytoskeleton. They expounded on the advantages and limitations of reprogramming technologies for disease modeling and drug development and conferred an outlook on future challenges and promises offered by this technology.

LRRK2 mutations are the most common genetic cause of PD. LRRK2 contains a functional kinase domain and G2019S, increases its kinase activity. LRRK2 regulates mitochondria morphology and ATG in neurons. LPS treatment increases LRRK2 and mitochondrial fission in microglia. The downregulation of LRRK2 expression or inhibition of its kinase activity attenuates microglia activation. Ho et al. (2018) evaluated the role of LRRK2 G2019S in mitochondrial dynamics in microglia. The observation of microglia in G2019S transgenic mice revealed a decrease in mitochondrial area and shortage of microglial processes compared with their littermates. The treatment of BV2 cells and primary microglia with LPS enhanced mitochondrial fission and increased Drp-1. Both phenotypes were rescued by treatment with GSK2578215A, a LRRK2 kinase inhibitor. The protein levels of CD68, microglia marker (Drp-1), and TNF-α were significantly higher in brain lysates of G2019S transgenic mice compared with their littermates, suggesting that LRRK2 promotes microglial mitochondrial alteration via Drp-1 in a kinase-dependent manner, resulting in the stimulation of pro-inflammatory responses. This mechanism in microglia might be a potential target to develop PD theranostics since inflammation by active microglia is a major characteristic of PD. Juárez-Flores et al. (2018) studied the role of mitochondria and ATG in LRRK2^{G2019S} -mutation, and its relationship with the PD-symptoms. Fibroblasts from six non-manifesting LRRK2^{G2019S} -carriers (NM-LRRK2^{G2019S}) and seven patients with LRRK2^{G2019S} -associated PD (PD-LRRK2^{G2019S}) were compared to eight healthy controls. Assessment of mitochondrial performance and ATG was performed after 24 hrs' exposure to a standard (glucose) or mitochondrial-challenging environment (galactose), where mitochondrial and ATG impairment are elevated. A similar mitochondrial phenotype of NM-LRRK2^{G2019S} and controls, except for an early mitochondrial depolarization (54.14% increased), was shown in the glucose medium. In response to galactose, the mitochondrial dynamics of NM-LRRK2^{G2019S} improved to maintain ATP levels. A CMB was suggested in PD-LRRK2^{G2019S} in glucose media. An inefficient response to galactose and worsened mitochondrial dynamics (–37.7% mitochondrial elongation) was revealed, leading to increased oxidative stress. ATG (SQTSM/P62) was upregulated in NM-LRRK2^{G2019S} when compared to controls (glucose + 118.4%, galactose + 114.44%) and APS formation increased in glucose media. Despite elevated SQSTM1/P62 levels of PD-NM^{G2019S} when compared to controls (glucose + 226.14%, galactose + 78.5%), APS formation was deficient in PD-LRRK2^{G2019S} when compared to NM-LRRK2^{G2019S} (–71.26%). The enhanced mitochondrial performance of NM-LRRK2^{G2019S} in mitochondrial-challenging conditions and upregulation of ATG suggested that CMB and CP/ATG aggregates may contribute to the development of PD in LRRK2^{G2019S} mutation carriers. LRRK-2 as a risk factor for PD is illustrated in Fig. 39.

Leucine-Rich Repeat Kinase 2 (LRRK2), As a Risk Factors for PD

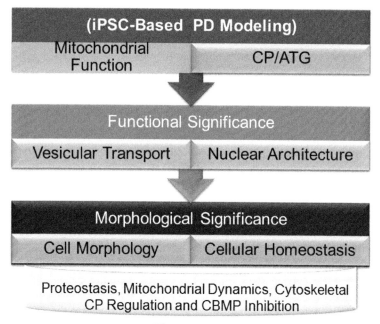

Figure 39

CP in Molecular Genetics of PD

GWAS have identified many genetic loci that associate with increased risk of developing diseases. However, translating genetic knowledge into an understanding of the molecular mechanisms relevant to disease remains a major challenge due to difficulties in precisely defining candidate genes at GWAS-risk loci. Ferrari et al. (2018) characterized candidate genes within GWAS loci using a protein-interactome-based approach and with PD data. They applied the Weighted Protein-Protein Interaction Network Analysis (WPPINA) to define impacted biological processes, risk pathways, and functional players by using Mendelian forms of PD to identify seed proteins, and to construct a protein network for genetic PD and carry out functional enrichment analyses. They isolated PD-specific processes indicating 'mitochondrial stressors mediated cell death', 'immune response and signaling', and 'waste disposal' mediated through 'CP/ATG'. It was confirmed that 10 candidate genes can nominate 17 candidate genes for sporadic PD. This study could better characterize the genetic and functional architecture of idiopathic PD, thus validating WPPINA for the *in silico* genetic and functional assessment of complex disorders.

Atrazine (2-chloro-4-ethylamino-6-isopropylamine-1, 3, 5-triazine; ATR) regulated ATG- and apoptosis-related proteins in DAergic neuronal damage. Ma et al. (2018) investigated the role of LC3-II in the ATR-induced degeneration of DAergic neurons. The *in vivo* DAergic neuron degeneration model was set up with ATR treatment and confirmed by the behavioral responses and pathological analysis. DAergic neurons were transfected with LC3-II siRNA and treated with ATR to observe cell survival and ROS release. After the ATR treatment, the grip strength of Wistar rats was decreased, and behavioral signs of anxiety were observed. The mRNA and protein levels of tyrosine hydroxylase, LC3-II, PINK1, and Parkin were decreased in ATR-induced DAergic neurons and PC-12 cells, while the mRNA expression and protein levels of SQSTM1/p62 and Parl were increased. Exposure to ATR also led to the accumulation of ATG lysosomes and ATG bodies along with decreased levels of DAergic neurons and alterations in mitochondrial homeostasis, which was reversed by LC3-II siRNA, suggesting that ATR affects the mitochondria-mediated DAergic cell death, which may be mediated by LC3-II and other ATG biomarkers through SQSTM1/p62 signaling pathway.

Recent data suggests that ATG is regulated by protein acetylation mediated by histone acetyltransferase (HAT) and histone deacetylase (HDAC). It also suggests that changes in histone acetylation are involved in PD pathogenesis, prompting an investigation of protein acetylation and HAT and HDAC activities in both idiopathic PD and G2019S-LRRK2 cell cultures (Banreti et al. 2013). Yakhine-Diop et al. (2018) used fibroblasts from PD patients (with or without the G2019S LRRK2 mutation) to assess the different phenotypes between idiopathic and genetic PD. This mutation display increased CP due to the activation of class III HDACs whereas idiopathic PD exhibits downregulation of clearance of defective mitochondria implicated in CBMP. The reduction in CP was accompanied by ROS overproduction. Parally, the acetylation protein levels of idiopathic and genetic individuals were different due to an upregulation in class I and II HDACs. Despite this upregulation, the total HDAC activity was decreased in idiopathic PD and the total HAT activity did not significantly vary. CP upregulation was beneficial for reducing the ROS-induced harm in genetic PD. The defective CP in idiopathic PD was inherent to the decrease in class III HDACs. Thus, there was an imbalance between total HATs and HDACs in idiopathic PD, which increased cell death. The inhibition of HATs in idiopathic PD cells displayed a protective effect.

There exists a new class of anti-diabetic insulin sensitizers in development that inhibit the mitochondrial pyruvate carrier (MPC), a protein which mediates the import of pyruvate across the IMM. Pharmacological inhibition of the MPC was neuroprotective in multiple neurotoxin-based and genetic models of PD. Quansah et al. (2018) summarized the neuroprotective effects of MPC inhibition and discussed the underlying mechanisms. These mechanisms involved the augmentation of ATG via attenuation of the activity of the mTOR in neurons, and inhibition of inflammation, which is mediated by direct inhibition of MPC in glia cells, suggesting that MPC is a novel theranostic target to slow PD progression.

Phospho-Ubiquitin in LB Disease and Aging

Two genes associated with recessive, early-onset PD encode the ubiquitin (Ub) kinase PINK1 and the E3 Ub ligase PRKN/PARK2/Parkin, which regulate a protective MQC pathway. Upon stress, both enzymes decorate CBs with phosphorylated poly-Ub (p-S65-Ub) chains. This label is subsequently recognized by ATG receptors that facilitate mitochondrial degradation in lysosomes to trigger CP. Hou et al. (2018) analyzed post-mortem brain specimens and identified distinct pools of p-S65-Ub-positive structures that co-localized with markers of mitochondria, ATG, lysosomes, and/or granulovacuolar degeneration bodies. They quantified levels and distribution of the 'CP tag' in two large cohorts of brain samples from normal aging and LB disease (LBD) cases, respectively. Somatic p-S65-Ub structures increased with age and disease in distinct brain regions and enhanced levels in LBD were age- and Braak tangle stage-dependent. A significant correlation between p-S65-Ub with LBs and neurofibrillary tangles was observed. The degree of co-existing p-S65-Ub signals and pathological PD hallmarks increased in the pre-mature stage, but decreased in the late stage of LB or tangle aggregation, indicating not only a potential pathogenic overlap among different forms of PD but also that p-S65-Ub can serve as a biomarker for mitochondrial damage involving CBMP in PD, AD, disease, and aging.

The Theranostic Significance of Antioxidants as CP Regulators in PD

Theranostic strategies are needed to protect DAergic neurons in PD patients. Oxidative stress caused by DA may play an important role in PD pathogenesis. CP, primarily regulated by PINK1 and Parkin, plays an important role in cellular homeostasis. Mutations in those genes cause accumulation of CBs, leading to nigral degeneration and early-onset PD. AMBRA1^ActA is a fusion protein expressed at the mitochondria, whose expression induces CP in mammalian cells. The pro-CP factor AMBRA1 restored CP in fibroblasts of PD patients carrying PINK1 and Parkin mutations. Di Rita et al. (2018) investigated the neuroprotective effect of AMBRA1-induced CP against 6-OH-DA and Rotenone-induced cell death in SH-SY5Y cells. AMBRA1^ActA overexpression induced mitochondrial clearance in SH-SY5Y cells. The apoptosis induced by 6-OHDA and Rotenone was reversed by AMBRA1-induced CP. Transfection of SH-SY5Y cells with a vector encoding AMBRA1^ActA reduced 6-OHDA and Rotenone-induced generation of ROS, indicating that AMBRA1^ActA induces CP to attenuate oxidative stress and apoptosis induced by both 6-OHDA and Rotenon. This, suggests that AMBRA1 may have promising neuroprotective properties in limiting ROS-induced DAergic cell death to prevent PD or other NDDs associated with oxidative stress involving CBMP. Wu et al. (2018b) investigated the effect of grape skin extract (GSE) when added to the daily food intake of a *Drosophila* model of PD associated with PINK1 loss-of-function. Consumption of GSE rescued mitochondrial morphological defects, caused an improvement in indirect flight muscle function and healthspan, and prolonged the lifespan of the PINK1 mutant flies. A link between the activation of CP and the beneficial effects of GSE was noticed, indicating that it can promote ATG, preserve mitochondria function, and attenuate PD pathogenesis by preventing CBMP, and that the beneficial effect of GSE in CP induction was not accounted for by Res alone. There is evidence from preclinical PD models that the activation of AMPK may have neuroprotective effects.

Curry et al. (2018) described the regulation and functions of AMPK and assessed the potential of targeting AMPK signaling as a neuroprotective treatment for PD. Numerous dietary supplements and pharmaceuticals (for example, Metformin) that increase AMPK activity are available, but clinical studies of their effects on PD patients are limited. AMPK is a serine/threonine kinase that is induced by falling energy levels and functions to restore cellular energy balance. However, in response to certain cellular stressors, AMPK activation may exacerbate neuronal atrophy and cell death. Díaz-Casado et al. (2018) analyzed *in vivo* mitochondrial respiration, which reflects changes in MB more precisely than *in vitro* mitochondrial preparations. These experiments were carried out in zebrafish embryos, which were treated with MPTP from 24 to 72 hrs post-fertilization (hpf). A reduction in electron transfer system capacity, ATP turnover, and increased proton leak were observed at 72 hpf in MPTP-treated embryos. These changes were followed by oxidative stress due to inhibition in antioxidant defense and ATG impairment. After removing MPTP from the treatment at 72 hpf, CMB persisted up to 120 hpf. The administration of Melatonin at 72 hpf, when mitochondrial dysfunction was already present, restored the respiratory capacity and ATP production, reduced oxidative stress, and normalized ATG after 48 hrs. Melatonin also counteracted MPTP-induced embryonic malformations and mortality, indicating the efficacy of Melatonin in restoring Parkinsonian phenotypes. Previous studies have shown that Melatonin can protect cells in Rotenone-induced cell death. Zhou et al. (2018) investigated the effects of Melatonin in inhibiting Rotenone-induced SH-SY5Y cells. These cells were treated with 0.3 or 1 µM Rotenone for 6 or 12 hrs. Melatonin inhibited Rotenone-induced SH-SY5Y cell death, mitochondrial dysfunction, increased Cyt-C expression, and inhibited Rotenone-induced Drp-1 expression, its translocation, and cell death. Drp-1 overexpression attenuated Melatonin-mediated protection in Rotenone toxicity in SH-SY5Y cells, indicating that Melatonin inhibited Rotenone-induced neuronal cell death by the transcriptional regulation of Drp-1 expression. In addition, mitochondrial dysfunction is considered as a critical mechanism in the pathogenesis of PD. Although, mitochondria-associated membranes (MAMs) have been implicated in the mitochondrial dysfunction, little is known about the role of MAMs-related proteins in the pathogenesis of PD. Wu et al (2018a) exposed nematode C. elegans to 0.5–10.0 µM Rotenone (RO) or 0.2–1.6 mM Paraquat (PQ) for 3 days. Both RO and PQ induced similar Parkinsonism including motor deficits and DAergic degeneration. RO/PQ caused mitochondrial damages characterized by the increase of vacuole areas and ATG vesicles, but the decrease of mitochondrial cristae. RO/PQ-induced mitochondrial dysfunction was also demonstrated by the decrease of ATP level and $\Delta\psi$. Additionally, the attachment or surrounding of ER to the CBs indicated ultrastructural alterations in MAMs. Using fluorescently labeled transgenic nematodes, these investigators discovered that the expression of tomm-7 and genes of Complex I, II and III was reduced, whereas the expression of PINK-1 was increased in the exposed animals. To determine MAMs in toxicity toward PD, they investigated the mutants of hop-1 and PINK-1, encoding presenilin and PTEN-induced putative kinase 1 (PINK1) in mitochondria-associated membranes, respectively. The mutation of both hop-1 and PINK-1 reduced the vulnerability of lethal, behavioral, and mitochondrial toxicity induced by RO/PQ, suggesting that presenilin and PINK1 play important roles in the RO/PQ-induced neurotoxicity through the mechanisms involved in MAMs.

Aging is associated with a gradual decline of cellular proteostasis, giving rise to protein mis-folding diseases, such as PD or AD, which exhibit a complex pathology involving non-cell autonomous proteotoxic effects. Using *C. elegans,* Sandhof et al. (2019) investigated how local protein misfolding is affecting neighboring cells and tissues by showing that misfolded PD-associated SNCA/α-Syn accumulates in endo-lysosomal vesicles. Irrespective of whether they were being expressed in muscle cells or DAergic neurons, accumulated proteins were transmitted into the hypodermis with increasing age, indicating that epithelial cells play a role in remote degradation when the local endo-lysosomal degradation capacity is compromised. The inter-tissue dissemination of SNCA was regulated by endo- and exocytosis (neuron/muscle to hypodermis) and basement membrane remodeling (muscle to hypodermis). Transferred SNCA conformers were inefficiently cleared and induced endo-lysosomal membrane permeability. Reducing IGF-1 signaling conferred protection by maintaining endo-lysosomal integrity, suggesting that the degradation of lysosomal substrates is coordinated across different tissues in metazoan organisms. Chronic dissemination of poorly degradable proteins into neighboring tissue exerts a non-cell autonomous toxicity. Hence, restoring endo-lysosomal function might help to halt disease progression in cells with pathological inclusions as well as in unaffected cells. In addition, Glucocerebrosidase (GBA1) mutations are the major genetic risk factor for PD. Alterations in lysosomal-ATG processes are implicated due to the reduction of mutated glucocerebrosidase (GCase) in lysosomes. Wild-type GCase activity is also decreased in sporadic PD brains. Small molecule chaperones that increase lysosomal GCase activity have the potential to be disease-modifying therapies for GBA1-associated and sporadic PD. Magalhaes et al. (2018) used mouse cortical neurons to explore the effects of the chaperone Ambroxol, which increased wild-type GCase mRNA, protein levels, and activity, as well as increased other lysosomal enzymes and LIMP2, the GCase transporter. Transcription factor EB (TFEB), the master regulator of the CLEAR pathway involved in lysosomal biogenesis was also increased upon Ambroxol treatment. macroATG flux was blocked and exocytosis increased in neurons treated with Ambroxol, suggesting that it blocks ATG and drives cargo towards the secretory pathway. Mitochondrial mass was also increased by Ambroxol via PGC1-α activation, suggesting that besides being a GCase chaperone, it also acts on other pathways, such as mitochondria, lysosomal biogenesis, and the secretory pathway to confer neuroprotection through the transcriptional regulation of CP.

CONCLUSION

Multiple signaling pathways have been proposed for CP dysregulation in PD, including impaired mitochondrial function and dysregulated ATG, which induced proteotoxicity, redox imbalance, and metabolic stress, whereas, the AAV-mediated expression of dominant-negative ULK1 provided neuronal survival and enhanced motoric performance in the MPTP mouse model of PD. Drp-1-dependent CB formation and ATG were observed in α-Syn overexpressing SH-SY5Y cells. USP14 inhibition resolved dysregulated CP/ATG. PINK1/Parkin and PGC-1α antagonism conferred mitochondrial homeostasis in Rotenone neurotoxicity. ER-mitochondrial interaction was regulated by Parkin via Mfn-2 pathways. Candidate genes were explored using a weighted protein-protein interaction analysis. *In vitro* and *in vivo* experimental models indicated that α-Syn-induced proteotoxicity implicated in CB formation, CP dysregulation, and eventually CBMP, to cause DAergic neurodegeneration. Modification of α-Syn by lipid peroxidation products derived from PUFA promoted toxic oligomerization, whereas small GTPase RAC1/CED-10 restored DAergic function. Phosphorylation of Parkin at serine 131 by p38 MAPK promoted CBMP neuronal death in the mutant A53T α-Syn model. The iPPCs-based LRRK2 mutation was linked to PD. LRRK2 kinase induced mitochondrial fission in microglia via Drp-1 and modulated inflammation. The exhaustion of mitochondrial and CP/ATG reserves were responsible for the development of LRRK2^{G2019S}-PD. LC3-II mediated ATR-induced CP in DAergic neurons through the SQSTM1/p62 pathway. Mfn-2 translocation boosted CP by uncoupling mitochondria from the ER. Mutation of Hop-1 and PINK1 attenuated neurotoxicity in *C. elegans*, confirming the crucial role of MAMs in Parkinsonism. Impaired CP and protein acetylation were observed in the fibroblasts of PD patients. Targeting the mitochondrial pyruvate carrier and transcription factors dFOXO and FER2 were proposed for the survival of DAergic neurons. Ambroxol provided neuroprotection through the ATG-lysosome pathway and mitochondria in primary cortical neurons. Endosomal Rab cycles regulated Parkin-mediated MTG and miR-5701 modulated mitochondrial-lysosomal crosstalk to attenuate neuronal demise. AMBRA1-mediated CP averted oxidative stress and apoptosis in SH-SY5Y cells, whereas GSE improved muscle function and extended the lifespan in a *Drosophila* model of PD through CP regulation. Targeting AMPK signaling was also explored. Melatonin as a CP regulator conferred neuroprotection in a MPTP-treated zebrafish model by restoring O/P and by attenuating Rotenone-induced death in SH-SY5Y cells through CP dysregulation and DRP-1 inhibition.

REFERENCES

Arduíno, D.M., A.R. Esteves and S.M. Cardoso. 2011. Mitochondrial fusion/fission, transport and autophagy in Parkinson's disease: When mitochondria get nasty. Parkinsons Dis 2011: 767230.

Balke, D., L. Tatenhorst, V. Dambeck, V.T. Ribas, et al. 2019. AAV-Mediated expression of dominant-negative ULK1 increases neuronal survival and enhances motor performance in the MPTP mouse model of Parkinson's disease. Mol Neurobiol 57: 685–697.

Basso, V., E. Marchesan, C. Peggion, J. Chakraborty, et al. 2018. Regulation of ER-mitochondria contacts by Parkin via Mfn-2. Pharmacol Res 138: 43–56.

Bánréti, A., M. Sass, Y. Graba. 2013. The emerging role of acetylation in the regulation of autophagy. Autophagy 9(6): 819–829.

Cackovic, J., S. Gutierrez-Luke, G.B. Call, A. Juba, et al. 2018. Mitochondrial aging, mitochondrial network loss and transiently reduced APS recruitment. Front Cell Neurosci 12: 39.

Chakraborty, J., S. von Stockum, E. Marchesan, F. Caicci, et al. USP14 inhibition corrects an *in vivo* model of impaired mitophagy. EMBO Mol Med 10: e9014.

Chen, J., Y. Ren, C. Gui, M. Zhao, et al. 2018. Phosphorylation of Parkin at serine 131 by p38 MAPK promotes mitochondrial dysfunction and neuronal death in mutant A53T α-Syn model of Parkinson's disease. Cell Death Dis 9: 700.

Chu, C.T. 2019. Multiple pathways for mitophagy: A neurodegenerative conundrum for Parkinson's disease. Neurosci Lett 697: 66–71.

Cornelissen, T., S. Vilain, K. Vints, N. Gounko, et al. 2018. Deficiency of Parkin and PINK1 impairs age-dependent MTG in *Drosophila*. eLife 7: e35878.

Cresto, N., C. Gardier, F. Gubinelli, M.C. Gaillard, et al. 2019. The unlikely partnership between LRRK2 and α-Syn in Parkinson's disease. Eur J Neurosci 49: 339–363.

Curry, D.W., B. Stutz, Z.B. Andrews and J.D. Elsworth. 2018. Targeting AMPK signaling as a neuroprotective strategy in Parkinson's disease. J Parkinsons Dis 8: 161–181.

Di Rita, A., P. D'Acunzo, L. Simula, S. Campello, et al. 2018. AMBRA1-mediated mitophagy counteracts oxidative stress and apoptosis induced by neurotoxicity in human neuroblastoma SH-SY5Y cells. Front Cell Neurosci 12: 92.

Díaz-Casado, M.E., I. Rusanova, P. Aranda, M. Fernández-Ortiz. et al. 2018. *In Vivo* determination of mitochondrial respiration in 1-Methyl-4-Phenyl-1,2,3,6-tetrahydropyridine-treated zebrafish reveals the efficacy of melatonin in restoring mitochondrial normalcy. Zebrafish 15: 15–26.

Doktór, B., M. Damulewicz and E. Pyza. 2019. Effects of MUL1 and Parkin on the circadian clock, brain and behaviour in *Drosophila* Parkinson's disease models BMC Neurosci 20: 24.

Esteves, A.R., D.M. Arduíno, D.F. Silva, C.R. Oliveira et al. 2011. Mitochondrial dysfunction: the road to alpha-syn oligomerization in PD. Parkinsons Dis 2011: 693761.

Ferrari, R., D.A. Kia, J.E. Tomkins, J. Hardy, et al. 2018. Stratification of candidate genes for Parkinson's disease using weighted protein-protein interaction network analysis. BMC Genomics 19: 452.

Ganguly, U., S.S. Chakrabarti, U. Kaur, A. Mukherjee, et al. 2018. Alpha-synuclein, proteotoxicity and parkinson's disease: search for neuroprotective therapy. Curr Neuropharmacol. 16(7): 1086–1097.

Gaudioso, A., P. Garcia-Rozas, M.J. Casarejos, O. Pastor, et al. 2019. Lipidomic alterations in the mitochondria of aged Parkin null mice relevant to ATG. Front Neurosci 13: 329.

Gómez-Suaga, P., J.M. Bravo-San Pedro, R.A. González-Polo, J.M. Fuentes, et al. ER-mitochondria signaling in Parkinson's disease. Cell Death Dis 9(3): 337.

Grassi, D., S. Howard, M. Zhou, N. Diaz-Perez, et al. 2018. Identification of a highly neurotoxic α-synuclein species inducing mitochondrial damage and mitophagy in Parkinson's disease. Proc Natl Acad Sci USA 115(11): E2634–E2643.

Ho, D.H., A.R. Je, H. Lee, I. Son, et al. 2018. LRRK2 Kinase activity induces mitochondrial fission in microglia via Drp-1 and modulates neuroinflammation. Exp Neurobiol 27: 171–180.

Hou, X., F.C. Fiesel, D. Truban, M. Castanedes Casey, et al. 2018. Age- and disease-dependent increase of the MTG marker phospho-ubiquitin in normal aging and lewy body disease. Autophagy 14: 1404–1418.

Juárez-Flores, D.L., I. González-Casacuberta, M. Ezquerra, M. Bañó, et al. 2018. Exhaustion of mitochondrial and autophagic reserve may contribute to the development of LRRK2 G2019S-Parkinson's disease. J Transl Med 16: 160.

Kim, H., C. Calatayud, S. Guha, I. Fernández-Carasa, et al. 2018. The Small GTPase RAC1/CED-10 is essential in maintaining dopaminergic neuron function and survival against α-synuclein-induced toxicity. Mol Neurobiol 55: 7533–7552.

Kim, S., H.S. Eun and E.K. Jo. 2019. Roles of autophagy-related genes in the pathogenesis of inflammatory bowel disease. Cells 8(1): 77.

Lee, S.H., S. Lee, J. Du, K. Jain, et al. 2019. Mitochondrial MsrB2 serves as a switch and transducer for mitophagy. EMBO Mol Med 11(8): e10409.

Li, G., J. Yang, C. Yang, M. Zhu, et al. 2018. PTENα regulates MTG and maintains mitochondrial quality control. Autophagy 14: 1742–1760.

Li, H., A. Ham, T.C. Ma, S-H. Kuo, et al. 2019. Mitochondrial dysfunction and mitophagy defect triggered by heterozygous GBA mutations. Autophagy 15(1): 113–130.

Ma, K., H. Wu, P. Li and B. Li. 2018. LC3-II may mediate ATR-induced mitophagy in dopaminergic neurons through SQSTM1/p62 pathway. ABBS 50: 1047–1061.

Magalhaes, J., M.E. Gegg, A. Migdalska-Richards and A.H. Schapira. 2018. Effects of ambroxol on the ATG-lysosome pathway and mitochondria in primary cortical neurons. Sci Rep 8: 1385.

Martinez, J.H., A. Alaimo, R.M. Gorojod, S. Porte Alcon, et al. 2018. Drp-1 dependent mitochondrial fragmentation and protective autophagy in dopaminergic SH-SY5Y cells overexpressing alpha-synuclein. Mol Cell Neurosci 88: 107–117.

McLelland, G.L. and E.A. Fon. 2018. Mfn-2 retrotranslocation boosts mitophagy by uncoupling mitochondria from the ER. Autophagy 14(9): 1658–1660.

McWilliams, T.G., A.R. Prescott, L. Montava-Garriga, G. Ball, et al. 2018. Basal mitophagy occurs independently of PINK1 in mouse tissues of high metabolic demand. Cell Metab 27: 439–449.

Park, J., S.B. Lee, S. Lee, Y. Kim, et al. 2006. Mitochondrial dysfunction in *Drosophila* PINK1 mutants is complemented by Parkin. Nature 441(7097): 1157–1161.

Peng, K., J. Xiao, L. Yang, F. Ye, et al. 2018. Mutual antagonism of PINK1/Parkin and PGC-1α contributes to maintenance of mitochondrial homeostasis in rotenone-induced neurotoxicity. Neurotox Res 35: 331–343.

Prajapati, P., L. Sripada, K. Singh, M. Roy, et al. 2018. Systemic analysis of miRNAs in PD stress condition: miR-5701 modulates mitochondrial-lysosomal cross talk to regulate neuronal death. Mol Neurobiol 55: 4689–4701.

Quansah, E., W. Peelaerts, J.W. Langston, D.K. Simon, et al. 2018. Targeting energy metabolism via the mitochondrial pyruvate carrier as a novel approach to attenuate neurodegeneration. Mol Neurodegener 13: 28.

Rango, M. and N. Bresolin. 2018. Brain mitochondria, aging, and Parkinson's disease. Genes 9(5): 250.

Rudenok, M.M., A.K. Alieva, M.A. Nikolaev, et al. 2019. Possible involvement of genes related to LSDs in the pathogenesis of Parkinson's disease. Mol Biol (Mosk) 53: 28–36.

Saiki, S., Y. Sasazawa, M. Fujimaki, K. Kamagata, et al. 2019. A metabolic profile of polyamines in Parkinson disease: A promising biomarker. Ann Neurol 86: 251–263.

Sandhof, C.A., S.O. Hoppe, S. Druffel-Augustin, C. Gallrein, et al. 2019. Reducing INS-IGF1 signaling protects against non-cell autonomous vesicle rupture caused by SNCA spreading. Autophagy 29: 878–899.

Shamoto-Nagai, M., S. Hisaka, M. Naoi and W. Maruyama. 2018. Modification of α-synuclein by lipid peroxidation products derived from polyunsaturated fatty acids promotes toxic oligomerization: Its relevance to Parkinson disease. J Clin Biochem Nutr 62(3): 207–212.

Sharma, S.K., E.C. Carlson and M. Ebadi. 2003. Neuroprotective actions of Selegiline in inhibiting 1-methyl, 4-phenyl, pyridinium ion (MPP+)-induced apoptosis in SK-N-SH neurons. J Neurocytol 32: 329–43.

Sharma, S. and Ebadi, M. 2013. *In vivo* molecular imaging in Parkinson's Disease. *In*: R.F. Pfeiffer, Z.K. Wszolek and M. Ebadi (eds), Parkinson's Disease, 2nd Ed. CRC Press Taylor & Francis Group, Boca Rotan, FL, U.S.A., pp. 787–802.

Sharma, S. 2019. The Charnoly Body: A Novel Biomarker of Mitochondrial Bioenergetics. CRC Press, Taylor & Francis Group, Boca Raton, FL, U.S.A.

Singh, A., L. Zhi and H. Zhang. 2018. LRRK2 and mitochondria: Recent advances and current views. Brain Res 1702: 96–104.

Strobbe, D., A.A. Robinson, K. Harvey, L. Rossi, et al. 2018. Distinct mechanisms of pathogenic DJ-1 mutations in mitochondrial quality control. Front Mol Neurosci 11: 68.

Surmeier, D.J. 2018. Determinants of dopaminergic neuron loss in Parkinson's disease. FEBS J 285: 3657–3668.

Tas, D., L. Stickley, F. Miozzo, R. Koch, et al. 2018. Parallel roles of transcription factors dFOXO and FER2 in the development and maintenance of dopaminergic neurons. PLoS Genet 14: e1007271.

Torrent, R., F. De Angelis Rigotti, P. Dell'Era, M. Memo, et al. 2015. Using iPS cells toward the understanding of Parkinson's disease. J Clin Med 4: 548–66.

Ugun-Klusek, A., T.S. Theodosi, J.C. Fitzgerald, F. Burté, et al. 2019. Monoamine oxidase-A promotes protective ATG in human SH-SY5Y neuroblastoma cells through Bcl-2 phosphorylation. Redox Biol 20: 167–181.

Valente, E.M., P.M. Abou-sleiman, V. Caputo, M.M. Muqit, et al. 2004. Hereditary early-onset Parkinson's disease caused by mutations in PINK1. Sci 304: 1158–60.

Wallings, R.L., S.W. Humble, M.E. Ward and R. Wade-Martins. 2019. Lysosomal dysfunction at the centre of Parkinson's disease and frontotemporal dementia/amyotrophic lateral sclerosis. Trends Neurosci 42: 899–912.

Wang, B., N. Abraham, G. Gao and Q. Yang. 2016. Dysregulation of autophagy and mitochondrial function in Parkinson's disease. Transl Neurodegener 5: 19.

Weil, R., E. Laplantine, S. Curic and P. Génin. 2018, Role of optineurin in the mitochondrial dysfunction: potential implications in neurodegenerative diseases and cancer. Front Immunol 9: 1243.

Weykopf, B., S. Haupt, J. Jungverdorben, L.J. Flitsch, et al. 2019. Induced pluripotent stem cell-based modeling of mutant LRRK2-associated Parkinson's disease. Eur J Neurosci 49: 561–589.

Wu, S., L. Lei, Y. Song, M. Liu, et al. 2018a. Mutation of hop-1 and PINK-1 attenuates vulnerability of neurotoxicity in *C. elegans*: The role of mitochondria-associated membrane proteins in Parkinsonism. Exp Neurol 309: 67–78.

Wu, Z., A. Wu, J. Dong, A. Sigears, et al. 2018b. Grape skin extract improves muscle function and extends lifespan of a *Drosophila* model of Parkinson's disease through activation of mitophagy. Exp Gerontol 113: 10–17.

Wu, J.Z., M. Ardah, C. Haikal, A. Svanbergsson, et al. 2019 Dihydromyricetin and salvianolic acid B inhibit alpha-synuclein aggregation and enhance chaperone-mediated autophagy. Translat Neurodeg 8: 18.

Yakhine-Diop, S.M.S., M. Niso-Santano, M. Rodríguez-Arribas, R. Gómez-Sánchez, et al. 2018. Impaired mitophagy and protein acetylation levels in fibroblasts from Parkinson's Disease patients. Mol Neurobiol 56(4): 2466–2481..

Yamano, K., C. Wang, S.A. Sarraf, C. Münch, et al. 2018. Endosomal rab cycles regulate Parkin-mediated mitophagy. eLife 7: e31326.

Zhang, J., M.L. Culp, J.G. Craver and V. Darley-Usmar. 2018. Mitochondrial function and ATG: Integrating proteotoxic, redox, and metabolic stress in Parkinson's disease. J Neurochem 144: 691–709.

Zhou, H., T. Cheang, F. Su, Y. Zheng, et al. 2018. Melatonin inhibits rotenone-induced SH-SY5Y cell death via the downregulation of Dynamin-Related Protein 1 expression. Eur J Pharmacol 819: 58–67.

26

Charnolophagy in Alzheimer's Disease

INTRODUCTION

Almost 50 million people in the world are affected by dementia; the most prevalent form of which is AD, characterized by the progressive loss of memory and cognitive impairment. Environmental factors contribute to the pathogenesis of AD which is characterized by mitochondrial dysfunction, abnormal accumulation of amyloid-β (1–42) peptide, neurofibrillary tangles, and hyper-phosphorylated tau. These inclusions inhibit normal axoplasmic transport through twisted neuro-tubules to cause impaired synaptic transmission, neurocybernetics, and cognitive impairment due to toxins release from destabilized CS. Since the etiology of AD remains unknown, it is extremely challenging to develop the effective drugs for preventing or slowing AD progression. CP/ATG dysfunction in AD is used as an important marker for evaluating the effects of potential candidate drugs. CP/ATG is a key pathway to clear abnormal protein aggregates, and is essential for protein homeostasis and NCF. CP deficits may occur in the early stages of AD. The accumulation of immature CP/ATG vacuoles and CS in the dystrophic neurites of AD brains suggested that CP/ATG is disrupted. Diversified stress (nutritional/environmental)-induced cortisol release augments CB formation, while MTs, IGF-1, and BDNF inhibit it, preventing neurodegeneration, early morbidity, and mortality in AD (Sharma 2019). Antioxidants and MTs inhibit CB formation as free radical scavengers through zinc-mediated transcriptional regulation of genes involved in growth, proliferation, differentiation, and development. Hence, drugs may be developed to prevent CB formation and/or enhance CP as a mechanism of ICD to avert cognitive impairments in AD. Brain regional MAO-specific CBs can be detected by ^{11}C or ^{18}F-labeled MAO-A or MAO-B inhibitors in vivo in addition to [18]FdG-PET neuroimaging to quantitatively assess and improve MB in AD. Recent studies indicated that Tau and mTOR induce CP dysregulation in AD. A study explored the impact of acute hypoxia on AD-like pathologies in APP[swe]/PS1[dE9] mice and their wild type littermates, indicated that acute hypoxia may induce AD-like pathology in the brain of APP[swe]/PS1[dE9] mice and WT mice to a certain extent.

This chapter highlights recent studies on AD with a special emphasis on CP/ATG regulation and TSE-EBPT strategies for the clinical management of AD. The theranostic significance of CP as an immediate and early biomarker of AD is emphasized.

Insulin-mediated Changes in Tau Phosphorylation

Although aging is the main risk factor for AD, epidemiological studies suggests that T2DM increases the risk of dementia including AD. Defective brain insulin signaling is suggested as an early event in AD and other tauopathies. Tau hyper-phosphorylation is a hallmark of neurofibrillary pathology and insulin resistance increases the number of neuritic plaques, particularly in AD. Utilizing a combination of *Drosophila* models of tauopathy (expressing the 2N4R-Tau) and neuroblastoma cells, Chatterjee et al. (2019) attempted to distinguish the pathways downstream of the insulin signaling cascade that lead to tau hyper-phosphorylation, aggregation, and ATG defects. Using cell-based, genetic, and biochemical approaches, they demonstrated that tau phosphorylation at AT8 and PHF1 residues is enhanced in an insulin-resistant microenvironment. Insulin-induced changes in total and phospho-tau are mediated by the interaction of Akt, GSK-3β, and ERK located downstream of the insulin receptor pathway. A significant change in the key proteins involved in the mTOR/ATG pathway indicated impaired aggregated protein clearance in the *Drosophila* models and cultured neuroblastoma cells. Tau and mTOR-PI3-Akt-mediated CP dysregulation in AD is presented in Fig. 40.

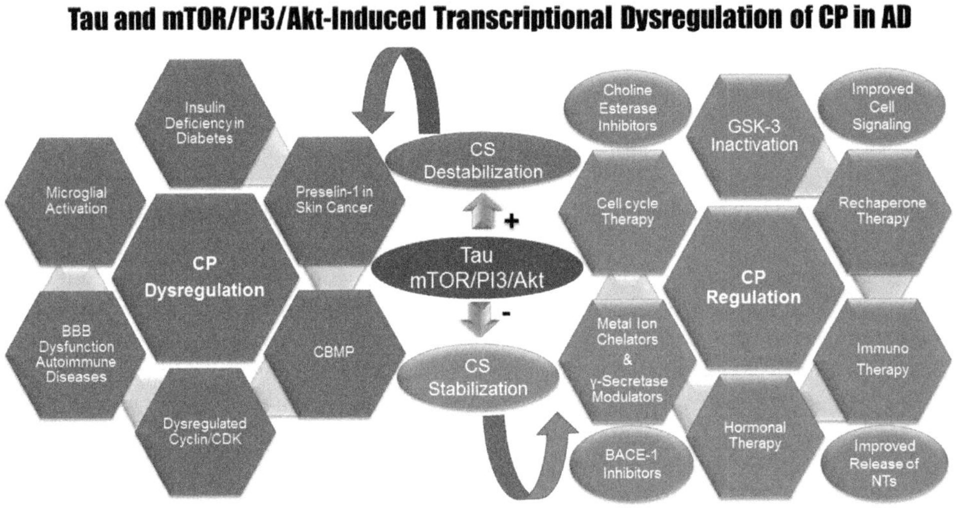

Figure 40

CP Dysregulation in AD

The hyper-phosphorylation of tau and the overexpression of mTOR proteins are the driving force behind Aβ plaques and neurofibrillay tangles (NFT's) formation in AD. Diabetes, autoimmune diseases, and cancer are correlated with AD. Mueed et al. (2019) studied the causes of AD and the association of tau and mTOR with other diseases. They emphasized that insulin deficiency in diabetes activated microglia, and the dysfunction of BBB in autoimmune diseases, presenilin 1 in skin cancer, increased ROS in mitochondrial dysfunction, and deregulated cyclins/CDKs. This in turn promoted CBMP in AD and the potential theranostics for AD such as GSK3 inactivation therapy, re-chaperoning therapy, immunotherapy, hormonal therapy, metal chelators, cell cycle therapy, γ-secretase modulators, and cholinesterase and BACE 1-inhibitors in combating pathological changes associated with AD. Recent research about the relationship between mTOR and aging and hepatic Aβ degradation offers promising opportunities to target AD. In future, we can develop novel drugs and modulators to improve cell-to cell signaling, prevent Aβ plaque formation and tau hyperphosphorylation, and promote better release of neurotransmitters by regulating CP/ATG and inhibit CBMP, implicated in progressive neurodegeneration in AD.

AD-Like Pathologies in APP^swe/PS1^dE9 Mice

Zhang et al. (2018) investigated the impact of acute hypoxia on Aβ and tau pathologies, neuro-inflammation, mitochondrial function, and ATG in the APP^{swe}/PS1^{dE9} mouse model of AD. Male APP^{swe}/PS1^{dE9} transgenic (Tg) mice and their age-matched wild type (WT) littermates were exposed to a single acute hypoxic episode (O$_2$ 7%) for 24 hrs. Acute hypoxia increased the expression of the amyloid precursor protein (APP), anterior pharynx-defective 1 (APH1), and cyclin-dependent kinase 5 (CDK5), and promoted tau phosphorylation at T181 and T231 residues in both Tg and WT mice. Acute hypoxia also induced ATG through mTOR signaling, eliciting abnormal mitochondrial function involved in CP dysregulation, neuro-inflammation, and CBMP in both Tg and WT mice, and suggesting that acute hypoxia induces AD-like pathogenesis in the APP^{swe}/PS1^{dE9} mice brain and WT mice to a certain extent.

Oleuropein Aglycone for AD

CP/ATG deficiency has been demonstrated in AD patients, impairing the elimination of denatured protein aggregates and damaged mitochondria participating in CBMP, leading to their accumulation and increasing their toxicity and oxidative stress. Cordero et al. (2018) demonstrated the downregulation of CP/ATG pathways in AD patients by a microarray analysis. The benefits of the Mediterranean diet on AD and cognitive impairment are well known, attributing this effect to several polyphenols, such as Oleuropein aglycone, which is present in extra virgin olive oil. OLE induces CP/ATG, achieving a decrease in aggregated proteins and a reduction of cognitive impairment *in vivo*. This effect is caused by the modulation of several pathways including the AMPK/mTOR axis and the activation of CP/ATG gene expression mediated by sirtuins and histone acetylation or the EB transcription factor. Hence, supplementation of diet with extra virgin olive oil might have benefits for AD patients via induction of CP/ATG as a mechanism of ICD for NCF.

Peripheral Biomarkers of AD

The classical amyloid cascade model for AD has been challenged by several findings. Morris et al. (2018) proposed an alternative molecular neurobiological model. The presence of the APOE ε4 allele, altered miRNA expression, and epigenetic dysregulation in the promoter region and exon 1 of TREM2, as well as ANK1 hyper-methylation and altered levels of histone post-translational methylation leading to increased transcription of TNFα, could explain the increased peripheral and central inflammation found in AD. Significantly increased activity of triggering receptor expressed on myeloid cells 2 (TREM2), presence of APOE4 isoforms, and altered ANK1 and miR-486 expression occur during AD progression. These changes induce alterations in protein kinase-B (Akt), mTOR, and STAT3 to trigger microglial activation, cell proliferation and cell survival. Microglial activation results in increased synthesis of cytokines, chemokines, NO, prostaglandins, ROS, iNOS, Cox-2, and other pro-inflammatory mediators to enhance further neurodegeneration in AD. These changes are associated with the amyloid and tau pathology, mitochondrial dysfunction (impaired ETC, $\Delta\Psi$ collapse, and oxidative damage to key TCA cycle enzymes), synaptic dysfunction, altered GSK-3 activity, mTOR activation, impaired CP/ATG, a compromised ubiquitin-proteasome system, iron dys-homeostasis, altered APP translation, amyloid plaque formation, tau hyper-phosphorylation, and neurofibrillary tangle formation in addition to CB formation, CP dysregulation, CS destabilization, impaired CS exocytosis/ endocytosis, CS permeability, CS sequestration, and CS fragmentation as a CBMP cascade in AD. Hence, novel CPTs (CB antagonists, CP regulators, CS stabilizers, CS exocytosis enhancers, and CBMP inhibitors) can be developed for the DSST-TSE-EBPT of AD. Potential peripheral biomarkers and originators of AD are presented in Fig. 41.

Potential Peripheral Biomarkers and Originators of AD

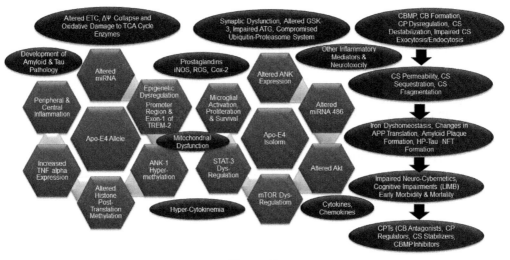

Figure 41

Inflammation and β-Amyloid

β-Amyloid peptide accumulation in the cortex and in the hippocampus results in neurodegeneration and memory loss. The inflammatory response triggered by β-Amyloid peptides promotes neuronal death and degeneration. In addition to inflammation, β-Amyloid peptides also induce alterations in neuronal CP/ATG, eventually leading to cell death. Álvarez-Arellano et al. (2018) evaluated whether the inflammatory response induced by the β-Amyloid peptides impairs memory via disrupting the ATG flux. Male mice overexpressing β-amyloid peptides (5XFAD) but lacking caspase-1, presented reduced β-amyloid plaques in the cortex and in the hippocampus; they had restored brain ATG flux and improved learning and memory. Inhibition of the inflammatory response in the 5XFAD mice restored LC3-II levels and prevented the accumulation of oligomeric p62 and ubiquitylated proteins. The caspase-1 deficiency reinstated the activation of the AMPK/Raptor pathway while downregulating the Akt/mTOR pathway. An inverse correlation was found between the increase of APS in the cortex of 5XFAD mice lacking caspase-1 and the presence of mitochondria with altered morphology implicated in CBMP, indicating that β-amyloid peptide-induced caspase-1 activation disrupts ATG in the cortex and in the hippocampus, resulting in neurodegeneration and memory loss.

CSF Endo-lysosomal Proteins and Ubiquitin

Increasing evidence implicates dysfunctional proteostasis and the involvement of CP, the endo-lysosomal system, and the ubiquitin-proteasome system in NDDs. Sjödin et al. (2019) reported that in AD, there is an accumulation of CP vacuoles within the neurons. In PD, susceptibility is linked to genes encoding proteins involved in CP and lysosomal function, as well as mutations causing lysosomal disorders. Both diseases are characterized by the accumulation of protein aggregates. Proteins associated with endocytosis, lysosomal function, and the ubiquitin-proteasome system were identified in the CSF and targeted by combining solid-phase extraction and parallel reaction monitoring mass spectrometry. In total, 50 peptides from

18 proteins were quantified in three cohorts, in five experimental groups including AD (N=61), PD (N=21), prodromal AD (N=10), stable mild cognitive impairment (N=15), and controls (N=68). A pilot study, including subjects selected based on their AD. CSF core biomarker concentrations, showed increased concentrations of several targeted proteins in subjects with core biomarkers indicating AD pathology compared to controls. Lower concentrations in CSF of proteins in PD were compared to subjects with prodromal AD. Significantly different peptide CSF concentrations were identified in proteins AP2B1, C9, CTSB, CTSF, GM2A, LAMP1, LAMP2, TCN2, and ubiquitin. The proteins having altered concentrations were AP2B1, CTSB, CTSF, GM2A, LAMP2, and ubiquitin. The CSF concentrations of CTSB, CTSF, GM2A, and LAMP2 were altered. However, differences in proteins associated with endocytosis (AP2B1) and the ubiquitin-proteasome system (ubiquitin), were observed. No difference in any peptide CSF concentration was found in clinically diagnosed subjects with AD compared to controls. The CSF analyses of subjects with PD suggested lysosomal dysfunction, which resonated well with recent genetic findings, while such changes were minor or absent in AD.

Dynamin-Related Protein 1 (Drp-1)

Recently, the mitochondrial protein, Drp-1, has been implicated in abnormal mitochondrial dynamics, mitochondrial fragmentation, CP/ATG, and neuronal loss in AD and other NDDs, including PD, HD, ALS, MS, diabetes, and obesity. Oliver and Reddy (2019) reported that DRP-1 is one of the evolutionarily conserved large families of GTPase proteins critical for mitochondrial division, size, shape, and distribution throughout the neuron, from cell body to axons, dendrites, and nerve terminals. Drp-1 is enriched at neuronal terminals and involved in synapse formation and synaptic sprouting. Different phosphorylated forms of Drp-1 act as both increased fragmentation and/or increased fusion of mitochondria for CP regulation. Increased levels of Drp-1 were found in diseased states which induced the excessive fragmentation of mitochondria, leading to mitochondrial dysfunction and neuronal damage implicated in CBMP. Recently, several Drp-1 inhibitors have been developed, including Mdivi-1, Dynasore, P110, and DDQ and their theranostic potential has been tested using cell cultures and mouse models of NDDs. Genetic-crossing studies revealed that a partial reduction of Drp-1 is protective in mutant protein(s)-induced mitochondrial and synaptic toxicities. It has been shown that reduced Drp-1 is a promising theranostic target for AD and other NDDs.

Endo-lysosomal Dysregulations

Van Acker et al. (2019) discussed the current knowledge about the risk genes APOE4, BIN1, CD2AP, PICALM, PLD3, and TREM2 and their impact on endolysosomal regulations in the late-onset AD pathology. Since cellular dysregulations in the degradative routes contribute to the initiation and progression of NDDs, including AD, CP/ATG and endolysosomal homeostasis need to be maintained throughout life as they are major cellular mechanisms involved in both the production of toxic amyloid peptides and the clearance of misfolded or aggregated proteins due to the oxidation of –SH moieties on cysteine and impaired electrostatic forces of attraction and repulsion in the amyloid peptides. As such, alterations in CP and CS, as a measure of degradation, may impact disease-related mechanisms such as amyloid-β clearance through the BBB and the inter-neuronal spreading of amyloid-β and/or Tau rudiments, affecting synaptic function, plasticity, and metabolism. The emergence of several genetic risk factors for late-onset AD that are related to endocytic transport regulation, including cholesterol metabolism and clearance, suggests that the CP/ATG/lysosomal flux might become more vulnerable during aging, thereby contributing to the onset of AD and other NDDs.

Bioactive Components of Salvia Miltiorrhiza Rhizome for AD

The rhizome of *Salvia miltiorrhiza* (Danshen), a traditional Chinese medicine, is used for the treatment of hyperlipidemia, stroke, and cardiovascular and cerebrovascular diseases. Chong et al. (2018) summarized studies regarding the effects of the bioactive component from Danshen on major characteristic features of AD in preclinical studies and explored the potential of Danshen components in the treatment of AD. The bioactive components of Danshen improved cognitive deficits in mice, protected neurons, reduced tau hyper-phosphorylation, and prevented amyloid-β fiber formation and disaggregation.

Intranasal Insulin Activates Akt2 in the Hippocampus

T2DM increases the risk for AD. Human AD brains show reduced glucose metabolism as measured by ^{18}FDG-PET. Gabbouj et al. (2019) used 14-month-old wild-type (WT) and APP$_{Swe}$/PS1$_{dE9}$ (APP/PS1) transgenic mice to investigate how a single dose of intranasal insulin modulates brain glucose metabolism and affects spatial learning and memory. They also assessed how insulin influences the activity of Akt1 and Akt2 kinases, the expression of glial and neuronal markers, and CP/ATG in the hippocampus. Intranasal insulin increased glucose metabolism and activated Akt2 and its downstream signaling in the hippocampus of the WT, but not APP/PS1 mice. Insulin differentially affected the expression of homeostatic microglia markers P2ry12 and Cx3cr1 and CP/ATG in the WT and APP/PS1 mice. There was no evidence that a single dose of intranasal insulin improves memory, suggesting that intranasal insulin exerts diverse effects on Akt2 signaling, CP/ATG, and the homeostatic status of microglia depending on the degree of AD-related pathogenesis. The potential TSE-EBPT strategies for AD are presented in Fig. 42.

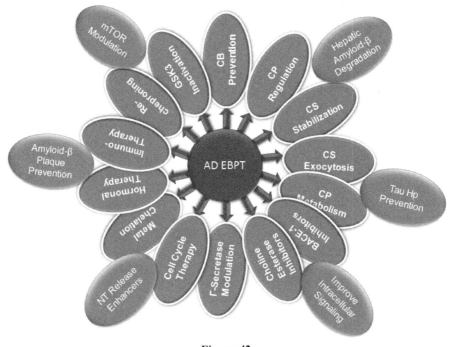

Figure 42

CONCLUSION

Recent studies explored the various peripheral biomarkers as originators of AD. The beneficial effects of *Oleuropein aglycone* and *Salvia miltiorrhiza* on AD through CP/ATG induction were reported. CP/ATG impairment by caspase-1-dependent inflammation in response to β-amyloid peptide accumulation in the cortex and hippocampus resulted in neurodegeneration and memory loss due to CP dysregulation and CBMP induction. Hence, in addition to naturally available antioxidants, specific CB antagonists, CP modulators/regulators, CS stabilizers, CS exocytosis enhancers, and CBMP antagonists can be developed as novel DSST-TSE-EBPT-CPTs to prevent and cure AD.

REFERENCES

Álvarez-Arellano, L., M. Pedraza-Escalona, T. Blanco-Ayala, N. Camacho-Concha, et al. 2018. ATG impairment by caspase-1-dependent inflammation mediates memory loss in response to β-Amyloid peptide accumulation. J Neurosci Res 96: 234–246.

Chatterjee, S., S.S. Ambegaokar, G.R. Jackson and A. Mudher. 2019. Insulin-mediated changes in tau hyperphosphorylation and autophagy in a *Drosophila* model of tauopathy and neuroblastoma cells. Front Neurosci 13: 801.

Chong, K., Z.A. Almsherqi, H.M. Shen and Y. Deng. 2018. Cubic membrane formation supports cell survival of amoeba Chaos under starvation-induced stress. Protoplasma. 255: 517–525.

Cordero, J.G., R. García-Escudero, J. Avila, R. Gargini, et al. 2018. Benefit of oleuropein aglycone for AD by promoting ATG. Oxid Med Cell Longev 2018: 5010741.

Gabbouj, S., T. Natunen, H. Koivisto, K. Jokivarsi, et al. 2019. Intranasal insulin activates Akt2 signaling pathway in the hippocampus of wild-type but not in APP/PS1 Alzheimer model mice. Neurobiol Aging 75: 98–108.

Morris, G., M. Berk, M. Maes and B.K. Puri. 2018. Could Alzheimer's disease originate in the periphery and if so how so? Mol Neurobiol. 56: 406–434.

Mueed, Z., P. Tandon, S.K. Maurya, R. Deval, et al. 2019. Tau and mTOR: The hotspots for multifarious diseases in Alzheimer's development. Front Neurosci 12: 101.

Oliver, D. and P.H. Reddy. 2019. Dynamics of dynamin-related protein 1 in Alzheimer's disease and other neurodegenerative diseases. Cells. 8(9): E961.

Sjödin, S., G. Brinkmalm, A. Öhrfelt, L. Parnetti, et al. 2019. Endo-lysosomal proteins and ubiquitin CSF concentrations in Alzheimer's and Parkinson's disease. Alzheimers Res Ther 11(1): 82.

Van Acker, Z.P., M. Bretou and W. Annaert. 2019. Endo-lysosomal dysregulations and late-onset Alzheimer's disease: Impact of genetic risk factors. Mol Neurodegener 14: 20.

Zhang, F., R. Zhong, H. Qi, S. Li, et al. 2018. Impacts of acute hypoxia on Alzheimer's disease-like pathologies in APPswe/PS1dE9 mice and their wild type littermates. Front Neurosci 12: 314.

27

Charnolophagy in Stroke

INTRODUCTION

CP/ATG is highly orchestrated, transcriptionally regulated, energy-driven, lysosomal-dependent, basic molecular mechanism of ICD which sustains NCF. Inflammatory cells, including microglia and vascular macrophages, play a pivotal role in secondary injury during AIS. CP/ATG confers neuroprotection by inducing anti-apoptotic and anti-inflammatory signal-transduction during the acute phase, and neurodegeneration during the chronic phase following acute brain injury. Dysregulated CP/ATG is involved in the stroke pathogenesis and has devastating clinical consequences. Hence, the timely charnolo-pharmacological modulation of CP/ATG may confer neuroprotection in AIS. AIS enhances CP/ATG by the transcriptional regulation of miR-200a/ FOXO3/ATG7 signaling pathway. The elevated homocysteine (Hcy) increases risk for the AIS. Homocysteine dysregulates the neural stem cell CP/ATG to augment NDD in AIS. CP/ATG is also induced following I/R injury in the brain. Nicotinamide phosphor-ribosyl-transferase is secreted from the microglia via exosome during AIS, whereas, Mdivi-1 alleviates BBB disruption and cell death in TBI by mitigating MTG induction and ATG dysfunction. The PINK1-PRKN/ PARK2 pathway of MTG is also induced to protect renal I/R injury during AIS. CP/ATG counteracts nutrient deprivation during starvation and hypoxia during hypo-perfusion and is slightly elevated even in baseline conditions, when it is useful to eliminate denatured proteins and dysfunctional organelles, particularly from the aging AIS patient. This is also critical when the mitochondria and/or proteins are damaged by toxic stimuli.

Recently, Ferrucci et al. (2018) suggested that the recruitment of CP/ATG is beneficial in counteracting brain hypo-perfusion while its hyper-activation may be detrimental for cell survival. While analyzing these opposite effects, the CP/ATG is not simply good or bad, but its role varies depending on the spatiotemporal context, suggesting the need for an appropriate CP/ ATG tuning to ascertain a beneficial effect for cell survival. Therefore, the accurate determination of signatures of CP/ATG induction/repression is highly crucial to define the appropriate spatio-temporal intensity and frequency of AIS. The need for finetuning the CP/ATG induction may explain why confounding outcomes occur when it is studied using a simplistic approach. By labeling bone marrow-derived stem cells (BMDSCs) with Cd/Se NPs, it was established that stem cells exhibit preferential chemotaxis and exponential elimination at the penumbral region in the middle cerebral artery occluded (MCAO) rats during AIS (Brenneman et al. 2010). Numerous stem cells derived from different biological sources are destroyed at the site of physico-chemical injury in the CNS via free radical-induced CB formation, CP induction, CS destabilization, and

CBMP, causing temporary or permanent impairment in sensorimotor performance depending on the brain region and intensity and frequency of the ischemic injury. The stem cell CS is exocytosed during AIS and is endocytosed in the penumbral region to confer trophic support for rejuvenating degenerating neurons to reduce the infarct size by releasing neurotrophic factors (BDNF, NGF), and anti-inflammatory (IL-4, IL-10) and angiogenic (VEGF and VWF) cytokines from endothelial progenitor cells. Whereas, the endocytosis of cancer stem cell-specific CS in the normal non-proliferating cell is involved in malignant transformation and/or transition from an aplastic to hyperplastic state due to the release of pro-inflammatory (Il-1β, IL-6, TNFα, NF-$\kappa\beta$, and TGF etc.) cytokines. It is important to emphasize that all three major forms of cellular demise can occur concomitantly including: (i) CP-mediated, (ii) MTG-mediated, and (iii) generalized ATG-mediated cell death, depending on the location and intensity of AIS. Hence, it will be highly prudent to regulate these fundamental events through physiological and/or pharmacological intervention to accomplish the TSE-EBPT of AIS. Currently, the exact spatio-temporal induction/repression of these highly crucial events remains uncertain. Further investigations in this direction employing specific nanotheranostic ATG biomarkers will facilitate AIS treatment with a better prognosis.

This chapter highlights the clinical significance of CP in developing promising TSE-EBPT-CPTs for the clinical management of AIS and the theranostic potential of natural and synthetic antioxidants for ameliorating the devastating symptoms suffered by stroke patients to improve their QOL.

NAMPT in Ischemic Injury

Nicotinamide phosphoribosyltransferase (NAMPT), as the key enzyme of the salvage pathway of nicotinamide adenine dinucleotide synthesis, is secreted and functions as a cytokine. Lu et al. (2019) showed that in the brain, NAMPT expression and secretion was induced in microglia upon neuro-inflammation and injury. NAMPT was secreted from microglia upon–O_2-glucose deprivation and recovery (OGD/R)-induced ischemia-like injury. The classical ER-Golgi pathway was not involved in NAMPT secretion. NAMPT secretion was further enhanced by ATP, and was mediated by the P2X$_7$ receptor and by $[Ca^{2+}]_i$. The phospholipase D inhibitor, n-Butanol, siRNA, and Wortmannin decreased OGD/R and the ATP-induced release of NAMPT in microglia, indicating that NAMPT is secreted via the exosome. Immune-EM identified NAMPT in extracellular vesicles with the size and morphology characteristics of exosome. Exosomal NAMPT was further confirmed by immunoblotting from vesicles harvested by ultra-centrifugation. However, the amount of NAMPT relative to exosomal protein markers remained unchanged upon treatment of OGD/R, suggesting a continuous load of exosomal NAMPT in microglia. This study identified NAMPT which is secreted via exosome from microglia during neuro-inflammation of ischemic injury.

Mdivi-1 Alleviates BBB Disruption

Drp-1 is a key regulator of mitochondrial fission. The inhibition of Drp-1 may attenuate TBI-induced functional outcome and cell death by maintaining normal mitochondrial morphology, and inhibiting CBMP and apoptosis. Wu et al. (2018a) investigated the role of the mitochondrial division inhibitor 1 (Mdivi-1), a small molecule inhibitor of Drp-1, as an underlying mechanism of CB-specific CP, generalized ATG, and MTG following TBI. The CPS/APS accumulated in cortical neurons at 24 hrs after TBI, owing to the enhanced ATG indicated by the accumulation in LC3 and the decrease in p62; but Mdivi-1 reversed the enhancement. Mdivi-1 alleviated the number of LC3 puncta and TUNEL-positive structures, indicating that it is involved in Mdivi-1's anti-apoptosis. TBI-induced mitochondrial fission (represented by Drp-1), mtDNA downregulation, and PINK1-Parkin-mediated MTG induction were inhibited by Mdivi-1. TBI-induced BBB disruption and MMP-9 expression were inhibited following the Mdivi-1 treatment. Mdivi-1 alleviated the scratch injury-induced cell death, $\Delta\Psi$ collapse, ROS production, and ATP depletion in primary cortical neurons. The lysosomal inhibitor, CQ, abrogated the Mdivi-1-induced decrease in APS accumulation and cell death within 24 hrs, suggesting that Mdivi-1 mitigates TBI-induced BBB disruption and cell death by regulating CP, MTG, and ATG.

Inhibition of Glutamine Transporter SNAT1

The pathophysiological role of mTORC1 in NDDs is well-established, but the theranostic targets responsible for its activation in neurons needs further investigation. Yamada et al. (2019) identified the solute carrier family 38a member-1 (SNAT1, *Slc38a1*) as a positive regulator of mTORC1 in neurons. Slc38a1$^{flox/flox}$ and Synapsin I-Cre mice were crossed to generate mutant mice in which Slc38a1 was deleted in neurons. The measurement of TTC or the MAP2-negative area in a mouse model of MCAO revealed that *Slc38a1* deficiency decreased infarct size. A transient increase in the phosphorylation of p70S6k1 (pp70S6k1) and a suppressive effect of Rapamycin on infarct size of the MCAO mice were identified. CP/ATG inhibitors mitigated the suppressive effect of the SNAT1 deficiency on neuronal cell death under *in vitro* stroke culture conditions, suggesting that SNAT1 promoted ischemic brain injury via the mTOR-ATG system.

Crotonaldehyde-Induced Endothelial Toxicity

Crotonaldehyde (CA) is a toxic α, β-unsaturated aldehyde found in cigarette smoke, and causes inflammation and vascular dysfunction. Lee et al. (2019) investigated the effect of CA-induced ATG in endothelial cells. Acute exposure to CA reduced cell viability and induced ATG and cell death. Inhibiting ATG promoted the viability of endothelial cells exposed to high concentrations of CA. CA activated the AMPK and p38 MAPK pathways, and pretreatment with inhibitors specific to these kinases demonstrated ATG inhibition and partial improvement in cell viability. An acute exposure to high concentrations of CA induced generalized ATG-mediated cell death. These results might be helpful in elucidating the mechanism of CA toxicity in the vascular system and environmental risk assessment.

The Theranostic Significance of Antioxidants and CP in Stroke

Naringin

Feng et al. (2018) tested the hypothesis that Naringin, a natural antioxidant, could inhibit ONOO⁻-mediated MTG and attenuate cerebral I/R injury. They found that Naringin possessed a potent ONOO⁻ scavenging capability and inhibited the production of superoxide and NO in SH-SY5Y cells exposed to 10 hrs of O_2-glucose-deprivation plus 14 hrs of re-oxygenation or ONOO⁻ donor 3-morpholinosydnonimine (SIN-1). Naringin inhibited the expression of NADPH oxidase subunits and iNOS in rat brains subjected to 2 hrs of Ischemia plus 22 hrs reperfusion. Naringin crossed the BBB, and decreased the neurological deficit score, reduced infarct size, and attenuated apoptotic cell death in the I/R rat brains. Naringin reduced 3-nitrotyrosine formation, decreased the ratio of LC3-II to LC3-I in mitochondrial fraction, and inhibited the translocation of Parkin to the mitochondria. Hence, it could be an effective theranostic agent to prevent the brain from I/R-induced injury via attenuating ONOO⁻-mediated excessive CP/ATG in AIS.

URB597

Su et al. (2018) investigated the protective effects of URB on CP/ATG in a CCH model. CCH decreased p62, CTSD, and LAMP1 and increased Beclin-1, Parkin, and Bnip-3, the LC3-II to LC3-I ratio, and the release of Cyt-C from mitochondria to cytoplasm. Furthermore, CCH induced the accumulation of ubiquitinated proteins in PSDs, which were reversed by URB. Besides, it inhibited the Beclin-1 from Beclin-1/Bcl-2 complex to whole-cell lysates, indicating that URB can inhibit impaired CP/ATG degradation and the disruption of Beclin-1/Bcl-2 complex and block Bnip-3-Cyt-C- and Parkin-required CP, preventing excessive CP/ATG. Hence, URB is a promising agent for the theranostic management of CCH.

p38 Inhibitor Attenuates Mitochondrial Dysfunction

p38 MAPK is a major player in mitochondrial dysfunction after subarachnoid hemorrhage (SAH). Huang et al. (2018) reported that DJ-1, which responds to oxidative stress and translocates to mitochondria, maintains MQC. Using an *in vitro* SAH model, alterations in p38, p-p38, DJ-1, and CP-related protein expression were detected. The p38 inhibitor blocked the enhanced expression of p38 and p-p38 after SAH, whereas total DJ-1 and mitochondrial DJ-1 were upregulated. The p38 inhibitor blocked oxyhemoglobin OxyHb)-induced CB formation, including $\Delta\Psi$ collapse and ROS release. In addition, the p38 inhibitor restored OxyHb-induced initially abnormal CB accumulation and CS formation by regulating Atg5, Beclin-1, the ratio of LC3-II/LC3-I, and p62 expression, suggesting that the overexpression of p38 induced mitochondrial dysfunction is involved in CBMP due to abnormal CP/ATG induction, which primarily relied on DJ-1 mitochondrial translocation.

Xiao-Xu-Ming Decoction

Lan et al. (2018) investigated whether the Xiao-Xu-Ming decoction reduced MTG activation and preserved mitochondrial function in cerebral I/R injury. Rats were divided into five groups: sham, IR, IR plus XXMD (60 g/kg/day) (XXMD60), IR plus Cyclosporin A (10 mg/kg/day) (CsA), and IR plus vehicle (Vehicle). Focal cerebral ischemia and reperfusion models were induced by MCAO. Cerebral infarct areas were measured by TTC staining. The MCAO rats showed worsened neurological score and ischemic damage, which were reversed by XXMD or CsA. XXMD/CsA downregulated MTG and attenuated cerebral ischemia and reperfusion-induced LC3, Beclin-1, and Lamp1 expression, demonstrating that XXMD exerted a neuroprotective effect via downregulating LC3, Beclin-1, Lamp1, and mitochondrial p62 expression by inhibiting enhanced MTG.

Rab9

Mitochondrial dysfunction is the characteristic of MTG, which is essential in MQC. However, excessive MTG contributes to cell death in AIS and hepatotoxicity. IGF-II and its receptor (IGF-IIR) play vital roles in the development of heart failure during hypertension. Huang et al. (2018) found that IGF-II triggers IGF-IIR receptor activation, causing mitochondria dysfunction, resulting in MTG, and cardiomyocyte cell death, indicating that IGF-IIR activation triggers mitochondria fragmentation, leading to APS formation, and loss of mitochondria. These results were associated with Parkin-dependent MTG. ATG proteins Atg5, and ATG7 deficiency did not suppress IGF-IIR-induced MTG. However, Rab9 knockdown reduced MTG and maintained mitochondrial function. These constitutive MTGs through IGF-IIR activation triggered mitochondrial loss and ROS accumulation to reduce cardiomyocyte viability, indicating that IGF-IIR induces MTG through the Rab9-dependent alternative ATG.

Hydrogen

Recently, Wu et al. (2018b) reported that H_2 can protect mitochondria function and have theranostic effects on cerebral IRI. In this study, OGD/R damaged hippocampal neurons were used to mimic cerebral IRI *in vivo* to detect the effect of H_2, Rap (ATG activator), and 3-MA (ATG inhibitor) on OGD/R neurons. H_2 and RAP increased cell viability after the OGD/R treatment, while 3-MA aggravated injury and inhibited the protection of H_2 and RAP. The ROS and apoptosis increased after OGD/R, H_2 and RAP restrained the increment of ROS and apoptosis ratio but its protective effect was attenuated by 3-MA. H_2 and RAP prevented $\Delta\Psi$ collapse and increased co-localization of mitochondria with GFP-LC3 while 3-MA exerted the opposite effect. The expression of LC3 was increased after OGD/R which was further enhanced by H_2 and RAP treatment, but treatment with 3-MA exhibited the opposite effect. H_2 and RAP induced, while 3-MA inhibited CP. H_2 and RAP-induced PINK1 and Parkin expression in OGD/R neurons was inhibited by 3-MA, indicating that H_2 confers neuroprotection in OGD/R damaged neurons by protecting mitochondrial function and by enhancing the CP-mediated PINK1/Parkin signaling pathway.

NaHS

Xu et al. (2018) explored the ability of NaHS, a H_2S donor, to provide neuroprotection in a mouse model of TBI and to discover the molecular mechanisms of these protective effects and found that administration of NaHS maintained the integrity of the BBB, protected neurons from apoptosis, promoted remyelination, axonal repair, and mitochondrial function. ATG was inhibited after treatment with NaHS following TBI, an effect that was induced by the activation of the PI3K/Akt/mTOR signaling, indicating that H_2S is beneficial for TBI and could be used as a potential theranostic target for treating TBI.

Intra-Carotid Cold Saline

Intra-carotid cold saline infusion (ICSI) confers neuroprotection in AIS. Wang et al. (2019) used the rat MCAO model to investigate the neuroprotective effects of ICSI and SGK1 in AIS rats. ICSI decreased infarct size and brain swelling, as determined by TTC staining and the dry wet weight method, respectively. The results of TUNEL and Nissl staining showed that ICSI also suppressed apoptosis and increased the relative integral optical density (IOD) of Nissl bodies in the rat MCAO model. ICSI upregulated SGK1 expression and downregulated Beclin-1 and LC-3 expression in the rat MCAO model of AIS. SGK1 knockdown increased ICSI-mediated infarct size and brain swelling, promoted apoptosis, and reduced the IOD values of Nissl bodies in the rat MCAO model. SGK1 knockdown upregulated Beclin-1 and LC-3 expression mediated by ICSI, which had a neuroprotective effect on AIS after reperfusion by upregulating SGK1 and inhibiting ATG.

Tetrahydrocurcumin

Vacek et al. (2018) hypothesized that Tetrahydrocurcumin (THC) may ameliorate Homocysteine (Hcy)-induced mitochondrial remodeling (MR) in mouse brain endothelial (bEnd3) cells. bEnd3 cells were exposed to Hcy in the presence or absence of THC. Cell viability and CP/ATG cell death were measured with MTT and a MDC staining assay. ROS production was determined using DCFH-DA staining by confocal microscopy. CP/ATG was assessed using a conventional GFP-LC3 dot assay. The interaction of the phagophore marker LC-3 with mitochondrial receptor NIX was observed by confocal imaging. Mitochondrial fusion and fission were evaluated by immunoblotting and RT-PCR. These studies indicated that Hcy causes cell toxicity, whereas supplementation of THC prevented the detrimental effects of Hcy on cell survival. Hcy induced fission marker (DRP-1), fusion marker (Mfn-2), ATG marker (LC-3), activated mitochondrial specific phagophore marker (LC-3), and co-localized with the mitochondrial receptor NIX. Pretreatment of bEnd3 with THC (15 µM) ameliorated Hcy-induced oxidative damage, mitochondrial fission/fusion, and MTG, suggesting its beneficial effects on MR and as a potential theranostic agent in homocysteinemia-induced mitochondrial dysfunction implicated in cerebrovascular diseases and CVDs.

CONCLUSION

Three types of cell death mechanisms were proposed in AIS: (i) CP-dependent, (iii) MTG-dependent, and (iii) ATG-dependent, which can be regulated at the transcriptional and translational level by developing spatiotemporally specific nanotheranostic probes to target these ATGs to accomplish TSE-EBPT of AIS. Transcriptionally regulated CP/ATG sustained MQC, ICD, and NCF, whereas dysregulated CP resulted in CBMP and neuro-apoptosis in AIS. The mitochondrial translocation of Ca^{2+} from the ER occurred during subarachnoid hemorrhage. The Xiao-Xu-Ming decoction improved mitochondrial function in cerebral I/R injury. BMDSCs and intra-carotid cold saline infusion conferred neuroprotection in the MCAO model of AIS via GSK and Rab9-dependent ATG in the IGF-IIR-mediated MTG to eliminate CB involved in CBMP and apoptosis. A natural antioxidant Naringin attenuated cerebral I/R injury by inhibiting $ONOO^-$-mediated CP/ATG dysregulation and CS destabilization. URB597 conferred neuroprotection in cerebral hypo-perfusion by inhibiting uncontrolled CP/ATG. Rab9 and NaHS as a p38 inhibitor prevented mitochondrial dysfunction through DJ-1 induction. H_2 provided neuroprotection in OGD/R-damaged rat hippocampal neurons by restoring MB through PINK1/Parkin-mediated CP regulation. NaHS restored mitochondrial function and dysregulated CP/ATG by activating the PI3K/Akt/mTOR signaling to improve neuronal recovery in TBI, whereas Tetrahydrocurcumin ameliorated Hcy-induced MR implicated in CBMP in the brain endothelial cells, suggesting CP as a promising biomarker for the development of novel DSST-TSE-EBPT-CPTs to prevent and cure AIS.

REFERENCES

Brenneman, M., S. Sharma, M. Harting, R. Strong, et al. 2010. Autologous bone marrow mononuclear cells enhance recovery after acute ischemic stroke in young and middle-aged rats. J Cereb Blood Flow Metab 30(1): 140–9.

Feng, J., X. Chen, S. Lu, W. Li, et al. 2018. Naringin attenuates cerebral ischemia-reperfusion injury through inhibiting peroxynitrite-mediated mitophagy activation. Mol Neurobiol. 55: 9029–9042.

Ferrucci, M., F. Biagioni, L. Ryskalin, F. Limanaqi, et al. 2018. Ambiguous effects of autophagy activation following hypoperfusion/ischemia. Int J Mol Sci 19(9): 2756.

Huang, C.Y., W.W. Kuo, T.J. Ho, S.F. Chiang, et al. 2018. Rab9-dependent ATG is required for the IGF-IIR triggering MTG to eliminate damaged mitochondria. J Cell Physiol 233: 7080–7091.

Lan, R., Y. Zhang, T. Wu, Y.Z. Ma. et al. 2018. Xiao-Xu-Ming decoction reduced MTG activation and improved mitochondrial function in cerebral ischemia and reperfusion injury. Behav Neurol 2018: 4147502.

Lee, S.E., H.R. Park, C.S. Park, H.J. Ahn, et al. 2019. ATG in crotonaldehyde-induced endothelial toxicity. Molecules 24: E1137.

Lu, Y.B., C.X. Chen, J. Huang, Y.X. Tian, et al. 2019. Nicotinamide phosphoribosyltransferase secreted from microglia via exosome during ischemic injury. J Neurochem 150: 723–737.

Su, S.H., Y.F. Wu, D.P. Wang and J. Hai. 2018. Inhibition of excessive autophagy and mitophagy mediates neuroprotective effects of URB597 against chronic cerebral hypoperfusion. Cell Death Dis 9(7): 733.

Vacek, J.C., J. Behera, A.K. George, P.K. Kamat, et al. 2018. Tetrahydrocurcumin ameliorates homocysteine-mediated mitochondrial remodeling in brain endothelial cells. J Cell Physiol 233: 3080–3092.

Wang, D., Z. Huang, L. Li, Y. Yuan, et al. 2019. Intracarotid cold saline infusion contributes to neuroprotection in MCAO-induced ischemic stroke in rats via serum and glucocorticoid-regulated kinase 1. Mol Med Rep 20(4): 3942–3950.

Wu, Q., C. Gao, H. Wang, X. Zhang. et al. 2018a. Mdivi-1 alleviates blood-brain barrier disruption and cell death in experimental traumatic brain injury by mitigating ATG dysfunction and MTG activation. Int J Biochem Cell Biol 94: 44–55.

Wu, X., X. Li, Y. Liu, N. Yuan, et al. 2018b. Hydrogen exerts neuroprotective effects on OGD/R damaged neurons in rat hippocampal by protecting mitochondrial function via regulating mitophagy mediated by PINK1/Parkin signaling pathway. Brain Res 1698: 89–98.

Xu, K., F. Wu, K. Xu, Z. Li, et al. 2018. NaHS restores mitochondrial function and inhibits ATG by activating the PI3K/Akt/mTOR signalling pathway to improve functional recovery after traumatic brain injury. Chem Biol Interact 286: 96–105.

Yamada, D., K. Kawabe, I. Tosa, S. Tsukamoto, et al. 2019. Inhibition of the glutamine transporter SNAT1 confers neuroprotection in mice by modulating the mTOR-ATG system. Commun Biol 2: 346.

Part-4

Charnolophagy in Inflammation, Cancer, Microbial Infections, and Aging

28

Charnolophagy in Inflammatory Diseases

INTRODUCTION

CB is implicated in the pathogenesis of inflammatory diseases, whereas CP/ATG regulates inflammation in the innate immunity. The selective clearance of CBs via CP can reverse pathological status in chronic inflammatory diseases. CP/ATG is a homeostatic process with diversified effects on immunity. A variety of internal and external factors regulate inflammatory diseases via altering the level of CP, which surveils mitochondrial population eliminating nonfunctional and undesired CBs by mediating cellular survival and viability in response to injury/trauma and infection. Compromised elimination of CB due to functionally-impaired CP leads to CBMP involving inflammasome (IS) activation in systemic inflammatory diseases as described in the author's featured book, *The Charnoly Body: A Novel Biomarker of Mitochondrial Bioenergetics* published by the CRC Press in U.S.A. CP/ATG is dysregulated in several autoimmune or auto-inflammatory diseases like SLE, rheumatoid arthritis, multiple sclerosis, and Crohn's disease. Certain treatments used in these pathologies impact CP/ATG, even if the causal link between their regulation and the efficiency of the treatments remains uncertain. CP/ATG plays critical roles in inflammation by influencing the development, homeostasis, and survival of inflammatory cells, including macrophages, neutrophils, and lymphocytes; effecting the transcription, processing, and secretion of cytokines; it is being regulated by cytokines. A pathogenic role of deregulated CP/ATG in rheumatoid arthritis (RA) has been suggested. A relationship between CP/ATG and inflammatory parameters in patients with RA receiving therapy has been established with severe clinical consequences. Gkikas et al. (2018) highlighted the molecular mechanisms of CP/ATG and its significance in the innate immune system homeostasis. A pivotal role of energy metabolism in innate immune cells function has been established. Hence, the maintenance of the mitochondrial network integrity and activity is a prerequisite for immune system homeostasis. Hu et al. (2018) identified the crucial role of nuclear receptor Nur77 and celastrol in priming inflamed mitochondria for ATG through its mitochondrial targeting and interaction with TNF-associated factor 2 (TRAF2) and the ATG adaptor p62/SQSTM1.

Inflammaging is involved in the development of sarcopenia, obesity, cardiomyopathy, and dysbiosis. ROS play an important role in mediating both physiological and pathophysiological signal transduction. Enzymes and subcellular compartments that produce ROS are associated with metabolic regulation, and diseases associated with metabolic dysfunction may be influenced by changes in redox balance. Forrester et al. (2018) described ROS and their role in metabolic and inflammatory regulation, focusing on signal transduction and its relationship to disease progression. They examined ROS production in the cytoplasm, mitochondria, peroxisome, and ER and their influence on proteasome function, ATG, inflammation, and regulation of metabolic/inflammatory diseases such as atherosclerosis, DM, and stroke. To develop theranostics that target oxidative signaling, it is important to understand the ROS signaling that plays a role in pathophysiology and its influence on cellular and tissue homeostasis. A better understanding of specific sources of ROS production and their influence on metabolism may help to treat CVDs more effectively. Zhao et al. (2018) focused on the inflammatory responses regulated by CP to elucidate its role in inflammation and provided guidelines for the TSE-EBPT of inflammatory diseases.

It is known that the ROS participate in both metabolic as well as inflammatory signaling. ROS and DAMPs activate ISs to induce inflammatory responses. Excessive inflammation induces tissue injuries, resulting in diversified diseases. CP specifically eliminates dysfunctional mitochondrial inclusion (CBs) to maintain IMD, ICD, and MQC to protect ROS-mediated inflammation and DAMPs. Deretic and Levine (2018) focused on the interaction between ATG and IS activation, ATG and interferons, and ATG and inflammation in infection. Harris et al. (2018) discussed the mechanisms through which MTG regulates inflammatory cytokine release. The loss of MTG/ATG can lead to a build-up of cytosolic ROS and mtDNA, which can activate immune signaling pathways that lead to the releases of inflammatory cytokines, including IL-1α, IL-1β, IL-18, type I IFN, and macrophage migration inhibitory factor (MIF). Moreover, release of these cytokines promote the release of others, including IL-23 and IL-17. Thus, MTG may represent regulatory mechanism controlling inflammatory responses in immune cells. Arbogast and Gros (2018) discussed the mechanisms linking ATG to lymphocyte subtype survival and the signaling pathways involved and the impact of ATG modulation in lymphocytes during the course of pro-inflammatory diseases. MacroATG leads to the integration of cytoplasmic proteins into vesicles named APSs that fuse with lysosomes. Chaperone-mediated ATG is in contrast to the direct translocation of protein in lysosomes. MacroATG is central to lymphocyte homeostasis. Although its role is controversial in lymphocyte development and in naive cell survival, it is involved in the maintenance of lymphocyte subtypes. Some effector cells like plasma cells rely on ATG for survival. ATG is central to glucose and lipid metabolism, and to the maintenance of mitochondria and ER. In addition, macroATG, or individual components of its machinery, are also involved in antigen presentation by B cells to receive help from T cells, this crosstalk favors their differentiation into memory or plasma cells.

This chapter describes the clinical significance of CP for the TSE-EBPT of acute and chronic inflammatory diseases such as inflammaging, sarcopenia, obesity, atherosclerosis, NFALD/NASH, hepatitis, gut dysbiosis, Crohon's disease, ulcerative colitis, lipotoxicity microbial septicemia, osteoarthritis, congestive heart failure, rheumatoid arthritis, fibromyalgia, gout, viral infections, and intracellular microbial infections. The thersanostic potential of some antioxidants (such as Resveratrol and Curcumin) as CP regulators and CBMP inhibitors is also described to treat the aforementioned inflammatory diseases.

Inflammaging and Sarcopenia

Sarcopenia, obesity and their coexistence, obese-sarcopenia (OBSP) as well as atherosclerosis-related CVDs (ACVDs), including chronic heart failure (CHF), are among the greatest public health concerns in the aging population. An age-dependent increased prevalence of sarcopenia and OBSP is noticed in CHF patients, suggesting mechanistic relationships. The development of OBSP is mediated by interaction between the visceral and s.c. adipose tissue (AT) and the skeletal muscle during low-grade local and systemic inflammation and inflammaging. Livshits and Kalinkovich (2019) highlighted that inflammaging is a basic mechanism governing the development of sarcopenia, OBSP, and ACVDs. Various immune cells release pro-inflammatory mediators in the skeletal muscle and myocardium. Subsequently, the endothelial structure is disrupted, and mitochondrial activity, CP/MTG, and ATG are impaired. Inflamed myocytes lose their contractile properties, which is characteristic of sarcopenia and CHF. Inflammation may increase the risk of ACVD in a hyperlipidemia-independent manner. Significant reduction of ACVD, without lowering of plasma lipids, following a specific targeting of key pro-inflammatory cytokines plays a key role of inflammation in ACVD pathogenesis. Gut dysbiosis, an imbalanced gut microflora is involved in the pathogenesis of age-associated sarcopenia and ACVDs by inducing inflammaging. Dysbiosis enhances the production of trimethylamine-N-oxide (TMAO), implicated in atherosclerosis, thrombosis, metabolic syndrome, and hypertension with poor CHF prognosis. In OBSP, ATG dysfunction, and inflammation in concert with dysbiosis, lipotoxicity, and other pathophysiological processes, exacerbating sarcopenia and CHF. Administration of specific, inflammation resolving CP-mediators may ameliorate the inflammatory manifestations. Hence, sarcopenia, OBSP, CHF, and dysbiosis are CP-dependent inflammaging-oriented disorders, whereby inflammaging is the causative mechanism driving their pathogenesis.

Mutation (R284S) in the STING

It is known that the cellular sensor stimulator of interferon genes (STING) initiates type I interferon (IFN) and cytokine production following association with cyclic dinucleotides (CDNs) generated from intracellular bacteria or via a synthase, cGAS, after binding microbial or self-DNA. Although essential for protecting the host against infection, unscheduled STING signaling is responsible for auto-inflammatory disorders. Konno et al. (2018) recently reported a gain-of-function mutation in STING (R284S), isolated from a patient who did not require CDNs to augment activity and who manifested an active phenotype. Control of the Unc-51-like ATG-activating kinase 1 (ULK1) pathway, which influences STING function, inhibited STING (R284S), alleviating cytokine production. These findings added to the growing list of inflammatory syndromes associated with STING signaling and provided a theranostic strategy for the treatment of STING-induced inflammatory disease.

CO-induced TFEB Nuclear Translocation

Recently, Kim et al. (2018) highlighted that CO can confer protection in cellular stress. The activation of protein kinase R (PKR)-like ER kinase (PERK) with CO increased the nuclear translocation of the transcription factor EB (TFEB). PERK activation by CO increased $[Ca^{2+}]_i$ and the phosphatase activity of calcineurin in TFEB. During the deficiency of the TFEB, CO could not recruit Parkin to the mitochondria and increase expression of lysosomal genes such as Lamp1, CathB, and TPP1, suggesting that CO increases CP through TFEB nuclear translocation by the PERK-calcineurin pathway. The inhibition of TFEB with siRNA in TFEB abrogated increase in mtDNA and biomarkers of MB (PGC1α, NRF1, and TFAM, and proteins COX II, COX IV, and Cyt-C). To investigate the effects of CO on mitochondrial homeostasis *in vivo*, they treated mice with LPS/D-galactosamine (D-GalN). CO inhalation reduced liver injury after challenge with LPS/GalN, increased TFEB activation, CP, and MB in mice, explaining novel mechanisms underlying CO-dependent cytoprotection in liver via activation of the TFEB-dependent CP and induction of both lysosomes and MB.

Annexin A1 Prevents Neuro-inflammation in Cardiac Arrest

Neuro-inflammation initiated by damage-associated molecular patterns, including HMGB1, has been implicated in adverse neurological outcomes following lethal hemorrhagic shock and trauma. EPR is a novel method for victims of exsanguinating cardiac arrest to improve survival with neurological recovery. Sirtuin 3 (SIRT3), the primary mitochondrial deacetylase, is a key regulator of metabolic and energy stress-response pathways in the brain to induce a neuronal pro-survival phenotype. Ma et al. (2019) examined whether systemic administration of an Annexin-A1 bioactive peptide (ANXA1sp) could resolve neuro-inflammation and induce sirtuin-3-regulated cytoprotection in a rat model of exsanguinating cardiac arrest and EPR. Adult male rats underwent hemorrhagic shock and ventricular fibrillation, profound hypothermia, followed by resuscitation and rewarming using cardiopulmonary bypass (EPR). ANXA1sp reduced cerebral HMGB1, IL-6, and TNFα and increased IL-10 expression, associated with improved neurological scores. ANXA1sp reversed EPR-induced increases in the expression of pro-apoptotic protein Bax and reduction in anti-apoptotic protein Bcl-2, with a corresponding decrease in cerebral levels of cleaved caspase-3. ANXA1sp induced ATG (increased LC3-II and reduced p62 expression) in the brain. These findings were accompanied by upregulation of the mitochondrial protein deacetylase Sirtuin-3, and its downstream targets, Foxo3a and Mn-SOD, in ANXA1sp-treated animals, indicating that Annexin-A1 biomimetic peptides can attenuate inflammation and enhance the neuroprotective effects of EPR after exsanguinating cardiac arrest.

IL-6 and IL-6/AMPK

IL-6 is a neuromodulation factor with complex biological activities. IL-6 activates AMPK, which regulates MB and CP/ATG. Chen et al. (2018) investigated the role of IL-6 in MB using astrocytes during the experimental septic condition and examined how the IL-6/AMPK signaling pathway affected this process. The primary cultures of cerebral cortical astrocytes were allocated into six groups: control group, LPS+IFN-γ group, IL-6 group (LPS+IFN-γ+IL-6), C group (LPS+IFN-γ+IL-6+Compound C), siRNA group (LPS+IFN-γ+IL-6+IL-6R siRNA), and siRNA+C group (LPS+IFN-γ+IL-6+IL-6R siRNA+Compound C). All groups were stimulated for 6 hrs. Cytokines and ROS analyses, detection of ATP, mtDNA, and cell viability, evaluation of the mitochondrial ultrastructure and volume density, and immunoblots of proteins associated with MB and p-AMPK were performed respectively. Compared with LPS+IFN-γ group, IL-6 group had milder damage to mitochondria, higher mtDNA content and mitochondrial volume, a higher expression of proteins was associated with MB (PGC-1α, NRF-1 and TFAM) and p-AMPK), and thus higher cell viability, whereas by blocking IL-6/AMPK signaling pathway, the protective effect of IL-6 was attenuated. IL-6 enhanced MB in astrocytes under an experimental septic condition through the IL-6/AMPK signaling pathway.

Sphingolipid-mediated Inflammation

Elevated levels of the pro-inflammatory cytokine TNFα inhibit erythropoiesis and cause anemia in patients with cancer and chronic inflammatory diseases. TNFα is also a potent activator of the sphingomyelinase (SMase)/ceramide pathway, leading to ceramide synthesis and regulating cell differentiation, proliferation, apoptosis, senescence, and ATG. Orsini et al. (2019) evaluated the implication of the TNFα/SMase/ceramide pathway on the inhibition of erythropoiesis in human CD34$^+$ hematopoietic stem/progenitor cells (CD34/HSPCs) from healthy donors. Synthetic C2- and C6-ceramide as well as bacterial SMase inhibited erythroid differentiation in erythropoietin-induced (Epo) CD34/HSPCs as shown by the analysis of various erythroid markers. The neutral SMase inhibitor GW4869 as well as the genetic inhibition of nSMase with siRNA against sphingomyelin phosphodiesterase 3 (SMPD3) prevented the inhibition by TNFα, but not the acid SMase inhibitor, Desipramine. Sphingosine-1-phosphate (S1P), a ceramide metabolite, restored erythroid differentiation, whereas TNFα inhibited sphingosine kinase-1, required for S1P synthesis. The erythropoiesis impairment was concomitant with a granulo-monocytic differentiation in TNFα- and ceramide-treated EpoCD34/HSPCs, which correlated to the modulation of hematopoietic transcription factors (TFs) GATA-1, GATA-2, and PU.1. The expression of miR)-144/451, miR-146a, miR-155, and miR-223 was also modulated by TNFα and ceramide, in line with cellular observations. CP/ATG plays an essential role during erythropoiesis and the TNFα/neutral SMase/ceramide pathway inhibits CP/ATG in EpoCD34/ HSPCs. TNFα- and ceramide-induced phosphorylation of mTOR^{S2448} and ULK1^{S758}, inhibited ATG13^{S355} phosphorylation, and blocked APS formation. Rapamycin prevented the inhibitory effect of TNFα and ceramides on erythropoiesis while inhibiting the induction of myelopoiesis. Bafilomycin A1, but not siRNA in Atg5, induced myeloid differentiation, while both impaired erythropoiesis, indicating that the TNFα/neutral SMase/ceramide pathway inhibits erythropoiesis to induce myelopoiesis via modulation of a hematopoietic TF/miR network and inhibition of the late steps of CP/ATG, suggesting its crucial role in erythroid vs. myeloid differentiation.

TLR-induced Antimicrobial Pathways

Macrophages are highly significant to innate immunity, responding to invading microorganisms by initiating inflammatory and antimicrobial programs. Immediate antimicrobial responses, such as NADPH-dependent ROS, are triggered upon phagocytic receptor engagement. Macrophages also detect and respond to microbial products through pattern recognition receptors (PRRs), such as TLRs, to influence multiple biological processes including antigen presentation, cell survival, inflammation, and direct antimicrobial responses. The latter enables macrophages to combat infectious agents that persist within the intracellular environment. Stocks et al. (2018) highlighted TLR-inducible direct antimicrobial responses that macrophages employ against bacterial pathogens, linking TLR signaling to reprogramming of mitochondrial functions to enable the production of direct antimicrobial agents such as ROS and itaconic acid. In addition, they described other TLR-inducible antimicrobial pathways, including ATG/MTG, modulation of nutrient availability, metal ion toxicity, RONS, immune GTPases (immunity-related GTPases and guanylate-binding proteins), and antimicrobial peptides. They also described mechanisms of evasion of such pathways by intra-macrophage pathogens, with a focus on Salmonella, Mycobacteria, and Listeria. An understanding of how TLR-inducible direct antimicrobial responses are regulated, as well as how bacterial pathogens subvert such pathways, may confer novel strategies for manipulating host defense to combat infectious diseases.

Regulation of B Cells

Recently, Sandoval et al. (2018) described the role of the APS and mitochondria in regulating B cell fate, survival, and function. They discussed the interaction between these two highly metabolic organelles during B cell development, maturation, and differentiation. B cells are responsible for protective antibody production after differentiation into antibody-secreting cells during humoral immune responses. From early B cell development in the bone marrow, to their maturation in the periphery, activation in the germinal center, and differentiation into plasma cells or memory B cells. ATG and mitochondria play important roles in B cell development, activation, and differentiation to accommodate the phenotypic and environmental changes encountered over the lifetime of the cell. Mitochondria and CP/ATG generate energy, mediate cell survival, and produce/eliminate RONS that can serve as signal molecules to regulate differentiation. As B cells mature and differentiate into plasma or memory cells, both CP/ATG and mitochondrial functions undergo significant changes.

TLR-3 Regulates Zika Virus Infection

The connection between ZIKV and neurodevelopmental defects is widely recognized. Ojha et al. (2019) showed that three strains of ZIKV, an African strain MR766 (Uganda) and two closely related Asian strains R103451 (Honduras) and PRVABC59 (Puerto Rico) infect human astrocytes, although Asian strains showed a higher infectivity and increased cell death compared to the African strain. The inhibition of AXL receptor attenuated the viral entry of MR766 and PRVABC59, and to a lesser extent, R103451, suggesting an important role of TAM receptors in ZIKV cell entry, irrespective of lineage. Infection by PRVABC59 elicited enhanced release of inflammatory molecules, with 8X increase in the release of RANTES, 10X increase in secretion of IP-10, and a 12X increase in IFN-β secretion compared to un-infected human astrocytes. Minor changes in the release of several growth factors, ERS response factors, and the transcription factor, NF-κB, were detected with the Asian strains, while significant increases in FOXO6, MAPK10, and JNK were detected with the African strain. Activation of the CP/ATG pathway was evident with increased expression of the ATG-related proteins Beclin-1, LC3B, and p62/SQSTM1 with all three strains of ZIKV. Pharmacological inhibition of the CP/ATG pathway and genetic inhibition of the Beclin-1 showed minimal effects on ZIKV replication. The expression of TLR3 was increased with all three strains; pharmacological and genetic inhibition of TLR3 caused a decrease in viral titers and in viral-induced inflammatory response in infected astrocytes, indicating that TLR3 plays a vital role in ZIKV replication and inflammatory responses, irrespective of the strains, while the CP/ATG protein Beclin-1 influenced host inflammatory responses. (For details, please refer to author's book, *Zika Virus Disease: Prevention & Cure* by Nova Science Publishers in New York, U.S.A. (2017)).

Sphingosine 1-phosphate Activates Microglia

Microglia mediated responses to neuronal damage as neuro-inflammation is a common mechanism propagating neuropathology. Karunakaran et al. (2019) investigated the microglial alterations occurring as a result of sphingosine 1-phosphate (S1P) accumulation in neural cells. There was increased microglial activation in the brains of neural S1P-lyase(SGPL1)-ablated mice (SGPL1$^{fl/fl/Nes}$) as shown by an activated and de-ramified morphology and increased activation markers on microglia. Increased pro-inflammatory cytokines in sorted and primary cultured microglia generated from SGPL1-deficient mice were noticed. Microglial inflammation was accompanied by defective ATG in SGPL1-ablated mice. Rescuing ATG by treatment with Rapamycin decreased IL-6 but not TNF secretion in cultured microglia. The Rapamycin-mediated decrease in IL-6 secretion suggested a microglia-specific mTOR-IL-6 link. Using inhibitors of the major receptors of S1P expressed in the microglia, S1P receptor 2 (S1PR2) was identified as the mediator of both impaired ATG and pro-inflammatory effects. The addition of exogenous administration of S1P to BV2 microglial cells showed similar effects as those observed in the genetic knockout of SGPL1 in the neural cells. Thus, a novel role of the S1P-S1PR2 axis in the microglia of mice was demonstrated with neural-targeted SGPL1 ablation and in BV2 microglial cell line treated with S1P.

IRGM Restrains NLRP3 IS Activation

IRGM is a genetic risk factor for Crohn disease (CD) and several other inflammatory disorders. Mehto et al. (2019) showed that IRGM regulates NLRP3 IS activation. IRGM employs two parallel approaches to constrain IS activation. IRGM interacts with NLRP3 and PYCARD/ASC, and mediates their SQSTM1/p62-dependent macroATG/ATG degradation. IRGM impedes IS assembly by blocking the polymerization of NLRP3 and PYCARD. IRGM suppressed NLRP3-mediated exacerbated outcomes of dextran sodium sulfate (DSS)-induced colitis in a mouse model, suggesting that it can directly regulate inflammation to protect from inflammatory diseases.

NLRP3 IS Activation in NASH

Activation of inflammation is an important mechanism in the development of NASH. Zhang et al. (2018) explored how CP affects NLRP3 IS-activation in hepatic lipo-toxicity. Mice were fed a high fat/calorie diet (HFCD) for 24 weeks. Primary rat hepatocytes were treated with palmitic acid (PA) for various periods of time. MTG was measured by protein levels of LC3-II and P62. NLRP3, caspase-1, IL-18, and IL-1β at mRNA and protein levels were used as indicators of IS activation. Along with steatotic progression in HFCD-fed mice, the ratio of LC3-II/β-actin was decreased with increased levels of liver P62, NLRP3, caspase-1, IL-1β, IL-18, and serum IL-1β levels in late-stage NASH. A PA treatment induced mitochondrial oxidative stress and triggered CP in hepatocytes. Cyclosporine A did not change LC3-II/Tomm20 ratios; but P62 levels were increased after an extended duration of PA exposure, indicating a defect in ATG. Along with impaired CP, mRNA and protein levels of NLRP3, caspase-1, IL-18, and IL-1β were upregulated by PA treatment. Pretreatment with MCC950, NAC, or Acetyl-L-carnitine reversed IS and pyroptotic cascade activation. CP was recovered as indicated by increases in the LC3-II/Tomm20 ratio, Parkin, and PINK1 expression, and decreased P62 expression, suggesting that impaired CP triggers hepatic NLRP3 IS activation in a murine NASH model and primary hepatocytes. The new insights into IS activation through CP has advanced our understanding of how fatty acids elicit lipo-toxicity through oxidant stress and ATG in mitochondria.

ATG in Eosinophilic Airway Inflammation

ATG is a homeostatic mechanism that discards not only invading pathogens but also damaged organelles and denatured proteins via lysosomal degradation. Lee and Kim (2019) studied the role of ATG in inflammatory diseases, including infectious diseases, Crohn's disease, cystic fibrosis, and pulmonary hypertension, and suggested that modulating CP/ATG could be a novel theranostic strategy for inflammatory diseases. Eosinophils are a major type of inflammatory cells, which aggravates airway inflammatory diseases, particularly corticosteroid-resistant inflammation. The eosinophil count is useful for assessing which patients may benefit from inhaled corticosteroid therapy. ATG plays a crucial role in eosinophilic airway inflammatory diseases by promoting airway remodeling and loss of function. Genetic variant in the ATG gene Atg5 is associated with asthma pathogenesis, and ATG regulates apoptotic pathways in epithelial cells in individuals with COPD. ATG dysfunction leads to severe eosinophilic inflammation, in chronic rhinosinusitis. However, the mechanism underlying the ATG-mediated regulation of eosinophilic airway inflammation remains uncertain. This review emphasized the role of ATG in eosinophilic airway inflammation and suggested that ATG may be a novel theranostic target for airway inflammation.

AGR2 Dimerization and ER Proteostasis in Inflammation

Anterior gradient 2 (AGR2) is a dimeric protein disulfide isomerase family member involved in the regulation of PQC in the ER. Mouse AGR2 deletion increases intestinal inflammation and promotes the development of IBD. Maurel et al. (2019) used a protein-protein interaction screen to identify cellular regulators of AGR2 dimerization, and unveiled specific enhancers, including TMED2, and inhibitors of AGR2 dimerization, that control AGR2 functions, and demonstrated that modulation of AGR2 dimer formation, whether by enhancing or inhibiting the process, yields pro-inflammatory phenotypes, through either ATG or secretion of AGR2, respectively. In IBD and Crohn's disease, the levels of AGR2 dimerization modulators were deregulated, which correlated with the severity of inflammatory disease, suggesting that AGR2 dimers act as sensors of ER homeostasis and are disrupted upon ERS and promote the secretion of AGR2 monomers. The latter might represent systemic alarm signals for pro-inflammatory responses in IBD.

Theranostic and Pathogenic Role of ATG

ATG is a complex cellular mechanism that maintains cellular and tissue homeostasis and integrity via the degradation of senescent, defective subcellular organelles, infectious agents, and misfolded proteins. ATG is involved in numerous immune processes, such as the removal of intracellular bacteria, cytokine production, autoantigen presentation, and survival of lymphocytes, indicating its important role in innate and adaptive immune responses. ATG-related gene polymorphisms are associated with the pathogenesis of autoimmune and inflammatory disorders, such as SLE, psoriasis, rheumatoid arthritis, IBD, and MS. The conditional knockdown of ATG-related genes in mice displayed theranostic effects on several autoimmune disease models by reducing inflammatory cytokines and autoreactive immune cells. However, the inhibition of ATG accelerated some inflammatory and autoimmune diseases via inflammatory cytokine production.

ATG Limits ISs Activation

Recently, Takahama et al. (2018) highlighted the crosstalk between IS activation and CP. Deficiencies in CP/ATG-related proteins induced the impaired activation of ISs, causing severe tissue damage. In contrast, CP inducers ameliorated symptoms of IS-related diseases. ISs are multiprotein complexes that control the maturation and production of IL-1 family members and play a crucial role in host defense against pathogens. However, dysregulated activation of ISs is associated with inflammation, leading to the development of inflammatory diseases. Therefore, ISs must be activated adequately to protect against infections and avoid tissue damage.

GIMAP6 for T Cell Maintenance

The GTPases of the immunity-associated proteins (GIMAP) are a family of proteins expressed in the adaptive immune system. Pascal et al. (2018) reported that in human cells, GIMAP6 interacts with the ATG8 family member GABARAPL2, and is recruited to APSs upon starvation, suggesting a role for GIMAP6 in the ATG. To study the function of GIMAP6 in the immune system, they established a mouse line in which the Gimap6 gene can be inactivated by Cre-mediated recombination. In mice bred to carry the CD2Cre transgene such that the Gimap6 gene was deleted within the T and B cell lineages, there was a 50–70% reduction in peripheral CD4+ and CD8+ T cells. The analysis of splenocyte-derived proteins from these mice indicated increased MAP1LC3B, particularly in the lipidated LC3-II form, and S405-phosphorylation of SQSTM1. TEM measurements of Gimap6–/– CD4+ T cells indicated an increased mitochondrial/ cytoplasmic volume ratio and increased numbers of APSs, consistent with ATG disruption in the cells. However, Gimap6–/– T cells were normal, could be activated *in vitro*, and supported T cell-dependent antibody production. The treatment of CD4+ splenocytes from GIMAP6fl/ flERT2Cre mice with 4-OH-Tamoxifen resulted in the disappearance of GIMAP6 within five days. Concomitantly increased phosphorylation of SQSTM1 and TBK1 indicated the requirement of GIMAP6 for normal peripheral adaptive immune system and a significant role for the protein in normal ATG processes. GIMAP6 was expressed in a cell-selective manner, indicating the existence of a cell-restricted mode of ATG regulation.

Carvedilol

The NLRP3 IS is a multiprotein complex that plays a key role in the innate immune system, and aberrant activation of this complex is involved in the pathogenesis of inflammatory diseases. Carvedilol (CVL) is an α-β-blocker used to treat hypertension and CHF; however, some benefits beyond decreased BP were observed, suggesting the potential anti-inflammatory activity of CVL. Wong et al. (2018) studied the inhibitory potential of CVL toward the NLRP3 IS. CVL attenuated

NLRP3 IS activation and pyroptosis in mouse macrophages, without affecting activation of the AIM2, NLRC4, and ISs. CVL prevented lysosomal and mitochondrial damage and reduced ASC oligomerization. CVL caused ATG induction through a Sirt1-dependent pathway, which inhibited the NLRP3 IS. In the mouse model of NLRP3-associated peritonitis, the oral administration of CVL reduced the (a) peritoneal recruitment of neutrophils, (b) the levels of IL-1β, IL-18, active caspase-1, ASC, IL-6, TNF-α, MCP-1, and CXCL1 in the lavage fluids, and (c) levels of NLRP3 and HO-1 in the peritoneal cells, indicating that CVL is a novel ATG inducer that inhibits the NLRP3 IS and can be used for ameliorating NLRP3-associated complications.

Interferon Regulatory Factor 8

Interferon regulatory factor 8 (IRF8) is a critical transcription factor in innate immune responses that regulates the development and function of myeloid cells. Human periapical lesions are caused by endodontic microbial infections. Yu et al. (2018) explored the expression of IRF8 in human periapical lesions and the association of IRF8 with macrophages, NF-κB signaling, and the ATG process. Thirty-nine human periapical tissues, including healthy control tissues ($n = 15$), radicular cysts (RCs, $n = 11$), and periapical granulomas (PG, $n = 13$), were examined. Double immunofluorescence assessment was performed to co-localize IRF8 with CD68, NF-κB p65, and LC3B. The expression of IRF8 was higher in RCs and PGs than in the healthy control group, but no significant difference was observed between RCs and PGs. There were more IRF8-CD68 double-positive cells in RCs and PGs than in the healthy control group, but no such difference was observed between RCs and PGs. The double-labeling analysis of IRF8 with NF-κB and LC3B indicated that IRF8 expression is associated with NF-κB signaling and the ATG during periapical lesions, suggesting that IRF8 might be involved in macrophages in the development of periapical lesions.

ATG

Protects PBMC in Diabetic Dyslipidemia. T2DM results in severe oxidative and nitrosative stress and inflammation when associated with hyperlipidemia. Chatterjee et al. (2019) explored the role of ATG in T2DM subjects with or without dyslipidemia. Experiments were conducted on isolated PBMC from study subjects and insulin-resistant HepG2 cells utilizing flow cytometry, confocal microscopy, immunoblotting, immunofluorescence, and real-time PCR. In case of T2DM with dyslipidemia, a higher population of ATG positive cells was detected compared to T2DM which may have been originated due to higher stress. Flow cytometric data indicated ATG to be triggered by RONS stress in PBMC of diabetic dyslipidemic patients. The expression of LC3 puncta, a hallmark of ATG was observed at the periphery of PBMC and Hep G2 cells in the diabetic dyslipidemic condition. An increased expression of Atg5, LC3B, and Beclin-1 supported the ATG pathway in both PBMC and Hep G2 cells. Upon blocking ATG by 3MA, the apoptotic cell population increased significantly. ATG-controlled oxidative stress mediated the upregulation of inflammatory markers like IL-6, TNF-α. Hence, the induction of ATG emerged as a protective mechanism for the diabetic cells coupled with dyslipidemia. Not only ROS, but also RNS were involved in ATG induction. ATG had a protective role in pro-inflammatory responses. Thus, enhancing ATG may be a novel theranostic strategy to restore glycemic regulation in T2DM.

Circulating mtDNA in Aging

Recently, Picca et al. (2018) highlighted that dysfunctional MQC and inflammation are hallmarks of aging and are involved in the pathogenesis of muscle-wasting disorders, including sarcopenia and cachexia. One of the consequences of failing MQC is the release of DAMPs. By virtue of their bacterial ancestry, these molecules can trigger an inflammatory response by interacting with receptors similar to those involved in pathogen-associated responses. Mitochondria-derived DAMPs, especially cell-free mtDNA, are associated with chronic inflammation, such as aging and degenerative diseases. These researchers highlighted the contribution of mitochondria-derived DAMPs to age-related systemic inflammation in order to further explore these signaling pathways for the TSE-EBPT of muscle wasting disorders.

Inflammasome (IS) Activation in RPE Cells

Piippo et al. (2018) demonstrated that blockade of the intracellular clearance systems in human RPE cells by MG-132 and Bafilomycin A1 (BafA) induces NLRP3 IS signaling. NLRP3 is an intracellular receptor detecting factors ranging from the endogenous alarmins and ATP to UV radiation and solid particles. Due to diversified triggers, the activation of NLRP3 is indirect and can be mediated through several alternative pathways. Potassium efflux, lysosomal rupture, and oxidative stress are currently the main mechanisms associated with many activators. NLRP3 ISs were activated in human RPE cells by blocking proteasomes and ATG using MG-132 and Bafilomycin A1 (BafA), respectively. The P2X7 inhibitor A740003 KCl, along with Glyburide, NAC, ammonium pyrrolidinedithiocarbamate (APDC), Diphenyleneiodonium chloride (DPI), and mito-TEMPO were added to cell cultures to study the role of K^+ efflux and oxidative stress, respectively. Elevated extracellular K^+ prevented the priming factor IL-1α from inducing the production of ROS. It also prevented IL-1β release after the exposure of primed cells to MG-132 and BafA. IS activation increased extracellular ATP levels, which did not trigger significant K^+ efflux. The activity of the lysosomal enzyme, cathepsin B, was reduced by MG-132 and BafA, suggesting that cathepsin B was not playing any role in this phenomenon. Instead, MG-132 triggered ROS production 30 min after exposure, but a treatment with antioxidants blocking NADPH oxidase and ROS prevented IL-1β release, suggesting that oxidative stress contributes to the NLRP3 IS activation upon dysfunctional cellular clearance. A clarification of IS activation mechanisms provided novel options for alleviating pathological inflammation in aggregation diseases, such as age-related macular disease (AMD) and AD.

Parkin and PINK1

Although serum from patients with PD contains elevated levels of pro-inflammatory cytokines including IL-6, TNF, IL-1β, and IFNγ, whether inflammation contributes to or is a consequence of neuronal loss remains unknown. Mutations in Parkin, an E3 ubiquitin ligase, and PINK1, a ubiquitin kinase, cause early onset PD. Both PINK1 and Parkin function within the same signaling pathway and eliminate damaged mitochondria from cells in culture and in animal models via CP. The *in vivo* role of CP, however, is unclear, because mice that lack either PINK1 or Parkin have no PD-relevant phenotypes. Mitochondrial stress can lead to the release of DAMPs that can activate innate immunity, suggesting that CP may mitigate inflammation. Sliter et al. (2018) reported an inflammatory phenotype in both PRKN$^{-/-}$ and PINK1$^{-/-}$ mice following exhaustive exercise and in PRKN$^{-/-}$ mutator mice, which accumulated mutations in mtDNA. Inflammation resulting from either exhaustive exercise or mtDNA mutation is rescued by the concurrent loss of STING, a regulator of the type I interferon response to cytosolic DNA. The loss of DAergic neurons from the SN and the motor deficits observed in aged PRKN$^{-/-}$ mutator mice were also rescued by loss of STING, suggesting that inflammation facilitates this phenotype. Humans with mono- and biallelic PRKN mutations also display elevated cytokines, supporting a role for PINK1- and Parkin-mediated CP/ATG in restraining innate immunity.

Pro-oxidant Adaptor p66SHC

MacroATG/ATG has emerged as a crucial process in lymphocyte homeostasis, activation, and differentiation. Based on the finding that the p66 isoform of SHC1 (p66SHC) pro-apoptotic ROS-elevating SHC family adaptor inhibits mTOR signaling in these cells, Onnis et al. (2018) investigated the role of p66SHC in B-cell ATG and showed that p66SHC disrupts mitochondrial function through its CYCS(Cyt-C, somatic)-binding domain, thereby impairing ATP production, which results in AMPK activation and enhanced ATG. While p66SHC binding to CYCS is adequate for triggering apoptosis, p66SHC-mediated ATG depends on its ability to interact with membrane-associated LC3-II through a specific binding motif within its N terminus. p66SHC also has an impact on MQC by inducing mitochondrial depolarization, protein ubiquitination at the OMM, and recruitment of active AMPK. These events initiate CP, whose execution relies on the role of p66SHC as an LC3-II receptor which brings phagophore membranes to mitochondria. p66SHC also promoted hypoxia-induced CP in B cells whereas p66SHC-deficiency enhanced B cell differentiation in plasma cells, which is controlled by ROS levels and the hypoxic germinal center environment, suggesting that mitochondrial p66SHC is a novel regulator of CP and ATG in B cells and p66SHC-mediated coordination of ATG and apoptosis in B cell survival and differentiation.

CP in Liver Injury

Toshihiko et al. (2017) summarized recent literature describing the versatile role of CP/ATG and its implications in the pathogenesis of sepsis in the liver. In animal models of sepsis induced by cecal ligation and puncture (CLP) or the systemic administration of LPS, CP/ATG is implicated in the activation and/or damage of various cells/organs, such as immune cells, heart, lung, kidney, and liver. Since sepsis is associated with an increased production of pro- as well as anti-inflammatory cytokines, hyper-cytokinemia is a fetal immune response leading to multiple organ failure (MOF) and mortality during sepsis. However, a recent paradigm illuminates the crucial roles of mitochondrial dysfunction as well as the perturbation of CP/ATG in the pathogenesis of sepsis. In the livers of animal models of sepsis, CP/ATG is involved in the elimination of damaged mitochondria to prevent the generation of ROS and the initiation of the mitochondrial apoptotic pathway involved in CBMP. In addition, many reports now indicate that the role of ATG is not restricted to the elimination of hazardous malfunctioning mitochondria, including CBs within the cells. CP/ATG is also involved in the regulation of IS activation and the release of cytokines as well as other inflammatory substances through CS destabilization.

The Theranostic Potential of Antioxidants as Anti-inflammatory CP Agonists

Resistin

Miao et al. (2018) reported that Resistin/TLR4 signaling pathway induces inflammation and insulin resistance in neuronal cells. They hypothesized that resistin-induced neuro-inflammation could be attributed to impaired ATG pathways in neuronal cells. Resistin decreased ATG as evidenced by the repression of the main ATG markers in the SH-SY5Y cell line. The silencing of TLR4 abolished these effects. Resistin also inhibited AMPK phosphorylation and increased Akt/mTOR contrasting with activated ATG where AMPK phosphorylation was augmented and mTOR inhibited. Resistin treatment inhibited the mRNA expression of ATG biomarkers in the hypothalamus of WT mice but not in *Tlr4−/−* mice. Resistin diminished LC3 (a marker of ATG) in the arcuate nucleus of WT mice, which was abolished in *Tlr4–/–* mice, suggesting Resistin/ TLR4 as a novel regulatory pathway of neuronal CP/ATG.

Arhalofenate Acid

Arhalofenate, is a non-agonist PPARγ ligand, with uricosuric activity via URAT1 inhibition. Phase II studies revealed that decreased acute arthritis flares in Arhalofenate-treated gout compared with Allopurinol alone. McWherter et al. (2018) investigated the anti-inflammatory effects and mechanisms of Arhalofenate and its active acid form for responses to monosodium urate (MSU) crystals. They assessed *in vivo* responses to MSU crystals in murine s.c. air pouches and *in vitro* responses in murine bone-marrow-derived macrophages (BMDMs). The oral administration of Arhalofenate (250 mg/kg) blunted total leukocyte ingress, neutrophil influx, and air pouch fluid IL-1β, IL-6, and CXCL1 in response to MSU crystal injection. Arhalofenate acid (100 μM) attenuated MSU crystal-induced IL-1β production in BMDMs via inhibition of NLRP3 IS activation. In addition, Arhalofenate acid increased activation (as assessed by phosphorylation) of AMPK. Studying AMPKα1 knockout mice, AMPK mediated the anti-inflammatory effects of Arhalofenate acid. Arhalofenate acid attenuated the potential of MSU crystals to suppress AMPK activity, regulated the expression of multiple downstream AMPK targets that modulate mitochondrial function and oxidative stress, preserved mitochondrial cristae and volume density, and promoted anti-inflammatory ATG flux, suggesting that Arhalofenate acid is anti-inflammatory and acts via AMPK activation, and its signaling in macrophages contribute to a reduction of gout flares.

Quercetin

Maternal restriction of dietary proteins during pregnancy and lactation induces renal disease in later life. High fructose intake causes metabolic syndrome, which results in an increased risk of developing CKD. Sato et al. (2019) investigated whether Quercetin intake during lactation affects inflammation and CP in the kidneys of high-fructose-diet-fed adult female offspring exposed to maternal normal-protein (NP) or low-protein (LP) diets. Pregnant Wistar rats received diets containing 20% (NP) or 8% (LP) casein, and 0 or 0.2% Quercetin containing NP diets (NP/NP or NP/NPQ) in experiment (Expt.) 1 and 0 or 0.2% Quercetin containing LP diets (LP/LP or LP/ LPQ) in Expt. 2 during lactation. At weaning, pups that received a diet of distilled water (Wa) or 10% fructose solution (Fr) were divided into six groups: NP/NP/Wa, NP/NP/Fr, NP/NPQ/Fr in Expt. 1, and LP/LP/Wa, LP/LP/Fr, LP/LPQ/Fr in Expt. 2. At week 12, macrophage infiltration, mRNA levels of TNF-α and IL-6, and markers of CP in the kidneys of male offspring were examined. The macrophage number, and TNF-α and IL-6 mRNA levels increased in the kidneys of the NP/NP/Fr and LP/LP/Fr, respectively. Conversely, macrophage number and IL-6 levels in the NP/NPQ/Fr and LP/LPQ/Fr decreased, respectively. LC3B-II levels were downregulated in the NP/NP/Fr and LP/LP/Fr rats. In contrast, LC3B-II levels were upregulated, while p62 levels were downregulated in the NP/NPQ/Fr and LP/LPQ/Fr rats, suggesting that maternal Quercetin intake during lactation may cause long-term alterations in inflammation and CP in the kidneys of high-fructose-diet-fed adult female offspring.

Resveratrol

Resveratrol (*Res*: 3,5,4′-trihydroxy stilbene) exerts an anti-inflammatory effect on collagen-induced arthritis and osteoarthritis in rats via activation of SIRT1. ATG can be induced by Res and leads to amelioration of IL-1β release *in vitro*. Yang et al. (2019) determined the anti-inflammatory role of Res in patients with gout. They obtained blood samples from patients with acute gout, inter-critical gout (IG), and healthy controls (HC). The mRNA and protein levels of

SIRT1 and NF-κB (p65) were determined in PBMCs lysate from these patients. In the *in vitro* experiment, SIRT1, ATG-related genes (Beclin-1 and microtubule-associated protein 1 light-chain 3), and genes involved in the gouty inflammatory pathway, including NF-κB p65, NLRP3, caspase-1, and IL-1β, were determined in PBMCs lysate or plasma from IG patients exposed to monosodium urate (MSU) crystals with or without Res. The mRNA and protein levels of SIRT1 were downregulated in PBMCs from gout patients in comparison with HC. The protein levels of SIRT1 were downregulated in PBMCs from IG patients exposed to MSU crystals and were restored by Res. High doses of Res ameliorated the release of the inflammatory cytokine IL-1β. The mRNA levels of NLRP3 and NF-κB p65 were regulated by Res, but caspase-1 and IL-1β were not. Res promoted MSU-induced CP/ATG in PBMCs from patients with gout, suggesting that it ameliorates gouty inflammation via upregulation of SIRT1 to promote CP/ATG in patients with gout. Resveratrol as a novel CPT for the TSE-EBPT of gout is illustrated in Fig. 43.

Resveratrol as a Novel CPT for the TSE-EBPT of Gout

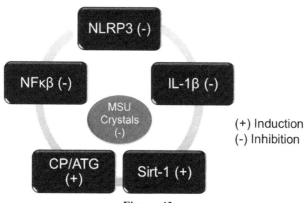

Figure 43

Curcumin as an Inflammasome Antagonist

Curcumin is the primary active ingredient in turmeric and inhibits inflammation. Turmeric is used as a spice and coloring in foods. Muhammad et al. (2018) demonstrated Curcumin intervention in AFB$_1$-induced hepatotoxicity. Besides, normal cellular morphology, APSs were found in the control and Curcumin control group. In contrast, fragmented and swollen mitochondria, irregular-shaped nuclei, and fat droplets were visible but APSs disappear in the AFB$_1$-treated group. The mRNA and protein expression of ATG-related genes indicated that AFB$_1$ inhibited ATG and induced inflammation. Nrf2 and HO-1 mRNA and protein level was reduced in AFB$_1$-fed group. Dietary curcumin modulated CP/ATG through the activation of Beclin-1, Atg5, Dynein, LC3a, LC3b-I/II, and downregulation of p53 & mTOR expression. Curcumin ameliorated AFB$_1$-induced inflammation, and elevated AFB$_1$-induced a decrease in Nrf2 and HO-1 mRNA and protein expression level. Thus, Curcumin activated CP/ATG and ameliorated inflammation involving the Nrf2 signaling pathway which may become a new TSE-EBPT strategy to prevent AFB$_1$-induced hepatotoxicity. Yin et al. (2018) reported that Curcumin inhibited caspase-1 activation and IL-1β secretion by suppressing LPS priming and the IS activation in mouse BMDMs. The inhibitory effect of Curcumin on IS activation was specific to the NLRP3, not to the NLRC4 or the AIM2 ISs. Curcumin inhibited the NLRP3 IS by preventing K$^+$ efflux and disturbing the downstream events, including the efficient spatial arrangement of mitochondria, ASC oligomerization, and speckle formation. ROS, ATG, sirtuin-2, or acetylated α-tubulin were ruled out as the mechanism by which Curcumin inhibits the IS. Curcumin attenuated IL-1β secretion and prevented HFD-induced insulin resistance in C57BL/6 mice but not in *Nlrp3*-deficient mice. Curcumin also repressed MSU crystal-induced peritoneal inflammation *in vivo*. Curcumin was identified as a common NLRP3 IS inhibitor. These findings revealed a mechanism through which Curcumin curbs inflammation and suggested its theranostic potential in NLRP3-driven diseases.

CONCLUSION

Pro-inflammation with a gain-of-function mutation (R284S) was observed in the innate immune sensor "STING". TFEB nuclear translocation enhanced CP and MB to ameliorate inflammatory hepatic injury. Sphingolipid-mediated inflammation caused ATG inhibition to convert erythropoiesis to myelopoiesis in hematopoietic progenitor cells. TLR-induced antimicrobial pathways were identified on the macrophages of MDR diseases. B cell fate, survival, and function were regulated by mitochondria, CP, MTG, and ATG. TLR-3 regulated Zika viral infection and inflammatory response in primary astrocytes. Sphingosine 1-phosphate accumulation induced microglial activation, inflammation, and impaired CP. IRGM attenuated NLRP3 IS activation by inducing SQSTM1/p62-dependent CP. GIMAP6 was required for T cell maintenance and efficient ATG in mice. The β-blocker Carvedilol served as a novel ATG inducer that inhibited the NLRP3 IS, whereas, ATG confined the IS activation. Impaired CP triggered NLRP3 IS activation during the progression of NAFLD to NASH. The interferon regulatory factor-8 was induced in human periapical lesions. ATG was induced to protect PBMCs in diabetic dyslipidemia involving RONS stress and eosinophilic airway inflammation. Circulating mtDNA, mitochondrial dysfunction, and inflammation involving CBMP were increased in aging and muscle wasting disorders. Oxidative stress enhanced IS activation in RPE cells with impaired proteasome profile and CP/ATG. Parkin and PINK1 mitigated STING-induced inflammation. CP/ATG participated in the lymphocyte homeostasis, activation, and inflammatory diseases. The pro-oxidant adaptor p66SHC promoted B cell CP by disrupting mitochondrial integrity and recruiting LC3-II. CP/ATG and MB were impaired during sepsis-induced liver injury. Resistin inhibited neuronal ATG through TLRs, whereas Arhalofenate acid inhibited MSU-induced gout by AMPK activation. MTG was involved in the release of inflammatory cytokines. Maternal Quercetin intake during lactation ameliorated neonatal inflammation. Reseveratrol ameliorated inflammation via sirtuin 1-induced CP/ATG in gout patients. Curcumin conferred hepatoprotection in AFB_1-induced toxicity by activating CP/ATG, ameliorating Nrf2/HO-1-mediated inflammation, suppressing IL-1β secretion, preventing inflammation, and inhibiting NLRP3 IS activation implicated in CBMP and apoptosis. The theranostic potential of natural and synthetic antioxidants as CP regulators in inflammatory diseases and microbial (bacteria, virus, and fungal) infections is currently being investigated.

REFERENCES

Arbogast, F. and F. Gros. 2018. Lymphocyte autophagy in homeostasis, activation, and inflammatory diseases. Front Immunol 9: 1801.

Chatterjee, T., R. Pattanayak, A. Ukil, S. Chowdhury, et al. 2019. Autophagy protects peripheral blood mononuclear cells against inflammation, oxidative and nitrosative stress in diabetic dyslipidemia. Free Radic Biol Med 143: 309–323.

Chen, X.L., Y. Wang, W.W. Peng, Y.J. Zheng, et al. 2018. Effects of interleukin-6 and IL-6/AMPK signaling pathway on MB and astrocytes viability under experimental septic condition. Int Immunopharmacol 59: 287–294.

Deretic, V. and B. Levine. 2018. ATG balances inflammation in innate immunity. Autophagy. 14: 243–251.

Forrester, S.J., D.S, Kikuchi, M.S. Hernandes, Q. Xu, et al. 2018. Reactive oxygen species in metabolic and inflammatory signaling. Circ Res 122: 877–902.

Gkikas, I., K. Palikaras and N. Tavernarakis. 2018. The role of mitophagy in innate immunity. Front Immunol 9: 1283.

Harris, J., N. Deen, S. Zamani, M.A. Hasnat. 2018. Mitophagy and the release of inflammatory cytokines. Mitochondrion 41: 2–8.

Hu, M., G. Alitongbieke, Y. Su, H. Zhou, et al. 2018. Moving nuclear receptor Nur77 to damaged mitochondria for clearance by mitophagy. Mol Cell Oncol 5: e1327005.

Karunakaran, I., S. Alam, S. Jayagopi, S.J. Frohberger, et al. 2019. Neural sphingosine 1-phosphate accumulation activates microglia and links impaired ATG and inflammation. Glia 67: 1859–1872.

Kim, Y.H., M.S. Kwak, J.M. Shin and R.A. Hayuningtyas. 2018. Inflachromene inhibits ATG through modulation of Beclin-1 activity. J Cell Sci 131(4): 211201.

Konno, H., I.K. Chinn, D. Hong, J.S. Orange, et al. 2018. Pro-inflammation associated with a gain-of-function mutation (R284S) in the innate immune sensor STING. Cell Rep 23: 1112–1123.

Lee, J. and H.S. Kim. 2019. The role of ATG in eosinophilic airway inflammation. Immune Net 19(1): e5.

Livshits, G. and A. Kalinkovich. 2019. Inflammaging as a common ground for the development and maintenance of sarcopenia, obesity, cardiomyopathy and dysbiosis. Ageing Res Rev 11: 100980.

Ma, Y., Z. Huang, Z. Zhou, X. He, et al. 2019. A novel antioxidant mito-tempol inhibits ox-LDL-induced foam cell formation through restoration of ATG flux. Free Radic Biol Med 129: 463–472.

Maurel, M., J. Obacz, T. Avril, Y.P. Ding, et al. 2019. Control of anterior GRadient 2 (AGR2) dimerization links endoplasmic reticulum proteostasis to inflammation. EMBO Mol Med 11: e10120.

McWherter, C., Y.J. Choi, R.L. Serrano, S.K. Mahata, et al. 2018. Arhalofenate acid inhibits monosodium urate crystal-induced inflammatory responses through activation of AMP-activated protein kinase (AMPK) signaling. Arthritis Res Ther 20: 204.

Mehto, S., S. Chauhan, K.K. Jena, N.R. Chauhan, et al. 2019. IRGM restrains NLRP3 IS activation by mediating its SQSTM1/p62-dependent selective ATG. Autophagy (9): 1645–1647.

Miao, J., Y. Benomar, S. Al-Rifai, G. Poizat, et al. 2018. Resistin inhibits neuronal ATG through toll-like receptor 4. J Endocrinol 238: 77–89.

Muhammad, I., X, Wang, S. Li, R. Li, et al. 2018. Curcumin confers hepatoprotection against AFB1-induced toxicity via activating ATG and ameliorating inflammation involving Nrf2/HO-1 signaling pathway. Mol Biol Rep 45: 1775–1785.

Ojha, C.R., M. Rodriguez, M.K.M. Karuppan, J. Lapierre, et al. 2019. Toll-like receptor 3 regulates Zika virus infection and associated host inflammatory response in primary human astrocytes. PLoS One 14: e0208543.

Onnis, A., V. Cianfanelli, C. Cassioli, D. Samardzic, et al. 2018. The pro-oxidant adaptor p66SHC promotes B cell MTG by disrupting mitochondrial integrity and recruiting LC3-II. Autophagy 14: 2117–2138.

Orsini, M., S. Chateauvieux, J. Rhim, A. Gaigneaux, et al. 2019. Sphingolipid-mediated inflammatory signaling leading to ATG inhibition converts erythropoiesis to myelopoiesis in human hematopoietic stem/progenitor cells. Cell Death Differ 26: 1796–1812.

Pascall, J.C., L.M.C. Webb, E.L. Eskelinen, S. Innocentin, et al. 2018. GIMAP6 is required for T cell maintenance and efficient ATG in mice. PLoS One 13: e0196504.

Picca, A., A.M.S. Lezza, C. Leeuwenburgh, V. Pesce, et al. 2018. Circulating mitochondrial DNA at the crossroads of mitochondrial dysfunction and inflammation during aging and muscle wasting disorders. Rejuvenation Res 21: 350–359.

Piippo, N., E. Korhonen, M. Hytti, K. Kinnunen, et al. 2018. Oxidative stress is the principal contributor to IS activation in retinal pigment epithelium cells with defunct proteasomes and ATG. Cell Physiol Biochem 49: 359–367.

Sandoval, II., S. Kodali and J. Wang. 2018. Regulation of B cell fate, survival, and function by mitochondria and ATG. Mitochondrion 41: 58–65.

Sato, S., T. Norikura and Y. Mukai. 2019. Maternal quercetin intake during lactation attenuates renal inflammation and modulates autophagy flux in high-fructose-diet-fed female rat offspring exposed to maternal malnutrition. Food Funct 10: 5018–5031.

Sliter, D.A., J. Martinez, L. Hao, X. Chen, et al. 2018. Parkin and PINK1 mitigate STING-induced inflammation. Nature 561: 258–262.

Stocks, C.J., M.A. Schembri, M.J. Sweet and R. Kapetanovic. 2018. For when bacterial infections persist: Toll-like receptor-inducible direct antimicrobial pathways in macrophages. J Leukoc Biol 103: 35–51.

Takahama, M., S. Akira and T. Saitoh. 2018. Autophagy limits activation of the inflammasomes. Immunol Rev 281: 62–73.

Toshihiko, A., K. Unuma and K. Uemura. 2017. Emerging roles of mitochondria and autophagy in liver injury during sepsis. Cell Stress 1: 79–89.

Wong, W.T., L.H. Li, Y.K. Rao, S.P. Yang, et al. 2018. Repositioning of the β-Blocker carvedilol as a novel ATG inducer that inhibits the NLRP3 IS. Front Immunol 9: 1920.

Yang, Q.B., Y.L. He, X.W. Zhong, W.G. Xie, et al. 2019. Resveratrol ameliorates gouty inflammation via upregulation of sirtuin 1 to promote ATG in gout patients. Inflammopharmacology 27: 47–56.

Yin, H., Q. Guo, X. Li, T. Tang, et al. 2018. Curcumin suppresses IL-1β secretion and prevents inflammation through inhibition of the NLRP3 IS. J Immunol 200: 2835–2846.

Yu, J., M. Liu, L. Zhu, S. Zhu, et al. 2018. The expression of interferon regulatory factor 8 in human periapical lesions. J Endod 44: 1276–1282.

Zhang, X., J. Du, Z. Guo, J. Yu, et al. 2018. Efficient near infrared light triggered nitric oxide release nanocomposites for sensitizing mild photothermal therapy. Adv Sci 6: 1801122.

Zhao, Y., S. Huang, J. Liu, X. Wu, et al. 2018. MTG contributes to the pathogenesis of inflammatory diseases. Inflammation 41: 1590–1600.

29

Charnolophagy in Cancer (A)

INTRODUCTION

In 1920, Otto Warburg observed that certain tumors display a metabolic shift towards glycolysis. This is referred to as the "Warburg effect", in which cancer cells produce energy via the conversion of glucose into lactate, even in the presence of O_2 (*aerobic glycolysis*). Initially, Warburg attributed this metabolic shift to mitochondrial dysfunction. Further studies showed that the hyper-proliferation in cancer cells is due to an overdrive in glycolysis (called a glycolytic shift), which leads to a decrease in O/P and mitochondrial density. As a consequence of the Warburg effect, cancer cells would produce large amounts of lactate, which is released to the extracellular environment to cause reduction in the extracellular pH. This micro-environmental acidification can lead to cellular stress, which in turn leads to CP/ATG, induced in response to DPCI including nutrient depletion, hypoxia, microbial infections, and oncogenes. CP/ATG suppresses tumorigenesis by inhibiting cancer-cell survival by inducing cell death, and facilitates tumorigenesis by promoting cancer-cell proliferation and tumor growth. Recently, scientists have focused on the mechanism of ATG in cancer. ATG is controlled by several proteins and depends on tumor type and stage. A multifaceted role of CP/ATG and microenvironment was assigned to cancer induction/repression. Folkerts et al. (2019) provided an overview of the facets of ATG in cancer cells and nonmalignant cells. ATG in fibroblasts induces tumorigenesis by supplying nutrients to cancer cells, whereas, in immune cells, it contributes to tumor-localized immune responses and regulates antigen presentation to and by immune cells among others. ATG also regulates T and NK cell activity and is required for T-cell memory responses. Thus, ATG has a multifaceted role that may facilitate tumorigenesis or support anticancer immune responses, which should be considered while designing CP/ATG-based cancer theranostics. Mechanisms by which ATG promotes cancer include the inhibition of the p53 tumor suppressor protein and sustain the metabolic function of mitochondria. p53 exerts cell responses to a variety of stresses by regulating cell cycle, apoptosis, ATG, and DNA damage. p53 in ATG-associated cell death can be induced by the activation of the photosensitizers. ATG facilitates cancer cell survival in metabolic stress and may confer MDR and radio resistance. The p53-dependent and -independent responses of cells challenged by photosensitization have been demonstrated. In the microenvironment of cancer cells, there is an increase in HIF-1A, which promotes Bnip-3 expression (Pavlides et al. 2012). ATG and mitochondrial metabolism are altered in chronic myeloid leukemia, whereas HUWE1 E3 ligase promotes PINK1/Parkin-independent CP by regulating AMBRA1 activation via IKKα, and

Artesunate-induced CP/ATG alters cellular redox status. CP/ATG demonstrates a dual response in the development of HCC. The inhibition of PI3K/mTOR increased the sensitivity of HCC cells to Cisplatin via interference with the mitochondrial-lysosomal crosstalk. A dual role of CP/ATG was also demonstrated in Docetaxel-sensitivity in prostate cancer cells and glucose-starvation-induced resistance to Metformin through the elevation of mitochondrial MDR-protein-1. Recently, Motegi et al. (2019) reported that Atg5 could be a differential biomarker between dermatofibrosarcoma protuberans and dermatofibroma. Abdel-Maksoud et al. (2019) described recent advances regarding the mechanism that involves mTOR in cancer, NDDs, and aging. The chemical and biological properties of small molecules that function as mTOR kinase inhibitors, including ATP-competitive inhibitors and dual mTOR/PI3K inhibitors, were highlighted. The mTOR regulates transcription, cell growth, and CP/ATG. Overstimulation of mTOR on the OMM by its ligands, amino acids, sugars, and/or growth factors trigger cancer and NDDs. Despite the development of selective BCR-ABL-targeting TK inhibitors (TKIs) transforming the management of chronic myeloid leukemia (CML), resistant leukemic stem cells (LSCs) persist after TKI treatment and present a serious challenge in its cure. Myelodysplastic syndromes (MDS) are a heterogeneous group of clonal stem cell disorders characterized by cytopenia and dysplasia. Anemia is the most common symptom in patients with MDS. Jiang et al. (2019) investigated CP dysregulation in erythroid precursors of MDS patients. NIX-mediated CP was impaired in bone-marrow-nucleated RBCs (NRBC) of MDS patients, associated with damaged mitochondria and ROS overproduction, leading to ineffective erythropoiesis and apoptosis through CBMP. The amount of mitochondria in GlycoA$^+$ NRBC positively correlated with the number of ring sideroblasts in bone marrow samples. The ATG-associated marker LC3B in GlycoA$^+$ NRBC had a positive correlation with hemoglobin (Hb), and the amount of mitochondria in GlycoA$^+$ NRBC had a negative correlation with Hb in high-risk MDS patients, indicating the involvement of CP/ATG in the pathogenesis of anemia associated with MDS, which could be utilized for the TSE-EBPT of these patients.

Dżugan et al. (2018) evaluated ultrastructural changes in the kidney and liver of chicken embryos exposed *in ovo* to Cd. The embryonated eggs were injected on the fourth day of incubation with Cd at the dose of 0, 2, 4, and 8 μg/egg (80 eggs/group), respectively. The samples of kidney and liver tissues were collected from embryos on the 14th and 18th days of incubation (E14 and E18) and on the hatching day (D1). Hepatocytes responded to damage caused by Cd toxicity with a disturbance in the mitochondria and lysososmes, while glomerular cells reacted with an increased proliferation of peroxisomes depending on the dose of Cd, stage of embryogenesis, and cell type. Baquero et al. (2018) focused on ATG and mitochondrial metabolism for LSCs' quiescence and survival, respectively. They discussed the theranostic potential of ATG and inhibition of mitochondrial metabolism to eliminate CML cells in patients where the resistance to TKI is driven by BCR-ABL-independent mechanism(s). Since cancer stem cells reside in their niches, these are not easily assessed by conventional therapeutic regimens and exhibit enhanced proliferation. These cells proliferate and are destroyed simultaneously due to efficient CP/ATG, which render them resistant to chemotherapy, radiotherapy, and surgery. Endogenously synthesized antioxidants such as glutathione, MTs, and HSPs facilitate MDR in cancer stem cells. Currently, it is challenging to exactly pinpoint and eradicate each and every cancer stem cell from the human body; hence, the great risk of cancer. Therefore, early cancer stem cell-specific CB formation, CP inhibition, CS destabilization, CS endocytosis/exocytosis, and CBMP induction is proposed to attenuate their MB by developing novel DSST-CPTs for the TSE-EBPT of MDR malignancies.

This chapter emphasizes the pathophysiological significance of CP during the acute and chronic phase of MDR in cancer involving concomitant CS destabilization, cell proliferation, apoptosis, and necrosis. It also focuses on the strategies to prevent/treat breast cancer, pancreatic cancer, and hepatic carcinoma by developing CBMP-based TSE-EBPT-CPTs.

Cancer Cell Mitochondria

Dysfunctional mitochondria enhance cancer cell proliferation, reduce apoptosis, and enhance MDR in patients with colorectal cancer, leading to a decrease in the therapeutic response. While cytochrome P450 (CYP)-mediated biosynthesis of arachidonic acid (AA) epoxides promotes tumor growth by driving angiogenesis, the intrinsic functions of cancer cell CYPs are less understood. CYP-derived AA epoxides, called epoxyeicosatrienoic acids (EETs), promote the growth of tumor epithelium. In cancer cells, CYP AA epoxygenase enzymes are associated with STAT3, mTOR signaling, and are localized in mitochondria to promote the ETC. Guo et al. (2018) found that Metformin inhibits CYP AA epoxygenase activity. This finding suggests that potent biguanides can be developed to target tumor growth. The biguanide inhibition of EET synthesis suppressed STAT3 and mTOR pathways, as well as the ETC. The convergence of biguanide activity and eicosanoids in cancer has shown a novel strategy to attack cancer metabolism and provides hope for improved treatments. Hence, inhibition of EET-mediated cancer metabolism and angiogenesis provides a dual approach for targeted cancer theranostics. Meyer et al. (2018) reported that AT 101 ([-]-Gossypol), a natural compound from cotton seeds, induced ACD in glioma cells as confirmed by the CRISPR/Cas9 knockout of Atg5 that rescued cell survival following AT 101 treatment. The proteomic analysis of AT 101-treated U87MG and U343 glioma cells revealed a decrease in mitochondrial protein clusters, whereas HMOX1 (heme oxygenase 1) was upregulated. AT 101 triggered mitochondrial membrane depolarization, engulfment of mitochondria within APSs, and a reduction of mitochondria and proteins that did not depend on the presence of BAX and BAK1. The AT 101-induced reduction of mitochondria could be reversed by inhibiting ATG with Wortmannin, Bafilomycin A_1, and CQ. The silencing of HMOX1 and the MTG receptors, Bnip-3 and BNIP3L, attenuated AT 101-dependent MTG and cell death, suggesting that early mitochondrial dysfunction and HMOX1 over-activation trigger lethal CP, which contributes to the cell killing effects of AT 101 in glioma.

Dhar et al. (2018) showed that DNA polymerase gamma (Polγ) deficiency activates a pro-survival ATG response via ROS and mTORC2 signaling. In keratinocytes, Polγ deficiency caused metabolic adaptation that triggered the cytosolic sensing of energy demand for survival. The knockdown of Polγ caused mitochondrial stress, CMB, enhanced glycolysis, ATG-associated genes, Akt phosphorylation, and cell proliferation. The deficiency of Polγ activated mTORC2 formation to increase ATG and cell proliferation, and knocking down Rictor abrogated these responses. Overexpression of Rictor, but not Raptor, reactivated ATG in Polγ-deficient cells. Inhibition of ROS scavengers abolished ATG and cell proliferation, suggesting Rictor as a crucial link between mitochondrial stress, ROS, and ATG. Huang et al. (2018a) found that in a conditioned medium, the release of HMGB1 from dying cells by chemotherapeutic drugs and resistant cells triggered Drp-1 phosphorylation via its receptor for advanced glycation end product (RAGE), which signaled ERK1/2 activation to phosphorylate Drp-1 at residue S616, triggering ATG for MDR and regrowth in the surviving cancer cells. Suppression of Drp-1 phosphorylation by the HMGB1 inhibitor and RAGE blocker enhanced sensitivity to the chemotherapeutic treatment by inhibiting ATG. Patients with high phospho-Drp-1[Ser616] were associated with a high risk for developing tumor relapse, poor five-year disease-free survival (DFS) and five-year overall survival after neoadjuvant chemo-radiotherapy (neoCRT) in advanced rectal cancer. Patients with RAGE-G82S polymorphism (rs2070600) were associated with high phospho-Drp-1[Ser616] within the tumor microenvironment, suggesting that the release of HMGB1 from dying cancer cells enhances MDR and regrowth via RAGE-mediated ERK/Drp-1 phosphorylation. Park et al. (2018) reported that an inhibitor of Hsp70, Apoptozole (Az), is translocated into lysosomes of cancer cells where it induces LMP, thereby promoting lysosome-mediated apoptosis. Az impairs ATG in cancer cells by disrupting the lysosomal function. However, the Az-triphenylphosphonium conjugate, Az-TPP-O3, localized mainly to the mitochondria of cancer cells where it inhibited the mortalin-p53 interaction and induced OMM permeabilization, leading to mitochondria-mediated apoptosis. Unlike Az, Az-TPP-O3 did not have an effect on ATG in cancer cells, indicating that inhibitors of lysosomal Hsp70 and mitochondrial mortalin enhance cancer cell death via different mechanisms. Hence, studies aimed at determining subcellular locations and functions of small-molecule modulators will provide a deeper understanding of their modes of action in cells.

CP/ATG in Breast Cancer

There is now evidence that the induction of ATG promotes survival of cancer cells. Zhao et al. (2019) studied the antitumor effects of arsenic disulfide (As2S2) on the proliferative, survival, and migratory ability of human BC MCF-7 and MDA-MB-231 cells, and its molecular mechanisms, with an emphasis on cell cycle arrest, apoptosis, ATG, and ROS generation. As2S2 inhibited the viability, survival, and migration of BC cells. As2S2 induced cell cycle arrest at the G2/M phase in the two BC cell lines by regulating the expression of cyclin B1 and cell division cycle protein 2. As2S2 induced apoptosis by activating the expression of pro-apoptotic proteins, caspase-7 and -8, and Bcl-2-associated X protein/Bcl-2 ratio, and decreased the expression of anti-apoptotic B-cell lymphoma. As2S2 stimulated the accumulation of LC3-II and increased the LC3-II/LC3-I ratio, indicating the occurrence of ATG. As2S2 treatment also inhibited the MMP-9 expression, but increased ROS, which may assist in alleviating metastasis and attenuating the progression of BC, suggesting that As2S2 inhibits the progression of BC cells through the regulation of cell cycle arrest, ROS generation, MMP-9 signaling, ATG, and apoptosis.

The protein XIAP possesses a critical role in promoting cell survival and maintaining cellular homeostasis. Elevated XIAP expression has been associated with malignancy, poor prognosis, and MDR. Schuetz et al. (2019) tested 206 SNPs in 54 genes related to inflammation, apoptosis, and ATG in a population BC study of women of European (658 cases and 795 controls) and East Asian (262 cases and 127 controls) descent. Logistic regression was used to estimate odds ratios for BC risk, and case-only analysis was implemented to compare BC subtypes (defined by ER/PR/HER2 status), with adjustment for confounders. They assessed statistical interactions between the SNPs and lifestyle factors (smoking status, physical activity, and BMI). Although no SNP was associated with BC risk among women of European descent, they found evidence for an association among East Asians for rs1800925 (IL-13) and BC risk, which remained significant after multiple testing corrections. This association was replicated in a meta-analysis of 4305 cases and 4194 controls in the *Shanghai BC Genetics Study*. An interaction between rs7874234 (TSC1) and physical activity among women of East Asian descent was noticed. Huang et al. (2019) examined the expression of XIAP and p62, two critical mediators of ATG, in breast and colon cancer. They observed a negative correlation between XIAP and p62 expression in normal and cancer tissues of breast and colon, and the ratio of XIAP and p62 expression determined the cancer phenotype. XIAP interacted with p62 and XIAP depletion increased the expression of p62. XIAP functioned as ubiquitination E3 ligase towards p62 and suppressed p62 expression through ubiquitin-proteasomal degradation. XIAP enhanced cancer cell proliferation, viability, and colony formation via the suppression of p62. XIAP-enhanced tumor growth was dependent on the depletion of p62. Hence, these investigators delineated a novel mechanism by which XIAP contributes to development and the progression of breast and colon carcinoma. In search of novel γ-secretase inhibitors (GSIs), Das et al. (2019a) screened triazole-based compounds to bind γ-secretase and observed that 3-(3′4′,5′-trimethoxyphenyl)-5-(*N*-methyl-3′-indolyl)-1,2,4-triazole compound (NMK-T-057) can bind to γ-secretase complex. NMK-T-057 inhibited proliferation, colony-forming ability, and motility in various BC cells such as MDA-MB-231, MDA-MB-468, 4T1 (triple-negative cells), and MCF-7 (estrogen receptor (ER)/progesterone receptor (PR)-positive cell line) with negligible cytotoxicity in noncancerous cells (MCF-10A and peripheral blood mononuclear cells). The induction of apoptosis and inhibition of epithelial-to-mesenchymal transition (EMT) and stem-ness were also observed in NMK-T-057-treated BC cells. The affinity of NMK-T-057 toward γ-secretase was validated by a fluorescence-based γ-secretase activity assay, which confirmed the inhibition of γ-secretase activity in NMK-T-057-treated BC cells. NMK-T-057-induced ATG in BC cells led to apoptosis. NMK-T-057 inhibited tumor progression in a 4T1-BALB/c mouse model; hence, it could be a potential drug candidate for BC as it can trigger ATG-mediated cell death by inhibiting γ-secretase-mediated activation of Notch signaling. Recently, Das et al. (2019b) highlighted that although estrogen receptor (ER) antagonist, tamoxifen is used routinely for the treatment of the ER-positive BC; the resistance to tamoxifen obstructs its successful treatment. So, there is a dire need to discover a novel theranostic target(s) for successful treatment of BC. These investigators demonstrated that acquired tamoxifen-resistant BC cell lines MCF-7 (MCF-7/ TAM-R) and T47D (T47D/TAM-R) exhibit higher apoptotic resistance accompanied with induction of pro-survival ATG compared to their parental cells. Tamoxifen resistance was associated with reduced ATP synthesis and induction of glycolytic pathways, leading to induced CP/ATG to meet the energy requirements. Lactate dehydrogenase-A (LDHA); one of the key molecules of glycolysis in association with Beclin-1 induced pro-survival CP/ATG in tamoxifen-resistant BC, whereas, pharmacological and genetic inhibition of LDHA reduced the pro-survival CP/ATG, with the restoration of apoptosis and reverting back the EMT like phenomena observed in tamoxifen-resistant BC. Hence, targeting LDHA offers a novel strategy to interrupt CP/ATG and tamoxifen resistance in BC

It is known that the extracellular matrix (ECM) affects cancer cell characteristics. Inability of normal epithelial cells to attach to the ECM induces anoikis. Cancer cells are anoikis-resistant, a prerequisite for their metastasis. Komemi et al. (2019) demonstrated that the placenta manipulates its surrounding ECM to prevent BC cells' (BCCL) attachment and induce their motility and aggregation. Although BC during pregnancy is often advanced, metastasis to the placenta is rarely observed. Placental inter-villous space provides suitable conditions for cancer cell arrival. Afore-mentioned (Komemi et al. 2019) investigators analyzed the effect of placental ECM on BCCL survival pathways and drug resistance. A microarray analysis suggested the activation of the NF-κB and stress response pathways. The placenta-conditioned ECM induced ATG in ERα + BCCL, inactivated the NF-κB inhibitor (IκB), and increased integrin α5 in the BCCL. The ATG mediated MCF-7 and T47D migration and the placental ECM-BCCL interactions reduced the BCCL sensitivity to Taxol. They also demonstrated that by using siRNA, the integrin α5 was responsible for the MCF-7 ATG and suggested this molecule as a suitable theranostic target.

The overexpression of Jumonji domain-containing 6 (JMJD6) has been associated with more aggressive BC characteristics. Liu et al. (2019) demonstrated that JMJD6 has TK activity and can utilize ATP and GTP as phosphate donors to phosphorylate Y39 of histone H2A.X (H2A.X^{Y39ph}). High JMJD6 levels promoted ATG in TNBC cells by regulating the expression of ATG-related genes. The JMJD6-H2A.X^{Y39ph} axis promoted TNBC cell growth via the ATG pathway. The concomitant inhibition of the JMJD6 kinase and ATG decreased TNBC growth, suggesting an effective strategy for TNBC treatment. Guo et al. (2019) discovered that excessive GSK-3β expression in BC tissues was correlated with worse prognosis. Progression of BC was suppressed by GSK-3β knockdown. Suppression of GSK-3β led to a decrease in ATP generation, associated with the stimulation of AMPK in T47D cells. The activation of AMPK, a typical sign of ATG stimulation, was triggered after the suppression of the GSK-3β function, in parallel with the increased generation of LC3 II, indicating that GSK-3β participates in regulation of migration as well as stimulation of ATG through activation of the AMPK pathway. This suggested that GSK-3β has potential as a predictor of clinical outcome and as a target for BC therapy. Romero et al. (2019) highlighted the role of microRNAs in the modulation of ATG in BC. They also summarized how TRAIL-mediated signaling and ATG operated in BC cells. The Akt/mTOR pathway is an upstream activator of ATG and is regulated by ATG-related genes signaling cascade. Wide ranging cell signaling pathways and non-coding RNAs play essential roles in ATG regulation. Since ATG behaved both as a cell death and a cell survival mechanism, it opened new horizons for a detailed analysis of cell type and context-dependent behavior in different types of cancers. Since ATG is primarily a mechanism to keep the cells alive, it may protect BC cells in stress conditions such as starvation and hypoxia. Hence, ATG is implicated in metastasis and MDR. TNBCs are more aggressive than other BC subtypes and lack effective theranostic options. Unraveling marker events of TNBCs may provide novel directions for targeted TNBC therapy. Zóia et al. (2019) reported that Annexin A1 (AnxA1) and Cathepsin D (CatD) are highly expressed in MDA-MB-231 (TNBC lineage), compared to MCF-10A and MCF-7. Since the proposed concept was that CatD has pro-tumorigenic activity associated with its ability to cleave AnxA1 (generating a 35.5 KDa fragment), they explored this mechanism using the inhibitor of CatD, Pepstatin A (PepA). Fourier Transform Infrared (FTIR) spectroscopy demonstrated that PepA inhibits CatD activity by occupying its active site; the OH bond from PepA interacts with a CO bond from carboxylic acids of CatD catalytic aspartate dyad, favoring the deprotonation of Asp[33] inhibiting CatD. Treatment of MDA-MB-231 cells with PepA induced ATG and apoptosis, while reducing the proliferation, invasion, and migration. *In silico* molecular docking demonstrated that catalytic inhibition comprises Asp[231] protonated and Asp[33] deprotonated, confirming all functional results. These findings elucidated critical CatD activity in the TNBC cell trough AnxA1 cleavage, indicating the inhibition of CatD as a possible strategy for TNBC treatment.

A study determined the effects of the overexpression of ATG3 on ATG and Salinomycin-induced apoptosis in BC cells. The ectonucleotidase CD73 is a cell surface enzyme involved in immunosuppression. Qiao et al. (2019) constructed the recombinant plasmid pET28a-CD73 and the CD73 protein was overexpressed in *E. coli* as an inclusion body that was subjected to refolding. The anti-CD73 monoclonal antibody (3F7) was obtained by hybridoma technology. The antibody subtype was identified as IgG2a with an affinity constant of 5.75 nM. The CD73 protein was located in the cytoplasm and distributed on the surface of TNB cancer cells, MDA-MB-231 and MDA-MB-468. The level of CD73 protein was associated with the survival rate. Although the anti-CD73 antibody could not inhibit tumor cell growth, it could enhance the cytotoxic effect of Dox to TNBC cells. The anti-CD73 mAb inhibited cell migration and invasion in both human TNB cancer and mouse 4T1 cell lines. Both the LC3-I/LC3-II ratio and p62 protein levels increased, indicating that the blockage of CD73 inhibits ATG, and cell migration and invasion are restored by Rapamycin. *In vivo*, anti-CD73 mAb inhibited the lung metastasis of 4T1 cells in a mouse xenograft model. Hence, this novel anti-CD73 antibody could be developed as an adjuvant drug for TNBC therapy and can be useful in tumor diagnosis. Li et al. (2019a) used the lentivirus approach to establish a BC cell line with stable overexpression of ATG3. Using the Akt/mTOR agonists, SC79 and MHY1485, they analyzed the effect of the Akt/mTOR signal pathway activation on ATG3-overexpression-induced ATG. ATG3 overexpression in MCF-7 cells promoted ATG, inhibited the Akt/mTOR signaling pathway, compromised Salinomycin-induced apoptosis, caused the reduction of pro-apoptotic proteins cleaved-caspase 3 and Bax, and enhanced the expression of the anti-apoptotic protein Bcl-2, suggesting that ATG3 overexpression promotes ATG by inhibiting the Akt/mTOR signaling pathway to decrease Salinomycin-induced apoptosis in MCF-7 cells, suggesting that ATG induction is one of the mechanisms of MDR in BC cells. Sirtuin-1 (SIRT1) is a class-III histone deacetylase (HDAC), an NAD+-dependent enzyme involved in gene regulation, genome stability maintenance, apoptosis, ATG, senescence, proliferation, aging, and tumorigenesis. Alves-Fernandes and Jasiulionis (2019) described the recent findings on the interaction among SIRT1, oxidative stress, and DNA repair machinery and its impact on normal and cancer cells. SIRT1 has a key role in the epigenetic regulation of tissue homeostasis and many diseases by de-acetylating both histone and non-histone targets. Different studies have shown the implications of SIRT1 as both a tumor suppressor and tumor promoter. However, this contradictory role is determined by the cell type and SIRT1 localization. SIRT1 upregulation has been demonstrated in AM, primary colon, prostate, melanoma, and non-melanoma skin cancers, while SIRT1 downregulation has been described in BC and HCC. Xu et al. (2019) performed transcriptome sequencing of 33 breast specimens to identify Ai-lncRNA EGOT. They also investigated the role of EGOT in the regulation of Paclitaxel sensitivity. The mechanism of EGOT-enhancing ATG sensitized Paclitaxel cytotoxicity via upregulation of ITPR1 expression by RNA-RNA and RNA-protein interactions was also investigated. Breast specimens in the cohort, TCGA and ICGC were applied to validate the role of EGOT in enhancing Paclitaxel sensitivity. EGOT enhanced APS accumulation via the upregulation of ITPR1 expression, thereby sensitizing cells to Paclitaxel toxicity. Although, EGOT upregulated ITPR1 levels via formation of a pre-ITPR1/EGOT dsRNA that induced pre-ITPR1 accumulation to increase ITPR1 protein expression in cis, EGOT recruited hnRNPH1 to enhance the alternative splicing of pre-ITPR1 in trans via two binding motifs in the EGOT segment 2 (324–645 nucleotides) in exon 1. EGOT is transcriptionally regulated by stress conditions. EGOT expression enhanced Paclitaxel sensitivity via assessment of BC specimens. Hence, regulation of EGOT may be a novel strategy for enhancing Paclitaxel sensitivity in BC therapy.

Glucose-6-phospate dehydrogenase (G6PD) is the limiting enzyme of the pentose phosphate pathway (PPP) correlated to cancer progression and drug resistance. G6PD inhibition leads to ERS being associated with ATG deregulation. The latter can be induced by target-based agents such as Lapatinib, an anti-HER2 TK inhibitor (TKI) mostly used in BC treatment. It was investigated whether G6PD inhibition causes ATG alteration, which can potentiate the Lapatinib effect on cancer cells (Mele et al. 2019). Immunofluorescence and flow cytometry for LC3B and lysosomes trackers were used to study ATG in cells treated with Lapatinib and/or G6PD inhibitors (Polydatin). Immunoblots for LC3B and p62 were performed to confirm ATG flux together with puncta and co-localization studies. They generated a cell line overexpressing G6PD and performed synergism studies on cell growth inhibition induced by Lapatinib and Polydatin. Synergism was validated with apoptosis analysis by Annexin V/PI staining in the presence or absence of ATG blockers. Inhibition of G6PD-induced ERS was responsible for the deregulation of ATG flux. The G6PD blockade increased mTOR-independent APSs formation. Cells engineered to overexpress G6PD became resilient to ATG and resistant to Lapatinib, whereas, G6PD inhibition increased the Lapatinib-induced cytotoxic effect on BC cells, while ATG blockade abolished this effect. *In silico* studies showed a significant correlation between G6PD expression and tumor relapse/resistance in patients. Hence, ATG and PPP are crucial in TKI resistance, and highlight the vulnerability of BC cells, where impairment in metabolic pathways and ATG could be used to reinforce TKI efficacy in BC treatment.

Tetrandrine is a bisbenzylisoquinoline alkaloid which exhibits anticancer activity in different cancers. Chandrasheka et al. (2019) evaluated the cytotoxic effect of Tetrandrine isolated from Cyclea peltata on pancreatic (PANC-1) and BC (MDA-MB-231) cells to understand its role on ROS generation and caspase activation. A cytotoxic effect of Tetradrine was observed on both MDA-MB-231 and PANC-1 cells. The treatment of MDA-MB-231 and PANC-1 cells with Tetrandrine showed the shrunken cytoplasm and damaged cell membrane. Tetrandrine enhanced ROS production and increased caspase-8, -9, and -3 activities, confirming the apoptosis of cells through both death receptor and caspase activation. Hence, the ROS-mediated caspase activation pathway may be targeted with the use of Tetrandrine to treat BC and PC. Chen et al. (2019) explored the mechanisms underlying the effects of Apoptin using recombinant adenoviruses expressing Apoptin. During the early stage of Apoptin stimulation (6 and 12 hrs), the expression of ATG pathway-associated proteins–Beclin-1, LC3, ATG-related 4B cysteine peptidase and ATG-related 5–were increased, suggesting that Apoptin upregulated ATG in MCF-7 cells. After 12 hrs of Apoptin stimulation, the apoptosis-associated protein was decreased, suggesting that apoptosis may be inhibited, indicating that Apoptin enhances ATG and inhibits apoptosis in MCF-7 cells at the early stage. Apoptin-induced cell death may involve both ATG and apoptosis. The induction of ATG may inhibit apoptosis, whereas apoptosis may inhibit ATG; however, occasionally both pathways operate simultaneously and involve Apoptin. Hence, Apoptin associated selection between cell survival and death may provide a theranostic strategy for BC.

Endocrine therapy is an essential component in the treatment of hormone receptor (HR)-positive BC. The addition of metronomic chemotherapy has been shown to improve therapeutic effects. Ueno et al. (2019) studied ATG-related markers, Beclin-1 and LC3, and apoptosis-related markers, TUNEL and M30, in pre- and post-treatment cancer tissues from a multicenter neoadjuvant trial, JBCRG-07, in which oral Cyclophosphamide plus Latrozole were administered to postmenopausal patients with HR-positive BC. Changes in the levels of markers were compared with those following neoadjuvant endocrine therapy according to their clinical response. Apoptosis, in addition to ATG-related markers, increased following metronomic CET and this increase was associated with a clinical response. Following endocrine therapy, the levels of apoptosis-related markers did not increase regardless of clinical response, whereas the ATG-related markers increased. Levels of the apoptosis-related marker, M30, decreased in responders of endocrine therapy, suggesting that the induction of apoptosis by metronomic CET was involved in the improved clinical outcome compared with endocrine therapy. Hence, metronomic CET induced a different cellular reaction from that of endocrine therapy, including the induction of apoptosis, which may contribute to improved efficacy compared with endocrine therapy alone. Velloso et al. (2019) undertook a global proteome profiling of TNBC-derived cells, ectopically expressing each one of these NOD receptors. They identified a total of 95 and 58 differentially regulated proteins in NOD1- and NOD2-overexpressing cells, respectively, and used bioinformatics to identify enriched molecular signatures aiming to integrate the differentially regulated proteins into functional networks. Overexpression of both NOD1 and NOD2 may disrupt immune-related pathways, particularly NF-κB and MAPK signaling cascades. Moreover, overexpression of either of these receptors may affect several stress response and protein degradation systems, such as ATG and the ubiquitin-proteasome complex. Several proteins associated to cellular adhesion and migration were also affected in these NOD-overexpressing cells. The proteomic analyses shed a new light on the molecular pathways that may be modulating tumorigenesis via NOD1 and NOD2 signaling in TNBC. Up- and downregulation of several proteins associated with the inflammation and stress response pathways may promote the activation of protein degradation systems, as well as modulate the cell cycle and cellular adhesion proteins. These signals modulated cell proliferation and migration via the NF-κB, PI3K/Akt/mTOR and MAPK-signaling pathways.

Sun et al. (2019) showed that Ambra1 inhibits Paclitaxel-induced apoptosis in BC cells. Moreover, Bim and mitochondria are key effectors of Ambra1 in this process. Thus, Ambra1 is a protein that makes BC cells MDR to apoptosis by modulating the Bim/mitochondrial pathway. Therefore, Ambra1 may be a potential target for the treatment of BC and CP/ATG can be employed as a theranostic biomarker to evaluate cardiotoxicity in TNBC (Li et al 2019a). ATG/Beclin-1 regulator 1 (Ambra1) is a pro-autophagic protein and plays an important role in the execution of apoptosis. TNBC is highly aggressive and Taxol-based chemoresistance remains a major therapeutic challenge. Verteporfin, a small molecular yes-associated protein 1

(YAP1)-inhibitor, is known as an antitumor drug for TNBC (Li et al 2019b). Over-expression of ATG-related-3 gene induced ATG and inhibited Salinomycin-induced apoptosis in MCF-1 cells (Li et al 2019c) and ATG/Beclin-1 regulator 1 (Ambra-1) a proautophagic protein played an important role in execution of apoptosis. McGrath et al. (2018) reviewed several roles for unfolded protein response (UPR) signaling in breast cancer (including TNBC), highlighting UPR-mediated therapeutic resistance and the potential for targeting the UPR alone or in combination with existing therapies. Accumulation of unfolded or misfolded proteins activates UPR signaling pathway, which acts to relieve ERS and, if remain unsuccessful, can be toxic and may lead to cell death. Prolonged expression of misfolded proteins triggers ERS, which initiates a cascade of reactions to induce UPR. Thus, UPR is a promising target for the development of novel breast cancer treatments. This pathway is activated in response to a disturbance in ER homeostasis but has diverse physiological and disease-specific functions. In breast cancer, UPR signaling promotes a malignant phenotype which can confer tumors with resistance to widely used therapies particularly in TNBC. ERS and the downstream UPR activation lead to changes in the levels and activities of key regulators of cell survival and ATG and this is finalized to restore metabolic homeostasis with the integration of pro-death or/and pro-survival signals. By contrast, the chronic activation of UPR in cancer cells is considered a mechanism of tumor progression. Sisinni et al. (2019) focused on the relationship between ERS, ATG, and apoptosis in human BC and the interplay between the activation of UPR and resistance to anticancer therapies to disclose novel therapeutic scenarios. Shinde et al. (2019) compared a reversible model of epithelial-mesenchymal transition (EMT) induced by TGF-β to a stable mesenchymal phenotype induced by the chronic exposure to the ErbB kinase inhibitor, Lapatinib. Only cells capable of returning to an epithelial phenotype resulted in skeletal metastasis. Gene expression analyses of the two mesenchymal states indicated similar transition expression profiles. A downregulated gene in both datasets was spleen TK (SYK). A similar diminution in mRNA, kinome analyses using a peptide array, and DNA-conjugated peptide substrates showed an increase in SYK activity upon TGF-β-induced EMT only. SYK was present in cytoplasmic RNA processing depots known as P-bodies formed during the onset of EMT, and SYK activity was required for the ATG-mediated clearance of P-bodies during mesenchymal-epithelial transition (MET). The genetic knockout of ATG7 or pharmacologic inhibition of SYK with Fostamatinib prevented P-body clearance and MET, inhibiting metastatic tumor outgrowth, suggesting the assessment of SYK activity as a biomarker for metastatic disease and the use of Fostamatinib to stabilize the latency of disseminated tumor cells. Hence, the inhibition of spleen TK can be utilized as a therapeutic option to limit BC metastasis by promoting systemic tumor dormancy. Beclin-1, as a key regulator of ATG, is associated with cancer cell resistance to chemotherapy. Wu et al. (2019) demonstrated that Paclitaxel suppressed cell viability and Beclin-1 expression in BT-474 BC cells. The knockdown of Beclin-1 enhanced BC cell death via the induction of caspase-dependent apoptosis following Paclitaxel treatment. In a BT-474 xenograft model, Paclitaxel achieved the inhibition of tumor growth in the Beclin-1 knockdown group, as compared with the control group. Analysis of the Gene Expression Omnibus datasets revealed a clinical correlation between Beclin-1 levels and the response to Paclitaxel therapy in patients with BC, suggesting that Beclin-1 protects BC cells from apoptotic death. Thus, the inhibition of Beclin-1 may be a novel strategy to improve the effect of Paclitaxel. Beclin-1 may function as a favorable prognostic biomarker for Paclitaxel treatment in patients with BC.

HER2/ErbB2 activation turns on transcriptional processes that induce local invasion and lead to systemic metastasis. Brix et al. (2019) linked ErbB2 activation to invasion via ErbB2-induced, SUMO-directed phosphorylation of a single serine residue, S27, of the transcription factor myeloid zinc finger-1 (MZF1). Utilizing an antibody against MZF1-pS27, they showed that the phosphorylation of S27 correlates with high-level expression of ErbB2 in primary invasive

BC. Phosphorylation of MZF1-S27 is an early response to ErbB2 activation and resulted in increased transcriptional activity of MZF1. It was needed for the ErbB2-induced expression of MZF1 target genes, CTSB and PRKCA, and invasion of single-cells from ErbB2-expressing BC spheroids. The phosphorylation of MZF1-S27 was preceded by poly-SUMOylation of K23, which could make S27 accessible to efficient phosphorylation by PAK4, suggesting a mechanism where phosphorylation of MZF1-S27 triggers MZF1 dissociation from its transcriptional repressors such as the CCCTC-binding factor (CTCF). In addition, SAHA is a class I HDAC/HDAC6 and an ATG co-inhibitor. Lee et al. (2016) found that SAHA is equally effective in targeting cells of different BC subtypes and Tamoxifen sensitivity. The downregulation of survivin plays an important role in SAHA-induced ATG and cell viability reduction in human BC cells. SAHA decreased survivin and XIAP gene transcription, and induced survivin protein acetylation and early nuclear translocation in MCF7 and MDA-MB-231 BC cells. It also reduced survivin and XIAP protein stability through modulating the expression and activation of the 26S proteasome and HSP90. Targeting HDAC3 and HDAC6 by siRNA/pharmacological inhibitors mimicked the effects of SAHA in modulating the acetylation, expression, and nuclear translocation of survivin and induced ATG in MCF7 and MDA-MB-231 cancer cells. Targeting HDAC3 also mimicked the effect of SAHA in upregulating the expression of proteasome, which might lead to the reduced protein stability of survivin in BC cells. This study provided insights into SAHA's molecular mechanism of actions in BC cells and emphasized their regulatory roles in different HDAC isoforms to assist in predicting the mechanism of novel HDAC inhibitors in targeted or combinational therapies. MTs-induced the transcriptional activation of genes by CS in MDR malignant cancer stem cells, which is presented in Fig. 44.

MTs-Induced Transcriptional Activation of Genes by Cancer Stem Cell-Specific CS in MDR Malignant Cells

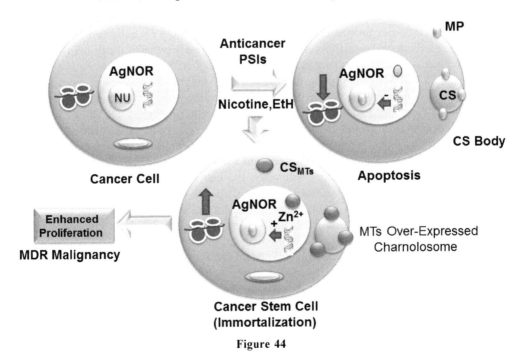

Figure 44

Transcriptional regulation of CP causes tumor suppression, whereas dysregulation augments tumor progression as presented in Fig. 45.

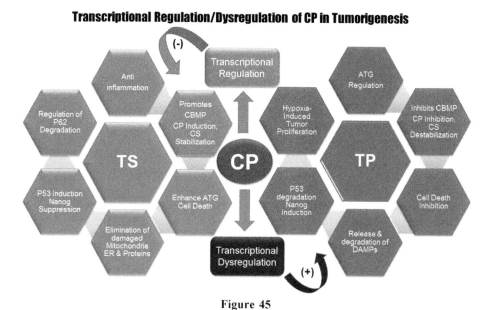

Figure 45

CP in Pancreatic Cancer

Pancreatic cancer (PC) is the leading cause of mortality, with limited theranostic targets. Alterations in ER-related proteostasis may be a potential target for PC therapy. Mitofusin2 (Mfn-2) plays a pivotal role in mitochondrial fusion and adjusting function. Xue et al. (2018) explored the effect of Mfn-2 on biological functions involving ATG in PC. The PC cell line, Aspc-1, was treated with Ad-Mfn-2 overexpression. Immunoblotting, caspase-3 activity, and CCK-8 and ROS assay were used to examine the effects of Mfn-2 on PC ATG, apoptosis, cell proliferation, oxidative stress, and PI3K/Akt/mTOR signaling. The expression of tissue Mfn-2 was detected by immuno-histochemical staining. The survival analysis of Mfn-2 was evaluated by OncoLnc. Mfn-2 improved the expression of LC3-II and Bax and downregulated the expression of p62 and Bcl-2 in PC cells. Mfn-2 inhibited the expression of p-PI3K, p-Akt, and p-mTOR in PC cells. In addition, Mfn-2 inhibited PC cell proliferation and ROS production. The assessment of Kaplan-Meier curves showed that Mfn-2$^-$ PC has a worse prognosis than Mfn-2$^+$ PC, suggesting that Mfn-2 induces CP/ATG of PC by inhibiting the PI3K/Akt/mTOR-signaling pathway. Mfn-2 also influenced the multiple biological functions of PC cells. Hence, Mfn-2 may act as a theranostic target in PC treatment. Li et al. (2018b) demonstrated that PINK1 and PARK2 suppressed pancreatic tumorigenesis through the control of mitochondrial iron-dependent metabolism. Using mouse models of PC, they showed that the depletion of PINK1 and PARK2 accelerates mutant Kras-driven pancreatic tumorigenesis. The PINK1-PARK2 pathway-mediated degradation of SLC25A37 and SLC25A28 increased mitochondrial iron accumulation, which induced the HIF-1A-dependent Warburg effect and AIM2-dependent APS activation in tumor cells. AIM2-mediated HMGB1 release further induced CD274/PD-L1 expression. Treatment of the mitochondrial iron chelator, anti-HMGB1 antibody, or genetic depletion of HIF-1A or Aim2 in PINK1$^{-/-}$ and PARK2$^{-/-}$ mice conferred protection in pancreatic tumorigenesis. Low PARK2 expression and high SLC25A37 and AIM2 expression were associated with poor prognosis in patients with PC, suggesting that disrupted mitochondrial iron homeostasis may contribute to cancer development and hence constitute a target for theranostic interventions. To ascertain the anti-cancer effects of P. suffruticosa on oncogenic functions, Liu et al. (2018) assessed the efficacy of the P. suffruticosa aqueous extracts (PS) *in vitro* using PC cells as a model system and *in vivo* in mouse xenograft tumors. The extracts were prepared and assessed using LC-MAS. For the xenograft model, AsPC1 cells were inoculated s.c. into immunocompromised mice and PS (oral) was administered over three weeks with or without Gemcitabine (GEM, i.p.) in a first-line advanced/metastatic PC therapy. PS stimulated ERS and affected $\Delta\Psi$ to increase APS number and block their degradation, followed by ATG induction and apoptosis. PS-mediated proteostasis impairment altered the dynamics of the actin cytoskeleton, cell motility, and cell cycle progression. The ROS scavenger reversed the PS-mediated degradation of peptidyl-prolyl cis-trans isomerase B (PPIB), an ER protein for protein folding, suggesting that ROS generation by PS may be involved in CP and apoptosis. The oral administration of PS, alone or in combination with GEM, delayed tumor growth in a xenograft model without affecting body weight. Cells in pancreatic ductal adenocarcinoma (PDAC) undergo ATG, but its effects vary with tumor stage and genetic factors. Görgülü et al. (2019) investigated the consequences of the varying levels of the ATG related 5 (Atg5) protein on pancreatic tumor progression. They raised mice that express oncogenic Kras in primary PC cells and had homozygous disruption of Atg5 (A5; Kras) or heterozygous disruption of Atg5 (A5+/–Kras), and compared them with mice with only oncogenic Kras (controls). A5+/– Kras mice, with reduced Atg5 levels, developed more tumors and metastases than the control mice, whereas the A5 Kras mice did not develop tumors. Cultured A5+/– Kras primary tumor cells were resistant to the induction and inhibition of ATG, and had altered mitochondrial morphology, CMB, changes in $[Ca^{2+}]_i$ oscillations, and increased activity of extracellular Cathepsin L and D. The tumors that formed in A5+/– Kras mice contained greater numbers of type 2 macrophages than control mice, and the primary A5+/– Kras tumor cells had an upregulated expression of cytokines (which regulate macrophage chemo-attraction and differentiation into M2 macrophage). The knockdown of Atg5 in PC cell lines increased their migratory and invasive capabilities, as well as the formation of metastases following their injection into mice. In human PDAC samples, lower levels of Atg5 were associated with tumor metastasis and shorter survival time. In mice that expressed oncogenic Kras in pancreatic cells, the heterozygous disruption of Atg5 and reduced protein levels promoted tumor development, whereas homozygous disruption of Atg5 blocked tumorigenesis. Hence, theranostic strategies to alter ATG in PDAC should consider the effects of Atg5 to avoid MDR in highly aggressive cells.

CP in Liver Cancer

Hepatocarcinogenesis comprises complex steps that occur after liver injury and involves telomere and cell cycle dysfunction, impaired WNT/β-catenin and Akt/mTOR signaling, oxidative stress mitochondria dysfunction, CP/ATG, and apoptosis implicated in CBMP. Wu et al. (2018) summarized the roles of hepatocarcinogenesis and the immune system in liver cancer. They studied basic and clinical findings to develop novel anti-carcinogenesis targets for theranostic interventions. Following liver injury, gene mutations, and accumulation of oxidative stress, local inflammation lead to cell proliferation, de-differentiation, apoptosis, and necrosis, to further enhance gene mutation and dysregulation of pro- and anti-inflammatory cytokines, such as IL-1β, IL-6, IL-10, IL-12, IL-13, IL-18, and TGF-β, resulting in immune escape through NF-κB and APS signaling. Zhu et al. (2018) investigated the proteomics response of HCC Hep3B cells to Danusertib (Danu), a pan-Aurora kinase inhibitor, and validated it based on stable-isotope labeling by amino acids in cell culture (SILAC). Danu modulated the expression of 542 protein molecules (279 upregulated, 260 downregulated, and 3 stable). An Ingenuity pathway analysis (IPA) and KEGG pathway analysis identified that 107 and 24 signaling pathways were regulated by Danu, respectively. The IPA analysis showed that the (i) growth (ii) proliferation, (iii) cell death, and (iv) survival were regulated by Danu. Danu inhibited the proliferation of Hep3B cells with a 24 hr IC_{50} value of 22.03 μM and arrested Hep3B cells in the G_2/M phase by regulating the expression of cell-cycle regulators and induced apoptosis via the mitochondria-dependent pathway. Danu induced ATG, while the inhibition of ATG enhanced the anticancer effects of Danu. The PI3K/Akt/mTOR signaling pathway was involved in Danu-induced ATG and apoptosis, suggesting that the Aurora kinases inhibition with Danu results in a global proteomic response and exerts anticancer effects on Hep3B cells, which involve regulation of the cell cycle, ATG, and apoptosis. Ma et al. (2018) discussed how DDR and mTOR pathways communicate to ensure an efficient protection of the cell against metabolic and genotoxic stresses, and how anticancer therapies benefit from targeting of these pathways. In eukaryotes, the highly conserved mTOR signaling integrated both intracellular and extracellular signals and served as a regulator of cellular metabolism, proliferation, and survival. mTOR signaling was related to the DNA damage response (DDR).

CP/ATG Regulation in Cancer

The author has proposed the CP-index (CPI) as a ratio of CP vs ATG, which can be quantitatively estimated by digital fluorescence imaging and several other analytical methods by using specific biomarkers as described in this manuscript to evaluate the chemo-sensitivity or resistance of cancer or any chronic MDR disease with poor prognosis. It is envisaged that cancers with relatively higher CPI will have a better prognosis, whereas those with lower CPI will have a poor prognosis, because CP occurs during the acute phase, whereas generalized ATG occurs during the chronic phase of disease progression and MDR. CP/ATG is an important recycling process in cancer initiation, cancer stem cell maintenance, and development of MDR in both solid and hematological malignancies. CP/ATG also plays an intricate role in the complex cancer microenvironment. The photosensitizer 1,9-dimethyl methylene blue (DMMB) has mitochondria and lysosomes as specific targets of cell death with CP/ATG. DMMB induces selective damage to mtDNA, saving nDNA. By challenging cells having different p53 content, Abrantes et al. (2019) investigated whether different p53 content modulates DMMB/light-induced phototoxicity and cell cycle dynamics. Cells lacking p53 were more resistant to photoactivated DMMB, with a smaller sub-G1 population, indicating reduced apoptosis. DMMB induced ATG-associated cell death and S-phase cell cycle arrest with replication stress, independent of the p53, indicating that p53 is not involved in either process. Li et al. (2019d) determined the interaction and co-localization of LC3 and lamin A/C. The role of the SUMO E2 ligase, UBC9, in the regulation of the SUMOylation of lamin A/C and nucleophagy was determined by the siRNA silencing of UBC9. The DNA damage induced nuclear accumulation of UBC9 ligase which resulted in SUMOylation of lamin A/C for the interaction between the ATG protein LC3 and lamin A/C for nucleophagy. The knockdown of UBC9 prevented the SUMOylation of lamin A/C and LC3-lamin A/C interaction. This attenuated nucleophagy which degraded nuclear components lamin A/C and leaked nDNA mediated by DNA damage, suggesting that nDNA leakage activates nucleophagy through the UBC9-mediated SUMOylation of lamin A/C, leading to degradation of nuclear components including lamin A/C and leaked nDNA. Defects in the basal ATG limit the nutrient supply from recycling of intracellular constituents. Lin et al. (2018) demonstrated that the conditional impairment of the ATG gene Atg5 (Atg5-KO) extends the survival of KRAS[G12V]-driven tumor-bearing mice by 38%. The Atg5-KO tumors spread more slowly during late tumorigenesis, despite a faster onset, displaying reduced mitochondrial function, and increased mitochondrial fragmentation involving CBMP. The metabolite profiles indicated a deficiency in the nonessential amino acid, asparagine, despite a compensatory overexpression of asparagine synthetase (ASNS), a key enzyme for asparagine synthesis. The inhibition of either ATG or

ASNS reduced KRAS[G12V]-driven tumor cell proliferation, migration, and invasion, which was rescued by asparagine supplementation or the knockdown of mitochondrial fission factor (MFF). These observations were reflected in human cancer-derived data, linking ASNS overexpression with poor clinical prognosis in multiple cancers. These data documented specific asparagine homeostasis control by ATG and ASNS, highlighting the significance of CP/ATG in suppressing the metabolic barriers of low asparagine and excessive CBMP to promote malignant KRAS-driven tumor progression. Wang et al. (2018) highlighted that the duration of stimulation and the cell type can influence PKC-dependent ATG. The subcellular localization of PKCs and their downstream regulators may influence ATG-regulation as well. Phase II studies on the PKC-β inhibitor, Enzastaurin, showed promising results in MCL, DLBCL, and recurrent high-grade gliomas. Rottlerin enhanced ATG in BC cells, which warrants further studies to verify PKC-δ as a theranostic target. Thus, identifying the function of PKC in modulating ATG and related clinical studies may provide novel targets for cancer chemotherapy.

Bgatova et al. (2018) studied structural changes in the liver of CBA mice during the development of tumor by inoculating HCC-29 cells in their pelvic region. A decrease in the volume density of hepatocyte cytoplasm, mitochondria, ER, and lipid inclusions and an increase in the volume density of lysosomal structures during tumor growth were observed. All the stages of ATG included the appearance of APSs and secondary lysosomes. Fragments of cytoplasm, glycogen rosettes, mitochondria, and ER with ribosomes were found in APSs, indicating the development of non-selective ATG during distant tumor growth aimed at the maintenance of intracellular homeostasis, ATP production, and homeostasis of organism. Although the Parkin/PINK1 axis is considered the main regulator of CP, this pathway is not unique and CP can still be functional in the absence of Parkin. Villa et al. (2018) described Parkin-independent CP and its role in cancer, representing potential novel targets to treat diseases affected by dysregulated CP. Wang et al. (2018) reported that PTEN-L, is a novel negative regulator of CP through the dephosphorylation of p-Ser65-Ub and a portion of PTEN-L localizes at the OMM and prevents PRKN's mitochondrial translocation, reduces the phosphorylation of PRKN, impairs its E3 ligase activity, and maintains PRKN in a closed/inactive status. PTEN-L dephosphorylated p-Ser65-Ub to disrupt the feedforward mechanism of CP, suggesting that PTEN-L acts as a brake in the regulation of CP. The ATG of mitochondria, that is, CP, plays a crucial role in coping with stressors in the aging process, metabolic disturbances, and neurological disorders. Impairments of the process might lead to the enhanced accumulation of aged and aggregated proteins and reduced cellular integrity in response to stress. Civelek et al. (2019) used the stress-sensitive mutant mev-1 of *C. elegans* to assess the effects of the knockdown of CP-relevant genes on survival under heat stress, the amount of APSs, and on protein aggregation. RNA interference for dct-1, drp-1, eat-3, fis-1, fzo1, glb-1, PINK1, and pgam-5 resulted in a reduction of the survival time at a temperature of 37°C. These effects were associated with a decrease in the APS flux of proteins, as indicated by the increased accumulation of GFP-tagged SQST-1, and reduced lysosomes indicating that ATG was impaired. The gene knockdowns led to increased levels of ROS and enhanced protein aggregation. Hence CP is important to sustain MQC in order to prevent ROS overproduction, protein aggregation, and reduction of survival during heat stress. To address whether macroATG/ATG inhibition will be effective in BRCA1-deficient mammary tumors, Yeo et al. (2018) generated mice with conditional deletion of an ATG gene, Rb1cc1, along with Brca1 and Trp53, through utilization of the K14-Cre transgene. Rb1cc1 deletion suppressed tumorigenesis in the BRCA1-deficient model when compared to wild type and heterozygous Rb1cc1 controls. However, in the mouse mammary tumor virus (MMTV)-polyoma middle T antigen (PyMT) model, tumor growth and the distribution of histological subtypes were not affected by the loss of RB1CC1. The loss of RB1CC1 decreased mitochondrial mass and O/P of these tumor cells, along with a decrease in the phosphorylation of mTOR substrates and transcript levels of genes involved in MB. An increased sensitivity to mitochondrial disrupting agents upon the loss of RB1CC1 was observed. A combination of an ATG inhibitor, Spautin-1, along with a mitochondrial complex I inhibitor, Metformin, was more effective in limiting oxidative respiratory capacity, colony-forming ability, and tumor growth, indicating that the inhibition of ATG can increase the benefits of Metformin in BRCA1-deficient BCs. Vu et al. (2018) used CRISPR/CAS9 to knockout the Atg5 gene, which is essential for APS formation, in tumor cells derived from GBM patients. While Atg5 disruption inhibited ATG, it did not change the phenotypes of glioma cells and did not alter their sensitivity to Temozolomide. Screening of an anticancer drug library identified compounds that showed greater efficacy in Atg5-knockout glioma cells, whereas, Nigericin and Salinomycin induced ATG. ATG-induced mTOR inhibition did not exhibit Atg5-dependent cytoprotective effects. Nigericin in combination with an Atg5 deficiency suppressed spheroid formation by glioma cells mitigated by Ca^{2+} chelation or CaMKK inhibition, indicating that, ATG inhibitors, in combination with calcium-mobilizing compounds contribute to efficient anticancer therapeutics. Atg5-knockout cells treated with Nigericin showed increased ROS and apoptosis compared to the controls. By using a patient-derived xenograft model, it was demonstrated that CQ enhanced the efficacy of Nigericin and Salinomycin. Hence, Ca^{2+}-mobilizing compounds combined with ATG inhibitors may be used as novel theranostic strategy to treat glioblastoma. Vera-Ramirez et al. (2018) showed that ATG is a crucial mechanism for the survival of disseminated dormant BC cells. Pharmacologic or genetic inhibition of ATG in dormant BC cells decreased cell survival and metastatic burden in mouse and human 3-D *in vitro* and *in vivo* preclinical models of dormancy. *In vivo* experiments identified ATG7 as essential for ATG induction. Inhibition of CP in dormant BC cells induced the accumulation of CB and ROS, resulting in apoptosis. CP-related 4C cysteine peptidase (ATG4C) is an ATG regulator responsible for the cleaving of pro-LC3 and de-lipidation of LC3 II. Wen et al. (2019) investigated the role of ATG4C in glioma progression and Temozolomide (TMZ) chemosensitivity. The association between ATG4C mRNA expression and prognosis of gliomas patients was analyzed using the TCGA datasets. The role of ATG4C in proliferation, apoptosis, ATG, and TMZ chemosensitivity were investigated by silencing ATG4C *in vivo*. An ectopic xenograft nude mice model was established to investigate the effects of ATG4C on glioma growth *in vivo*. The median survival (OS) time of patients with higher ATG4C expression was reduced. ATG4C mRNA expression was increased with the rising of the glioma grade. Knockdown ATG4C suppressed glioma cells proliferation by inducing cell cycle arrest at the G1 phase. ATG4C depletion suppressed ATG and triggered apoptosis through ROS accumulation. Depletion of ATG4C suppressed TMZ-activated ATG and promoted sensitivity of glioma cells to TMZ. ATG4C knockdown suppressed the growth of glioma in nude mice, indicating that ATG4C is a potential prognostic predictor for glioma patient and its targeting may provide promising theranostic strategies for gliomas. There remains a high demand for highly specific and novel agents which can be used to study the regulation of CP/ATG to discover novel pharmacophores for cancer theranostics. ATG has a prominent role in the survival, proliferation, and MDR of tumors in metabolic and chemotherapeutic stress. Clinical trials with CQ–a known CP/ATG inhibitor–were unable to achieve complete ATG inhibition *in vivo*, warranting the search for more potent CP/ATG inhibitors. Konstantinidis et al. (2019) described a cell-based quantitative high-content screening (HCS) for ATG inhibition using a human breast adenocarcinoma MCF7 cell line stably expressing EGFP-LC3, a biomarker of ATG. In addition, Guntuku et al. (2019) discovered that both IITZ-01 and IITZ-02 act as potent ATG inhibitors. Treatment with these compounds induced a vacuolated appearance of cells due to their accumulation in lysosomes. These compounds de-acidified lysosomes as evidenced by the decrease in Lysotracker red staining and the inhibited maturation of lysosomal enzymes leading to lysosomal dysfunction. IITZ-01 and IITZ-02 enhanced APS accumulation but inhibited APS degradation by impairing lysosomal function, resulting in the inhibition of ATG. Compound IITZ-01 exhibited >10X potent ATG inhibition along with 12–20X better cytotoxic action than

CQ. IITZ-01 and IITZ-02 abolished ΔΨ and triggered apoptosis through the mitochondrial-mediated pathway. Furthermore, IITZ-01 and IITZ-02 displayed antitumor action through ATG inhibition and apoptosis induction in MDA-MB-231 BC xenografts with IITZ-01 exhibiting superior anticancer efficacy, indicating that IITZ-01 is potent ATG inhibitor with single-agent anticancer activity. Cutaneous melanoma is one of the most common malignant skin tumors and advanced melanoma is usually associated with a poor prognosis. Wang et al. (2019) demonstrated the tumor suppressing role of epithelial membrane protein-2 (EMP2) by inducing apoptosis in A375 human melanoma cell line. The low expression of EMP2 in melanoma is due to ATG protein degradation mediated by the mTOR pathway, suggesting regulation of ATG as well as EMP2 levels as a novel TSE-EBPT strategy for melanoma.

Prostate cancer (PC) is one of the leading causes of death in males. Existing treatments lead to MDR and metastases. Within tumor mass, ATG may promote cell survival by enhancing cancer cells tolerability to different cell stresses, like hypoxia, starvation, or those triggered by chemotherapeutic agents. ATG has been implicated, either as pro-death or pro-survival factor, in aggressive tumors. Cristofani et al. (2018) used LNCaP, PC3, and DU145 cells to test how different ATG inducers modulate Docetaxel-induced apoptosis. They selected the mTOR-independent Trehalose and the mTOR-dependent Rapamycin as CP/ATG inducers. In castration-resistant PC (CRPC) PC3 cells, Trehalose prevented apoptosis in Docetaxel-treated cells. Trehalose reduced the release of Cyt-C triggered by Docetaxel and the formation of aberrant mitochondria, by enhancing the turnover of damaged mitochondria via CP. Trehalose increased LC3 and p62 expression, LC3-II and p62 (p62 bodies) accumulation, and the induction of LC3 puncta. In Docetaxel-treated cells, Trehalose induced perinuclear mitochondrial aggregation (CS), and co-localization with LC3 and p62-positive CPS. In PC3 cells, Rapamycin activated ATG without evidence of MTG, even in the presence of Docetaxel. These results were confirmed in LNCaP cells. Trehalose and Rapamycin did not modify the response to Docetaxel in the Atg5-deficient (ATG resistant) DU145 cells. Hence, depending on the cancer cell type and signaling pathway, CP/ATG may modify the chemotherapy response. Zhang et al. (2018) showed that Artisunate (ART) enhances lysosomal function and ferritin degradation as an anti-cancer agent. ART targeted mitochondria, which also improves its efficacy. ART localized in the mitochondria and binds to mitochondrial proteins to cause mitochondrial fission. It induced ATG and decreased mitochondrial proteins. When ATG was inhibited, the decrease in mitochondrial proteins was reversed, indicating that the degradation of mitochondrial proteins is through MTG. ART stabilized the PINK1 on the mitochondria and activated the PINK1-dependent pathway, leading to the recruitment of Parkin, sequestosome 1 (SQSTM1), ubiquitin, and LC3 to induce MTG. When PINK1 was knocked down, ART-induced MTG was suppressed. The PINK1 knockdown altered the cellular redox status in ART-treated cells, decreased GSH, and increased ROS and lactate. PINK1 knockdown increased mitochondrial depolarization and apoptosis by ART, suggesting that MTG protects from ART-induced cell death through the PINK1-dependent pathway, and that its inhibition may augment the anti-cancer activity of ART. Towers et al. (2019) developed a CRISPR/Cas9 assay with live-cell imaging to measure the acute effects of the knockout (KO) of ATG genes. Some cancer cells require ATG, in addition to DNA replication, mRNA transcription, and protein translation for their growth and proliferation. However, even these highly ATG-dependent cancer cells evolve to circumvent the loss of ATG by upregulating NRF2, which is necessary for ATG-dependent cells to circumvent ATG7 KO and maintain protein homeostasis. This adaptation increased susceptibility of ATG-dependent cells to protease inhibitors, identified a mechanism of resistance to ATG inhibition, and showed that selection to avoid tumor cell dependency on ATG creates potentially-targeted cancer cell susceptibilities.

Dysregulation of ATG results in neurodegeneration, microbial infections, and cancer. Singh et al. (2018a) summarized how ATG is involved at various stages of tumorigenesis. They addressed the link between ATG and hallmarks of cancer to provide a better understanding of tumor dependence on ATG and discussed how therapeutics targeting ATG can inhibit transformations in tumorigenesis and proposed a novel insight into the mutational landscapes of ATG-related genes, using genetic information collected from an array of cancers. Yazdani et al. (2019) summarized the dual role of ATG in the development of HCC and elucidated theranostic strategies for anti-HCC therapy. ATG was both upregulated and downregulated in different cancers indicating that it plays a dual role in suppressing and promoting cell survival.

Mitochondrially-targeted Anticancer Drugs

Molecules designed to target the mitochondria are novel theranostic approaches for cancer and microbial infections. These redox agents induce mitochondrial damage and ATG in cancer cells. Using BC cell lines and targeted molecules, mitochondrial dysfunction and ATG was selective for MDA-MB-231 cancer cells as compared to the non-cancerous MCF-12A cells (Biel and Rao 2017). The mitochondrial dysfunction precedes the activation of ATG in these cancer cells. To determine the onset of MTG, stably expressing *mKeima*, a mitochondrial pH sensor, the cell-lines were generated to demonstrate that these drugs activate lysosomal-dependent mitochondrial degradation in MDA-MB-231 cells. MTG was confirmed by identifying the accumulation of a PINK1, APSs, and the formation of an APS-mitochondria protein (Mfn-2-LC3-II) complex, demonstrating that mitochondrial redox agents induce MTG in a BC cell line, thus indicating their potential in cancer theranostics. Metabolism is a key component of the melanoma response to BRAF and/or MEK inhibitors. Mitochondrial targeting may offer novel theranostic approaches to overwhelm the mitochondrial addiction that limited the efficacy of BRAF and/or MEK inhibitors. These theranostic approaches might be applicable to the clinical situation. Besides its influence on survival, growth, proliferation, invasion and metastasis, cancer cell metabolism also influences the cellular responses to molecular-targeted therapies (Li et al. 2019e). To review the recent advances in elucidating the metabolic effects of BRAF and MEK inhibitors (inhibitors of the MAPK/ERK pathway) in melanoma and discuss the mechanisms involved in the way metabolism can influence melanoma cell death and resistance to BRAF and MEK inhibitors, Marchetti et al. (2018) emphasized the theranostic potential of innovative drug combinations. Besides its influence on survival, growth, proliferation, invasion and metastasis; cancer cell metabolism also influences the cellular responses to molecular-targeted therapies. Metabolism is a central component of the melanoma response to BRAF and/or MEK inhibitors. These investigators elucidated the metabolic effects of BRAF and MEK inhibitors in melanoma and discussed the underlying mechanisms involved in the way metabolism can influence melanoma cell death and resistance to BRAF and MEK inhibitors. They also highlighted the therapeutic perspectives in terms of innovative drug combinations. Particularly, a combination of BRAF and MEK inhibitors inhibits "aerobic glycolysis and induces metabolic stress leading to cell death by apoptosis in BRAF-mutated cancer cells. An increase in "MAPK/ERK pathway inhibitors and the cells that survive to these inhibitors are characterized by mitochondrial OXPHOS phenotype. Consequently, mitochondrial inhibition could be combined with oncogenic "drivers" as inhibitors of the MAPK/ERK pathway for improving the clinical efficacy of molecular-targeted cancer therapy. Novel drugs can be developed to regulate MAP/ERK pathways for the successful treatment of cancer. In view of the above, mitochondrial-targeting may offer novel therapeutic approaches to overwhelm the mitochondrial addiction that limits the efficacy of BRAF and/or MEK inhibitors. Hence, innovative therapeutic combinations targeting cancer-specific mitochondrial metabolism, MAPK/ERK pathway inhibitors, and mitochondrial inclusion (CB-specific) agonists, CP antagonists, and CBMP agonists will be beneficial for the TSE-EBPT of cancer as highlighted in this edition. BRAF and MEK inhibitors attenuated aerobic glycolysis and induced metabolic stress leading to apoptosis in BRAF-mutated cancer cells. An increase in mitochondrial metabolism was required to survive the MAPK/ERK pathway inhibitors and the cells that survived to these inhibitors were characterized by the mitochondrial O/P phenotype. Consequently, mitochondrial inhibition could be combined with oncogenic "drivers" inhibitors of the MAPK/ERK pathway for improving the efficacy of molecular-targeted therapy. Mutations in the KRAS proto-oncogene are present in 50% of colorectal cancers and are associated with MDR to frontline drugs. The overactive KRAS mutations play a crucial role in the metabolic reprogramming from O/P to aerobic glycolysis in cancer cells. Boyle et al. (2018) exploited the more negative membrane potential of cancer cell mitochondria for interfering with energy metabolism in KRAS variant-containing and KRAS WT colorectal cancer cells. Mitochondrial function, ATP, cellular uptake, energy sensor signaling, and functional effects on cancer cell proliferation were assayed. 3-Carboxyl proxyl nitroxide (*Mito-CP*) and *Mito-Metformin*, two mitochondria-targeted compounds, depleted ATP and inhibited ATP-linked O_2 consumption in both KRAS WT and KRAS variant-containing colon cancer cells and had only limited effects on non-transformed intestinal epithelial cells. These anti-proliferative effects reflected in the activation of AMPK and the phosphorylation-mediated suppression of the mTOR target ribosomal protein S6 kinase B1 (RPS6KB1 or p70S6K). *Mito-CP* and *Mito-Metformin* released Unc-51-like ATG-activating kinase 1 (ULK1) from mTOR-mediated inhibition, affected mitochondrial morphology, and decreased $\Delta\Psi$. The pharmacological inhibition of the AMPK mitigated the anti-proliferative effects of *Mito-CP* and *Mito-Metformin*, suggesting that these drugs selectively target mitochondria and induce MTG in cancer cells. Hence, targeting bioenergetics with mitochondrial-targeted drugs to stimulate MTG provides an attractive approach for theranostic intervention in KRAS WT and overactive mutant-expressing colon cancer.

Conway et al. (2019) demonstrated a caspase-independent mechanism of cell death in p53-mutated GBM cells exposed to plasma. They elucidated the molecular mechanisms in caspase-independent cell death induced by plasma treatment. Plasma induced cell death in GBM cells, independent of caspases. The accumulation of vesicles was observed in plasma-treated cells that stained positive with Acridine orange. ATG was not activated following plasma treatment. Acridine orange intensity correlated with the lysosomal marker *Lyso TrackerTM Deep Red*. Isosurface visualization of confocal imaging confirmed that lysosomal accumulation occurred in plasma-treated cells. The accumulation of lysosomes was associated with cell death following plasma treatment. These investigators observed the accumulation of acidic vesicles and cell death following CAP treatment in GBM cells and determined that a rapid accumulation of late stage endosomes/lysosomes precedes membrane permeabilization, $\Delta\Psi$ collapse, and caspase independent cell death. Mendonca et al. (2019) highlighted a methodology to measure the most abundant non-histone nuclear protein HMGB1 and determine its subcellular localization, which governs many HMGB1's functions. To promote DNA repair and apoptosis, it restricts the transcriptional access to unfold chromatin and limit DNA release. When HMGB1 is translocated to the cytosol with DPCI, it induces CP/ATG. It can also be released by activated immune cells and damaged or dying cells into the extracellular space, where it acts as a DAMP molecule, contributing to the progression of cancer. Metastatic melanoma cells rely on glutaminolysis rather than aerobic glycolysis for their MB needs through the TCA cycle. Vara-Perez et al. (2019) compared the effects of glucose or glutamine on melanoma cell proliferation, migration, and O/P *in vitro*. The glutamine-driven melanoma cell's aggressive traits positively correlated with the increased expression of HIF-1α and its pro-ATG target, Bnip-3. Bnip-3 silencing reduced glutamine-mediated effects on melanoma cell growth, migration, and bioenergetics. Hence, Bnip-3 is a vital component of the MQC for glutamine-driven melanoma aggressiveness.

As the modulation of CP/ATG can be beneficial to cancer theranostics, the identification of novel CP/ATG enhancers is direly needed. However, current CP/ATG-inducing anticancer agents exert undesired side effects owing to their non-specific bio-distribution in off-target tissues. Huang et al. (2018b) synthesized mitochondrial-targeting near-infrared (NIR) fluorophores and screened and identified their ATG-inducing ability. They identified a new NIR ATG-enhancer, IR-58, which exhibited tumor-selective demise. IR-58 accumulated in the mitochondria of colorectal cancer (CRC) cells and xenografts, a process that was glycolysis and organic anion transporter polypeptide-dependent. IR-58 induced apoptosis via augmenting ATG through the ROS-Akt- mTOR signaling pathway. RNA sequencing, mass spectrometry, and siRNA analyses demonstrated that translocase of IMM-44 (TIM44)-SOD2 pathway inhibition was responsible for the excessive ROS, ATG, and apoptosis induced by IR-58. TIM44 expression correlated with CRC development and poor prognosis in patients. Although, Metformin, a drug for T2DM has shown therapeutic effects for various cancers, it has no beneficial effects on the survival rate of human malignant mesothelioma (HMM) patients. Hwang et al. (2019) elucidated the mechanism of Metformin resistance in HMM cells. Glucose-starved HMM cells had enhanced resistance to Metformin, demonstrated by decreased apoptosis, induced CP, and increased cell survival. These cells showed mitochondrial abnormalities (decreased ATP synthesis, elongation, altered permeability transition pore, and hyperpolarization of $\Delta\Psi$) implicated in CBMP. Mdr1 was upregulated in mitochondria but not in cell membrane and was reversed by treatment with CCCP, $\Delta\Psi$ depolarization inducer. CP and apoptosis were increased in MDR protein 1 knockout HMM cells cultured under glucose starvation with Metformin treatment, suggesting that mitochondrial Mdr1 plays a critical role in the chemoresistance to Metformin in HMM cells for improving its theranostics. The pro-ATG molecule, AMBRA1 (ATG/Beclin-1 regulator-1), is also a novel CP regulator in both PINK1/Parkin-dependent and -independent systems. Di Rita et al. (2018) identified the E3 ubiquitin ligase HUWE1 as a key inducing factor in AMBRA1-mediated CP, a process that takes place independently of the main CP receptors. The CP function of AMBRA1 is post-translationally controlled, upon HUWE1 activity, by phosphorylation on its serine 1014, mediated by the IKKα kinase and induces structural changes in AMBRA1, thus promoting its interaction with LC3/GABARAP (mATG8) proteins, indicating that AMBRA1 regulates CP through a pathway, in which HUWE1 and IKKα are key factors, shedding new insights on the regulation of MQC and homoeostasis in mammalian cells. Martins et al. (2018) addressed the concept that a parallel damage in the mitochondrial membranes and lysosomes leads to ATG malfunction that can improve the efficiency of the photosensitizers to cause cell death. Damage to these organelles was induced by irradiation of cells pretreated with 2 phenothiazinium salts, methylene blue (MB), and 1,9-dimethyl methylene blue (DMMB). At a low concentration (10 nM), only DMMB could induce mitochondrial damage, leading to CP induction, which did not progress to completion because of the damage in lysosome, triggering cell death. MB-induced photo-damage was perceived after irradiation, in response to nonspecific oxidative stress at a higher concentration (2 μM). The parallel damage in mitochondria and lysosomes activated and inhibited CP, respectively, leading to a late and more efficient cell death, offering a significant advantage over photosensitizers that cause unspecific oxidative stress. This concept could be used to develop better light-activated drugs. ATG is an essential cellular process implicated in cellular homeostasis and is downregulated by mTOR, whose activity can be modulated by Rapamycin, a lipophilic macrolide antibiotic, through forming a complex with immunophilin FKBP12 which is essential for mTOR regulation. Therefore, Rapamycin is used as a neuroprotective agent. The FKBP12-binding ligand, FK506, is as an immunosuppressive agent and inhibits calcineurin expression. Ding et al. (2018) synthesized compounds based on the FKBP12-binding moiety as the binding structure of Rapamycin and FK506. They removed other binding regions of the complex that had the property of immunosuppression and found that a small molecule, TH2849, from these derivatives, which has a significant binding connection with mTOR as compared to calcineurin. The effects of TH2849 on calcineurin/NFAT were not as significant as FK506, and weak effects on the IL2/p34^{cdc2}/cyclin signaling pathway were also found. TH2849 showed a mitochondrial-protective effect through stabilizing its structure and $\Delta\Psi$ and rescued DAergic neurons in MPTP-treated zebrafishes as well as in mouse models without significant immunosuppressive effect, suggesting that TH2849 serves as a neuroprotective agent by inducing ATG and having an immunosuppressive effect. Both the QC process of CP and the defensive process of intracellular pathogen-engulfment (Xenophagy) are facilitated via protein assemblies which have shared molecules, a prime example being the Tank-Binding Kinase 1 (TBK1), which plays a pivotal role in the immune response driven by Xenophagy as an amplifying mechanism in CP/ATG, indicating the potential crosstalk between the two processes. Singh et al. (2018b) draw parallels between Xenophagy and CP/ATG, speculating on the inhibitory mechanisms of 18 kDa protein TSPO, and how the preferential sequestering toward one of the two pathways may undermine the other, and thus impair cellular response to pathogens and cellular immunity. Further studies in this direction may present an opportunity to develop CP-targeted TSE-EBPT-CPTs for the clinical management of cancer. UVA (315–400 nm) is the most abundant form of UV radiation in sunlight and indoor tanning beds. Sample et al. (2018) showed that UVA, but not the shorter wave band UVB (280–315 nm), upregulates adaptor protein p62 in an Nrf2- and ROS-dependent manner, suggesting a UVA-specific effect on p62 regulation. UVA-induced p62 upregulation was inhibited by a mitochondria-targeted antioxidant or Nrf2 knockdown. In addition, p62 knockdown inhibited UVA-induced ROS production and Nrf2 upregulation. These investigators also reported a novel regulatory feedback loop between p62 and PTEN in melanoma cells. PTEN overexpression reduced p62 protein, and p62 knockdown increased PTEN protein. As compared with normal human skin, p62 was upregulated in human nevus, malignant melanoma, and metastatic melanoma. Furthermore, p62 was upregulated in melanoma cells relative to normal human epidermal melanocytes, independent of their BRAF or NRAS mutation status. UVA upregulated p62 and induced a p62-Nrf2 positive feedback loop to counteract oxidative stress and p62 formed a feedback loop with PTEN in melanoma cells, suggesting p62 functions as an oncogene in UVA-associated melanoma development and progression. Salidroside has diversified pharmacological activities, including antitumor, anti-inflammatory, analgesic, antibacterial, antiviral, and anti-fertility abilities. Li et al. (2018c) examined the effects of Salidroside on the viability and apoptosis of bladder cancer cells. Treatment with Salidroside reduced cell viability and induced apoptosis and caspase-9/3 activation in the T24 human bladder carcinoma cell line. Salidroside induced ATG, promoted the protein expression of nucleoporin p62 and the LC3B, suppressed PI3K and p-Akt expression, inhibited MMP-9 expression, and increased Bcl-2-associated X protein, which functions as an apoptosis regulator in T24 cells. Salidroside reduced the viability and induced the apoptosis of bladder cancer cells through the ATG/PI3K/Akt and MMP-9 signaling pathways.

CONCLUSION

Concomitant damage occurring in mitochondria and lysosomes was proposed as an efficient strategy to photo-induce cancer cell death. XIAP facilitated BC and colon carcinoma growth by p62 depletion through ubiquitination-dependent proteasomal degradation. mTOR and its involvement in pathological aspects and inhibitors were investigated for the cancer theranostics. Placenta-conditioned ECM activated BC cell survival for metastases. JMJD6 regulated histone H2A.X phosphorylation and promoted ATG in TNBC cells via TK activity. IITZ-01, a novel lysosomotropic ATG inhibitor, had antitumor efficacy in TNBC. GSK-3β promoted cell migration and inhibited ATG by mediating the AMPK pathway in BC. Bnip-3 contributed to the glutamine-driven aggressive behavior of melanoma cells. Novel ATG inhibitors were identified via cell-based high-content screening. The theranostic potential of CP was explored for the early detection of cancer stem cells. Resistance to endocrine therapy in BC, molecular mechanisms, and future goals for its clinical management were highlighted. EMP2 suppressed melanoma and was negatively regulated by mTOR-mediated ATG. Adult stem cell deficits induced Slc29a3 disorders in mice. SIRT1 on DNA damage occurred in response to epigenetic alterations in cancer. Ai-lncRNA EGOT-enhanced ATG sensitized Paclitaxel toxicity via upregulation of ITPR1 expression through RNA-RNA and RNA-protein interactions in human cancer. Tetrandrine isolated from Cyclea peltata induced cytotoxicity and apoptosis through ROS and caspase pathways in BC and PC cells. Recombinant adenoviruses expressing Apoptin suppressed the growth of MCF-7 BC cells and affected CP/ATG. Overexpression of ATG-related gene 3 promoted ATG and inhibited Salinomycin-induced apoptosis in MCF-7 cells. Inhibition of TNBC cell aggressiveness by Cathepsin D blockage and the role of Annexin A1 was explored. LDH regulated ATG in Tamoxifen-resistance in BC. Ambra1 inhibited Paclitaxel-induced apoptosis in BC cells by modulating the Bim/mitochondrial pathway. Variants in genes were related to inflammation, CP/ATG, and apoptosis in BC risk. In addition, CPI has been proposed to evaluate chemo-sensitivity or resistance of cancer.

REFERENCES

Abdel-Maksoud, M.S., M.I. El-Gamal, D.R. Benhalilou, S. Ashraf, et al. 2019. Mechanistic/mammalian target of rapamycin: Recent pathological aspects and inhibitors. Med Res Rev 39: 631–664.

Abrantes, A.B.P, G.C. Dias, N.C. de Souza-Pinto, M.S. Baptista. 2019. p53-Dependent and -independent responses of cells challenged by photosensitization. Photochem Photobiol 95: 355–363.

Alves-Fernandes, D.K. and M.G. Jasiulionis. 2019. The role of SIRT1 on DNA damage response and epigenetic alterations in cancer. Int J Mol Sci 20(13): E3153.

Baquero, P., A. Dawson and G.V. Helgason. 2018. ATG and mitochondrial metabolism: insights into their role and therapeutic potential in chronic myeloid leukaemia. FEBS J 286: 1271–1283.

Bgatova, N.P., S.A. Bakhbaeva, Y.S. Taskaeva, V.V. Makarova, et al. 2018. ATG in hepatocytes during distant tumor growth. Bull Exp Biol Med 165: 390–393.

Biel, T.G. and V.A. Rao. 2017. Mitochondrial dysfunction activates lysosomal-dependent MTG selectively in cancer cells. Oncotarget 11: 995–1011.

Boyle, K.A., J. Van Wickle, R.B. Hill, A. Marchese, et al. 2018. Mitochondria-targeted drugs stimulate MTG and abrogate colon cancer cell proliferation. J Biol Chem 293: 14891–14904.

Brix, D.M., S.A. Tvingsholm, M.B. Hansen, K.B. Clemmensen, et al. 2019. Release of transcriptional repression via ErbB2-induced, SUMO-directed phosphorylation of myeloid zinc finger-1 serine 27 activates lysosome redistribution and invasion. Oncogene 38: 3170–3184.

Chandrashekar, K.R., A. Prabhu and P.D. Rekha. 2019. Tetrandrine isolated from cyclea peltata induces cytotoxicity and apoptosis through ROS and caspase pathways in breast and PC cells. In Vitro Cell Dev Biol Anim 55: 331–340.

Chen S, Y.-Q. Li, X.-Z. Yin, S.-Z. Li, et al. 2019. Recombinant adenoviruses expressing apoptin suppress the growth of MCF-7 breast cancer cells and affect cell autophagy. Oncol Rep 1(5): 2818–2832.

Civelek, M., J.F. Mehrkens, N.M. Carstens, E. Fitzenberger, et al. 2019. Inhibition of MTG decreases survival of Caenorhabditis elegans by increasing protein aggregation. Mol Cell Biochem 452: 123–131.

Conway, G.E., Z. He, A.L. Hutanu, G.P Cribaro, et al. 2019. Cold Atmospheric Plasma induces accumulation of lysosomes and caspase-independent cell death in U373MG glioblastoma multiforme cells. Sci Rep 9: 12891.

Cristofani, R., M.M. Marelli, M.E. Cicardi, F. Fontana, et al. 2018. Dual role of autophagy on docetaxel-sensitivity in prostate cancer cells. Cell Death Dis 9: 889.

Das, A., M.K. Narayanam, S. Paul, P. Mukhnerjee, et al. 2019a. A novel triazole, NMK-T-057, induces autophagic cell death in BC cells by inhibiting γ-secretase-mediated activation of notch. J Biol Chem 294: 6733–6750.

Das, C.K., A. Parekh, P.K. Parida, S.K. Bhutia, et al. 2019b. Lactate dehydrogenase a regulates autophagy and tamoxifen resistance in breast cancer. Biochim Biophys Acta Mol Cell Res 1866: 1004–1018.

Dhar, S.K., V. BAkthavatchalu, B. Dhar, J. Chen, et al. 2018. DNA polymerase gamma (Polγ) deficiency triggers a selective mTORC2 prosurvival ATG response via mitochondria-mediated ROS signaling. Oncogene 37: 6225–6242.

Di Rita, A., A.D. Peschiaroli, P. Acunzo, D. Strobbe, et al. 2018. HUWE1 E3 ligase promotes PINK1/Parkin-independent MTG by regulating AMBRA1 activation via IKKα. Nat Commun 9: 3755.

Ding, L.Y., M. Chu, Y.S. Jiao, Q. Hao, et al. 2018. TFDP3 regulates the apoptosis and ATG in BC cell line MDA-MB-231. PLoS One 13: e0203833.

Dżugan, M., W. Trybus, M. Lis, M. Wesołowska, et al. 2018. Cadmium-induced ultrastructural changes in primary target organs of developing chicken embryos (Gallus domesticus). J Trace Elem Med Biol 50: 167–174.

Folkerts, H., S. Hilgendorf, E. Vellenga, E. Bremer, et al. 2019. The multifaceted role of ATG in cancer and the microenvironment. Med Res Rev 39: 517–560.

Görgülü, K., K.N. Diakopoulos, J. Ai, B. Schoeps, et al. 2019. Levels of the ATG related 5 protein affect progression and metastasis of pancreatic tumors in mice. Gastroenterology 156: 203–217.

Guntuku, L., J.K. Gangasani, D. Thummuri, R.M. Borkar, et al. 2019. IITZ-01, a novel potent lysosomotropic ATG inhibitor, has single-agent antitumor efficacy in TNB cancer *in vitro* and *in vivo*. Oncogene 38: 581–595.

Guo, Z., V. Johnson, J. Barrera, M. Porras, et al. 2018. Targeting cytochrome P450-dependent cancer cell mitochondria: Cancer associated CYPs and where to find them. Cancer Metastasis Rev 37: 409–423.

Guo, L., D. Chen, X. Yin and Q. Shu. 2019. GSK-3β promotes cell migration and inhibits ATG by mediating the AMPK pathway in BC. Oncol Res 27: 487–494.

Huang, C.Y., S.F. Chiang, W.T. Chen, T.W. Ke, et al. 2018a. HMGB1 promotes ERK-mediated mitochondrial Drp-1 phosphorylation for chemoresistance through RAGE in colorectal cancer. Cell Death Dis. 9(10): 1004.

Huang, Y., J. Zhou, S. Luo, Y. Wang, J. He, et al. 2018b. Identification of a fluorescent small-molecule enhancer for therapeutic autophagy in colorectal cancer by targeting mitochondrial protein translocase TIM44. Gut 67(2): 307–319.

Huang, X., Z.N. Wang, X.D. Yuan, W.Y. Wu, et al. 2019. XIAP facilitates breast and colon carcinoma growth via promotion of p62 depletion through ubiquitination-dependent proteasomal degradation. Oncogene 38: 1448–1460.

Hwang, S.H., M.C. Kim, S. Ji, Y. Yang, et al. 2019. Glucose starvation induces resistance to metformin through the elevation of mitochondrial multidrug resistance protein 1. Cancer Sci 110: 1256–1267.

Jiang, G.M., Y. Tan, H. Wang, L. Peng, et al. 2019. The relationship between ATG and the immune system and its applications for tumor immunotherapy. Mol Cancer 18(1): 17.

Komemi, O., G.E. Shochet, M. Pomeranz, A. Fishman, et al. 2019. Placenta-conditioned extracellular matrix (ECM) activates BC cell survival mechanisms: A key for future distant metastases. Int J Cancer 144: 1633–1644.

Konstantinidis, G., S. Sievers and Y.W. Wu. 2019. Identification of novel ATG inhibitors via cell-based high-content screening. Methods Mol Biol 1854: 187–195.

Lee, J.Y.C., C.W. Cu, S.L, Tsai, S.M. Cheng, et al. 2016. Inhibition of HDAC3- and HDAC6-promoted survivin expression plays an important role in SAHA-induced autophagy and viability reduction in breast cancer cells. Front Pharmacol 7: 81.

Li, H., A. Ham, T.C. Ma, S.H. Kuo, et al. 2018a. Mitochondrial dysfunction and MTG defect triggered by heterozygous GBA mutations. Autophagy 12: 1–18.

Li, C., Y. Zhang, X. Cheng, H. Yuan, et al. 2018b. PINK1 and PARK2 suppress pancreatic tumorigenesis through control of mitochondrial iron-mediated immunometabolism. Dev Cell 46: 441–455.

Li, T., K. Xu and Y. Liu. 2018c. Anticancer effect of salidroside reduces viability through autophagy/PI3K/Akt and MMP-9 signaling pathways in human bladder cancer cells. Oncol Lett 16: 3162–3168.

Li, M., M. Russo, F. Pirozzi, C.G. Tocchetti, et al. 2019a. Autophagy and cancer therapy cardiotoxicity: From molecular mechanisms to therapeutic opportunities. Biochim Biophys Acta Mol Cell Res 1867(3): 118493.

Li, Y., S. Wang, X. Wei, S. Zhang, et al. 2019b. Role of inhibitor of yes-associated protein 1 in TNB cancer with Taxol-based chemoresistance. Cancer Sci 110: 561–567.

Li, F., G. Huang, P. Peng, Y. Liu, et al. 2019c. Overexpression of autophagy-related gene 3 promotes autophagy and inhibits salinomycin-induced apoptosis in breast cancer MCF-7 cells. Nan Fang Yi Ke Da Xue Xue Bao 39: 162–168.

Li, Y., X. Jiang, Y. Zhang, Z. Gao, et al. 2019d. Nuclear accumulation of UBC9 contributes to SUMOylation of lamin A/C and nucleophagy in response to DNA damage. J Exp Clin Cancer Res 38(1): 67.

Li, S., Y. Song, C. Quach, H. Guo, et al. 2019e. Transcriptional regulation of autophagy-lysosomal function in BRAF-driven melanoma progression and chemoresistance. Nat Commun 10: 1693. https://doi. org/10.1038/s41467-019-09634-8.

Lin, H.H., Y. Chung, C.T. Cheng, C. Ouyang, et al. 2018. Autophagic reliance promotes metabolic reprogramming in oncogenic KRAS-driven tumorigenesis. Autophagy 14: 1481–1498.

Liu, Y.H., Y.P, Weng, H.Y. Tsai. C.J. Chen, et al. 2018. Aqueous extracts of *Paeonia suffruticosa* modulates mitochondrial proteostasis by reactive oxygen species-induced endoplasmic reticulum stress in pancreatic cancer cells. Phytomedicine 46: 184–192.

Liu, E.A. and A.P. Lieberman. 2019. The intersection of lysosomal and endoplasmic reticulum calcium with autophagy defects in lysosomal diseases. Neurosci Lett 697: 10–16.

Liu, Y., Y.H. Long, S.Q. Wang, Y.Y. Zhang, et al. 2019. JMJD6 regulates histone H2A.X phosphorylation and promotes ATG in TNB cancer cells via a novel TK activity. Oncogene 38: 980–997.

Ma, Y., Y. Vassetzky and S. Dokudovskaya. 2018. mTORC1 pathway in DNA damage response. Biochim Biophys Acta Mol Cell Res 1865: 1293–1311.

Marchetti, P., A. Trinh, R. Khamari and J. Kluza. 2018. Melanoma metabolism contributes to the cellular responses to MAPK/ERK pathway inhibitors. Biochim Biophys Acta Gen Subj. 1862: 999–1005.

Martins, W.K., N.F. Santos, C.S. Rocha, I.O.L. Bacellar, et al. 2018. Parallel damage in mitochondria and lysosomes is an efficient way to photoinduce cell death. Autophagy 25: 1–21.

Mele, L., M. la Noce, F. Paino, T. Regad, et al. 2019. Glucose-6-phosphate dehydrogenase blockade potentiates tyrosine kinase inhibitor effect on breast cancer cells through autophagy perturbation. J Exp Clin Cancer Res 38: 160.

Mendonça Gorgulho, C., P. Murthy, L. Liotta, V. Espina, et al. 2019. Different measures of HMGB1 location in cancer immunology. Methods Enzymol 629: 195–217.

Meyer, N., S. Zielke, J.B. Michaelis, B. Linder, et al. 2018. AT 101 induces early mitochondrial dysfunction and HMOX1 (heme oxygenase 1) to trigger mitophagic cell death in glioma cells. Autophagy 14: 1693–1709.

Motegi, S.I., C. Fujiwara, A. Sekiguchi, S. Yamazaki, et al. 2019. Possible contribution of PDGF-BB-induced autophagy in dermatofibrosarcoma protuberans: Autophagy marker Atg5 could be a differential marker between dermatofibrosarcoma protuberans and dermatofibroma. J Dermatol Sci 93: 139–141.

Park, S.H., K.H. Baek, I. Shin and I. Shin. 2018. Subcellular Hsp70 inhibitors promote cancer cell death via different mechanisms. Cell Chem Biol 25: 1242–1254.

Pavlides, S., I. Vera, R. Gandara, S. Sharon, S. Sneddon, et al. 2012. Warburg meets autophagy: Cancer-associated fibroblasts accelerate tumor growth and metastasis via oxidative stress, mitophagy, and aerobic glycolysis. Antioxidants & Redox Signaling. 16: 1264–1284.

Qiao, Z., X. Li, N. Kang, Y. Yang, et al. 2019. A novel specific Anti-CD73 antibody inhibits TNB cancer cell motility by regulating ATG. Int J Mol Sci 20(5): E1057.

Romero, M.A., E.O. BayrAktar, B.G.O, Bagca, C.B. Avci, et al. 2019. Role of ATG in BC development and progression: Opposite sides of the same coin. Adv Exp Med Biol 1152: 65–73.

Sample, A., B. Zhao, C. Wu, S. Qian, et al. 2018. The ATG receptor adaptor p62 is Up-regulated by UVA radiation in melanocytes and in melanoma cells. Photochem Photobiol 94: 432–437.

Schuetz, J.M., A. Grundy, D.G. Lee, A.S. Lai, et al. 2019. Genetic variants in genes related to inflammation, apoptosis and ATG in BC risk. PLoS One 14(1): e0209010.

Sheng, J., L. Shen, L. Sun, X. Zhang, et al. 2019. Inhibition of PI3K/mTOR increased the sensitivity of hepatocellular carcinoma cells to Cisplatin via interference with mitochondrial-lysosomal crosstalk. Cell Prolif 52: e12609.

Shinde, A., S.D. Hardy, D. Kim, S.S. Akhand, et al. 2019. Spleen TK-mediated ATG is required for epithelial-mesenchymal plasticity and metastasis in BC. Cancer Res 79: 1831–1843.

Singh, S.S., S. Vats, A.Y. Chia, T.Z. Tan, et al. 2018a. Dual role of ATG in hallmarks of cancer. Oncogene 37: 1142–1158.

Singh, A., S.L. Kendall, M. Campanella. 2018b. Common traits spark the Mitophagy/Xenophagy interplay. Front Physiol 9: 1172.

Singh, R. and S. Singh. 2019. Redox-dependent catalase mimetic cerium oxide-based nanozyme protect human hepatic cells from 3-AT induced acatalasemia. Colloids Surf B Biointerfaces 175: 625–635.

Sisinni, L., M. Pietrafesa, S. Lepore, F. Maddalena, et al. 2019. Endoplasmic reticulum stress and unfolded protein response in breast cancer: The balance between apoptosis and autophagy and its role in drug resistance. Int J Mol Sci 20(4): 857.

Sun, W.L., L. Wang, J. Luo, H.W. Zhu, et al. 2019. Ambra1 inhibits Paclitaxel-induced apoptosis in BC cells by modulating the Bim/mitochondrial pathway. Neoplasma 66: 377–385.

Towers, C.G., B.E. Fitzwalter, D. Regan, A. Goodspeed, et al. 2019. Cancer cells upregulate NRF2 signaling to adapt to ATG inhibition. Dev Cell 50: 690–703.

Ueno, T., N. Masuda, S. Kamigaki, T. Morimoto, et al. 2019. Differential involvement of ATG and apoptosis in response to chemoendocrine and endocrine therapy in BC: JBCRG-07TR. Int J Mol Sci 20(4): E984.

Vara-Perez, M., H. Maes, S. Van Dingenen and P. Agostinis. 2019. Bnip-3 contributes to the glutamine-driven aggressive behavior of melanoma cells. Biol Chem. 400(2): 187–193. doi: 10.1515/hsz-2018-0208.

Velloso, F.J., A.R. Campos, M.C. Sogayar and R.G. Correa. 2019. Proteome profiling of triple negative BC cells overexpressing NOD1 and NOD2 receptors unveils molecular signatures of malignant cell proliferation. BMC Genomics 20(1): 152.

Vera-Ramirez, L., S.K. Vodnala, R. Nini, K.W. Hunter, et al. 2018. ATG promotes the survival of dormant BC cells and metastatic tumour recurrence. Nat Commun 9: 1944.

Villa, E., S. Marchetti and J.E. Ricci. 2018. No Parkin zone: MTG without Parkin. Trends Cell Biol 28: 882–895.

Vu, H.T., M. Kobayashi, A.M. Hegazy, Y. Tadokoro, et al. 2018. ATG inhibition synergizes with calcium mobilization to achieve efficient therapy of malignant gliomas. Cancer Sci 109: 2497–2508.

Wang, X.Z., Z. Jia, H.H. Yang and Y.J. Liu. 2018. Dibenzoxanthenes induce apoptosis and autophagy in HeLa cells by modeling the PI3K/Akt pathway. J Photochem Photobiol B 187: 76–88.

Wang, L., C. Guo, X. Li, X. Yu, et al. 2019. Design, synthesis and biological evaluation of bromophenol-thiazolylhydrazone hybrids inhibiting the interaction of translation initiation factors eIF4E/eIF4G as multifunctional agents for cancer treatment. Eur J Med Chem 177: 153–170.

Wen, Z.P., W.J. Zeng, Y.H. Chen, H. Li, et al. 2019. Knockdown ATG4C inhibits gliomas progression and promotes temozolomide chemosensitivity by suppressing autophagic flux. J Exp Clin Cancer Res 38: 298.

Wu, M.Y., G.T. Yang, P.W. Cheng, P.Y. Chu, et al. 2018. Molecular targets in hepatocarcinogenesis and implications for therapy. J Clin Med 7(8): 213.

Wu, N.N. and J. Ren. 2019. Aldehyde dehydrogenase 2 (ALDH2) and aging: Is there a sensible link? Adv Exp Med Biol 1193: 237–253.

Wu, C.L., J.F. Liu, Y. Liu, Y.X. Wang, et al. 2019. Beclin1 inhibition enhances Paclitaxel-mediated cytotoxicity in BC *in vitro* and *in vivo*. Int J Mol Med 43: 1866–1878.

Xu, S., P. Wang, J. Zhang, H. Wu, et al. 2019. Ai-lncRNA EGOT enhancing ATG sensitizes paclitaxel cytotoxicity via upregulation of ITPR1 expression by RNA-RNA and RNA-protein interactions in human cancer. Mol Cancer 18(1): 89.

Xue, R., Q. Meng, D. Lu, X. Liu, et al. 2018. Mitofusin2 induces cell ATG of PC through inhibiting the PI3K/Akt/mTOR signaling pathway. Oxid Med Cell Longev 2018: 2798070.

Yazdani, H.O., H. Huang and A. Tsung. 2019. ATG: Dual response in the development of hepatocellular carcinoma. Cells 8(2): E91.

Yeo, S.K., R. Paul, M. Haas, C. Wang, et al. 2018. Improved efficacy of mitochondrial disrupting agents upon inhibition of ATG in a mouse model of BRCA1-deficient BC. Autophagy 14: 1214–1225.

Zhang, J., X. Sun, L. Wang and Y.K. Wong. 2018. Artesunate-induced MTG alters cellular redox status. Redox Biol 19: 263–273.

Zhao, Y., K. Onda, K. Sugiyama, B. Yuan, et al. 2019. Antitumor effects of arsenic disulfide on the viability, migratory ability, apoptosis and ATG of BC cells. Oncol Rep 41: 27–42.

Zóia, M.A.P., F.V.P. Azevedo, L. Vecchi, S.T.S. Mota, et al. 2019. Inhibition of Triple-Negative Breast cancer cell aggressiveness by cathepsin D blockage: Role of annexin A1. Int J Mol Sci 20(6): 1337.

30

Charnolophagy in Cancer (B)

INTRODUCTION

Mitochondrial dysfunction has potential implications in NDDs, CVDs, and cancer. In earlier studies, the author described that drugs may be developed specifically to enhance CB formation, inhibit CP, and destabilize CP in cancer stem cells to cure MDR malignancies and chronic infections. The TSE-EBPT of chronic MDR malignancies can be accomplished by augmenting cancer-stem-cell-specific CP and destabilizing CS and vice-versa for the clinical management of NDDs, MDDs, multiple drug abuse, and CVDs. Nonspecific induction of CB formation, CP inhibition, and CS destabilization causes undesirable adverse effects in MDR malignancies. Hence, cancer stem cell-specific CB, CP, and CS agonists/antagonists can be developed as novel TSE-EBPT-CPTs for the clinical management of MDR malignancies. Impaired CP of nucleated erythroid cells causes anemia in patients with myelodysplastic syndromes. ATG promotes metabolic reprogramming in KRAS-driven tumorigenesis. Hence, a CP-driven metabolic switch can reprogram stem cell fate in malignancies. PP2A-like protein phosphatase Ppg1 serves as a negative regulator of CP in yeast and 2-deoxy-D-glucose augments photodynamic therapy by inducing mitochondrial caspase-independent ATP-driven CP/ATG and apoptosis. Recently, Naik et al. (2019) described MTG and its association with cellular programming through alteration in the MB. The metabolic shift post MTG was suggested as a crucial factor in the cell fate transition during differentiation and de-differentiation. "Cellular reprogramming" facilitates the generation of desired cellular phenotype through transition by affecting the mitochondrial dynamics and metabolic reshuffle in the embryonic and somatic stem cells. Both differentiation and de-differentiation of cells lead to the alteration in the morphology, number, distribution, and O/P capacity of mitochondria, regulated by the fission/fusion cycle, and clearance through CP/ATG following their fission. CP and CPI are essential in the differentiation of stem cells into various lineages such as RBCs, eye lenses, neurites, myotubes, and M1 macrophages. CP also plays a crucial role in the de-differentiation of a terminally differentiated cells into an iPPC and in the acquisition of 'stemness' in cancer cells. CP-induced alteration in the mitochondrial dynamics facilitates a metabolic shift, either into a glycolytic phenotype or into an O/P phenotype, depending on the cellular demand. CP-induced rejuvenation of mitochondria regulates the transition of bioenergetics and metabolome remodeling to facilitate an alteration in their cellular developmental capability. Kruppa and Buss (2018) reported that intracellular homeostasis is maintained by removing dysfunctional, undesired, ubiquitinated mitochondria from the network via PRKN-dependent CP/ATG. MYO6, a myosin that moves towards the minus ends of actin filaments, forms a complex with PRKN and is recruited to CBs by binding to ubiquitin. On the mitochondrial surface, a myosin motor initiates the assembly of F-actin cages, which serve as a MQC mechanism to isolate CBs, thereby preventing their refusion with the neighboring population of normal mitochondria. MYO6 also plays a role in the later stages of the CP pathway by tethering endosomes to actin filaments facilitating CS maturation and APS-lysosome fusion. Furukawa and Kanki (2017) showed that the protein phosphatase 2A-like protein phosphatase Ppg1 and its associated complex inhibit CP by counteracting casein kinase 2-mediated phosphorylation of the CP receptor ATG32. In the yeast S, cerevisiae, receptor proteins for the cytoplasm-to-vacuole targeting pathway, CP, and pexophagy are regulated by kinases, which facilitate interaction with the scaffold/adaptor protein ATG11, recruiting ATG proteins to initiate APS formation.

The chapter describes novel CP/ATG inhibitors, CP regulators, antioxidants, and CPTs for the TSE-EBPT of MDR malignancies.

Chloroquine as a CP Antagonist in Cancer Theranostics

A lysosomotropic agent Chloroquine (CQ) exhibits antitumor activity in several tumors including lung cancer as mono- or add-on therapy by augmenting CPI. The antitumor effect of CQ depend on the tumor type, stage, and genetic background. A study identified the antitumor effect of CQ monotherapy. CQ suppressed human A549 cell growth by targeting PI3K/Akt pathway, thus, inducing mitochondria-mediated apoptosis at relatively higher concentrations by downregulating Bcl-2, upregulating Bax, decreasing $\Delta\Psi$, releasing Cyt-C from the mitochondria into the cytosol, activating caspase-3 and cleaving PARP, providing a rationale for using CQ as an adjuvent lung cancer therapy. Similarly, Hydroxy-CQ (HCQ) disrupted ATG and sensitized cancer cells to radiation and chemotherapeutics. However, the optimal method of delivery, dose, and tumor concentrations required for these effects remain uncertain due to the lack of sensitive and reproducible analytical methods for HCQ estimation.

Chhonker et al. (2018) developed a selective and sensitive LC-MS/MS method for the estimation of HCQ and its metabolites in blood and tissue samples. The chromatographic separation and detection of analytes were achieved on a reversed phase Thermo Aquasil C_{18} (50×4.6 mm, 3 µ) column, with gradient elution using 0.2% formic acid and 0.1% formic acid in methanol as mobile phase at a flow rate of 0.5 mL/min. Protein precipitation was utilized for the extraction of analytes, which were identified and quantitated using MS/MS with an electrospray ionization source in positive multiple reaction monitoring (MRM) mode. The method was applied to a preclinical PKs study involving low volume blood and tissue samples for HQ and metabolites. GBM, often referred to as a grade IV astrocytoma, is the most invasive tumor arising from glial cells with poor prognosis due to MDR to standard therapy. The main treatment options for GBM include surgery, radiation, and chemotherapy, which tend to be only palliative rather than curative. Currently, Temozolomide (TMZ), an alkylating agent is used for the treatment of GBM. However, GBM cells can repair TMZ-induced DNA damage and diminish the therapeutic efficacy. The potential to evade apoptosis by GBM cells accentuates the need to target the non-apoptotic pathway and/or inhibit pro-survival strategies that contribute to its high resistance to conventional therapies. HDAC inhibitors, such as Vorinostat (suberoyl anilide hydroxamic acid; SAHA) can induce ATG in cancer cells, thereby stimulating APS formation. CQ can result in accumulation of ATG vacuoles by inhibiting APS-lysosome fusion, which can drive the cell towards apoptosis. Hence, a combination treatment with SAHA and CQ may lead to the increased formation of APSs, resulting in its accumulation and ultimately, cell death in GBM cells. CQ co-treatment enhanced SAHA-mediated GBM cell apoptosis. Hence, the combined effect of SAHA and CQ can be developed as a novel theranostic strategy for the treatment of GBM. Similarly, Vorinostat, a pan-histone deacetylase (HDAC) inhibitor, exerts anticancer activity in a variety of solid and hematologic malignancies. However, the efficacy of Vorinostat monotherapy is unsatisfactory. Jing et al. (2018) showed that Quinacrine (QC), an anti-malaria drug with ATG inhibitory activity, could synergistically enhance Vorinostat-induced cell death. Compared to the single treatment, QC plus Vorinostat induced apoptosis, disrupted $\Delta\Psi$, and decreased Mcl-1 and Bcl-2/Bax ratio. The application of QC plus Vorinostat resulted in a CP blockade, as reflected by the increase in the K63-linked ubiquitination of mitochondria protein and the formation of CPS/CS. QC plus Vorinostat increased the ROS whereas the ROS scavenger NAC abrogated QC plus Vorinostat-induced ROS, decreased the ubiquitination of mitochondrial proteins, and cell death. In a xenograft mouse model, QC plus Vorinostat reduced cell proliferation and induced cell death *in vivo*, indicating that the combination of QC with Vorinostat may represent a novel regimen for the TSE-EBPT of T-cell acute lymphoblastic leukemia (ALL). ATG inhibition is crucial for improving the efficacy of cancer radiotherapy. A study determined the potential therapeutic value of ATG and its correlation with mitochondria in human esophageal carcinoma cells following treatment with ionizing radiation (IR). ATG in Eca-109 cells was induced under poor nutrient conditions. A nude mouse xenograft model was also employed to verify the effects and mechanisms underlying ATG *in vivo*. The formed ATG vesicles and increased LC3 II/LC3 I ratio indicated induction of ATG by Earle's balanced salt solution (EBSS) in Eca-109 cells. 3-MA or LY294002 antagonized EBSS-induced ATG and increased apoptosis of irradiated cells, suggesting that ATG inhibition conferred radio-sensitivity *in vitro*. IR induced release of Cyt-C and Bax activation, and decreased Bcl-2 and $\Delta\Psi$ in Eca109 cells under poor nutrient conditions. These changes were more prominent following pretreatment with ATG inhibitors. IR treatment delayed tumor growth, but the radio-therapeutic effect was improved by abolishing ATG. Furthermore, mitochondrial signaling was investigated in the Eca109 xenograft nude mice model, and the results were consistent with the *in vitro* study. Therefore, the mitochondrial pathway may be associated with improvement of radio-sensitivity in Eca109 cells. GBM cells are characterized by high phagocytosis, lipogenesis, exocytosis, low CP/ATG and high lysosomal demand are necessary for survival and invasion. The lysosome is implicated in lipid biosynthesis, transporting, sorting between exogenous and endogenous cholesterol. Hsu et al. (2018) hypothesized that the ATG inducer, Sirolimus (Rapamycin, Rapa), the ATG inhibitor, CQ, and DNA alkylating, Temozolomide (TMZ) could synergize in GBM. Triple therapy induced GBM apoptosis *in vitro* and inhibited GBM xenograft growth *in vivo*. Cytotoxicity was caused by induction of LMP and the release of hydrolases, and could be rescued by cholesterol supplementation. Triple treatment inhibited lysosomal function, prevented cholesterol extraction from LDL, and caused clumping of LAMP-1 and LD accumulation. Co-treatment with inhibitor of caspases and Cathepsin B only partially reversed cytotoxicities, while NAC was more effective. A combination of ROS generation from cholesterol depletion was the underlying mechanism. Cholesterol repletion abolished the ROS production and reversed the cytotoxicity from the QRT treatment. The shortage of free cholesterol destabilized lysosomal membranes, converting aborted ATG to apoptosis through either direct mitochondrial damage or Cathepsin B release. This triple therapy combination decreased mitochondrial function, induced lysosome-dependent apoptotic cell death, and could be evaluated for the TSE-EBPT of GBM. Yan et al. (2018a) prepared lup-20(29)-en-3β,28-di-yl-nitrooxy acetate (NBT), a derivative of Betulin (BT), that was chemically modified at position 3 of ring A and C-28 by introducing a NO-releasing moiety to explore the mechanism of NBT in treating BC through the crosstalk between apoptosis and ATG in mitochondria. NBT possessed a potent anti-proliferative activity in MCF-7 cells, both *in vitro* and *in vivo*. NBT affected cell death through the mitochondrial apoptosis pathway and ATG. NBT induced cell-cycle arrest in the G_0/G_1 phase by decreasing the expression of cyclin D1. It also induced mitochondrial apoptosis by increasing the expression of Bax, caspase-9, PARP cleavage, $\Delta\Psi$ collapse, and leakage of Cyt-C from mitochondria in MCF-7 cells and decreasing the expression of Bcl-2. These investigators further investigated whether CQ, which inhibits the degradation of APS induced by NBT, affects the proliferation of MCF-7 cells compared with NBT. A combination of NBT and CQ promoted MCF-7 cell mitochondria to divide and Cyt-C to be released from mitochondria to the cytoplasm, resulting in an enhanced apoptosis. NBT inhibited the growth of MCF-7 tumor via the apoptotic pathway similar to 5-fluorouracil. Bai et al. (2018) showed that 5-(3, 4, 5-trimethoxybenzoyl)-4-methyl-2-(p-tolyl) imidazol (BZML) is a novel Colchicine-binding-site inhibitor with anti-cancer activity in apoptosis resistant A549/Taxol cells through mitotic catastrophe (MC). The different functional forms of ATG were distinguished by determining the impact of ATG inhibition on drug sensitivity. BZML also exhibited anti-cancer activity against MDR-NSCLC by showing ROS overproduction and $\Delta\Psi$ collapse followed by Cyt-C release from the mitochondria to cytosol in both A549 and A549/Taxol cells. However, the ROS-mediated apoptotic pathway involving mitochondria induced by BZML was activated in A549 cells but not in A549/Taxol cells. ATG remained non-protective during BZML-induced apoptosis in A549 cells, whereas it conferred protection against BZML-induced MC in A549/Taxol cells, suggesting that this anti-apoptotic property originated from a defect in the activation of the mitochondrial apoptotic pathway, and ATG inhibitors like CQ can potentiate BZML-induced MC to overcome resistance to mitochondrial apoptosis. Tamoxifen is used to treat patients with ESR/ER-positive BC, but its theranostic potential is limited by the development of MDR. Recently, alterations in the macroATG/ATG function were demonstrated as potential mechanism for Tamoxifen resistance (Mishra et al. 2020). Lee et al. (2018) reported that the level of MTA1 expression was upregulated in the Tamoxifen resistant BC cell lines MCF7/TAMR and T47D/TR, and the knockdown of MTA1 sensitized the cells to 4-Hydroxy-Tamoxifen (4OHT). The knockdown of MTA1 decreased the enhanced ATG flux in the Tamoxifen-resistant cell lines. To confirm the role of MTA1 in the development of Tamoxifen resistance, they established a cell line, MCF7/MTA1, which expressed MTA1. Compared with parental MCF7, MCF7/MTA1 cells were more resistant to 4OHT-induced growth inhibition, and exhibited enhanced ATG and higher numbers of APSs. The knockdown of ATG7 or co-treatment with OH-CQ restored sensitivity to 4OHT in both the MCF7/MTA1 and Tamoxifen resistant cells. AMPK was activated because of an increased AMP: ATP ratio and decreased expression of ETC components. BC patient data indicated that MTA1 levels correlate with poor prognosis and development of recurrence in patients treated with Tamoxifen, indicating that MTA1 induces AMPK activation and subsequent ATG could contribute to Tamoxifen resistance in BC.

CP-targeted Cancer Theranostics

ING4 in Cancers and Non-Neoplastic Disorders

Inhibitors of growth 4 (ING4), a member of the ING family, act as tumor suppressors and are downregulated in various human cancers. ING4 is responsible for characteristic cancer hallmarks: cell-cycle arrest, apoptosis, ATG, contact inhibition, hypoxic adaptation, tumor angiogenesis, invasion, and metastasis, associated with regulation through chromatin acetylation by binding histone H3 trimethylated at lysine 4 (H3K4me3) and through the transcriptional activity of P53 and NF-κB. Abnormalities in ING4 expression and function play key roles in non-neoplastic disorders. Du et al. (2019) provided an overview of ING4-modulated chromosome remodeling and transcriptional function, as well as the functional consequences of different genetic variants and current understanding regarding the role of ING4 in the development of neoplastic and non-neoplastic diseases for pursuing novel TSE-EBPT of various cancers. The role of NGL-4 in various neoplastic and non-neoplastic diseases is presented in Fig. 46.

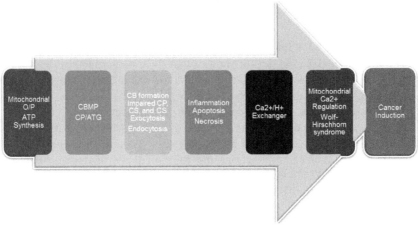

Figure 46

Leucine Zipper EF-hand Transmembrane Protein-1

Lin et al. (2019) provided an overview of the current understanding of the LETM1 structure and function and highlighted the lacunae in the present knowledge to unravel the basic molecular function of LETM1 in health and disease. Mitochondrial Ca^{2+} uptake shapes cytosolic Ca^{2+} signals in numerous cellular processes and regulates mitochondrial functions, including ATP production, CP/ATG, and apoptosis. Given the intimate link to both life and death processes, it is imperative that mitochondria regulate their Ca^{2+} levels with a high degree of precision. Among the Ca^{2+} handling tools of mitochondria, the leucine EF-hand (containing transmembrane protein-1 (LETM1), a transporter protein is a Ca^{2+} regulating tool of mitochondria, which is localized to the IMM and constitute a Ca^{2+}/H^+ exchanger. The significance of LETM1in mitochondrial Ca^{2+} regulation is evident from Wolf-Hirschhorn syndrome patients that harbor a haplo-deficiency in LETM1 expression, leading to impaired mitochondrial Ca^{2+} handling and from various cancer cells that show an upregulation of LETM1 expression. I have proposed LETM1 as a molecular switch in the induction and repression of CBMP involving CB formation, CP dysregulation, CS stabilization, and impaired CS exocytosis/endocytosis in health and disease as illustrated in Fig. 47.

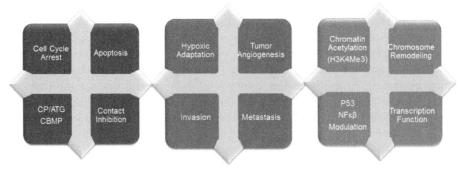

Figure 47

Omics Characterization

Cavadas et al. (2018) conducted omics study of the oncocytic phenotype in 488 papillary thyroid carcinomas (PTC) from *The Cancer Genome Atlas* (Weinstein et al. 2013). Oncocytic phenotype is secondary to PTC, being unrelated to several pathologic scores. The nuclear genome had low impact on this phenotype (except in specific copy number variation), which was driven by the accumulation of mtDNA non-synonymous and frameshift mutations at high heteroplasmy levels. ATP and mitochondrial-related pathways were enriched in oncocytic tumors that also displayed an increased expression of genes involved in ATG and fusion of mitochondria, confirming that ATG is increased and remains functional while CP is decreased in these tumors.

Photodynamic Therapy

The ability of photosensitizing agents to create photo-damage at specific subcellular sites is useful for characterizing pathway(s) to cell death and for selecting optimal targets for anti-tumor efficacy. ER photo-damage involves extensive cytoplasmic vacuole formation but does not represent ATG. This is termed "paraptosis" due to the appearance of misfolded ER proteins. Kessel (2018) summarized current knowledge relating to death pathways and information relating to paraptosis as a PDT response. ATG and apoptosis occur after photodamage directed at mitochondria, lysosomes, or the ER. Hence, a combination of lysosomal + mitochondrial targets may enhance efficacy.

Cis-Khellactone

Jung et al. (2018) introduced cis-khellactone (c-Kh) as a new anti-cancer agent, which was isolated from the chloroform soluble fraction of the rhizomes of *Angelica amurensis*. It was at first tested in MCF7 and MDA-MB-231 breast cell lines. MCF7 is resistant to many anti-cancer drugs. MCF10A normal breast cell line was used as a control. c-Kh suppressed cell growth and proliferation at low concentrations (<5 µg/ml) and decreased cell viability at high concentrations (>10 µg/ml) in both cancer cell lines. The anti-cancerous effect was also checked in an additional 16 different types of normal and cancer cell lines. c-Kh suppressed cell proliferation and enhanced cell death in all tested cancer cell lines. c-Kh induced three types of cell death (CD): apoptosis, ATG-mediated, and necrosis/necroptosis, and decreased cell viability by increasing ROS and decreasing $\Delta\Psi$, related to all three types of CD. c-Kh induced the translocation of BAX and BAK into mitochondria as well as the overexpression of VDAC1, which accelerated $\Delta\Psi$ disruption and finally, cell death. *In vivo* studies with xenograft model confirmed anticancer properties of c-Kh without any deleterious effect on the normal tissue. These findings suggested that c-Kh may have TSE-EBPT potential for the treatment of cancer.

Interferon-γ

Colorectal cancer (CRC) is the second most commonly diagnosed cancer in females and the third in males. Wang et al. (2018a) investigated the possible anti-cancer effects of IFN-γ on CRC cells. IFN-γ induced ROS production in SW480 and HCT116 cell lines. The IFN-γ-induced ROS generation was dependent on the activation of phospholipase A2 (cPLA2). A mitochondria-targeted antioxidant SS31 and/or cPLA2 inhibitor AACOCF3 abolished the IFN-γ-induced ROS production and subsequent ATG and apoptosis. Suppression of ATG by CQ reduced IFN-γ-induced cell apoptosis. Beclin-1 gene silencing resulted in caspase-3 inactivation, a decreased Bax/Bcl-2 ratio, and less population of apoptotic cells, suggesting that IFN-γ induces ATG-associated apoptosis in CRC cells via inducing cPLA2-dependent ROS production.

Hydrogel and Monolayer Cultures

TNBC is a devastating breast carcinoma that is unresponsive to targeted receptor therapies. The development of new treatment strategies would benefit from an expanded repertoire of *in vitro* cell culture systems, such as those that support 3D growth in the presence of hydrogel scaffolds. Jogalekar and Serrano (2018) established protocols for maintenance of the TNBC cell line HCC70 in monolayer culture and in a commercially available basement membrane matrix hydrogel. They evaluated the general morphology of cells grown in both conditions with LM, and examined their subcellular organization using TEM. Phase contrast and confocal microscopy showed the prevalence of irregularly shaped flattened cells in monolayer cultures, while cells maintained in hydrogel organized into multi-layered spheroids. The cells that formed spheroids comprised a greater number of mitochondria, ATG vacuoles, and intercellular junctions than their monolayer counterparts, within the equivalent area of sampled tissue, suggesting that TMBC cells in culture can alter their organelle content, as well as their morphology, in response to their microenvironment. These methods may be useful for those who intend to image cell cultures with TEM, and to implement diverse *in vitro* models in the search for a TSE-EBPT for TNBC.

Polyamine Conjugate of Flavonoid

Polyamine conjugated flavonoid with a naphthalene moiety (ZYY14) displayed therapeutic activity against HCC. Li et al. (2018) designed three series of novel flavonoid-polyamine conjugates and screened them in tumor cell lines. The structure-activity relationship demonstrated the importance of the naphthalene moiety (as the B-ring), the basic side chains in the A-ring, and the methoxy group linked to the C-ring. The optimized compound 9b displayed better antitumor potency *in vitro* and *in vivo* than the lead compound ZYY14. Fluorescent assays revealed that 9b could enter cancer cells via polyamine transporter (PAT) and locate in mitochondria and ER. Compound 9b and ZYY14 demonstrated similar apoptotic mechanisms of cytotoxicity and induced apoptosis-related proteins, such as p-p38, p-JNK, p53, and Bax. In addition, 9b could initiate ATG which inhibited apoptosis. Thus, 9b can be used for the development of antitumor agents.

Inonotus Taiwanensis Polysaccharide

Chao et al. (2018) evaluated the anti-cancerous efficacy of a water-soluble polysaccharide extract from *Inonotus taiwanensis* (WSPIS) on human acute monocytic leukemia THP-1 and U937 cell lines *in vitro*. WSPIS elicited dose-dependent growth retardation and induced apoptotic cell death. The WSPIS induced a mitochondrial apoptotic pathway, ($\Delta\Psi$ collapse, caspase-9, caspase-3 activation, and PARP cleavage). However, a caspase inhibitor, Z-VAD.fmk, could not prevent WSPIS-induced apoptosis, indicating mechanism(s) other than caspase might be involved. Thus, the involvement of endonuclease G (endoG), a mediator arbitrating caspase-independent oligonucleosomal DNA fragmentation, was examined. WSPIS elicited the nuclear translocation of endoG. MMP disruption after WSPIS treatment was accompanied by ROS generation. However, pretreatment with NAC could not attenuate WSPIS-induced apoptosis. WSPIS inhibited ATG while the activation of ATG by Rapamycin decreased WSPIS-induced apoptosis and cell death, suggesting that cell-cycle arrest, endonuclease G-mediated apoptosis, and ATG inhibition contribute to the anti-cancerous effect of WSPIS.

Peroxisomal Changes with 7-Ketocholesterol

To study the role of peroxisomes in cell death, Nuri et al. (2018) treated 158 N murine oligo-dendrocytes with 7-ketocholesterol (7 KC: 25–50 μM, 24 hrs). The highest concentration induced oxiapoptophagy (OXIdative stress + APOPTOsis + ATG), whereas the lowest concentration did not induce cell death. In those conditions, (with KC: 50 μM), morphological, topographical, and functional peroxisomal alterations were associated with modification of the cytoplasmic distribution of mitochondria. These modifications were accompanied with mitochondrial dysfunction, characterized by $\Delta\psi$ collapse, decreased cardiolipin, and oxidative stress. During oxidative stress, peroxisomes appeared abnormal in size and shapes, similar to those observed in Zellweger fibroblasts. Lower cellular level of ABCD3 was used as a marker of peroxisomal mass employing flow cytometry. Lower mRNA and protein levels of ABCD1 and ABCD3 (two ATP-dependent peroxisomal transporters) and of ACox1 and MPP2 enzymes, and of DHAPT, involved in peroxisomal β oxidation and plasmalogen synthesis, respectively were estimated. Increased levels of very long chain fatty acids (VLCFA:C24:0, C24:1, C26:0, C26:1) were quantitatively estimated by gas chromatography coupled with mass spectrometry. In the presence of 7 KC (25 μM), slight mitochondrial dysfunction and oxidative stress were found, and no induction of apoptosis was detected; however, modifications of the cytoplasmic distribution of mitochondria and clusters of mitochondria were detected. The peroxisomal alterations observed with 7 KC (25 μM) were similar to those with 7 KC (50 μM). TEM and immunofluorescence microscopy by dual staining with antibodies raised against p62, involved in ATG, and ABCD3, supported that 7 KC (25–50 μM) induces pexophagy. 7 KC (25–50 μM)-induced side effects were attenuated by α-Tocopherol but not by α-Tocotrienol, whereas the anti-oxidant properties of these molecules determined with the FRAP assay were in the same range, indicating that 7 KC triggers morphological, topographical, and functional peroxisomal alterations associated with mitochondrial changes.

Peroxisomes in Dox Chemotherapy

Doxorubicin (Dox), a commonly used anti-neoplastic agent, causes severe neurotoxicity by cortical atropyy and accelerates brain aging, leading to cognitive impairment due to the unspecific induction of CBMP. Oxidative stress induced by Dox contributes to cellular damage. In addition to mitochondria, peroxisomes also generate ROS and promote cell senescence. Moruno-Manchon et al. (2018) demonstrated that the number of peroxisomes was increased in Dox-treated neurons and in the brains of mice which underwent Dox-based chemotherapy. Pexophagy (ATG of peroxisomes) was downregulated in neurons, and peroxisomes produced more ROS. 2-Hydroxypropyl-β-cyclodextrin (HPβCD), an activator of the transcription factor TFEB, which regulates gene expression involved in ATG and lysosome function, mitigated pexophagy damage and decreased Dox-induced ROS production, indicating that peroxisome-associated oxidative stress induced by Dox may contribute to neurotoxicity, cognitive dysfunction, and accelerated brain aging in cancer patients and survivors. Hence, peroxisomes might be a valuable target for alleviating neurotoxicity caused by chemotherapeutic drugs and for slowing down brain aging in general.

Gambogic Acid

Pan et al. (2018) treated PTEN$^{-/-}$/p53$^{-/-}$ PC cells and Los Angeles prostate cancer-4 (LAPC-4) cells with GA for 24 hrs and 48 hrs, and determined cell viability by cell proliferation assay to investigate its effect on the growth and death of castrate-resistant prostate cancer (PC) with PTEN and p53 genes deleted cells. The PTEN$^{-/-}$/p53$^{-/-}$ PC cells' organoids number was calculated via a GA treatment for 1 week. A cell titer glo assay was performed to analyze the 3-D cell viability of patients-derived xenografts (PDX) 170.2 organoids. Flow cytometry was used to detect apoptotic cells. Apoptotic-cell-death-related protein levels were measured in GA-treated cells and organoids. The treatment of GA reduced the cell viability of PTEN$^{-/-}$/p53$^{-/-}$ PC cells and LAPC-4. In organoids, GA showed inhibition towards organoids' numbers and diameters and led to a complete inhibition of organoids with GA 150 nmol/L. *Ex vivo* results validated that GA 1 μmol/L inhibited 44.6% PDX170.2 organoids' growth. Flow cytometry detected increased apoptosis under GA treatment. In addition, the mitochondrial fragmentation that emerged in GA-treated cells indicated the mitochondrial apoptotic pathway might be involved. Furthermore, WB detected caspases-3, -9 activation and LC-3 conversion with GA treatment. WB revealed decreased activity of the MAPK pathway and downregulation of the downstream *c-fos* oncogene RNA level was detected before undergoing apoptosis. GA was a potent anti-tumor compound for PTEN$^{-/-}$/p53$^{-/-}$ PC, which contributed to apoptosis via inhibition of the MAPK pathway and *c-fos*.

Bromophenol-thiazolylhydrazone Hybrids

The eukaryotic initiation factor 4E (eIF4E) is an emerging anticancer drug target for specific anticancer therapy to overcome drug resistance and promote antitumor efficacy. Wang et al. (2019) synthesized a series of bromophenol-thiazolylhydrazone hybrids and evaluated for their antitumor activities. The most potent compound 3E (EGPI-1) could inhibit the eIF4E/eIF4G interaction. EGPI-1 played an antitumor role in multiple modes of action including regulating the activity of eIF4E by inhibiting the phosphorylation of eIF4E and 4EBP1, disrupting mitochondrial function through the mTOR/4EBP1 signaling pathway, and inducing ATG, apoptosis, and ROS generation. EGPI-1 showed good safety and favorable Pks properties *in vivo*, indicating that it may serve as a lead compound for the development of new anticancer drugs that target the eIF4E/eIF4G interface and as a genetic probe to investigate its role in biological processes and human diseases.

7-Acetylsinumaximol B

The 7-Acetylsinumaximol B (7-AB), a bioactive cembranoid, was discovered from aquaculture soft coral *Sinularia sandensis*. Tsai et al. (2018) investigated the anti-proliferative property of 7-AB in NCI-N87 human gastric cancer cell line. 7-AB-induced anti-proliferation towards NCI-N87 cells was associated with the release of Cyt-C from the mitochondria, activation of pro-apoptotic proteins (such as caspase-3/-9, Bax and Bad), and inhibition of anti-apoptotic proteins (Bcl-2, Bcl-xL, and Mcl-1). The 7-AB treatment triggered ERS, leading to the activation of the PERK/eIF2α/ATF4/CHOP apoptotic pathway. Furthermore, 7-AB initiated ATG in NCI-N87 cells and induced the expression of ATG-related proteins, including ATG3, Atg5, ATG7, ATG12, LC3-I, and LC3-II, suggesting that 7-AB may be developed as a useful anti-cancer agent for the treatment of gastric cancer. Activation of afore-mentioned apoptotic pathway also induced ERS in Lead-induced nephrotoxicity (Wang et al. 2019b).

2-Deoxy-D-Glucose and Photodynamic Therapy

To assess the combined impact of the glycolysis inhibitor 2-deoxy-D-glucose (2-DG) and photodynamic therapy (PDT) on ATG and apoptosis on human BC cells, Feng et al. (2018) used calcium-AM/PI double staining to evaluate cell viability. Combined 2-DG+PDT resulted in higher cytotoxicity in the three BC cell lines (MDA-MB-231, MCF-7, and 4T1), consistent with tumor growth regression seen in the 4T1 xenograft model. A synergistic augmentation of mitochondrial dysfunction (that is, ROS generation, ΔΨ collapse, and PGC-1α downregulation, and ATP depletion) was seen in cells receiving 2-DG and PDT. The nuclear translocation of AIF and DNA damage indicated that the cytotoxic effects were mediated by a caspase-independent mechanism, which was relieved by the ROS scavenger, NAC. ATG via AMPK was also observed following 2-DG+PDT, and reversed upon pre-treatment with the CP/ATG inhibitor 3-MA. The anti-cancer effects of 2-DG+PDT were mediated by both AMPK-mediated CP/ATG and mitochondria-triggered apoptosis.

Dibenzoxanthenes

Wang et al. (2018) synthesized dibenzoxanthene derivatives which showed anti-tumor activity in A549, Eca-109, HeLa, HepG2, and SGC-7901 cell lines. Compounds 4a-4d could inhibit the migration and invasion of HeLa cells in wound healing and trans-well assays. Compounds induced specifically DNA damage, arrested cell cycle distribution at the G0/G1 phase, and ATG of HeLa cells, and upregulated the expression of LC3-II and Beclin-1. Treatment with the ATG inhibitor, 3-MA, induced a decrease in apoptosis, indicating that ATG promoted apoptosis. Compounds 4a-4d enhanced the intracellular Ca^{2+} and ROS. The $\Delta\Psi$ was depolarized and the Cyt-C was released from mitochondria into cytoplasm. These compounds decreased the expression of PI3K and Akt and exhibited anti-cancer activity via ATG and apoptosis through the inhibition of the PI3K/Akt signaling pathway.

Oxazolinoanthracyclines

Rogalska et al. (2018) reported the ability of oxazoline analogs of Dox (O-DOX) and Daunorubicin (O-DAU) to induce apoptosis and ATG in ovarian and liver cancer cells. RONS, together with $[Ca^{2+}]_i$ are essential for the anticancer effect of these anthracycline analogs. The changes of $\Delta\Psi$ and induction of the ceramide pathway suggested that these compounds induce apoptosis. A significant increase of APS formation was observed by fluorescence assay and Acridine orange staining, indicating that these analogs also induce ATG. Compared to free DOX- and DAU-treated cells, they observed the inhibition of colony formation and migration, a time-dependency between ROS/RNS levels and $\Delta\Psi$ collapse. This study broadened the basis of oxazolinoanthracyclines targets and revealed that derivatives mediated oxidative stress, ceramide production, and increase in $[Ca^{2+}]_i$ by mitochondria, highlighting the importance of mitochondria as inducers of CP/ATG as well as apoptotic signals.

Bnip-3 in Glutamine-driven Melanoma Cells

Vara-Perez et al. (2019) compared the effects of glucose or glutamine on melanoma cell proliferation, migration, and oxidative phosphorylation *in vitro*. The glutamine-driven melanoma cell's aggressive traits positively correlated with an increased expression of HIF-1α and its pro-ATG (CP) target, Bnip-3. Bnip-3 silencing reduced glutamine-mediated effects on melanoma cell growth, migration, and bioenergetics, indicating that Bnip-3 is a vital component of the MQC for glutamine-driven melanoma aggressiveness.

Endorepellin

Regulation of ATG by proteolytically cleaved fragments of heparan sulfate proteoglycans is a now research focus in tumor biology. Endorepellin (EndoR) is the C-terminal angiostatic fragment of the heparan sulfate proteoglycan perlecan and induces ATG in endothelial cells. Neill et al. (2018) used NanoString, a digital PCR for measuring pre-defined transcripts in biological samples to analyze a custom subset of 95 ATG-related genes in umbilical vein endothelial cells treated with recombinant EndoR. They discovered an EndoR-evoked pro-CP and pro-ATG gene expression, which included two up-regulated mitochondrial-associated genes encoding the E3 ubiquitin protein ligase, Parkin, and the tumor suppressor, mitostatin. Induction of both proteins required the TK activity of VEGFR2. EndoR evoked mitochondrial depolarization in endothelial cells via a specific interaction between its two proximal LG1/2 domains and VEGFR2. Following $\Delta\Psi$ collapse, mitostatin and Parkin interacted and mitostatin associated with the Parkin receptor, mitofusin-2.

Pt(II) Complexes

Rahman et al. (2019) conducted a study to demonstrate ONS-donor ligand based Pt(II) complexes with anticancer potency showed a higher anticancer effect as compared to Cisplatin. Pt(II) (R-salicylaldimine)Cl (C1a-C4a) (R = 5-H, 5-CH$_3$, F, 3-CH$_3$O) complexes were prepared from commercially available materials. The chloride ancillary ligand of "a" series (C1a-C4a) was replaced with 4-picoline and "b" series of four complexes Pt(II)(R-salicylaldimine)(4-picoline) BF$_4$ (C1b-C4b) (R = 5-H, 5-CH$_3$, F, 3-CH$_3$O) was obtained. Among these, the structures of C1a, C2a, C2b, and C3b were determined in solid state by a single crystal X-ray analysis. A quick aquation of "a" series of complexes in the DMSO/water mixture was found that was wel-l investigated by ^{1}H NMNR, LCMS, and ESI-MS, while "b" series of these complexes remained stable over a month as described by the ^{1}H NMNR in the DMSO/D$_2$O mixture. This ONS-donor ligand based class of Pt(II) complexes showed anticancer potency in non-small cell lung cancer A549, colorectal cancer HT-29, and TNB cancer MDA-MB-231 cells. These Pt(II) complexes induced PARP cleavage and the inhibited colony-formation ability of cancer cells. Reduced aggressive growth of cancer cells was observed by the induction of ATG cell death via LC3-I/LC3-II expression and recruitment of LC3B to the APS membrane. These complexes induced p21 expression, suggesting their potentials to suppress cell cycle progression. Activation of Caspase3/7-dependent apoptotic signaling was observed in cancer cells treated with these Pt(II) complexes. Morphological changes of cancer cells suggested their potentials to modulate epithelial-mesenchymal-transition (EMT)-like features of cancer cells. Gel electrophoresis revealed their interaction with plasmid DNA. Similarly, a strong growth retardation effect and filamentous morphology was observed in *E. coli*. These ONS-donor Pt(II) complexes possessed an anticancer effect on multiple human cancer cells via activation of multiple pathways for ATG and apoptotic cell death.

MAL-PDT Inhibits Oral Precancerous Cells

Oral cancer is very common with a high mortality rate. Although surgery is the most effective treatment, it causes deformity and dysfunction in the orofacial region. In a study, methyl aminolevulinate photodynamic therapy (MAL-PDT) as a prevention tool in the progression of precancerous lesion to oral cancer was explored (Wang et al. 2019b). MAL-PDT induced ATG cell death in DOK oral precancerous cells. The ATG-related markers LC3-II and p62/SQSTM1 and APS formation in DOK cells were increased after the MAL-PDT treatment. *In vivo*, Metvix®-PDT treatment decreased tumor growth and enhanced LC3-II expression in hamster buccal pouch tumors induced by DMBA, suggesting that MAL-PDT may provide an effective therapy for oral precancerous lesions through ATG-induced cell death.

HMGB1-mediated ATG in Thyroid Cancer Cells

It is known that sodium/iodide symporter (NIS)-mediated iodide uptake plays an important role in regulating thyroid gland function, as well as in diagnosing and treating Graves' disease and thyroid cancer. High-mobility group box 1 (HMGB1), a highly conserved nuclear protein, is a positive regulator of ATG conferring MDR, radiotherapy, and immunotherapy in cancer cells. Chai et al. (2019) identified the role of HMGB1 in Hank's balanced salt solution (HBSS)-induced ATG, explored NIS protein degradation through an ATG-lysosome pathway in thyroid cancer cells, and elucidated on the possible molecular mechanisms. HMGB1 was a critical regulator of ATG-mediated NIS degradation in HBSS-treated FTC-133/TPC-1 cells. HMGB1 up-egulation was prevalent in thyroid cancer tissues and correlated with worse lymph node metastasis and clinical stage. The HMGB-knockdown suppressed ATG and NIS degradation and increased iodide uptake in HBSS-treated cells. HBSS enhanced ROS-sustained ATG and promoted the cytosolic translocation of HMGB1. A knockdown of HMGB1 suppressed LC3-II conversion and NIS degradation via an AMPK/mTOR-dependent signal pathway through regulation of ROS generation, rather than ATP. The xenografts formed by HMGB1 knockdown cells reverted the uptake of $^{99m}TcO4^-$ as compared with control shRNA-transfected cells in the hungry group, suggesting that as a regulator of ATG-mediated NIS degradation via ROS/AMPK/mTOR pathway, HMGB1 may serve as a target of radioiodine therapy in thyroid cancer.

H_2Se in HepG2 Cells

Pan et al. (2018) revealed a novel anti-cancer mechanism of selenite by employing a H_2Se fluorescent probe. HepG2 cells were cultured under a simulated tumor hypoxic microenvironment. The H_2Se and H_2O_2 levels were detected by fluorescent probes in living cells and in mice. After pharmacological doses of Na_2SeO_3 treatment of HepG2 cells under hypoxic conditions, high levels of H_2Se were produced before cell death, which resulted in reductive stress instead of oxidative stress, and was induced under normoxic conditions. H_2Se targeted the HMGB1 protein and induced ATG. H_2Se interrupted the disulfide bond in HMGB1 and promoted its secretion. The reduced HMGB1 outside the cells stimulated ATG by inhibiting the Akt/mTOR axis. Thus, mild ATG inhibited apoptosis, while excessive ATG led to cell death, suggesting that H_2Se plays a key role during HepG2 cell death induced by selenite.

Pentamethinium Salt

Krejcir et al. (2019) showed that salt 1-3C, a quinoxaline unit (with cytotoxic activity) incorporated into a meso-substituted pentamethinium salt (with mitochondrial selectivity and fluorescence properties), displayed potent cytotoxic effects without significant toxic effects on normal tissues. They investigated the cytotoxic mechanism of salt 1-3C compared to its analogue, salt 1-8C, with an extended side carbon chain. Live cell imaging demonstrated that salt 1-3C, but not 1-8C, was incorporated into mitochondria, correlating with its increased cytotoxicity. The accumulation in mitochondria led to their fragmentation and loss of function, accompanied by increased CP/ATG. Salt 1-3C activated AMPK and inhibited mTOR signaling pathways (sensors of cellular metabolism), but did not induce apoptosis, indicating that salt 1-3C cytotoxicity involves mitochondrial perturbation and disintegration involving CBMP, and such compounds are promising candidates for mitochondria as a vulnerable target of cancer.

Cold PSM

Room temperature cold atmospheric plasma (CAP) has shown promising efficacy for the treatment of cancer. Both apoptosis and necrosis have been implicated as the mode of cell death in various cancer cells. TNF-related apoptosis-inducing ligand (TRAIL) and cold plasma-stimulated medium (PSM) are promising anticancer and tumor-selective tools. Ito et al. (2018) demonstrated that PSM and TRAIL may trigger ATG in human malignant melanoma and osteosarcoma cells. Even under nutritional and stress-free conditions, these cells possessed APSs, localized in the cytoplasm in addition to tubular mitochondria. In response to cytotoxic levels of PSM, the mitochondria became highly fragmented, aggregated, and co-localized with the APSs. The cytotoxic effects of PSM were suppressed in response to ATG inhibitors, including 3-MA and Bafilomycin A1, indicating the induction of ATG cell death (ACD). Lethal levels of PSM also resulted in non-apoptotic, non-autophagic cell death in a ROS-dependent manner under certain circumstances. TRAIL exhibited only a modest cytotoxicity toward these tumor cells, and did not induce ACD and mitochondrial aberration. The combined use of TRAIL and of 3-MA decreased basal ATG, increased mitochondrial aberration and co-localization with APSs and apoptosis, indicating that PSM may induce ACD, whereas, TRAIL may trigger protective ATG that compromises apoptosis, providing a rationale for the advantage of PSM over TRAIL in the destruction of apoptosis-resistant melanoma and osteosarcoma cells.

Mitochondrially-Trageted Metal Complexes in Cancer Theranostics

Iridium(III) Complexes

He et al. (2018) synthesized and characterized four cyclometalated Ir(iii) complexes with good photophysical properties and potent anticancer activity. Activation of afore-mentioned apoptotic pathway also triggered ERS in lead-induced nephrotoxicity (Wang et al 2019b). They were taken up by human lung adenocarcinoma A549 cells efficiently and specifically targeted mitochondria. IrM2 induced paraptosis accompanied with mitochondria-derived cytoplasmic vacuoles. IrM2 also affected the UPS and MAPK signaling and induced mitochondria-related dysfunctional events, including $\Delta\Psi$ collapse, ATP depletion, mitochondrial O/P inhibition, and ROS overproduction. The loss of mitochondrial functions, elevation of ROS, and impaired UPS induced by IrM2 resulted in $\Delta\Psi$ collapse and the subsequent cytoplasmic vacuolation before the CP/ATG and/pre-apoptosis. Among the ROS, superoxide anion radicals played a critical role in IrM2-mediated cell death. IrM2 inhibited tumor growth in a mouse model. In addition, Zhang et al. (2018) conducted the cell cycle distribution in BEL-7402 cells by flow cytometry of three iridium complexes [Ir (ppy)$_2$ (ipbc)](PF$_6$) (1), [Ir (bzq)$_2$ (ipbc)](PF$_6$) (2), and [Ir (piq)$_2$ (ipbc)](PF$_6$) (3). They were tested for anticancer activity using the MTT method. The complexes showed no cytotoxic activity toward cancer BEL-7402, SGC-7901, Eca-109, A549, HeLa, and HepG2 cells. However, upon irradiation with white light, the complexes display high cytotoxicity against BEL-7402 cells. AO/EB staining and a comet assay revealed that the complexes can induce apoptosis in BEL-7402 cells. The complexes increased intracellular ROS and Ca^{2+} levels and decreased $\Delta\Psi$. ATG assays exhibited that the complexes induce ATG and regulate the expression of Beclin-1 and LC3 proteins. The complexes released Cyt-C and inhibited the polymerization of α-tubulin. Complexes inhibited the cell growth in BEL-7402 cells through ROS-mediated mitochondrial dysfunction and targeting tubules pathways for the development of multi-target anticancer drugs.

Selenium-containing phycocyanin (Se-PC) has been proved to have anti-inflammatory and antioxidant effects. Liu et al. (2018) investigated the photodynamic therapy (PDT) effects of Se-PC in liver tumor. Se-PC location migration from lysosomes to mitochondria was time-dependent. In *in vivo* experiments, the tumor inhibition rate was 75.4% in the Se-PC PDT group, compared to 52.6% in PC PDT group. The tumor cells outside the tissue showed cellular necrosis, and those inside the tissue exhibited apoptotic nuclei and digested vacuoles in the cytoplasm after a Se-PC PDT treatment. An antioxidant enzyme analysis indicated that GSH-Px activity was linked to the selenium content of Se-PC, and SOD activity was affected by PC PDT. Hence, Se-PC PDT could induce cell death through the free radical production of PDT in tumors and enhanced the activity of antioxidant enzymes with selenium *in vivo*. The mechanism of Se-PC PDT against liver tumor involved hematocyte damage and mitochondria-mediated apoptosis accompanied with ATG inhibition during the early stage of tumor development, which displayed new prospects and offered a relatively safe way for cancer therapy. Huang et al. (2018) synthesized two organometallic gold (III) complexes harboring C^N ligands that structurally resemble tetrahydroisoquinoline (THIQ): Cyc-Au-1 (AuL^{1}Cl$_2$, L^1 = 3,4-dimethoxyphenethylamine) and Cyc-Au-2 (AuL^{2}Cl$_2$, L^2 = methylenedioxyphenethylamine). Both gold complexes exhibited lower toxicity, lower resistance factors, and better anticancer activity than those of Cisplatin. The organometallic gold (III) complexes accumulated in mitochondria and induced elevated ROS and ERS through mitochondrial dysfunction, resulting in simultaneous CP/ATG and apoptosis.

Compared to Cisplatin, Cyc-Au-2 exhibited lower toxicity and better anticancer activity in a murine tumor model. The Cyc-Au-2 compound induced ATG and apoptotic death; hence, it can be a promising anticancer agent or lead compound for further anticancer drug development.

CP/ATG and MDR in Cancer

As an estrogen receptor (ER) antagonist, Tamoxifen, has been used for the treatment of the ER-positive BC; however, the emergence of resistance to Tamoxifen obstructs the successful treatment of this cancer. So, there is need to search for a novel therapeutic target for treatment of BC. Recently, Szostakowska et al. (2019) reported that the majority of BCs are characterized by the expression of estrogen receptor alpha (ERα+). ERα acts as ligand-dependent transcription factor for genes associated with cell survival, proliferation, and tumor growth. Thus, blocking the estrogen agonist's effect on ERα is the main strategy in the treatment of ERα+ BCs. However, despite the development of targeted anti-estrogen therapies for ER+ BC, around 30–50% of early BC patients relapse. Anti-estrogen resistance is a consequence of molecular changes, which allow tumor growth irrespective of estrogen presence. These changes may be associated with ERα modifications either at the genetic, regulatory, or protein level. The activation of alternate growth pathways and/or cell survival mechanisms can lead to estrogen-independence and endocrine resistance. Thus, genetic alterations, stress responses, cell survival mechanisms, and cell reprogramming are associated with resistance to the anti-estrogen therapy of BC. Acquired Tamoxifen-resistant BC cell lines MCF-7 (MCF-7/TAM-R) and T47D (T47D/TAM-R) showed apoptotic resistance accompanied by induction of pro-survival ATG. Tamoxifen resistance was also associated with reduced production of ATP and with overexpression of glycolytic pathways, leading to induced ATG to meet the energy demand. Das et al. (2019) demonstrated that LDHA, one of the key molecules of glycolysis, in association with Beclin-1 induced pro-survival ATG in Tamoxifen-resistant BC. The pharmacological and genetic inhibition of LDHA reduced the pro-survival ATG, with the restoration of apoptosis and reverting back the EMT-like phenomena noticed in Tamoxifen-resistant BC, indicating that targeting LDHA may be a novel strategy to interrupt ATG and Tamoxifen resistance in BC. Li et al. (2019a) showed that in BRAF^{V600E}-melanoma, ATG is induced by BRAF inhibitor (BRAFi), as part of a transcriptional program coordinating lysosome biogenesis/function, mediated by the TFEB transcription factor. TFEB is phosphorylated and thus inactivated by BRAF^{V600E} via its downstream ERK independently of mTORC1. BRAFi disrupts TFEB phosphorylation, allowing its nuclear translocation, which is synergized by increased phosphorylation/inactivation of the ZKSCAN3 transcriptional repressor by JNK2/p38-MAPK. The blockade of BRAFi-induced the transcriptional activation of ATG-lysosomal function in melanoma xenografts caused by enhanced tumor progression, EMT-trans-differentiation, metastatic dissemination, and MDR, was associated with elevated TGF-β levels and enhanced TGF-β signaling. Inhibition of TGF-β signaling restored tumor differentiation and drug responsiveness in melanoma cells. Thus, the "BRAF-TFEB-ATG-lysosome" axis represented an intrinsic regulatory pathway in BRAF-mutant melanoma, coupling BRAF signaling with TGF-β signaling to drive tumor progression and MDR. Furthermore, Li et al. (2019b) showed that YAP1 expression was associated with relapse in tissue samples of patients with TNBC Taxol CR. Verteporfin reduced migration and enhanced ATG and apoptosis of a Taxol-resistant MDA-MB-231 cell line. Knockdown of YAP1 increased epithelial-mesenchymal transition response in a Taxol-resistant TNBC cell line. Verteporfin c shrunk tumor weight and volume and decreased Ki67 expression in a Taxol-resistant mouse model, providing evidence that Verteporfin could be a chemosensitizer for TNBC patients with Taxol-based treatment. Oral lichen planus (OLP) is a common T lymphocyte-mediated autoimmune disease of unknown etiology. The mTOR can regulate proliferation, apoptosis, and ATG of T lymphocytes, therefore impacting the T lymphocyte-mediated immunity. Wang et al. (2019) characterized the roles of two miRNAs, miR122 and miR199, in OLP. miRNA microarray analysis was performed to detect potential miRNAs involved in OLP, while insilicon analysis, RTqPCR, immunoblot, and IHC analyses were utilized to explore the molecular mechanisms underlying the roles of miR199 and miR122 in OLP. The results from the microarray and RTqPCR analyses demonstrated that the expression of miR122 and miR199 were decreased in the PBMCs from the OLP group compared with the control group. In addition, miR122 and miR199 targeted Akt1 and mTOR, respectively, by binding to their 3′ UTRs. Akt1 and mTOR were highly expressed in PBMCs derived from OLP patients. A negative regulatory relationship was observed between miR122 and Akt1, and between miR199 and mTOR. The protein levels of Akt1, mTOR, and LC3B were upregulated in the OLP group compared with the control group. Overexpression of miR122 inhibited the Akt1 and LC3B expression, while miR199 overexpression reduced mTOR and LC3B, suggesting that miR199 and miR122 are implicated in the pathogenesis of OLP by regulating mTOR and Akt1 expression. In addition, Wang et al. (2019) investigated the association between Akt/mTOR/4E-BP1 (eIF4E-binding protein 1) signaling, phospholipase D (PLD), and Hif-1α in peripheral T lymphocytes of OLP and the correlation of their expression with the disease severity. RAE (reticular, atrophic, and erosive lesion) scores were used to assess the disease severity of OLP. Akt, mTOR, 4E-BP1, PLD1, PLD2, and Hif-1α expression in peripheral T lymphocytes were measured by using qRT-RT-PCR. Associations of Akt/mTOR/4E-BP1 expression with PLD1, PLD2, and Hif-1α expression were also assessed, in addition to correlations of their expression with RAE scores. Expressions of mTOR, 4E-BP1, PLD2, and Hif-1α mRNA were reduced in peripheral T lymphocytes of OLP patients. mTOR expression was positively correlated with PLD2 and Hif-1α expression. mTOR, PLD2 and Hif-1α expression were negatively correlated with RAE scores. Hence, dysregulated PLD2/mTOR/Hif-1α may contribute to the development of OLP and severity of the disease. Abunimer et al. (2018) described the process by which mitochondria donate their membranes for the formation of APSs, and showed that the same process could be involved in drug sequestration and exocytosis resulting in MDR cancerous cells. They examined the implications of mitochondrial vesicle formation of mito-APS (MAPS) in response to the drug MKT-077, which targets mortalin, in a MDR-BC cell line overexpressing P-glycoprotein (P-gp). The BC cell line MCF-7Adr is derived from MCF-7, but differs from its ancestral line in tolerance of MKT-077-induced mitochondrial toxicity. ATG in the MCF-7Adr cells entailed regional sequestration of MKT077 in multi-lamellar LC3-labeled MAPS, which separate from their mitochondria, and fuse with or engulf each other. MAPS migrated through the cytoplasm and fuse with the plasma membrane, thus carrying out exocytotic secretion. This mechanism provided a resistance mechanism for MKT-077 by enhancing the efflux process of the cells. After 8 hrs of MKT-077 exposure, a fraction of the resistant cells appeared viable and contained a larger number of smaller sized mitochondria. Similar to CS, MAPS provide a potentially novel model for MDR in cancer cells and may contribute to the P-gp efflux process.

Cisplatin Resistance in Cancer

Chemo-resistance (CR) remains a challenge in the effective treatment of solid tumors, including oral squamous cell carcinoma (OSCC). Mitochondrial dynamics and ATG is implicated in the CR of cancer cells due to significantly reduced CPI. The neutralization of ceramide is also associated with MDR, and ceramide synthase 6 (CerS6) induces apoptosis. Li et al. (2018) investigated the role of CerS6 in the susceptibility of OSCC cells to Cisplatin. They observed that Cisplatin-resistant OSCC cells process lower levels of fission-state mitochondria and apoptosis than Cisplatin-sensitive cells, and ATG was activated in Cisplatin-resistant OSCC cells. Lower CerS6 expression was detected in Cisplatin-resistant OSCC cells. Overexpression of CerS6 with lentivirus-encoded CerS6 complementary DNA in Cisplatin-resistant OSCC cells increased Cisplatin sensitivity. Overexpression of CerS6 enhanced mitochondrial fission and apoptosis and attenuated Cisplatin-induced ATG in Cisplatin-resistant OSCC cells. Hence, CerS6 might function through altering calpain expression to enhance Cisplatin sensitivity (Li et al. 2018). Cisplatin-resistant OSCC cells xenografted onto a nude mouse model confirmed that CerS6 enhanced Cisplatin sensitivity to reduce tumor volume, indicating that CerS6 could mediate an effective response to Cisplatin in chemoresistant OSCC. Wang et al. (2018b) synthesized two mono-functional platinum complexes containing 8-substituted quinoline derivatives. In comparison to Cisplatin, n-Mon-Pt-1 exhibited a greater cytotoxicity, was more effective in resistant cells, and elicited a better anticancer effect. n-Mon-Pt-1 accumulated in the mitochondria, and stimulated TrxR inhibition, ROS release, and an ERS response, resulting in a simultaneous induction of CP/ATG and apoptosis. Compared to Cisplatin, n-Mon-Pt-2 exhibited lower toxicity and better anticancer activity in a murine tumor model. Abdrakhmanov et al. (2018) reported that CP induction suppressed Cisplatin-induced apoptosis, while CP inhibition enhanced ATG and apoptosis. Suppression of CP enhanced ROS production, and the fate of the cell was dependent on the interaction between ERS and ATG. The genotoxicity of Cisplatin towards nDNA is insufficient to explain the Cisplatin resistance of HCC cells which interacts with many organelles to influence the cell's sensitivity. Sheng et al. (2019) explored the role of mitochondrial-lysosomal crosstalk in the Cisplatin resistance in Huh7 and HepG2 cells. Flow cytometry was performed to detect ROS, mitochondrial mass, lysosomal function, $\Delta\Psi$, and apoptosis, and immunoblotting was used to evaluate protein levels. The O_2 consumption rate was measured to evaluate mitochondrial function. Cisplatin activated CP and lysosomal biogenesis, resulting in crosstalk between mitochondria and lysosomes and its resistance in HCC cells. A combination of Cisplatin with the PI3K/mTOR inhibitor PKI-402 induced LMP to change the role of lysosomes from a protective one to that of a cell death promoter, destroying the mitochondrial-lysosomal crosstalk and enhancing the chemosensitivity of HCC cells to Cisplatin, which could be developed for the TSE-EBPT of HCC.

CP/ATG Induction in CBMP and MDR Malignancies

Therapeutic resistance of tumor cells is a major obstacle in efficient anticancer treatment and has been attributed to tumor heterogeneity as well as genetic and epigenetic changes. Tumor cell adhesion to the extracellular matrix acts as an additional factor conferring resistance to both radio- and chemotherapeutic intervention. Vehlow and Cordes (2019) demonstrated that (discoidin domain receptor TK 1 (DDR1) elicits therapy resistance of GBM stem-like and bulk cells through its adhesion to the extracellular matrix and modulation of macroATG/ATG. DDR1 associated with a YWHA/14-3-3-BECN1-Akt1 multiprotein complex favoring pro-survival/anti-autophagic and resistance-mediating Akt-MTOR signaling. Inhibition of DDR1 sensitized glioblastoma cells to radio- and chemotherapy by inducing CP, suggesting that DDR1 may be a potential target for sensitizing glioblastoma cells to combination therapies through its efficient induction of ATG cell death. Bhat et al. (2018) highlighted the dynamic relationship between the rate of protein degradation through ATG, that is, ATG flux, and the susceptibility of tumors to undergo apoptosis remains uncertain. Currently, it is challenging to target ATG to overcome tumor CR. Hence, the author proposed transcriptional regulation of DSST-CP in this edition to control cancer stem cell-specific CS destabilization in MDR malignancies, involved in cancer invasion and metastasis. ATG protects cells from chemotherapeutic agents by scavenging CBs implicated in CBMP. Yan and Li (2018) summarized the current knowledge on the dual role of MTG in cancer drug resistance. Modulation of anticancer drug resistance plays a slightly beneficial role in clinical prognosis due to complex MDR mechanisms. MTG degrades excessive or damaged mitochondria by CP/ATG. Dysregulation of MTG contributes to neoplastic progression and MDR in various types of tumors. MTG was originally thought to be an onco-suppressor that maintains cellular homeostasis and prevents oncogenic transformation, while it promotes cancer cell survival during cytotoxic stress by degrading damaged mitochondria and reducing mitochondrial ROS. Therefore, induction and inhibition of MTG in cancer drug resistance are controversial. Nevertheless, disease-specific spatio-temporal regulation of CB formation, CP induction, CS stabilization, and CBMP provides unique opportunities to develop novel TSE-EBPT of MDR malignancies. Yan et al. (2018b) used plasmid transfection and shRNA to regulate SHP-2 expression. In cervical cancer, SHP-2 suppressed apoptosis induced by Oxaliplatin and 5-FU. SHP-2 protected against mitochondrial damage, which was associated with the activation of ATG. SHP-2 degraded impaired mitochondria depending on the ubiquitin ligase function of Parkin, suggesting that SHP-2 inhibits the apoptosis induced by drugs through activating ATG to degrade damaged mitochondria and ubiquitin ligase Parkin involved in SHP-2-induced ATG. $\Delta\Psi$ collapse is considered the initiation of regulated cell death (RCD). Several cell stress responses such as CP, ATG and MTG, MB, and the ubiquitin proteasome system may differentially contribute to restrain the initiation of RCD depending on the extent of mitochondrial damage. Lombardo et al. (2018) induced graded mitochondrial damage after $\Delta\Psi$ collapse with CCCP in Burkitt's lymphoma cells, and evaluated the effect of drugs targeting cell stress responses over RCD at 72 hrs using flow cytometry. CCCP caused $\Delta\Psi$ collapse after 30 min., massive mitochondrial fission, oxidative stress, and increased MTG within the 5–15 µM low-dose range (LDR) of CCCP. Within the 20–50 µM high-dose range (HDR), CCCP caused lysosomal destabilization and rupture, precluding MTG and ATG. Cell death after 72 hrs was <20%, with increased mitochondrial mass (MM). The inhibitors of MTG3-(2,4-dichloro-5-methoxyphenyl)-2,3-dihydro-2-thioxo-4(1H)-quinazolinone (Mdivi-1) and Vincristine (VCR) increased cell death from CCCP within the LDR, while Valproic acid (an inducer of MB) also increased MM and cell death within the LDR. The proteasome inhibitor, MG132, increased cell death only in the HDR. Dox, an antibiotic that disrupts MB, had no effect on cell survival, while Iodoacetamide, an inhibitor of glycolysis, increased cell death at the HDR, suggesting that MTG influenced RCD of lymphoma cells after $\Delta\Psi$ collapse by CCCP only within the LDR, while proteasome activity and glycolysis contributed to survival in the HDR under extensive mitochondrial and lysosomal damage.

Theranostic Potential of CP/ATG Regulators in Cancer (Experimental Studies)

Stem Cell Deficit in Slc29a3 Disorders

Mutations in equilibrative nucleoside transporter 3 (ENT3), the intracellular nucleoside transporter within the solute carrier 29 (SLC29) gene family, cause human genetic disorders (for example, H syndrome, PHID syndrome, and SHML/RDD syndrome). Nair et al. (2019) identified adult stem cell deficits that drive ENT3-related abnormalities in mice. ENT3 deficiency alters hematopoietic and mesenchymal stem cell fates; the former leads to stem cell exhaustion, and the latter leads to breaches of mesodermal tissue integrity. The molecular pathogenesis stems from the loss of lysosomal adenosine transport, which impedes ATG-regulated stem cell differentiation programs via dysregulation of the AMPK-mTOR-ULK axis. Mass spectrometry-based metabolomics and bioenergetics studies identified defects in fatty acid utilization and alterations in MB, which can induce stem cell deficits (Nair et al. 2019). Genetic, pharmacologic, and stem cell interventions ameliorated ENT3-disease pathologies and extended the lifespan of ENT3-deficient mice. These findings delineated a pathogenic basis for the development of ENT3 spectrum disorders and conferred theranostic strategies to treat human ENT3-related disorders.

ATG and Immune System for Tumor Immunotherapy

Currently, tumor immunotherapy is a promising treatment strategy. ATG controls immune responses by modulating the functions of immune cells and the production of cytokines. Some cytokines and immune cells have a significant effect on the function of ATG. Jiang et al. (2018) discussed the possible mechanisms of an ATG-regulating immune system, and its applications in tumor immunotherapy. ATG is a cellular process that is genetically controlled by a set of ATG-related genes. ATG can promote or suppress tumor progression, depending on the cell and tissue types and the stages of tumor. Therapies aiming at ATG to enhance the immune responses and anti-tumor effects of immunotherapy have become the prospective strategy, with enhanced antigen presentation and higher sensitivity to CTLs. However, the induction of ATG may also benefit tumor cells' escape from immune surveillance and result in intrinsic resistance against anti-tumor immunotherapy. The optimal use of either ATG inducers or inhibitors can restrain tumor growth and progression by enhancing immune responses and overcoming the immune resistance in combination with immunotherapeutic strategies, indicating that the induction or inhibition of ATG might develop a TSE-EBPT strategy combined with immunotherapy.

Activin A and Cancer Cachexia

The majority of patients with advanced cancer develop cachexia, a weight-loss disorder that reduces QOL and limits survival. Several tumor-derived factors and inflammatory mediators contribute to weight loss in cachectic patients. Activin A and IL-6 are among the best studied factors, and several studies support their role in cachexia. Pettersen et al. (2019) investigated the interaction between activin A and IL-6 in the cachexia-inducing TOV21G cell line, both in culture and in tumors in mice. The human TOV21G cells secrete IL-6 that induces ATG in reporter cells and cachexia in mice. Using this cachexia cell model, they targeted autocrine activin A by genetic, chemical, and biological approaches. The secretion of IL-6 from the cancer cells was determined in both culture and tumor-bearing mice by ELISA. ATG reporter cells were used to monitor the culture medium for ATG-inducing activities, and muscle mass changes were evaluated in tumor-bearing mice. Activin A acted in an autocrine manner to promote the synthesis and secretion of IL-6 from cancer cells. By inhibiting activin A signaling, the production of IL-6 from the cancer cells was reduced by 40–50%. Reduced IL-6 secretion from the cancer cells was observed when using biological, chemical, and genetic approaches to interfere with the autocrine activin A loop inhibiting activin signaling which also attenuated ATG in non-cancerous cells. The use of an anti-activin receptor 2 antibody in cachectic tumor-bearing mice reduced serum levels of cancer cell-derived IL-6 by 62%, and, reversed cachexia and counteracted loss of all muscle groups, supporting a functional link between activin A and IL-6 signaling and indicated that interference with activin A-induced IL-6 secretion from the tumor has theranostic potential for cancer-induced cachexia.

The Theranostic Significance of Antioxidants as CP Regulators and CP Inhibitors in MDR Malignancies

Curcuminoids

It will be promising to develop CP regulators rather than simply CP inhibitors for the TSE-EBPT of MDR malignancies because of their heterogeneous nature. Numerous studies support the use of herbal medicines or natural products for cancer chemotherapy (Yin et al. 2013). Reports have associated curcumin (CUR), dimethoxy curcumin (DMC), and bisdemethoxycurcumin (BDMC) with anticancer properties. Hsiao et al. (2018a) investigated the effect of CUR, DMC, and BDMC on cell viability, apoptotic cell death, ROS, Ca^{2+}, $\Delta\Psi$, and caspase activities using flow cytometry and ATG by Monodansyl Cadaverine (MDC) and Acridine Orange (AO) staining in oral cancer SAS cells. CUR, DMC, and BDMC decreased viable cell numbers through ATG induction and apoptosis in SAS cells. Cells were pretreated with NAC, 3MA, Rapamycin, and Carbobenzoxy-valyl-alanyl-aspartyl-[O-methyl]-fluoro-methylketone (Z-VAD-fmk) and then were treated with CUR, DMC, and BDMC that led to increased total viable cell numbers when compared to CUR, DMC, and BDMC treatments alone. Apoptotic cell death occurred through ROS overproduction, mitochondria-dependent pathway, and CP/ATG induction, suggesting that CUR, DMC, and BDMC could be used as an anticancer agent in oral cancer. Furthermore, Hsiao et al. (2018b) investigated the effects of Gefitinib with or without CUR, DMC, or BDMC co-treatment on the cell viability, apoptotic cell death, ATG, $\Delta\Psi$, and caspase-3 activities in oral cancer SAS cells. Gefitinib co-treated with CUR, DMC, or BDMC decreased viable cell numbers through the induction of cell apoptosis and ATG and decreased $\Delta\Psi$ and increased caspase-3 activities in SAS cells. Gefitinib combined with CUR, DMC, or BDMC decreased Bcl-2 expression and increased Atg5, Beclin-1, p62/SQSTM1, and LC3 expression associated with ATG in SAS cells. Gefitinib combined with CUR and DMC led to reduced tumor weights and volumes in SAS cell xenograft nude mice but did not affect the total body weights, suggesting that this combination can be a potential anticancer strategy for oral cancer.

Resveratrol

Resveratrol (Res), a natural polyphenolic compound is considered as a potent anticancer agent. TRAIL is a promising anticancer agent that has the potential to sensitize a wide variety of cancer or transformed cells by inducing apoptosis. However, resistance to TRAIL is a growing concern. Rasheduzzaman et al. (2018) employed a combination treatment to investigate Res-induced TRAIL sensitization in NSCLC. A549 and HCC-15 cells were used in an experimental design. Res is capable of the activation of tumor suppressor p53 and its pro-apoptotic modulator, PUMA. p53-independent apoptosis by decrease in the expression of phosphorylated Akt-mediated suppression of NF-κB is also substantiated with the downregulation of anti-apoptotic factors Bcl-2 and Bcl-xl in NSCLC, resulting in the attenuation of TRAIL resistance in combined treatment. Apoptosis was induced in TRAIL-resistant lung cancer cells with a co-treatment of Res and TRAIL assessed by $\Delta\Psi$ collapse, ROS generation, and translocation of Cyt-C from the mitochondria into the cytosol. ATG flux was not affected by Res-induced TRAIL-mediated apoptosis in NSCLC. Targeting the NF-κB (p65) pathway via Res attenuated TRAIL resistance and induced TRAIL-mediated apoptosis which could be an effective TRAIL-based cancer therapy regimen. Li et al. (2018) demonstrated that Res displayed anti-proliferative activity in MM cell lines. A low concentration of Res was synergistic with a low dose of the proteasome inhibitor, Carfilzomib (CFZ), to induce apoptosis in myeloma cells. Mitochondria was the key regulatory site after the Res/CFZ combination treatment. Res induced the release of second mitochondria-derived activator of caspase (Smac) and kept the Smac in a high level after combination with CFZ. Also, Res was additive with CFZ to increase ROS production. A stress sensor SIRT1, with deacetylase enzyme activity, was downregulated after Res/CFZ combination, thereby decreasing its target protein, survivin in MM cells. ATG was invoked after the Res/CFZ combination treatment in myeloma cells. Inhibition of ATG enhanced ROS production and apoptosis, indicating the linkage between ATG and proteasome to modulate the oxidative stress, suggesting that induction of multiple stress responses after Res/CFZ combination is a major mechanism to synergistically inhibit MM cell growth and reduce the toxicity of CFZ in MM cells. This indicated a rationale to consider an ATG inhibitor for the combination therapy in MM patients. Nutrient-deprivation ATG factor-1 (NAF-1), which is an OMM protein, plays important roles in Ca^{2+} metabolism, anti-apoptosis, and antiATG.

Cheng et al. (2018) demonstrated that Res suppresses the expression of NAF-1 in PC cells by inducing ROS accumulation and activating Nrf2 signaling. The knockdown of NAF-1 activated apoptosis and inhibited the proliferation of PC cells. Hence, targeting of NAF-1 by Res can improve the sensitivity of PC cells to Gemcitabine.

Berberine

Sun et al. (2018) showed that Berberine, a natural compound that is used as an antibacterial agent, could reduce cellular viability and induce oncotic-like death, characterized by cell swelling, cytoplasmic vacuoles, and plasma membrane blebbing, in gliomas, and that these effects were correlated with ATP depletion. Berberine induced CP/ATG as a protective effect and decreased the O_2 consumption rate, which could inhibit mitochondrial aerobic respiration by repressing p-ERK1/2. The downregulation of mitochondrial p-ERK1/2 by Berberine inhibited aerobic respiration and led to glycolysis, an inefficient energy production pathway. Berberine reduced tumor growth and inhibited Ki-67 and p-ERK1/2 expression *in vivo*, indicating that it decreases metabolic activity by reducing ERK1/2 activity.

Aleuritolic Acid

Aleuritolic acid (AA) is a triterpene that is isolated from the root of *Croton crassifolius* Geisel. Yi et al. (2018a) evaluated the cytotoxic effects of AA on HCC cells. AA exerted cytotoxicity by inducing mitochondria-dependent apoptosis in the HCC cell line, HepG2. Treatment with AA dysregulated ATG, as evidenced by enhanced conversion of LC3-I to LC3-II, p62 accumulation, and co-localization of GFP and mCherry-tagged LC3 puncta. Blockage of APS formation by Atg5 knockdown or inhibitors of PI3-kinase (3-MA or Ly294002), reversed AA-mediated cytotoxicity, indicating that AA retarded the clearance of ATG cargos, resulting in the production of cytotoxic factors and led to apoptosis in HCC cells.

Lycopene

Lycopene, a carotenoid, has an inhibitory function on tumor cell migration. Bi et al. (2019) assessed the biological effects of Lycopene on cSCC cell line COLO-16, human epidermal keratinocytes (HEKs), and the immortalized human keratinocyte cell line HaCaT. Lycopene inhibited the cell proliferation and migration of COLO-16 cells but not normal keratinocytes. In addition, Lycopene upregulated the protein levels of ZO-1 in COLO-16 and HaCaT cells but not in HEKs. Lycopene upregulated the protein level of claudin-1 in HEKs but downregulated claudin-1 in COLO-16 cells. Lycopene induced MTORC1-dependent decrease in ATG flux in COLO-16 cells. ATG inhibition contributed to the Lycopene-induced regulation on ZO-1 and claudin-1 in COLO-16 cells. JNK inhibitor (SP600125) and MEK inhibitor (U0126) treatment abolished the increase in phosphorylated MTOR and ribosomal protein S6 as well as the increase in ZO-1 and decrease in claudin-1 in Lycopene-treated COLO-16 cells. The gene silencing of JNK and ERK prohibited ZO-1 upregulation and claudin-1 downregulation. Lycopene upregulated ZO-1 expression and downregulated claudin-1 expression through ERK, JNK, and MTORC1 activation and inhibition of CP/ATG in cSCC cells, suggesting that CP/ATG plays a key role in Lycopene-mediated pharmacological effects and might be a useful chemo-preventive agent in cSCC as a CPI inducer.

Deep-sea Water

Lee et al. (2019) investigated the effect of deep-sea water (DSW) in HaCaT keratinocyte exposed by UVB ($\lambda = 290{\sim}320$ nm). UVB-induced cell death was reinforced by DSW treatment in a hardness-dependent manner. The increased cell death by DSW was associated with the downregulation of survivin and RAD51 expressions induced by UVB. There was inhibition of H2A.X phosphorylation, a marker for double-stranded DNA damage, and the enhancement of LC3-II and SQSTM1/p62 expressions by DSW administration in UVB-radiated HaCaT keratinocyte, indicating that the enhancement of UVB-induced cell death by DSW is associated with ATG. Therefore, they further explored the regulation of ATG-regulating proteins and apoptosis-related factors expression. Phosphorylation of mTOR, ribosomal protein S6, and S6 kinase by UVB radiation were regressed via DSW treatment, causing the increase in AMPK phosphorylation. UVB-induced NF-κB and JNK phosphorylations were increased with DSW treatment, whereas DSW lessened the Ser15 phosphorylation of p53 and cleavage of PARP-induced by UVB radiation. DSW enhanced UVB-damaged skin cell clearance through the activation of CP/ATG-induced cell death through the regulation of AMPK/mTOR signaling as well as NF-κB and JNK phosphorylation, suggesting that DSW prevents UV-induced skin cancer.

Herbal Medicine in Cancer Theranostics

Tea is one of the most widely consumed beverages worldwide and is available in various forms. Green tea is richer in antioxidants compared to other forms of tea. Prasanth et al. (2019) reported anti-photo-aging, stress resistance, neuroprotective, and ATG-regulating properties of one of the most widely known functional foods: green tea. Tea is composed of polyphenols, caffeine, minerals, and trace amounts of vitamins, amino acids, and carbohydrates. The composition of the tea varies depending on the fermentation process employed to produce it. The phytochemicals present in green tea stimulate the CNS and maintain overall health in humans. A cup of tea contains between 25–45 mg of caffeine, whereas a cup of coffee contains between 60–80 mg of caffeine depending on the natural content. Caffeine is methyl xanthine derivative and activates brain regional adenyate cyclase to synthesize cAMP as a second messenger from ATP. Caffeine is also a mild phosphodiesterase inhibitor, which promotes cAMP buildup in the neurons to serve as a nerve tonic. If we consume coffee or tea during the day or night, it will keep us alert. Skin-aging is a complex process mediated by intrinsic factors such as senescence, along with extrinsic damage induced by external factors such as chronic exposure to UV irradiation—a process known as photo-aging-which can lead to erythema, edema, sunburn, hyperplasia, premature aging, and the development of non-melanoma and melanoma skin cancers. UV can cause skin damage either directly, through the absorption of energy by biomolecules, or indirectly, by the increased production of RONS. Green tea phytochemicals could nullify excess endogenous ROS and RNS inside the body, and thereby diminish the impact of photo-aging. Green tea increases the collagen and elastin fiber content, and suppresses the collagen-degrading enzyme, MMP-3's production in the skin, conferring an anti-wrinkle effect. Green-tea-mediated lifespan extension depends on the DAF-16 pathway. Green tea has stress resistance and neuroprotective properties. Its ROS scavenging activity makes it a potent stress mediator, as it can also regulate the stress induced by metal ions. Tea polyphenols can induce the expression of different antioxidant enzymes and hinder the DNA-oxidative damage. Green tea can also be used to mediate NDDs, including AD. EGCG, an abundant Catechin in tea, suppress the neurotoxicity induced by Aβ as it activates GSK-3β, along with inhibiting c-Abl/FE65-the cytoplasmic non-receptor TK which is involved in the development of the CNS and in nuclear translocation. Additionally, green tea polyphenols induce ATG, thereby revitalizing the overall health of the organism, and activates ATG in HL-60 xenographs by increasing the activity of PI3 kinase and BECLIN-1 by modulating CP and by preventing free radical-mediated CBMP implicated in CVDs, NDDs, and MDR malignancies. Nevertheless, readers should not be carried with the notion that consumption of tea or coffee will cure these devastating diseases.

In addition, Astragalus membranaceus (AM), also named Huangqi, is one of the most important herbs in traditional Chinese medicine and its extracts possess many biological activities related to ATG, including anti-oxidation, anti-inflammation, anticancer, anti-photoaging, and improvement of cardiomyocyte function. The AM extracts can have therapeutic potential in ATG-dysregulation-associated diseases because of their clinically-beneficial effects. Shan and Zheng (2019) highlighted the effects of AM extracts on aforementioned ATG dysregulation-associated diseases. Recent studies on ATG, mediated by subsets of ATG proteins, are emerging in many physiological and pathological processes. AM extracts can have theranostic potential in ATG dysregulation-associated diseases because of their positive biological effects. Furthermore, F3 is a novel fraction isolated from Valeriana jatamansi Jones, which is a traditional Chinese medicine. Zhu et al. (2019) investigated the anti-cancer effects of F3 on human BC cell lines. F3 inhibited the growth of BC cells by inducing apoptosis and had no inhibitory effect of the growth on MCF-10A cells. F3-induced apoptosis was mediated by DNA damage as presented by DNA strand breaks and γ-H2AX activation that might be attacked by ROS accumulation. This triggered several key molecular events involving the activation of the MAPKs pathway. F3 induced ATG with the APS formation and increased LC3-II levels. F3 exhibited an antitumor effect and induced DNA damage in MDA-MB-231 xenografts, suggesting that it may be used for the treatment of BC. Antrodia cinnamomea (AC) is a medicinal fungus due to its potent hepato-protective and cytotoxic activities. Chen et al. (2019) evaluated the anti-proliferative activity of the ethanol extract of artificially cultured AC (EEAC) on BC cells (T47D cells). EEAC inhibited T47D cells' proliferation mediated by cell-cycle arrest at G1 phase as well as induced ATG. EEAC decreased the expression of the cell-cycle-related proteins and increased the expression of the transcription factor FOXO1, ATG marker LC3 II, and p62. EEAC AC mediated ERS by promoting the expression of (IRE 1α), (glucose regulating protein 78 (GRP78/Bip), and C/EBP homologous protein (CHOP). Apart from previous studies, (histone deacetylases (HDACs) activity was inhibited. The *in vivo* studies demonstrated that EEAC decreased tumor volume and inhibited tumor growth without any significant side effects, suggesting that this extract may be developed as a potential dietary supplement targeting BC. Yi et al. (2018b) explored the anti-proliferative activity and mechanism of 5β-spirost-25(27)-en-1β,3β-diol-1-O-α-L-rhamnopyranosyl-(1→2)-β-D-xylopyranosyl-3-O-α-L-rhamnopyranoside (SPD), a Spirostanol saponin from R. chinensis, in human HL-60 cells. The antiproliferative activity of SPD *in vitro* was evaluated by MTT assay compared with cis-dichlorodiammineplatinum (II). Treatment of HL-60 cells with SPD resulted in growth inhibition and induction of apoptosis and ATG. Results from an Annexin V-FITC/PI double-staining assay and $\Delta\Psi$ confirmed apoptosis after SPD treatment. The regulation of caspase-3, Bax, Bcl-2, and PARP following SPD treatment contributed to the induction of mitochondria-dependent apoptosis. SPD induced ATG related with Akt/mTOR/p70S6K signaling and activation of the AMPK signaling pathway. Blocking ATG with Bafilomycin A1 reduced the cytotoxicity of SPD. The anti-proliferative, apoptosis and pro-death ATG activities of SPD suggested that Spirostanol saponins would be a potential therapeutic for acute promyelocytic leukemia.

CONCLUSION

This chapter systematically described recently emerging pharmaceutical drugs, synthetic antioxidants, natural antioxidants, and herbal medicines as CP/ATG regulators for the TSE-EBPT of cancer. A brief description of Chloroquine (CQ) as a CP/ATG antagonist is provided as an adjunct anticancer therapy. Pathological significance of ING-4 in cancers and nonneoplastic disorders; role of leucine zipper EF-hand transmembrane protein-1, omic characterization of tumors, photodynamic therapy, cis-Khellactone as a new anticancer drug, therapeutic potential of interferon-γ in colorectal cancer, clinical significance of hydrogels and monolayer cultures to develop novel theranostic agents for TBNC, polyamine conjugated flavonoids, Inonotus, Taiwanensis polysaccharide, peroxisomal changes with 7-ketocholesterol and Dox chemotherapy, Gambogic acid, bromophenol-thiazolylhydazone hydrids, 7-acetylsinumaximol-B, role of 2-deoxyglucose and photodynamic therapy, dibenzoxanthines-oxazolinoanthracyclines and BNIP-3 as a molecular target in glutamine-driven melanoma cells, regulation of CP/ATG by endorepellin, inhibition of oral precancerous cells by MAL-PDI, role of HMGB-1-mediated CP/ATG in thyroid cancer cells, and the therapeutic potential of H2Se in HepG2 cells, pantamethonium salts, and cold PSM is described. In addition, mitochondrially-targeted metal complexes are described in cancer theranostics, including Pt (II) complexes, Irridium-III complexes; and cisplatin resistance in cancer. Furthermore, CP/ATG induction in CBMP and MDR malignancies, theranostic potential of CP/ATG regulators in cancer; pathophysiological role of CP/ATG in MDR malignancies, experimental studies to explore stem cell deficit in SLC 29a3 disorders, CP/ATG as a theranostic tool in the development of tumor immunotherapy, and the role of activin-A in cancer cachexia are highlighted. Particularly, antioxidants as CP regulators and CP inhibitors in MDR malignancies including: Curcuminoids, Resveratrol, Berbarine, Aleuritolic acid, Lycopenes, deep sea water, and herbal medicines are described with currently limited theranostic success in cancer cure. Hence, there is ample scope to develop disease-specific CP/ATG and CBMP regulators for the TSE-EBPT of MDR malignancies and other chronic diseases as emphasized in this edition.

REFERENCES

Abdrakhmanov, A., A.V. Kulikov, E.A. Luchkina, B. Zhivotovsky, et al. 2018. Involvement of MTG in cisplatin-induced cell death regulation. Biol Chem 400: 161–170.

Abunimer, A.N., H. Mohammed, K.L. Cook, D.R. Soto-Pantoja, et al. 2018. Mitochondrial autophagosomes as a mechanism of drug resistance in breast carcinoma. Ultrastruct Pathol 42(2): 170–180.

Bai, Z., M. Gao, X. Xu, H. Zhang, et al. 2018. Overcoming resistance to mitochondrial apoptosis by BZML-induced mitotic catastrophe is enhanced by inhibition of ATG in A549/Taxol cells. Cell Prolif 51: e12450.

Bhat, P., J. Kriel, B. Shubha Priya, N.S. Basappa, N.S. Shivananju, et al. 2018. Modulating ATG in cancer therapy: Advancements and challenges for cancer cell death sensitization. Biochem Pharmacol 147: 170–182.

Bi, S., L. Li, H. Gu, M. Li, et al. 2019. Lycopene upregulates ZO-1 and downregulates claudin-1 through ATG inhibition in the human cutaneous squamous cell carcinoma cell line COLO-16. J Cancer 10: 510–521.

Cavadas, B., J.B. Pereira, M. Correia, V. Fernandes, et al. 2019. Genomic and transcriptomic characterization of the mitochondrial-rich oncocytic phenotype on a thyroid carcinoma background. Mitochondrion 46: 123–133.

Chai, W., F. Ye, L. Zeng, Y. Li, et al. 2019. HMGB1-mediated ATG regulates sodium/iodide symporter protein degradation in thyroid cancer cells. J Exp Clin Cancer Res 38: 325.

Chao, T.L., T.Y. Wang, C.H. Lee, S.J. Yiin, et al. 2018. Anti-cancerous effect of inonotus taiwanensis polysaccharide extract on human acute monocytic leukemia cells through ROS-independent intrinsic mitochondrial pathway. Int J Mol Sci 19(2): 393.

Chen, Y.C., Y.C. Liu, M. El-Shazly, T.Y. Wu, et al. 2019. *Antrodia cinnamomea*, a treasured medicinal mushroom, induces growth arrest in breast cancer cells, T47D cells: New mechanisms emerge. Int J Mol Sci 20(4): 833.

Cheng, L., B. Yan, K. Chen, Z, Jiang, et al. 2018. Resveratrol-induced downregulation of NAF-1 enhances the sensitivity of pancreatic cancer cells to gemcitabine via the ROS/Nrf2 signaling pathways. Oxid Med Cell Longev 2018: 1–16. Article ID 9482018.

Chhonker, Y.S., R.L. Sleightholm, J. Li, D. Oupický, et al. 2018. Simultaneous quantitation of hydroxy-chloroquine and its metabolites in mouse blood and tissues using LC-ESI-MS/MS: An application for pharmacokinetic studies. J Chromatogr B Analyt Technol Biomed Life Sci 1072: 320–327.

Das, C.K., A. Parekh, P.K. Parida, S.K. Bhutia, et al. 2019. Lactate dehydrogenase a regulates autophagy and tamoxifen resistance in breast cancer. Biochim Biophys Acta Mol Cell Res 1866: 1004–1018.

Du, Y., Y. Cheng and G. Su. 2019. The essential role of tumor suppressor gene ING4 in various human cancers and non-neoplastic disorders. Biosci Rep 39: BSR20180773.

Feng, J., X. Chen, S. Lu, W. Li, et al. 2018. Naringin attenuates cerebral ischemia-reperfusion injury through inhibiting peroxynitrite-mediated MTG activation. Mol Neurobiol 55: 9029–9042.

Furukawa, K. and T. Kanki. 2018. Mitophagy in yeast: A screen of mitophagy-deficient mutants. *In*: N. Hattori and S. Saiki (eds), Mitophagy: Methods and Protocols. Series: Methods in Molecular Biology, vol 1759. Humana Press, New York, NY, pp. 95–104. https://doi.org/10.1007/7651_2017_13

He, L., K.N. Wang, Y. Zheng, J.J. Cao, et al. 2018. Cyclometalated iridium(iii) complexes induce mitochondria-derived paraptotic cell death and inhibit tumor growth *in vivo*. Dalton Trans 47: 6942–6953.

Hsiao, Y.T., C.L. Kuo, J.J. Lin, W. Huang, et al. 2018a. Curcuminoids combined with gefitinib mediated apoptosis and autophagy of human oral cancer SAS cells *in vitro* and reduced tumor of SAS cell xenograft mice *in vivo*. Environ Toxicol. 33: 821–832.

Hsiao, Y.T., C.L. Kuo, F.S. Chueh, K.C. Liu, et al. 2018b. Curcuminoids induce reactive oxygen species and ATG to enhance apoptosis in human oral cancer cells. Am J Chin Med 46: 1145–1168.

Hsu, S.P.C, J.S. Kuo, H.C. Chiang, H.E. Wang, et al. 2018. Temozolomide, sirolimus and chloroquine is a new therapeutic combination that synergizes to disrupt lysosomal function and cholesterol homeostasis in GBM cells. Oncotarget 9: 6883–6896.

Huang, K.B., F.Y. Wang, X.M. Tang, H.W. Feng, et al. 2018. Organometallic gold(III) complexes similar to tetrahydroisoquinoline induce ER-stress-mediated apoptosis and pro-death autophagy in A549 cancer cells. J Med Chem 61: 3478–3490.

Ito, T., T. Ando, M. Suzuki-Karasaki, T. Tokunaga, et al. 2018. Cold PSM, but not TRAIL, triggers autophagic cell death: A therapeutic advantage of PSM over TRAIL. Int J Oncol 53: 503–514.

Jiang, H., L. Yang, L. Guo, N. Cui, et al. 2018. Impaired mitophagy of nucleated erythroid cells leads to anemia in patients with myelodysplastic syndromes. Oxid Med Cell Longev 2018: 6328051.

Jing, B., J. Jin, R. Xiang, M. Liu, et al. 2018. Vorinostat and quinacrine have synergistic effects in T-cell acute lymphoblastic leukemia through reactive oxygen species increase and MTG inhibition. Cell Death Dis 9(6): 589.

Jogalekar, M.P. and E.E. Serrano. 2018. Morphometric analysis of a triple negative BC cell line in hydrogel and monolayer culture environments. Peer J 6: e4340.

Jung, S., H.I. Moon, B.S. Lee, S. Kim, et al. 2018. Anti-cancerous effect of cis-khellactone from angelica amurensis through the induction of three programmed cell deaths. Oncotarget 9: 16744–16757.

Kessel, D. 2019. Apoptosis, paraptosis and ATG: Death and survival pathways associated with photodynamic therapy. Photochem Photobiol 95: 119–125.

Krejcir, R., L. Krcova, P. Zatloukalova, T. Briza, et al. 2019. A cyclic pentamethinium salt induces cancer cell cytotoxicity through mitochondrial disintegration and metabolic collapse. Int J Mol Sci 20(17): 4208.

Kruppa, A.J. and F. Buss. 2018. Actin cages isolate damaged mitochondria during mitophagy. Autophagy 14: 1644–1645.

Lee, M.H., D. Koh, H. Na, N.L. Ka, et al. 2018. MTA1 is a novel regulator of ATG that induces tamoxifen resistance in BC cells. Tophagy 14: 812–824.

Lee, K.S., M.G. Lee, Y.J. Woo, K.S. Nam. 2019. The preventive effect of deep sea water on the development of cancerous skin cells through the induction of autophagic cell death in UVB-damaged HaCaT keratinocyte. Biomed Pharmacother 111: 282–291.

Li, S., Y. Wu, Y. Din, M. Yu, Z. Ai. 2018a. CerS6 regulates cisplatin resistance in oral squamous cell carcinoma by altering mitochondrial fission and ATG. Cell Physiol 233: 9416–9425.

Li, Q., Y. Yue, L. Chen, C. Xu, et al. 2018b. Resveratrol sensitizes carfilzomib-induced apoptosis via promoting oxidative stress in multiple myeloma cells. Front Pharmacol 9: 334.

Li, Q., Z.X. Zhu, X. Zhang, W. Luo, et al. 2018c. The lead optimization of the polyamine conjugate of flavonoid with a naphthalene motif: Synthesis and biological evaluation. Eur J Med Chem 146: 564–576.

Li, S., Y. Song, C. Quach, H. Guo, et al. 2019a. Transcriptional regulation of autophagy-lysosomal function in BRAF-driven melanoma progression and chemoresistance. Nat Commun 10: 1693. https://doi.org/10.1038/s41467-019-09634-8.

Li, Y., S. Wang, X. Wei, S. Zhang, et al. 2019b. Role of inhibitor of yes-associated protein 1 in TNB cancer with Taxol-based CR. Cancer Sci 110: 561–567.

Lin, S., L. Li, M. Li, H. Gu, et al. 2019. Raffinose increases ATG and reduces cell death in UVB-irradiated keratinocytes. J Photochem Photobiol B 201: 111653.

Liu, Z., X. Fu, W. Huang, C. Li, et al. 2018. Photodynamic effect and mechanism study of selenium-enriched phycocyanin from spirulina platensis against liver tumours. Photochem Photobiol B 180: 89–97.

Lombardo, T., M.G. Folgar, L. Salaverry, E. Rey-Roldán, et al. 2018. Regulated cell death of lymphoma cells after graded mitochondrial damage is differentially affected by drugs targeting cell stress responses. Basic Clin Pharmacol Toxicol 122: 489–500.

Mishra, A., A. Pateriya, A.K. Mishra, A. Shrivastava, et al. 2020. Prognostic significance of autophagy related genes in estrogen receptor positive Tamoxifen treated breast cancer. Bioinformation 16: 710–718.

Moruno-Manchon, J.F., N.E. Uzor, S.R. Kesler, J.S. Wefel, et al. 2018. Peroxisomes contribute to oxidative stress in neurons during dox-based chemotherapy. Mol Cell Neurosci 86: 65–71.

Naik, P.P., A. Birbrair and S.K. Bhutia. 2019. Mitophagy-driven metabolic switch reprograms stem cell fate. Cell Mol Life Sci 76: 27–43.

Nair, S., A.M. Strohecker, A.K. Persaud, B. Bissa, et al. 2019. Adult stem cell deficits drive Slc29a3 disorders in mice. Nat Commun 10: 2943.

Neill, T., E. Andreuzzi, Z.X. Wang, S.C. Peiper, et al. 2018. Endorepellin remodels the endothelial transcriptome toward a pro-autophagic and pro-mitophagic gene signature. J Biol Chem 293: 12137–12148.

Nury, T., R. Sghaier, A. Zarrouk, F. Ménétrier, et al. 2018. Induction of peroxisomal changes in oligodendrocytes treated with 7-ketocholesterol: Attenuation by α-tocopherol. Biochimie 153: 181–202.

Pan, H., LY. Lu, X.O. Wang, B.X. Li, et al. 2018. Gambogic acid induces cell apoptosis and inhibits MAPK pathway in PTEN–/–/p53–/– prostate cancer cells *in vitro* and *ex vivo*. Chin J Integr Med 24: 109–116.

Pettersen, K., S. Andersen, A. van der Veen, U. Nonstad, et al. 2019. Autocrine activin A signalling in ovarian cancer cells regulates secretion of interleukin 6, autophagy, and cachexia. J Cachexia Sarcopenia Muscle 11(1): 195–207.

Prasanth, M.I., B.S. Sivamaruthi, C. Chaiyasut and T. Tencomnao. 2019. A review of the role of green tea (*Camellia sinensis*) in antiphotoaging, stress resistance, neuroprotection, and autophagyagy. Nutrients 11(2): 474.

Rahman, F.U., A. Ali, H.Q. Duong, I.U. Khan, et al. 2019. ONS-donor ligand based Pt(II) complexes display extremely high anticancer potency through autophagic cell death pathway. Eur J Med Chem 164: 546–561.

Rasheduzzaman, M., J.K. Jeong and S.Y. Park. 2018. Resveratrol sensitizes lung cancer cell to TRAIL by p53 independent and suppression of Akt/NF-κB signaling. Life Sci 208: 208–220.

Rogalska, A., A. Gajek, M. Łukawska, I. Oszczapowicz, et al. 2018. Novel oxazolinoanthracyclines as tumor cell growth inhibitors-Contribution of ATG and apoptosis in solid tumor cells death. PLoS One 13(7): e0201296.

Sanchez, A.M.J. 2018. MTG flux in skeletal muscle during chronic contractile activity and ageing. J Physiol 596: 3461–3462.

Shan, H., X. Zheng and M. Li. 2019. The effects of astragalus membranaceus active extracts on ATG-related diseases. Int J Mol Sci 20(8): E1904.

Sheng, J., L. Shen, L. Sun, X. Zhang, et al. 2019. Inhibition of PI3K/mTOR increased the sensitivity of hepatocellular carcinoma cells to cisplatin via interference with mitochondrial-lysosomal crosstalk. Cell Prolif 52: e12609.

Sun, Y., J. Yu, X. Liu, C. Zhang, et al. 2018. Oncosis-like cell death is induced by berberine through ERK1/2-mediated impairment of mitochondrial aerobic respiration in gliomas. Biomed Pharmacother 102: 699–710.

Szostakowska, M., A. Trębińska-Stryjewska, E.A. Grzybowska, A. Fabisiewicz. 2019. Resistance to endocrine therapy in BC: molecular mechanisms and future goals. BC Res Treat 173: 489–497.

Tsai, T.C., K.H. Lai, J.H. Su, Y.J. Wu, et al. 2018. 7-Acetylsinumaximol B induces apoptosis and autophagy in human gastric carcinoma cells through mitochondria dysfunction and activation of the PERK/eIF2α/ATF4/CHOP signaling pathway. Mar Drugs 16(4): 104.

Vara-Perez, M., H. Maes, S. van Dingenen, P. Agostinis. 2019. Bnip-3 contributes to the glutamine-driven aggressive behavior of melanoma cells. Biol Chem 400(2): 187–193. doi: 10.1515/hsz-2018-0208.

Vehlow, A. and N. Cordes. 2019. DDR1 (discoidin domain receptor TK 1) drives glioblastoma therapy resistance by modulating ATG. Autophagy 15: 1487–1488.

Wang, Q.S., S.Q. Shen, H.W. Sun, Z.X. Xing, et al. 2018a. Interferon-gamma induces ATG-associated apoptosis through induction of cPLA2-dependent mitochondrial ROS generation in colorectal cancer cells. Biochem Biophys Res Commun 498: 1058–1065.

Wang, F.Y., Tang, X.M., X. Wang, K.B. Huang, et al. 2018b. Mitochondria-targeted platinum(II) complexes induce apoptosis-dependent autophagic cell death mediated by ER-stress in A549 cancer cells. Eur J Med Chem 155: 639–650.

Wang, M.G., R.F. Fan, W.H. Li, D. Zhang, et al. 2019a. Activation of PERK-eIF2α-ATF4-CHOP axis triggered by excessive ER stress contributes to lead-induced nephrotoxicity. Biochim Biophys Acta Mol Cell Res 1866: 713–726.

Wang, Y.Y., Y.K. Chen, C.S. Hu, L.Y. Xiao, et al. 2019b. MAL-PDT inhibits oral precancerous cells and lesions via autophagic cell death. Oral Dis 25: 758–771.

Weinstein, J.N., E.A. Collison, G.B. Mills, K.R.M. Shaw, et al. 2013. The cancer genome Atlas Pan-Cancer analysis project. Nature Genetics. 45: 1113-1120.

Yan, C. and T.S. Li. 2018. Dual role of mitophagy in cancer drug resistance. Anticancer Res 38: 617–621.

Yan, X., L. Yang, G. Feng, Z. Yu, et al. 2018a. Lup-20(29)-en-3β,28-di-yl-nitrooxy acetate affects MCF-7 proliferation through the crosstalk between apoptosis and autophagy in mitochondria. Cell Death Dis 9: 241.

Yan, D., D. Zhu, X. Zhao and J. Su. 2018b. SHP-2 restricts apoptosis induced by chemotherapeutic agents via Parkin-dependent autophagy in cervical cancer. Cancer Cell Int 18: 8.

Yi, H., K. Wang, B. Du, L. He, et al. 2018a. Aleuritolic acid impaired autophagic flux and induced apoptosis in hepatocellular carcinoma HepG2 cells. Molecules 23: 1338.

Yi, X., L. Xiang, Y. Huang, Y. Wang, et al. 2018b. Apoptosis and pro-death ATG induced by a spirostanol saponin isolated from Rohdea chinensis (Baker) N. Tanaka (synonym Tupistra chinensis Baker) on HL-60 cells. Phytomedicine 42: 83–89.

Yin, S.Y, W.C. Wei, F.Y. Jian, N.S. Yang, et al. 2013. Therapeutic applications of herbal medicines for cancer patients. Evid Based Complement Alternat Med 2013: 302426.

Zhang, W.Y., Q.Y. Yi, Y.J. Wang, F. Du, et al. 2018. Photoinduced anticancer activity studies of iridium(III) complexes targeting mitochondria and tubules. Eur J Med Chem 151: 568–584.

Zhu, Q., X. Yu, Z.W. Zhou, M. Luo, et al. 2018. A quantitative proteomic response of hepatocellular carcinoma Hep3B cells to danusertib, a pan-Aurora kinase inhibitor. J Cancer 9: 2061–2071.

Zhu, Z., W. Shen, S. Tian, B. Yang, et al. 2019. F3, a novel active fraction of Valeriana jatamansi Jones induces cell death via DNA damage in human BC cells. Phytomedicine 57: 245–254.

31

Charnolophagy in Microbial Infections

INTRODUCTION

Infectious diseases are caused by pathogenic microorganisms, such as bacteria, viruses, parasites, or fungi. The diseases can spread, directly or indirectly, from one person to another. Zoonotic diseases are infectious diseases of animals that can cause disease when transmitted to humans. CP/ATG is emerging as a central component of antimicrobial host defense against microbial infections (from zoonotic diseases as well) and is an evolutionary conserved ATP-driven catabolic process that allows the degradation of intracellular microbes (including COVID-19) by lysosomes in the macrophages. CP/ATG can be triggered by nutrient deprivation, microbial infections, or other challenges to promote cell survival under stressful conditions, is critical in protecting cells from microbial infections, and intertwines with different infectious diseases. However, basal CP/ATG is also crucial for the maintenance of cellular homeostasis by ensuring the selective removal of protein aggregates and dysfunctional organelles (particularly mitochondria, as these are naturally-abundant in a physiologically and metabolically active cell). A strict regulation of this process is essential for NCF and organismal health. CP is also associated with diversified pathologies including cardiovascular disorders, gastrointestinal disorders, skin disorders, musculo-skeletal disorders, neurodegenerative disorders, inflammatory disorders, nutritional disorders, and cancer, in addition to microbial (bacteria, viral, fungal, and parasitic) infections. Ubiquitination and de-ubiquitination of CP substrates, as well as components of the CP machinery, are critical regulatory mechanisms of CP. Recently Jacomin et al. (2018) reviewed the de-ubiquitinating enzymes (DUBs) in the regulation of CP and discussed how they may constitute novel theranostic opportunities for the treatment of pathologies such as NDDs, CVDs, cancers, and infections. In addition to pathogen degradation, ATG has other functions during infection such as innate and adaptive immune activation. ATG also plays a crucial role in combating the infection and pathogenesis by regulating inflammation, which is the basis for a movement in infectious-disease research that hopes to exploit CP/ATG, a process by which cells recycle needed nutrients, to eliminate dangerous pathogens from the body.

Recent studies reported an intricate interaction between vitamin D and viral infections (Razdan et al. 2020, Xu et al. 2020, Martineau and Forouhi 2020, Bilezikian et al. 2020, Abdel-Mohsen and Ahmed 2018, Shaoping and Sun 2011). Human immunodeficiency virus-associated nephropathy (HIVAN) induced tubular pathology was associated with ERS, mitochondrial changes, and CP/ATG. It was shown that IRF5 is required for bacterial clearance in human M1-polarized macrophages. Fecal microbiota transplantation regulated intestinal mucosal CP and alleviated gut barrier injury. The Hepatitis C viral infection was associated with mitochondrial damage and dysregulation of iron metabolism in the liver. Iron depletion also induced MTG in pathogenic yeast. Genetic variations in innate immunity genes affected response to *Coxiella burnetii* and were associated with susceptibility to Q fever. ATG and inflammasomes (IS) complex assembly are physiological processes that control homeostasis, inflammation, and immunity. Seveau et al. (2018) highlighted that ATG is a ubiquitous pathway that degrades cytosolic macromolecules or organelles, as well as intracellular pathogens. Inflammasomes are multi-protein complexes that assemble in the cytosol of cells upon detection of pathogens or DAMPS. IS assembly triggers caspase-1 activation, which activates the pro-inflammatory cytokine precursors, pro-IL-1β and pro-IL-18. Studies on chronic inflammatory diseases, heart diseases, AD, and MS revealed that CP and ISs interact with and regulate each other. In infectious diseases, less is known about the interaction between ATG and IS assembly, although pathogens have evolved strategies to inhibit and/or subvert these pathways and to take advantage of their intricate crosstalk. An improved understanding of these pathways and their subversion by diverse pathogens will help in designing anti-infective theranostic strategies. Disease-specific CPTs can be developed to prevent viral attack during acute phase and inhibit its deleterious consequences during chronic phase of infection and disease progression. This can be accomplished by preventing (i) viral attachment with the mitochondrial membrane; (ii) viral entry in the mitochondrial matrix; (iii) viral activity as an uncoupler of O/P by developing novel therapeutic antioxidants as potent free radical scavengers; (iv) by enhancing inactivation and efflux of viral spike proteins, envelop proteins, and nucleic acid from the infected cell cytoplasm and mitochondria to sustain IMD and ICD; (v) by inhibiting incorporation of viral genome with the host cell mtDNA and nDNA to sustain mitochondrial growth, proliferation, regeneration, and network establishment so that it may not compromise MB and highjack physiologically-significant O/P and CP/ATG (implicated in IMD and ICD for NCF) of immune or any other highly vulnerable cell upon infection. During chronic phase, viral-induced persistent mitochondrial attack can trigger extensive CB formation and CP deregulation to increase ICT, toxemia, and multiple organ failure resulting in early morbidity and mortality. Hence, we can develop novel CPTs to enhance CP, prevent CS destabilization (through permeation, perforation, and fragmentation), enhance CS exocytosis for efficient detoxification and elimination of its toxic metabolites through liver and kidney, respectively to prevent viral-mediated CBMP implicated in CMB, generalized fatigue, and weakness. This can be accomplished by developing novel DSST-CB, CP, and CBMP-targeted CPTs in diversified chronic diseases in addition to viral infection, as highlighted in this edition. Recent strategies are attempting to target different phases of CBMP including CB formation, CP inhibition, CS destabilization, and CS exocytosis in the infectious microorganism for their radical elimination from the human body in light of emerging CP/ATG involvement in infectious diseases (Sharma 2017a, 2019b). Hence, stem-cell-specific CB, CP, and CS agonists/antagonists can be developed for the successful treatment of infectious diseases even during intrauterine life. In *C. elegans* embryos, paternally inherited mitochondria and their mtDNA are degraded via selective ATG called allophagy (allogeneic organelle ATG: CP). CP can also be identified as mitochondrial-specific inclusionophagy. This is a developmentally programmed ATG and, combined with *C. elegans* genetics and *in vivo* imaging, provides a unique opportunity to analyze selective ATG (including CP) under physiological conditions.

This chapter describes basic molecular mechanism of microbial (viral, bacterial, and fungal) infections involved in CP deregulation and its restoration by specific therapeutic antioxidants as free radical scavengers to cure these diseases.

CP In Viral Infections

Virus Compromises iPPCs Pluripotency

Maternal viral infections (including influenza, Zika, rubella, CMV) during pregnancy were reported as the possible cause of many defects and congenital anomalies (Chan and Smith 2018). Apart from several cases of influenza-related miscarriage during various trimesters of pregnancy, some epidemiological data suggest a link between maternal influenza infection and genetic abnormalities in offspring (Memoli et al. 2013). Zahedi-Amiri et al. (2019) used proteomic approaches and utilized hiPSCs for modeling intra-blastocyst infection with influenza virus to not only investigate the vulnerability and responses of pluripotent stem cells to this virus but also to determine the possible impacts of influenza on pluripotency and signaling pathways controlling differentiation and embryogenesis, indicating that viral protein production in influenza A virus (IAV)-infected hiPSCs. Although, viral replication was restricted in these cells, cell viability and pluripotency were negatively affected. These events occurred simultaneously with an excessive level of IAV-induced CP as well as cytopathic effects. Quantitative SOMA scan screening also indicated that changes in the proteome of hiPSCs corresponded to abnormal differentiation in these cells, suggesting that IAV-modulated reduction in hiPSC pluripotency is associated with activation of CP/ATG. A viral infection causes physiological alterations in the host cell, and many of these alterations can affect the host mitochondrial network, including aspects such as CB formation and CP induction. Zhang et al. (2018) discussed virus-regulated CP and its functional relevance in the pathogenesis of viral infection and disease. Some viruses trigger CP directly or indirectly and control CP via different mechanisms. This enables viruses to promote persistent infection and attenuate the innate immune responses as the author described in his book, *Zika Virus Disease: Prevention and Cure*, published by Nova Science Publishers in New York, U.S.A. The ATG signaling pathway is involved in cellular homeostasis, developmental processes, cellular stress responses, and immune pathways. Recently, Abdoli et al. (2018) summarized the relationship between ATG and viruses. They focused on the interaction of ATG and viruses and explored how human viruses exploit multiple steps in the ATG pathway to help viral propagation and escape immune response. They discussed the role of macroATG in cells infected with hepatitis C virus, hepatitis B virus, rotavirus gastroenteritis, immune cells infected with HIV virus, and respiratory tract infections including influenza virus and other coronaviruses. These investigators described a cross-talk between ATG and viral infections. They summarized the multifaceted roles of ATG in normal physiology and viral infection and pathogenesis, and described recent advances in understanding the relationship between ATG and viral infection, and how ATG plays dual roles in the disease progression. These data provided an overview of the molecular mechanisms that underlie ATG, the role of this pathway in the pathogenesis of viruses, and strategies for therapeutic interventions. Manipulation of ATG heralds the potential for highly effective treatments for a wide range of clinical diseases, including both bacterial and viral infections as well as autoimmune and inflammatory disease states which deserve attention as highlighted in this edition. Major highlights of this review were: (i) HCV NS4B triggers a stress response that induces ATG and leads to the lipidation of LC3 and forms complexes with Rab5, Vps34, and Beclin-1 (ii) HCV causes mitochondrial damage and oxidative stress, and impaired mitochondria are selectively eliminated by MTG; (iii) NS5B/Atg5 interaction could be necessary for the establishment of HCV replication; (iv) HCV-NS3 induces ATG in an IRGM-dependent pathway; (v) HCV activates a selective ATG for lipids (lipophagy) protects cells from an excessive lipid accumulation; (vi) HCV triggers lipoprotein degradation through lipophagy. In this edition, I have described in the introduction that lipid droplets start accumulating in the severely protein malnourished rat Purkinje neurons due to compromised CP and lipophagy. Hence there seems to be an intricate relationship between viral infection, CP/ATG, and malnutrition which needs further investigations. These investigators also highlighted that although knowledge of the ATG pathway is quickly progressing, there is still much to be learned regarding the specific molecules that regulate this pathway and the mechanisms by which viruses target these molecules to facilitate their replication. Hence, further studies are needed to be evaluated in preclinical and clinical trials.

RIG-I-Mediated Antiviral Signaling

ATG has been implicated in innate immune responses in various intracellular pathogens. ATG can be triggered by pathogen-recognizing sensors, including TLRs and cGMP-AMP synthase, to participate in innate immunity. Lee et al. (2018a) examined whether the RIG-I signaling pathway, which detects viral infections by recognizing viral RNA, triggers ATG. The introduction of polyI:C into the cytoplasm, or Sendai virus infection, induced ATG in normal cells but not in RIG-I-deficient cells. PolyI:C transfection or the Sendai virus infection induced ATG in the cells lacking type-I interferon signaling, suggesting that the effect was not due to interferon signaling. RIG-I-mediated ATG diminished by the deficiency of mitochondrial antiviral signaling protein (MAVS) or tumor necrosis factor receptor-associated factor (TRAF)6, showing that the RIG-I-MAVS-TRAF6 signaling axis was critical for RIG-I-mediated ATG. Beclin-1 was translocated to the mitochondria, and it interacted with TRAF6 upon RIG-I activation. Beclin-1 underwent K63-polyubiquitination upon RIG-I activation, and the ubiquitination decreased in TRAF6-deficient cells, suggesting that the RIG-I-MAVS-TRAF6 axis induced the K63-linked poly-ubiquitination of Beclin-1, implicated in triggering ATG. As deficient ATG increases the type-I interferon response, the induction of ATG by the RIG-I pathway might also contribute to preventing an excessive interferon response as a negative-feedback mechanism.

Influenza-viral Infection

Influenza-associated mortality continues to occur despite available antiviral therapies. Novel therapies that improve host immunity could reduce the influenza virus disease burden. Targeting the macrophage migration inhibitory factor (MIF) has improved the outcomes of inflammatory diseases. Smith et al. (2019) showed that during the influenza viral infection, Mif-deficient mice have less inflammation, viral load, and mortality compared with WT control mice; conversely, Tg mice, which overexpressed Mif in alveolar epithelial cells, had higher inflammation, viral load, and mortality. An antibody-mediated blockade of MIF in WT mice during the influenza viral infection improved their survival. Mif-deficient murine lungs showed reduced levels of Parkin, a CP protein that negatively regulates antiviral signaling, prior to infection and augments antiviral type I/III IFN levels in the airspaces after infection. *In vitro* assays with human lung epithelial cells showed that treatment with rMIF increased the percentage of the influenza-virus-infected cells, indicating that MIF impairs antiviral host immunity and increases inflammation during the influenza infection; hence, targeting MIF could be theranostically beneficial in the influenza viral infection.

CP and Corona Viral Infection

Coronavirus can be transmitted from man to man, with an incubation period of 1–14 days, and induces mild to severe respiratory diseases, inflammation, high fever, dry cough, xerostomia, acute respiratory tract infection, diarrhea, hyposmia, hypogeusia, and dysfunction of internal organs that may lead to death. Coronavirus attacks immune cells including mast cells (MCs), which are located in the submucosa of the respiratory tract and in the nasal cavity. The virus activates MCs which release early inflammatory mediators including histamine and protease, while late activation provokes pro-inflammatory IL-1 and IL-33. Inflammation by coronavirus may be inhibited by anti-inflammatory cytokines belonging to IL-1 family members (Kritas et al. 2020). CP/ATG is an essential process affecting viral infection and other diseases and Beclin-1 (BECN1) is one of its key regulators. Studies with Sindbis virus and herpes simplex virus-1 have indicated that CP/ATG may be a defense mechanism against an infection with these viruses. CP/ATG is a mechanism of replication complex formation for the positive-sense RNA viruses, corona virus, poliovirus, equine arteritis virus (EAV), and mouse hepatitis virus (MHV). Replication complexes of these viruses as double-membrane vesicles (DMVs) in the cytoplasm, is suggestive of CP/ATG origin. For poliovirus and MHV, multiple organelle biomarkers co-localize or co-fractionate with replication complexes, consistent with CP/ATG-like process. Poliovirus and MHV replication complexes acquire lysosomal markers similar to the maturation of inflammasome (APS), which share features of APS. Recently, markers for CP/ATG vacuoles in mammalian cells have been described: LC3 and Apg12, which provide theranostic approaches to investigate the role of CP/ATG in viral infections. Coronaviruses are enveloped, positive-sense RNA viruses that replicate in the cytoplasm; they are important causes of disease in many domesticated animals, and for up to 30% of human colds. A human coronavirus is the causative agent of severe acute respiratory syndrome (SARS). Coronaviruses and arteriviruses are the two families within the order Nidovirales. Viruses in this order have a similar genome organization and express the proteins required for RNA replication as polyproteins. Thus, studies of the mechanisms of the coronavirus replication complex may be critical to understanding the pathogenesis, treatment, and vaccine development for the prevention of infection. Mouse hepatitis virus (MHV) is a coronavirus used for studies of replication complex formation and function. MHV replication complexes form in the cytoplasm of infected cells and are first detectable at 4–5 hrs p.i. by immunofluorescence in MHV-infected DBT cells. Replication complexes appear as punctate perinuclear foci, with the number and size of replication complexes increasing as a function of time. These complexes are active in viral RNA synthesis and contain replicase, and the structural nucleocapsid protein (N). Components of the replication complex, the helicase (hel) and N proteins, translocate between 6 and 8 hrs p.i. from the sites of RNA.

Coronaviruses induce the rearrangement of cellular membranes upon infection of a host cell for the assembly of replication complexes, improving RNA synthesis (Maier and Britton 2012). Coronavirus induces membrane rearrangements and CP/ATG or LC3 during replication. Several human coronaviruses cause mild respiratory infections, with the exception of SARS-CoV. The avian coronavirus, infectious bronchitis virus (IBV), causes infectious bronchitis (IB), a mild respiratory infection, but has serious effects on the poultry industries due to poor weight gain in chickens, reduced egg production, and subpar egg quality. Some strains of IBV are nephron-pathogenic while others cause severe pathology in the reproductive organs. BCoV causes respiratory infection and diarrhea in cattle; transmissible gastroenteritis virus (TGEV) and porcine epidemic diarrhea virus (PEDV) cause diarrhea in pigs and the porcine hemagglutinating encephalomyelitis virus (PHEV) causes vomiting and wasting disease in pigs. Coronavirus mouse hepatitis virus (MHV) performs RNA replication on double membrane vesicles (DMVs) in the cytoplasm of the host cell (Prentice et al. 2003). Replication complexes co-localize with the ATG proteins, LC3 and Apg12. The MHV infection induced ATG that was resistant to 3-MA inhibition. MHV replication was impaired in ATG knockout, APG5−/−, embryonic stem cell lines, but MHV replication was restored by expression of APG5 in the APG5−/− cells. In MHV-infected APG5−/− cells, DMVs were not detected; rather, the RER was swollen, suggesting that CP/ATG is required for the formation of double-membrane bound MHV replication complexes, and that DMV formation enhances replication. The RER was implicated as a source of membranes for replication complexes.

Recently, Gassen et al. (2019) identified S-phase kinase-associated protein 2 (SKP2) as an E3 ligase that executes lysine-48-linked poly-ubiquitination of BECN1, thus promoting its proteosomal degradation. SKP2 activity is regulated by phosphorylation in a hetero-complex involving FKBP51, PHLPP, Akt1, and BECN1. The genetic or pharmacological inhibition of SKP2 decreased BECN1 ubiquitination, decreased BECN1 degradation. and enhanced CP/ATG. MERS-CoV multiplication resulted in reduced BECN1 and blocked the fusion of APS and lysosomes. Inhibitors of SKP2 enhanced ATG and reduced the replication of MERS-CoV up to 28,000X. The SKP2-BECN1 link constitutes a promising target for host-directed antiviral drugs and other ATG-sensitive conditions. ATG-inducing, FDA-approved drugs have become available for treatment in humans. Valinomycin (VAL) targets SARS-CoV *in vitro* as an SKP2 inhibitor. Niclosamide (NIC) and VAL were efficient in enhancing BECN1, LC3B-II/I, and ATG. NIC and VAL reduce MERS-CoV multiplication by up to 1000-X in 48 hrs p.i.

The SARS-CoV E protein consists of three domains, that is, the amino (N)-terminal, the transmembrane (TM), and the C-terminal domain. With sequence homology 96.3% with BatCoV, RaTG13, shows discordant clustering with the Bat SARS-like coronavirus sequences. Specifically, in the 5′-part spanning the first 11,498 nucleotides and the last 3′-part spanning 24,341–30,696 positions, COVID-19 and RaTG13 formed a single cluster with Bat SARS-like coronavirus sequences, whereas in the middle region spanning the 3′-end of ORF1a, the ORF1b and almost half of the spike regions, COVID-19 and RaTG13 grouped in a separate distant lineage within the sarbecovirus branch. The genetic similarity between the COVID-19 and RaTG13 suggested that the latter does not provide the exact variant that caused the outbreak in humans, but the presumption that COVID-19 has originated from bats is very likely. COVID-19 is not-mosaic consisting in almost half of its genome of a distinct lineage within the beta-coronavirus (Paraskevis et al. 2020).

A high diversity of corona- and paramyxoviruses have been detected in different bat species worldwide. Recently, samples from bats collected from caves in Ruhengeri, Rwanda, were tested for the presence of corona- and para-myxoviral RNA using RT-PCR. Results were characterized by DNA sequencing and phylogenetic analysis. In addition to the morphological identification of bat species, they also did confirmation of species identities, contributing to the known genetic database available for African bat species and detected a novel *Betacoronavirus* in two Geoffroy's horseshoe (*Rhinolophus clivosus*) bats and detected several paramyxoviral species from insectivorous bats. One of these viral species was homologous to the genomes of viruses belonging to the *Jeilongvirus* genus. Additionally, a *Henipavirus*-related sequence was detected in an Egyptian rousette fruit bat (*Rousettus aegyptiacus*) (Markotter et al. 2019).

MERS-coronavirus was first identified in 2012 in Saudi Arabia. Capable of causing severe pneumonia, the pathogen resulted in death in ~30% of infections. There are currently no effective treatments for MERS. ATG-inducing substances have demonstrated efficacy in reducing the rate at which the virus replicates. The MERS virus can only replicate efficiently if it inhibits CP/ATG. Several viruses have evolved to combat this defense. A MERS pathogen benefits from an attenuation of the cellular recycling process. A molecular switch that regulates the CP/ATG is the SKP2 protein. The MERS virus activates this molecular switch to slow down the cell's recycling processes and avoid degradation; hence, SKP2 inhibitors conferred a therapeutic benefit. Niclosamide, a treatment for helminthes as an SKP2 inhibitor, reduced the replication of the MERS virus in cell culture. Whether SKP2 inhibitors could be effective against SARS or the 2019-nCoV that has currently emerged is yet to be established. CP/ATG plays important roles in modulating viral replication and an antiviral immune response. Although a coronavirus infection is associated with CP/ATG, little is known about the mechanisms of its induction and contribution to regulation of the host's innate responses. The membrane-associated papain-like protease PLP2 (PLP2-TM) of coronaviruses acts as a novel CP/ATG-inducing protein. Intriguingly, PLP2-TM induces partial CP/ATG by increasing the accumulation of APS but blocks the fusion of APS with lysosomes. PLP2-TM interacts with the key CP/ATG regulators, LC3 and Beclin-1, and promotes Beclin-1 interaction with STING, the key regulator for antiviral

IFN signaling. The knockdown of Beclin-1 reversed PLP2-TM's inhibitory effect on innate immunity resulting in decreased coronavirus replication, suggesting that its papain-like protease induces partial CP/ATG by interacting with Beclin-1, which modulates its replication and innate immunity (Chen et al. 2014). APS induced by CoV PLP2-TM/PLpro-TMs may provide a platform for viral targeting Beclin-1 to sequester STING and other innate signaling components to impede downstream antiviral responses, thereby promoting viral replication. Further studies are needed to elucidate the precise mechanisms of CPS/APS induction by CoV PLPs and the exact roles of CP/ATG in coronavirus replication, antiviral innate immune responses, and disease pathogenesis.

Schoeman and Fielding (2019) reported that CoVs cause enzootic infections in birds and mammals but, in the last few decades, is capable of infecting humans as well. The outbreak of SARS in 2003 and MERS has demonstrated the lethality of CoVs when they crossed the species barrier and infected humans. Interest in coronaviral research has led to the discovery of several novel human CoVs and progress has been made in understanding the CoV life cycle. The CoV envelope (E) protein is involved in the viral life cycle, such as assembly, budding, envelope formation, and pathogenesis. Recent studies have expanded on its structural motifs and topology, its functions as an ion-channeling *viroporin,* and its interactions with other CoV proteins and host cell proteins, particularly in SARS-CoV E, regarding specific structural requirements for its functions in its life cycle as well as mechanisms of pathogenesis. E is involved in the viral life cycle and CoVs lacking E make promising vaccine candidates. The high mortality rate of certain CoVs, along with their ease of transmission, highlights the need for more research into its molecular biology which can aid in the production of effective agents for both human CoVs and enzootic CoVs. Niclosamide (NIC) and VAL were efficient in enhancing BECN1, LC3B-II/I and CP/ATG flux. NIC and VAL reduced MERS-CoV multiplication by up to 1000X at 48 hrs p.i. Both drugs enhanced ATG14 oligomerization by about 2X and increased the number of APS >2X. NIC also affected the ATG flux in the infected cells similar to SKP2i. Therefore, these three compounds were tested for their effect in a MERS-CoV infection. BECN1 as a target of the E3 ligase SKP2. SKP2 executed K48-linked ubiquitination at K402 of BECN1, resulting in proteosomal degradation. This action of SKP2 was counteracted by FKBP51, which regulates SKP2 phosphorylation through complexes with Akt1 and PHLPP. Inhibition of SKP2 increased BECN1 levels, enhanced the assembly of lysosomal SNARE proteins and ATG, and reduced the replication of MERS-CoV. FKBP51 is a pivotal element of molecular feedback loops of the cellular and physiological stress reaction. It emerges as a scaffolder that chaperones various regulatory protein interactions. FKBP51 recruits SKP2 in its inactive form to BECN1, by virtue of its interaction with the kinase Akt1 and the phosphatase PHLPP. Similarly, FKBP51-directed protein interactions increase BECN1 phosphorylation and decrease phosphorylation and the activity of Akt1. Thus, FKBP51 impacts BECN1 via two mechanisms, phosphorylation of BECN1 and of its regulatory E3 ligase SKP2. Both mechanisms involve Akt1, exhibiting yet another way of influencing BECN1 by phosphorylating USP14, which removes K63-linked ubiquitins from BECN1. In addition to K48-linked poly-ubiquitination by SKP2, BECN1 undergoes ubiquitination by other E3 ligases, at different sites, and with different types of poly-ubiquitination linkage. NEDD4 produces both K63- and K11-linkages at certain sites of BECN1. Decoration of BECN1 with the non-canonical K11-linked ubiquitins by NEDD4 leads to its proteasomal degradation. K63-linked ubiquitination of the BH3 domain of BECN1 at K117 by TRAF6 enhances ATG, by reducing the interaction of BECN1 with BCL.

AMBRA1 is another positive regulator of CP/ATG. As a substrate receptor for the DDB1-cullin4 E3 ligase complex, it forms K63-linked ubiquitin chains at K437 of BECN1, enhancing the association between BECN1 and Vps34/PI3K3C, and thus stimulating CP/ATG promoting lipid kinase. Thus, BECN1 activity is regulated by ubiquitination in multiple ways, both stimulatory and inhibitory. The polyQ domain protein ataxin 3 interacts with BECN1 and removes K48-linked polyubiquitin, which was competitively inhibited by longer polyQ mutation in a disease protein. Together with the discovery of SKP2 as a K48-linking E3 ligase of BECN1, it is suggested that inhibiting SKP2 using small molecule inhibitors might counteract the deleterious effects of soluble proteins with polyQ expansions for causing NDDs such as HD and ataxin 3 in spinocerebellar ataxia (SCA) (Gassen et al. 2019, Ashkenazi et al. 2017).

Due to the variability of viral proteins, there is considerable interest in host cell-encoded pathways that could be exploited for fighting viral infection. CP/ATG can serve as a pivotal component of virus-host interaction and potential broad-spectrum antiviral target. For MERS-CoV replication, it remains to be elucidated whether blocking basal CP/ATG is mandatory or only auxiliary; nevertheless, the virus encodes three proteins that limit CP/ATG when expressed ectopically: NSP6, p4b, and p5. MERS-CoV NSP6 may also play a role in inhibiting the expansion of APS as in other beta-coronaviruses. MERS-CoV p4b has a phosphodiesterase function which inhibits the activation of RNAse L, which can activate ATG. MERS-CoV p5 is located in the ER-Golgi compartment and inhibits IFN-β, which may constitute another link to ATG. Deletion of p4b or p5 resulted in reduced MERS-CoV growth. In addition, a very low MOI and a type I IFN-deficient cell line (VeroB4) was used, which allows researchers to determine minor growth differences (Gassen et al. 2019). The absence of p4b and p5 during MERS-CoV replication may also result in lower LC3B compared to MERS-CoV in wild-type-infected mice but also as compared to the mock-infected control cells. This points to a more complex interaction between virus replication and ATG; p4b and p5 may counteract a response of the host to viral infection, but the functional relevance of their link to CP/ATG requires further investigation. Several CoV proteins collaborate to reprogram the membrane traffic in the cell for DMV formation serving as compartments of viral genome replication and transcription. MERS-CoV blocks CP/ATG not only to evade degradation but also to improve membrane availability. Most of the treatments arising from the reduction of viral replication upon ATG stimulation are not easily applicable *in vivo* because of side effects and inefficient peptide delivery. Examples are Rapamycin and Vitamin D which restricted the replication of HIV in primary human macrophages, and the CP/ATG-inducing BECN1-derived peptide which limited the replication of a number of viruses *in vitro*. The therapeutic induction of CP/ATG by inhibition of SKP2 has emerged as a promising approach. The antiviral effects of compounds can be evaluated by targeting BECN1, which is a client of SKP2. Nevertheless, future experiments should assess the effect of these drugs on CP/ATG-defective cells such as the Atg5 knockout cells. Whether inhibiting SKP2 will affect all ATG-sensitive viruses remains uncertain. SINV, which was not influenced by Atg5 knockout despite the indications of degradation of viral components through CP/ATG, reacted primarily to SKP2i. It may relate to the involvement of other immune pathways influencing SINV, for example the JAK/STAT pathway or stress granule formation, or to CP/ATG functioning in the absence of Atg5.

FDA-approved drugs as SKP2 inhibitors are also available. Some of these drugs are effective in reducing MERS-CoV replication *in vitro*, for example Niclosamide and Pyrvinium pamoate. Recently, Gassen et al. (2020) reported that the antiviral effect of compounds targeting BECN1 is related to SKP2. SARS0CoV-2 infection downregulates ATG-inducing spermidine, and facilitates Akt1/SKP2-dependent degradation of ATG-initiating Beclin-1 (BECN1). Targeting these pathways by exogenous administration of spermidine, Akt inhibitor MK-2206, and the Beclin-1 stabilizing, antihelminthic drug Niclosamide inhibited SARS-CoV-2 propagation, indicating that SARS-CoV-2 infection inhibits ATG. A clinically-approved and well-tolerated ATG-inducing compounds including colchicine revealed potential for evaluation as a treatment against SARS-CoV-2. Recently, Levin et al. (2015) reported several FDA-approved ATG inhibitors including Carbamazepine, Clonidine, Lithium, Metformin, Rapamycin, Rilmenide, Sodium Valproate, Verapamil, Trifluprazine, Statins, and Tyrosine Kinase Inhibitors. Compound BH3 is in investigational stage. Some nutritional supplements including Caffeine, Omega-3 Polyunsaturated Fatty Acids (PUFA), Resveratrol, Curcumin, Spermidine, Vitamin-D, and

Trehlose also exhibit CP/ATG-inducing properties as described in this edition. Furthermore, ATG gene transgenic expression, ATG gene therapy, and ATG-inducing peptides are currently under investigation. Even though there are reports of low absorption of these drugs, others found that considerable absorption and serum levels of Niclosamide reached 1–20 µM, to limit MERS-CoV replication. Inhalable formulations of Niclosamide have been developed as well. SKP2-targeting compounds also may have theranostic potential in other infections and conditions that are influenced by CP/ATG induction/inhibition. Recent clinical trials with HCQ and Ramdesivir provided limited success in the TSE-EBPT of COVID-19. Further studies are needed to develop CP, CS, and CBMP-targeted safe and effective vaccine(s) and therapeutics to nullify the deleterious consequences of novel COVID-19 and other viruses on human health and quality of life.

CP and HIV Infection

HIV Type-1 Gp120 and Tat Induce CBMP

HIV enters the CNS during the early stages of infection and can cause neurological dysfunction, including neurodegeneration and neurocognitive impairment. Specific CP/ATG are responsible for the removal of CBs and mitochondrial dynamics which constitute MQC mechanisms, and are impaired in NDDs and numerous other diseases. The release of HIV proteins, gp120 and Tat, from infected cells play an important role in HIV-associated neurocognitive disorders (HAND). Teodorof-Diedrich and Specter (2018) reported that exposure of human primary neurons (HPNs) to HIV gp120 and Tat accelerate the balance of mitochondrial dynamics toward fission and induced perinuclear aggregation of mitochondria and Drp-1 mitochondrial translocation, leading to mitochondrial fragmentation involving CBMP. HIV gp120 and Tat increased LC3 protein expression, and induced Parkin/SQSTM1 selective recruitment to the CBs. Using a dual fluorescence reporter system expressing mito-mRFP-EGFP or a tandem LC3 vector (mRFP-EGFP-LC3), both HIV proteins inhibit mitophagic flux in human primary neurons. HIV gp120 and Tat induced mitochondrial damage and altered mitochondrial dynamics by decreasing $\Delta\Psi$, indicating that HIV gp120 and Tat initiate activation and recruitment of MTG markers to CBs in neurons, but impair the delivery of mitochondria to the lysosomal compartment. Altered mitochondrial dynamics associated with HIV infection and impaired neuronal CP may play a significant role in the development of HAND and accelerate aging associated with HIV infection. Despite viral suppression by anti-retrovirals, HIV proteins continue to be detected in infected cells and neurologic complications remain common in infected people. Although HIV is unable to infect neurons, viral proteins including gp120 and Tat, can enter neurons and cause neurodegeneration and neurocognitive impairment. Neuronal health is dependent on the functional integrity of mitochondria and CBs are subjected to MQC mechanisms. Specific elimination of CBs through CP and mitochondrial dynamics play an important role in CNS diseases. Human primary neurons, gp120 and Tat, favor the balance of mitochondrial dynamics toward enhanced fragmentation through the activation of mitochondrial translocation of Drp-1 to the CBs implicated in CBMP-induced apoptosis and hence, disease progression. CP fails to go to completion leading to neuronal damage. These findings support a role for altered CP in HIV-associated NDDs and provide novel targets to develop TSE-EBPT-CPTs to cure HIV infection.

HIV-1 Patients with CD4+ T Cell Decline

The goal of antiretroviral therapy (ART) is to suppress HIV-1 replication and restore CD4+ T cells. Lisco et al. (2019) reported on HIV-infected individuals who had a decline in CD4+ T cells despite the ART-mediated suppression of plasma HIV-1 load (pVL). They defined such an immunological outcome as extreme immune decline (EXID). EXID's clinical and immunological characteristics were compared to immunological responders (IRs), immunological non-responders (INRs), healthy controls (HCs), and idiopathic CD4+ lymphopenia (ICL) patients. T cell immune-phenotyping and assembly/activation of ISs were evaluated by flow cytometry. PBMC transcriptome analysis and genetic screening for pathogenic variants were performed. Cytokines/ chemokines were measured by electro-chemiluminescence. The luciferase immunoprecipitation system and NK-mediated antibody-dependent cellular cytotoxicity (ADCC) assays were used to identify anti-lymphocyte autoantibodies. EXIDs were infected with non-B HIV-1 subtypes and after 192 weeks of consistent ART-mediated pVL suppression, had a median CD4+ decrease of 157 cells/µl, compared with CD4+ increases of 193 cells/µl and 427 cells/µl in INR and IR, respectively. EXID had reduced naive CD4+ T cells, but had similar proportions of cycling CD4+ T cells and HLA-DR+CD38+CD8+ T cells compared with IR and INR. Levels of inflammatory cytokines were also similar in EXID and INR, but the IL-7 axis was significantly perturbed compared with HC, IR, INR, and ICL. Genes involved in T cell and monocyte/macrophage function, ATG, and cell migration were differentially expressed in EXID. Two of the five EXIDs had autoantibodies causing ADCC, while two different EXIDs had an increased IS/caspase-1 activation despite ART-suppressed pVL. EXID is a distinct immunological outcome compared with previously described INR. Anti-CD4+ T cell autoantibodies and aberrant IS/caspase-1 activation despite suppressed HIV-1 viremia are among the mechanisms responsible for EXID.

HIV-1 TAT-mediated Microglial Activation

Although the advent of combination antiretroviral therapy (cART) has increased the life expectancy of HIV-1 infected individuals, the prevalence of HIV-1-associated neurocognitive disorders is on the rise. Based on the premise that the cytotoxic HIV-1 protein, transactivator of transcription (TAT), a known activator of glial cells that is found to persist in the CNS despite cART, Thangaraj et al. (2018) explored the role of defective CP in HIV-1 TAT-mediated microglial activation. The exposure of mouse primary microglia to HIV-1 TAT resulted in activation involving altered $\Delta\Psi$ that was accompanied by accumulation of damaged mitochondria participating in CBMP. Exposure of microglia to HIV-1 TAT resulted in an increased expression of CP-signaling proteins, PINK1, PRKN, and DNM1L, with a concomitant increase in the formation of CPS, as evidenced by the increased expression of BECN1 and MAP1LC3B-II. The exposure of cells to HIV-1 TAT also increased the expression of SQSTM1, a possible blockade of the CP, resulting in the accumulation of CPS. HIV-1 TAT-mediated activation of microglia was associated with a decreased rate of extracellular acidification and mitochondrial O_2 consumption and increased expression of pro-inflammatory cytokines, such as Tnf, Il1b, and Il6. HIV-1 TAT-mediated defective CP leading to microglial activation was further validated *in vivo* in the brains of HIV-1 transgenic rats, suggesting that HIV-1 TAT activates microglia by increasing mitochondrial damage via defective CP.

HIVAN-associated Nephropathy

HIV-associated nephropathy (HIVAN) is a unique form of a renal parenchymal disorder. Katuri et al. (2019) highlighted mechanisms in HIVAN, related to the renal tubules' association with ERS, MTS, and ATG. This disease and its characteristics can be accredited to the incorporation of DNA and mRNA of HIV-1 into the renal parenchymal cells. A proper understanding of the HIVAN and the mechanisms associated with renal function and disorders is vital for the development of a reliable treatment for HIVAN. Specifically, the renal tubule segment of the kidney is characterized by its transport capabilities and its ability to reabsorb water and salts into the blood. However, the segment is also known for certain disorders, such as renal tubular epithelial cell infection and micro-cyst formation, linked to HIVAN. Organelles, like the ER, mitochondria, and lysosome, are vital for certain mechanisms in kidney cells. A paradigm of the importance of these organelles can be seen in of HIVAN cases where the renal disorder increases ERS due to HIV viral propagation. This balance can be restored through the synthesis of secretory proteins, but the secretion requires more energy; therefore, there is an increase in MRS. The increased ER changes and MRS upregulate CP/ATG, which involves the lysosomes and ATP. The ERS and MTS are associated in the Tg26 animal model of HIVAN, which may shed light on improved treatment of HIVAN.

mtDNA Depletion by Zidovudine

The nucleoside reverse transcriptase inhibitor Zidovudine (AZT), used in HIV infection treatment, induces mtDNA depletion. A relationship between mtDNA status alterations and ATG has been reported. Both events are common in liver diseases, including HCC. Santos-Llamas et al. (2018) studied ATG activation in rat liver with mtDNA depletion induced by AZT administration in drinking water for 35 days. AZT at a concentration of 1 mg/ml, but not 0.5 mg/ml in the drinking water, decreased mtDNA levels in rat liver and extrahepatic tissues. In the liver, mtDNA-encoded cytochrome c oxidase 1 protein levels were decreased. Although the serum biomarkers of liver and kidney toxicity remained unaltered, β-hydroxybutyrate levels were increased in the liver of AZT-treated rats. ATG was dysregulated at two levels: (i) decreased induction signaling of this process as indicated by increases in ATG inhibitors activity (Akt/mTOR), and absence of changes (Beclin-1, Atg5, ATG7) or decreases (AMPK/ULK1) in the expression/activity of pro-ATG proteins; and (ii) reduced APS degradation as indicated by decreases in the lysosome abundance (LAMP2 marker) and the transcription factor TFEB controlling lysosome biogenesis, resulting in increased APS abundance (LC3-II marker) and accumulation of the protein degraded by ATG p62, and the transcription factor Nrf2 in liver of AZT-treated rats. Nrf2 was activated as indicated by the upregulation of the antioxidant target genes Nqo1 and Hmox-1. Rat liver with AZT-induced mtDNA depletion presented dysregulations in APS formation and degradation balance, which resulted in accumulation of these structures in parenchymal liver cells, favoring hepato-carcinogenesis.

CP and Other Viral Infections

HPV Infection and ATG-Related Genes

Condylomata acuminata are benign ano-genital warts caused by a human papillomavirus (HPV) infection with a high recurrence rate. CP/ATG plays an important role in maintaining internal environmental stability. However, the role of CP/ATG regulation in the ano-genital warts caused by HPV infection remains unknown. Jiang et al. (2019) identified the CP/ATG gene fingerprint involved in ano-genital warts arising from infections with different HPV genotypes. Human ATG-PCR arrays were performed on the initial 18 participants grouped by their different HPV genotypes for gene expression-profiling. The negative control was skin samples collected during plastic surgery on the chest from a group of individuals who showed none of the clinical symptoms or evidence of HPV infection. qPCR was performed to validate the microarray results in another 24 individuals. Out of 84 genes involved in ATG, different responses were noticed among the 29 genes that encode ATG machinery components, and expression levels of 13 of these genes were downregulated. The expression levels of two key genes that participate in the formation of APS, ATG3, and -Beclin-1, were downregulated in the HPV infection groups, suggesting that the HPV infection downregulated ATG expression in CA and there were no differences in the ATGs between the different HPV genotype infection groups. This study provided new insights into the ATG response to HPV infection.

HSV-1 Infection and ESCRT-Related ATPase Vps4

Interferons (IFNs) and ATG are critical neuronal defenses against viral infection. IFNs alter neuronal ATG by promoting the accumulation of IFN-dependent LC3-decorated ATG structures, termed LC3 clusters. Cabrera et al. (2019) analyzed LC3 clusters in sensory ganglia following a herpes HSV-1 infection. In the vicinity of acutely infected neurons, antigen-negative neurons contained structures resembling accumulated APS and autolysosomes that culminated in LC3 clusters. This accumulation reflects a delayed completion of ATG. The endosomal sorting complexes required for transport (ESCRT) machinery participates in APS closure and is also required for HSV-1 replication. An HSV-1 infection *in vivo* and in primary neurons caused a decrease in Vps4 (a key ESCRT pathway ATPase) RNA and protein with concomitant Stat1 activation and LC3 cluster induction. The IFNs decreased RNA and protein levels of Vps4 in primary neurons and in other cell types. The accumulation of ubiquitin was also observed at the LC3 cluster sites. IFNs modulated the ESCRT machinery in neurons in response to HSV-1 infections. Neurons rely on IFNs and ATG as major defenses against viral infections, and HSV must overcome such defenses in order to replicate. In addition to controlling host immunity, HSV must also control host membranes to complete its life cycle. HSV uses the host ESCRT membrane scission machinery for viral production and transport. These researchers presented evidence of a new IFN-dependent mechanism used by the host to prevent ESCRT subversion by HSV. This activity also impacted the dynamics of ATG, explaining the presence of LC3 clusters in the HSV-infected nervous system. The induced accumulations of ubiquitin in LC3 clusters resembled those observed in certain NDDs, suggesting a possible interaction between these conditions.

Varicella-zoster Virus Capsids Exit

Varicella-zoster virus (VZV) is an alpha herpesvirus that lacks the herpes viral neuro-virulence protein ICP34.5 because inhibitors of ATG reduce VZV infectivity. Girsch et al. (2019) selected the vacuolar proton ATPase inhibitor Bafilomycin A1 for analysis because of its antiATG property of impeding acidification during the late stage of ATG. Bafilomycin treatment from 48–72 hrs post-infection lowered VZV titers. Capsids were observed in the nucleus, in the perinuclear space, and in the cytoplasm adjacent to Golgi apparatus vesicles. Many of the capsids had an aberrant appearance, as has been observed in infections not treated with Bafilomycin. In contrast to prior untreated infections, the secondary envelopment of capsids was not seen in the *trans*-Golgi network, nor were prototypical enveloped particles with capsids (virions) seen in cytoplasmic vesicles after the Bafilomycin treatment. Instead, multiple particles with varying diameters without capsids (light particles) were seen in large virus assembly compartments near the disorganized Golgi apparatus. Bafilomycin increased the numbers of multi-vesicular bodies in the cytoplasm, some of which contained remnants of the Golgi apparatus and disrupted the site of secondary envelopment of VZV capsids by altering the pH of the *trans*-Golgi network and thereby preventing the correct formation of virus assembly compartments. This study emphasized the importance of the Golgi apparatus/*trans*-Golgi network in the α-herpesvirus life cycle. VZV induces ATG in human skin, a major site of VZV assembly. Bafilomycin impaired assembly of VZV capsids after primary envelopment/de-envelopment but before secondary re-envelopment. This study complemented prior herpes simplex virus 1 and pseudorabies virus studies investigating two other inhibitors of ER/Golgi apparatus function: Brefeldin A and Monensin (Wild et al. 2017). Studies with porcine herpesvirus demonstrated that primary enveloped particles accumulated in the perinuclear space in the presence of Brefeldin A, while studies with herpes simplex virus 1 revealed an impaired secondary assembly of enveloped viral particles in the presence of Monensin (Girsch et al. 2019).

STING-dependent Translation Inhibition

In mammalian cells, IFN responses that occur during RNA and DNA virus infections are activated by distinct signaling pathways. The RIG-I-like-receptors (RLRs) bind viral RNA and engage the adaptor MAVS (mitochondrial antiviral signaling) to promote IFN expression, whereas cGAS (*cGMP-AMP synthase*) binds viral DNA and activates an analogous pathway via the protein STING (stimulator of IFN *genes*). Franz et al. (2018) confirmed that STING was not necessary to induce IFN expression during the RNA virus infection but also found that STING was required to restrict the replication of diverse RNA viruses. The antiviral activities of STING were not linked to its ability to regulate the basal expression of IFN-stimulated genes, activate transcription, or ATG. Using vesicular stomatitis virus as a model, these investigators identified STING to inhibit translation during infection and upon transfection of synthetic RLR ligands. This inhibition occurred at the level of translation initiation and restricted the production of viral and host proteins. The inability to restrict translation rendered STING-deficient cells 100X more likely to support productive viral infections than wild-type counterparts. Genetic analysis linked RNA-sensing by RLRs to STING-dependent translation inhibition, independent of MAVS. Thus, STING has a dual role in host defense: regulating protein synthesis to prevent an RNA virus infection and regulating IFN expression to restrict DNA viruses.

CP in Hepatitis C Viral Infection

Although an HCV infection is expected to decrease due to the high rate of HCV eradication via the rapid dissemination and use of directly acting antivirals, its infection remains a leading cause of HCC. Hepatitis C virus (HCV) infection often leads to chronic hepatitis that can progress to liver cirrhosis and HCC. Hino et al. (2019) discussed the mechanisms by which HCV induces mitochondrial damage and iron accumulation in the liver and offer new insights concerning CBMP and iron accumulation linked to the development of HCC. Although the mechanisms underlying the HCC development are not fully understood, oxidative stress is present in HCV infection and has been proposed as a mechanism of liver injury in patients with hepatitis C. Hepatocellular mitochondrial alterations and iron accumulation are well-known in patients with chronic hepatitis C and are related to oxidative stress, since the mitochondria are the main site of ROS generation, and iron produces $ONOO^-$ ions in the presence of ·OH and NO· radicals via the Fenton reaction, which induce oxidative as well as nitrative stress and CBMP in a cell. In addition, phlebotomy is an iron reduction approach that aims to lower serum transaminase levels in patients with chronic hepatitis C. Recently, Mori et al. (2018) investigated the characteristics of CP induced by an HCV infection. To examine the involvement of ATG-related gene (ATG) proteins in HCV-induced LC3 lipidation, they established Atg5, ATG13, or ATG14 knockout (KO) Huh7.5.1 cell lines and confirmed that the accumulation of lipidated LC3 was induced in an ATG13- and ATG14-independent manner. HCV infectivity was not influenced by deficiencies in these genes. LC3-positive dots were co-localized with ubiquitinated aggregates, and a deficiency of Atg5 or ATG14 enhanced the accumulation of ubiquitinated aggregates as compared to the restored cells, suggesting that HCV infection induces Atg5- and ATG14-dependent CP. Moreover, LC3-positive ubiquitinated aggregates accumulated near the site of the replication complex. The researchers examined CP flux in cells replicating HCV RNA using Bafilomycin or E64d, and found that the increase in LC3 lipidation by treatment with Bafilomycin or E64d was impaired in HCV-replicating cells, suggesting that CP is inhibited by the progress of HCV infection, and that HCV RNA replication induces CP and the HCV infection impairs ATG flux.

STAT3 in Newcastle Disease Virus-induced Melanoma

Oncolytic viruses (OVs) are emerging as inducers of immunogenic cell death, releasing DAMPs that induce anticancer immunity. Oncolytic Newcastle disease virus (NDV) induces immunogenic cell death in both glioma and lung cancer cells. Shao et al. (2019) investigated whether oncolytic NDV induces ICD in melanoma cells and how it is regulated. Various time points were actuated to check the expression and release of ICD markers induced by the NDV strain, NDV/FMW, in melanoma cell lines. The expression and release of ICD markers induced by oncolytic NDV strain, NDV/FMW, in melanoma cell lines at various time points were determined. Surface-exposed calreticulin (CRT) was inspected by confocal imaging. The supernatants of NDV/FMW infected cells were collected and concentrated for the determination of ATP secretion by ELISA, HMGB1, and HSP70/90 expression by immunoblotting (IB). The pharmacological inhibition of apoptosis, ATG, necroptosis, ERS, and STAT3 was achieved by treatment with small molecule inhibitors. Melanoma cell lines depleted of STAT3 were established with lentiviral constructs. Supernatants from NDV-infected cells were injected to mice bearing melanoma cells-derived tumors. Oncolytic NDV induced CRT exposure, the release of HMGB1 and HSP70/90, as well as secretion of ATP in melanoma cells. Inhibition of apoptosis, ATG, and necroptosis or ERS attenuated the NDV/FMW-induced release of HMGB1 and HSP70/90. NDV/FMW-induced ICD markers in melanoma cells were also suppressed by either treatment with a STAT3 inhibitor or shRNA-mediated depletion of STAT3. Treatment of mice bearing melanoma cells-derived tumors with supernatants from NDV/FMW-infected cells inhibited tumor growth, confirming that oncolytic NDV/FMW might be a potent inducer of ICD in melanoma cells, which is accompanied with several forms of cell death. STAT3 played a role in NDV/FMW-induced ICD in melanoma cells, highlighting oncolytic NDV as propitious for cancer theranostics by stimulating an anti-melanoma immune response.

Innate Immune Responses in Poliomyelitis

Poliovirus (PV) is one of the most studied viruses. Because of the rare disease phenotype of paralytic poliomyelitis (PPM), Andersen et al. (2019) hypothesize that a genetic etiology may contribute to the disease course and outcome. They used whole-exome sequencing (WES) to investigate the genetic profile of 18 patients with PPM. Functional analysis was performed on PBMC and monocyte-derived macrophages (MdMs). They identified rare variants in host genes involved in interferon signaling, viral replication, apoptosis, and CP. Upon the PV infection of MdMs, a tendency toward increased viral burden in patients compared to controls was seen, suggesting the reduced control of PV infection. In MdMs from patients, the IFNβ response correlated with the viral burden, suggesting that genetic variants in innate immune defenses and cell death pathways contribute to the clinical presentation of PV infection. This study identified the genetic profile in patients with PPM combined with immune responses and viral burden in primary cells.

Ectromelia Virus and Mitochondrial Network

Mitochondria are multifunctional organelles that participate in numerous processes in response to viral infection, but they are also a target for viruses. Gregorczyk et al. (2018) defined subcellular events leading to alterations in mitochondrial morphology and function during infection with ectromelia virus (ECTV). Early on in the infection of L929 fibroblasts and RAW 264.7 macrophages, mitochondria gathered around viral factories. Later, the mitochondrial network became fragmented, forming punctate mitochondria that co-localized with the progeny virions. ECTV-co-localized mitochondria associated with the cytoskeleton components. $\Delta\Psi$, mitochondrial fission-fusion, mass, and generation of ROS were altered later in ECTV infection leading to damage of mitochondria involving CBMP, suggesting an important role of mitochondria in supplying energy for virus replication and morphogenesis. Mitochondria participate in the transport of viral particles inside and outside of the cell and/or they are a source of membranes for viral envelope formation. Hence, observed changes in the mitochondrial network organization and physiology in ECTV-infected cells may provide suitable conditions for viral replication and morphogenesis. Mitochondria are the safe haven for viral un-coating, incorporation of their genome with the mitochondrial genome, preparing coat proteins, assembly, and MDR. The viruses remain hidden in the non-dividing terminally differential cells such as neurons, cardiomyocytes, and skeletal muscles, and liver highly rich in mitochondria, and can be a part of an outbreak in response to favorable inducers and microenvironment any time later in life to cause early morbidity and mortality. The viral burden in an infected cell can be easily estimated in CBs utilizing fluorescently labeled viral specific antigen/antibody. CBs derived from the infected neuron are highly rich in viral coat proteins and their nucleic acid (DNA/RNA). Hence, the primary symptoms of any viral infection are generalized fatigue and/or cognitive impairment accompanied with learning, intelligence, memory, and behavioral disorders due to induction of viral-induced CBMP and apoptosis implicated in defective neuro-cybernetics due to CS destabilization at the neuronal synaptic terminals. In addition, viruses need lipids, proteins, carbohydrates, and nucleic acid as building blocks; those are readily available while residing in the mitochondria as compared to cytosol and nucleus because the cytosol is highly acidic and nucleus is highly basic and compact with very little space for their exponential growth and replication. Somehow, viruses escape from the deleterious effects of a mitochondrial free radical attack, which needs further investigation.

Vitamin D and Viral Infections

The pleiotropic role of vitamin D has been explored and there is epidemiological evidence for an association between poor vitamin D status and a variety of viral diseases. Teymoori-Rad et al. (2019) indicated a complex interaction between viral infections and vitamin D, including the induction of an anti-viral state, functional immune-regulatory features, inter action with cellular and viral factors, induction of CP and apoptosis, and genetic and epigenetic alterations. While crosstalk between vitamin D and intracellular signaling pathways may provide an essential modulatory effect on viral gene transcription, the immunomodulatory effect of vitamin D on viral infections is transient. The interactions between vitamin D and viral infections are presented in Table 15.

Table 15 Interactions between Vitamin D and Viral Infections

S.No	Interaction
1.	Immuno-regulation
2.	Immunomodulation
3.	Viral Gene Transcription
4.	CB Formation, Genetic & Epigenetic Alterations
5.	CP/ATG/Inflammation, Apoptosis, Necrosis
6.	Interaction with Cellular & Viral Factors
7.	Inhibition of Virus-induced CBMP

CP in Molecular Mechanisms of Bacterial Infections

Glutamine Donor

The protein cross-linking enzyme transglutaminase from Streptomyces mobaraensis (MTG) is used to modify theranostic proteins. To reveal the binding mode of glutamine donor substrates,

Juettner et al. (2018) crystallized MTG covalently linked to large inhibitory peptides. They examined peptide structures but DIPIGSKMTG, which was chloro-acetylated at serine, was the only inhibitory molecule that resulted in an interpretable density map. Besides the warhead (modified Ser6), Ile4 and Gly5 of the inhibitory peptide occupied the tight but extended hydrophobic bottom of the MTG-binding cleft. Both termini of the peptide protrude along the cleft walls perpendicular to the bottom of the extended cleft, suggesting a zipper-like cross-linking mechanism of self-assembled substrate proteins by MTG.

Basal and Starvation-Induced ATG

The precise role of CP/ATG in *P. falciparum* remains unknown. Although a limited number of ATG genes have been identified in this apicomplex, only *Pf*ATG8 has been characterized. On the basis of the expression of *Pf*ATG8 and the putative *Pf*Atg5, Joy et al. (2018) reported that the basal ATG in this parasite is robust and mediates the intra-erythrocytic development and fresh invasion of RBCs in the subsequent cycles. The basal ATG responded to both inducers and inhibitors of ATG. The parasite survival upon starvation was governed by the ATG status. Brief periods of starvation, which induce ATG, helped survival while prolonged starvation decreased ATG leading to stalled parasite growth and reduced invasion. Thus, starvation-induced ATG seems context-dependent. These investigators characterized another ATG marker in this parasite, the putative *Pf*Atg5 (*Pf*3D7_1430400), which is expressed in all the intra-erythrocytic stages and co-localizes within ER, mitochondria, apicoplast and *Pf*ATG8. It was also present on the double membrane-bound vesicles. These studies pave way for developing new theranostics as antimalarials.

N^ε-Fatty Acylation

It is known that Shigella flexneri, an intracellular Gram-negative bacterium causative for shigellosis, employs a type III secretion system to deliver virulence effectors into host cells. One such effector, IcsB, is critical for S. flexneri intracellular survival and pathogenesis. Liu et al. (2018) discovered that IcsB is an 18-carbon fatty acyltransferase catalysing lysine N^ε-fatty acylation. IcsB disrupted the actin cytoskeleton in eukaryotes, resulting from N^ε-fatty acylation of Rho-GTPases on lysine residues in their polybasic region. Chemical proteomic profiling identified ~60 additional targets modified by IcsB during infection, which were validated by biochemical assays. Most IcsB targets are membrane-associated proteins bearing a lysine-rich polybasic region, including members of the Ras, Rho, and Rab families of small GTPases. IcsB also modifies SNARE proteins and other non-GTPase substrates, suggesting an extensive interplay between S. flexneri and host membrane trafficking. The IcsB protein is localized in the vacuoles containing Shigella and is involved in the fatty acid acylation of its target molecules. Knockout of CHMP5—one of the IcsB targets and a component of the ESCRT-III complex—specifically affected *S. flexneri's* escape from host ATG. The unique N^ε-fatty acyltransferase activity of IcsB and its altering of the fatty acylation landscape of host membrane proteomes represents a mechanism in bacterial pathogenesis.

Intracellular Microbial Pathogens

The macrophages are pillars of innate immunity, responding to invading microorganisms by initiating inflammatory and antimicrobial programs. Antimicrobial responses, such as NADPH-dependent ROS, are triggered upon phagocytic receptor engagement. Macrophages also detect and respond to microbial products through pattern recognition receptors (PRRs), such as TLRs, whose signaling influences multiple biological processes including antigen presentation, cell survival, inflammation, and direct antimicrobial responses. The latter enables macrophages to combat infectious agents that persist within the intracellular environment. Stocks et al. (2018) recently summarized the current understanding of TLR-inducible antimicrobial responses that macrophages employ against bacterial pathogens, with a focus on emerging evidence linking TLR signaling to reprogramming of mitochondrial functions to enable the production of direct antimicrobial agents such as ROS and itaconic acid. In addition, they described other TLR-inducible antimicrobial pathways, including CP/ATG, modulation of nutrient availability, metal ion toxicity, RNS, immune GTPases (immunity-related GTPases and guanylate-binding proteins), and antimicrobial peptides. They also described mechanisms of evasion of such pathways by intracellular pathogens, with a focus on *Salmonella, Mycobacteria,* and *Listeria.* These investigators highlighted how TLR-inducible antimicrobial responses are regulated, and bacterial pathogens subvert such pathways, which may confer new opportunities for manipulating host defense to combat infectious diseases. Septins are cytoskeletal proteins implicated in cytokinesis and host-pathogen interactions. During the CP/ATG of *Shigella flexneri,* septins assemble into cage-like structures to entrap actin-polymerizing bacteria and restrict their dissemination. Krokowski et al. (2018) discovered that mitochondria support septin cage assembly to promote the ATG of Shigella. Consistent with roles for the cytoskeleton in mitochondrial dynamics, DNM1L/Drp-1 (dynamin 1 like) interact with septins to enhance mitochondrial fission. Shigella fragment mitochondria and escape from septin cage entrapment to avoid ATG, indicating a close relationship between mitochondria and septin assembly, and a new role of mitochondria in bacterial ATG. Septins are cytoskeletal proteins implicated in cytokinesis and host-pathogen interactions. During the CP/ATG of *Shigella flexneri,* septins assemble into cage-like structures to entrap actin-polymerizing bacteria and restrict their dissemination. These investigators discovered that mitochondria support septin cage assembly to promote the ATG of Shigella. Consistent with roles for the cytoskeleton in mitochondrial dynamics, DNM1L/Drp-1 (dynamin 1 like) can interact with septins to enhance mitochondrial fission. Shigella fragment mitochondria and escape from septin cage entrapment to avoid ATG, demonstrating a close relationship between mitochondria and septin assembly, and a new role for mitochondria in bacterial ATG. Recently, Kim et al. (2018) demonstrated that GABAergic activation enhances antimicrobial responses in intracellular bacterial infection which decreased GABA levels *in vitro* in macrophages and *in vivo* in sera. Treatment of macrophages with GABA or GABAergic drugs promoted ATG, and enhanced APS maturation and antimicrobial responses in mycobacterial infection. In macrophages, the GABAergic defense was mediated via macrophage type A GABA receptor (GABA$_A$R), [Ca^{2+}]$_i$ release, and the GABA type A receptor-associated protein-like 1 (GABARAPL1; an ATG8 homolog). Finally, GABAergic inhibition increased bacterial loads in mice and zebrafish *in vivo,* suggesting that the GABAergic defense plays an essential role in metazoan host defenses. This study identified a role for GABAergic signaling in linking antibacterial ATG to enhance host innate defense in intracellular bacterial infection. It is known that CASP4/caspase-11-dependent IS activation is important for the clearance of Gram-negative bacteria entering the host cytosol. CASP4 modulates the actin cytoskeleton to promote the maturation of phagosomes harboring intracellular pathogens such as Legionella pneumophila but not those enclosing nonpathogenic bacteria. MacroATG/ATG, a catabolic process within eukaryotic cells, is also implicated in the elimination of intracellular pathogens such as *Burkholderia cenocepacia.* Krause et al. (2018a) showed that CASP4-deficient macrophages exhibit a defect in APS formation in response to *B. cenocepacia* infection. The absence of CASP4 caused an accumulation of the small GTPase RAB7, reduced colocalization of B. cenocepacia with LC3 and acidic compartments accompanied by increased bacterial replication. These data revealed a novel role of CASP4 in regulating ATG in response to *B. cenocepacia* infection.

Phagocytic cells are the first line of innate defense against intracellular pathogens, and yet *Toxoplasma gondii* is renowned for its ability to survive in macrophages, although this paradigm is based on virulent type I parasites. Matta et al. (2018) found that avirulent type III parasites are preferentially cleared in naive macrophages, independent of IFN-γ activation. The ability of naive macrophages to clear type III parasites was dependent on enhanced activity of NADPH oxidase (Nox)-generated ROS and induction of guanylate-binding protein 5 (Gbp5). Macrophages infected with type III parasites (CTG strain) showed a time-dependent increase in ROS generation that was higher than that induced by type I parasites (GT1 strain). The absence of Nox1 or Nox2 (gp91 subunit isoforms of the Nox complex) reversed the ROS-mediated clearance of CTG parasites. Consistent with this finding, both Nox1$^{-/-}$ and Nox2$^{-/-}$ mice showed higher susceptibility to CTG infection than wild-type mice. Gbp5 expression was induced upon infection and the enhanced clearance of CTG-strain parasites was reversed in Gbp5$^{-/-}$ macrophages. Expression of a type I ROP18 allele in CTG prevented clearance in naive macrophages, suggesting that it plays a role counteracting Gbp5. Although ROS and Gbp5 have been linked to the activation of the NLRP3 IS, clearance of CTG parasites did not rely on the induction of pyroptosis. Not all strains of *T. gondii* are adept at avoiding clearance in macrophages and define new roles for ROS and Gbps in controlling this intracellular pathogen. *Toxoplasma* infections in humans and other mammals are controlled by IFN-γ produced by the activated adaptive immune system. This work identified intrinsic activities in naive macrophages in counteracting *T. gondii* infection. Using an avirulent strain of *T. gondii*, these investigators highlighted the importance of Nox complexes in conferring protection in parasite infection and also identified Gbp5 as a novel macrophage factor involved in limiting intracellular infection by avirulent strains of *T. gondii*. The rarity of human infections caused by type III strains suggested that these mechanisms may be important in controlling human toxoplasmosis. Once pathogens have breached the mechanical barriers to infection, survived extracellular immunity, and successfully invaded host cells, cell-intrinsic immunity becomes the last line of defense to protect the mammalian host against viruses, bacteria, fungi, and protozoa. Coers et al. (2018) highlighted that many cell-intrinsic defense programs act as high-precision weapons that specifically target intracellular microbes or cytoplasmic sites of microbial replication while leaving endogenous organelles unharmed. Critical executioners of cell-autonomous immunity include interferon-inducible dynamin-like GTP-ases and ATG proteins, which act in locating and antagonizing intracellular pathogens. These investigators discussed possible mechanistic models to account for the functional interactions that occur between these two distinct classes of host defense proteins.

Brucella spp. are intracellular vacuolar pathogens that causes brucellosis, a worldwide zoonosis of great importance. Pandey et al. (2018) demonstrated that the activity of host UPR sensor IRE1α (inositol-requiring enzyme 1) and ER-associated ATG confer susceptibility to *Brucella melitensis* and *Brucella abortus* intracellular replication. By employing a diverse array of molecular approaches, including biochemical analyses, fluorescence microscopy imaging, and infection assays using primary cells derived from *Ern1* (encoding IRE1) conditional knockout mice, these investigators demonstrated that a novel IRE1α to ULK1, which is an important component for ATG initiation signaling, confers susceptibility to the intracellular parasitism of *Brucella*. Deletion or inactivation of key signaling components along this axis, including IRE1α, BAK/BAX, ASK1, and JNK as well as components of the host ATG system ULK1, ATG9a, and Beclin 1, resulted in disruption of *Brucella* intracellular trafficking and replication. Host kinases in the IRE1α-ULK1 axis, including IRE1α, ASK1, JNK1, and/or AMPKα as well as ULK1, were also phosphorylated in an IRE1α-dependent fashion upon the pathogen infection, demonstrating that the IRE1α-ULK1 signaling axis is subverted by the bacterium to promote intracellular parasitism, and provide new insight into our understanding of the molecular mechanisms of intracellular lifestyle of *Brucella*.

CP in Bacterial Infections

Fecal Microbiota Transplantation

The gut microbiota plays a crucial role in human and animal health, and its disorder causes multiple diseases. Fecal microbiota transplantation (FMT) is one of the most effective ways to regulate the gut microbiota. FMT has gained increasing attention due to the success in treating the Clostridium difficile infection (CDI) and IBD. Recently, Cheng et al. (2018) investigated the effect of exogenous fecal microbiota on gut function for the analysis of the mucosal proteomes in a piglet model. They selected newborn piglets and *E. coli* K88-infected piglets to explore the interaction between host and gut microbiota following FMT. FMT triggered intestinal mucosal CP/ATG and alleviated gut barrier injury caused by *E. coli* K88, conferring a basis for the use of FMT as a bio-therapeutic method for gut microbial regulation. A total of 289 differentially expressed proteins were annotated with 4,068 gene ontology (GO) function entries in the intestinal mucosa, and the levels of CP-related proteins in the FoxO signaling pathway were increased whereas the levels of proteins related to inflammatory response were decreased in the recipient. To assess the alleviation of epithelial injury in the *E. coli* K88-infected piglets following FMT, intestinal microbiome-metabolome responses were determined. 16S rRNA gene sequencing showed that the abundances of beneficial bacteria, such as *Lactobacillus* and *Succinivibrio*, were increased whereas those of *Enterobacteriaceae* and *Proteobacteria* bacteria were decreased in the infected piglets following FMT. Metabolomic analysis revealed that levels of 58 metabolites, such as lactic acid and succinic acid, were enhanced in the intestinal lumen and that seven metabolic pathways (including the branched-chain amino acid metabolic pathways), were upregulated in the infected piglets following FMT. Metagenomics prediction analysis also demonstrated that FMT modulated the metabolic functions of gut microbiota associated with linoleic acid metabolism. Intestinal morphology was improved, which coincided with protective CP/ATG and alleviated gut barrier injury through alteration of the gut microbial structure with the decrease in intestinal permeability and the enhanced mucins and mucosal expression of tight junction proteins in the recipient, suggesting that FMT triggers intestinal mucosal CP/ATG to confer therapeutic benefit.

IRF5 for Bacterial Clearance

Common IFN regulatory factor 5 (*IRF5*) variants associated with multiple immune-mediated diseases are a major determinant of variability in pattern recognition receptor (PRR)-induced cytokines in macrophages. PRR-initiated pathways also contribute to bacterial clearance, and dysregulation of bacterial clearance can contribute to immune-mediated diseases. Hedl et al. (2019) found that IRF5 was required for bacterial clearance in PRR-stimulated, M1-differentiated human macrophages. Mechanisms regulated by IRF5 included inducing ROS through p40phox, p47phox, and p67phox, NOS2, and CP/ATG through Atg5. Complementing these pathways in IRF5-deficient M1 macrophages restored bacterial clearance. These antimicrobial pathways required the activation of IRF5-dependent MAPK, NF-κB, and Akt2 pathways. Relative to high IRF5-expressing rs2004640/rs2280714 TT/TT immune-mediated disease risk-carrier human macrophages, M1-differentiated GG/CC carrier macrophages demonstrated less ROS, NOS2, and CP/ATG pathway induction and reduced bacterial clearance. Increasing IRF5 expression to the rs2004640/rs2280714 TT/TT levels restored these antimicrobial pathways. These investigators defined mechanisms wherein common *IRF5* genetic variants modulate bacterial clearance, hence immune-mediated disease risk *IRF5* carriers might be relatively protected from microbial-associated diseases.

Genetic Variations to Chronic Q Fever

Chronic Q fever is a persistent infection, mostly of aortic aneurysms, vascular prostheses, or damaged heart valves, caused by the intracellular bacterium *Coxiella burnetii*. Only a fraction of C. burnetii-infected individuals at risk develop chronic Q fever. In these individuals, a defective innate immune response may contribute to the development of chronic Q fever. Jansen et al. (2019) assessed whether variations in genes involved in the apoptotic machinery for C. burnetii by macrophages contribute to the progression to chronic Q fever. The prevalence of 66 SNPs in 31 genes in APSS maturation, bacterial killing, and ATG was determined in 173 chronic Q fever patients and 184 controls with risk factors for chronic Q fever and serological evidence of a C. burnetii infection. Associations were detected with univariate logistic regression models. To assess the effect of these SNPs on innate responses to C. burnetii, cytokine production and the basal ROS production of healthy volunteers were determined. RAB7A (rs13081864) and P2RX7 loss-of-function SNP (rs3751143) were more common in chronic Q fever patients than in controls. RAB5A (rs8682), P2RX7 gain-of-function SNP (rs1718119), MAP1LC3A (rs1040747) and Atg5 (rs2245214) were more common in controls. In healthy volunteers, RAB7A (rs13081864) and MAP1LC3A (rs1040747) influenced the C. burnetii-induced cytokine production. RAB7A (rs13081864) modulated basal ROS production. RAB7A (rs13081864) and P2RX7 (rs3751143) are associated with the development of chronic Q fever, whereas RAB5A (rs8682), P2RX7 (rs1718119), MAP1LC3A (rs1040747), and Atg5 (rs2245214) may have theranostic benefits.

Stress Responses to Bacterial Pathogenesis

Recently, Rodrigues et al. (2018) reviewed the evidence demonstrating a role for the ISR as an integral part of the innate immune response to bacterial pathogens. They highlighted that activation of an appropriate innate immune response to bacterial infection is critical to limit microbial spread and generate cytokines and chemokines to instruct appropriate adaptive immune responses. Recognition of bacteria or bacterial products by pattern recognition molecules is crucial to initiate this response. However, the context in which this recognition occurs can dictate the quality of the response and determine the outcome of an infection. The crosstalk established between host and pathogen results in profound alterations in cellular homeostasis, triggering specific cellular stress responses. Particularly, the highly conserved integrated stress response (ISR) shape the host's response to bacterial pathogens by sensing cellular insults resulting from infection and modulating the transcription of key genes, translation of new proteins, and cell autonomous antimicrobial mechanisms such as ATG.

Porphyromonas Gingivalis

Porphyromonas gingivalis, an opportunistic pathogen usurps gingival epithelial cells (GECs) for its colonization in the oral mucosa. Lee et al. (2018b) employed high-resolution 3D-TEM to determine the subcellular location of P. gingivalis in human primary GECs upon invasion. Serial sections of infected-GECs and their tomographic reconstruction depicted ER-rich-double-membrane APS-vacuoles harboring P. gingivalis. P. gingivalis induces LC3-lipidation in a time-dependent-manner and co-localizes with LC3, ER-lumen-protein Bip, or ER-tracker, which are major components of the phagophore membrane. GECs that were infected with FMN-green-fluorescent transformant-strain (PgFbFP) and selectively permeabilized by Digitonin showed large numbers of double-membrane-vacuolar-P. gingivalis over 24 hrs of infection with a low-ratio of cytosolic free-bacteria. Inhibition of ATG using 3-MA or Atg5 siRNA reduced the viability of intracellular P. gingivalis in GECs as determined by an antibiotic-protection assay. The lysosomal marker, LAMP-1, showed a low-degree co-localization with P. gingivalis (~20%). PgFbFP was used to investigate the fate of vacuolar- versus cytosolic-P. gingivalis by their association with ubiquitin-binding-adaptor-proteins, NDP52 and p62. Only cytosolic-P. gingivalis had a significant association with both markers, suggesting that cytosolically-free bacteria are involved in the lysosomal-degradation pathway whereas the vacuolar-P. gingivalis survives. These results revealed a novel mechanism for P. gingivalis's survival in GECs by the harnessing of host ATG machinery to establish a replicative niche and persistence in the oral mucosa.

β_2 Integrin Mac-1

Gluschko et al. (2018) demonstrate that Listeria monocytogen (L.m) infection of macrophages *in vivo* evokes LC3-associated phagocytosis (LAP), but not canonical ATG, and that targeting of L.m. by LAP is required for anti-listerial immunity. The pathway leading to LAP induction in response to a L.m. infection emanates from the β_2 integrin Mac-1 (CR3, integrin $\alpha_M\beta_2$), a receptor recognizing diverse microbial ligands. Interaction of L.m. with Mac-1 induces acid sphingomyelinase-mediated changes in the membrane lipid composition, which facilitates the assembly and activation of the phagocyte NAPDH oxidase Nox2. Nox2-derived ROS then triggers LC3's recruitment to L.m.-containing phagosomes by LAP. By promoting the fusion of L.m.-containing phagosomes with lysosomes, LAP increases the exposure of L.m. to bactericidal acid hydrolases, thereby enhancing the anti-listerial activity of macrophages and immunity of mice.

Streptomyces Metabolite

In cervical cancer, the association between HPV infection and dysregulation of the PI3K/Akt/mTOR pathway places mTOR as an attractive theranostic target. The failure of the current treatment in advanced stages of this cancer and drawbacks of the available mTOR inhibitors have increased the demand for novel drug candidates. Recently, Dan et al. (2018) identified the presence of an mTOR inhibitor Streptomycin ethyl acetate fraction-4 (SEA-4) in an active fraction of the ethyl acetate extract of Streptomyces sp OA293. The metabolites in the active fraction completely inhibited mTORC1 and suppressed the activation of both of its downstream targets, 4E-BP1 and P70S6k, in *cervical* cancer cells. It also suppressed the Akt activation via inhibition of mTORC2. The mechanism of mTOR inhibition overcomes the drawbacks of mTOR inhibitors such as Rapamycin and Rapalogs. The active fraction induced ATG and Bax-mediated apoptosis, suggesting that mTOR inhibition resulted in the apoptosis of cancer cells. The molecular weight determination of the components in the active fraction confirmed the absence of any previously known natural mTOR inhibitor.

Epithelial Mitochondrial Function and IL-8

The uncoupling of O/P in epithelial mitochondria results in decreased epithelial barrier function as characterized by increased internalization of non-invasive *E. coli* and their translocation across the intestinal epithelium. Saxena et al. (2018) hypothesized that the increased burden of intracellular commensal bacteria would activate the enterocyte to promote inflammation. The treatment of human colon-derived epithelial cell lines with Dinitrophenol (DNP) and commensal *E. coli* (strains F18, HB101) provoked the increased production of IL-8, which was not observed with conditioned medium derived from bacteria, LPS, or inert beads. The IL-8 response was inhibited by co-treatment with Cytochalasin-D (which blocks F-actin rearrangement), CQ (which blocks phagosome acidification), and a MyD88 inhibitor (which blocks TLR signaling), consistent with TLR-signaling mediating IL-8 synthesis subsequent to bacterial internalization. Use of the mitochondrial-targeted antioxidant, mitoTEMPO, or U0126 to block ERK1/2 MAPK signaling inhibited DNP + *E. coli*-evoked IL-8 production. Mutations in the NOD2 (the intracellular sensor of bacteria) or ATG16L1 (ATG protein) genes are susceptibility traits for Crohn's, and epithelia lacking either protein displayed enhanced IL-8 production in comparison to wild-type cells when exposed to DNP + *E coli*. Thus, metabolic stress perturbs the normal epithelial-bacterial interaction, resulting in increased IL-8 production due to the uptake of bacteria into the enterocyte: this pro-inflammatory event is enhanced in cells lacking NOD2 or ATG16L1 that favor the increased survival of bacteria within the enterocyte. By increasing epithelial permeability and IL-8 production, reduced mitochondrial function in the enteric epithelium contributes to the initiation, pathophysiology, and reactivation of the inflammatory disease in the gut via CP dysregulation and CBMP induction.

Bacillus subtilis Lipopeptides

The lipopeptide iturin from Bacillus subtilis has a potential inhibitory effect on BC, alveolar adenocarcinoma, renal carcinoma, and colon adenocarcinoma. Zhao et al. (2018) evaluated the potential of B. subtilis lipopeptides (a mixture of iturin homologues, concentration of 42.75%) to inhibit chronic myelogenous leukemia (CML) using K562 myelogenous leukemia cells. The lipopeptides could inhibit the growth of K562. The lipopeptides inhibited the profile of K562 via three pathways: (1) induction of paraptosis indicated by the occurrence of cytoplasmic vacuoles, and swelling of the mitochondria and ER without membrane blebbing in the presence of a caspase inhibitor; (2) inhibition of ATG illustrated by the upregulated expression of LCII and p62; and (3) induction of apoptosis by causing ROS burst, and induction of the intrinsic pathway indicated by the upregulated expression of Cyt-C, bax, and bad, together with downregulated Bcl-2 expression. The ROS-dependent apoptosis and caspase-independent paraptosis were verified using the ROS inhibitor and caspase inhibitor, respectively. The extrinsic apoptosis pathway was not involved in the lipo-peptide's effects on K562. The B. subtilis lipo-peptides (consisting of a majority of iturin) exhibited potential in inhibiting CML *in vitro* via paraptosis, apoptosis, and the inhibition of ATG.

Pyoverdine from Pseudomonas Aeruginosa

Pseudomonas aeruginosa, a re-emerging, opportunistic human pathogen, encodes a variety of virulence determinants. Pyoverdine, a siderophore produced by this bacterium, is essential for pathogenesis in mammalian infections due to its roles in acquiring iron and/or regulating other virulence factors. Kang et al. (2018) reported that pyoverdine translocates into the host, where it binds and extracts iron. Pyoverdine-mediated iron-extraction-damaged host mitochondria, disrupting their function and triggering mitochondrial turnover via ATG. The host detects this damage via a conserved mitochondrial surveillance pathway mediated by the ESRE network.

(+)-Spectaline and Iso-6-Spectaline

Lim et al. (2018), while searching for new trypanocidal lead compounds from Malaysian plants, two known piperidine alkaloids (1) (+)-spectaline and (2) iso-6-spectaline were isolated from the leaves of Senna spectabilis (sin. Cassia spectabilis). Analysis of the ^{1}H and ^{13}C NMR spectra showed that Compound 1 and Compound 2 presented analytical and spectroscopic data in full agreement with those published in the literature. Both the compounds were screened *in vitro* against Trypanosoma brucei rhodesiense in comparison to the standard drug Pentamidine. Both, Compound 1 and 2 inhibited the growth of T. b. rhodesiense without a toxic effect on L6 cells. These data showed that piperidine alkaloids constitute a class of natural products that feature a broad spectrum of biological activities, and are potential templates for the development of new trypanocidal drugs. These compounds had inhibitory effects on T. b. rhodesiense. The ultrastructural alterations in the trypanosome induced by Compounds 1 and 2, leading to apoptosis, were characterized using TEM. These alterations included wrinkling of the trypanosome surface, formation of ATG vacuoles, disorganization of kinetoplast, and swelling of the mitochondria, suggested CP/ATG-mediated cell death.

CP/ATG in Mussels Infections

Balbi et al. (2018) reported that in invertebrates that lack acquired immunity, ATG may play a crucial role in the protection against potential pathogens. In aquatic molluscs, evidence has been provided for the induction of ATG by starvation and different environmental stressors; however, no information is available on ATG in the hemocytes of the marine bivalve, the mussel Mytilus galloprovincialis. The effects of classical inducers/inhibitors of mammalian ATG were first tested. Rapamycin induced a decrease in lysosomal membrane stability-LMS that was prevented by the ATG inhibitor, Wortmannin. Increased MDC fluorescence and expression of LC3-II were also observed. Cellular responses to *in vitro* challenge with the bivalve pathogen Vibrio tapetis were evaluated. Mussel hemocytes activated the immune response towards V. tapetis. However, the bacterial challenge induced a moderate decrease in LMS, corresponding to lysosomal activation but no cytotoxicity; this effect was prevented by Wortmannin. V. tapetis resulted in rapid formation of APS and autolysosomes. Increased LC3-II expression and decreased levels of phosphorylated mTor and of p62 were observed, demonstrating CP/ATG in bivalve hemocytes in response to bacterial challenge, as a protective mechanism against pathogenic vibrios.

Immunopathology in Acute Infection

The mechanisms protecting from immunopathology during acute bacterial infections are not properly known yet. In response to apoptotic immune cells and live or dead L.m scavenger receptor BI (SR-BI), an anti-atherogenic lipid exchange mediator, activated internalization mechanisms with characteristics of macro-pinocytosis assisted by Golgi fragmentation induce ATG. This was supported by scavenger receptor-induced local increases in membrane cholesterol which generated lipid domains in cell extensions and the Golgi. SR-BI is a key driver of Beclin-1-dependent ATG during an acute bacterial infection of the liver and spleen. ATG-regulated tissue infiltration of neutrophils suppressed the accumulation of Ly6C$^+$ (inflammatory) macrophages, and prevented hepatocyte necrosis in the core of infectious foci. Peri-focal levels of Ly6C$^+$ macrophages and Ly6C$^-$ macrophages were unaffected, indicating predominant regulation of the focus core. SR-BI-triggered ATG promoted co-elimination of apoptotic immune cells and dead bacteria but barely influenced bacterial sequestration and survival or IS activation, thus exclusively counteracting damage inflicted by immune responses. Hence, SR-BI- and ATG promoted a surveillance pathway that partially responded to products of antimicrobial defenses and selectively prevented immunity-induced damage during an acute infection, suggesting that control of infection-associated immunopathology can be based on a unified defense operation.

CP in LM Theranostics

Leishmaniasis are infectious diseases caused by protozoa of the Leishmania (LM) genus. Its treatment presents high toxicity, long-term administration, many adverse effects, and is expensive, besides the risk of resistant parasites. Neutrophils, the essential components of the innate immune system, are recruited in large numbers to the pathogen site of entry. Several pathogens induce neutrophil ATG; however, its functional significance during LM parasite infection remain unknown. Pitale et al. (2019) reported a finding of how LM-induced human poly-morpho-nuclear neutrophil (hPMN) ATG regulates the silent mode of parasite transfer to macrophages by influencing the engulfment of infected cells. An LM infection induced a time-dependent ATG response which was blocked by 3-MA, but was sensitive to ULK1/2 inhibition only after 3 hrs, suggesting that canonical ATG is induced during later hrs, ULK1/2 inhibition blocked only canonical ATG. The interaction of Rubicon and Beclin-1 at 1 hr post-infection affirmed the prevalence of noncanonical ATG during early infection. There was a reduction in the macrophage uptake of parasite-exposed hPMNs treated with 3-MA or ULK1/2 inhibitor, suggesting the involvement of ATG in neutrophils. The ATG inducer, Rapamycin, augmented neutrophil engulfment by macrophages. The redistribution of hPMN surface CD47 enhanced neutrophil uptake. Activation of ERK, PI3-kinase, and NADPH oxidase-mediated ROS generation were induced after parasite binding. The *lpgl*-knockout parasites expressing defective lipo-phosphoglycan did not induce ATG, indicating that lipophosphogly is necessary for interaction with the neutrophils. ATG induction was TLR2/4-independent because the receptor blockade did not interfere with infection-induced ATG. The engulfment of neutrophils by the macrophages was influenced by the escalation of hPMN-ATG, which is an important event during a LM infection. Currently, there is no satisfactory treatment for LM, owing to the cost, mode of administration, side effects, and increasing MDR. As a consequence, the proteins involved in LM apoptosis seem a target of choice for the development of new therapeutic tools against these tropical diseases. LM cell death, while similar to mammalian apoptosis, involves no homologue of the key mammalian apoptotic proteins such as caspases and death receptors. Basmaciyan et al. (2019) identified a protein involved in LM apoptosis from a library of genes overexpressed during its differentiation when ATG occurs. The gene was overexpressed when L. major cell death was induced by Curcumin or Miltefosine. Its overexpression increased L. major Curcumin-and Miltefosine-induced apoptosis. This gene, named LmjF.22.0600, whose expression is dependent on the expression of the metacaspase, another apoptotic protein, encodes acetyltransferase. This new protein, involved in LM apoptosis, may contribute to a better understanding of LM death, owing to the absence of a satisfactory treatment in LM. It will also allow for a better understanding of the original apoptotic pathways of eukaryotes in general.

Among different LM infections, visceral LM if not treated is the most severe form with high mortality rates. In India, it is caused by the protozoan LM donovani. The therapy of visceral LM is limited due to high toxicity, resistance to existing drugs, and increasing cases of LM co-infections. Hence, there is a need to identify novel drug and targets to overcome these hindrances. miRNAs are a class of small non-coding RNAs (~22–24 nucleotide in length) that regulate gene expression in various biological processes and play the role of intracellular mediators, which are essential for different biological processes. Singh and Chauhan (2018) explored the impact of the anti-LM role of trans-dibenzalacetone (*DBA,* a synthetic monoketone analog of Curcumin) on the expression profile of miRNA in intracellular amastigotes of LM donovani. Small RNA libraries of samples (macrophages-infected with LM amastigotes; and infected macrophages treated with DBA) were prepared by using a Illumina Trueseq Small RNA kit. Using the miRDIP database, they identified the target gene of differentially expressed miRNAs (target miRNAs: hsa-mir-15b, hsa-mir-671, hsa-mir-151a, and has-mir-30c), which was confirmed by real time stem-loop PCR. Ten KEGG pathways were enriched with these target miRNA genes and related to the MAPK pathway. These investigators established the anti-proliferative and apoptotic effect of trans-dibenzalacetone on the LM donovani parasites. By using the GFP-ATG8 gene as a marker for tracking APS, the researchers confirmed that vacuolization may lead to ATG cell death in the DBA-treated parasites, indicating that Curcumin analog DBA regulated the balance between ATG and apoptosis and triggered imbalance between two known phenotypes of cell death viz CP/ATG and apoptosis.

Calixto et al. (2018) evaluated the anti-LM activity of *quinoline derivative salts* (QDS), toxicity on mammalian cells, and the mechanism of action. Only the compound QDS3 showed activity against promastigotes and amastigotes of LM spp., being more active against the intracellular amastigotes of LM-GFP. This value was very close to the one observed for Miltefosine, used as a control drug. The compound QDS3 exhibited a selective effect, being 40.35 times more toxic to the amastigote form than to the host cell. Promastigotes of LM treated with this compound exhibited characteristics of apoptosis represented by mitochondrial membrane depolarization, mitochondrial swelling, ROS overproduction, PS externalization, reduced and rounded shape, and cell cycle alteration. The integrity of the plasma membrane remained unaltered, excluding necrosis in treated promastigotes. The compound QDS3 inhibited the formation of ATG vacuoles, which may have contributed to parasite death by preventing ATG mechanisms in the removal of damaged organelles, intensifying the damage caused by the treatment, and thus, highlighting the anti-LM effect of this compound. Treatment with QDS3 induced increased ROS levels in LM-infected macrophages, but not in the uninfected host cell, suggesting that the induction of oxidative stress is one of the main toxic effects caused by the treatment with the compound QDS3 in LM, causing irreversible damage and triggering a selective death of intracellular parasites, thus, confirming the biological activity of quinoline derivatives.

Cavalcanti de Queiroz et al. (2019) investigated the anti-LM activity of synthetic compounds, containing a semicarbazone scaffold as a peptide mimetic framework. The anti-LM effect against amastigotes of LM amazonensis was also evaluated at concentration of 100 µM–0.01 nM. The derivatives 2e, 2f, 2g, and 1g, beyond the standard Miltefosine and Pentamidine, diminished the number of LM amastigotes in macrophages which were also active against amastigotes of LM. As 2g presented potent anti-LM activity against the amastigotes of LM in macrophages, they also investigated the anti-LM activity of this compound against LM. Approximately 10^5 LM promastigotes were inoculated s.c. into the dermis of the right ear of BALB/c mice, which were treated with 2g (p.o. or i.p.), Miltefosine (p.o.) or Glucantime (i.p.) at 30 µmol/kg/day × 28 days. A similar reduction in the lesion size was observed after the administration of 2g through oral and i.p. routes. A larger effect was observed after treatment with Miltefosine, and Glucantime did not exhibit activity after the dose was administered. With respect to the ear parasite load, 2g diminished the number of parasites by p.o. and i.p. administration. In addition, 2g induced *in vitro* apoptosis, ATG, and cell-cycle alterations in LM promastigotes, suggesting that the derivative 2g might represent a lead candidate for anti-LM drugs.

CP in Trypanosoma Theranostics

Jabłoński et al. (2017) reported the synthesis of four cymantrene-5-fluorouracil derivatives (1–4) and two cymantrene-adenine derivatives (5 and 6). All these compounds were characterized by spectroscopic analysis and the crystal structure of two derivatives (1 and 6), together with the cymantrene-adenine compound C, which was determined by X-ray crystallography. While the compounds 1 and 6 crystallized in the triclinic P-1 space group, compound C crystallized in the monoclinic $P2_1/m$ space group. The newly-synthesized compounds 1–6 were tested together with the two previously described cymantrene derivatives B and C to guage their *in vitro* anti-proliferative activity against seven cancer cell lines (MCF-7, MCF-7/DX, MDA-MB-231, SKOV-3, A549, HepG2m, and U-87-MG), five bacterial strains *Staphylococcus aureus* (methicillin-sensitive, methicillin-resistant, and vancomycin-intermediate strains), *Staphylococcus epidermidis*, and *Escherichia coli*, including clinical isolates of *S. aureus* and *S. epidermidis*, as well as against the protozoan parasite *Trypanosoma brucei*. The most cytotoxic compounds were derivatives 2 and C for A549 and SKOV-3 cancer cell lines, respectively, with IC_{50} values of about 7 µM. The anticancer activity of the cymantrene compounds was determined to be due to their ability to induce oxidative stress and to trigger ATG and apoptosis in cancer cells. Three derivatives (1, 4, and 5) displayed anti-trypanosomal activity, with GI_{50} values at 3–4 µM. The introduction of the 5-Fluorouracil moiety in 1 enhanced the trypanocidal activity when compared to the activity previously reported for the corresponding uracil derivative. The antibacterial activity of cymantrene compounds 1 and C was within the range of 8–64 μg/mL and seemed to be the result of induced cell shrinking.

CP in Toxoplasma Infection

Toxoplasma gondii is a ubiquitous pathogen that can cause encephalitis, congenital defects, and ocular disease. *T. gondii* has also been implicated as a risk factor for mental illness in humans. *Toxoplasma gondii*, the etiological agent of toxoplasmosis, infects nucleated cells and then resides and multiplies within a parasitophorous vacuole. The parasite secretes virulence factors for invading and subverting the host microbicidal defenses to facilitate its survival in the intracellular milieu. The parasite persists in the brain as slow-growing bradyzoites contained within intracellular cysts. No treatments exist to eliminate this form of parasite. Although proteolytic degradation within the parasite lysosome-like vacuolar compartment (VAC) is critical for bradyzoite viability, whether other aspects of the VAC are important for parasite persistence remains unknown. An ortholog of *Plasmodium falciparum* CQ resistance transporter (CRT), TgCRT, has been identified in *T. gondii*. To determine the function of TgCRT in chronic-stage bradyzoites and its role in persistence, Kannan et al. (2019) knocked out TgCRT in a cystogenic strain and assessed VAC size, VAC digestion of host-derived proteins and parasite APS, and the viability of *in vitro* and *in vivo* bradyzoites. Whereas parasites deficient in TgCRT exhibited normal digestion within the VAC, they displayed distended VAC and their viability was compromised. Impairing VAC proteolysis in TgCRT-deficient bradyzoites restored VAC size, consistent with the role of TgCRT as a transporter of products of digestion from the VAC. These findings suggested a functional link between TgCRT and VAC proteolysis. This study provided further evidence of a crucial role for the VAC in bradyzoite persistence and a new potential VAC target to abate a chronic *Toxoplasma* infection. Individuals chronically infected with the *Toxoplasma gondii* are at increased risk of experiencing a reactivated disease that can result in a progressive loss of vision. A study showed that a *T. gondii* transporter is linked to protein digestion within the parasite lysosome-like organelle and that this transporter is necessary to sustain chronic infection in culture and in infected mice. Ablating the transporter resulted in severe bloating of the lysosome-like organelle, suggesting that this organelle is vital for parasite survival, thus rendering it a potential target for diminishing infection and reducing the risk of reactivated disease. Essential metals are structural components of proteins and enzymes or cofactors of enzymatic reactions responsible for these parasitic survival mechanisms. However, an excess of non-essential or essential metals can lead to parasite death. de Carvalho and de Melo (2018) incubated infected host cells with 20 μM $ZnCl_2$ in conjunction with 3 μM $CdCl_2$ or $HgCl_2$ for 12 hrs to investigate cellular events and organelle damage related to parasite death and elimination. In the presence of these metals, the tachyzoites experienced lipid uptake and transport impairment, functional and structural mitochondrial disorders, DNA condensation, and acidification of the parasitophorous vacuole, thus leading to their death. The lysosome-vacuole fusion was involved in parasite elimination since acid phosphatases were found inside the parasitophorous vacuole, and vacuoles containing parasites were also positive for CP/ATG, indicating that low concentrations of $CdCl_2$, $HgCl_2$, and $ZnCl_2$ can cause damage to *Toxoplasma gondii* organelles, leading to a loss of viability, organelle death, elimination of the microorganism *Toxoplasma gondii* without causing toxic effects to the host cells. Pernas (2018) showed that fatty acid uptake of the intracelllar parasite *Toxoplasma gondii* was inhibited by their fusion with the host mitochondria. A combination of genetics and imaging of FA trafficking indicated that Toxoplasma infection triggers lipophagy, the ATG of host LDs, to secure cellular FAs essential for its proliferation. Fatty acid siphoning and growth of Toxoplasma were reduced in the host cells those were genetically-deficient for ATG or trigylceride depots. Toxoplasma FA uptake and proliferation are increased in host cells lacking mitochondrial fusion, which is required for efficient mitochondrial FA oxidation, or where mitochondrial FA oxidation is pharmacologically inhibited. Thus, mitochondrial fusion involving CB formation can be regarded as a cellular defense mechanism against intracellular parasites, by limiting Toxoplasma access to host nutrients liberated by lipophagy.

CP in Cystic Fibrosis

Cystic fibrosis (CF) is a multi-organ disorder characterized by chronic sino-pulmonary infections and inflammation. Many patients with CF suffer from repeated pulmonary exacerbations that are predictors of worsened long-term morbidity and mortality. There are no reliable markers that associate with the onset or progression of an exacerbation or pulmonary deterioration. Thymosin-α-1 (Tα1) is a naturally occurring polypeptide of 28 amino acids, whose mechanism of action is related to its ability to signal through innate immune receptors. Stincardini et al. (2018) reported that Tα1 (ZADAXIN®) is used for treating viral infections, immune-deficiencies, and malignancies. Owing to its ability to activate the tolerogenic pathway of tryptophan catabolism via the immune-regulatory enzyme indoleamine 2,3-dioxygenase, Tα1 potentiates immune tolerance mechanisms, breaking the vicious circle that perpetuates chronic inflammation in response to a variety of infectious noxae. Tα1 has never been studied in cystic fibrosis (CF) in which the hyper-inflammatory state is associated with early and non-resolving activation of innate immunity, which impairs microbial clearance and promotes a self-sustaining condition of progressive lung damage. Optimal CF treatments should rescue CF transmembrane conductance regulator protein localization and functionality and alleviate the associated hyper-inflammatory pathology. Because of the complexity of the pathogenetic mechanisms, a multidrug approach is required. By providing an attack against CF, that is, by restraining inflammation and correcting the basic defect, Tα1 opposed CF symptomatology in preclinical relevant disease settings, suggesting its possible exploitation for 'real-life' clinical efficacy in CF. This could represent a major advance in the CF field, namely a drug with the unique activity to correct CFTR defects through regulation of inflammation. Krause et al. (2018b) found that the Mirc1/Mir17-92a cluster, which is comprised of six microRNAs (Mirs), is highly expressed in CF mice and negatively regulates CP/ATG to improve CF transmembrane conductance regulator (CFTR) function. They examined the expression of individual Mirs within the Mirc1/Mir17-92 cluster in human cells and biological fluids and determined their role as biomarkers of pulmonary exacerbations and response to treatment. Mirc1/Mir17-92 cluster expression was measured in human CF and non-CF plasma, blood-derived neutrophils, and sputum samples. Values were correlated with pulmonary function, exacerbations, and use of CFTR modulators. The Mirc1/Mir17-92 cluster expression was not significantly elevated in CF neutrophils nor plasma when compared to the non-CF cohort. The Cluster expression in CF sputum was higher than its expression in plasma. Elevated CF sputum Mirc1/Mir17-92 cluster expression positively correlated with pulmonary exacerbations and negatively correlated with lung function. Patients with CF undergoing treatment with the CFTR modulator Ivacaftor/Lumacaftor did not demonstrate a significant change in the expression of the Mirc1/Mir17-92 cluster after six months of treatment, indicating that Mirc1/Mir17-92 cluster expression was a promising biomarker of respiratory status in patients with CF including pulmonary exacerbation.

　　Skeletal muscle function is compromised in many illnesses, including chronic infections. The *Pseudomonas aeruginosa* quorum sensing (QS) signal, 2-amino acetophenone (2-AA), is produced during acute and chronic infections and excreted in human tissues, including the lungs of CF patients. Bandyopadhaya et al. (2019) showed that 2-AA facilitates pathogen persistence, via its ability to promote the formation of bacterial per-sister cells, and that it acts as an immunomodulatory signal that epigenetically reprograms innate immune functions. Moreover, 2-AA compromises muscle contractility and impacts the expression of genes involved in ROS homeostasis in skeletal muscle and in mitochondrial functions. They elucidated the molecular mechanisms of 2-AA's impairment of skeletal muscle function and ROS homeostasis. Murine *in vivo* and differentiated C2C12 myotube cells showed that 2-AA promotes ROS generation via the modulation of xanthine oxidase (XO) activity, NAD(P)H oxidase2 (NOX2) protein level, and the activity of antioxidant enzymes. ROS accumulation triggers the activity of AMPK, upstream of the observed locations of induction of ubiquitin ligases *Muscle RING Finger 1 (MuRF1)* and *Muscle Atrophy F-box (MAFbx),* and induces ATG-related proteins. The perturbation in SIRT1, PGC-1, and UCP3 was rescued by the antioxidant NAC. These results unveiled a novel form of action of a QS bacterial molecule and provided insights into the 2-AA-mediated skeletal muscle dysfunction caused by *P. aeruginosa*, a bacterium that is resistant to treatment, causing serious acute, persistent, and relapsing infections in humans. Bacterial-excreted small molecules play a critical role during infection. A quorum-sensing (QS)-regulated excreted small molecule, 2-AA, produced by *P. aeruginosa*, promotes persistent infections, dampens host inflammation, and triggers mitochondrial dysfunction in skeletal muscle implicated in CBMP. QS is a cell-to-cell communication system utilized by bacteria to promote collective behaviors. The significance of this study in identifying a mechanism that leads to skeletal muscle dysfunction, via the action of a QS molecule, is that it may open new avenues in the control of muscle loss as a result of infection and sepsis. Given that QS is a common characteristic of prokaryotes, 2-AA-like molecules promoting similar effects may exist in other pathogens.

CP in Fungal Infections

Tanabe and Nagi (2018) described methods to monitor MTG in the pathogenic yeast Candida under iron-depleted conditions but not under nitrogen starvation, which may provide clues to elucidate the physiological roles of MTG in eukaryotes. Methods for detection of MTG have been reported for several fungal cells, including budding yeast, methylotrophic yeast, and filamentous fungi. MTG in yeast is activated under nitrogen-poor conditions; however, the regulatory mechanism of MTG as well as CP/ATG in most fungi remains to be elucidated. Transporters are transmembrane proteins that mediate the selective translocation of solutes, ions, or drugs across biological membranes. Their function is related to cell nutrition, communication, stress resistance, and homeostasis. Their malfunction is associated with genetic or metabolic diseases and drug sensitivity or resistance. A characteristic of transporters is their translocation and folding in a membrane bilayer: this being the ER in eukaryotes or the cell membrane in prokaryotes. In the former case, transporters exit the ER packed in secretory vesicles and traffic via unconventional, rather than Golgi-dependent, sorting routes to their final destination, the plasma membrane (PM). Proper folding is a prerequisite for ER exit and further trafficking. Misfolded transporters, either due to mutations or high temperature of chemical agents (for example, DMSO, DTT) are blocked in the ER. The accumulation of ER-retained transporters elicits ER-associated degradation, but also ubiquitination-dependent, chaperone-mediated CP. The function of PM transporters is regulated at the cellular level, in response to physiological or stress signals that promote, via α-arrestin-assisted ubiquitination, their endocytosis and vacuolar/lysosomal degradation, and in some cases recycling to the PM. Transporter oligomerization and specific interactions with membrane lipids are important players in transporter expression, function, and turnover.

CP in Amoebic Infections

The soil-dwelling social amoeba *Dictyostelium discoideum* feeds on bacteria. Each meal is a potential source of infection because some bacteria have evolved mechanisms to resist predation. To survive such a hostile environment, *D. discoideum* has evolved efficient antimicrobial responses that are intertwined with phagocytosis and CP/ATG, its nutrient acquisition pathways. The core machinery and antimicrobial functions of these pathways are conserved in the mononuclear phagocytes of mammals, which mediate the initial, innate-immune response to infection. Recently, Dunn et al. (2018) discussed the relevance of *D. discoideum* as a model phagocyte to study cell-autonomous defenses. They covered the antimicrobial functions of phagocytosis and CP/ATG and described the processes that create a microbicidal phagosome: acidification and delivery of lytic enzymes, generation of ROS, and the regulation of Zn^{2+}, Cu^{2+}, and Fe^{2+} availability. High concentrations of metals poisoned microbes while metal sequestration inhibited their metabolic activity. They also described microbial interference with these defenses and highlighted observations made in *D. discoideum*. Finally, they discussed galectins, TNF receptor-associated factors, tripartite motif-containing proteins, and STATs (microbial restriction factors characterized in mammalian phagocytes) that have either homologs or functional analogs in *D. discoideum*.

CP in Plant Infections

In animals, the contribution of ATG and the UPS to antibacterial immunity is well documented and several bacteria have evolved measures to target and exploit these systems to the benefit of the infection. In plants, the UPS has been established as a hub for immune responses and is targeted by bacteria to enhance virulence. Recently, Wang et al. (2018) investigated the ATG-mediated plant defense responses against Verticillium dahliae (V. dahliae) infection by comparative proteomics and cellular analyses. An assessment of the ATG activity and disease development showed that the CP/ATG processes were related to the tolerance of the Arabidopsis plant to Verticillium wilt. An isobaric tag for relative and absolute quantification (iTRAQ)-based proteomics analysis was performed. A total of 780 differentially accumulated proteins (DAPs) between wild-type and mutant atg10-1 Arabidopsis plants upon V. dahliae infection were identified, of which, 193 ATG8-family-interacting proteins were identified *in silico* and their associations with ATG were verified for selected proteins. Three important aspects of ATG-mediated defense against V. dahliae infection were revealed: 1) CP/ATG was required for the activation of upstream defense responses; 2) CP/ATG-mediated mitochondrial degradation (CP) occurred and was an important player in the defense process; and 3) CP/ATG promoted the differentiation of perivascular cells and the formation of xylem hyperplasia, crucial for protection in this vascular disease, suggesting the functional association between CP/ATG and plant immune responses. CP/ATG and the ubiquitin-proteasome system (UPS) are major proteolytic pathways that are recognized as battlegrounds during host-microbe interactions in eukaryotes. In plants, the UPS has emerged as a central component of innate immunity and is manipulated by bacterial pathogens to enhance virulence. CP/ATG has been ascribed a similar importance for anti-bacterial immunity in animals, but the contribution of ATG to host-bacteria interactions remains enigmatic in plants. Recently, Üstün et al. (2018a) identified both pro-and antibacterial functions of ATG upon infection of *Arabidopsis thaliana* with virulent *Pseudomonas syringae* pv *tomato* DC3000 (*Pst*). *Pst* activated ATG in a type III effector (T3E)-dependent manner and stimulated the autophagic removal of proteasomes (*proteaphagy*) to support bacterial proliferation. The T3E Hrp outer protein M1 (HopM1) was identified as a principle mediator of ATG-inducing activities during infection. In contrast to the probacterial effects of

Pst-induced *proteaphagy*, neighbor of BRCA1-dependent CP counteracts disease progression and limits the formation of HopM1-mediated water-soaked lesions, indicating that distinct CP/ATG pathways contribute to host immunity and bacterial pathogenesis during *Pst* infection and there exists a crosstalk between proteasome and CP/ATG in plant-bacterial interactions. Furthermore, Üstün et al. (2018b) revealed anti- and pro-bacterial roles of ATG pathways during bacterial infection in the plant *Arabidopsis thaliana.* Selective ATG mediated by the ATG cargo receptor AT4G24690/NBR1 limits growth of Pseudomonas syringae pv. Tomato DC3000 (Pst) by suppressing the establishment of an aqueous extracellular space ('water-soaking'). In turn, Pseudomonas employed the effector protein HopM1 to activate ATG and proteasome degradation (*proteaphagy*), thereby enhancing its pathogenicity, demonstrating that distinct selective CP/ATG pathways contribute to host immunity and bacterial pathogenesis during a *Pst* infection and provided evidence for an association between the proteasome and CP/ATG system in plant-bacterial interactions.

CONCLUSION

This chapter systematically describes the molecular pathology of various microbial (viral, bacterial, fugal, and parasitic) infections (including COVID-19) and the clinical significance of mitochondrially-targeted CP/ATG for the development of targeted, safe and effective vaccines and therapeutics for human health, BQL, and control pandemics. CP/ATG is a multi-purpose connection between microbial infections and host cells. Various checks and balances between CP/ATG and IS have been identified during microbial infections. CB formation followed by CP induction prevents the dissemination of toxic microbial as well as degenerated mitochondrial metabolites of an infected cell to sustain IMD, ICD, and MQC for NCF, as a mechanism of minimizing the deleterious effect of microbial infections which cause intracellular invasion such as, CMV, Rubella, HIV, Ebola, Zika, Corona, Influenza, Plasmodium, Toxoplasma, and Mycobacteria. Viral strategies for triggering and manipulating CP/ATG have been proposed. HIV type-1 gp120 and Tat induce mitochondrial fragmentation and incomplete CP involving CMBP in human neurons. Although, ART therapy is associated with a significant increase in the CD4–4 T cells in the HIV-1-infected patients, ART-induced viral suppression was unable to restore CD4+ T2 counts to normal in extreme cases of HIV-1 infection. HIV-1 TAT-mediated microglial activation involved CBMP. Dysregulation of CP/ATG was observed in rat liver with mtDNA depletion induced by the nucleoside analogue, Zidovudine. STING-dependent translation inhibition restricted RNA virus replication. CP/ATG was induced in cells replicating hepatitis C viral genome. The influenza virus-induced CP/ATG compromised the pluripotency of human-iPPCs. HPV infection downregulated the expression of ATG-related genes in condylomata acuminata. Varicella-zoster virus capsids exit the nucleus but never undergo secondary envelopment during ATG inhibition by Bafilomycin A1.Viral (Zika, CMV, and rubella)-induced CP/ATG compromised the pluripotency of human iPPCs to cause microcephaly and arthrogryposis in the developing fetus. Ectromelia virus affected mitochondrial network morphology, distribution, and physiology in murine fibroblasts and macrophage cell line. Host genetics, innate immune responses, and cellular death pathways were explored in poliomyelitis patients. Reduced intestinal epithelial mitochondrial function enhanced IL-8 production in response to commensal *E. coli.* The theranostic potential of Bacillus subtilis lipopeptides as an anti-cancer agent was confirmed by the induction of apoptosis, paraptosis, and inhibition of ATG in K562 cells. The structure of a glutamine donor mimicked inhibitory peptide shape by the catalytic cleft of microbial transglutaminase. GABAergic signaling linked to ATG enhanced host protection against intracellular bacterial infections. CASP4/Caspase-11 promoted APS formation in response to bacterial infection. Cellular proteostasis forms a new twist in the action of

Thymosin $\alpha 1$ during microbial infection and N^ε-fatty acylation of multiple membrane-associated proteins by Shigella IcsB effector modulates the host function. Interferon-inducible GTPases and ATG proteins were identified in host defense. Mitochondria promoted septin assembly into cages that entrap Shigella for ATG. The activation of host IRE1α-dependent signaling contributed to the intracellular parasitism of Brucella melitensis. *Porphyromonas gingivalis* traffics ER-rich-APS for survival in human gingival epithelial cells, whereas β_2 integrin Mac-1 induced LC3-associated phagocytosis of Listeria monocytogenes. Streptomyces Sp metabolite(s) promoted Bax-mediated intrinsic apoptosis and ATG involving inhibition of the mTOR pathway in cervical cancer cell lines. iTRAQ-based proteomics of ATG-mediated immune responses was conducted in the vascular fungal pathogen Toll-like receptors-induced antimicrobial pathways in macrophages, whereas activation of RIG-I-mediated antiviral signaling triggered ATG through the MAVS-TRAF6-Beclin-1 signaling. The Pseudomonas aeruginosa quorum-sensing molecule alters skeletal muscle protein homeostasis by perturbing the antioxidant defense. The effects of Vibrio tapetis on ATG was investigated in Mytilus galloprovincialis hemocytes. The role of Toxoplasma gondii CQ-resistance transporter in bradyzoite viability and digestive vacuole maintenance was investigated. Toxoplasma could be eliminated from the host with metal ions. The expression of Mircl/Mir17-92 in sputum samples correlated with pulmonary exacerbations in cystic fibrosis patients. Paternal mitochondrial degradation was monitored in the nematode *C. elegans*. NADPH oxidase and guanylate binding protein 5 restricts the survival of avirulent type III strains of Toxoplasma gondii in naive macrophages. Basal and starvation-induced ATG mediated parasitic survival during intra-erythrocytic stages of Plasmodium falciparum. The microRNA expression of dibenzalacetone-treated intracellular amastigotes of LM was conducted for its safe and effective treatment. LM donovani induces ATG in neutrophils. Acetyltransferase was involved in LM's cell death. Quinoline derivatives triggered apoptosis by inhibiting ATG in LM. Semicarbazone derivatives were also developed as therapeutic alternatives in LMsis. The inhibitory effects of (+)-spectaline and iso-spectaline extracted from Senna spectabilis were demonstrated by evaluating the growth and ultrastructure of human infective species of *C. elegans*. Mitochondria restricted the growth of the intracellular parasite *Toxoplasma gondii* by limiting its uptake of fatty acids. Pyoverdine, a siderophore from *Pseudomonas aeruginosa*, translocated into *C. elegans*, removed iron, and activated a host cell response. Transporter membrane traffic in mold was investigated to discover the TSE-EBPT of fungal infections. A fungus, *Verticillium dahliae* is a soil-borne vascular pathogen that causes wilt symptoms in many plants. Co-culture of *V. dahliae* with Arabidopsis roots for 24 hrs induces changes in the gene expression profiles of both partners, even before defense-related phytohormone levels are induced in the plant. Dictyostelium discoideum was selected to investigate cellular-autonomous defenses. Bacteria exploit CP/ATG for proteasome degradation and enhance virulence in plants. The anti and pro-microbial roles of CP/ATG were reported in plant-bacterial interactions as well.

REFERENCES

Abdel-Mohsen, M. Ahmed, A. Abd-Allah El-Braky, A. Abd El-Rahim Ghazal, M. Mohammed Shamseya. 2018. Autophagy, apoptosis, vitamin D, and vitamin D receptor in hepatocellular carcinoma associated with hepatitis C virus. Medicine 97(12): e0172.

Abdoli, A., M. Alirezaei, P. Mehrbod and F. Forouzanfar. 2018. Autophagy: The multi-purpose bridge in viral infections and host cells. Rev Med Virol 28: e1973.

Andersen, N.B., S.M. Larsen, S.K. Nissen, S.E. Jørgensen, et al. 2019. Host genetics, innate immune responses, and cellular death pathways in poliomyelitis patients. Front Microbiol 10: 1495.

Ashkenazi, A., C. Bento, T. Ricketts, M. Vicinanza, et al. 2017. Polyglutamine tracts regulate beclin 1-dependent autophagy. Nature 545: 108–111.

Balbi, T., K. Cortese, C. Ciacci, G. Bellese, et al. 2018. Autophagic processes in *Mytilus galloprovincialis* hemocytes: Effects of *Vibrio tapetis*. Fish Shellfish Immunol 73: 66–74.

Bandyopadhaya, A., A.A. Tzika and K.G. Rahme. 2019. *Pseudomonas aeruginosa* quorum sensing molecule alters skeletal muscle protein homeostasis by perturbing the antioxidant defense system. MBio 10: e02211–19.

Basmaciyan, L., N. Azas and M. Casanova. 2019. A potential acetyltransferase involved in LM major metacaspase-dependent cell death. Parasit Vectors 12(1): 266.

Bilezikian, J.P., D. Bikle, M. Hewison, M. Lazaretti-Castro, et al. 2020. Mechanisms in endocrinology: Vitamin D and COVID-19. Eur J Endocrin 183(5): R133–R147.

Cabrera, J.R., R. Manivanh, B.J. North and D.A. Leib. 2019. The ESCRT-related ATPase Vps4 is modulated by interferon during herpes simplex Virus 1 infection. 10(2): e02567–18.

Calixto, S.L., N. Glanzmann, M.M. Xavier Silveira, J. da Trindade Granato, et al. 2018. Novel organic salts based on quinoline derivatives: The *in vitro* activity trigger apoptosis inhibiting autophagy in *Leishmania* spp. Chem Biol Interact 293: 141–151.

Cavalcanti de Queiroz, A., M.A. Alves, E.J. Barreiro, L.M. Lima, et al. 2019. Semicarbazone derivatives as promising therapeutic alternatives in leishmaniasis. Exp Parasitol 201: 57–66.

Chan, M.Y. and M.A. Smith. 2018. Infections in pregnancy. Comprehensive Toxicology 2018: 232–249.

Chen, X., K. Wang, Y. Xing, J. Tu, et al. 2014. Coronavirus membrane-associated papain-like proteases induce autophagy through interacting with Beclin1 to negatively regulate antiviral innate immunity. Protein Cell 5(12): 912–927.

Cheng, S., X. Ma, S. Geng, X. Jiang, et al. 2018. Fecal microbiota transplantation beneficially regulates intestinal mucosal autophagy and alleviates gut barrier injury. mSystems 3(5): e00137–18.

Coers, J., H.M. Brown, S. Hwang and G.A. Taylor. 2018. Partners in *anti-crime*: How interferon-inducible GTPases and autophagy proteins team up in cell-intrinsic host defense. Curr Opin Immunol 54: 93–101.

Dan, V.M., B. Muralikrishnan, R. Sanawar, B.B. Burkul, et al. 2018. *Streptomyces* sp metabolite(s) promotes Bax mediated intrinsic apoptosis and autophagy involving inhibition of mTOR pathway in cervical cancer cell lines. Sci Rep 8: 2810.

de Carvalho, L.P. and E.J.T. de Melo. 2018. Further aspects of *Toxoplasma gondii* elimination in the presence of metals. Parasitol Res 117: 1245–1256.

Dunn, J.D., C. Bosmani, C. Barisch, L. Raykov, et al. 2018. Eat prey, live: *Dictyostelium discoideum* as a model for cell-autonomous defenses. Front Immunol 8: 1906.

Franz, K.M., W.J. Neidermyer, Y.J. Tan, S.P.J. Whelan, et al. 2018. STING-dependent translation inhibition restricts RNA virus replication. Proc Natl Acad Sci U.S.A. 115: E2058–E2067.

Gassen, N.C., D. Niemeyer, D. Muth, V.M. Corman, et al. 2019. SKP2 attenuates autophagy through Beclin1-ubiquitination and its inhibition reduces MERS-Coronavirus infection. Nat Commun 10, 5770.

Girsch, J.H., K. Walters, W. Jackson and C. Grose. 2019. Progeny varicella-zoster virus capsids exit the nucleus but never undergo secondary envelopment during autophagic flux inhibition by bafilomycin A1. J Virol 93(17): e00505–19.

Gluschko, A., M. Herb, K. Wiegmann, O. Krut, et al. 2018. The β_2 Integrin Mac-1 Induces Protective LC3-Associated Phagocytosis of *Listeria monocytogenes*. Cell Host Microbe 23: 324–337.

Gregorczyk, K.P., Z. Wyżewski, J. Szczepanowska, F.N. Toka, et al. 2018. Ectromelia virus affects mitochondrial network morphology, distribution, and physiology in murine fibroblasts and macrophage cell line. Viruses 10(5).

Hedl, M., J. Yan, H. Witt and C. Abraham. 2019. IRF5 is required for bacterial clearance in human M1-polarized macrophages, and IRF5 immune-mediated disease risk variants modulate this outcome. J Immunol 202: 920–930.

Hino, K., S. Nishina, K. Sasaki and Y. Hara. 2019. Mitochondrial damage and iron metabolic dysregulation in hepatitis C virus infection. Free Radic Biol Med 133: 193–199.

Jabłoński, A., K. Matczak, A. Koceva-Chyła, K. Durka, et al. 2017. Cymantrenyl-nucleobases: Synthesis, anticancer, antitrypanosomal and antimicrobial activity studies. Molecules 22(12): 2220. doi: 10.3390/molecules22122220.

Jacomin, A.C., E. Taillebourg, M.O. Fauvarque. 2018. Deubiquitinating enzymes related to autophagy: New therapeutic opportunities? Cells 7(8): 112.

Jansen, A.F.M., T. Schoffelen, C.P. Bleeker-Rovers, P.C. Wever, et al. 2019. Genetic variations in innate immunity genes affect response to *Coxiella burnetii* and are associated with susceptibility to chronic Q fever. Clin Microbiol Infect 25(5): 631.e11–631.e15.

Jiang, M., M. Ju, W. Bu, K. Chen, et al. 2019. HPV Infection downregulates the expression of autophagy-related genes in condylomata acuminata. Dermatology 235: 418–425.

Joy, S., L. Thirunavukkarasu, P. Agrawal, A. Singh, et al. 2018. Basal and starvation-induced autophagy mediates parasite survival during intraerythrocytic stages of *Plasmodium falciparum*. Cell Death Discov 4: 43.

Juettner, N.E., S. Schmelz, A. Kraemer, S. Knapp, et al. 2018. Structure of a glutamine donor mimicking inhibitory peptide shaped by the catalytic cleft of microbial transglutaminase. FEBS J 285: 4684–4694.

Kang, D., D.R. Kirienko, P. Webster, A.L. Fisher, et al. 2018. Pyoverdine, a siderophore from Pseudomonas aeruginosa, translocates into *C. elegans*, removes iron, and activates a distinct host response. Virulence 9: 804–817

Kannan, G., M. Di Cristina, A.J. Schultz, M.H. Huynh, et al. 2019. Role of *Toxoplasma gondii* chloroquine resistance transporter in bradyzoite viability and digestive vacuole maintenance. MBio 10(4): e01324–19.

Katuri, A., J.L. Bryant, D. Patel, V. Patel, et al. 2019. HIVAN associated tubular pathology with reference to ER stress, mitochondrial changes, and autophagy. Exp Mol Pathol 106: 139–148.

Kim, J.K., Y.S. Kim, H.M. Lee, H.S. Jin, et al. 2018. GABAergic signaling linked to ATG enhances host protection against intracellular bacterial infections. Nat Commun 9: 4184.

Krause, K., K. Caution, A. Badr, K. Hamilton, et al. 2018a. CASP4/caspase-11 promotes APS formation in response to bacterial infection. Autophagy 14: 1928–1942.

Krause, K., B.T. Kopp, M.F. Tazi, K. Caution, et al. 2018b. The expression of Mirc1/Mir17-92 cluster in sputum samples correlates with pulmonary exacerbations in cystic fibrosis patients. J Cyst Fibros 17: 454–461.

Kritas, S.K., G. Ronconi, A. Caraffa, C.E. Gallenga, et al. 2020. Mast cells contribute to coronavirus-induced inflammation: new anti-inflammatory strategy. J Biol Regul Homeost Agents 34(1): 9–14.

Krokowski, S., D. Lobato-Márquez and S. Mostowy. 2018. Mitochondria promote septin assembly into cages that entrap *Shigella* for autophagy. Autophagy 14: 913–914.

Lee, N.R., J. Ban, N.J. Lee, C.M. Yi, et al. 2018a. Activation of RIG-I-Mediated antiviral signaling triggers autophagy through the MAVS-TRAF6-Beclin-1 signaling axis. Front Immunol 9: 2096.

Lee, K., J.S. Roberts, C.H. Choi, K.R. Atanasova, et al. 2018b. Porphyromonas gingivalis traffics into endoplasmic reticulum-rich-APS for successful survival in human gingival epithelial cells. Virulence 9: 845–859.

Lim, K.T., A. Amanah, N.J.-Y. Chear, Z. Zahari, et al. 2018. Inhibitory effects of (+)-spectaline and iso-6-spectaline from *Senna spectabilis* on the growth and ultrastructure of human-infective species *Trypanosoma brucei rhodesiense* bloodstream form. Exp Parasitol 184: 57–66.

Lisco, A., C.S. Wong, S.L. Lage, I. Levy, et al. 2019. Identification of rare HIV-1-infected patients with extreme CD4+ T cell decline despite ART-mediated viral suppression. JCI Insight 4: 127113.

Liu, W., Y. Zhou, T. Peng, P. Zhou, et al. 2018. N^ε-fatty acylation of multiple membrane-associated proteins by *Shigella* IcsB effector to modulate host function. Nat Microbiol 3: 996–1009.

Maier, H.J. and P. Britton. 2012. Involvement of ATG in Coronavirus Replication. Viruses 4(12): 3440–3451.

Markotter, W., M. Geldenhuys, P. Jansen van Vuren, A. Kemp, et al. 2019. Paramyxo- and coronaviruses in rwandan bats. Trop Med Infect Dis 4(3): 99.

Martineau, A.P. and N.G. Forouhi. 2020. Vitamin-D for COVID-19: A Case to Answer. Lancet 8: 735–736.

Matta, S.K., K. Patten, Q. Wang, B.H. Kim, et al. 2018. NADPH oxidase and guanylate binding protein 5 restrict survival of avirulent type III strains of *Toxoplasma gondii* in naive macrophages. MBio 9: e01393–18.

McGrath, E.P., S.E. Logue, K. Mnich, S. Deegan, et al. 2018. The unfolded protein response in breast cancer. Cancers (Basel) 10(10): 344.

Memoli, M.J., H. Harvey, D.M. Morens, J.K. Taubenberger, et al. 2013. Influenza in pregnancy. Influenza Other Respir Viruses 7(6): 1033–1039.

Mori, H., T. Fukuhara, C. Ono, T. Tamura, et al. 2018. Induction of selective ATG in cells replicating hepatitis C virus genome. J Gen Virol 99: 1643–1657.

Pandey, A., F. Lin, A.L. Cabello, L.F. da Costa, et al. 2018. Activation of host IRE1α-dependent signaling axis contributes the intracellular parasitism of *Brucella melitensis*. Front Cell Infect Microbiol 8: 103.

Paraskevis, D., E.G. Kostaki, G. Magiorkinis, G. Panayiotakopoulos, et al. 2020. Full-genome evolutionary analysis of the novel corona virus (2019-nCoV) rejects the hypothesis of emergence as a result of a recent recombination event. Infect Genet Evol 79: 104212.

Pernas, L., C. Bean, J.C. Boothroyd and L. Scorrano. 2018. Mitochondria restrict growth of the intracellular parasite *Toxoplasma gondii* by limiting its uptake of fatty acids. Cell Metab 27: 886–897.

Pitale, D.M., N.S. Gendalur, A. Descoteaux and C. Shaha 2019. *Leishmania donovani* induces autophagy in human blood–derived neutrophils. J Immunol 202: 1163–1175.

Prentice, E., W.G. Jerome, T. Yoshimori, N. Mizushima, et al. 2003. Coronavirus replication complex formation utilizes components of cellular autophagy. J Biol Chem 279: 10136–10141.

Razdan, K., K. Singh and D. Singh. 2020. Vitamin D levels and COVID-19 susceptibility: Is there any correlation? Medicine in Drug Discovery 7: 100051.

Rodrigues, L.O.C.P., R.S.F. Graça and L.A.M. Carneiro. 2018. Integrated stress responses to bacterial pathogenesis patterns. Front Immunol 9: 1306.

Santos-Llamas, A., M.J. Monte, J.J.P. Marin, M.J. Perez, et al. 2018. Dysregulation of ATG in rat liver with mitochondrial DNA depletion induced by the nucleoside analogue Zidovudine. Arch Toxicol 92: 2109–2118.

Saxena, A., F. Lopes and D.M. McKay. 2018. Reduced intestinal epithelial mitochondrial function enhances in vitro interleukin-8 production in response to commensal *Escherichia coli*. Inflamm Res 67: 829–837.

Schoeman, D. and B.C. Fielding. 2019. Coronavirus envelope protein: Current knowledge. Virol J 16: 69.

Seveau, S., J. Turner, M.A. Gavrilin, J.B. Torrelles, et al. 2018. Checks and balances between ATG and ISs during infection. J Mol Biol 430: 174–192.

Shao, X., X. Wang, X. Guo, K. Jiang, et al. 2019. STAT3 contributes to oncolytic newcastle disease virus-induced immunogenic cell death in melanoma cells. Front Oncol 9: 436.

Shaoping, W. and J. Sun. 2011. Vitamin D, vitamin D receptor, and macroautophagy in inflammation and infection. Discovery Medicine. 59: 325–335.

Singh, N. and I.S. Chauhan. 2018. MicroRNA expression profiling of dibenzalacetone (DBA) treated intracellular amastigotes of LM donovani. Exp Parasitol 193: 5–19.

Smith, C.A., D.J. Tyrell, U.A. Kulkarni, S. Wood, et al. 2019. Macrophage migration inhibitory factor enhances influenza-associated mortality in mice. JCI Insight 4(13): 128034.

Stincardini, C., G. Renga, V. Villella, M. Pariano, et al. 2018. Cellular proteostasis: A new twist in the action of thymosin α1. Expert Opin Biol Ther 18(sup1): 43–48.

Stocks, C.J., M.A. Schembri, M.J. Sweet and R. Kapetanovic. 2018. For when bacterial infections persist: Toll-like receptor-inducible direct antimicrobial pathways in macrophages. J Leukoc Biol 103: 35–51.

Tanabe, K. and M. Nagi. 2018. Monitoring of iron depletion-induced MTG in pathogenic yeast. Methods Mol Biol 1759: 161–172.

Teodorof-Diedrich, C. and M.A. Spector. 2018. Human immunodeficiency virus type-1 gp120 and Tat induce mitochondrial fragmentation and incomplete MTG in human neurons. J Virol 92(22).

Teymoori-Rad, M., F. Shokri, V. Salimi, S.M. Marashi, et al. 2019. The interplay between vitamin D and viral infections. Rev Med Virol 29: e2032.

Thangaraj, A., P. Periyasamy, K. Liao, V.S. Bendi, et al. 2018. HIV-1 TAT-mediated microglial activation: Role of mitochondrial dysfunction and defective mitophagy. Autophagy 14: 1596–1619.

Üstün, S. and D. Hofius. 2018a. Anti-and pro-microbial roles of ATG in plant-bacteria interactions. Autophagy 14: 1465–1466.

Üstün, S., A. Hafrén, Q. Liu, R.S. Marshall, et al. 2018b. Bacteria exploit ATG for proteasome degradation and enhanced virulence in plants. Plant Cell 30: 668–685.

Wang, F.X., Y.M. Luo, Z.Q. Ye, X. Cao, et al. 2018. iTRAQ-based proteomics analysis of autophagy-mediated immune responses against the vascular fungal pathogen *Verticillium dahliae* in *Arabidopsis*. Autophagy 14: 598–618.

Wild, P., A. Kaech, E.M. Schraner, L. Walser, et al. 2017. Endoplasmic reticulum-to-Golgi transitions upon herpes virus infection. F1000 Research 6: 1804.

Xu, Y., D.J. Baylink, C.S. Chen. M.E. Reeves, et al. 2020. The importance of vitamin d metabolism as a potential prophylactic, immunoregulatory and neuroprotective treatment for COVID-19. J Transl Med 18(1): 322.

Zahedi-Amiri, A., G.L. Sequiera, S. Dhingra and K.M. Coombs. 2019. Influenza a virus-triggered ATG decreases the pluripotency of human-induced pluripotent stem cells. Cell Death Dis 10: 337.

Zhang, L., Y. Qin and M. Chen. 2018. Viral strategies for triggering and manipulating mitophagy. Autophagy 14: 1665–1673.

Zhao, H., L. Yan, X. Xu, C. Jiang, et al. 2018. Potential of *Bacillus subtilis* lipopeptides in anti-cancer I: induction of apoptosis and paraptosis and inhibition of autophagy in K562 cells. AMB Express 8: 78.

32

Charnolophagy in Aging

INTRODUCTION

Recently, the molecular mechanism of nutrition and longevity for CP/ATG regulation, and mitochondria-associated membranes in aging and senescence have been explored (Sharma and Ebadi 2014a, b, Sharma 2019c, Leidal et al. 2018). CP/ATG declines during aging. Failure of ATG worsens aging-associated diseases, including CVDs NDDs, microbial infections, and MDR malignancies. Mitochondria are involved in crucial cellular functions, such as lipid metabolism, Ca^{2+} buffering, and apoptosis in addition to ATP production. Their malfunction can be detrimental to normal cellular physiology and homeostasis. Charmpilas et al. (2018) presented procedures for quantitative *in vivo* monitoring of MTG in the nematode *C. elegans*, which can reveal the basic cellular, molecular, genetic and epigenetic basis of aging and longevity and associated chronic diseases. Potential anti-aging roles of CP modulators, inhibitors of apoptotic proteins, and double knockouts of Akt2 and AMPK predisposed cardiac aging without affecting the lifespan. The CP/ATG correlation between cell senescence and idiopathic pulmonary fibrosis, aldehyde dehydrogenase 2 (ALDH2) in aging, and Nix-mediated MTG regulation of platelet activation and lifespan and aging in *Drosophila* have been explored. We highlighted the TSE-EBPT significance of CP/ATG in the clinical management of aging and associated chronic diseases to remain healthy and enjoy better QOL by MTs' induction and hypothesized that MTs-regulated CP transcriptionally regulates telomere length by preventing free radical-induced mitochondrial and nuclear DNA oxidation to sustain intra-nuclear detoxification and thus the lifespan of a biological system (Sharma and Ebadi 2014a, b).

This chapter provides important information about longest living animals, along with their natural habitat and life style, the significance of CP/ATG for the TSE-EBPT of aging, and age-associated comorbidities, and promising strategies to increase the lifespan and enhance productivity for a better QOL of humans and all other living organisms. Molecular mechanisms and the theranostic significance of antioxidants and CPTs as CP/ATG regulators, CS stabilizers, and CS exocytosis enhancers to accomplish longevity are described without compromising on fertility and fecundity. The chapter also highlights the predominant role of sex hormones in CP/ATG regulation, and CS/APS stabilization and exocytosis to increase the lifespan.

Longest-Living Animals

The longest-lived animals are the Greenland shark, bowhead whale, Galapagos giant tortoise, African elephant, macaw, long-finned eel, and koi fish. Generally, koi fish live for 25–30 years but some of them have reached >200 years. They live in artificial rock pools and decorative ponds. The oldest koi was Hanako that died at the age of 226 years. There are tortoises presently living that were 25–50 years old when Charles Darwin was born. There are current-day cold-water sponges that were filter-feeding during the days of the Roman Empire. There are large saltwater clams native to the Puget Sound which have been alive for at least 160 years. They have necks, or siphons, which can grow to >1 meter long. The two species of currently alive tuatara are the only surviving members of an order that flourished ~200 million years ago—they are living fossils of 100–200 years. There are colorful deep-sea creatures called tube worms that live along hydrocarbon vents on the ocean floor. They have been known to live 170 years, but some have lived >250 years. The red sea urchin is found in the Pacific Ocean along the West Coast of North America. It lives in shallow, rocky waters from the low-tide line down to 90 meters, but stay out of extremely wavy areas. They crawl along the ocean floor, using their spines as stilts. There are sharks which live in Arctic waters and grows to an average length of 16 feet. These scavenge for their food and are attracted to the smell of rotting meat in the deep ocean. Radiocarbon testing on the eye lens of female sharks determined their lifespan >272 years. The Greenland shark is the longest-living vertebrae. Some specimens are >200 years old. The bowhead Arctic whale is the longest living mammal. Some of them have been found with the tips of ivory spears lodged in their flesh from failed attempts by whalers 200 years ago. The oldest known bowhead whale was at least 211 years old. One of the oldest known Galápagos tortoise – Harriet – died of heart attack at the age of 175 years in a zoo owned by the late Steve Irwin. An Aldabra giant tortoise named Adwaita died at the age of 250 years. The ocean quahog is a species of clam that is exploited commercially. The dark concentric rings or bands on the shell are annual marks, just as a tree has rings. Some specimens have been calculated to be >400 years old. Due to the extremely low temperature of the Antarctic Ocean, this immobile creature has an extremely slow growth rate. The oldest known specimens are 1,550 years. Some species of jellyfish can recycle from a mature adult stage to an immature polyp stage and back again to remain almost immortal. Hence, there seems to be no natural limit to their lifespan. Because they can bypass death, their number is currently spiking in the ocean. Active memory-enhancing molecules have been extracted from them and exploited for the treatment of AD and other age-related dementias to enhance cognition. Efficient CP regulation and antioxidants implicated in CBMP suppression might play a crucial role in improving the MQC and ICD for NCF of these long-lived animals as described in this manuscript.

The Anti-aging Role of CP

Aging is a complex biological process affecting almost all living organisms. Although its detrimental effects on animals' physiology have been extensively documented, several aspects of the biology of aging are insufficiently understood. Aging is an irreversible biological process associated with the increased prevalence of chronic diseases and healthcare liabilities. Several theories have been proposed for the biology of aging, including free radical accumulation, DNA damage, telomere shortening, stem cell decline, genetic, epigenetic, and acquired mutations, unhealthy lifestyle (high salt, sugar, and saturated fat intake, and lack of exercise), social, physical, mental, economical, and psychological crisis, hurries, worries, curries, malnutrition, substance abuse, extreme hostile environment, chronic infections, serious accidents, repeated surgeries, repeated hospitalization, diverse physico-chemical injuries, disturbed autonomic response, and CMB (CB formation, CP dysregulation, CS destabilization, CBMP induction, and apoptosis) are implicated in early morbidity and mortality. Mitochondria, the central energy producers of the cell, play pivotal roles in diversified cellular processes, including the regulation of MB, Ca^{2+} signaling, metabolic responses, and cell death, among others. Thus, proper mitochondrial function is a prerequisite for the maintenance of cellular and organismal homeostasis. Recently, Markaki et al. (2018) highlighted the molecular signaling pathways that regulate and coordinate MB, critical factors that hold promise for the development of pharmacological interventions towards enhancing human health and QOL throughout aging. Several MQC mechanisms have evolved to allow adaptation to different metabolic conditions, thereby preserving cellular homeostasis and survival. A transcriptionally-regulated molecular interaction of MB, CP, MTG, and ATG is extremely essential for NCF to enjoy BQL and longevity. A dynamic balance between cell proliferation and apoptosis regulates stress resistance, health, and lifespan. MB and CP regulation decline with age due to CMB and an inefficient/inadequate lysosomal enzyme system, leading to the progressive accumulation of damaged and/or unwanted CBs implicated in early morbidity and mortality. Several regulatory factors that contribute to energy homeostasis have been implicated in the development and progression of pathological conditions, such as metabolic diseases, CVDs, and NDDs, among others. Therefore, CP/ATG modulation may serve as an early theranostic strategy to tackle age-associated pathologies. Hrdinka and Yabal (2019) provided an overview of mechanisms of action of various inhibitors of apoptosis proteins (IAPs), and focused on their specific role in mediating innate immunity. They evaluated the distinct phenotypes related to the dysregulation of the IAPs, and pathologies associated with human IAP. The IAPs regulate cell survival and death. IAPs also act as innate immune sensors and modulate multiple pathways, such as CP/ATG and cell division. Many of these IAP functions are non-redundant even though they are based on the same molecular mechanism of action. IAPs can be used as target-specific substrates for ubiquitination and/or proteolytic cleavage. They have unique cellular localizations, cell type, and tissue-specific expression. In humans, the IAP family comprises eight distinct members. Genetic evidence from human pathologies confirms that diverse diseases arise upon aberrant IAP expression. Hence, further studies to determine the exact role of IAPs in CP induction/repression will confer the TSE-EBPT of aging.

Increased age often leads to a gradual deterioration in cardiac geometry, contractility, elasticity, rhythmicity, and elasticity. Both Akt and AMPK play a crucial role in the maintenance of cardiac homeostasis. Wang et al. (2019a) examined the impact of the ablation of Akt2 (the main cardiac isoform of Akt) and AMPKα2 on development of cardiac aging and the mechanisms involved with a primary focus on ATG. Cardiac geometry, contractility, and $[Ca^{2+}]_i$ were evaluated in young (4-month-old) and old (12-month-old) wild-type (WT) and Akt2-AMPK double knockout mice using echocardiography, IonOptix® edge-detection, and fura-2 techniques. Levels of CP and ATG were evaluated using immunoblotting. Increased age (12 months) did not elicit any notable effects on cardiac geometry, contractile function, morphology, ultrastructure, CP or ATG, although Akt2-AMPK double knockout predisposed aging-related changes in geometry (heart weight, LVESD, LVEDD, cross-sectional area, and interstitial fibrosis), TEM ultrastructure, and function (fractional shortening, peak shortening, maximal velocity of shortening/relengthening, time-to-90% relengthening), $[Ca^{2+}]_i$ release and clearance rate. Double knockout of Akt2 and AMPK unmasked age-induced cardiac ATG loss, including decreased Atg5, ATG7, Beclin-1, LC3BII-to-LC3BI ratio, and increased p62. These genotypes also unmasked age-related loss in CP markers PTEN-induced putative kinase 1 (PINK1), Parkin, Bnip-3, and FundC1, the MB cofactor PGC-1α, and lysosomal biogenesis factor TFEB, indicating that Akt2-AMPK double ablation predisposes cardiac aging in relation to compromised CP and ATG.

Zhao et al. (2019) outlined the role and mechanism of cellular senescence in IPF. Cellular senescence is a key factor driving age-related diseases. The senescence-associated secretory phenotype, telomere attrition, epigenetic changes, and CP damage may mediate the pathogenesis of senescence-related idiopathic pulmonary fibrosis (IPF). Reducing the level of cellular senescence or clearing senescent cells can downregulate the expression of fibrosis factors and alleviate the symptoms of IPF. Downregulation of lamin B1 is recognized as a crucial step for the development of senescence. Accelerated cellular senescence linked to impaired mTOR signaling and accumulation of mitochondrial damage is implicated in COPD pathogenesis. Saito et al. (2019) hypothesized that lamin B1 protein levels are reduced in COPD lungs, contributing to the cigarette smoke (CS)-induced cellular senescence via dysregulation of mTOR and MQC. To illuminate the role of lamin B1 in COPD pathogenesis, lamin B1 protein levels, mTOR activation, mitochondrial mass, and cellular senescence were evaluated in CS extract (CSE)-treated human bronchial epithelial cells (HBEC), CS-exposed mice, and COPD lungs. Lamin B1 was reduced by exposure to CSE and ATG was responsible for lamin B1 degradation in HBEC. Lamin B1 reduction was linked to mTOR activation through DEP domain-containing mTOR-interacting protein (DEPTOR) downregulation, resulting in accelerated cellular senescence. Aberrant mTOR activation was associated with increased mitochondrial mass, due to PPAR-γ coactivator-1β-mediated MB. CS-exposed mouse lungs and COPD lungs also showed reduced lamin B1 and DEPTOR protein levels, along with mTOR activation accompanied by increased mitochondrial mass and cellular senescence. Metformin prevented CSE-induced HBEC senescence and mitochondrial accumulation via increased DEPTOR expression, suggesting that lamin B1 reduction is a hallmark of lung aging and is involved in the progression of cellular senescence during COPD pathogenesis through impaired mTOR signaling. Wu and Ren (2019) highlighted the relationship between ALDH2 and cardiovascular aging. Aging is also associated with the progressive deterioration of cardiovascular and neurological functions. Linkage, GWAS, and NGS analysis confirmed a number of susceptibility loci for aging, in particular, AD. A link between the genetic mutation of mitochondrial aldehyde dehydrogenase (ALDH2) and lifespan as well as cardiovascular aging has been established. ALDH2 represents a gene with the greatest polymorphism and is an important enzyme for the detoxification of reactive aldehydes.

Experimental Studies on CP and Aging

It is well-known that genes, environment, and lifestyle can influence our lifespan. Although it is impossible to choose the best parents, we can definitely select a better environment and lifestyle to enjoy healthy aging and longevity. Aging is a complex and multifactorial process driven by genetic, environmental, and stochastic factors that lead to the progressive decline in the biological system. The mechanisms of aging have been investigated in nematode *C eligans*, fruit fly (*Drosophila*), and yeast. Studies on yeast aging have made relevant contributions to the progress in this field. Different longevity factors and pathways in yeast regulate aging in invertebrate and mammalian models as well. Currently used potential anti-aging drugs such as *Spermidine* and *Resveratrol* or anti-aging interventions such as *CR* were first discovered in yeast. The yeast model has been used to study the effects of proteins associated with age-related PD, HD, or AD. Maruzs et al. (2019) highlighted the recent progress made in understanding the relationship of ATG and aging in *Drosophila*, which involves the lysosome-mediated breakdown and recycling of material, as it degrades obsolete or damaged intracellular constituents (primarily mitochondria) and confers building blocks for biosynthetic and energy producing reactions. Defective CP/ATG lead to a rapid decline in neuromuscular function, neurodegeneration, sensitivity to stress (starvation or oxidative damage), and stem cell decline. Human ATG gene mutations cause similar symptoms including ataxia and mental retardation.

Physiologically, CP/ATG degradation decreases during aging, which may contribute to the development of age-associated diseases. Many manipulations that extend lifespan (including CR, reduced TOR kinase signaling, exercise, or treatment with anti-aging substances) require CP/ATG for their beneficial effect on longevity as an ICD process. Genetic (ATG8a overexpression in either neurons or muscle) or pharmacological (feeding Rapamycin or Spermidine to animals), and CP/ATG induction has been used to extend lifespan in *Drosophila*, suggesting that this primary housekeeping pathway can rejuvenate cells and organisms, having an impact on their longevity. CP/ATG is involved in cellular homeostasis and maintenance and may play a crucial role in cardio-metabolic and general health. Portilla-Fernandez et al. (2019) elucidated the role of ATG in cardio-metabolic traits by investigating genetic variants and DNA methylation in ATG-related genes in relation to CVDs and related traits. They implemented a multidirectional approach using molecular epidemiology tools, including genetic association analysis with GWAS, exome sequencing, and differential DNA methylation analysis. They investigated 21 ATG-related genes in relation to coronary artery disease and cardio-metabolic traits (blood lipids, BP, glycemic traits, T2DM) and used data from the largest GWAS as well as DNA methylation and exome sequencing from *The Rotterdam Study*. SNP rs110389913 in AMBRA1 was associated with blood proinsulin levels, whereas rs6587988 in ATG4C and rs10439163 in ATG4D were associated with lipid traits. The rs7635838 in ATG7 was associated with HDL. Rs2447607 located in ATG7 showed association with systolic BP and pulse pressure. Rs2424994 in MAP1LC3A was associated with CAD. An association of an exonic variant located in ATG3 with diastolic BP was identified. Using DNA methylation data, two CpGs located in ULK1 and two located in ATG4B were associated with both systolic and diastolic BP. In addition, one CpG in ATG4D was associated with HDL, indicating the role of ATG in glucose and lipid metabolism, and BP regulation. It is recognized that platelet activation requires functional mitochondria to provide an energy source and control their lifespan. Previous reports have shown that both CP and general ATG are essential for platelet function. Zhang et al. (2019) showed that Nix, as a CP receptor, plays an important role in RBCs maturation; it also mediates CP in platelets. The genetic ablation of Nix impairs MQC, platelet activation, and $FeCl_3$-induced carotid arterial thrombosis without affecting the expression of platelet glycoproteins (GPs) such as GPIb, GPVI, and $\alpha_{IIb}\beta_3$. A metabolic analysis revealed decreased $\Delta\Psi$, enhanced ROS level, diminished O_2 consumption rate, and compromised ATP production in $Nix^{-/-}$ platelets. Transplantation of wild-type (WT) bone marrow cells or transfusion of WT platelets into Nix-deficient mice rescued defects in platelet function and thrombosis, suggesting a platelet-autonomous role of Nix in platelet activation. The loss of Nix increased the lifespan of platelets *in vivo*, by preventing the CP degradation of Bcl-xL, indicating a link between Nix-mediated CP, platelet lifespan, and platelet physiopathology. Hence, targeting platelet CP and Nix might confer novel antithrombotic strategies in aging.

Molecular Mechanisms of Aging and CP

Sites of contact between mitochondria and the ER are known as mitochondria-associated membranes (MAM) or mitochondria-ER contacts (MERCs), and play pivotal role in cellular pathophysiology. Janikiewicz et al. (2018) highlighted the current knowledge of basic MAM biology, composition, and discussed the connections supporting MAM that are significant molecules in longevity. Changes observed in the molecular composition of MAM and in the number of MERCs predisposes MAM to be considered a dynamic structure. Its involvement in lipid biosynthesis and trafficking, Ca^{2+} homeostasis, ROS production, and ATG has been confirmed. MAM has also been studied in AD, PD, ALS, T2DM, and GM1-gangliosidosis. These findings linked MAM with aging or senescence (Paillusson et al. 2016). Aging is usually accompanied with overt structural and functional changes as well as compromised CP/

ATG. Wang et al. (2018a) evaluated the role of the innate pro-inflammatory mediator TLR4 in cardiac aging with a focus on ATG. Cardiac geometry and function were monitored in young or old wild-type (WT) and TLR4 knockout (TLR4$^{-/-}$) mice using echocardiography, IonOptix® edge-detection, and Fura-2 techniques. ATG, MTG, nuclear receptor corepressor 1 (NCoR1), and histone deacetylase I (HDAC1) were examined by immunoblotting. TEM was employed to monitor the myocardial ultrastructure. TLR4 ablation alleviated advanced aging (24 months)-induced changes in myocardial remodeling (increased heart weight, chamber size, cardiomyocyte cross-sectional area), contractile function and [Ca^{2+}]$_i$ handling as well as CP and ATG [Beclin-1, Atg5, LC3B, PINK1, Parkin, and p62]. Aging downregulated NCoR1 and HDAC1 as well as their interaction, the effects of which were attenuated or negated by TLR4 ablation. Advanced aging disturbed myocardial ultrastructure as evidenced by the loss of myofilament alignment and swollen mitochondria, which was obliterated by TLR4 ablation. Aging suppressed ATG (GFP-LC3B puncta) in neonatal mouse cardiomyocytes, the effect of which was negated by the TLR4 inhibitor, CLI-095. Inhibition of HDCA1 using Apicidin attenuated the CLI095-induced beneficial response of GFP-LC3B puncta, indicating a role for TLR4-mediated ATG in cardiac remodeling and contractile dysfunction in aging through a HDAC1-NCoR1-dependent mechanism. Various life-extending factors have been proposed, including CR without malnutrition, methionine restriction, low protein intake, and Spermidine intake. These metabolic and physiological interventions can influence the lifespan. In addition, high intake of whole grains, vegetables, fruits, and nuts, low IGF-1 levels, the Mediterranean diet, and a reduced intake of red meat and coffee can also increase the lifespan. Lifestyle modifications such as moderate exercise, yoga, prayer, pranayama, sex, and sleep regulation can also influence longevity. The author has proposed that mTOR/PI3/Akt-regulated CP/ATG can influence IMD, ICD, and MQC for NCF. The molecular mechanism of nutrition and longevity by CP/ATG regulation is presented in Fig. 48.

Molecular Mechanism of Nutrition and Longevity by CP/ATG Regulation

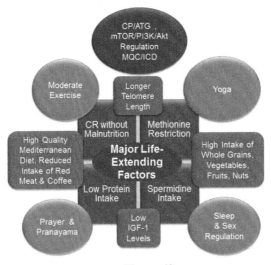

Figure 48

One of the hallmarks of aging is mitochondrial dysfunction. Recently, Madeo et al. (2019) highlighted that we associate getting older with a loss of energy, and at the molecular level, this is literally true. As we age, mitochondria become less efficient in generating the ATP we need for various cellular and biochemical processes. Just like bacteria, mitochondria engage in repeated cycles of fission and fusion. Both these processes are essential, but they need to be kept in balance. As we age, mitochondrial fusion predominates, and fission is compromised.

This leads to the accumulation of gigantic, condensed, and impaired mitochondria (collectively classified as CBs) that can't function efficiently, but are too large to be recycled through CP. The detrimental effects of CBs become most evident in tissues that need lots of energy, such as the brain, heart, and skeletal muscle. Hence, poor mitochondrial function is linked to compromised CV performance, reduced muscular strength, and slow gait in elderly individuals. If we could find a way to increase mitochondrial fission – and thus boost CP during the acute phase and ATG during the chronic phase, we could retain mitochondrial function throughout our life. It was found that small molecules that bind mRNA can regulate the fate or function of the bound RNA after transcription cells from elderly animals were screened to identify RNA-binding proteins that are altered by the aging process (Borbolis and Syntichaki 2015). Pumilio2 (PUM2) protein was highly expressed in older animals. PUM2 binds an mRNA which encodes for a mitochondrial fission factor (MFF), which in turn regulates mitochondrial fission. Higher levels of MFF increases the division of mitochondria into multiple smaller organelles, and facilitates the removal of CBs through CP and MTG. When PUM2 binds to its target, it inhibits the translation of MFF. Hence, more PUM2 should mean less MFF in the muscles and brain tissue of old animals. The tissue samples contained abundant PUM2, and less MFF proteins. The reduction in MFF was accompanied by less CP/MTG, and poorer MQC. Worms with better mitochondria were healthier and were moving faster and lived longer. Interfering with PUM2 could be the key to reversing this trend. CRISPR-Cas9 were used to selectively inactivate the gene that encodes for PUM2 in the skeletal muscle of older animals. By depleting this gene, the translation of MFF was augmented to increase MTG, resulting in improved MQC and an increased lifespan. Currently, there is no way to repress PUM2 in humans. However, there are ways to enhance CP. Naturally derived bio-actives could reverse age-related sarcopenia and cachexia by modulating mitochondrial functioning.

A lead bioactive, *Urolithin A,* induces MTG in model organisms. *Urolithin A* results from the biotransformation of dietary *Ellagitannins* via the gut microbiota. Ellagic acid and Ellagitannins in the diet can be derived from from pomegranate, walnuts, and berries. However, individuals vary in the extent to which they can convert these phenolic compounds into *Urolithin A*. If we do not have the adequate gut microbes, we could eat all of the aforementioned diet, and still fail to generate this metabolite, indicating that it is highly prudent to supplement the compound directly, in order to obtain its full benefit. In animal models, *Urolithin A* has shown promising effects. It increased the lifespan of nematodes by as much as 45%. Older mice that were administered *Urolithin A* exhibited a 40% improvement in endurance while running. Oral administration of *Urolithin A* in healthy elderly subjects was safe and effective in improving mitochondrial health, by upregulating mitochondrial gene expression in skeletal muscle. Currently, there are no effective treatments for age-related decline in muscle function except moderate exercise and CR.

Aged Horses' Skeletal Muscle

Aging is associated with decreased mitochondrial content and function in skeletal muscle due to CMB, lysosomal downregulation, and inefficient removal of CBs through CP. Li et al. (2018a) compared markers of mitochondrial content and biogenesis and of ATG between skeletal muscle from young and aged American quarter horses. The citrate synthase and mtDNA copy number were decreased in triceps brachii (TB) muscle from aged horses, suggesting an age-related induction of CBs as the primary culprit of CMB and reduced performance in horse race. Concomitantly, the mRNA expression of PGC-1α and TFAM, regulators of MB, was lower in aged compared to young TB. The expression of biomarkers suggested an age-associated decline in CP/ATG. The CPS/APS cargo protein, SQSTM/p62, accumulated with age in both muscles. Expression of the ATG-related protein Atg5 and the APS-bound form of LC3-II were lower in aged compared to young TB. While the LC3 transcript was elevated in aged compared to young GM, protein expression of LC3-II remained unaffected. Although, the gene expression of LAMP2 was not affected by age in either muscle, LAMP2 protein expression declined with age, suggesting a decline in APS-lysosome fusion, indicating that equine skeletal muscle mitochondrial content and biogenesis are impaired with age due to the induction of CBMP. The APS formation and lysosomal degradation were negatively affected in aged TB and GM, respectively. Recently, Medeiros and Graef (2019) reported that ATG determines mtDNA copy number during starvation, primarily implicated in aging. Further research is needed to explore whether interventions targeting CP/ATG processes can prolong health and performance of aging American quarter horses.

Sarcopenia in Chronic Heart Failure

Sarcopenia is an age-related geriatric syndrome that is characterized by a progressive loss of muscle mass, strength, and function. CHF, the final stage of various CVDs, may be correlated with the occurrence of sarcopenia. Yin et al. (2019) highlighted the latest progress in the pathogenesis of sarcopenia in patients with CHF which promotes the development of sarcopenia through multiple pathophysiological mechanisms, including malnutrition, inflammation, hormonal changes, oxidative stress, CP/ATG, and apoptosis. CHF can aggravate the adverse outcomes associated with sarcopenia, including falls, osteoporosis, frailty, cachexia, repeated hospitalization, and mortality. Sarcopenia and CHF are mutually interacting clinical syndromes. Patients with these syndromes endure a double burden, with no effective way to hinder their progression. However, physical exercise, nutritional supplements, antioxidants, and drug therapy may counteract the development of these maladies as CP regulators.

Epigenetics in Vascular Aging

Vascular aging is a major risk factor and driver of age-related CVD. Atherosclerosis, hypertension, and other CVDs lead to vascular dysfunction that involves multiple pathological processes such as oxidative stress, endothelial dysfunction, inflammation, and CP/ATG (Jin et al. 2019). Epigenetics refers to genetic changes that occur when the DNA remains unchanged; these include DNA methylation, histone modification, and non-coding RNA. Epigenetics plays a regulatory role in CVD and affects cardiovascular repair. Presently, drugs targeting epigenetics have applications in malignant tumors and inflammation. Therefore, exploration of epigenetic mechanisms in vascular aging facilitate understanding the pathogenesis of diseases related to vascular aging. The pathological changes in vascular aging and the relationship between vascular aging and epigenetics has been reported. The pathogenesis of vascular aging-related diseases to develop epigenetic-based TSE-EBPT strategies have been proposed for patients with age-related CVDs.

Neuronal Preconditioning of HSC70-interacting Protein

Lizama et al. (2018) demonstrated that the C-terminus of the HSC70-interacting protein (CHIP) is critical for neuronal responses to stress. CHIP upregulation and localization to mitochondria is required for CP. Unlike other disease-associated E3 ligases such as Parkin and Mahogunin, CHIP controls the homeostatic and stress-induced removal of CBs. Although CHIP deletion resulted in greater numbers of mitochondria, these organelles had distorted IMM without distinct cristae. Neuronal cultures derived from animals lacking CHIP were more vulnerable to acute injuries, and the transient loss of CHIP rendered neurons incapable of mounting a protective response following low-level stress, suggesting that CHIP is an essential regulator of mitochondrial number, cell signaling, and survival. The C-terminus of HSC70-interacting protein (CHIP, *STUB1*) is a ubiquitously expressed cytosolic E3-ubiquitin ligase. CHIP-deficient mice exhibited cardiovascular stress and motor dysfunction prior to premature death. This phenotype was more consistent with animal models in which master regulators of ATG are affected rather than with the mild phenotype of classic E3-ubiquitin ligase mutants. CHIP deficiency was associated with greater numbers of mitochondria, but these organelles were swollen and misshapen due to the induction of CBMP. Acute bio-energetic stress triggered CHIP induction and re-localization to mitochondria where it played a role in the removal of damaged organelles including CBs following low-level bio-energetic stress in neurons. CHIP expression overlapped with stabilization of the redox stress sensor PINK1 and was associated with increased LC3-mediated CP. Introducing human promoter-driven vectors with mutations in either the E3 ligase or TPR domains of CHIP in primary neurons derived from CHIP-null animals enhanced CHIP accumulation in the mitochondria. Exposure to ATG inhibitors suggested that increase in mitochondrial CHIP was due to the diminished clearance of CHIP-tagged organelles. A proteomic analysis of WT and CHIP KO mouse brains revealed proteins essential for maintaining energetic, redox, and mitochondrial homeostasis, which undergo significant genotype-dependent expression changes, suggesting the use of CHIP-deficient animals as a predictive model of age-related degeneration with selective neuronal proteo-toxicity and CMB involving CBMP.

The Theranostic Significance of Antioxidants in CP Regulation and Longevity

López-Lluch et al. (2018) highlighted the importance of mitochondria in aging and the repercussion in the progression of age-related diseases and metabolic syndromes. Mitochondria are essential for generating ATP from glucose and fatty acids but also in many other essential functions, including amino acid metabolism, pyridine synthesis, phospholipid modifications, and Ca^{2+} regulation. Mitochondrial activity is also the principal source of ROS. Aging and age-related diseases are associated with the dysfunction of mitochondria and deregulation of cell metabolism involving CBMP. Cell metabolism is regulated by three major nutritional sensors: mTOR, AMPK and Sirtuins, which control MQC by fusion, fission and turnover through CP, MTG, and ATG. A complex interaction between the activity of these nutritional sensors, MB, and dynamics exists and affects aging, and age-related diseases including metabolic diseases. Furthermore, mitochondria maintain communication with nuclear modulating gene expression and modifying epigenetics. Among all cellular organelles, mitochondria and lysosomes undergo initial senescence-related alterations. These organelles undergo gradual structural changes associated with reduced function. Lysosomes exhibit deteriorated function along with the accumulation of lipofuscins. Lysosomal dysfunction induces the deterioration of mitochondrial turnover by downregulating CP, resulting in the generation of more ROS, which target lysosomes. This vicious feedback loop between lysosomes and mitochondria involving dysregulated CP and CBMP aggravates senescence phenotypes. Hence, compromised lysosomal activity due to mitochondrial oxidative stress correlated with CBMP triggers cell senescence. Park et al. (2018) investigated the interaction between lysosomes and mitochondria during senescence and proposed the lysosomal-mitochondrial axis as an inducer of senescence alleviation. Thus, learning how to control the lysosomal-mitochondrial axis should represent an important area for developing the TSE-EBPT-CPTs of aging and related diseases. Further research in this direction will enhance our knowledge regarding aging, age-related pathologies, and novel TSE-EBPT strategies for anti-aging intervention.

MTs in Aging Brain

Aging is an inevitable biological process, associated with gradual and spontaneous biochemical and physiological changes, and increased susceptibility to diseases. Chronic inflammation and oxidative stress are hallmarks of aging. MTs are low molecular weight, zinc-binding, anti-inflammatory, and antioxidant proteins which provide neuroprotection in the aging brain through the zinc-mediated transcriptional regulation of genes involved in cell growth, proliferation, and differentiation. In addition to Zn^{2+} homeostasis, the antioxidant role of MTs is routed through -SH moieties on cysteine residues. MTs are induced in the aging brain as a defensive mechanism to attenuate RONS-induced oxidative and nitrative stress implicated in broadly classified neurodegenerative charnolopathies. In addition, MTs as free radical scavengers inhibit CB formation and CP induction to provide mitochondrial neuroprotection in the aging brain. In general, MT-1 and MT-2 induce cell growth and differentiation, whereas MT-3 is a growth inhibitory factor, which is reduced in AD. MTs are downregulated in wv/wv mice, exhibiting progressive neurodegeneration, early aging, morbidity, and mortality. These neurodegenerative changes were attenuated in MTs overexpressing wv/wv mice, suggesting the neuroprotective role of MTs in aging. Recent knowledge regarding the theranostic potential of MTs in NDDs such as PD, AD, and drug addiction was provided by the author's research team (Sharma et al. 2016). MTs are downregulated in long-lived dwarf mice and CR-fed mice. Particularly, Snell/Ames mutation, GHRKO mutation, a long-term CR diet, and a short-term CR diet exert a significant impact on the longevity of dwarf mice and CR-fed mice. MTs, as potent free radical scavengers, inhibit CB formation, and augment CP induction, CS stabilization, and CS exocytosis/endocytosis to safeguard functionally intact the mitochondrial population and their bioenergetics potential to synthesize ATP by the most vulnerable cell. MTs dysregulation in long-lived dwarf mice and CR-fed mice is presented in Fig. 49.

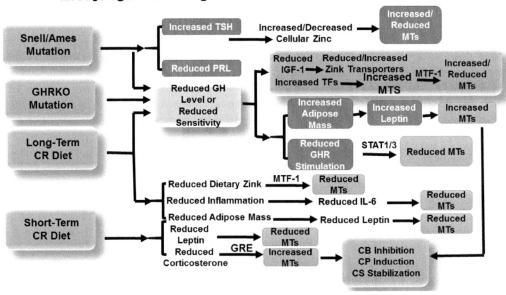

Figure 49

Sestrin-like Protein in Starvation

Sestrins are highly conserved, stress inducible proteins that maintain metabolic homeostasis and protect cells during stress. They are induced during stress and influence AMPK and mTOR pathways. Rafia et al. (2019) investigated the role of Sestrin from Dictyostelium discoideum (Dd), a eukaryote where starvation stress initiates multicellular development. The single DdSesn-like gene was expressed and its endogenous functions were characterized. Both the knockout and constitutively-expressing strains were made and their involvement in starvation-induced CP was analyzed by monitoring the ROS levels. Overexpression of DdSesn decreased cell growth and exhibited a prolonged lag phase. During starvation, both DdSesn and ROS were increased. Sesn^{OE} showed reduced ROS levels while sesn$^-$ showed increased ROS levels compared to the wild type, suggesting that increased sesn expression may be beneficial in reducing ROS levels during starvation. Deletion of sesn exhibited reduced CP and increased p4EBP1, indicating that DdSesn promotes CP in D. discoideum during starvation.

Acetyl-CoA Transport

The membrane transporter AT-1/SLC33A1 translocates cytosolic acetyl-CoA into the ER lumen, participating in QC mechanisms within the secretory pathway. Mutations and duplication events in AT-1/SLC33A1 are highly pleiotropic and have been linked to diseases such as spastic paraplegia, developmental delay, autism spectrum disorder, intellectual disability, propensity to seizures, and dysmorphism. Recently, Peng et al. (2018) showed that the systemic overexpression of AT-1 in the mouse leads to a segmental form of progeria with dysmorphism and metabolic alterations. The phenotype included delayed growth, short lifespan, alopecia, skin lesions, rectal prolapse, osteoporosis, cardiomegaly, muscle atrophy, reduced fertility, and anemia. In terms of homeostasis, the AT-1 overexpressing mouse displays hypocholesterolemia, altered glycemia, and increased indices of systemic inflammation. The phenotype is caused by a block in ATG9a-Fam134b-LC3β and ATG9a-Sec62-LC3β interactions, and defective reticulo-phagy, the ATG recycling of the ER. Inhibition of ATase1/ATase2 acetyltransferase enzymes downstream of AT-1 restored reticulo-phagy and rescued the phenotype of the animals, suggesting that abnormally elevated acetyl-CoA flux into the ER, inducing defects in CP/ATG and the recycling of subcellular structures. This diversion of acetyl-CoA from cytosol to ER is causal in the progeria phenotype, suggesting cytosol-to-ER flux of acetyl-CoA as a novel event that governs the pace of aging phenotypes and acetyl-CoA-dependent homeostasis linked to metabolism and inflammation.

Sex Hormones and Lifespan

While, it remains uncertain whether the intensity and frequency of CP is relatively higher in women as compared to men, the lifetime incidence and frequency of CP as a mechanism of ICD seems relatively higher in women as compared to men. In general, women live longer, as evidenced by the relatively higher number of centenarian women as compared to men due to the hormone estrogen which plays a significant role in regulating CP during the development of secondary sex characteristics, follicular maturation, oogenesis, menstrual cycle, endometrial desquamation, and spiral arteries sequestration during mensturation. Other hormones such as progesterone, follicle-stimulating hormone (FSH), and human chorionic-gonado-torphic hormone (β-HCG) also play important roles in maintaining pregnancy and regulates growth and development of the embryo during intrauterine life. The total number of sex hormones is relatively higher in women as compared to men. Moreover, efficient CP during menstruation, pregnancy, delivery, and milk ejection are potential mechanisms of MQC and ICD in a woman with a reproductive capacity. Nevertheless, during the postmenopausal period, women become equally susceptible to increased risk of osteoporosis, CVDs, and NDDs due to depletion of estrogen reserves and other hormones due to compromised CP; this is also noticed in men during aging. However, the estrogen-regulated CP-based hypothesis of female longevity needs further confirmation with experimental evidence. Using the age of female sexual maturation as a biomarker, Wang et al. (2018b) identified Nrip1 as a candidate gene that may regulate aging and longevity. They discovered that the deletion of Nrip1 extended the longevity of female mice. Nrip1 expression was altered differentially in various tissues during aging and diet restriction.

Nrip1 expression was induced with aging in visceral white adipose tissue (WAT), but reduced after four months of CR. In gastrocnemius muscle, particularly, Nrip1 expression was induced following CR. In mouse embryonic fibroblasts, the deletion of Nrip1 could suppress fibroblast proliferation, enhance CP under normal culture or amino acid starvation conditions, and delay oxidative and replicative senescence. In WAT of old animals, the deletion of the Nrip enhanced CP and reduced the number of senescent cells, suggesting that deleting Nrip1 can extend female longevity, but tissue-specific deletion may have varying effects on health and longevity. Hence, the deletion of Nrip1 in WAT may delay senescence in WAT and extend NCF for normal health and wellbeing.

Nutrition and Longevity

Various genetic, environmental, and lifestyle factors determine the lifespan of humans. Nutrition is a key component affecting our health, and studies on rodent models have shown that nutrition can increase the lifespan. Ekmekcioglu (2019) discussed the most important nutritional components and diets associated with longevity. They presented mechanistic factors involved, like mTor, IGF-1, CP and ATG. The association of foods and diets with all-cause mortality were summarized by conducting a meta-analyses. CR without malnutrition, methionine restriction, lower protein intake, or supplementation of Spermidine are major life-extending factors, in model organisms or rodents. In humans, certain healthy foods are associated with longer telomere length, and reductions in protein intake with lower IGF-1 levels, respectively, associated with longer lifespan. High intake of whole grains, vegetables, fruits, and nuts is associated with a reduced risk for all-cause mortality whereas a high intake of (red) meat and especially processed meat is positively related to all-cause mortality. The Mediterranean and high-quality diets are associated with reduced all-cause mortality risk. In recent years, there has been a great deal of attention toward the molecular mechanisms relevant to age-related progression controlled through the external intervention of polyphenols—an epigenetic-modulating diet. Cătană et al. (2018) highlighted that natural antioxidants Sirtuins, Rutins, Polyphenols, Resveratrol, Catechin, Lycopenes, and LSDs modulate cellular longevity through histone post-translational modification which boost MB by preventing CB formation and by regulating CP, thus reducing the level of acetyl coenzyme A (AcCoA). In addition, the effect of CR on cancer-related chronic inflammation is of great significance in aging. In line with this, SIRT1 protein levels have been expanded in response to CRM, by acting as CP regulators in cancer prevention (Lin and Fang 2013).

Changes in mitochondrial structure and function involving CBMP are the initial factors of cell senescence. Spermidine has an antiaging effect, but its effect on neuronal aging and mitochondrial mechanisms remains uncertain. Recently, Madeo et al. (2018) emphasized that interventions that delay aging and protect from age-associated disease are approaching clinical implementation. Such interventions include CRM, defined as agents that mimic the beneficial effects of DR/CR while limiting its detrimental effects. One such agent, Spermidine, has cardio-protective and neuroprotective effects and stimulates anticancer immune-surveillance in rodent models. Dietary polyamine uptake correlated with reduced cardiovascular and cancer-related mortality in human epidemiological studies. Spermidine augmented MB, exhibited anti-inflammatory properties, and prevented stem cell senescence. It shared the molecular pathways engaged by other CRM, induced protein deacetylation, and was dependent on CP regulation. Based on these findings, it was proposed that because Spermidine is already present in daily human nutrition, clinical trials aiming at increasing the uptake of polyamine seem promising for longevity and cancer prevention (Madeo et. al 2018). Jing et al. (2018) treated mouse neuroblastoma (N2a) cells with d-galactose (d-Gal) to establish cell aging and investigate the antiaging effect of Spermidine. Changes in the cell cycle and β-galactosidase activity were analyzed to evaluate cell aging. Stabilities of mitochondrial mRNA and $\Delta\Psi$ were evaluated in cellular aging under different treatments. The mitochondrial function was also evaluated using the seahorse metabolic analysis combined with ATP production. The UPR of the N2a cells was analyzed under different treatments. Spermidine delayed cell aging and maintained the mitochondrial stability during d-Gal treatment. Spermidine increased the proportion of cells in the S phase and maintained the $\Delta\Psi$. The O_2 utilization and ATP production in the N2a cells were reduced by d-Gal treatment but were partially rescued by the Spermidine pretreatment, which ameliorated the N2a cell aging by promoting ATG and inhibiting the apoptosis except the UPR, suggesting that it could ameliorate the N2a cell aging by maintaining the mitochondrial mRNA transcription, $\Delta\Psi$, and O_2 utilization potential during the d-Gal treatment. Recently, Zhou et al. (2016) showed that soon after fertilization, paternal mitochondria are depolarized and lose their inner membrane integrity, which marks them for degradation by ATG (more specifically, CP). The inner membrane breakdown triggers the entry of the intermembrane CPS-6 into the matrix to degrade mtDNA, which encodes 12 mitochondrial proteins, two rRNAs, and 22 tRNAs for normal functions and MQC. Degradation of mtDNA accelerates the breakdown of mitochondria and promotes externalization of signals recognized by the CP/ATG or proteasome machinery, leading to PME. Loss of paternal cps-6 delays the internal breakdown of paternal mitochondria, their enclosure, and degradation by the CP/ATG machinery. Delayed removal of either mutant or slightly different wild-type paternal CBs results in embryonic lethality in hetero-plasmic animals, due to incompatibility in cellular signaling between the mitochondrial and nuclear genomes, indicating that persistence of paternal CB compromises animal development and may be the impetus for the maternal inheritance of mitochondria. Endonuclease G mediated the degradation of sperm mtDNA during *Drosophila* spermatogenesis before fertilization to prevent paternal mtDNA transmission. In *C. elegans*, cps-6 served even after fertilization to mediate degradation of both paternal CBs and mtDNA to facilitate their elimination through CP. These findings imply a conserved role of endonuclease G in paternal mtDNA elimination and expand the roles of this nuclease beyond MQC and apoptosis as described in the author's book, *Fetal Alcohol Spectrum Disorder: Prevention and Cure,* published by Nova Science Publishers in New York, U.S.A.

Psyllium Seed Husk

Vascular dementia (VaD) develops through a pre-VaD step during which blood vessels narrow due to atherosclerosis attributed to risk factors, including hyperlipidemia. This is followed by a VaD progression step during which inadequate blood supply results in white matter damage and cognitive impairment. Furthermore, administration of Arabinoxylan attenuated white matter damage in a rat model of VaD. Lim et al. (2019) hypothesized that consumption of psyllium seed husk (PSH), containing Arabinoxylan (~60%), could inhibit the VaD progression step. To test this hypothesis, rats were supplemented with PSH at various dosages for 33 days in a model of bilateral common carotid artery occlusion. PSH supplementation decreased astrocytic and microglial activation in the optic tract (opt) and attenuated white matter damage in the opt. Attenuation of white matter damage resulted in the improvement of the pupillary light reflex, an indicator reflecting intactness of the opt. In addition, PSH treatment improved the survival of glial cells cultured under hypoxic and glucose-deprived conditions by inhibiting both apoptosis and ATG, suggesting that PSH consumption can inhibit the VaD progression through a decrease in white matter damage. This supported the researchers' hypothesis that PSH consumption prevents VaD due to the high Arabinoxylan content in the rat model. PSH consumption reduce risk factors, thereby inhibiting the pre-VaD step. Consequently, PSH consumption can contribute to the prevention of VaD by inhibiting both the pre-VaD and VaD progression steps. Hence, PSH might be a candidate to explore its use to reduce VaD.

NDP52 Mitochondrial RNA Poly(A) Interaction

Parkin-mediated CP is a QC pathway that selectively removes damaged mitochondria through ATG. ATG receptors, which interact with ubiquitin and Atg8 family proteins, contribute to the recognition of CBs by APS. NDP52, an ATG receptor, is required for ATG engulfment of CBs during the mitochondrial un-coupler treatment. The N-terminal SKICH domain and C-terminal zinc finger motif of NDP52 are required for CP/s function in ATG as CP occurs earlier than generalized ATG during DPCI in the most vulnerable cell. While the zinc finger motif contributes to poly-ubiquitin binding, the function of the SKICH domain remains unclear. Furuya (2018) showed that NDP52 interacts with mitochondrial RNA poly(A) polymerase (MTPAP) via the SKICH domain. During CP, NDP52 invades depolarized mitochondria and interacts with MTPAP dependent on the proteasome but independent of ubiquitin binding. Loss of MTPAP reduced NDP52-mediated CP, and the NDP52-MTPAP complex attracted more LC3 than NDP52 alone, indicating that NDP52 and MTPAP form an ATG receptor complex, which enhances ATG elimination of CBs implicated in early morbidity and mortality.

RedMIT/GFP-LC3 Mouse Model

Autosomal dominant optic atrophy (ADOA) due to the OPA1Q285STOP mutation is usually caused by mutations in the essential gene, OPA1. This encodes a ubiquitous protein involved in mitochondrial dynamics; hence, tissue specificity in this case is not understood. Dysregulated CP is implicated in ADOA, as it is increased in OPA1 patient fibroblasts. Furthermore, ATG may be increased in retinal ganglion cells (RGCs) of the OPA1^{Q285STOP} mouse model. Diot et al. (2018) developed a mouse model for studying mitochondrial dynamics to investigate MTG in ADOA. They crossed the OPA1^{Q285STOP} mouse with a RedMIT/GFP-LC3 mouse, harboring red fluorescent mitochondria and green fluorescent APSs. Co-localization between mitochondria and APSs, the hallmark of CP, was quantified in fluorescently labeled organelles in primary cell cultures, using two high throughput imaging methods: Image-stream (Amnis) and In Cell Analyzer 1000 (*GE Healthcare Life Sciences*). They examined co-localization between mitochondria and APSs using confocal microscopy. They validated imaging methods for RedMIT/GFP-LC3 mouse cells, showing that co-localization is a useful indicator of CP. Co-localization increased when lysosomal processing was impaired. Co-localization of mitochondrial fragments and APSs was increased in cultures from the OPA1^{Q285STOP}/RedMIT/GFP-LC3 mice compared to RedMIT/GFP-LC3 control mouse cells that were wild type for OPA1. This was apparent in both mouse embryonic fibroblasts (MEFs) using IN Cell 1000 and in splenocytes using Image-Stream imaging flow cytometer (*Amnis*). This represented increased CP flux using lysosomal inhibitors. The researchers also investigated the level of CP in the retina from the OPA1^{Q285STOP}/RedMIT/GFP-LC3 mice and the RedMIT/GFP-LC3 control mice. However, the fluorescent protein expression and the signal-to-background ratios precluded the detection of co-localization so they were unable to show any difference between these mice. Co-localization of fluorescent mitochondria and APSs in cell cultures could be used to detect CP. This model was used to confirm that CP is increased in a mouse model of ADOA. Hence, it can be useful for cell-based studies of diseases caused by impaired mitochondrial dynamics involving CBMP.

Ubiquinone (CoQ$_{10}$)-mediated Longevity

Mutations in the *clk-1* gene impair mitochondrial ubiquinone biosynthesis and extend lifespan in *C. elegans*. Molenaars et al. (2018) demonstrated that this life extension is linked to the repression of cytoplasmic mRNA translation, independent of the alleged nuclear form of *Clk-1*. *Clk-1* mutations inhibit polyribosome formation, similar to *daf-2* mutations that dampen insulin signaling. Comparisons of total versus polysomal RNAs in *clk-1(qm30)* mutants revealed a reduction in the translational efficiencies of mRNAs coding for elements of the translation machinery and an increase in those coding for the oxidative phosphorylation and ATG pathways. Knocking down the transcription initiation factor TAF-4, a protein that becomes sequestered in the cytoplasm during early embryogenesis to induce transcriptional silencing, ameliorated the *clk-1* inhibition of polyribosome formation, emphasizing a prominent role of the repression of cytoplasmic protein synthesis in eukaryotic lifespan extension and suggested that mutations impairing mitochondrial function can exploit this repression in a similar manner to reductions of insulin signaling.

p53 Inhibition and Aging

Recently, Fu et al. (2019) reported that aging of white adipose tissue (WAT) is associated with reduced insulin sensitivity, which contributes to whole-body glucose intolerance. WAT aging in mice impairs cold-induced beige adipocyte recruitment (beiging), which has been attributed to the senescence of adipose progenitor cells. Tumor suppressor p53 has also been implicated in WAT aging. p53 increased in adipose tissues of 28-weeks-old (aged) mice with impaired beiging capability. Cold exposure decreased p53 in beiging WAT of young mice but not in aged mice. In aged mice, inducible p53 ablation in differentiated adipocytes restored cold-induced WAT beiging and augmented whole-body energy expenditure and insulin sensitivity. The pharmacological inhibition of p53 rendered similar beneficial effects. Cold exposure repressed ATG in beiging WAT of young mice yet increased ATG in aged WAT. P53-ablation reduced LC3-mediated CP and facilitated the increase in mitochondria during beiging, suggesting that p53-induced CP in aged WAT impedes beiging and may be theranostic target to improve insulin sensitivity in aged WAT.

Skeletal Muscle Affected by Aging and Lifelong Exercise

Exercise training prevent the age-induced decline in muscle mass and fragmentation of mitochondria implicated in CB formation to affect CP/ATG. Dethlefsen et al. (2018) tested the hypothesis that cellular degradation pathways, including CP/ATG and apoptosis, are regulated in mouse and human skeletal muscle during aging and lifelong exercise training through a PGC-1α-p53 axis. Muscle samples were obtained from young untrained, aged untrained, and aged lifelong-exercise-trained men, and from whole-body PGC-1α knockout mice and their littermate controls that were either lifelong-exercise-trained or sedentary young and aged. Lifelong exercise training prevented the aging-induced reduction in PGC-1α, p53, and p21 mRNA as well as caused increases in LC3-II and Bnip-3 proteins in mouse skeletal muscle, while the Bax/Bcl2 ratio, LC3-I, and Bax protein were decreased in the aging muscle without any significant effect on life-long exercise training. In humans, aging was associated with reduced PGC-1α mRNA as well as decreased p62 and p21 protein in skeletal muscle, while lifelong exercise training increased Bnip-3 protein and decreased p53 mRNA. There was a regulation of CP/ATG and apoptosis in mouse muscle with aging and lifelong exercise training, whereas healthy aged human skeletal muscle seemed robust during changes in CP/ATG and apoptosis markers compared with mouse muscle at the investigated age.

S-Nitrosylation

S-nitrosylation, a prototypic redox-based posttranslational modification, is dysregulated in disease. *S*-nitrosoglutathione reductase (GSNOR) regulates protein *S*-nitrosylation by functioning as a protein denitrosylase. Deficiency of GSNOR results in tumorigenesis and disrupts cellular homeostasis, including metabolic, cardiovascular, and immune function. Rizza and Filomeni (2018) demonstrated that GSNOR expression decreases in primary cells undergoing senescence, as well as in mice and humans during their lifespan. Exceptionally long-lived individuals maintained GSNOR levels. GSNOR deficiency promoted mitochondrial nitrosative stress, including excessive *S*-nitrosylation of Drp-1 and Parkin, thereby impairing mitochondrial dynamics and CP, implicating GSNOR in longevity, suggesting a molecular link between protein *S*-nitrosylation and MQC in aging, and a redox-based perspective on aging with direct theranostic implications. Mitochondrial dynamics are required to adapt the manifold functions of mitochondria to cell needs and regulate their turnover by CP. This is possible only if CBs involved in CBMP are engulfed by phagophores, the precursors to CPS, and subsequently degraded to maintain a correct and healthy number of mitochondria that otherwise might be harmful as they participate in deleterious CBMP. They represent the main source of RONS that— according to the free radical theory of aging—can cause aging when chronically overproduced. Furthermore, Rizza et al. (2018) demonstrated that *S*-nitrosylation, the reversible modification of cysteine residues by NO, induces CB formation by targeting DNM1L/Drp-1 (dynamin 1-like) at Cys644, but inhibits CP, driving cell senescence and aging characterized by an epigenetically-driven decrease in alcohol dehydrogenase 5 [class III], chi polypeptide (ADH5/GSNOR), suggesting that ADH5 may serve as a novel longevity gene.

Aged Kidney

Jankauskas et al. (2018) discussed critical elements which determine the difference between young and old phenotypes and provide directions to prevent or cure lesions occurring in aged organs including the kidney. The term "aging" covers organisms, cells, cellular organelles and their constituents. In general terms, the aging system admits the existence of nonfunctional structures which by some reasons have not been removed by a clearing system, for example, through CP/MTG/ATG labeling and eliminating unwanted cells or CBs. This is particularly relevant to old kidney where normal function is highly critical for the viability of an organism. One of the main problems in biomedical studies is that in their majority, young organisms serve as a standard to investigate the aged system. Some protective systems, which demonstrate their efficiency in young systems, lose their beneficial effect in aged organisms. It may be more pertinent for the ischemic preconditioning of the kidney and may not be useful for an old kidney with compromised MB. The pharmacological intervention employing novel CPTs could correct the defects of the senile system provided that the complete understanding of all elements involved in aging will be achieved.

Loss of UBE2E3

Cellular senescence plays essential roles in tissue homeostasis as well as diseases ranging from cancers to NDDs. Various molecular pathways can induce senescence and dictate the phenotypic and metabolic changes that accompany the transition to, and maintenance of the senescence. Plafker et al. (2018) described a novel senescence phenotype induced by the depletion of UBE2E3, a highly-conserved, metazoan ubiquitin conjugating enzyme. Cells depleted of UBE2E3 become senescent in the absence of overt DNA damage and have a distinct senescence-associated secretory phenotype, increased mitochondrial and lysosomal mass, an increased sensitivity to mitochondrial and lysosomal poisons, and an increased basal ATG. The senescence phenotype can be suppressed by co-depletion of either p53 or its cognate target gene, p21[CIP1/WAF1], or by co-depleting the tumor suppressor p16[INK4a]. These findings highlighted a link between ubiquitin-conjugating enzymes and cellular senescence, and emphasized the consequences of disrupting the integration between the ubiquitin proteolysis system and ATG.

Mitochondria, ATG, and Inflammation

As mitochondria age, they become progressively inefficient and potentially toxic, and acute damage can trigger the permeabilization of their membranes to initiate apoptosis or necrosis through the induction of CBMP. Moreover, mitochondria have an important role in pro-inflammatory signaling. Green et al. (2011) highlighted that alterations of mitochondrial functions are linked to acute or chronic degenerative diseases. ATG turnover of cellular constituents, be it general (ATG) or specific for mitochondria (CP), eliminates dysfunctional or damaged mitochondria, thus counteracting degeneration, attenuating inflammation, and preventing undesired cell loss through CBMP. Decreased expression of genes that regulate CP/ATG can cause degenerative diseases where compromised MQC results in inflammation and the death of cell populations. Thus, a combination of CB formation and impaired CP/ATG involving CBMP may contribute to multiple aging-associated pathologies.

SIRT3 Deficiency

Mitochondrial dynamics play critical roles in aging, and their impairment represents a risk factor for myocardial dysfunction. Mitochondrial deacetylase sirtuin (SIRT)3 contributes to the prevention of redox stress and cell aging. Li et al. (2018b) explored the role of SIRT3 in myocardial aging. SIRT3 expression was significantly lower in the myocardia of aged mice compared with young mice. The activity of mitochondrial MnSOD and PGC-1α was reduced in the aged heart. To further explore the association between SIRT3 and myocardial senescence, SIRT3 heart-specific knockout (SIRT3–/–) mice were used. Obvious features of aging were present in the myocardium of SIRT3–/– mice, including mitochondrial protein dysfunction, enhanced oxidative stress, and energy metabolism dysfunction. The SIRT3 deficiency impaired Parkin-mediated MTG by increasing p53-Parkin binding and blocking the mitochondrial translocation of Parkin in cardiomyocytes. An injection of ATG agonist, CCCP, increased the mitochondrial Parkin in young wild-type hearts but not in aged hearts; the effect was less pronounced in SIRT3–/– hearts, suggesting that CCCP-induced Parkin translocation was reduced in aged and SIRT3–/– hearts. CCCP-induced mitochondrial clearance, which could be rescued by ATG antagonist BafilomycinA1, was attenuated in aged and SIRT3–/– hearts vs. young hearts. The SIRT3 deficiency exacerbated p53/Parkin-mediated MTG inhibition and disrupted MQC, suggesting that loss of SIRT3 may increase the susceptibility of aged hearts to cardiac dysfunction. The theranostic activation of SIRT3 and improved mitochondrial function may ameliorate the symptoms of cardiac aging.

PGC-1α in Aging Muscle

PGC-1α is a transcriptional co-activator known as the master regulator of MB. Its control over the metabolism exerts a critical influence on the aging process. Garcia et al. (2018) used aged mice overexpressing PGC-1α in skeletal muscle to determine whether the transcriptional changes reflected a pattern of expression observed in younger muscle. Analyses of muscle proteins showed that Pax7 and several ATG markers were increased. In general, the steady-state levels of several muscle proteins resembled that of muscle from young mice. Age-related mtDNA deletion levels were not increased by the PGC-1α-associated increase in MB. Age-related changes in the neuromuscular junction were minimized by PGC-1α overexpression. RNA-Seq showed that several genes overexpressed in the aged PGC-1α transgenics were expressed at higher levels in young skeletal muscle as opposed to when they were compared to aged skeletal muscle. There was an increased expression of genes associated with energy metabolism but also of pathways associated with muscle integrity and regeneration. PGC-1α overexpression had a significant effect on longevity, suggesting that its overexpression in aged muscle leads to molecular changes that resemble the patterns observed in skeletal muscle in younger mice.

PQC and the Stress of Aging

There exists a phenomenon in aging research whereby early life stress can have positive impacts on longevity. Higuchi-Sanabria et al. (2018) provided an overview of the PQC mechanisms which determine MQC that operate in the cytosol, mitochondria, and ER, and discussed how they affect cellular health and viability during stress and aging, suggesting a robust, long-lasting induction of cellular defense mechanisms. These include various unfolded protein responses (UPR) of the ER, cytosol, and mitochondria. Induction of UPR pathways, in the absence of stress, increases lifespan in organisms as diverse as yeast, worms, and flies.

Senotherapy

Senotherapy is an anti-aging strategy and refers to the selective elimination of senescent cells by senolytic agents and CP agonists, boosting the activity of immune cells (macrophages) that eliminate senescent cells or alleviates the secretory phenotype (SASP) of senescent cells. As senescent cells accumulate with age and are implicated in age-related disorders, senotherapy seems to be promising in improving the healthspan. Genetic approaches, which allowed researchers to selectively induce death of senescent cells in transgenic mice, indicated that elimination of senescent cells can be a potential theranostic strategy for treating age-related diseases. Recently, Paez-Ribes et al. (2019) proposed primarily four different strategies to prevent the deleterious effects of cellular senescence. Targeting pro-survival pathways involving the BCl2 family proteins, the P53 or PI3/Akt pathways is currently the leading strategy to promote senescent cell elimination in the degenerated or aged tissue. The inhibition of pro-survival pathways can be achieved by using apoptosis-inducing drugs to enhance CP/ATG and ICD. The first and second generation of inhibitors of the BCL-2 cell death regulator family of proteins can induce apoptosis of senescent cells by selectively targeting senescence metabolism through glycolysis blockade and attenuation of ATM, HDAC, FOXO4 activities as well as the PI3K cascade as clinically-significant approaches. A second strategy is the activation of the immune system against senescent cells to stimulate their clearance by enhancing the cytotoxic activity of NK cells against senescent cells, and manipulating the humoral innate immunity by using antibodies against receptors, such as DPP4 and vimentin. Thirdly, manipulation of the SASP without compromising the cell cycle arrest of senescent cells has also proven beneficial. A large number of molecules can interfere with NF-κB and C/EBPβ transcriptional activities or their upstream regulators, attenuating the expression of senescence-associated secretory phenotype (SASP) factors, such as IL-1, IL-6 and IL-8, and thus reducing the senescence-derived inflammatory milieu. SASP is a phenotype associated with senescent cells wherein those cells secrete high levels of inflammatory cytokines, immune modulators, growth factors, and proteases. Lastly, genetic and epigenetic manipulation of cells, including the induction of reprogramming, to bypass or revert cellular senescence has been proposed. These investigators emphasized that all these approaches should be taken with extreme caution given the potential risk of cancer induction. It is important to emphasize that DSST-CP/ATG regulation will be extremely important to accomplish afore-mentioned theranostic strategies to prevent early morbidity and mortality and improve the quality of life which is the primary message of this edition. Translating these results into humans is based on searching for synthetic and natural compounds to exert such beneficial effects. The major challenge is to demonstrate efficacy, safety, and tolerability of senotherapy in humans. How these DSST-TSE-EBPT-CPTs can influence the senescence of non-dividing post-mitotic cells (particularly neurons and muscles) is yet to be established. Another issue concerns the senescence of cancer cells induced during therapy as there is a risk of resumption of senescent cell division that could result in cancer renewal. Thus, development of effective senotherapeutics as novel CPTs is also an urgent issue in cancer theranostics.

Dark-induced Leaf Senescence in Barley

A barley crop model was analyzed for early and late events during the dark-induced leaf senescence (DILS) as well as for deciphering the critical time limit for reversal of the senescence. Sobieszczuk-Nowicka et al. (2018) determined the chlorophyll fluorescence vitality index RFD that correlated with the cessation of photosynthesis prior to microATG symptoms, initiation of DNA degradation, and increase in the endonuclease *BNUC1*. DILS was characterized by upregulation of processes that enable recycling of degraded macromolecules and metabolites, including increased NH_4^+ remobilization, gluconeogenesis, glycolysis, and partial upregulation of glyoxylate and TCA cycles. The most evident differences in genes between DILS and developmental senescence included hormone-activated signaling pathways, lipid catabolism, carbohydrate metabolism, low-affinity ammonia remobilization, and RNA methylation. The mega-ATG symptoms were apparent on day 10 of DILS, when disruption of organelles-nucleus and mitochondria became evident. Also, during this latter-stage apoptosis, represented by shrinking of the protoplast, tonoplast interruption, vacuole breakdown, chromatin condensation, DNA fragmentation, and disintegration of the cell membrane were prominent. Reversal of DILS by re-exposure of the plants from dark to light was possible until but not later than day 7 of dark exposure and was accompanied by regained photosynthesis, increase in chlorophyll, and reversal of RFD, despite the induction of macro-ATG-related genes.

CONCLUSION

The ablation of TLR-4 attenuated aging-induced MR and contractile dysfunction through NCoRI-HDAC1-mediated regulation of CP/ATG. Yeast was used for research on aging and age-related diseases. CP/ATG-related genes with CVDs and intermediate vascular traits were explored in addition to epigenetic regulation of vascular aging. Mitochondrial metabolic dysfunction and aging, adjustment of the lysosomal-mitochondrial axis for control of cellular senescence, significance of MTs in aging brain and longevity, sestrin-like protein in CP during starvation, increased transport of acetyl-CoA into the ER causing a progeria-like phenotype, deletion of Nrip1 for extending longevity, and enhancing CP to delay cellular senescence are described. The mechanism of natural products with anti-aging potential, such as Curcumin, Retinol, Hyaluronic acid, chondroitin Suphate, glucosamine, Collagen, Vitamin C (Ascorbic acid), Vitamin-E, Vitamin-D, Epigallocatechin gallate (PGCE), Green Tea (Catechin), Biotin, Pentapeptide-48, Nicotinamide Riboside, Theanine, Rhodiola, Nicotinamide Mononucleotide, Crocin, Garlic, Astraglus, Fesetin, Reseveratrol, and several others as described in the introduction of this edition. Majority of these natural and synthetic products are used in skin and hair care industry as well as potent CP/ATG regulators. Spermidine in health, disease, and aging as a CP regulator, and the mitochondrial-endonuclease-G-mediated breakdown of paternal mitochondria upon fertilization are described. Protective effects of ATG were observed in blue light-induced retinal degeneration of aged mice. The ubiquinone-mediated longevity was marked by reduced cytoplasmic mRNA translation. Transient p53 inhibition sensitized aged WAT during beige adipocyte recruitment by blocking CP. *S*-Nitrosylation derived cell senescence and aging by regulating MQC and CP. CP/ATG and apoptosis can be regulated in mouse and human skeletal muscle with aging through lifelong exercise and by de-nitrosylation, whereas ADH5/GSNOR linked CP/ATG to aging.

Skeletal muscle from aged American quarter horses exhibited compromised MQC and CP/ATG biomarkers. The effect of CP/ATG, mitochondria, and mechanisms of ischemic preconditioning were investigated in the aged kidney. The loss of the ubiquitin-conjugating enzyme, UBE2E3, induced cellular senescence. Mitochondria, CP/ATG–inflammation–cell death axis, and telomere shortening were implicated in aging. SIRT3 deficiency exacerbated p53/Parkin-mediated MTG inhibition and promoted CBMP in aging hearts. A young-like molecular pattern was observed by over-expression of PGC-1α in the aging muscle, whereas chronic stress compromised MQC in accelerated aging due to compromised CP accompanied with CBMP induction. Hence, targeting normal, cancerous, and senescent cells could be a potential TSE-EBPT strategy for senotherapy. Dark-induced leaf senescence and its reversal in barley was also transcriptionally regulated by CP/ATG.

REFERENCES

Borbolis, F. and P. Syntichaki. 2015. Cytoplasmic mRNA turnover and ageing. Mech Ageing Dev 152: 32–42.

Cătană, C.S., A.G. Atanasov and I. Berindan-Neagoe. 2018. Natural products with anti-aging potential: Affected targets and molecular mechanisms. Biotechnol Adv 36: 1649–1656.

Charmpilas, N., K. Kounakis and N. Tavernarakis. 2018. Monitoring mitophagy during aging in caenorhabditis elegans. Methods Mol Biol 1759: 151–160.

Dethlefsen, M.M., J.F. Halling, H.D. Møller, P. Plomgaard, et al. 2018. Regulation of apoptosis and ATG in mouse and human skeletal muscle with aging and lifelong exercise training. Exp Gerontol 111: 141–153.

Diot, A., T. Agnew, J. Sanderson, C. Liao, et al. 2018. Validating the RedMIT/GFP-LC3 mouse model by studying MTG in autosomal dominant optic atrophy due to the OPA1Q285STOP mutation. Front Cell Dev Biol 6: 103.

Ekmekcioglu, C. 2019. Nutrition and longevity–From mechanisms to uncertainties. Crit Rev Food Sci Nutr 21: 1–20.

Fu, W., Y. Liu, C. Sun and H. Yin. 2019. Transient p53 inhibition sensitizes aged white adipose tissue for beige adipocyte recruitment by blocking mitophagy. 33: 844–856.

Furuya, N. 2018. Short overview. Methods Mol Biol 1759: 3–8.

Garcia, S., N. Nissanka, E.A. Mareco, S. Rossi, et al. 2018. Overexpression of PGC-1α in aging muscle enhances a subset of young-like molecular patterns. Aging Cell 17(2): e12707.

Green, D.R., L. Galluzi and G. Kroemer. 2011. Mitochondria and the autophagy-inflammation-cell death axis in organismal aging. Science 333: 1109–1112.

Higuchi-Sanabria, R., P.A. Frankino, J.W. Paul III, S.U. Tronnes, et al. 2018. A futile battle? Protein quality control and the stress of aging. Dev Cell 44: 139–163.

Hrdinka, M. and M. Yabal. 2019. Inhibitor of apoptosis proteins in human health and disease. Genes Immun 20: 641–650.

Janikiewicz, J., J. Szymański, D. Malinska, P. Patalas-Krawczyk, et al. 2018. Mitochondria-associated membranes in aging and senescence: Structure, function, and dynamics. Cell Death Dis 9(3): 332.

Jankauskas, S.S., D.N. Silachev, N.V. Andrianova, I.B. Pevzner, et al. 2018. Aged kidney: Can we protect it? ATG, mitochondria and mechanisms of ischemic preconditioning. Cell Cycle 17: 1291–1309.

Jin, J., Y. Liu, L. Huang and H. Tan. 2019. Advances in epigenetic regulation of vascular aging. Rev Cardiovasc Med 20(1): 19–25.

Jing, Y.H., J.L. Yan, Q.J. Wang, H.C. Chen, et al. 2018. Spermidine ameliorates the neuronal aging by improving the mitochondrial function *in vitro*. Exp Gerontol 108: 77–86.

Leidal, A.M., B. Levine and J. Debnath. 2018. Autophagy and the cell biology of age-related disease. Nat Cell Biol 20: 1338–1348.

Li, C., S.H. White, L.K. Warren, S.E. Wohlgemuth. 2018a. Skeletal muscle from aged american quarter horses shows impairments in mitochondrial biogenesis and expression of autophagy markers. Exp Gerontol 102: 19–27.

Li, Y., Y. Ma, L. Song, L. Yu, et al. 2018b. SIRT3 deficiency exacerbates p53/Parkin-mediated mitophagy inhibition and promotes mitochondrial dysfunction: Implication for aged hearts. Int J Mol Med 41: 3517–3526.

Lim, S.H., M.J. Kim and J. Lee. 2019. Intake of psyllium seed husk reduces white matter damage in a rat model of chronic cerebral hypoperfusion. Nutr Res 67: 27–39.

Lin, Z. and D. Fang. 2013. The roles of SIRT1 in cancer. Genes Cancer 4: 97–104.

Lizama, B.N., A.M. Palubinsky, V.A. Raveendran, A.M. Moore. 2018. Neuronal preconditioning requires the mitophagic activity of C-terminus of HSC70-interacting protein. J Neurosci 38: 6825–6840.

López-Lluch, G., J.D. Hernández-Camacho, D.J.M. Fernández-Ayala and P. Navas. 2018. Mitochondrial dysfunction in metabolism and aging: Shared mechanisms and outcomes? Biogerontology 19: 461–480.

Madeo, F., D. Carmona-Gutierrez, S.J. Hofer and G. Kroemer. 2019. Caloric restriction mimetics against age-associated disease: Targets, mechanisms, and therapeutic potential. Cell Metab 29: 592–610.

Markaki, M., K. Palikaras and N. Tavernarakis. 2018. Novel insights into the anti-aging role of mitophagy. Int Rev Cell Mol Biol 340: 169–208.

Maruzs T., Z. Simon-Vecsei, V. Kiss, T. Csizmadia, et al. 2019. On the fly: Recent progress on autophagy and aging in *Drosophila*. Front Cell Dev Biol 7: 140.

Medeiros, T.C and M. Graef. 2019. ATG determines mtDNA copy number dynamics during starvation. Autophagy 15: 178–179.

Molenaars, M., G.E. Janssens, T. Santermans, M. Lezzerini, et al. 2018. Mitochondrial ubiquinone-mediated longevity is marked by reduced cytoplasmic mRNA translation. Life Sci Alliance 1(5): e201800082.

Paillusson, S., R. Stoica, P. Gomez-Suaga, D.H.W. Lau, et al. 2016. There's something wrong with my MAM; The ER-mitochondria axis and neurodegenerative diseases. Trends Neurosci 39(3): 146–157.

Park, J.T., Y.S. Lee, K.A. Cho and S.C. Park. 2018. Adjustment of the lysosomal-mitochondrial axis for control of cellular senescence. Aging Res Rev 47: 176–182.

Peng, Y., S.L. Shapiro, V.C. Banduseela, I.A. Dieterich, et al. 2018. Increased transport of acetyl-CoA into the endoplasmic reticulum causes a progeria-like phenotype. Aging Cell 17(5): e12820.

Plafker, K.S., K. Zyla, W. Berry and S.M. Plafker. 2018. Loss of the ubiquitin conjugating enzyme UBE2E3 induces cellular senescence. Redox Biol 17: 411–422.

Portilla-Fernandez, E., M. Ghanbari, J.B.J. van Meurs, A.H.J. Danser, et al. 2019. Dissecting the association of autophagy-related genes with cardiovascular diseases and intermediate vascular traits: A population-based approach. PLoS One. 14: e0214137.

Rafia, S. and S. Saran. 2019. Sestrin-like protein from *Dictyostelium discoideum* is involved in autophagy under starvation stress. Microbiol Res 220: 61–71.

Rizza, S. and G. Filomeni. 2018. Denitrosylate and live longer: How ADH5/GSNOR links MTG to aging. Autophagy 14: 1285–1287.

Rizza, S., S. Cardaci, C. Montagna, G. Di Giacomo, et al. 2018. S-nitrosylation drives cell senescence and aging in mammals by controlling mitochondrial dynamics and mitophagy. Proc. Natl Acad Sci U.S.A. 115: E3388–E3397.

Saito, N., J. Araya, S. Ito, K. Tsubouchi, et al. 2019. Involvement of lamin B1 reduction in accelerated cellular senescence during chronic obstructive pulmonary disease pathogenesis. J Immunol 202: 1428–1440.

Sharma, S. and M. Ebadi. 2014a. Significance of metallothioneins in aging brain. Neurochem Int 65: 40–48.

Sharma, S. and M. Ebadi. 2014b. Charnoly body as a universal biomarker of cell injury. Biomarkers & Genomic Medicine 6: 89–98.

Sharma, S., J. Choga, V. Gupta, F. N-Kalala, et al. 2016. Charnoly body as novel biomarker of nutritional stress in Alzheimer's disease. Functional Foods in Health & Disease 6: 344–370.

Sharma, S. 2019. The Charnoly Body: A Novel of Mitochondrial Bioenergetics. CRC Press, Taylor & Francis Group, Boca Raton, FL, U.S.A.

Sobieszczuk-Nowicka, E., T. Wrzesiński, A. Bagniewska-Zadworna, S. Kubala, et al. 2018. Physio-genetic dissection of dark-induced leaf senescence and timing its reversal in barley. Plant Physiol 178: 654–671.

Wang, S., W. Ge, C. Harns, X. Meng, et al. 2018a. Ablation of toll-like receptor 4 attenuates aging-induced myocardial remodeling and contractile dysfunction through NCoRI-HDAC1-mediated regulation of autophagy. J Mol Cell Cardiol 119: 40–50.

Wang, J., X. Chen, J. Osland, S.J. Gerber, et al. 2018b. Deletion of Nrip1 extends female mice longevity, increases autophagy, and delays cell senescence. J Gerontol A Biol Sci Med Sci 73: 882–892.

Wang, D., Z. Huang, L. Li, Y. Yuan, et al. 2019. Intracarotid cold saline infusion contributes to neuroprotection in MCAO-induced ischemic stroke in rats via serum and glucocorticoid-regulated kinase 1. Mol Med Rep 20: 3942–3950.

Wang, S., M.R. Kandadi and J. Ren. 2019a. Double knock out of Akt2 and AMPK predisposes cardiac aging without affecting life-span: Role of Autophagy and Mitophagy. Biochimia et Biophisica Acta. (Molecular Basis of Disease). 1865: 1865–1875.

Wei, W., Z.T. Rosenkrans, Q.Y. Luo, X. Lan, et al. 2019. Exploiting nanomaterial-mediated autophagy for cancer therapy. Small Methods 3(2): 1800365.

Wu, N.N. and J. Ren. 2019. Aldehyde dehydrogenase 2 (ALDH2) and aging: Is there a sensible link? Adv Exp Med Biol 1193: 237–253.

Yin, J., X. Lu, Z. Qian, W. Xu, et al. 2019. New insights into the pathogenesis and treatment of sarcopenia in chronic heart failure. Theranostics 9(14): 4019–4029.

Zhao, S., X. Zhang and Y. Ke. 2019. Progress on correlation between cell senescence and idiopathic pulmonary fibrosis. J Zhejiang Univ (Med Sci) 48(1): 111–115.

Zhang, W., Q. Ma, S. Siraj, P.A. Ney, et al. 2019. Nix-mediated mitophagy regulates platelet activation and life span. Blood advances, 3(15): 2342–2354.

Zhou, Q., H. Li, A. Nakagawa, J.L. Lin, et al. 2016. Mitochondrial endonuclease G mediates breakdown of paternal mitochondria upon fertilization. Science 353: 394–399.

Part-5

Charnolophagy in Nanomedicine

33

Charnolophagy in Nanotheranostics
(Part-1)

INTRODUCTION

Nanotechnology has conferred clinically significant information at the cellular, molecular, and genetic level to facilitate the TSE-EBPT of chronic MDR diseases. Many theranostic nanomaterials have been developed by integrating therapeutic and diagnostic agents in a single platform. Recently, the author highlighted advances in the safe, economical, and effective management of NDDs, CVDs, and cancer by adopting emerging nanotheranostic strategies (Sharma 2014). Efficient drug delivery systems are very important for the discovery of novel CPTs. The EBPM promises to deliver the right drug to the right patient at appropriate time because it takes into consideration clinically-significant genetic predisposition, chronopharmacological, and charnolopharmacological aspects of nanotheranostics. The real-time visualization of nano-drug carrier bio-distributions, drug release processes, and theranostic responses can render information needed for optimizing real-time personalized treatment as described by Jo et al. (2016). Nanotheranostic imaging can be utilized for: (i) monitoring drug bio-distribution, (ii) visualizing drug release, (iii) assessing therapeutic efficacy, (iv) simultaneous optical imaging, photodynamic therapy, and (v) NPs for optical imaging. Nanotheranostic MRI is performed by Gd-based theranostic agents; Magnetic NPs-based theranostic agents; nanotheranostic X-ray, CT; nanotheranostic PET; nanotheranostic US imaging; *in situ* gas-generating materials; and high-intensity focused ultrasound-triggered controlled release of drugs. Multifunctional NPs possessing both theranostic and imaging properties for NDDs, CVDs, and MDR malignancies are currently being developed. Particularly, drug encapsulation in pegylated liposomes has improved the pharmacodynamics (PDs) of these diseases. NPs are particularly promising for cancer theranostics due to their tumor-targeting capability induced by the enhanced permeability and retention (EPR) effect. Long-circulating liposomes and block copolymers concentrate slowly via EPR in the solid tumors and are highly significant for efficient drug delivery in MDR cancer chemotherapeutics. NPs can be easily surface-modified to make them stealthy for the immune system, to increase their blood circulation times, and avoid the retention of drug-loaded NPs in the reticuloendothelial (lungs, liver, and spleen) system. NPs can be used as promising platforms for constructing "All-in-One" delivery systems in which all functions (therapeutic, imaging, targeting, controlled release) are integrated. All-in-one NPs enable researchers to combine diagnosis, therapy, and monitoring operations for the treatment of cancer to save considerable time, money, and energy of the hospital and patient. Theranostic NPs can be used for image-guided cancer therapy. Real-time non-invasive visualization of the tumor accumulation behavior of drugs can help define the limits of the drug's influence zone, while visualization of the drug release and apoptosis can help optimize the dose and schedule of the drug treatment, and monitoring of theranostic responses can provide immediate feedback regarding how well the treatment works for each patient and can thus enable researchers to modify treatment strategies as needed. Nanotheranostics will accomplish these goals toward realizing personalized cancer care.

The selective targeting of siRNA, miRNA, and oligonucleotides to tumor cells with a potential to inhibit MDR malignancies has also shown promise. In addition, implantable drug delivery devices have improved the theranostic potential of several chronic diseases. Recently, the author proposed microRNA, MTs, α-Syn index, and CB, CP, and CS as novel drug discovery biomarkers in nenotheranostics. Particularly, ROS-scavenging antioxidant-loaded targeted NPs can be developed as CB and CP regulators for the TSE-EBPT of NDDs and CVDs. The nonspecific induction of CBs in the hyper-proliferative cells may cause alopecia, GIT symptoms, myelosuppression, neurotoxicity, and infertility. Therefore, nanoformulations may be designed to augment cancer stem cell specific CB formation and regulate CP and CS to eradicate MDR malignancies with minimum or no adverse effects as highlighted in this chapter.

Recently, nanocarriers for nanotheranostic applications including: polymer conjugations, dendrimers, micelles, liposomes, metal and inorganic NPs, carbon nanotubes, and NPs of biodegradable polymers for sustained, controlled, and targeted co-delivery of diagnostic and therapeutic agents for superior theranostics with fewer side effects have been summarized (Muthu et al. 2014, Mei et al. 2014). NPs-induced CP/ATG is currently being exploited for biomedical and toxicological applications (Peynshaert et al. 2014, Reynold et al. 2017, Sharma 2014), and as CQ-modified NPs (Sleightholm et al. 2017) for the treatment of CNS, CVD, and MDR malignancies and enhanced drug delivery (Zhang et al. 2014a,b). The CP/ATG targeted nanotheranostics can achieve systemic circulation, evade host defenses, and deliver the theranostic agents at the targeted site to diagnose and treat the disease at the cellular, molecular, genetic, and epigenetic levels simultaneously. The therapeutic and diagnostic agents, nano-formulated as a single platform, can be further conjugated to a biological ligand for drug targeting. Nanotheranostics can also promote stimuli-responsive release, synergetic and combinatory therapy, siRNA co-delivery, multimodality therapies, oral delivery, delivery across the blood-brain barrier, as well as modulation of intracellular CP/ATG. The fruition of nanotheranostics will confer DSST-TSE-EBPT-CPTs with a promising prognosis, which would render even the fatal diseases curable or at least treatable at an earliest stage.

Recently, it has been highlighted that the modulation of the mTOR, the principal regulator of cellular homeostasis (Papadopolim et al. 2019), underlies the biological effects of engineered NPs, including the regulation of cell death/survival and metabolic responses (Lunova et al. 2019). Hence, the basic understanding of the mechanisms and biological actions of NP-mediated mTOR modulation may help in developing safe and efficient nanotherapeutics to cure human disease. CP/ATG is a transcriptionally regulated catabolic process which maintains ICD and homeostasis. It plays a crucial role in the clearance of damaged cellular organelles (mitochondria), misfolded or aggregated proteins like α-Syn, β-amyloid peptides, and Tau proteins, and infectious pathogens (bacteria, virus, fungus, and parasites). Dysfunction in CP/ATG leads to the development of NDDs, CVDs, MDR malignancies, chronic infection, aging, and other diseases. Therefore, modulation of CP/ATG has theranostic significance in that it can successfully cure chronic intractable diseases including using external stimuli. Recently, researchers proposed small molecules such as CQ, 3-MA, Rapamycin, etc. for the treatment of cancer through CP/ATG regulation. However, these molecules have side effects which limit their clinical application. Hence, the nanotheranostic approach could stand as an alternative treatment option to induce selective and spatiotemporal CP/ATG for the TSE-EBPT of cancer. Several investigators developed a variety of nanomaterials as CP/ATG inducers or inhibitors. Recently, Zheng et al. (2017) highlighted the impacts of various NMs on CP/ATG and their functional consequences. They discussed the underlying mechanisms for NM-modulated CP/ATG. Nanomaterials (NMs) have CP/ATG-modulating effects, thus predicting a valuable and promising application of NMs in the diagnosis and treatment of almost all CP/ATG-related diseases. NMs exhibit unique physico-chemical and bio-functional properties, which may endow NMs to modulate CP/ATG via various mechanisms. Particularly, CP elucidates and resolves many intricate nanotheranostic mechanisms involved in CP, MTG, and generalized ATG, and confers a detailed understanding of the basic events involved in MQC and ICD for NCF.

Despite the extensive genetic and phenotypic variations present in the different tumors, they frequently share common metabolic alterations, such as CP/ATG, a self-degradative process in response to stresses by which damaged macromolecules and organelles are targeted by vesicles to lysosomes and then eliminated. CP/ATG dysfunctions can promote tumorigenesis and cancer development, but, its overstimulation by cytotoxic drugs may also induce cell death and chemo-sensitivity. Hence, the possibility to modulate CP/ATG may represent a valid theranostic approach to treat different types of cancers using CP/ATG modulators, are currently employed. Recent progress in nanotechnology offers unique opportunities to fight cancer with innovative and efficient therapeutic agents by overcoming obstacles encountered with traditional drug therapy regimens. Nanomaterials can modulate CP/ATG and have been exploited as theranostic agents against cancer. Recently, investigators highlighted advances in the application of metallic nanostructures as potent modulators of CP/ATG through multiple mechanisms, emphasizing their theranostic application in cancer. Hence, CP/ATG modulation with NP-based strategies would gain clinical relevance as a complementary therapy for the TSE-EBPT of cancers and other chronic MDR diseases.

The current therapeutic strategies for brain diseases are based on symptomatology and most of these diseases are incurable. Nanotechnology has the potential to facilitate the transport of drugs across the blood-brain barrier (BBB) and enhance their PKs profile. However, to reach clinical application, the precise understanding of nano-neurotoxicity in terms of oxidative stress and inflammation is required. Emerging evidence has shown that NPs have the potential to alter CP/ATG, which can induce inflammation and oxidative stress, or vice versa. Catalan-Figueroa et al. (2016) emphasized how nanomaterials may induce neurotoxicity focusing on neurodegeneration, and how these effects could be exploited toward brain cancer treatment. Feng et al. (2015) discussed the dual effect of NMs on the CNS. NMs are used for the therapy, diagnosis, and monitoring of disease- or drug-induced mechanisms in a biological system. In view of their small size, after certain modifications, NMs have the potential to bypass or cross the BBB. Nanotechnology is particularly advantageous in the field of neurology. For example, the utilization of NP-based drug carriers to readily cross the BBB to treat CNS tumors, nano-scaffolds for axonal regeneration, and nano-electromechanical systems in neurological operations, and NPs in CNS molecular imaging. However, NPs can also be potentially hazardous in terms of neurotoxicity via oxidative stress, CP, ATG, lysosome dysfunction, and the activation of signaling pathways involved in CP dysregulation and CBMP.

Generally, NPs can be classified into two broad categories: (i) inorganic (metallic) and (ii) organic (nonmetallic). In this chapter, a brief description of inorganic (metallic) and organic (nonmetallic) NPs for the TSE-EBPT of chronic MDR diseases is provided. The chapter also highlights recent developments and the theranostic significance of CP/ATG in nanomedicine with a primary focus on the treatment of MDR malignancies, in addition to CVDs and NDDs. Molecular mechanisms of NPs-mediated CP/ATG induction/inhibition, developing new strategies to fight against chronic diseases, microbial infections, CP/ATG inhibition/induction, and future challenges are described. The chapter also highlights the theranostic significance of MTs and their versatility as early and sensitive biomarkers in cell-based therapy and nanomedicine.

The Theranostic Significance of MTs as CP Regulators

Recently, the author described that MTs are low molecular weight (6–7 kDa) cysteine-rich proteins that are specifically induced by metal NPs. MT induction in cell-based therapy may provide better protection by serving as potent antioxidant, anti-inflammatory, and anti-apoptotic agents, and by augmenting the zinc-mediated transcriptional regulation of genes involved in cell proliferation and differentiation (Sharma et al. 2013). A liposome-encapsulated MT-1 promoter has been used extensively to induce GH or other genes in culture and gene-manipulated animals. MTs are induced as a defensive mechanism in chronic inflammatory conditions including NDDs, CVDs, cancer, and microbial infections; hence, they can serve as early and sensitive biomarkers of environmental safety and effectiveness of newly developed NPs for theranostic applications. A microarray analysis has suggested that MTs are significantly induced in MDR malignancies and during radiation treatment. Nutritional stress and environmental toxins (Kainic acid and Domoic acid) also induce MTs and the aggregation of multi-lamellar electron-dense membrane stacks (CBs) due to mitochondrial degeneration. MTs enhance the MB of reduced nicotinamide adenine dinucleotide-ubiquinone oxidoreductase (complex-1), a rate-limiting enzyme complex involved in the O/P. Monoamine oxidase-B inhibitors (Selegiline, Rasagiline) inhibited α-Syn nitration, implicated in Lewy body formation, and inhibited MPP^+ and SIN-1-induced apoptosis in cultured human DAergic (SK-N-SH and SH-S-Y5Y)) neurons and mesencephalic fetal stem cells. MTs as potent free radical scavengers inhibit CB formation, enhance CP, and stabilize CS and neurodegenerative charnolopathies; hence, CB formation, CP induction/repression, CS stabilizers/destabilizers, and the α-Syn index may be used as early and sensitive biomarkers to assess NP effectiveness and toxicity to discover better drug delivery and surgical interventions. Furthermore, pharmacological interventions augmenting MTs may facilitate the theranostic potential of NP-labeled cells and other theranostic agents. In addition, the author has proposed three types of NPs for the TSE-EBPT of chronic MDR diseases, including (i) toxic NPs, (ii) neutral NPs, and (iii) protective NPs. Toxic NPs enhance CB formation, impair CP, and destabilize CS to induce IS activation and apoptosis/nectrosis through the induction of CBMP; neutral NPs neither enhance CB formation nor CP induction, repression, or CS destabilization, whereas protective NPs enhance MTs, inhibit CB formation, regulate CP, and stabilize CS and its exocytosis as a mechanism of MQC and ICD for NCF by preventing CBMP. These unique characteristics of MTs might be helpful in the synthesis, characterization, and functionalization of emerging NPs for theranostic applications (Sharma and Ebadi 2014a, b).

Cancer Stem Cell-specific CS Targeted Therapies for MDR Malignancies

The author proposed cancer-stem-cell-specific CB agonists, CP antagonists, and CS destabilizers for the TSE-EBPT of MDR malignancies (Sharma 2014, Sharma and Ebadi 2014a, b, 2016a, b, 2017, 2019). Recently, Singh et al. (2017) focused on the biological processes regulating cancer stem cells' (CSCs) drug resistance and strategies to deal with them. They also reviewed various nano-theranostic approaches to overcome CSCs-related issues and their future perspectives. CSCs exhibit distinctive self-renewal, proliferation, and differentiation capabilities, and play a significant role in cancer. CSCs have significant impacts on the progression of tumors, drug resistance, recurrence and metastasis in different malignancies. Due to their primary role, most researchers have focused on developing anti-CSC theranostic strategies, and extensive efforts have been made to explore methods for the selective eradication of MDR cells. Many reports have shown that the use of CSCs-specific approaches such as ATP-binding cassette (ABC) transporters, blockade of self-renewal and survival of CSCs, CSCs-surface-markers-targeted drugs delivery, and eradication of the tumor microenvironment. Small molecule drugs, such as nucleic acids and antibodies can destroy CSCs selectively. Xie et al. (2016) provided the latest information to summarize the concept, strategies, mechanisms, and current status as well as future promises of nanotheranostic strategies for the eradication of CSCs. These are original cancer cells that have characteristics associated with normal stem cells. CSCs are highly resistant against various treatments and thus responsible for cancer metastasis and recurrence. Therefore, the development of specific and effective treatments for CSCs plays a key role in improving the survival and QOL of cancer patients, especially those in the metastatic stage. Nanomedicine strategies, which include prodrugs, micelles, liposomes, and NPs of biodegradable, nonimmunogenic, biocompatible, and disease-specific polymers, could improve the theranostic index of conventional therapeutics due to sustained, controlled, targeted delivery, and high transportation efficiency across the cell membrane and low elimination by intracellular CP/ATG, thus providing a promising solution to solve the problem encountered in CSCs treatment.

The Nanotheranostic Significance of CP in MDR Malignancies

Nanomaterial-induced ATG in MDR Malignancies

The theranostic strategies to counteract cancer imply killing off specifically malignant cells. The most exploited cell death mechanism in cancer therapies is apoptosis, but recently, other mechanisms, mainly CP, MTG, and ATG, could represent a novel approach in the fight against cancer. Panzarini and Dini (2014) published the relationship between MDR reversal and NMs or ATG pointing to hypothesize a pivotal role of ATG modulation induced by NMs in counteracting MDR which enables the cancer cells to develop MDR, especially for chemotherapy. The MDR mechanisms include: (a) the decreased uptake of the drug, (b) reduced intracellular drug concentration by efflux pumps, (c) altered cell cycle checkpoints, (d) altered drug targets, (e) increased metabolism of drugs, (f) induced emergency response genes to impair the apoptotic pathway, and (g) altered drug detoxification. Great efforts have been made to reverse MDR. Currently, CP/ATG and nanosized drug delivery systems (DDSs) confer alternative strategies to circumvent MDR. Nanosized DDSs accumulate chemotherapeutics at the target sites and control the spatiotemporal drug release into tumor cells. Similarly, CP/ATG could overrule MDR upon its activation by ensuring cell death via switching its pro-survival role to a pro-death one or by mediating cell death, that is, apoptosis or necrosis. Hence, CP/ATG inhibition could counteract MDR by sensitizing the cells to anticancer molecules, that is, the Src family TK (SFK) inhibitors or 5-Fluorouracil. CP/ATG is a common cellular response to NMs, corroborating the fascinating idea of exploitation of NM-induced CP, MTG, and ATG in nanotheranostics. An overview of CP regulation and CBMP nenotheranostics in chronic MDR diseases is presented in Fig. 50.

AIEgens for Biological Process and Nanotheranostics

Monitoring biological processes and the diagnosis of diseases based on fluorescent techniques would provide comprehensive knowledge about the mechanism of pathogenesis of diseases, and precisely evaluating the therapeutic potential of novel CPTs in nanotheranostics. It relies on fluorophores with excellent photostability, large Stokes shift, high S/N ratio, and free of aggregation-caused quenching (ACQ). Luminogens with aggregation-induced emission characteristic (AIEgens) could serve for biological process monitoring and disease theranostics.

Gu et al. (2017) discussed the recent results in monitoring biological processes such as CP, MTG, ATG, mitochondrial dynamics, mitosis, long-term cellular tracing of CP/ATG, and apoptosis as well as the diagnosis of diseases based on AIEgens in real time. As part of AIEgens and AIEgen-based NPs with the functionalities of drugs, photosensitizers, and adjuvants accompanied with imaging, these NPs confer image-guided chemotherapy, photodynamic therapy, and radiotherapy, indicating their potential for understanding disease pathogenesis, for drug development, and the evaluation for EBPT. Hence, future research efforts focused on developing long-wavelength excitable and phosphorescence-emissive AIEgens with improved depth-penetration and minimum Bkg interference for fluorescence and photoacoustic imaging, will extend the theranostic applications of AIEgens.

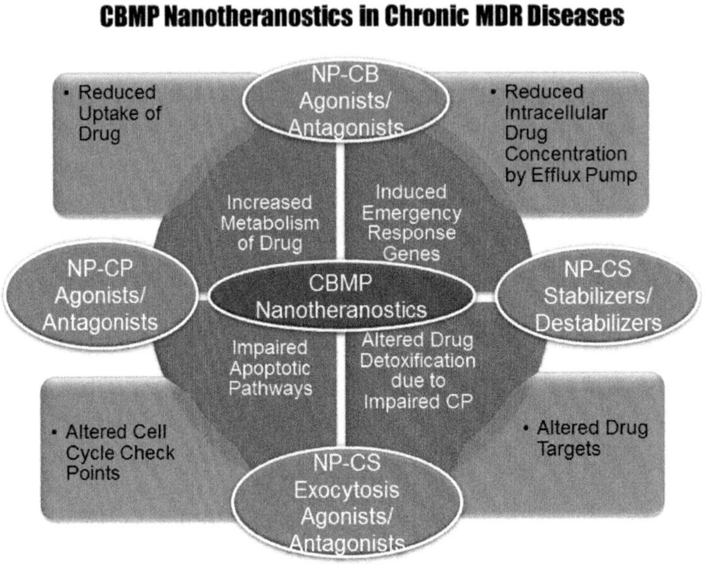

CBMP Nanotheranostics in Chronic MDR Diseases

Figure 50

Folate-appended Methyl-β-Cyclodextrin

Kameyama et al. (2017) revealed that folate-appended methyl-β-cyclodextrin (FA-M-β-CyD) provides selective antitumor activity in folate receptor-α (FR-α)-expressing cells by the induction of ATG. To gain insight into the detailed mechanism of this antitumor activity, they induced MTG by the treatment of FR-α-expressing tumor cells with FA-M-β-CyD. In contrast to methyl-β-cyclodextrin, FA-M-β-CyD entered KB cells and human epithelial cells from a fatal cervical carcinoma (FR-α (+) through FR-α-mediated endocytosis. The transmembrane potential of isolated mitochondria after treatment with FA-M-β-CyD was elevated. In addition, FA-M-β-CyD lowered ATP production and promoted ROS production in KB cells (FR-α (+)). FA-M-β-CyD enhanced LC3 conversion (LC3-I to LC3-II) in KB cells (FR-α (+)) and induced PINK1 protein expression, involved in the induction of MTG. Furthermore, FA-M-β-CyD had potent antitumor activity in BALB/c *nu/nu* mice xenografted with KB cells (FR-α (+)) without any significant side effects, demonstrating that the ATG cell death by FA-M-β-CyD could be associated with CP, MTG, and ATG induced by an impaired mitochondrial function.

Nanozymes in Biology and Medicine

Golchin et al. (2017) developed metal NPs and explored their theranostic potential in modern medicine. Nanozymes are artificial enzymes and have widespread applications including targeted cancer therapy, diagnostic medicine, and bio-sensing (even environmental toxicology). These applications are a novel research field in medicine, and are growing fast. Enzyme-based applications such as ELISA are expensive because of the complexity of producing enzymes and antibodies. Some NPs can mimic these enzymes such as superoxides and can manipulate biological pathways directly like CP, MTG, and ATG, which make them a suitable alternative for nanotheranostics.

Nanoporous Microstructures and Osteogenesis

The osteo-immune environment plays an indispensable role in bone regeneration because the early immune environment that exists during the regenerative process promotes the recruitment and differentiation of osteoblastic lineage cells. The response of immune cells growing on nano-topographic surfaces and the microenvironment they generate should be considered when evaluating nano-topography-mediated osteogenesis. Chen et al. (2017) investigated the modulatory effects of nano-porous anodic alumina with different sized pores on macrophage responses and their subsequent effects on the osteogenic differentiation of BMSCs. The nanopore structure and the pore size proved important adhesive cues for macrophages, which affected their spreading and cell shape, regulated the expression and activation of ATG pathway components (LC3A/B, Beclin-1, Atg3, Atg7, and p62), and modulated the inflammatory response, osteoclastic activities, and release of osteogenic factors. The osteogenic pathways (Wnt and BMP) of BMSCs were regulated by different nanopore-induced inflammatory environments, which affected the osteogenic differentiation. This study emphasized the effects of immune cells on nano-topography-mediated osteogenesis, which could lead to novel strategies for the development of advanced nano-biomaterials for tissue engineering, nanomedicine, and immunotherapeutic applications.

Cationic PEGylated Liposomes in MDR Malignancies

Antimicrobial peptides (AMPs) have been recently evaluated as a new generation of adjuvants in cancer chemotherapy. Juang et al. (2016) designed PEGylated liposomes encapsulating Epirubicin as an antineoplastic agent and tilapia Hepcidin 2–3, an AMP, as a MDR transporter suppressor and an apoptosis/ATG modulator in human cervical cancer HeLa cells. The co-treatment of HeLa cells with the PEGylated liposomal formulation of Epirubicin and Hepcidin 2–3 significantly increased the cytotoxicity of Epirubicin. The liposomal formulations of Epirubicin and/or Hepcidin 2–3 escalated the intracellular H_2O_2 and O_2^- levels of cancer cells. These treatments reduced the mRNA expressions of MDR protein 1, MDR-associated protein (MRP) 1, and MRP2. The addition of Hepcidin 2–3 in liposomes enhanced the Epirubicin uptake and localized into the nucleus and triggered CP/ATG and apoptosis in HeLa cells, as confirmed by $\Delta\Psi$ collapse, LC3-II, caspase-3, caspase-9 activation, PARP cleavage. The apoptosis was also confirmed by the rise in the sub-G1 phase of the DNA cell cycle and apoptosis percentage of annexin V/propidium iodide flow cytometric assays. The liposomal Epirubicin and Hepcidin 2–3 augmented the accumulation of GFP-LC3 puncta amplified by CQ, implying the involvement of CP/ATG. The partial inhibition of necroptosis and the epithelial-mesenchymal transition by this combination was also verified, indicating that co-incubation with PEGylated liposomes of Hepcidin 2–3 and Epirubicin causes cervical cancer cells' demise through the modulation of multiple signaling pathways, including MDR transporters, CP/ATG, apoptosis, and/or necroptosis. Thus, this nano-formulation may provide a platform for the combined treatment of traditional chemotherapy and Hepcidin 2–3 as a novel adjuvant for effective MDR reversal.

Caveolin-1 Contributes to Realgar NP Therapy

Chronic myelogenous leukemia (CML) is characterized by the t(9;22) (q34;q11)-associated Bcr-Abl fusion gene, which is an essential element of clinical diagnosis. As a traditional Chinese medicine, Realgar has been used for the treatment of various diseases for >1,500 years. Realgar NPs were prepared with an average particle size of <100 nm (Tian et al. 2014). Compared with coarse Realgar, the Realgar NPs have higher bioavailability. As a principal constituent protein of caveolae, caveolin-1 (Cav-1) participates in regulating various cellular physiological and pathological processes, including tumorigenesis and tumor development. Shi et al. (2016) found that Realgar NPs inhibit cell proliferation of K562 cells and degrade Bcr-Abl fusion protein. Both apoptosis and ATG were activated in Realgar-NPs-treated cells, and the induction of ATG was associated with the class I PI3K/Akt/mTOR pathway. A morphological analysis indicated that Realgar NPs induced differentiation in CML cells. Hence Cav-1 might play a crucial role in Realgar nanotheranostics. To study the effects of Cav-1 on K562 cells during the Realgar NP treatment, a Cav-1 overexpression cell model was established by using transient transfection. Cav-1 overexpression inhibited K562 cell proliferation, promoted endogenic ATG, and increased the sensitivity of K562 cells to Realgar NPs, demonstrating that they degrade Bcr-Abl oncoprotein, while the underlying mechanism might be related to apoptosis and ATG, and Cav-1 might be considered as a potential target for comprehensive therapy of CML.

Barriers of PC

Pancreatic ductal adenocarcinoma (PDAC) is one of the leading causes of cancer-related deaths. PDAC remains one of the most difficult-to-treat cancers, owing to its unique patho-physiological features: a nearly impenetrable desmoplastic stroma, and hypovascular and hypo-perfused tumor vessels which render most treatment options ineffective (Orth et al. 2019). These investigators studied the theranostic approaches that have been pursued to date and those that are the focus of ongoing research. They also outlined the therapeutic potential nanomedicines in PDAC and key challenges those must be overcome. Progress in understanding the pathobiology and signaling pathways involved in disease progression is helping to develop novel ways to fight PDAC, including improved nanotechnology-based drug-delivery platforms that have the potential to overcome the biological barriers that underlie persistent drug resistance. Nanomedicine strategies have the potential to enable targeting of the Hedgehog signaling pathway, the ATG pathway, and specific RAS-mutant phenotypes, among other pathological processes of the disease. These novel therapies, alone or in combination with agents designed to disrupt the patho-biological barriers of the disease, could result in superior treatments, with increased efficacy and reduced off-target toxicities compared with the current standard-of-care regimens. By overcoming drug-delivery challenges, advances can be made in the treatment of PDAC.

ABHD5 Interacts with BECN1

ATG contributes to metabolic reprogramming and chromosomal stability. The monoallelic loss of the essential ATG gene, BECN1 (encoding BECN1/Beclin-1), promotes cancer development and progression. However, the mechanism by which BECN1 is inactivated in malignancy remains elusive. Peng et al. (2016) reported the tumor suppressor role of ABHD5 (abhydrolase domain containing 5), a co-activator of PNPLA2 (patatin like phospholipase domain containing 2) in colorectal carcinoma (CRC). A noncanonical role of ABHD5 was reported in regulating ATG and CRC tumorigenesis. ABHD5 directly competes with CASP3 for binding to the cleavage sites of BECN1, and prevents BECN1 from being cleaved by CASP3. ABHD5 deficiency provides CASP3 an advantage to cleave and inactivate BECN1, thus impairing BECN1-induced ATG flux and augmenting genomic instability, which promotes tumorigenesis. Clinical data also confirms that ABHD5 proficiency is correlated with the expression of BECN1, LC3-II, and CASP3 in human CRC tissues, suggesting that ABHD5 possesses a PNPLA2-independent function in regulating ATG and tumorigenesis, further establishing the tumor suppressor role of ABHD5, and offering an opportunity to develop novel theranostic strategies aimed at preventing CRC carcinogenesis.

Intracellular Trafficking of Protein Nanocapsules

The inner membrane vesicle system is a complex transport system that includes endocytosis, exocytosis, and CP/ATG. Zhang et al. (2016a) investigated the intracellular trafficking pathway of protein nanocapsules using >30 Rab proteins as markers of multiple trafficking vesicles in endocytosis, exocytosis, and CP/ATG. FITC-labeled protein NPs were internalized by the cells primarily through Arf6-dependent endocytosis and Rab34-mediated micropinocytosis. Two novel transport pathways: the micropinocytosis (Rab34 positive)-LEs (Rab7 positive)-lysosome pathway and the EEs-liposome (Rab18 positive)-lysosome pathway were identified. The cells used a slow endocytosis recycling pathway (Rab11 and Rab35 positive vesicles) while GLUT4 exocytosis vesicles (Rab8 and Rab10 positive) transported the protein nano-capsules out of the cells. Protein NPs were observed in APSs, which received protein nano-capsules through multiple endocytosis vesicles. Using an ATG inhibitor to block these transport pathways could prevent the degradation of NPs through lysosomes, and Rab proteins as vesicle markers to investigate the detailed intracellular trafficking of the protein nano-capsules, will provide unique targets to interfere with the cellular behavior of NPs, and improve the theranostic potential of nanomedicine.

The Theranostic Potential of Organic NPs as CP Regulators in Chronic MDR Diseases

Co-delivery of Salinomycin and CQ by Liposomes

To improve the suboptimal therapeutic efficacy of SAL toward liver cancer cells using CQ combination by the liposomes co-delivering SAL and CQ (SCNL), Xie et al. (2016) evaluated the synergy of these two drugs in liver cancer cells (HepG2) and liver cancer stem cells (LCSCs) by a median-effect analysis. SCNL with an optimized ratio were developed. The cytotoxic effect and basal ATG flux (measure of autophagic degradation activity) of various formulations were evaluated. CQ increased the cytotoxic effect of SAL in HepG2 cells, but not in HepG2-LCSCs, due to the increased basal ATG flux in HepG2 cells, supporting the promising role of combination therapy for eradicating LCSCs and providing an effective treatment of liver cancer.

Polymeric CQ as an Inhibitor of Cancer

CQ is a widely used antimalarial drug with potential in anticancer therapies due to its inhibitory effects on the CXCR4 chemokine receptor, ATG, and cholesterol metabolism. Yu et al. (2016) reported on polymeric CQ (pCQ) as a drug with antimetastatic activity. The pCQ polymers were synthesized by the copolymerization of methacryloylated hydroxy-CQ (HCQ) and N-(2-hydroxypropyl)methacrylamide (HPMA). pCQ inhibited cancer cell migration and invasion when compared with the parent HCQ by inhibiting cell migration mediated by the CXCR4/CXCL12 pathway. The pCQ also demonstrated superior inhibitory activity over HCQ when tested in a mouse model of experimental lung metastasis. pCQ translocates to the cytoplasm while exhibiting lower cytotoxicity than HCQ, supporting pCQ as a promising polymeric drug platform for the combination of anti-metastatic strategies and cytoplasmic drug delivery.

Nanomaterials and ATG in Cancer Theranostics

Panzarini et al. (2013) summarized the effects of nanomaterials on autophagic processes in cancer, considering the therapeutic outcome of synergism between nanomaterials and ATG to improve cancer nanotheranostics. Recent evidences support a relationship between several classes of nanomaterials and ATG perturbation (both induction and blockade) in biological models. In fact, the autophagic mechanism represents a common cellular response to nanomaterials. On the other hand, the dynamic nature (Wang et al. 2017b) of ATG in cancer biology is an intriguing approach for cancer theranostics, since during tumor development and therapy, ATG triggers both an early cell survival and a late cell death. The use of nanomaterials to deliver chemotherapeutic drugs and target tumors is well known. Recently, ATG modulation mediated by nanomaterials has become fascinating in nanotherapeutics, since it can be exploited as adjuvant in chemotherapy or in the development of cancer vaccines or as a potential anti-cancer agent.

Anticancer Activities of Self-assembled Molecular Bowls

Kim et al. (2015) described the coordination-driven self-assembly and anticancer activities of three organometallic tetranuclear Ru(II) molecular bowls. [2+2] Coordination-driven self-assembly of 3, 6-bis(pyridin-3-ylethynyl) phenanthrene (bpep) (1) and one of the three dinuclear arene ruthenium clips, [(η6-p-iPrC6H4Me)2Ru2-(OO\OO)][OTf]2 (OO\OO = 2, 5-dioxido-1, 4-benzoquinonato, OTf = triflate) (2), 5, 8-dioxido-1, 4-naphthoquinonato (3), or 6, 11-dioxido-5, 12-naphthacenediona (4), resulted in three molecular bowls (5–7) having a general formula [{(η6-p-iPrC6H4Me)2Ru2-(OO\OO)}2(bpep)2][OTf]4. All molecular bowls were obtained as triflate salts in >90% yields and were characterized using multinuclear NMR, electrospray ionization-mass spectrometry (ESI-MS), and elemental analysis. The structure of the representative molecular bowl 5 was confirmed by single-crystal X-ray diffraction analysis. The anticancer activities of molecular bowls 5–7 were determined by MTT, ATG, and immunoblot analysis. Bowl 6 showed cytotoxicity in AGS human gastric carcinoma cells and was more cytotoxic than Dox. In addition, ATG activity and the ratio of apoptotic cell death increased in AGS cells by treatment with bowl 6, which also induced APS formation via upregulation of p62 and promotion of the conversion of LC3-I to LC3-II. Bowl 6 promoted apoptotic cell death through the downregulation of Akt/mTOR activation, followed by increased caspase-3 activity, suggesting that it induces gastric cancer cell death via modulation of ATG and apoptosis. Hence, molecular bowl 6 was a potent anticancer agent and a potential treatment for human gastric cancer which requires further investigations. Molecular bowl 7 was not as effective as molecular 6. Hence, was not not studied in detail.

Ceria NPs Enhance Radiotherapy

Radiotherapy is one of the main strategies for cancer treatment but has significant challenges, such as cancer cell resistance and radiation damage to normal tissue. Radiosensitizers that selectively increase the susceptibility of cancer cells to radiation can enhance the effectiveness of radiotherapy. Chen et al. (2015) developed a novel radiosensitizer consisting of monodispersed ceria NPs (CNPs) encapsulated with the anticancer drug Neogambogic acid (NGA-CNPs) that were used in conjunction with radiation in MCF-7 BC cells, and the efficacy and mechanisms of action of this combined treatment were evaluated. NGA-CNPs potentiated the toxic effects of radiation, leading to a higher rate of cell death than either treatment used alone and inducing the activation of ATG and cell cycle arrest at the G2/M phase, while pretreatment with NGA or CNPs did not improve the rate of radiation-induced cancer cells death. However, NGA-CNPs decreased both endogenous and radiation-induced ROS formation, unlike other nanomaterial, suggesting that the adjunctive use of NGA-CNPs can increase the effectiveness of radiotherapy in BC treatment by lowering the radiation doses required to kill cancer cells and thereby minimize collateral damage to healthy adjacent tissue.

Quinoxaline-Containing Peptide

Zamudio-Vázquez et al. (2015) described the synthesis of a new small library of quinoxaline-containing peptides. After cytotoxic evaluation in four human cancer cell lines, as well as detailed biological studies, the most active compound, RZ2, was found to promote the formation of acidic compartments, where it accumulated, blocking the progression of ATG. Further disruption of the $\Delta\Psi$ and an increase in ROS was observed, causing cells to undergo apoptosis. Given its cytotoxic activity and protease-resistant features, RZ2 could be a potential drug candidate for cancer treatment and provide a basis for future research into the crosstalk between ATG and apoptosis and the relevance of Quinoxaline-containing peptide in cancer theranostics.

Antitumor Efficacy of Dribble Vaccine

Vaccines play important roles in antitumor biotherapy. ATG in tumor cells plays a critical role in depredating proteins, including tumor-specific antigens and tumor-associated antigens. Su et al. (2015) induced and collected tumor-derived APSs (DRibbles) from tumor cells as a novel antitumor vaccine by inhibiting the functions of proteasomes and lysosomes. DRibbles were prepared and their morphological and ATG properties characterized. Dendritic cells (DCs) generated from the bone marrow monocytes of mice were co-cultured with DRibbles, then surface molecules of DCs and B cells, as well as apoptosis of DCs, were determined by flow cytometry. The functional properties of the DRibble-DCs were examined by mixed lymphocyte reactions and animal experiments. The diameter of autophagic NPs with spherical and double-membrane structures was 200–500 nm. DRibbles resulted in the upregulation of costimulatory molecules CD40 and CD86, as well as MHC-I molecules on DCs, but not MHC-II. The expressions of CD40, CD80, and CD86 and that of MHC-II molecules on B cells were upregulated. Suppression of tumor growth and lifetime prolongation was observed in DRibble-DC-vaccinated tumor-bearing mice, demonstrating that naïve T cells can be activated by DC cross-presenting antigens on upregulated MHC-I, suggesting that DRibbles be deployed as an effective antitumor vaccine for head and neck cancer immunotherapy in clinical trials.

Polycation-mediated Integrated Cell Death

One of the major challenges in the field of nucleic acid delivery is the design of delivery vehicles which render them safe as well as efficient in transfection. Polycationic vectors have been investigated with native polyethylenimines (PEIs) being the gold standard. PEIs are efficient transfectants, but depending on their architecture and size, they induce cytotoxicity. Parhamifar et al. (2014) reviewed dynamic and integrated cell death processes and pathways, and discussed considerations in cell death assay design and their interpretation in relation to PEIs and PEI-based vectors, which are also translatable for the design and studying the safety of other transfectants.

microRNA Therapeutics and Anticancer Drugs

Dai and Tan (2015) summarized the mechanisms and advantages for the combination therapies involving miRNAs and small-molecule drugs, as well as the recent advances in the co-delivery nanocarriers for these agents. miRNAs regulate multiple molecular pathways for the hallmarks of cancer with a high biochemical specificity and potency. By restoring tumor suppressive miRNAs or ablating oncomiRs, miRNA-based therapies can sensitize cancer cells to conventional cytotoxins and the molecularly targeted drugs by promoting apoptosis and ATG, reverting epithelial-to-mesenchymal transition, suppressing tumor angiogenesis, and downregulating efflux transporters. The development of miRNA-based therapeutics in combination with small-molecule anticancer drugs confer the opportunity to counteract MDR and improve the TSE-EBPT of human cancers.

Fumagillin Prodrug Nanotheranostics

Anti-angiogenesis has been explored for the treatment of a variety of cancers and certain inflammatory processes. Fumagillin, a mycotoxin produced by Aspergillus fumigatus that binds methionine aminopeptidase 2 (MetAP-2), is a potent antiangiogenic agent. Zhou et al. (2014) developed a lipase-labile Fumagillin prodrug (Fum-PD) that eliminated the photo-instability of the compound. Using $\alpha v \beta 3$-integrin-targeted perfluorocarbon nanocarriers to deliver Fum-PD specifically to angiogenic vessels, they suppressed clinical disease in an experimental model of rheumatoid arthritis (RA). Fum-PD nanotheranostics suppressed inflammation through the local production of eNO. Fum-PD-induced NO-activated AMPK, which modulates macrophage inflammatory response. *In vivo*, NO-induced AMPK activation inhibits mTOR activity and enhances ATG flux, as evidenced by p62 depletion and increased autolysosome formation. ATG mediates the degradation of the Ikappaβ kinase (IKK), suppressing the NF-$\kappa\beta$ p65 signaling pathway and inflammatory cytokine release. Inhibition of NO production by N(G)-nitro-L-arginine methyl ester (L-NAME), a NOS inhibitor, reversed the suppression of NF-$\kappa\beta$-mediated inflammatory response induced by Fum-PD nanotherapy, indicating that Fum-PD nanotherapy may be further explored in the treatment of angiogenesis-dependent diseases.

Docetaxel-loaded Dendritic NPs in BC

Dendrimers are synthetic nanocarriers that comprise a highly branched spherical polymer and are efficient tools for drug delivery. Zhang et al. (2014) prepared Docetaxel-loaded dendritic copolymer H40-poly(D,L-lactide) NPs, referred to as "DTX-H40-PLA NPs", to evaluate whether these were sequestered by ATG and fused with lysosomes. Besides being degraded through the endolysosomal pathway, the DTX-loaded H40-PLA NPs were also sequestered by APSs and degraded through the autolysosomal pathway. DTX-loaded H40-PLA NPs may stop exerting beneficial effects after inducing ATG of human MCF-7 cancer cells. The co-delivery of the ATG inhibitors CQ and DTX by dendritic copolymer NPs enhanced cancer cell killing *in vitro*, and decreased both the volume and weight of the tumors in SCID mice, providing evidence for the development of dendritic copolymer NPs for BC nanotheranostics.

ATG Promotes Degradation of Polyethyleneimine-alginate NPs

Polyethyleneimine (PEI)-alginate (Alg) NP is a safe and effective vector for the delivery of siRNA or DNA. Wang et al. (2017a) isolated CD34$^+$VEGFR-3$^+$ endothelial progenitor cells from rat bone marrow which were treated with 25 kDa branched PEI-NPs modified by Alg. Morphological changes and distribution of the NPs in the cells were examined with scanning and TEM. Cytotoxicity of the NPs was analyzed by ROS production, LDH leakage, and induction of apoptosis. The ATG was assessed by evaluating the expression of Beclin-1 and LC3 and formation of ATG structures and amphisomes. Colocalization of LC3-positive puncta and the NPs was determined by LC3-GFP tracing. The cytotoxicity of PEI NPs was reduced after modification with Alg. PEI-Alg NPs were distributed in mitochondria, RER, and nuclei as well as cytoplasm. After their phagocytosis, the expression of Beclin-1 mRNA and LC3 protein was upregulated, and the number of LC3-positive puncta, ATG structures, lysosomes, and amphisomes increased. There were LC3-positive puncta in nuclei, and some puncta were colocalized with the NPs, indicating that the ATG induction promotes the degradation of PEI-Alg NPs via multiple pathways.

Edelfosine Lipid NPs Overcome MDR in K-562 Leukemia Cells

The antitumor ether lipid Edelfosine is the prototype of a promising anticancer drug that has been shown to be an effective antitumor agent in numerous malignancies. However, several cancer types display resistance to antitumoral compounds due to MDR, a major drawback in anticancer therapy. The leukemic cell line K-562 shows resistance to Edelfosine, which is overcome by the use of nanotechnology. Aznar et al. (2014) described the rate and mechanism of the internalization of free and nano-encapsulated Edelfosine. The molecular mechanisms underlying cell death were described by the characterization of several molecules implied in the apoptotic and ATG pathways (PARP, LC3-IIB, caspases-3, -9 and -7), and their pattern of expression was compared with the cell induction in a sensitive cell line HL-60. Results showed different internalization patterns in both cells. Clathrin and lipid-raft-mediated endocytosis were observed in Edelfosine uptake, whereas these mechanism were not visible in the uptake of lipid NPs, which might suffer phagocytosis and macropinocytosis. Both treatments induced caspase-mediated apoptosis in HL-60 cells, whereas this cell death mechanism was unnoticeable in K-562 cells. Moreover, increase in ATG vesicles was visible in K-562 cells. Thus, this mechanism might be implicated in overcoming K-562 resistance with the treatment by lipid NPs.

Atg5 Deficit Augments Lysosome Formation

Paul and Munz (2016) described the role of immune response, viral replication, and CP/ATG in mammalian viruses. CP/ATG is one of the key mechanism mammalian cells utilize to get rid of intracellular pathogens including viruses. CP/ATG plays an important role during viral infection. Initially, CP/ATG regulates the immune response through selective degradation of immune components by preventing the deleterious pro-inflammatory response. Subsequently, CP/ATG delivers virus-derived antigens to antigen-loading compartments for presentation to T lymphocytes and may participate in the viral lytic cycle by facilitating its release from the infected cells. Furthermore, virus may compromise and/or high jack CP/ATG for its own advantage as described in this manuscript. These investigators described important steps involved during viral infection in which CP/ATG plays a pivotal role by selecting examples of some important viruses (including herpes virus and influenza virus) and described their molecular mechanism of virulence and intricate relationship with CP/ATG as a consequence of host-pathogen coevolution. Lu et al. (2014) investigated the role of ATG-lysosome signaling in the brain after the application of NPs. Lipid NPs (LNs) induced elevations of Atg5, p62, LC3, and Cathepsin B in mice brains. The TEM revealed a dramatic elevation of lysosome vacuoles co-localized with LNs cluster inside the neurons in mice brain. The abnormal expression of Cathepsin B was observed in brain cortex following LNs injection, which was further elevated in Atg5(+/–) mice. The importance of Atg5 in the LNs-induced ATG-lysosome cascade was supported by exaggerated neurovascular response in Atg5(+/–) mice. In addition, the siRNA knockdown of Atg5 blunted the increasing of LC3 and p62 in LNs-treated Neuro-2a cells, suggesting that LNs induce ATG-lysosome signaling and neurovascular response via an Atg5-dependent pathway. These authors investigated ATG-lysosome signaling in the mouse brain after the application of lipid NPs and reported that these NPs induce ATG-lysosome signaling and neurovascular response via an Atg5-dependent pathway.

Rapamycin NPs Target Defective ATG in Muscular Dystrophy

Duchenne muscular dystrophy (DMD) in boys progresses rapidly to severe impairment of muscle function and death in the second or third decade of life. Current therapy with corticosteroids results in a modest increase in strength as a consequence of a general reduction in inflammation, albeit with potential long-term side effects and ultimate failure of the agent to maintain strength. Bibee et al. (2014) demonstrated that alternative approaches that rescue defective ATG in mdx mice, a model of DMD, with the use of Rapamycin-loaded NPs induce increase in both skeletal muscle strength and cardiac contractile performance not achievable with conventional oral Rapamycin, even in pharmacological doses. The increase in physical performance occurred in both young and adult mice, and, even in aged wild-type mice for systemic therapies to facilitate improved cell function by the ATG disposal of toxic byproducts of cell death and regeneration.

Cytotoxicity of Fullerene

Nanomaterials translocate into the circulation and directly affect vascular endothelial cells (ECs), causing vascular injury for the development of atherosclerosis. To explore the direct effects of nanomaterials on endothelial toxicity, Yamawaki and Iwai (2006) treated human umbilical vein ECs with 1–100 μg/ml hydroxyl fullerene [C60(OH)24; mean diameter, 7.1 +/– 2.4 nm] for 24 hrs. C60(OH)24 induced cytotoxic morphological changes such as cytosolic vacuole formation and decreased cell density in a dose-dependent manner. An LDH assay revealed that a maximal dose of C60(OH)24 (100 μg/ml) induced cytotoxic injury. A proliferation assay also showed that a maximal dose of C60(OH)24 inhibited EC growth. C60(OH)24 did not induce apoptosis but caused the accumulation of polyubiquitinated proteins and facilitated autophagic cell death. Formation of APSs was confirmed using a specific marker, LC3 antibody, and TEM. Chronic treatment with low-dose C60(OH)24 (10 μg/ml for 8 days) inhibited cell attachment and delayed EC growth. Although fullerenes changed morphology, only maximal doses caused cytotoxic injury and/or death and inhibited cell growth. EC death was caused by the activation of ubiquitin-ATG cell death pathways. Although exposure to NMs represent a risk for CVDs, further *in vivo* validations are necessary.

Mitochondria-Homing Peptide NPs

One of the major challenges in the treatment of hearing loss is the reduced efficacy of theranostic agents. To achieve the optimum drug efficacy, Zhou et al. (2018) designed a novel peptide (D-Arg-Dmt-Arg-Phe-NH$_2$)-mediated mitochondrial targeted delivery nanosystem, geranylgeranylacetone (GGA). The zebrafish lateral line system, a model for mammalian hair cells, was used to identify the efficacy of GGA against Gentamycin, a well-known ototoxic agent. The nanosystem facilitated lysosomal escape and mitochondrial accumulation, and conferred superior protection against a wide range of Gentamicin compared with unmodified NPs and free drugs. Peptides-modified NPs' internalized hair cells via both dynamin-dependent and independent routes, following a classic endocytic or ATG pathway. Although, extracellular action via MET channels, the primary protective mechanism underlying peptides-modified NPs, was revealed due to their intracellular interaction providing a general strategy to enhance the clinical efficacy of a broad range of drugs in the treatment of hearing loss.

Survivin in Colon Cancer

Endogenous survivin expression is related with cancer survival, MDR, and metastasis. Therapies targeting survivin inhibit tumor growth and recurrence. Roy et al. (2015) found out that a cell-permeable dominant negative survivin (SurR9-C84A, referred to as SR9) competitively inhibited endogenous survivin and blocked the cell cycle at the G1/S phase. Nanoencapsulation in mucoadhesive chitosan NPs (CHNP) increased the bioavailability and serum stability of SR9. The mechanism of NP uptake was studied to confirm that CHNP-SR9 protected primary cells from ATG and induced tumor-specific apoptosis via both extrinsic and intrinsic apoptotic pathways. CHNP-SR9 reduced the tumor spheroid size (3-D model) by ~7X. The effects of SR9 and CHNP-SR9 on 35 key molecules involved in the apoptotic pathway were studied. A significant (4.26X) reduction in tumor volume was observed using an *in vivo* mouse xenograft colon cancer model. Apoptotic (6.25X) and necrotic indexes (3.5X) were higher in CHNP-SR9 when compared to void CHNP and CHNP-SR9 was internalized more in cancer stem cells (4.5X). Nanoformulation of SR9 did not reduce its theranostic potential; however, it provided SR9 with enhanced stability and superior bioavailability. This study presented a tumor-specific protein-based cancer therapy that had several advantages over the conventionally used chemotherapeutics.

Cationic Liposomes Induce Cell Necrosis

The application of cationic liposomes (CLs) as nonviral vectors is hampered by their cellular toxicity. Yang et al. (2016) investigated the mechanisms underlying the cellular toxicity of CLs. The effect of CLs on the ATG flux, APS-lysosome fusion, lysosome membrane permeabilization, and cell necrosis of liver cells was investigated. They revealed a novel mechanism of CL-induced cell necrosis involving the induction of lysosome membrane permeabilization and late-stage ATG flux inhibition that resulted in the cytoplasmic release of Cathepsin B, mitochondrial dysfunction, and ROS production, as the key mediators of cell necrosis. This study was important for revealing the cellular toxicity of CLs and designing safer gene delivery systems.

^{188}Re-Liposomes Induce CP

Despite standard treatment, about 70% of ovarian cancer recur. CSCs have been implicated in the MDR mechanism. Several drug resistance mechanisms have been proposed, and CP/ATG plays a crucial role for the maintenance and tumorigenicity of CSCs. CSCs display a higher level of ATG flux. CP and MTG, specific types of ATG that selectively degrade excessive or damaged mitochondria contribute to cancer progression and recurrence in several types of tumors. Nanomedicine tackle the CSCs by overcoming MDR. Chang et al. (2017) developed ^{188}Re-liposome, which targeted CP/ATG and MTG in the tumor microenvironment. The inhibition of CP/ATG and MTG could lead to significant tumor inhibition in two xenograft animal models. They presented two cases of recurrent ovarian cancer, both in drug-resistance status that received a level I dose from a phase I clinical trial. Both the MDR cases showed drug sensitivity to ^{188}Re-liposome, suggesting that inhibition of CP, MTG, and/or ATG by a nanomedicine may be a novel strategy to overcome MDR in ovarian cancer.

The Theranostic Potential of Inorganic NPs as CP Regulators in Chronic MDR Diseases

Platinum NPs

Despite the fact that nanoparticulate platinum (nano-Pt) has been validated to act as a platinum-based prodrug for anticancer therapy, the factor controlling its cytotoxicity remains to be clarified. Cheng et al. (2016) found that the corrosion susceptibility of nano-Pt can be triggered by inducing oxidation of superficial Pt atoms, which can kill both Cisplatin-sensitive/resistance cancer cells. Direct evidence in the oxidation of superficial Pt atoms is validated to observe the formation of platinum oxides by X-ray absorption spectroscopy. The cytotoxicity is originated from the dissolution of nano-Pt followed by the release of highly toxic Pt ions during the corrosion process. The limiting ATG induction by nano-Pt might prevent cancer cells from acquiring ATG-related MDR. With such advantages, the possibility of further ATG-related MDR could be reduced or even eliminated in cancer cells treated with nano-Pt. Nano-Pt killed Cisplatin-resistant cancer cells by inducing apoptosis as well as necrosis implicated in pro-inflammatory/inflammatory responses. Thus, nano-Pt treatment might bring theranostic benefits by regulating immunological responses in the tumor microenvironment, suggesting that nano-Pt might benefit patients with Cisplatin resistant chemotherapy.

Gold NPs

GNPs are widely used nanomaterials and induce APS accumulation. Ma et al. (2011) found that GNPs can be taken into cells through endocytosis in a size-dependent manner. The internalized GNPs accumulate in lysosomes and cause impairment of lysosome degradation through alkalinization of lysosomal pH. GNPs induces APS accumulation and processes LC3, an APS marker protein. However, degradation of the ATG substrate p62 is blocked in GNPs-treated cells, indicating that APS accumulation results from the blockade of ATG flux, rather than induction of ATG. These findings clarified the mechanism by which GNPs induce APS accumulation and revealed their effect on lysosomes. Iron core-gold shell NPs (Fe@Au) possess cancer-preferential cytotoxicity in oral and colorectal cancer (CRC) cells. However, CRC cell lines are less sensitive to Fe@Au treatment when compared with oral cancer cell lines. Recently, Sun et al. (2018) highlighted that generation of new cell death regulators is urgently needed for disease treatment. Exhibiting stability and ease of decoration, GNPs could be used in diagnosis and disease treatment. Upon entering the human body, GNPs contact human cells in the blood, targeting organs and the immune system, which results in the disturbance of cell function and even cell death. Therefore, GNPs may act as powerful cell death regulators. GNPs' size, shape, and surface properties play key roles in regulating various cell death modalities and related signaling pathways, which could guide the design of GNPs for nanomedicine. Wu et al. (2013) found, Fe@Au to decrease the cell viability of CRC cell lines, including Caco-2, HT-29, and SW480, through growth inhibition rather than the induction of cell death. The cytotoxicity induced by Fe@Au in CRC cells uses different subcellular pathways to the CP found in Fe@Au-treated oral cancer cells called OECM1. The Caco-2 cell line showed a similar response to OECM1 cells and was more sensitive to Fe@Au treatment than the other CRC cell lines. They investigated the mechanism of cell resistance of Fe@Au-treated CRC cells. The resistance of CRC cells to Fe@Au did not result from the amount of Fe@Au internalized. The different amounts of Fe and Au internalized determined the different response to treatment with Fe-only NPs in Fe@Au-resistant CRC cells compared with the Fe@Au-sensitive OECM1 cells. The only moderately cytotoxic effect of Fe@Au NPs on CRC cells, when compared to the highly sensitive OECM1 cells, appears to arise from the CRC cells' relative insensitivity to Fe, as demonstrated by Fe-only. The Au coatings enhanced the cytotoxicity of Fe@Au in certain CRC cells. Hence, both the Fe and Au in these core-shell NPs are essential for the anticancer properties. GNPs can be deposited in the kidneys, particularly in renal tubular epithelial cells. Chronic hypoxia is inevitable in CKD, and results in renal tubular epithelial cells that are susceptible to different types of injuries. Ding et al. (2014) characterized the cytotoxic effects of GNPs in hypoxic renal tubular epithelial cells. Both 5 nm and 13 nm GNPs were synthesized and characterized using TEM, dynamic light scattering, and UV-visible spectrophotometry. The cytotoxicity of GNPs (0, 1, 25, and 50 nM) was tested in human renal proximal tubular cells (HK-2) by a Cell Counting Kit-8 assay and a LDH release assay. The toxic effects of 5nm (particle size) GNPs were observed only at 50 nM dose of GNPs under hypoxic condions. GNPs were either localized in vesicles or in the lysosomes in 5 nm GNPs-treated HK-2 cells, and their cellular uptake in the hypoxic cells was higher than that in normoxic cells. In normoxic HK-2 cells, 5 nm GNPs (50 nM) treatment caused ATG and cell survival. However, in hypoxic conditions, these GNP induced ROS overproduction, $\Delta\Psi$ collapse, and an increase in apoptosis and autophagic cell death, demonstrating that renal tubular epithelial cells presented different responses under normoxic and hypoxic conditions, which provide the basis for understanding the risks associated with GNP use-especially for the potential GNP-related therapies in CKD patients. To investigate the effect of GNPs on retinal angiogenesis, Shen et al. (2018) used the seed growth method to synthesize GNPs. The size, zeta potential, absorption spectrum, and morphology of GNPs were identified using Malvern Nano-ZS, multimode reader (BioTek synergy2), and TEM. Cell viability was analyzed using the Cell Counting Kit-8 method and cell growth was assessed with an EdU kit. The trans-well chamber was used to investigate cell migration. The tube formation method was used to assess the angiogenic property *in vitro*. An O_2-induced retinopathy (OIR) model was used to investigate the effect of GNPs on retinal angiogenesis. A confocal microscope and immunoblot were used to study the mechanism of GNPs-induced inhibition of angiogenesis. These GNPs were uniform and well dispersed. GNPs of 10 µg/mL and 20 µg/mL inhibited the proliferation, migration, and tube formation of human umbilical vein endothelial cells. GNPs improved the retinopathy in an OIR model, suggesting that GNPs inhibit retinal neovascularization *in vitro* and *in vivo* as a potential nanomedicine for the TSE-EBPT of retinal angiogenesis.

Tian et al. (2019) investigated the biotransformation mechanism of Au(III) in GNPs using a hydroxylated tetraterpenoid deinoxanthin (DX) from the extremophile Deinococcus radiodurans. Au(III) was reduced to Au(I) and Au(0) by deprotonation of the hydroxyl head groups of the tetraterpenoid. The oxidized, deprotonated form 2-ketodeinoxanthin (DX3) served as a surface-capping agent to stabilize the GNPs. The functionalized DX- GNPs demonstrated stronger inhibitory activity against cancer cells compared with sodium citrate-GNPs and were nontoxic to normal cells. DX- GNPs accumulated in the cytoplasm, organelles, and nuclei, and induced ROS generation, DNA damage, and apoptosis in MCF-7 cancer cells. In cells treated with DX- GNPs, 374 genes, including the RRAGC gene, were upregulated; and 135 genes, including the genes encoding FOXM1 and NR4A1, were downregulated (these genes are involved in metabolism, cell growth, DNA damage, oxidative stress, ATG, and apoptosis). The anticancer activity of the DX- GNPs was attributed to the alteration of gene expression and induction of apoptosis. These GNPs were functionalized with natural tetraterpenoids to enhance their anticancer potential. Wan et al. (2015) investigated the effects of different aspect ratios and surface modifications on the cytotoxicity and cellular uptake of GNPs in cultured cells and in mice. The surface chemistry (but not the aspect ratio) of GNPs mediated their biological toxicity. CTAB- GNPs with various aspect ratios induced similar apoptosis and ATG by mitochondrial degeneration and by ROS overproduction. However, GNPs coated with CTAB/PSS, CTAB/PAH, CTAB/PSS/PAH or CTAB/PAH/PSS displayed low toxicity and did not induce cell death. CTAB/PAH-coated GNPs caused minimally abnormal cell morphology compared with CTAB/PSS- and CTAB/PSS/PAH-coated GNPs. The i.v injection of CTAB/PAH GNPs enabled the GNPs to reach tumor tissues through blood circulation in animals and remained stable, with a longer half-life compared to the other GNPs, suggesting that further coating can prevent cytotoxicity and cell death with better biocompatibility and minimal cytotoxicity.

No currently available HER2-targeted therapeutic agent is effective in Trastuzumab (Tmab)-resistant gastric cancer. GNPs are promising drug carriers with unique characteristics of a large surface area for attachment with antibodies. Kubota et al. (2018) created HER2-targeted GNPs (T-GNPs) and examined their theranostic potential and cytotoxic mechanisms using HER2-postive Tmab-resistant (MKN7) or Tmab-sensitive (NCI-N87) gastric cancer cell lines. *In vitro*, T-GNPs showed stronger cytotoxic effects than controls against MKN7 and NCI-N87 cells although Tmab had no effect on MKN7 cells. ATG played an important role in T-GNPs cytotoxic mechanisms, which was driven by internalization of T-GNPs and displayed potent antitumor effects in NCI-N87 and MKN7 s.c. tumors in mouse models. Hence, HER2-targeted GNPs with conjugated Tmab is a promising strategy for the development of the TSE-EBPT to overcome Tmab resistance in gastric cancer. Tsai et al. (2017) modified GNPs with the nuclear localization signal from the Simian Virus 40 large T antigen (GNP-PEG/SV40), which accumulated on the cytoplasmic side of the nuclear membrane in HeLa cells. Accumulation of GNP-PEG/SV40 around the nucleus blocked nucleocytoplasmic transport and prevented RNA export and nuclear shuttling of signaling proteins, resulting in cell death. This cell death was not caused by apoptosis or necrosis because caspases 3 and 9 were not activated, and the expression of annexin V/propidium iodide was not enhanced in HeLa cells. APSs and autolysosomes were seen after 72 hrs of treatment with GNP-PEG/SV40. Increasing levels of enhanced GFP-microtubule-associated protein 1 light chain 3 (EGFP-LC3)-positive punctate and LC3-II confirmed the presence of GNP-PEG/SV40-induced ATG. In SiHa cells, this treatment did not induce accumulation of GNP-PEG/SV40 around the nucleus and ATG. Treating cells with wheat germ agglutinin, a nuclear pore complex inhibitor, induced ATG in both HeLa and SiHa cells. GNP-PEG/SV40-induced ATG plays a role in cell death, not survival, and virus-mediated small hairpin RNA silencing of Beclin-1 attenuated cell death, indicating that a long-term blockade of nucleocytoplasmic transport results in ATG cell death. Haynes et al. (2016) developed a small molecule inhibitor SMI#9 for Rad6, a protein overexpressed in aggressive BCs and involved in DNA damage tolerance. SMI#9 induced cytotoxicity in cancerous cells but spared normal breast cells; however, its therapeutic efficacy was limited by poor solubility. They modified SMI#9 to enable its conjugation and hydrolysis from GNPs. SMI#9-GNP and parent SMI#9 activities were compared in mesenchymal and basal triple negative BC (TNBC) subtype cells. Whereas SMI#9 is cytotoxic to all TNBC cells, SMI#9-GNP is endocytosed and cytotoxic only in mesenchymal TNBC cells. SMI#9-GNP endocytosis in basal TNBCs was compromised by aggregation. However, when combined with Cisplatin, SMI#9-GNP was imported and synergistically increases Cisplatin sensitivity. Like SMI#9, SMI#9-GNP spared normal breast cells. The released SMI#9 was active and induced cell death via mitochondrial dysfunction and PARP-1 stabilization/hyperactivation. This work signified the development of a nanotechnology-based Rad6-targeting therapy for TNBCs. Protein Rad6 is overexpressed in BC cells and its blockade may provide a new treatment in TNBC. The researchers conjugated a small molecule inhibitor SMI#9 for Rad6 to GNPs and showed that this new formulation specifically targeted MDR-BC cells and highlighted the importance of nanotechnology in drug carrier development.

Although TRAIL and its agonistic receptors have been identified as promising antitumor agents that preferentially eliminate cancer cells with minimal damage, the emergence of TRAIL resistance contributes to theranostic failure. Thus, there is an urgent need for novel approaches to overcome TRAIL resistance. AuNPs are one of the most promising nanomaterials that show immense antitumor potential via targeting various cellular and molecular processes. Ke et al. (2017) found that AuNPs combined with TRAIL exhibited a greater potency in promoting apoptosis in non-small-cell lung cancer (NSCLC) cells compared with TRAIL alone, suggesting that AuNPs sensitize cancer cells to TRAIL. The combination of TRAIL and AuNPs was more effective in inducing excessive mitochondrial fragmentation in cancer cells accompanied by an increase in the mitochondrial recruitment of Drp-1, mitochondrial dysfunctions, and ATG induction involving CBMP. The siRNA silencing of Drp-1 or inhibition of ATG alleviated apoptosis in cells exposed to TRAIL combined with GNPs, which augmented TRAIL sensitivity in tumor-bearing mice, indicating the GNPs' potentiate apoptotic response to TRAIL in NSCLC cells through Drp-1-dependent mitochondrial fission, and that TRAIL combined with AuNPs can be a potential chemotherapeutic strategy for the treatment of NSCLC.

Sliver NPs

Nanosilver ranges from 1–100 nm in diameter. Smaller particles more readily enter cells and interact with the cellular components. The exposure dose, particle size, coating, and aggregation state of the nanosilver, as well as the cell type or organism on which it is tested, are all determining factors on the effect and potential toxicity of nanosilver. A high exposure dose to nanosilver alters the cellular stress responses and triggers organelle ATG and apoptosis. Radiotherapy performs an important function in the treatment of cancer, but the resistance of tumor cells to radiation still remains a serious concern. Liu et al. (2016) evaluated and compared the radio-sensitizing efficacies of GNPs and AgNPs on glioma at clinically relevant megavoltage energies. Both GNPs and AgNPs potentiated the antiglioma effects of radiation. AgNPs showed a more powerful radiosensitizing ability than AuNPs at the same mass and molar concentrations, leading to a higher rate of apoptotic cell death. The combination of AgNPs with radiation increased ATG as compared with GNPs plus radiation, suggesting the potential application of AgNPs as a highly effective nano-radiosensitizer for the treatment of glioma. Cameron et al. (2018) summarized the current knowledge of the effects of nanosilver on cellular metabolic function and response to stress. Both the causative effects of nanosilver on oxidative stress, ERS, and hypoxic stress—as well as the effects on the responses to such stresses—were investigated. The interactions and effects of nanosilver on cellular uptake, RONS stress, inflammation, hypoxic response, mitochondrial function, ER function and the UPR, ATG and apoptosis, angiogenesis, epigenetics, genotoxicity, cancer development and tumorigenesis, as well as other pathway alterations were highlighted. Yuan and Gurunathan (2017) investigated the combined effect of Cis and a reduced graphene oxide-silver NP nanocomposite (rGO-AgNPs) on HeLa cells. They synthesized AgNPs, rGO, and rGO-AgNP nanocomposites using C-phycocyanin. The anticancer properties of the Cis, rGO-AgNPs, and the combination of Cis and rGO-AgNPs were evaluated using cell viability, cell proliferation, LDH leakage, ROS generation, and cellular levels of oxidative and antioxidative stress markers such as malondialdehyde, glutathione, SOD, and CAT assays. The expression of proapoptotic, anti-apoptotic, and ATG genes were measured using real-time rtPCR. The AgNPs were well dispersed, homogeneous, and spherical, with an average size of 10 nm and uniformly distributed on graphene sheets. Cis, GO, rGO, AgNPs, and rGO-AgNPs inhibited cell viability. The combination of Cis and rGO-AgNPs showed significant effects on cell proliferation, cytotoxicity, and apoptosis and had more pronounced effects on the ATG and apoptotic genes, and also induced the accumulation of APSs, associated with the generation of ROS, authenticating that rGO-AgNPs potentiate Cis-induced cytotoxicity, ATG, and apoptosis in HeLa cells. Hence, this combination could be applied to cervical cancer treatment as a synergistic agent with Cis or any other chemotherapeutic agents. Buttacavoli et al. (2017) embedded AgNPs into a specific polysaccharide (EPS), were biogenerated by employing the bacteria *Klebsiella oxytoca* DSM 29617 under aerobic (AgNPs-EPS[aer]) and anaerobic conditions (AgNPs-EPS[anaer]). Both AgNPs-EPS matrices were tested by an MTT assay for cytotoxicity against human breast (SKBR3 and 8701-BC) and colon (HT-29, HCT 116, and Caco-2) cancer cell lines, revealing AgNPs-EPS[aer] as the most active, with pronounced efficacy against BC cell lines. Colony forming capability, morphological changes, generation of ROS, induction of ATG and apoptosis, inhibition of migratory and invasive capabilities, and proteomic changes were investigated using SKBR3 –BC cells to elucidate the AgNPs-EPS[aer] mode of action. AgNPs-EPS[aer] induced a significant decrease of cell motility and MMP-2 and MMP-9 activity and increased ROS generation, supporting cell death through ATG and apoptosis. Ag^+ accumulated preferentially in mitochondria and in smaller concentrations in the nucleus to interact with DNA as confirmed by a differential proteomic analysis that highlighted important pathways involved in AgNPs-EPS[aer] toxicity, including ERS, oxidative stress, and mitochondrial impairment triggering CP/ATG or apoptotic cell death.

Usually viral infections create a conducive microenvironment for enhanced bacterial infections. For example, HIV/AIDs infected patients are highly prone to aspergillosis, candidiasis, streptococcal and staphylococcal pneumonia, and tuberculosis due to viral-induced reduction in CD-4 and CD-8 T-lymphocytes involved in the immune response. AgNPs are also microbicidal agents which could be used as an alternative to antivirals to treat human infectious diseases, especially influenza virus infections where antivirals have generally proven unsuccessful. Villere et al. (2018) showed in the context of an influenza virus infection of lung epithelial cells, that AgNPs downregulated influenza-induced CCL-5 and IFN-β release (two cytokines important in antiviral immunity) through RIG-I inhibition, while enhancing IL-8 production, a cytokine important for mobilizing host antibacterial responses. AgNPs activity was independent of coating and was not observed with GNPs. AgNPs disorganized the mitochondrial network and prevented the antiviral IRF-7 transcription factor influx into the nucleus. The modulation of the RIG-I-IRF-7 pathway was concomitant with the inhibition of either classical or alternative ATG (Atg5- and Rab-9 dependent, respectively), depending on the epithelial cell type. AgNPs-mediated functional dichotomy (down-]regulation of IFN-dependent antiviral responses and upregulation of IL-8-dependent antibacterial responses) may have TSE-EBPT implications for their use in the clinic. Polydopamine-coated branched Au-Ag NPs (Au-Ag@PDA NPs) exhibit structural stability, biocompatibility, and photothermal performance, along with potential anticancer efficacy. Zhao et al. (2018) investigated the cytotoxicity of Au-Ag@PDA NPs in human bladder cancer cells (T24 cells), and the molecular mechanisms of photothermal therapy-induced T24 cell death. T24 cells were treated with different doses of Au-Ag@PDA NPs followed by 808 nm laser irradiation, and the effects on cell proliferation, cell cycle, apoptosis, and ATG were analyzed. Real-time PCR and immunoblotting were used to evaluate markers of cell cycle, CP/ATG apoptosis, and the Akt/ERK signaling pathway. They evaluated the effects of the treatment on $\Delta\Psi$ and ROS generation to confirm the mechanisms of inhibition. They tested the T24 tumor inhibitory effects of Au-Ag@PDA NPs plus laser irradiation *in vivo* using a xenograft mouse model. Au-Ag@PDA NPs, with appropriate laser irradiation, inhibited the proliferation of T24 cells, altered the cell cycle distribution by increasing the proportion of cells in the S phase, induced apoptosis by activating the mitochondria-mediated intrinsic pathway, and triggered an ATG response in T24 cells. Au-Ag@PDA NPs decreased the expression of phosphorylated Akt and ERK and promoted the production of ROS that function upstream of ATG and apoptosis. In addition, Au-Ag@PDA NP-mediated photothermolysis also suppressed tumor growth *in vivo*. This study provided a mechanistic basis for Au-Ag@PDA NP-mediated photothermal therapy in the treatment of bladder cancer. Ovarian cancer is one of the most important malignancies, and the origin, detection, and pathogenesis of epithelial ovarian cancer remain elusive. Although many cancer drugs have been developed to reduce the size of tumors, most cancers relapse, posing a problem to overcome. Hence, it is necessary to identify possible alternative therapeutic approaches to reduce the mortality rate of this devastating disease. Zhang et al. (2016b) synthesized AgNPs using a bacterium *Bacillus clausii*. The synthesized AgNPs were homogenous and spherical in shape, with an average size of 16–20 nm, which are known to cause cytotoxicity in various types of human cancer cells, whereas Salinomycin (Sal) kills cancer stem cells. Hence, they selected both Sal and AgNPs to study their combined effect on apoptosis and ATG in ovarian cancer cells. The cells treated with either Sal or AgNPs showed a dose-dependent effect with IC_{50} values of 6.0 μM and 8 μg/mL for Sal and AgNPs, respectively. To determine the combination effect, they measured the IC_{25} values of both Sal and AgNPs (3.0 μM and 4 μg/mL), which showed a more inhibitory effect on cell viability and cell morphology than either Sal or AgNPs alone. The combination of Sal and AgNPs had a more pronounced effect on cytotoxicity and expression of apoptotic genes and induced the accumulation of APS, associated with mitochondrial dysfunction and loss of cell viability involving CBMP. There was a synergistic interaction between Sal and AgNPs in cancer cells. The combination treatment increased the theranostic potential and demonstrated the relevant targeted therapy for the treatment of ovarian cancer. Manshian et al. (2017) exploited the degradation of Ag NPs to treat s.c. tumor models in mice. To investigate the impact of the immune system, they used the same tumor cell type (KLN 205 murine squamous cell carcinoma) in a xenograft model in NOD SCIDγ immune-deficient mice and as a syngeneic model in immune-competent DBA/2 mice. The Ag NPs are screened for their cytotoxicity on various cancer cell lines, indicating the induction of oxidative stress, mitochondrial damage, and ATG in all cell types. At sub-cytotoxic concentrations, prolonged cellular exposure to the Ag NPs induced toxicity due to NP degradation and the generation of toxic Ag$^+$ ions. At these conditions, the NPs caused inflammation *in vitro*. Similar results were obtained in the immune-competent mouse model, where inflammation was observed after treatment of the implanted tumors with Ag NPs. The inflammation induced an anti-tumoral effect, resulting in a significantly reduced tumor growth compared to Ag NP-treated tumors in an immune-deficient model.

CuO NPs

Ahamed et al. (2015) assessed the current findings of the toxicity of CuO NPs (CONPs) in the lung. *In vitro* studies indicated that CuO NPs induce cytotoxicity, oxidative stress, and genetic toxicity in cultured human lung cells. Leaching of Cu ions, ROS generation, and ATG were the mechanisms of Cu NP toxicity in lung cells. Some studies showed that intra-tracheal instillation of ONPs induced oxidative stress, inflammation, and neoplastic lesions in rats. Cervical carcinoma is one of the main causes of women's cancer, and side effects from standard treatment (including platinum-based chemotherapy) limit the options for escalation. Using cervical cancer cell lines and tumor-bearing mice as models, Xia et al. (2017) reported that CONPs inhibit the proliferation of cancer cells *in vitro* and *in vivo*. CONPs inhibited tumor growth as Cisplatin without weight loss and induced ATG through the Akt/mTOR pathway, suggesting their theranostic application in cervical cancer. To investigate the biological fate of ONPs and their potential in uveal melanoma therapy, Song et al. (2019) investigated the protein corona, cellular uptake mechanism, and localization of ONPs. Furthermore, the effect of ONPs on uveal melanoma cell proliferation, migration, and invasion, and possible mechanisms were studied in detail. ONPs adsorbed serum proteins in a cell culture medium, which were internalized by uveal melanoma cells through the lipid raft-mediated endocytosis. ONPs inhibited cancer cell growth and impaired the ability of uveal melanoma cell migration, invasion, and the cytoskeleton assembly. ONPs were located in the damaged mitochondria involved in CBMP, leading to elevated ROS and CP/ATG and apoptosis. This study conferred detailed information of ONPs for uveal melanoma therapy.

ZnO NPs

To characterize molecular mechanisms underlying photocatalytic cell death of head and neck squamous cell carcinoma (HNSCC) by ZnO-NPs, Hackenberg et al. (2014) incubated human HNSCC-derived FaDu cells with ZnO-NPs followed by UVA-1 irradiation. Apoptosis-independent cytotoxic effects were induced by 0.2- and 2-µg/ml ZnO-NPs and UVA-1. FaDu cells promoted APS formation. Significantly elevated light chain 3 II and ROS were observed after the combined application of both ZnO-NPs and UVA-1 as a photocatalytic treatment. ATG mediated cell survival under UVA-1 or ZnO-NP exposure alone but induced self-digestive cell death after combined treatment. The effect of ATG on HNSCC viability after the NPs-induced photocatalytic treatment seemed to depend on the impact of the physicochemical trigger. To characterize molecular mechanisms underlying photocatalytic cell death of head and neck squamous cell carcinoma (HNSCC) by ZnO-NPs, Gehrke et al. (2017) incubated human HNSCC-derived FaDu cells with ZnO-NPs followed by UVA-1 irradiation. Cytotoxicity was assessed by MTT assay and annexin-V propidium iodide test. ATG was detected by APS accumulation, conversion of LC-3 I to LC-3 II, and lysosomal activity. The generation of ROS was measured using the 2′,7′-dichlorofluorescein-diacetate test. The effect of ATG on HNSCC viability after NP-induced photocatalytic treatment seemed to depend on the impact of the physicochemical trigger. Bai et al. (2017) investigated the effect of ZnO NPs on ATG, cytotoxicity, and apoptosis in human ovarian cancer cells (SKOV3). ZnO NPs with a size of 20 nm were characterized with various analytical techniques, including UV-VIS spectroscopy, X-ray diffraction, TEM, Fourier transform infrared spectroscopy, and atomic force microscopy. The cytotoxicity, apoptosis, and ATG were examined using a series of cellular assays. ZnO NPs resulted in a dose-dependent loss of cell viability, and the characteristic apoptosis was represented by rounding and the loss of adherence, ROS overproduction, and $\Delta\Psi$ collapse were observed in the ZnO NP-treated cells. The cells treated with ZnO NPs showed double-strand DNA breaks, as evidenced from significant number of γ-H2AX and Rad51 expressed cells. ZnO NP-treated cells showed upregulation of p53 and LC3, indicating that these can upregulate ATG and apoptosis. Upregulation of Bax, caspase-9, Rad51, γ-H2AX, p53, and LC3 and downregulation of Bcl-2, indicated that ZnO NPs can induce significant cytotoxicity, ATG, and apoptosis in human ovarian cells through ROS generation and oxidative stress, suggesting that ZnO NPs are suitable anticancer agents due to their favorable band gap, electrostatic charge, surface chemistry, and potentiation of redox cycling cascades. He et al. (2018) found that the ZnO NPs induce crosstalk between ATG and apoptosis, which leads to osteosarcoma cell death. The NP uptake promotes ATG by inducing accumulation of APSs along with impairment of lysosomal functions. The ATG caused the NPs to release zinc ions by promoting their dissolution. These intracellular zinc ions, together with those that are originally released from the extracellular NPs flowed into the cells, collectively targeted mitochondria to induce ROS overproduction and CB formation to inhibit cell proliferation by arresting S phase and trigger apoptosis by extrinsic and intrinsic pathways, leading to cell death. Suppression of the early stage ATG restores cell viability by abolishing apoptosis whereas blockade of the late stage ATG inversely enhances apoptosis. In contrast, inhibition of apoptosis showed a limited ability to restore cell viability but enhance ATG. Cell viability was ameliorated by the combination of inhibitors for both the late stage ATG and the apoptosis. Tongue squamous cell carcinoma is one of the most common malignancies in the oral maxillofacial region. The tumor easily relapses after surgery, and the prognosis remains poor. ZnO NPs target multiple cancer cell types. Wang et al. (2018) elucidated the anticancer effect of ZnO NPs on CAL 27 human tongue cancer cells and identified the role of PINK1/Parkin-mediated MTG in this effect. They analyzed the cytotoxic effects of ZnO NPs on CAL 27 cells. Cells were cultured in media containing ZnO NPs for 24 hrs. They examined the intracellular ROS levels, monodansylcadaverine intensity, and $\Delta\Psi$ following the administration of 25 µg/mL ZnO NPs for 4, 8, 12, or 24 hrs and investigated the role of PINK1/Parkin-mediated MTG in ZnO NP-induced toxicity in CAL 27 cells. The viability of CAL 27 cells decreased after treatment with increasing ZnO NP concentrations. The IC_{50} of the ZnO NPs was calculated as 25 µg/mL. The ZnO NPs increased the intracellular ROS levels and $\Delta\Psi$ collapse as well as activated the PINK1/Parkin-mediated MTG in CAL 27 cells. Babele et al. (2018) investigated the toxic effects of ZnO NPs on budding yeast, S. cerevisiae, to elucidate the underlying mechanism of toxicity. They observed cell wall damage and accumulation of ROS leading to cell death upon ZnO-NPs exposure. A significant change in the cellular distribution of lipid biosynthetic enzymes (Fas1 and Fas2) was detected. Exposure of ZnO-NPs altered the architecture of ER and mitochondria as well as the ER-mitochondria encounter structure (ERMES) complex causing toxicity due to lipid disequilibrium and proteostasis involving CBMP. A significant change in heat shock and UPR, monitored by Hsp104-GFP localization and cytosolic Hac1 splicing, respectively, was observed. Activation of MAP kinases of CWI (Mpk1) and HOG (Hog1) pathways upon exposure to ZnO-NPs was noticed. Transcriptional analyses showed the induction of chitin synthesis and redox homeostasis genes. The induction in LDs formation distorted vacuolar morphology and induction of CP as monitored by localization of ATG8p. However, no significant change in epigenetic markers was noticed as evaluated by immunoblotting, indicating that exposure of ZnO-NPs results in cell death by affecting cell wall integrity and ER homeostasis as well as accumulation of ROS and saturated free fatty acids. To investigate the antitumor effects and action mechanism of Zn-doped CuO nanocompostes (Zn-CuONPs), Xu et al. (2019) investigated the theranostic effects and mechanisms of Zn-CuONPs both *in vitro* and *in vivo*. Zn-CuONPs inhibited tumor growth both *in vitro* and *in vivo*, resulted in cytotoxicity, ROS production, DNA damage, apoptosis, and ATG. The ROS scavenger NAC attenuated all aforementioned effects. NAC also restored the effects of Zn-CuONPs on protein expressions related to apoptosis, ATG, and NF-κB pathways. The NF-κB pathway inhibitor pyrrolidine dithiocarbamate attenuated Zn-CuONPs-induced apoptosis and ATG. Hence, Zn-CuONPs could inhibit tumor growth by ROS-dependent apoptosis and ATG cross-linked by NF-κB pathways. Mitochondrial damage was reported in the toxicity of ZnO NPs. PINK1/Parkin-mediated CP and MTG are emerging additional functions of ATG that selectively degrade impaired mitochondria. Wei et al. (2017) established a PINK1 gene knockdown BV-2 cell model to determine whether PINK1/Parkin-mediated MTG was involved in ZnO NP-induced toxicity in BV-2 cells. The expression of total Parkin, mito-parkin, cyto-parkin, and PINK1 both in wild type and PINK1$^{-/-}$ BV-2 cells was evaluated using immunoblotting after the cells were exposed to 10 μg/mL of 50 nm ZnO NPs. The downregulation of PINK1 resulted in a reduction in the survival rate after ZnO NP exposure was compared with that of control cells. ZnO NPs induced the transportation of Parkin from the cytoplasm to the mitochondria, implying the involvement of MTG in ZnO NP-induced toxicity. The deletion of the PINK1 gene inhibited the recruitment of Parkin to the mitochondria, causing failure of the cell to trigger MTG, demonstrating that apart from ATG, PINK1/Parkin-mediated MTG plays a protective role in ZnO NP-induced cytotoxicity.

Iron Oxide NPs

Magnetite (iron oxide, Fe_3O_4) NPs have been used for drug delivery and MRI. Many metal-based NPs including Fe_3O_4 NPs can induce APS accumulation in treated cells. To investigate the biosafety of Fe_3O_4 and PLGA-coated F_e3O_4 NPs, experiments related to the mechanism of ATG induction by these NPs were conducted. Zhang et al. (2016c) showed that Fe_3O_4, PLGA-coated Fe_3O_4, and PLGA NPs could be taken up by the cells through cellular endocytosis. Fe_3O_4 NPs impair lysosomes and lead to the accumulation of LC3-positive APSs, while PLGA-coated Fe_3O_4 NPs reduce this destructive effect on lysosomes. Fe_3O_4 NPs also caused mitochondrial damage and ER and Golgi body stresses, which induce ATG, while PLGA-coated Fe_3O_4 NPs reduce the destructive effect on these organelles. Thus, the Fe_3O_4 NP-induced APS accumulation may be caused by multiple mechanisms. The APS accumulation induced by Fe3O4 was also investigated. The Fe_3O_4, PLGA-coated Fe_3O_4, and PLGA NP-treated mice were sacrificed to evaluate the toxicity of these NPs on the mice. Fe_3O_4 NP treated mice demonstrated accumulation of APSs in the kidney and spleen in comparison to the PLGA-coated Fe_3O_4 and PLGA NPs. These findings may have an important impact on the clinical application of Fe_3O_4 based NPs. Wu et al. (2017) focused on dextran-coated iron oxide NPs and their induced ATG in human monocytes. NPs are endocytosed by human monocytes where these may be localized within the vesicles or exist freely in the cytoplasm. APS formation was observed with an increased expression of the LC3-II protein, the specific marker of ATG. The ATG substrate p62 was degraded, and ATG was blocked by ATG (or lysosome) inhibitors alone or along with iron oxide NPs, indicating that APS accumulation was due to ATG induction. Iron oxide NPs increased the viability of human monocytes. Inhibition of ATG attenuated the survival of cells, with acceleration of the inflammation induced by these NPs. Thus, ATG activation in monocytes may play a protective role in the Fe_3O_4 NPs' toxicity. He et al. (2019) performed a high-content analysis (HCA) to detect the increase in PINK1, a protein controlling CP, in hepatic cells treated with NPs.

PINK1 immunofluorescence-based HCA was more sensitive than assays and detections for cell viability and mitochondrial functions. Superparamagnetic iron oxide (SPIO)-NPs or graphene oxide-quantum dots (GO-QDs) was selected as a positive or negative inducer of CP. SPIO-NPs, but not GO-QDs, activated PINK1-dependent CP as demonstrated by the recruitment of Parkin to mitochondria and the degradation of injured mitochondria. SPIO-NPs caused $\Delta\Psi$ collapse, decreased ATP, and increased ROS and Ca^{2+} implicated in CBMP. Blocking CP with Parkin siRNA aggravated the cytotoxicity of SPIO-NPs, indicating that PINK1 immunofluorescence-based HCA was be an early, sensitive, and reliable approach to evaluate safety of NPs. Shi et al. (2015) found that Fe_3O_4 NPs induced ATG in blood cells. Both naked and modified Fe_3O_4 NPs induced LC3 lipidation and degraded p62, a monitor of ATG flux, which could be abolished by ATG inhibitors. Fe_3O_4 NP-induced ATG was accompanied with increased Beclin-1 and VPS34 and decreased Bcl-2, thus promoting the formation of the critical complex in ATG initiation. Fe_3O_4 NPs attenuated cell death induced by the anticancer drugs Bortezomib and Dox, suggesting that these NPs can induce pro-survival ATG in blood cells by modulating the Beclin l/Bcl-2/VPS34 complex. Hence, caution should be taken when Fe_3O_4 NPs are used in blood cancer patients. Kuroda et al. (2014) demonstrated the epidermal growth factor receptor (EGFR)-targeted hybrid plasmonic magnetic NPs (225-NP) to produce a therapeutic effect on human lung cancer cell lines *in vitro*. They investigated the molecular mechanism of 225-NP-mediated antitumor activity both *in vitro* and *in vivo* using the EGFR-mutant HCC827 cell line. The growth inhibitory effect of 225-NP on lung tumor cells was determined by cell viability and cell-cycle analysis. Protein expression related to ATG, apoptosis, and DNA-damage were determined by immunoblotting and immunofluorescence. An *in vivo* efficacy study was conducted using a human lung tumor xenograft mouse model. The 225-NP treatment reduced tumor cell viability at 72 hrs compared with the cell viability in control treatment groups. The Cell-cycle analysis showed that the percentage of cells in the G2/M phase was reduced when treated with 225-NP, with a concomitant increase in the number of cells in the Sub-G1 phase, indicative of cell death. LC3B and PARP cleavage indicated that 225-NP-treatment induced both ATG- and apoptotic cell death. The 225-NP induced γH2AX and phosphorylated histone H3, markers indicative of DNA damage and mitosis, respectively. Significant γH2AX foci formation was observed in 225-NP-treated cells compared with control treatment groups, suggesting 225-NP-induced cell death by triggering DNA damage, involving abrogation of the G2/M checkpoint by inhibiting BRCA1, Chk1, and phospho-Cdc2/CDK1 protein expression. Treatment with 225-NP reduced EGFR phosphorylation, increased γH2AX foci, and induced tumor cell apoptosis, resulting in the suppression of tumor growth, providing a rationale for combining 225-NP with other DNA-damaging agents to accomplish enhanced anticancer activity.

Titanium Dioxide (TiO₂) NPs

It has been shown that miR34a acts as a tumor suppressor gene by targeting many oncogenes. Bai et al. (2016) observed the activation of Titanium dioxide (TiO2) NPs(TNPs)-induced ATG through monodansylcadaverine staining and LC3-I/LC3-II conversions and detected the expression of miR34a and B-cell lymphoma/leukemia-2 (Bcl-2). The mechanism of TNP-induced ATG was investigated using the overexpression of miR34a by a lentivirus vector transfection. TNPs induced ATG generation. Typical morphological changes in the process of ATG were observed and LC3-I/LC3-II conversion increased in TNP-treated cells. TNPs induced the downregulation of miR34a and increased the expression of Bcl-2. Overexpressed miR34a decreased the expression of Bcl-2 both at the mRNA and protein, following which the level of ATG and cell death rate increased after the transfected cells were incubated with TNPs for 24 hrs, providing the evidence that overexpressed miR34a enhance CP/TNP-induced ATG and cell death through targeted downregulation of Bcl-2 in BEAS-2B cells.

TiO$_2$ NPs exist in many nano-products and concerns have been raised about their potential toxicity for human beings. Zhang et al. (2018) employed human trophoblast HTR-8/SVneo cells to investigate the effects of TiO$_2$ NPs on trophoblast. TiO$_2$ NPs could enter cells and were distributed in lysosomes, with some in the cytoplasm. TiO$_2$ NPs and protein aggregation were found in both fetal bovine serum (FBS) in culture medium and cytoplasm of HTR-8/SVneo cells. Proteostasis of HTR-8/SVneo cells was disrupted and ERS-related markers including PERK, IRE1-α were increased. After high speed centrifugation, the proteins PERK and IRE1-α were decreased in the highest TiO$_2$ NPs treatment group, which indicated interactions between TiO$_2$ NPs and these two proteins. The protein expressions of LC3-II/LC3-I and p62, the ATG biomarkers, were increased and the ATG flux was not blocked. Cellular ROS stress increased and CP-related genes including PINK and Parkin increased along with the increased co-localization of LC3 and mitochondria indicated that TiO$_2$ NPs interacted with intracellular proteins and activated ERS and CP in HTR-8/SVneo cells, which might impair placental function.

Quantum Dots (Cd/SeO$_2$) NPs

QDs are different from the materials with the micrometer scale. Owing to the superiority in fluorescence and optical stability, QDs act as theranostic tools for application in biomedical field. However, potential threats of QDs to human health hamper their wide utilization in life sciences. Wang and Tang (2018) highlighted that oxidative stress and inflammation are involved in toxicity caused by QDs. Disturbance of subcellular structures plays a significant role in cytotoxicity of QDs. Diverse organelles would collapse during QD treatment, including DNA damage, ERS, mitochondrial dysfunction, and lysosomal rupture. Different forms of cellular end points on the basis of recent research have been concluded. Apart from ATG and apoptosis, a new form of cell death termed 'pyroptosis', which is orchestrated by an IS complex and gasdermin family with secretion of IL-1β and IL-18, was also highlighted. Several potential cellular signaling pathways were also listed. Activation of TLR-4/myeloid differentiation primary response 88, NF-$\kappa\beta$-light-chain-enhancer of activated B cells and NACHT, LRR and PYD domains-containing protein 3 IS pathways by QD exposure were associated with regulation of cellular processes. Gladkovskaya et al. (2019) described the interplay of various cell death mechanisms triggered by Q-dots as a consequence of particle parameters and experimental conditions. Experiments were conducted to track the bone-marrow-derived MNCs in a rat model of acute ischemic stroke by MCAO. QDs labelled MNCs were injected i.v through the femoral vein to track their PKs (Brenneman et al. 2010). MNCs exhibited preferential chemotaxis at the site of cerebral ischemic injury and were exponentially eliminated as a function of time. MNCs conferred neuroprotection by releasing anti-inflammatory cytokines such as IL-4 and IL-10., and thus by performing *in vitro* cell culture, their molecular mechanism of neuroprotection was determined. In the *in vitro* model of AIS by glucose and O$_2$ deprivation in the developing rat brain embryonic neuronal culture, it was discovered that IL-10 receptors are localized on the cortical neurons (Sharma et al. 2011). The time window to determine their theranostic potential in the MCAO model of control and IL-10 knockout mice was investigated. The theranostic window of bone marrow-derived MNCs could be extended to 72 hrs and IL-10 provided neuroprotection in both *in vitro* and *in vivo* experimental models of AIS (Yang et al. 2011). In addition, Fan et al. (2016) evaluated the toxicity of CdTe QDs of different sizes and their mechanism of toxicity in the yeast. A growth inhibition assay revealed that orange-emitting CdTe (O-CdTe) QDs were more toxic than green-emitting CdTe QDs. Further studies on toxicity using a TEM and GFP-tagged ATG8 processing assay revealed that O-CdTe QDs inhibit ATG at a late stage, which differs from the results reported in mammalian cells. ATG inhibited at a late stage by O-CdTe QDs could be recovered by Rapamycin, combined with an increased number of living cells, indicating that the inhibition of ATG acts as a toxicity mechanism of CdTe QDs. Recently, Huang et al. (2018) highlighted that *Helicobacter pylori* (Hp) is a Gram-negative pathogenic bacterium that colonizes and causes a wide range of gastric diseases. Once Hp penetrates into parietal cells, the currently available triple or quadruple therapy often loses effectiveness. ATG is associated with an Hp infection, and can play an important role in the eradication of Hp. QDs can induce and modulate cellular CP/ATG, and developed into nanoconjugates making potential candidates as new anti-Hp agents.

Nano Rare-earth Oxides

Generally, four rare earth oxides induce ATG. Zhang et al. (2010) observed that vacuolization was not always involved in this autophagic process. They investigated three other rare-earth elements, including Yttrium (Y), Ytterbium (Yb), and Lanthanum (La). ATG could be induced by all of them but only Y_2O_3 and Yb_2O_3 induced vacuolization. Y_2O_3 and Yb_2O_3 treated by sonication or centrifugation to reduce particle size were used to test vacuolization level in HeLa cell lines. Rare earth oxides-induced vacuolization that was size-dependent and differed from autophagic pathway. To further clarify the characteristics of this ATG, they used the MEF Atg5 knockout cell line. ATG induced by rare earth oxides was Atg5-dependent and the observed vacuolization was independent from ATG. Similar results were observed in experiments on 3-MA, an ATG inhibitor. This study clarified the relationship between vacuolization and ATG induced by rare earth oxide NPs and pointed out their size's effect on the formation of vacuoles, which conferred clues for the further investigation of the mechanisms underlying their biological effects.

Alumina NPs

Exposure to nanoalumina, but not to nanocarbon, induced $\Delta\Psi$ collapse, increased the ATG of brain endothelial cells, and decreased expression of the tight-junction proteins occludin and claudin-5. Chen et al. (2013) focused on BBB disruption and neurovascular damage induced by NMs. Inhibition of ATG by pretreatment with Wortmannin attenuated the effects of nanoalumina on decreased claudin-5 expression; however, it did not affect the disruption of occludin. These findings were confirmed in mice by administration of nanoalumina into the cerebral circulation. Systemic treatment with nanoalumina induced ATG-related genes and ATG in the brain, decreased tight-junction protein expression, and elevated BBB permeability. Exposure to nanoalumina, but not to nanocarbon, increased brain infarct volume in mice subjected to a focal ischemic stroke model, suggesting that ATG constitutes an important mechanism involved in nanoalumina-induced neurovascular toxicity in the CNS. This study reported the effects of nanoalumina on the permeability of the BBB, suggesting ATG as a primary mechanism in nanoalumina-induced neurovascular toxicity.

MoS$_2$ NPs

Emerging 2D nanomaterials, such as transition-metal dichalcogenide (TMD) nanosheets (NSs), have shown potential for use in cancer nanotheranostics. The interaction of nanomaterials with bio-systems is of critical importance for their safe and efficient application. Zhu et al. (2018) chose molybdenum disulfide (MoS$_2$) NSs as representative 2D nanomaterials to investigate their mechanisms of action in cancer cells. MoS$_2$ NSs was internalized through three pathways: clathrin $\rightarrow$ early endosomes $\rightarrow$ lysosomes, caveolae $\rightarrow$ early endosomes $\rightarrow$ lysosomes, and macropinocytosis $\rightarrow$ late endosomes $\rightarrow$ lysosomes. ATG-mediated accumulation in the lysosomes and exocytosis-induced efflux. Based on these findings, they developed a strategy to achieve effective and synergistic *in vivo* cancer therapy with MoS$_2$ NSs loaded with low doses of drug through inhibiting exocytosis pathway-induced loss.

Tantalum NPs

Porous tantalum (Ta) implants are corrosion-resistant and biocompatible, and possess better stability than conventional titanium (Ti) implants. During loading wear, Ta-NPs that were deposited on the surface of a porous Ta implant are released and come into direct contact with peri-implant osteoblasts. The debris may influence cell behavior and implant stabilization. Kang et al. (2017) investigated the effect of Ta-NPs on cell proliferation. The Cell Counting Kit-8 (CCK-8) assay was used to measure the cell viability of MC3T3-E1 mouse osteoblasts and showed that Ta-NP treatment increased cell viability. Confocal microscopy, immuo-blotting, and TEM were used to confirm the ATG induced by Ta-NPs, and evidence of ATG induction as positive LC3 puncta, high-LC3-II expression, and autophagic vesicle ultrastructures. The CCK-8 assay revealed that the cell viability was increased and decreased by the application of an ATG inducer and inhibitor, respectively. Pre-treatment with the ATG inhibitor 3-MA inhibited the Ta-NP-induced ATG, indicating that the Ta-NPs can promote cell proliferation and that an ATG inducer can further strengthen this effect while an ATG inhibitor can weaken this effect, indicating that ATG is involved in Ta-NP-induced cell proliferation and has a growth-promoting effect.

Europium Hydroxide NPs

Wei et al. (2014) demonstrated that europium hydroxide [Eu(III)(OH)3] nanorods can reduce huntingtin protein aggregation (EGFP-tagged huntingtin protein with 74 polyQ repeats), responsible for NDDs. These nanorods induced ATG flux in Neuro 2a, PC12, and HeLa cell lines through the expression of ATG marker protein LC3-II and the degradation of selective ATG substrate/cargo receptor p62/SQSTM1. Depression of protein aggregation clearance through the ATG blockade was observed by using specific inhibitors (Wortmannin and CQ), indicating that ATG is involved in the degradation of huntingtin protein aggregation. Since [Eu(III)(OH)3] nanorods can enhance the degradation of huntingtin aggregation via ATG induction, these nanorods would be useful for the development of theranostic strategies for various NDDs using nanomedicine approach.

Silica NPs

Silicon-based materials and their oxides are used in drug delivery, dietary supplements, implants, and dental fillers. SiNPs interact with immunocompetent cells and induce immunotoxicity. Chen et al. (2018) highlighted that the toxicity of SiNPs to the immune system depends on their physicochemical properties and the cell type. Assessments of immunotoxicity include determining cell dysfunctions, cytotoxicity, and genotoxicity. The main mechanisms were pro-inflammatory responses, oxidative stress, and ATG. Considering the toxicity of SiNPs, surface and shape modifications may mitigate the toxic effects of SiNPs, providing a new way to produce these nanomaterials with less toxic impaction. Environmental exposure to SiNPs is inevitable due to their widespread application in industrial, commercial, and biomedical fields. Recently, Guo et al. (2016) explored the interaction of SiNPs with endothelial cells, and investigated the effects of ROS on the signaling molecules and cytotoxicity involved in SiNPs-induced endothelial injury. Significant cytotoxicity as well as oxidative stress, apoptosis, and ATG was observed in human umbilical vein endothelial cells. The oxidative stress was induced by ROS generation, leading to redox imbalance and lipid peroxidation. SiNPs induced mitochondrial dysfunction, characterized by $\Delta\Psi$ collapse, and elevated Bax and declined bcl-2 expression, leading to apoptosis, and an increased number of APSs and ATG biomarkers, such as LC3 and p62 involving CBMP. Phosphorylated ERK, PI3K, Akt, and mTOR were decreased, but phosphorylated JNK and p38 MAPK were increased in SiNPs-exposed endothelial cells, which were suppressed by NAC through inhibition of apoptosis and ATG via MAPK/Bcl-2 and PI3K/Akt/mTOR signaling, and the suppression of ROS via activating antioxidant enzyme and Nrf2 signaling. SiNPs triggered ATG and apoptosis via ROS-mediated MAPK/Bcl-2 and PI3K/Akt/mTOR signaling in endothelial cells, and disturbed the endothelial homeostasis, providing evidence for CVDs triggered by SiNPs.

The application of antioxidant may provide a novel way for safer use of nanomaterials. Silica NPs embedded in a biodegradable scaffold offer several advantages when used in laser-tissue-soldering of blood vessels in the brain. During degradation, these NPs are released into the surrounding brain tissue. A study investigated cellular uptake mechanism(s) of the two silica NP types in microglial cells as well as their effect on ATG and inflammatory cytokines. The NP uptake was analyzed using high-content analysis. NP incubation did not modulate cytokine secretion and ATG. The NPs were taken up by the microglia cells. The maximal uptake was reached after 4 hrs and they were found in the ER and lysosomes. Macropinocytosis and phagocytosis were responsible for the uptake, whereas clathrin- and caveolin-independent endocytosis were involved to a certain extent. The pulmonary delivery of NPs is a promising approach in nanomedicine. For the efficient and safe use of inhalable NPs, the understanding of NP interference with lung surfactant metabolism is needed. A lung surfactant is predominantly a phospholipid substance, synthesized in alveolar type II cells (ATII), where it is packed in special organelles, lamellar bodies (LBs). NPs impact on surfactant homeostasis. Kononenko et al. (2017) showed that in ATII-like A549 human lung cancer cells, silica-coated superparamagnetic iron oxide NPs (SiO$_2$-SPIONs), caused an increased number of acid organelles and phospholipids. In SiO$_2$-SPION treated cells, elevated multi-vesicular bodies (MVBs) organelles were involved in LB biogenesis. In spite of the results indicating increased surfactant production, the cellular quantity of LBs was diminished and the majority of the remaining LBs were filled with SiO$_2$-SPIONs. LBs were detected inside abundant ATG vacuoles (AVs) and destined for degradation. There were changes in mRNA expression for proteins involved in lipid metabolism, demonstrating that non-cytotoxic concentrations of SiO$_2$-SPIONs interfere with surfactant metabolism and LB biogenesis, leading to a compromised ability to reduce hypo-phase surface tension. To ensure the safe use of NPs for pulmonary delivery, it was proposed that potential NP interference with LB biogenesis is highly essential. Wang et al. (2017b) confirmed the effects of SiNPs on ATG dysfunction. Cell-internalized SiNPs exhibited cytotoxicity in both L-02 and HepG2 cells. SiNPs induced ATG even at the noncytotoxic level and blocked the ATG flux at higher doses. SiNPs impaired the lysosomal function by damaging their ultrastructure, increasing membrane permeability, and downregulating the expression of lysosomal proteases, cathepsin B (as evidenced by TEM), acridine orange staining, quantitative rtPCR, and immunoblotting, suggesting that SiNPs inhibited APS degradation via lysosomal impairment in hepatocytes, resulting in ATG dysfunction. Herd et al. (2011) studied the influence of geometry of silica nanomaterials on cellular uptake and toxicity on epithelial and phagocytic cells. Three types of amine-terminated silica nanomaterials were prepared and characterized via the modified Stober method, namely spheres (178±27 nm), worms (232±22 nm × 1348±314 nm) and cylinders (214±29 nm × 428±66 nm). In this size range and for the cell types studied, geometry did not play a dominant role in the modes of toxicity and uptake of these particles. Rather, a concentration threshold and cell-type-dependent toxicity of all particle types was observed. This correlated with confocal microscopy observations, as all nanomaterials were taken up in both cell types, with a greater extent in phagocytic cells. There appears to be a concentration threshold at ~100 µg/mL, below which there is no impact of the NPs on membrane integrity, mitochondrial function, phagocytosis, or cell death. Analysis of cell morphology by TEM, co-localization experiments with intracellular markers, and immunoblotting provided evidence of lysosomal escape, ATG-like activity, compartmental fusion, and recycling in response to intracellular NPs accumulation. These processes could be involved in cellular coping or defense mechanisms. The manipulation of physicochemical properties to enhance or reduce toxicity paved the way for the safe design of silica-based NPs for use in nanomedicine. Mesoporous silica NPs (MSNPs) are excellent candidates for biomedical applications and drug delivery to different organs, including the brain. Orlando et al. (2017) used an *in vitro* approach to clarify relationships among size, dose, and time of exposure of MSNPs (0.05–1 mg/mL dose range), and cellular responses by analyzing the morphology, viability, and functionality of human vascular endothelial cells and neurons. 24 hrs of exposure of endothelial cells to 250 nm MSNPs exerted greater toxicity in terms of mitochondrial activity and membrane integrity than 30 nm MSN at the same dose. This was due to induced cell ATG, probably consequent to MSNP cellular uptake (>20%). After 24 hrs of treatment with 30 nm MSNPs, very low MSNP uptake (<1%) and an increase in NO production (30%) were measured, suggesting that MSNPs affect endothelial functionality from outside the cells. These differences could be attributed to the different protein-corona composition of the MSNPs used, as suggested by the SD-PAGE analysis of the plasma proteins covering the MSNP surface. Doses of MSNPs up to 0.25 mg/mL perturbed network activity by increasing excitability, as detected by the multi-electrode-array technology, without affecting neuronal cell viability, suggesting that MSNPs may be low-risk if prepared with a diameter <30 nm and if they reach human tissues at doses <0.25 mg/mL. These findings could help the rational design of NPs for theransotic applications. Hence, careful toxicity evaluation is necessary before using MSNPs in patients. Duan et al. (2014) clarified the biological behavior and influence of silica NPs (Nano-SiO$_2$) on endothelial cell function. The Nano-SiO$_2$ were internalized into endothelial cells. Monodansylcadaverine staining, autophagic ultrastructural observation, and LC3-I/LC3-II conversion were employed to verify ATG activation induced by Nano-SiO$_2$, and the generalized ATG was also observed in endothelial cells. In addition, the level of NO, the activities of NOS and eNOS were decreased, while the activity of inducible (i) NOS was increased. The expression of C-reactive protein, and the production of pro-inflammatory cytokines (TNFα, IL-1β, and IL-6) were elevated. Nano-SiO$_2$ had an inhibitory effect on the PI3K/Akt/mTOR signaling pathway, suggesting that Nano-SiO$_2$ disturb the NO/NOS system, induce inflammatory response, activate ATG, and eventually lead to endothelial dysfunction via the PI3K/Akt/mTOR pathway. Hence, exposure to Nano-SiO$_2$ is a potential risk factor for CVDs.

CeO$_2$ NPs

Hussain and Garantziotis (2013) described that an environmentally and theranostically relevant nano metal (cerium dioxide) can affect primary human monocyte viability and interact with cell death pathways leading to ATG and apoptosis. CeO$_2$ NPs-induced ATG acts as a pro-death mechanism, which lead to the increased cytotoxicity of human monocytes. A better understanding of the biological significance of CeO$_2$ NPs-induced ATG and apoptosis will help us understand the risks associated with its uses and develop safer nanomedicine.

The Theranostic Potential of Organic NPs as CP Regulators in MDR Diseases

Carbon NPs

Identification of pharmacological and toxicological profiles is of critical importance for the use of NPs as drug carriers in nanomedicine and for the biosafety evaluation of environmental NPs in nanotoxicology. Yang et al. (2010) showed that lysosomes are the target organelles for single-walled carbon nanotubes (SWCNTs) and that mitochondria arc the target organelles for their cytotoxicity. The GIT-absorbed SWCNTs were lysosomotropic but also entered mitochondria at higher doses. Genes encoding PI-3-kinase and LAMP-2 were involved in such an organelle preference. SWCNT induced $\Delta\Psi$ collapse, ROS overproduction, leading to mitochondrial damage, which was followed by lysosomal and cellular injury implicated in CBMP. Based on the dosage differences in target organelles, SWCNTs were used to deliver ACh into the brain for the treatment of experimentally induced AD with a moderate safety range by precisely controlling the doses, ensuring that SWCNTs preferentially enter lysosomes, the target organelles, and not mitochondria.

The induction of ATG by NPs causes nanotoxicity but appropriate modulation of ATG by NPs may have theranostic potential. MWCNTs interact with cell membranes and membrane-associated molecules before and after internalization. These interactions alter cellular signaling and impact major cell functions such as cell cycle, apoptosis, and ATG. Wu et al. (2014) demonstrated that MWCNT-cell interactions can be modulated by varying densely distributed surface ligands on them. Using a fluorescent ATG-reporting cell line, they evaluated the ATG induction capability of 81 surface-modified MWCNTs and identified strong and moderate ATG-inducing MWCNTs as well as those that did not induce ATG. Variation of the surface ligand structure of ATG nano-inducers led to the induction of different ATG-activating signaling pathways through their different interactions with cell surface receptors. Orecna et al. (2014) reported that carboxylated MWCNTs induce a decrease in the viability of cultured human umbilical vein endothelial cells (HUVECs) associated with the accumulation of APSs which was mTOR-kinase-independent and was induced by blockade of the ATG flux rather than by activation of ATG. Stimulation of the ATG flux with Bafilomycin A1 (1 nmol/L) attenuated the cytotoxicity of carboxylated MWCNTs in HUVECs and was associated with the extracellular release of the nanomaterial in ATG microvesicles. Thus, pharmacological stimulation of the ATG flux may represent a new method of cytoprotection against the toxic effects of NMs. This study concluded that the pharmacological stimulation of ATG flux may represent a new method of cytoprotection against the toxic effects of these NMs. The fullerene C60 NPs (nC60) induce ATG and sensitize the chemotherapeutic killing of cancer cells. Wei et al. (2010) showed that water-dispersed NPs of derivatized-fullerene C60, C60(Nd) NPs (nC60(Nd)), has greater potential in inducing ATG and sensitizing chemotherapeutic killing of both normal and MDR cancer cells than nC60 does in an ATG-dependent fashion. Additionally, ATG induced by nC60/C60(Nd) and Rapamycin had different roles in cancer chemotherapy. These results revealed a novel and more potent derivative of the C60 NP in enhancing the cytotoxicity of chemotherapeutic agents and reducing drug resistance through ATG modulation, which may lead to novel TSE-EBPT strategies in cancer therapy. Many studies have focused on the neuroprotective effects of C(60) fullerene-derived nanomaterials. The peculiar structure of C(60) fullerene, capable of "adding" multiple radicals per molecule, serves as a "free radical sponge," and can be an effective antioxidant by reducing cytotoxic effects caused by oxidative stress. Lee et al. (2011) investigated PEG-C (60)-3, a C (60) fullerene derivative incorporating poly (ethylene glycol), and its Pentoxifylline-bearing hybrid (PTX-C (60)-2) were investigated against β-amyloid ($A\beta$) (25–35)-induced toxicity toward Neuro-2A cells. PEG-C (60)-3 and PTX-C (60)-2 reduced $A\beta$ (25–35)-induced cytotoxicity, with comparable activities in decreasing ROS and maintaining the $\Delta\Psi$. $A\beta$ (25-35) treatment elicited AMPK-associated ATG. Cytoprotection by PEG-C(60)-3 and PTX-C(60)-2 was partially diminished by an ATG inhibitor, indicating that the elicited ATG and antioxidative activities protect cells from $A\beta$ damage. PTX-C(60)-2 was more effective than PEG-C(60)-3 in enduring the induced ATG. These findings offered novel insights into theranostic drug design using C(60) fullerene-PTX dyad NPs in $A\beta$-associated diseases. The neuroprotective effects of C60 fullerene-derived NMs are known and thought to be related to their capacity of scavenging free radicals. C(60) fullerene-PTX dyad NPs may enhance the ATG of the β-amyloid peptide, which could minimize the damaging effects of this peptide. NMs (including MWCNT) and rare earth oxide (REO) NPs, which are capable of activating the NLRP3 IS and inducing IL-1β production, may cause chronic lung toxicity. Although it is known that lysosome damage is an upstream trigger in initiating this pro-inflammatory response, the same organelle is also an important homeostatic regulator of activated NLRP3 IS complexes, which are engulfed by APSs and then destroyed in lysosomes after fusion. These investigators used a myeloid cell line (THP-1) and bone-marrow-derived macrophages (BMDM) to compare the role of ATG in regulating IS activation and IL-1β production by MWCNTs and REO NPs. THP-1 cells expressed a constitutively active ATG pathway and also mimicked NLRP3 activation in pulmonary macrophages. Li et al. (2014) demonstrated that while activated NLRP3 complexes could be effectively removed by APS fusion in cells exposed to MWCNTs, REO NPs interfered in APS fusion with lysosomes. This leads to the accumulation of the REO-activated ISs, resulting in sustained IL-1β production. REO NP interfered in ATG as demonstrated by disrupted lysosomal phosphoprotein function and interference in the acidification for lysosome fusion with APSs. The binding of LaPO4 to the REO NP surfaces led to urchin-shaped NPs collecting in the lysosomes, demonstrating that REOs interfere in ATG, thereby disrupting the homeostatic regulation of activated NLRP3 complexes.

Graphene Oxide NPs

Graphene-based materials (GBMs) are widely used in many fields, including Nanomedicine. Ou et al. (2017) presented the recent literature regarding the impact of GBMs on apoptosis. CP, ATG, apoptosis, and necrosis are four major PCDs. The mitochondrial pathways, MAPKs (JNK, ERK, and p38), and TGF-β-related signaling pathways were implicated in GBMs-induced ATG and apoptosis. CP/ATG and necroptosis play a vital role in the cell homeostasis, hence their role in cell death should be carefully considered. GBMs induced unrestrained ATG accelerating cell death through APS accumulation and lysosome impairment. Mitochondrial dysfunction, ERS, TLRs signaling pathways, and p38 MAPK and NF-κB pathways participate in GBMs-induced ATG. Necrosis was activated by RIP kinases, PARP, and TLR-4 signaling in macrophages after GBMs exposure. Although ATG, apoptosis, and necroptosis are distinguished by some characteristics, their signaling pathways comprised a network and correlated with each other, such as the TLRs, p53 signaling pathways, and the Beclin-1 and Bcl-2 interaction. A better understanding of the mechanisms of PCD induced by GBMs may allow the thorough study of the toxicology of GBMs and a more precise determination of the consequences of human exposure to GBMs, which will benefit safety assessments for the theranostic applications of GBMs. Yue et al. (2015) explored a vaccine based on the 2D graphene oxide (GO). Without addition of bio/chemical stimulators, the micro-sized GO imparted immune activation tactics to improve the antigen immunogenicity. A high antigen adsorption was acquired, and the mechanism was revealed to be a combination of electrostatic, hydrophobic, and π-π stacking interactions. The *"folding GO"* served as a cytokine self-producer and antigen reservoir and showed a CP, which promoted the activation of APCs and subsequent antigen cross-presentation. Such a modality induced a high level of anti-tumor responses and resulted in efficient tumor regression. This work may shed light on the potential use of a new dimensional nano-platform in the development of cancer vaccines. GO and AgNPs are valuable for the development of nanocomposites, permitting the combination of nanomaterials with different physicochemical properties to generate novel materials with improved and effective functionalities in a single platform. Therefore, Yuan et al. (2017) synthesized an environmentally friendly, facile, reliable, and simple method for the synthesis of GO-AgNPs nanocomposites using Quercetin and evaluated their potential cytotoxicity and theranostic potential in SH-SY5Y cells. The potential toxicities of GO-AgNPs were evaluated using biochemical and cellular assays. GO-AgNPs exhibited higher cytotoxicity toward SH-SY5Y cells than GO by the loss of cell viability, inhibition of cell proliferation, increased leakage of LDH, $\Delta\Psi$ collapse, reduced numbers of mitochondria, enhanced ROS generation, increased pro-apoptotic gene expression, and decreased expression of anti-apoptotic genes. GO-AgNPs induced caspase-9/3-dependent apoptosis via DNA fragmentation and accumulation of APSs and ATG vacuoles. miR-101 is a potent cancer suppressor with a special algorithm to target a wide range of pathways and genes indicating its ability to regulate apoptosis, cellular stress, metastasis, CP/ATG, and tumor growth. Silencing of some genes such as *Stathmin1* with miR-101 can be interpreted as apoptotic accelerator and CP/ATG suppressor. Assali et al. (2018) hypothesized that hybrid miRNA delivery structures based on cationized GO could take superiority of targeting and photo-thermal therapy to suppress the cancer cells. GO nano-platforms were covalently decorated with PEG and poly-l-arginine (P-l-Arg) that reduced the surface of GO and increased the near infrared absorption ~7.5X higher than nonreduced GO. The nanoplatform [GO-PEG-(P-l-Arg)] showed a higher miRNA payload and greater internalization and facilitated endosomal escape into the cytoplasm in comparison with GO-PEG. Applying P-l-Arg, as a targeting agent, improved the selective transfection of nanoplatform in cancer cells (MCF7, MDA-MB-231) in comparison with immortalized breast cells and fibroblast primary cells. Treating cancer cells with GO-PEG-(P-l-Arg)/miR-101 and incorporating near infrared laser irradiation induced 68% apoptosis and suppressed Stathmin1 protein, indicating that GO-PEG-(P-l-Arg) would be a highly suitable targeted delivery system of miR-101 transfection that could downregulate ATG and conduct thermal stress to activate apoptotic cascades when combined with photo-thermal therapy. CQ has shown its potential in cancer therapy and GO exhibited tumor-targetability, biocompatibility, and low toxicity. Arya et al. (2018) conjugated CQ to GO sheets and investigated the former's nonproliferative action on A549 cell lines along with cell signaling pathways. Cytotoxicity, ATG flux, and cell death induced by GO-CQ were investigated on A549 cell lines. GO-CQ induced accumulation of APSs (monodansylcadaverine staining, GFP-tagged LC3 plasmid, and TEM observations) in A549 cells through the blockade of ATG flux that serves as scaffold for necrosome assembling and activates necroptotic cell death. GO-Chl nanoconjugate could be used as an effective cancer therapeutic agent, by targeting the ATG-necroptosis axis. Tang et al. (2018) evaluated the toxicity of GO on two osteosarcoma (OSA) cancer cell lines, MG-63 and K_7M_2 cells. MG-63 and K_7M_2 cells were treated by GO (0–50 µg/mL) for various time periods. Cell viability was tested by MTT and Live/Dead assays. A ROS Detection Kit based on DHE oxidative reaction was used for ROS detection. Dansylcadaverine (MDC) dyeing was applied for seeking unspecific APSs. K_7M_2 cells were more sensitive to GO compared with MG-63 cells. The mechanism was attributed to the different extent of the generation of ROS. In K_7M_2 cells, ROS was stimulated and the apoptosis was activated, accompanied by an elevated expression of pro-apoptosis proteins (caspase-3) and decreased expression of anti-apoptosis proteins (Bcl-2). A ROS inhibitor (*NAC*) alleviated the cytotoxic effects of GO in K_7M_2 cells. However, the production of ROS in MG-63 cells was inhibited by the activation of an antioxidant factor, *nuclear factor-E2-related factor-2 (NRF-2)*, which translocated from the cytoplasm to the nucleus after GO treatment, while a NRF-2 inhibitor (ML385) increased ROS production in MG-63 cells when combined with GO. In addition, ATG was stimulated by APS formation and ATG flux, and increased the expression of ATG-related proteins (LC3-I to LC3-II conversion, Atg5, and ATG7).

Chitosan/Alginate NPs

Chitosans (derived from crustacean chitin) are +vely charged, whereas alginates (derived from algae and sea kelp) are –vely charged. Hence, in combination, they can be used for the encapsulation of large molecules for theranostic applications including nucleic acid (DNA, RNA), miRNA, enzymes, polypeptides hormones (insulin, GH, BDNF, IGF-1, GM-CSF etc), and vaccines. Moreover, these nano-formulations are nontoxic, biocompatible, biodegrading, non-immunogenic, and do not produce any toxic effects to the biological system. The development of resistance toward anticancer drugs results in ineffective therapy leading to increased morbidity and mortality. Therefore, overriding resistance and restoring sensitivity to anticancer drugs will improve therannostic efficacy. Recent studies implicated a role for proteasome and the ATG regulatory protein p62/SQSTM1 (p62) in MDR. Specifically, reduction in the expression of the $\beta 5$ subunit of the proteasome and/or enhanced p62 protein expression contributes to MDR such as Cisplatin (CDDP) in ovarian cancer cells. Therefore, Babu et al. (2014) hypothesized that restoration of $\beta 5$ expression and/or suppression of p62 protein expression in CDDP-resistant ovarian cancer cells will lead to restoration of sensitivity to CDDP and enhance cell killing. They developed a biodegradable multifunctional NP (MNP) system that co-delivered p62siRNA, $\beta 5$ plasmid DNA, and CDDP and tested its efficacy in CDDP-resistant 2008/C13 ovarian cancer cells. MNP consisted of CDDP-loaded polylactic acid NP as the inner core and cationic chitosan (CS), consisting of ionically linked p62siRNA (siP62) and/or $\beta 5$ expressing plasmid DNA (p$\beta 5$) as the outer layer. The MNPs were spherical in shape with a hydrodynamic diameter in the range of 280–350 nm, and demonstrated encapsulation efficiencies of 82% and 78.5% for CDDP and siRNA, respectively. MNPs protected the siRNA and showed superior serum stability compared to naked siRNA as measured by gel retardation and spectrophotometry. The MNPs delivered siP62 and p$\beta 5$, causing p62 knockdown and restoration of $\beta 5$ expression in 2008/C13 cells. The combined delivery of siP62, p$\beta 5$, and CDDP using the MNPs resulted in a marked reduction in the IC_{50} value of CDDP in 2008/C13 cells from 125 ± 1.3 µM to 98 ± 0.6 µM (21.6% reduction) when compared to the reduction in the IC_{50} of CDDP that had only siP62 delivered ($IC_{50} = 106 \pm 1.1$ µM; 15.2% reduction) or p$\beta 5$ delivered ($IC_{50} = 115 \pm 2.8$ µM; 8% reduction) via MNPs. Finally, the CDDP resistance index in 2008/C13 cells was reduced from 4.62 for free CDDP to 3.62 for MNP treatment. This study demonstrated the efficacy of MNP in overcoming CDDP resistance in ovarian cancer cells.

The Theranostic Potential of Antioxidant-loaded NPs

Lin et al. (2017) used Res-loaded NPs (Res NPs) for improving the PKs properties of Res and analyzed their effect on CKD. They coupled anti-kidney injury molecule-1 antibodies to Res NPs and analyzed safety and efficacy. Res NPs had low toxicity, induced ATG, and inhibited the NLRP3 IS and IL-1β secretion. Higher NLRP3 expression was observed in the PBMCs of CKD patients than in healthy individuals. Treatment with kidney injury molecule-1-Res NPs reduced creatinine and protected in tubule-interstitial injury in a murine model, suggesting their theranostic potential in CKD. Hence, Res NPs, through NLRP3 IS attenuation and ATG induction, may be a novel strategy to prevent CKD. In addition, Quercetin induced apoptosis in a number of cancer cell lines. Wang et al. (2012) examined if Quercetin-loaded liposomes (QUE-NL) has enhanced cytotoxic effects and if such effects involve type III cell death in C6 glioma cells. C6 glioma cells were treated with QUE-NL and assayed for cell survival, apoptosis, and necrosis. The levels of ROS production and $\Delta\Psi$ collapse were determined by flow cytometry. ATP levels and LDH activity were measured, and immunoblotting was used to assay Cyt-C release and caspase expression. QUE-NL induced necrotic cell death in C6 glioma cells. High concentrations of QUE-NL induced necrosis, which were distinct from apoptosis and ATG, whereas liposomes administered alone induced neither apoptosis nor necrosis. QUE-NL-induced $\Delta\Psi$ collapse and Cyt-C release had no effect on caspase activation, but decreased ATP and increased LDH activity, indicating that QUE-NL stimulated necrotic cell death.

CONCLUSIONS

Limited information is available to evaluate the exact theranostic potential of antioxidant-loaded NPs for enhanced drug delivery. Various antioxidants can pass through the BBB without any adverse effect, however, they have low potency; hence, they need to be consumed in bulk quantity through fruits, vegetables, and nuts, which may cause gastric upset (Sharma and Ebadi 2013). Hence, ROS-scavenging antioxidant-loaded NPs are proposed. Three types of NPs were proposed based on their response to CB formation, CP modulation/inhibition/regulation, CS stabilization/destabilization, CS exocytosis/endocytosis agonists/antagonists, and CBMP inhibition/or induction to enhance the MQC and ICD for NCF. Toxic NPs augment CB formation and participate in CBMP and are involved in chronic MDR diseases; neutral NPs neither induce nor inhibit CP or CBMP, whereas cyto-protective NPs enhance the efficacy and potency of endogenous and exogenously-administered antioxidants to confer theranostic benefit in various NDDs, CDs, and MDR malignancies to prevent MDR and invasion implicated in early morbidity and mortality. Particularly, NPs used in theranostics must be biocompatible, biodegradable, non-immunogenic, targetable, and easily detectable with an increased signal to noise ratio for molecular imaging to evaluate their safe and effective TSE-EBPT potential to cure chronic MDR diseases, including invasive MDR malignancies. The chapter also highlighted the theranostic and toxic potential of broadly classified (i) organic (including chitosan and alginate) and (ii) inorganic NPS (including Q-Dots) to accomplish the TSE-EBPT of chronic MDR diseases with currently limited therapeutic success. In addition to CP/ATG inhibitors such as CQ and 3-MA, special properties including pegylation, EPR, and tumor angiogenesis utilizing $\alpha5\beta3$ integrin antagonists, block copolymers, dendrimers, aptamers, carbon nanotubes, and exogenously IR-heated gold nano-shells as CP modulators/regulators are other novel strategies which are being investigated for the TSE-EBPT of cancer.

REFERENCES

Ahamed, M., M.J. Akhtar, H.A. Alhadlaq and S.A. Alrokayan. 2015. Assessment of the lung toxicity of copper oxide nanoparticles: Current status. Nanomedicine (Lond) 10(15): 2365–2377.

Arya, B.D., S. Mittal, P. Joshi, A.K. Pandey, et al. 2018. Graphene oxide-chloroquine nanoconjugate induce necroptotic death in A549 cancer cells through ATG modulation. Nanomedicine (Lond) 13: 2261–2282.

Assali, A., O. Akhavan, F. Mottaghitalab, M. Adeli, et al. 2018. Cationic graphene oxide nanoplatform mediates miR-101 delivery to promote apoptosis by regulating ATG and stress. Int. J. Nanomed 13: 5865–5886.

Aznar, M.A., B. Lasa-Saracíbar and M.J. Blanco-Prieto. 2014. Edelfosine lipid NPs overcome multidrug resistance in K-562 leukemia cells by a caspase-independent mechanism. Mol Pharmaceutics 8: 2650.

Babele, P.K., P.K. Thakre, R. Kumawat and R.S. Tomar. 2018. Zinc oxide nanoparticles induce toxicity by affecting cell wall integrity pathway, mitochondrial function and lipid homeostasis in Saccharomyces cerevisiae. Chemosphere 213: 65–75.

Babu, A., Q. Wang, R. Muralidharan, M. Shanker, et al. 2014. Chitosan coated polylactic acid nanoparticle-mediated combinatorial delivery of cisplatin and siRNA/Plasmid DNA chemosensitizes cisplatin-resistant human ovarian cancer cells. Mol Pharm 11: 2720–2733.

Bai, W., Y. Chen, P. Sun, A. Gao. 2016. Downregulation of B-cell lymphoma/leukemia-2 by overexpressed microRNA 34a enhanced titanium dioxide nanoparticle-induced autophagy in BEAS-2B cells. Int J Nanomed 11: 1959–1971. https://doi.org/10.2147/IJN.S99945

Bai, D.P., X.F. Zhang, G.L. Zhang, Y.F. Huang, et al. 2017. Zinc oxide NPs induce apoptosis and ATG in human ovarian cancer cells. Int J Nanomed 12: 6521–6535.

Bibee, K.P., Y.J. Cheng, J.K. Ching, J.N. Marsh, et al. 2014. Rapamycin nanoparticles target defective autophagy in muscular dystrophy to enhance both strength and cardiac function. FASEB J. 28(5): 2047–2061.

Brenneman, M., S. Sharma, M. Harting, R. Strong, et al. 2010. Autologous bone marrow mononuclear cells enhance recovery after acute ischemic stroke in young and middle-aged rats. J Cereb Blood Flow Metab 30(1): 140–149.

Buttacavoli, M., N.N. Albanese, G. Di Cara, R. Alduina, et al. 2017. Anticancer activity of biogenerated silver NPs: An integrated proteomic investigation. Oncotarget 9(11): 9685–9705.

Cameron, S.J., F. Hosseinian and W.G. Willmore. 2018. A current overview of the biological and cellular effects of nanosilver. Int J Mol Sci 19(7): 2030. doi.org/10.3390/ijms19072030

Catalan-Figueroa, J., S. Palma-Florez, G. Alvarez, H.F. Fritzm, et al. 2016. Nanomedicine and nanotoxicology: The pros and cons for neurodegeneration and brain cancer. Nanomedicine (Lond) 11(2): 171–87.

Chang, C.M., K.L. Lan, W.S. Huang, Y.J. Lee, et al. 2017. [188]Re-Liposome can induce mitochondrial autophagy and reverse drug resistance for ovarian cancer: From bench evidence to preliminary clinical proof-of-concept. Int J Mol Sci 18(5): 903. doi.org/10.3390/ijms18050903

Chen, L., B. Zhang and M. Toborek. 2013. ATG is involved in nanoalumina-induced cerebrovascular toxicity. Nanomedicine 9: 212–221.

Chen, F., X.H, Zhang, X.D. Hu, W. Zhang, et al. 2015. Enhancement of radiotherapy by ceria nanoparticles modified with neogambogic acid in breast cancer cells. Int J Nanomedicine 10: 4957–4969.

Chen, Z., S. Ni, S. Han, R. Crawford, et al. 2017. Nanoporous microstructures mediate osteogenesis by modulating the osteo-immune response of macrophages. Nanoscale 9: 706–718.

Chen, L., J. Liu, Y. Zgang, G. Zhang, et al. 2018. The toxicity of silica nanoparticles to the immune system. Nanomedicine (Lond). 13(15): 1939–1962.

Cheng, H.J., T.H. Wu, C.T. Chien, H.W. Tu, et al. 2016. Corrosion-activated chemotherapeutic function of nanoparticulate platinum as a cisplatin resistance-overcoming prodrug with limited autophagy induction. Small 12: 6124–6133.

Dai, X. and C. Tan. 2015. Combination of microRNA therapeutics with small-molecule anticancer drugs: Mechanism of action and co-delivery nanocarriers. Adv Drug Deliv Rev 81: 184–97.

Ding, F., Y. Li, J. Liu, L. Liu, et al. 2014. Overendocytosis of gold NPs increases ATG and apoptosis in hypoxic human renal proximal tubular cells. Int J Nanomed 9: 4317–30.

Duan, J., Y. Yu, Y. Yu, Y. Li, et al. 2014. Silica nanoparticles induce autophagy and endothelial dysfunction via the PI3K/Akt/mTOR signaling pathway. Int J Nanomed 9: 5131–5141.

Fan, J., M. Shao, L. Lai, Y. Liu, et al. 2016. Inhibition of autophagy contributes to the toxicity of cadmium telluride quantum dots in Saccharomyces cerevisiae. Int J Nanomed 11: 3371–3383.

Feng, X., A. Chen, Y. Zhang, J. Wang, et al. 2015. Central nervous system toxicity of metallic NPs. Int J Nanomed 10: 4321–4340.

Gehrke, T., A. Scherzad, P. Ickrath, P. Schendzielorz, et al. 2017. Zinc oxide nanoparticles antagonize the effect of Cetuximab on head and neck squamous cell carcinoma *in vitro*. Cancer biology & therapy, 18(7): 513–518.

Gladkovskaya, O., Y.K. Gun'ko, G.M. O'Connor, V. Gogvadze, et al. 2019. In one harness: The interplay of cellular responses and subsequent cell fate after quantum dot uptake. Nanomedicine 11:(19) 2603–2615.

Golchin, J., K. Golchin, N. Alidadian and S. Ghaderi. 2017. Nanozyme applications in biology and medicine: an overview. Artif Cells Nanomed Biotechnol 45: 1–8.

Gu, X., R.T.K. Kwok, J.W.Y. Lam and B.Z. Tang. 2017. AIEgens for biological process monitoring and disease theranostics. Biomaterials 146: 115–135.

Gukovskaya, A.S., F.S. Gorelick, G.E. Groblewski, Q.A. Mareninova, et al. 2019. Recent insights into the pathogenic mechanism of pancreatitis: Role of acinar cell organelle disorders. Pancreas 48: 459–470.

Guo, C., M. Yang, L. Jing, J. Wang, et al. 2016. Amorphous silica nanoparticles trigger vascular endothelial cell injury through apoptosis and autophagy via reactive oxygen species-mediated MAPK/Bcl-2 and PI3K/Akt/mTOR signaling. Int J Nanomed 11: 5257–5276.

Hackenberg, S., A. Scherzed, A. Gohla, A. Technau, et al. 2014. NP-induced photocatalytic head and neck squamous cell carcinoma cell death is associated with autophagy. Nanomedicine (Lond) 9: 21–33.

Haynes, B., Y. Zhang, F. Liu, J. Li, et al. 2016. Gold NP conjugated Rad6 inhibitor induces cell death in triple negative BC cells by inducing mitochondrial dysfunction and PARP-1 hyperactivation: Synthesis and characterization. Nanomedicine 12: 745–757.

He, G., Y. Ma, Y. Zhu, L. Yong, et al. 2018. Crosstalk between autophagy and apoptosis contributes to ZnO nanoparticles-induced human osteosarcoma cell death. Adv Healthc Mater. 7(17): e1800332.

He, C., S. Jiang, H. Yao, L. Zhang, et al. 2019. High-content analysis for mitophagy response to nanoparticles: A potential sensitive biomarker for nanosafety assessment. Nanomedicine 15: 59–69.

Herd, H.L., A. Malugin and H. Ghandehari. 2011. Silica nanoconstruct cellular toleration threshold *in vitro*. J Control Release 153: 40–48.

Huang, Y., X. Deng, J. Lang, X. Liang, et al. 2018. Modulation of quantum dots and clearance of *Helicobacter pylori* with synergy of cell autophagy. Nanomedicine 14(3): 849–861.

Hussain, S. and S. Garantziotis. 2013. Interplay between apoptotic and ATG pathways after exposure to cerium dioxide NPs in human monocytes. Autophagy 9: 101–103.

Jo, S.D., S.H. Ku, Y.Y. Won, S.H. Kim, et al. 2016. Targeted nanotheranostics for future personalized medicine: Recent progress in cancer therapy. Theranostics 6(9): 1362–1377.

Juang, V., H.P. Lee, A.M. Lin and Y.L. Lo. 2016. Cationic PEGylated liposomes incorporating an antimicrobial peptide tilapia hepcidin 2–3: an adjuvant of epirubicin to overcome multidrug resistance in cervical cancer cells. Int J Nanomed 11: 6047–6064.

Kameyama, K., K. Motoyama, N. Tanaka, Y. Yamashita, et al. 2017. Induction of mitophagy-mediated antitumor activity with folate-appended methyl-β-cyclodextrin. Int J Nanomed 12: 3433–3446.

Kang, C., L. Wei, B. Song, L. Chen, et al. 2017. Involvement of autophagy in tantalum nanoparticle-induced osteoblast proliferation. Int J Nanomed 12: 4323–4333.

Ke, S., T. Zhou, P. Yang, Y. Wang, et al. 2017. Gold NPs enhance TRAIL sensitivity through Drp-1-mediated apoptotic and autophagic mitochondrial fission in NSCLC cells. Int J Nanomed 12: 2531–2551.

Kim, I., Y.H. Song, N. Singh, Y.J. Jeong, et al. 2015. Anticancer activities of self-assembled molecular bowls containing a phenanthrene-based donor and Ru(II) acceptors. Int J Nanomed 10(Spec Iss): 143–153.

Kononenko, V., A. Erman, T. Petan, I. Križaj, et al. 2017. Harmful at non-cytotoxic concentrations: SiO$_2$-SPIONs affect surfactant metabolism and lamellar body biogenesis in A549 human alveolar epithelial cells. Nanotoxicology 11: 419–429.

Kubota, T., S. Kuroda, N. Kanaya, T. Morihiro, et al. 2018. HER2-targeted gold NPs potentially overcome resistance to trastuzumab in gastric cancer. Nanomedicine 14: 1919–1929.

Kuroda, S., J. Tam, J.A. Roth, K. Sokolov, et al. 2014. EGFR-targeted plasmonic magnetic NPs suppress lung tumor growth by abrogating G2/M cell-cycle arrest and inducing DNA damage. Int J Nanomed 9: 3825–39.

Lee, C.M., S.T. Huang, S.H. Huang, H.W. Lin, et al. 2011. C60 fullerene-pentoxifylline dyad NPs enhance ATG to avoid cytotoxic effects caused by the β-amyloid peptide. Nanomedicine 7: 107–14.

Li, R., Z. Ji, H. Qin, X. Kang, et al. 2014. Interference in APS fusion by rare earth NPs disrupts autophagic flux and regulation of an interleukin-1β producing IS. ACS Nano 8: 10280–92.

Lin, Y.F., Y.H. Lee, Y.H. Hsu, Y.J. Chen, et al. 2017. Resveratrol-loaded nanoparticles conjugated with kidney injury molecule-1 as a drug delivery system for potential use in chronic kidney disease. Nanomedicine (Lond) 12: 2741–2756.

Liu, P., H. Jin, Z. Guo, J. Ma, et al. 2016. Silver nanoparticles outperform gold nanoparticles in radiosensitizing U251 cells in vitro and in an intracranial mouse model of glioma. Int J Nanomed 11: 5003–5014.

Lu, N.N., J. Liu, Y. Tian, M.H. Liao, et al. 2014. Atg5 deficit exaggerates the lysosome formation and cathepsin B activation in mice brain after lipid NPs injection. Nanomedicine 10: 1843–52.

Lunova, M., B. Smolková, A. Lynnyk, M. Uzhytchak, et al. 2019. Targeting the mTOR signaling pathway utilizing nanoparticles: A critical overview. Cancers (Basel) 11(1): 82.

Ma, X., Y. Wu, S. Jin, Y. Tian, et al. 2011. Gold NPs induce APS accumulation through size-dependent NP uptake and lysosome impairment. ACS Nano 5: 8629–39.

Manshian, B.B., J. Jimenez, U. Himmelreich and S.J. Soenen. 2017. Presence of an immune system increases anti-tumor effect of Ag nanoparticle treated mice. Adv Healthc Mater 6(1): 1601099.

Mei, L., X. Zhang and S.S. Feng. 2014. Autophagy inhibition strategy for advanced nanomedicine. Nanomedicine 9(3): 377–380.

Muthu, M.S., D.T. Leong, L. Mei and S.S. Feng. 2014. Nanotheranostics—application and further development of nanomedicine strategies for advanced theranostics. Theranostics 4: 660–77

Orecna, M., S.H. De Paoli, O. Janouskova, T.Z. Tegegn, et al. 2014. Toxicity of carboxylated carbon nanotubes in endothelial cells is attenuated by stimulation of the autophagic flux with the release of nanomaterial in autophagic vesicles. Nanomedicine 10: 939–48.

Orlando, A., E. Cazzaniga, M. Tringali, F. Gullo, et al. 2017. Mesoporous silica NPs trigger MTG in endothelial cells and perturb neuronal network activity in a size- and time-dependent manner. Int J Nanomed 12: 3547–3559.

Orth, M., P. Metzger, S. Gerum, J. Mayerle, et al. 2019. Pancreatic ductal adenocarcinoma: Biological hallmarks, current status, and future perspectives of combined modality treatment approaches. Radiat Oncol 14: 141.

Ou, L., S. Lin, B. Song, J. Liu, et al. 2017. The mechanisms of graphene-based materials-induced programmed cell death: A review of apoptosis, autophagy, and programmed necrosis. Int J Nanomed 12: 6633–6646

Panzarini, E., V. Inguscio, B.A. Tenuzzo, E. Carata, et al. 2013. Nanomaterials and ATG: New insights in cancer treatment. Cancers (Basel) 5: 296–319.

Panzarini, E. and L. Dini. 2014. Nanomaterial-induced ATG: A new reversal MDR tool in cancer therapy? Mol Pharm 11: 2527–38.

Papadopolim, D., K. Boulay, L. Kazak, M. Pollak, et al. 2019. mTOR as a central regulator of lifespan and aging. F1000Research 2019, 8(F1000 Faculty Rev): 998. https://doi.org/10.12688/f1000research.17196.1

Parhamifar, L., H. Andersen, L. Wu, A. Hall, et al. 2014. Polycation-mediated integrated cell death processes. Adv Genet 88: 353–98.

Paul, P. and C. Münz. 2016. Autophagy and mammalian viruses: Roles in immune response, viral replication, and beyond. *In*: M. Kielian, K. Maramorosch and T.C. Mettenleiter (eds), Advances in Virus Research, Vol. 95. Academic Press, Elsevier, Burlington, pp. 149–195.

Peng, Y., M. Hongming, W. Shuang, Y. Weiwen, et al. 2016. ABHD5 interacts with BECN1 to regulate autophagy and tumorigenesis of colon cancer independent of PNPLA2. Autophagy 12(11): 2167–2182.

Peynshaert, K., B.B. Manshian, F. Joris, K. Braeckmans, et al. 2014. Exploiting intrinsic NP toxicity: The pros and cons of NP-induced ATG in biomedical research. Chem Rev 15: 7581–7609.

Reynolds, J.L. and R.I. Mahato. 2017. Nanomedicines for the treatment of CNS diseases. J Neuroimmune Pharmacol 12: 1–5.

Roy, K., R.K. Kanwar, S. Krishnakumar, C.H. Cheung, et al. 2015. Competitive inhibition of survivin using a cell-permeable recombinant protein induces cancer-specific apoptosis in colon cancer model. Int J Nanomed 10: 1019–43.

Sharma, S., B. Yang, X. Xi, J.C. Grotta, et al. 2011. IL-10 directly protects cortical neurons by activating PI-3 kinase and STAT-3 pathways. Brain Res 1373: 189–194.

Sharma, S. and M. Ebadi. 2013. Antioxidants as potential therapeutics in neurodegeneration. *In*: I. Laher (ed.), Systems Biology of Free Radicals and Antioxidants. Springer Verlag, Heidelberg, pp. 2191–2273.

Sharma, S., A. Rais, R. Sandhu, W. Nel, et al. 2013. Clinical significance of metallothioneins in cell therapy and nanomedicine. Int J Nanomed 8: 1477–1488.

Sharma, S. and M. Ebadi. 2014a. Charnoly body as a universal biomarker of cell injury. Biomarkers & Genomic Medicine. 6: 89–98.

Sharma, S. and M. Ebadi. 2014b. Significance of metallothioneins in aging brain. Neurochem Int 65: 40–48.

Sharma, S. 2014. Nanotheranostics in evidence based personalized medicine. Curr Drug Targets 15: 915–930.

Sharma, S. 2016a, Personalized Medicine (Beyond PET Biomarkers). Nova Science Publishers, New York, U.S.A.

Sharma, S. 2016b. PET radiopharmaceuticals for personalized medicine. Curr Drug Targets 17(999): 1894–1907.

Sharma, S. 2017. Zika Virus Disease: Prevention and Cure. Nova Science Publishers, New York, U.S.A.

Sharma, S. 2018. Nicotinism and Emerging Role of eCigarettes (with special reference to adolescents). Vol. 1–4, Nova Science Publishers. New York, U.S.A.

Sharma, S. 2019. The Charnoly Body: A Novel Biomarker of Mitochondrial Bioenergetics. CRC Press, Taylor & Francis Group, Boca Raton, FL, U.S.A.

Shen, N., R. Zhang, H.R. Zhang, H. Luo, et al. 2018. Inhibition of retinal angiogenesis by gold nanoparticles via inducing autophagy. Int J Ophthalmology 11(8): 1269–1276.

Shi, M., L. Cheng, Z. Zhang, Z. Liu, et al. 2015. Ferroferric oxide NPs induce prosurvival ATG in human blood cells by modulating the Beclin-1/Bcl-2/VPS34 complex. Int J Nanomed 10: 207–216.

Shi, D., Y. Liu, R. Xi, W. Zou, et al. 2016. Caveolin-1 contributes to realgar NP therapy in human chronic myelogenous leukemia K562 cells. Int J Nanomed 11: 5823–5835.

Singh, V.K., A. Saini and R. Chandra. 2017. The implications and future perspectives of nanomedicine for cancer stem cell targeted therapies. Front Mol Biosci 4: 52.

Sleightholm, R., B. Yang, F. Yu, Y. Xie, et al. 2017. Chloroquine-modified hydroxyethyl starch as a polymeric drug for cancer therapy. Biomacromolecules 18: 2247–2257.

Song, Y., Z. Huang, X. Liu, Z. Pang, et al. 2019. Platelet membrane-coated NP-mediated targeting delivery of Rapamycin blocks atherosclerotic plaque development and stabilizes plaque in apolipoprotein E-deficient (ApoE–/–) mice. Nanomedicine 15: 13–24.

Su, H., Q. Luo, H. Xie, X. Huang, et al. 2015. Therapeutic antitumor efficacy of tumor-derived autophagosome (DRibble) vaccine on head and neck cancer. Int J Nanomed 10(1): 1921–1930.https://doi.org/10.2147/IJN.S74204.

Sun, H., J. Jia, C. Jiang and S. Zhai. 2018. Gold nanoparticle-induced cell death and potential applications in nanomedicine. Int J Mol Sci 19(3): 754.

Tang, Z., L. Zhao, Z. Yang, Z. Liu, et al. 2018. Mechanisms of oxidative stress, apoptosis, and autophagy involved in graphene oxide nanomaterial anti-osteosarcoma effect. Int J Nanomed 13: 2907–2919.

Tian, Y., X. Wang, R. Xi, W. Pan, et al. 2014. Enhanced antitumor activity of realgar mediated by milling it to nanosize. Int J Nanomed 9: 745–757.

Tian, Z., M. Wang, N. Yao, S. Yang, et al. 2019. Expression of autophagy-modulating genes in peripheral blood mononuclear cells from familial clustering patients with chronic hepatitis B virus infection. Arch Virol 164: 2005–2013.

Tsai, T.L., C.C. Hou, H.C. Wang, Z.S. Yang, et al. 2017. Nucleocytoplasmic transport blockage by SV40 peptide-modified gold nanoparticles induces cellular autophagy. Int J Nanomed 7: 5215–5234.

Villeret, B., A. Dieu, M. Straube, B. Solhonne, et al. 2018. Silver NPs impair retinoic acid-inducible gene I-mediated mitochondrial antiviral immunity by blocking the autophagic flux in lung epithelial cells. ACS Nano 12: 1188–1202.

Wan, J., J.H. Wang, T. Liu, Z. Xie, et al. 2015. Surface chemistry but not aspect ratio mediates the biological toxicity of gold nanorods *in vitro* and *in vivo*. Sci Rep 5: 11398.

Wang, G., J.J. Wang, G.Y. Yang, S.M. Du, et al. 2012. Effects of quercetin nanoliposomes on C6 glioma cells through induction of type III programmed cell death. Int J Nanomed 7: 271–80

Wang, G.D., Y.Z. Tan, H.J. Wang and P. Zhou. 2017a. Autophagy promotes degradation of polyethyleneimine-alginate nanoparticles in endothelial progenitor cells. Int J Nanomed 12: 6661–6675.

Wang, J., Y. Yu, K. Lu, M. Yang, et al. 2017b. Silica nanoparticles induce autophagy dysfunction via lysosomal impairment and inhibition of autophagosome degradation in hepatocytes. Int J Nanomed 12: 809–825.

Wang, Y. and M. Tang. 2018. Dysfunction of various organelles provokes multiple cell death after quantum dot exposure. Int J Nanomed 3: 2729–2742.

Wang, F., X. Xia, C. Yang, J. Shen, et al. 2018. $SMAD_4$ gene mutation renders pancreatic cancer resistance to radiotherapy through promotion of autophagy. Clin Cancer Res 24: 3176–3185.

Wei, P., L. Zhang, Y. Lu, N. Manm, et al. 2010. C60(Nd) nanoparticles enhance chemotherapeutic susceptibility of cancer cells by modulation of autophagy. Nanotechnology 21(49): 495101.

Wei, P.F., L. Zhang, S.K. Nethi, A.K. Barui, et al. 2014. Accelerating the clearance of mutant huntingtin protein aggregates through ATG induction by europium hydroxide nanorods. Biomaterials 35: 899–907.

Wei, L., J. Wang, A. Chen, J. Liu, et al. 2017. Involvement of PINK1/Parkin-mediated mitophagy in ZnO nanoparticle-induced toxicity in BV-2 cells. Int J Nanomed 12: 1891–1903.

Wu, Y.N., P.C. Wu, L.X. Yang, K.R. Ratinac, et al. 2013. The anticancer properties of iron core-gold shell NPs in colorectal cancer cells. Int J Nanomed 8: 3321–3331.

Wu, L., Y. Zhang, C. Zhang, X. Cui, et al. 2014. Tuning cell autophagy by diversifying carbon nanotube surface chemistry. ACS Nano 8: 2087–99.

Wu, Q., R. Jin, T. Feng, L. Liu, et al. 2017. Iron oxide nanoparticles and induced autophagy in human monocytes. Int J Nanomed 12: 3993–4005.

Xia, L., Y. Wang, Y. Chen, J. Yan, et al. 2017. Cuprous oxide nanoparticles inhibit the growth of cervical carcinoma by inducing autophagy. Oncotarget 8: 61083–61092.

Xie, F.Y., W.H. Xu, C. Yin, G.O. Zhang, et al. 2016. Nanomedicine strategies for sustained, controlled, and targeted treatment of cancer stem cells of the digestive system. World J Gastrointest Oncol 8(10): 735–744.

Xu, H., R. Yuan, X. Liu, X. Li, et al. 2019. Zn-doped CuO nanocomposites inhibit tumor growth by NF-κB pathway cross-linked autophagy and apoptosis. Nanomedicine (Lond) 14: 131–149.

Yamawaki, H. and N. Iwai. 2006. Cytotoxicity of water-soluble fullerene in vascular endothelial cells. Am J Physiol Cell Physiol 290: C1495–502.

Yang, Z., Y. Zhang, Y. Yang, L. Sun, et al. 2010. Pharmacological and toxicological target organelles and safe use of single-walled carbon nanotubes as drug carriers in treating Alzheimer disease. Nanomedicine 6: 427–41.

Yang, K., Y. Lu, F. Xie, H. Zou, et al. 2016. Cationic liposomes induce cell necrosis through lysosomal dysfunction and late-stage autophagic flux inhibition. Nanomedicine (Lond) 23: 3117–3137.

Yu, X, T. Ian, R. Muqing, D. Kayla, et al. 2016. Design of nanoparticle-based carriers for targeted drug delivery. J. Nanomater 2016: 1087250. doi:10.1155/2016/1087250.

Yuan, Y.G. and S. Gurunathan. 2017. Combination of graphene oxide-silver nanoparticle nanocomposites and cisplatin enhances apoptosis and autophagy in human cervical cancer cells. Int J Nanomed 12: 6537–6558.

Yuan, Y.G., Y.H. Wang, H.H. Xing and S. Gurunathan. 2017. Quercetin-mediated synthesis of graphene oxide-silver nanoparticle nanocomposites: A suitable alternative nanotherapy for neuroblastoma. Int J Nanomed 12: 5819–5839.

Yue, H., W. Wei, Z. Gu, D. Ni, et al. 2015. Exploration of graphene oxide as an intelligent platform for cancer vaccines. Nanoscale 7: 19949–19957.

Zamudio-Vázquez, R., S. Ivanova, M. Moreno and M.I. Hernandez-Alvarez. 2015. A new quinoxaline-containing peptide induces apoptosis in cancer cells by ATG modulation. Chem Sci 6: 4537–4549.

Zhang, Y., C. Yu, G. Huang, C. Wang, et al. 2010. Nano rare-earth oxides induced size-dependent vacuolization: An independent pathway from ATG. Int J Nanomed 5: 601–9.

Zhang, X., Y. Dong, X. Zeng, X. Liang, et al. 2014. The effect of ATG inhibitors on drug delivery using biodegradable polymer NPs in cancer treatment. Biomaterials 35: 1932–43.

Zhang, X., Y. Yang, X. Liang, X. Zeng, et al. 2014a. Enhancing therapeutic effects of docetaxel-loaded dendritic copolymer nanoparticles by co-treatment with autophagy inhibitor on breast cancer. Theranostics 4(11): 1085–1095.

Zhang, X., X. Zeng, X. Liang, Y. Yang, et al. 2014b. The chemotherapeutic potential of PEG-b-PLGA copolymer micelles that combine chloroquine as autophagy inhibitor and docetaxel as an anti-cancer drug. Biomaterials 35: 9144–9154.

Zhang, J., X. Zhang, G. Liu, D. Chang, et al. 2016a. Intracellular trafficking network of protein nanocapsules: endocytosis, exocytosis and autophagy. Theranostics 6(12): 2099–2113.

Zhang, X.F., Z.G. Liu, W. Shen and S. Gurunathan. 2016b. Silver nanoparticles: Synthesis, characterization, properties, applications, and therapeutic approaches. Int J Mol Sci 17: E1534.

Zhang, X., H. Zhang, X. Liang, J. Zhang, et al. 2016c. Iron oxide nanoparticles induce autophagosome accumulation through multiple mechanisms: Lysosome impairment, mitochondrial damage, and ER stress. Mol Pharm 13(7): 2578–2587.

Zhang, Y., B. Xu, M. Yao, T. Dong, et al. 2018. Titanium dioxide nanoparticles induce proteostasis disruption and autophagy in human trophoblast cells. Chemico Biol Interact 296: 124–133.

Zhao, X., T. Qi, C. Kong, M. Hao, et al. 2018. Photothermal exposure of polydopamine-coated branched Au-Ag nanoparticles induces cell cycle arrest, apoptosis, and autophagy in human bladder cancer cells. Int J Nanomed 13: 6413–6428.

Zhao, S., X. Zhang and Y. Ke. 2019. Progress on correlation between cell senescence and idiopathic pulmonary fibrosis. J Zhejiang Univ (Med Sci) 48(1): 111–115.

Zheng, Y., C. Su, L. Zhao, Y. Shi. 2017. Chitosan nanoparticle-mediated co-delivery of shAtg-5 and gefitinib synergistically promoted the efficacy of chemotherapeutics through the modulation of autophagy. J Nanobiotechnol 15: 28. https://doi.org/10.1186/s12951-017-0261-x

Zhou, H.F., H. Yan, Y. Hu, L.E. Springer, et al. 2014. Fumagillin prodrug nanotherapy suppresses macrophage inflammatory response via endothelial nitric oxide. ACS Nano 8: 7305–17

Zhou, S., Y. Sun, X. Kuang, S. Hou, et al. 2018. Mitochondria-homing peptide functionalized NPs performing dual extracellular/intracellular roles to inhibit aminoglycosides induced ototoxicity. Artif Cells Nanomed Biotechnol Mar 29: 1–10.

Zhu, X., X. Ji, N. Kong, Y. Chen, et al. 2018. Intracellular mechanistic understanding of 2D MoS2 Nanosheets for anti-exocytosis-enhanced synergistic cancer therapy. ACS Nano 12(3): 2922–2938.

34

Charnolophagy in Nanotheranostics
(Part-2)

INTRODUCTION

NPs have been widely used in cosmetics, ceramics, semiconductor, and the pharmaceutical industry for improved drug delivery, diagnostic imaging, and as anti-microbial agents because of their unique physicochemical characteristics such as ultrastructure, dispersity, cellular uptake, biodegradability, biocompatibility, target ability, non-immunogenicity, CP/ATG, and CBMP-modulating capabilities. Tremendous progress in nanotechnology and nanomaterials has raised serious concerns regarding their safety and toxicity for theranostic applications in chronic MDR diseases. Several mechanisms have been proposed in NPs-induced toxicity, including apoptosis, necrosis, and oxidative stress, CP, MTG, and ATG. CP was recently recognized as an important cell death mechanism in NPs-induced toxicity, but the exact cellular, molecular, genetic, and epigenetic mechanism of nanotoxicity currently remain uncertain. Li et al. (2018) reviewed generalized ATG, its roles in NP-treated *in vitro/in vivo* models, and mechanisms of their toxicity. The physicochemical mechanisms include dispersity, size, charge, and surface chemistry; cellular mechanisms focus on lysosomal impairment, mitochondria dysfunction, CP/MTG, ERS and ATG; while the molecular mechanisms include signaling pathways, HIF, and oxidative stress. Hence, the significance of CP/ATG as a primary molecular event in evaluating their toxicity and developing novel NPs for theranostic applications cannot be overemphasized. NPs-induced LMP through overloading or direct damage to the lysosomes in the blockade of APS-lysosome fusion, CP/ATG dysfunction, and IS activation are emerging mechanisms of toxicity. These molecular mechanisms of nanotoxicity may be utilized in TSE-EBPT applications (Gulumian and Andraos 2018).

Recently, Wei et al. (2019) focused on the role of NMs utilizing ATG inhibitors for cancer theranostics. Despite their dichotomous roles in health and diseases, CP, MTG, and ATG promote growth and progression of chronic MDR diseases, including malignancies. Clinical trials using CQ and OH-CQ have suggested that the pharmacological inhibition of ATGs can be a promising strategy for treating advanced malignancies and/or overcoming MDR as a molecularly-targeted therapy. The efficient delivery of CP/ATG inhibitors may enhance theranostic potential, reduce systemic toxicity, and overcome MDR in chronic malignancies. Nanocarriers-based drug delivery systems have several distinct advantages over free CP/ATG inhibitors including: increased circulation of the drugs, reduced off-target systemic toxicity, increased drug delivery, and increased solubility and stability. With their versatile drug encapsulation and surface-functionalization capabilities, nanocarriers can be developed to deliver tumor-specific ATGs inhibitors specifically. This unique strategy can be employed for the successful treatment of MDR malignancies with minimum or no adverse effects. Considerable attention in cancer theranostics has been focused on the mTOR inhibition implicated in CP/ATG cell death. Although a combination of CP/ATG inducers with chemotherapeutic agents is being investigated, nanomedicine-based therapy for ACD remains in its infancy. With a primary objective to trigger ACD for synergistic chemotherapy, Mei et al. (2014) incorporated the ATG-inducer, Rapamycin (RAP), into 7pep-modified PEG-DSPE polymer micelles (7pep-M-RAP) to target and prime ACD of Michigan Cancer Foudation-7 Breast Cancer (MCF-7 BC) cell line with a high expression of transferrin receptors (TfR). Paclitaxel (PTX)-loaded micelle (7pep-M-PTX) was considered as a drug model. With superior intracellular uptake *in vitro* and more tumor accumulation of micelles *in vivo*, 7pep-M-RAP exhibited ATG induction and synergistic antitumor efficacy with 7pep-M-PTX. 7pep-M-RAP and 7pep-M-PTX in combination conferred enhanced efficacy through the induction of CP and apoptosis, suggesting that the targeted CP/ATG may confer a rational TSE-EBPT strategy to improve the treatment outcome of BC, and that the simultaneous induction of ACD and apoptosis may be a promising anticancer theranostic strategy.

Recently, the author proposed disease-specific spatio-temporal CB antagonists, CP agonists, CS stabilizers, CS exocytosis enhancers, and CBMP inhibitors as novel CPTs for the TSE-EBPT of CVDs and NDDs, and vice versa for the theranostic management of MDR malignancies. Various CP, MTG, and ATG inhibitors/regulators/modulators such as Rapamycin, CQ, and 3-MA are being clinically tried alone or in combination with conventional anticancer chemotherapeutic regimens with mixed results. The currently available CP, MTG, and ATG modulators induce adverse effects due to unspecific drug delivery. Hence, organelle-specific (particularly mitochondria, ER, lysosomes, peroxisomes, CS, and IS) stable NPs hold a promising future for their targeted delivery to cancer stem cell-specific CB formation/inhibition, CP regulation, and CS stabilization/destabilization as the most promising strategy for the TSE-EBPT of chronic MDR diseases.

This chapter describes various NPs and their theranostic significance as diversified ATGs regulators/modulators. The chapter also highlights synthesis, functional characterization, and the TSE-EBPT potential of NPs for chronic MDR diseases with currently limited theranostic options. Particularly, CQ-modified multifunctional NPs have been introduced to improve their target-ability, drug delivery, and therapeutic benefit. Novel concepts and mechanisms of their theranostic potential, toxicity, and bio-safety are also highlighted based on the author's own experimental findings and from several other investigators across the globe.

Numerous publications have highlighted that ATGs are highly significant in scavenging nonfunctional macromolecules or degenerated organelles for IMD and ICD to maintain NCF and homeostasis in a biological system. ATG is a term generally used to represent lysosomal-mediated elimination of ubiquinated macromolecules or degenerated intracellular organelles such as E.R membranes, peroxisomes, proteasomes, Golgi body, nuclear membranes, in addition to mitochondria. It is important to emphasize that no other intracellular membrane or macromolecule is as cytotoxic as compared to degenerated mitochondria which exist in different pleomorphic forms as CBs and their metabolites in the destabilized CS following ATP-driven, lysosomal-dependent CP. The CS membranes are readily hydrolyzed by the lysosomal lipases and proteases. A starving cell proteolytically-degrades labile CS membanes at the cost of protein-rich diet. Hence, it is conceivable to assume that following ATG, a resulting CPS or APS may pose a specific threat to the MB and ICD. However, this scenario is not so simple, particularly when a CB is phagocytosed by lysosomal-dependent ATP-driven CP. Following CP, a CPS is formed, which is transformed to CS when the phagocytosed CB is degraded by the lysosomal releases, lipases, and nucleases. Numerous mitochondrial metabolites in the CS remain un-hydrolyzed and are highly toxic even after CP. These toxic metabolites include but are not limited to Cyt-C, ammonia, H_2O_2, lactate, acetaldehyde, ammonia, caspase-3, AIF-1, GAPDH, 8-OH, 2dG (mtDNA oxidation product), and 2,3, dihydroxy nonenal (a lipid peroxidation production) as described in this manuscript. The translocation of these toxic metabolites in the nucleus triggers nDNA damage, causing cellular demise involving apoptosis and pyroptosis (pyroptosis is an inflammatory form of PCD that occurs most frequently). Cell death by pyroptosis results in plasma-membrane rupture, release of damage-associated molecular pattern (DAMP), and free-radical-mediated denaturation of proteins, CB-based charnoptosis, apoptosis, necrosis, necro-apoptosis, paraptosis, and/or oncosis (cell death due to ions pump failure). The CS is structurally and functionally labile. It is a single layered intracellular organelle, with a life span of 3–4 hrs in a hostile microenvironment of free radicals generated during oxidative and nitrative stress in the degenerating mitochondria and is readily degraded if it is not stabilized by steroid hormones and/or antioxidants such as MTs, glutathione, SOD, catalase, HSPs, HIF, HSFs, thioredoxine, and HO, which provide structural and functional stability to CS as free radical scavengers and chaperons. Hence, it is highly prudent to stabilize a CS membrane till it is completely exocytosed from the physico-chemically-injured cell for IMD, ICD, and NCF. Following CS exocytosis, the toxic metabolites are released in the systemic circulation to be detoxified in the liver through the hepato-portal system via first pass effect. Water-soluble end products of CS metabolites are excreted through kidneys during phase-1 metabolism with cytochrome-P-450 enzymes and phase-II metabolism with acetylases, glucronidases, and sulphatases. The lipophilic products (such as lipoproteins) are emulsified by the bile. The water insoluble CS products are excreted through fecal matter. The exocytosis of CS requires structurally and functionally intact CS membranes as well as energy (ATP), which is possible only if a physico-chemically injured cell still possesses sufficient structurally and functionally intact mitochondria so that they could generate sufficient energy (ATP) and anti-inflammatory steroid hormones (such as cortisol, testosterone, estrogen, and progesterone from its precursor, cholesterol). A constant mitochondrial biosynthesis of steroid hormones is highly essential to stabilize inner mitochondrial membrane (cristae) which is noncovalently studded with toxic Cyt-C. Hence, the cholesterol transporter (TSPO: 18 kDa channel protein) must be structurally and functionally intact during oxidative and nitrative stress to resist free radical-induced lipid peroxidation which causes the breakdown of PUFA (linoleic acid, linolinic acid, and arachidonic acid), and downregulation of omega-3 fatty acids including icosatrienoic acid, icosatetraenoic acid, icosapentaenoic acid (IPA), exohexaenoic acid, ecosaheptanoic acid, ecosadecanoic acid, and hexosapentanoic acid, icosahetpanoic acid, and docosohexaneoic acid (DHA) to cause structural and functional breakdown of the mitochondrial and other membranes. If TSPO (a 17 kDa protein for cholesterol transport) is delocalized, it becomes incapable of translocating cholesterol in the mitochondria to synthesize steroid hormones. As a consequence, cholesterol goes on accumulating and crystalizing in the mitochondria particularly in the adipocytes due to compromised lipophagy to impair MB in patients suffering from syndrome-X (insulin resistance, hyperlipidemia, hypercholesterolemia, and hypertriglyceridemia), truncal (pumpkin-shaped) obesity, chronic inflammatory diseases, and atherosclerosis. There are at least 21 steroid hormones synthesized in the mitochondria, not only to stabilize their own membranes but also other organelle membranes, including peroxisome, lysosomes, CS, Golgi body, ER, and proteasome for NCF. The Delocalization of TSPO and/or inability of mitochondrial enzymes to synthesize steroid hormones triggers CS destabilization, characterized by increased permeability, sequestration, and fragmentation to induce a pro-inflammatory cascade involving ISs, apoptosomes, and necro-apoptosome activation in MDR malignancies and impaired or delayed wound healing in chronic T2DM resulting in dry or wet gangrene requiring amputations. Hence, novel theranostic interventions involving CB prevention and/or inhibition, CP induction, CS stabilization, CS exocytosis, and CBMP agonists/antagonists will be beneficial for the TSE-EBPT of progressive NDDs, CVDs, microbial infections, chronic inflammatory diseases, and MDR malignancies. This intricate cycle of CB formation, CP induction, CS formation, CS exocytosis, and CS entry in the systemic circulation, CS metabolites detoxification in the liver, and excretion through kidney occurs constantly even in an healthy individual. A typical example includes the GIT system, hematopoietic system, and reproductive system. Every day at least 10^{-6} cells from the intestinal mucosa are destroyed during defecation and the similar number is replaced simultaneously for normal GIT functioning. Any physicochemical or drug-induced disturbance in this GIT cellular dynamic can induce either constipation (Opioids) or diarrhea (microbial infections) to disturb systemic detoxification which can induce toxicity and chronic MDR diseases such as Crohn's disease, inflammatory bowel disease (ulcerative colitis), myelosuppression, infertility, NDDs, CVDs, MDR malignancies, and microbial (bacterial, viral, and fungal) infections, septicemia, hyper-cytokinemia, multiple organ failure, and eventually, mortality. Any physicochemical, physiological, biochemical, and pharmacological perturbation can induce genetic and epigenetic change initially in the mtDNA, followed by nDNA, to induce deleterious CBMP, involving CP dysregulation, CS destabilization, and compromised CS exocytosis to increase ICT and disease progression. Microbes (particularly viruses) prefer to reside within the mitochondria, because they can readily utilize ATP for their growth and proliferation, membranes for encapsulation, and incorporation of their genome with the mtDNA to compromise MB, IMD, ICD, and enhance inflammation. Viruses also escape from the lysosomal phagocytosis while dwelling in the mitochondria. Hence viral infections are usually accompanied with severe rhinorrhea, diarrhea, weakness, and fatigue as noticed in the COVID-19 infection. A structurally and functionally intact circulating CScsc is capable of fusing with any normal non-proliferating cell of a human body to cause malignant transformation. The CScsc is responsible for metastasis and malignancies, as it triggers MTs-mediated Zn and microRNA-regulated genes involved in the DNA cell cycle, cell proliferation, differentiation, migration, development, and growth in uncontrolled MDR malignancies. These malignancies pose a significant theranostic challenge because we lack DSST-CScsc inhibitors/antagonists in acute stages and CScsc stabilizers for the safe and effective management during the chronic stage. Hence, any physicochemical, physiological, biochemical, and/or pharmacological intervention to prevent or inhibit CBMP of toxic CS metabolites from CScsc through the liver and kidneys will be beneficial for the TSE-EBPT of chronic MDR diseases. Nevertheless, CS derived from hematopoitic stem cells or from other biological sources may provide trophic support for growth and regeneration to render theranostic benefit in AIS and in several chronic MDR diseases.

CP as a Biomarker for Enhanced Delivery of Nanoformulations

The conventional CSCs-specific therapeutics, suffer from limited water solubility, reduced circulation time, and inconsistent stability with limited theranostic potential. Targeted drug delivery holds the key to the success of most of the anti-CSCs-based drugs/therapies. Recent advances have demonstrated that specially-designed nanocarrier-based drug delivery approaches (nanomedicine) can be useful in delivering adequate drug molecules even in the most interiors of CSCs niches to overcome the limitations of conventional free drug delivery systems. The nanomedicine has also been promising in designing a therapeutic regimen against pump-mediated drug resistance and reduces its detrimental effects on normal stem cells. To gain a better understanding of the intracellular processing of nanomedicines, Vercauteren et al. (2011) employed quantitative live-cell fluorescence co-localization microscopy to study the endosomal trafficking of polyplexes in RPE cells. A dynamic co-localization algorithm was developed, based on particle tracking and trajectory, allowing spatiotemporal characterization of internalized polyplexes in comparison with endosomal compartments labeled with EGFP constructs. This revealed early trafficking of the polyplexes, specifically to Rab5- and flotillin-2-positive vesicles, and subsequent delivery to Rab7 and LAMP1-labeled endo-lysosomes where the major fraction of the polyplexes remains entrapped for days, suggesting the functional loss of these nanomedicines. The co-localization of polyplexes with the ATG marker LC3 suggested that xenophagy plays a significant role in the persistent endosomal entrapment of nanomedicines. Although treatments of malignant glioma include surgery, radiotherapy, and chemotherapy, the prognosis of patients with glioma remains poor. Ding et al. (2017) developed a PEG-dipalmitoylphosphatidyle-thanoiamine (mPEG-DPPE) calcium phosphate NP injectable thermos-responsive hydrogel (nanocomposite gel) for sustained and local delivery of Paclitaxel (PTX) and Temozolomide (TMZ). In addition, the proportion of PTX and TMZ for the optimal synergistic anti-glioma effect on C6 cells was 1:100 (w/w). The ATG induced by PTX:TMZ NPs play a significant role in regulating tumor cell death, while ATG inhibition reversed the antitumor effect of PTX: TMZ NPs, suggesting that anti-proliferative ATG occurs in response to PTX: TMZ NPs treatment.

Targeting and delivering macromolecular therapeutics to the CNS has been a major challenge. The BBB is the main obstacle that must be overcome to allow compounds to reach their targets in the brain. Therefore, much effort has been made to improve the transport of nano-formulations across the BBB, including the use of NPs. Therefore, much effort has been made to improve the transport of nano-formulations across the BBB, and the use of NPs for delivery of siRNA, specific to a key ATG protein in the microglia, and NP delivery of a soluble mediator to suppress neuro-inflammation in HIV/AIDs patients. Gene therapy for neurological diseases, enhanced drug targeting CNS tumors, NPs functionalization, drugs targeting the brain tumor by overcoming BBB, and the use of macrophages as a delivery vehicle to CNS tumors have been explored. The antitumor efficacy of the PTX:TMZ NP-loaded gel was evaluated *in situ* using C6 tumor-bearing rats, and the PTX:TMZ NP-loaded gel exhibited a superior antitumor performance. The antitumor potential of the nanocomposite gel correlated with ATG cell death. Some anti-cancer drugs induce protective ATG and reduce cell apoptosis. ATG can adversely affect apoptosis, and its blockade may increase the sensitivity of cells to apoptosis. Zheng et al. (2017) designed chitosan NPs to promote the co-delivery of Gefitinib (an anti-cancer drug) and shRNA-expressing plasmid DNA that targets the Atg5 gene (shAtg5) as an ATG inhibitor to improve anti-cancer effects. Chitosan NPs facilitated the intracellular distribution of NPs, and improved the transfection efficiency of the gene *in vitro*. The co-delivery of Gefitinib and shAtg5 increased cytotoxicity, induced significant apoptosis through ATG inhibition, and inhibited tumor growth *in vivo*. The co-delivery of Gefitinib/shAtg5 in chitosan NPs produced superior anti-cancer efficacy via the internalization of NPs, while blocking ATG with shAtg5 enhanced the synergistic antitumor efficacy of Gefitinib.

Osteoarthritis (OA) is a major cause of disability and morbidity in the aging population. Joint injury leads to cartilage damage, a known determinant for the subsequent development of posttraumatic OA, which accounts for 12% of all OA. Understanding the early molecular and cellular responses may provide targets for theranostic interventions that limit articular degeneration. Yan et al. (2016) used a murine model of controlled knee joint impact injury to evaluate cartilage responses to injury at specific time points, and intraarticular delivery of a peptidic NP complexed to NF-κB siRNA which significantly reduced early chondrocyte apoptosis and reactive synovitis. These investigators suggested that NF-κB siRNA nanotherapy maintains cartilage homeostasis by enhancing AMPK signaling while suppressing mTORC1 and Wnt/β-catenin activity. An extensive crosstalk between NF-κB and signaling pathways that govern cartilage responses suggested that delivery of NF-κB siRNA to attenuate early inflammation may limit the chronic consequences of joint injury. siRNA nanotherapy may also be applied to primary OA, in which NF-κB activation mediates chondrocyte catabolic responses. The peptide-siRNA nanocomplexes were non-immunogenic, could freely penetrant to human OA cartilage, and remained in the chondrocyte lacunae for at least 2 weeks. The peptide-siRNA platform thus provided a theranostically promising approach to facilitate drug delivery to the highly-inaccessible chondrocytes.

CP/ATG Antagonist in Cancer Nanotheranostics (NPs in Drug Delivery)

Recently, the author described advances on safe, economical, and effective treatment of NDDs, CVDs, and cancer by adopting emerging nanotheranostic strategies to accomplish EBPT (Sharma 2014). Efficient drug delivery systems are exceedingly important for novel drug discovery. The EBPT promises to deliver the right drug at the right time to a right patient as it covers clinically significant genetic predisposition, chronopharmacological, and charnolopharmacological aspects of nanotheranostics. Recently, nanotechnology provided clinically significant information at the cellular, molecular, and genetic level to facilitate the TSE-EBPT of chronic MDR diseases. Particularly, drug encapsulation in pegylated liposomes has improved PKs and PDs of cancer, CVDs, and NDDs. Long-circulating liposomes and block copolymers concentrate slowly via the EPR effect in the solid tumors and are highly significant for the drug delivery in cancer nanotheranostics. The selective targeting of siRNA and oligonucleotides to tumor cells with a potential to inhibit MDR malignancies has also shown promise. In addition, implantable drug delivery devices have improved the treatment of several chronic diseases. Particularly, microRNA, MTs, α-Syn index, and CB have emerged as novel drug discovery biomarkers. Hence, CB-antagonists-loaded ROS-scavenging targeted NPs may be developed for the treatment of aforementioned diseases. In addition, selective CB agonists may be developed to augment cancer-stem-cell-specific CB formation to eradicate MDR malignancies with minimum or no adverse effects.

Targeted drug delivery systems that combine imaging and therapeutic functions in a single structure have now become popular in nanomedicine; however, many challenges remain for the optimal use of conventional and NP-based therapies in oncology owing to poor drug delivery, rapid clearance, and drug resistance. CQ mitigates some of these challenges by modulating cancer cells and the tissue microenvironment. ATG represents an important cellular response to NPs, whose modulation holds great promise for developing nanomedicine. To enhance ATG in cancer cells, Zhang et al. (2014a) used Docetaxel in the cholic acid-conjugated poly(lactic-co-glycolic acid (PLGA) NPs. Co-administration of ATG inhibitors (3-MA and CQ) enhanced the theranostic potential of this nano-formulation. The volume and weight of the tumor was noticed after a 20 days treatment with the PLGA in mice. NPs formulation combined with 3-MA or CQ were only 50% in comparison with the PLGA NPs formulation alone. Clinically approved cancer therapies include small molecules, antibodies, and NPs. Pelt et al. (2018) discussed the use of CQ as a combination therapy to improve cancer theranostics. CQ reduced immunological clearance of NPs by resident macrophages in the liver, leading to the increased tumor accumulation of nano-formulations. CQ improved drug delivery and efficacy through normalization of the tumor vasculature by suppressing various oncogenic and stress-tolerance pathways, such as ATG, that protected cancer cells from cytotoxic agents. Although limited success has been achieved in atherosclerosis treatment, tremendous challenges remain in developing efficient strategies for its treatment. Platelets have an inherent affinity for plaques and a natural home in atherosclerotic sites. Rapamycin has a potent anti-atherosclerosis effect, but its theranostic utility is limited by its low concentration at the atherosclerotic site and systemic toxicity. Song et al. (2019) used platelet membrane-coated NPs (PNP) to treat atherosclerosis. PNP displayed ~5X greater efficiency than control NPs in atherosclerotic arterial trees, indicating its effective homing in on atherosclerotic plaques. In an atherosclerosis model established in Apo E-deficient mice, PNP-encapsulating Rapamycin attenuated the progression and stabilized atherosclerotic plaques, confirming the efficacy and theranostic potential of PNP as a TSE-EBPT of atherosclerosis. Thomas et al. (2018) highlighted that pharmacologic agents that affect ATG are tested to enhance macrophage nano-formulated antiretroviral drug (ARV) depots and their slow release. These agents included URMC-099, Rapamycin, Metformin, Desmethylclomipramine, 2-Hydroxy-β-cyclodextrin (HBC), and Clonidine. Each was administered with nano-formulated Atazanavir (ATV) NPs to human macrophages. ARV retention, antiretroviral activity, and autophagosomal formation were evaluated. URMC-099, HBC, and Clonidine retained ATV. HBC, URMC-099, and Rapamycin improved intracellular ATV retention and proved superior in affecting antiretroviral activities. As an ATG-inducing agent, URMC-099 facilitated nanoformulated ARV depots, sustained their release, and improved antiretroviral responses. Hence, these NPs should be considered for tbe development of long acting antiretroviral therapeutic regimens.

Mild photothermal therapy (PTT) suffers from limited theranostic accuracy and side-effects due to uneven heat distribution. Therefore, Jiang et al. (2020) constructed nanocomposites based on bismuth sulfide (Bi_2S_3) NPs and bis-N-nitroso compounds (BNN) for NO-enhanced mild PTT. High photothermal conversion efficiency and on-demand NO release were observed upon 808 nm irradiation. The enhanced antitumor efficacy of mild PTT based on BNN-Bi_2S_3 nanocomposites was achieved *in vitro* and *in vivo*. The exogenous NO from BNN-Bi_2S_3 impaired the ATG self-repairing ability of tumor cells, and diffused to the surrounding cells to overcome the limitations of mild PTT, indicating that this nano-formulation could be employed for NO-sensitized synergistic photo-dynamic cancer therapy. Duman et al. (2019) developed PEGylated Ag_2S QDs functionalized with Cetuximab (Cet) antibody and loaded with an anticancer drug, 5-Fluorouracil (5FU). These theranostic QDs were used for targeted NIR imaging and the treatment of lung cancer using low (H1299) and high (A549) EGFR overexpressing cell lines. The Cet conjugated QDs selectively delivered 5FU to A549 cells and induced enhanced apoptotic cell death. While treatment of cells with free 5FU activated ATG, a cellular mechanism conferring resistance to cell death, the EGFR-targeting multimodal QDs overcame drug resistance compared to 5FU treatment alone. The improved therapeutic outcome of 5FU delivered to A549 cells by Cet conjugated Ag_2S QDs was suggested as the synergistic outcome of enhanced receptor-mediated uptake of NPs. Hence, the NPs-loaded drug suppressed CP/ATG even in the absence of an ATG inhibitor. Kong et al. (2018) studied ATG responses elicited by the diverse protein corona types surrounding NPs with different sizes, shapes, and compositions. The physicochemical properties of NP-protein coronas exerted a remarkable influence on cell ATG responses. Surface protein modulation of ATG was correlated with the type of protein adsorbed on the Fe_3O_4 NPs. The ATG in response could be modulated at various levels of protein adsorption, providing novel strategies by the rational design of NP protein complexes to facilitate the TSE-EBPT of cancer. By using confocal microscopy, Sipos et al. (2018) assessed the uptake, processing, and egress of NIR-labeled carboxylated polystyrene NPs (PNP) in live alveolar epithelial cells (AEC) during the former's interactions with primary rat AEC monolayers (RAECM). PNP fluorescence intensity and co-localization with intracellular vesicles in a cell were determined via z stacking. Isotropic cuvette-based micro-fluorimetry was used to determine PNP concentration. PNP uptake kinetics and steady-state intracellular concentration decreased as the diameter increased from 20 to 200 nm. For 20-nm PNP, the uptake rate and steady-state intracellular content increased with increased apical [PNP] but were unaffected by the inhibition of endocytic pathways. PNP co-localized with APS and/or lysosomes. PNP egress exhibited fast Ca^{2+} release and a slower diffusion. The inhibition of microtubule polymerization curtailed rapid PNP egress, resulting in elevated vesicular and intracellular PNP content. The interference with APS formation led to slower PNP uptake and decreased intracellular content. The cytosolic [PNP] was higher than apical PNP, and vesicular PNP (~80% of intracellular PNP content) exceeded both cytosolic and intracellular PNP, consistent with the hypotheses: 1) ATG processing of NPs is essential for the maintenance of AEC integrity; 2) altered ATG and/or lysosomal exocytosis may lead to AEC injury; and 3) intracellular PNP in AEC can be regulated, suggesting strategies to enhance NP-driven AEC gene/drug delivery and/or ameliorate AEC NP-related cellular toxicity.

Understanding the mechanism of radioresistance could help develop strategies to improve the theranostic response of patients with PDAC. The SMAD4 gene is frequently mutated in PC. Wang et al. (2018a) investigated the role of SMAD4 deficiency in PC cells' response to radiotherapy. SMAD4 expression was downregulated with SMAD4 siRNA or SMAD4 shRNA; overexpressed SMAD4 in SMAD4 mutant PC cells were evaluated by a clonogenic survival assay to evaluate their effects on radio-resistance. To study the mechanism of radio-resistance, the effects of SMAD4 loss on RO) and ATG were determined by flow cytometry and immunoblot analysis, respectively. The radio-resistance was measured by the clonogenic survival assay after treatment with ATG inhibitor (CQ) and ROS inhibitor (NAC) in SMAD4-depleted PC cells. The effects of SMAD4 on radio-resistance were confirmed in an orthotopic tumor model derived from SMAD4-depleted Panc-1 cells. The SMAD4-depleted PC cells were resistant to radiotherapy based on the clonogenic survival assay. The overexpression of wild-type SMAD4 in SMAD4-mutant cells rescued their radio-sensitivity. Radio-resistance mediated by SMAD4 depletion was associated with higher levels of ROS and radiation-induced ATG. SMAD4 depletion induced *in vivo* radio-resistance in the Panc-1-derived orthotopic tumor model. The protein level of SMAD4 was inversely correlated with ATG in orthotopic tumor tissue samples, indicating that defective SMAD4 was responsible for radio-resistance in PC through ROS overproduction and increased radiation-induced ATG.

Sorafenib is a first-line drug for HCC. ATG facilitates Sorafenib resistance, whereas miR-375 is an inhibitor of ATG. Zhao et al. (2018) loaded miR-375 and Sorafenib into calcium carbonate NPs with lipid coating (miR-375/Sf-LCC NPs). The NPs had a high loading efficiency and were ~50 nm in diameter. NPs increased the stability and residence time of both drugs. ATG was activated by Sorafenib but not by miR-375/Sf-LCC NPs. *In vitro*, miR-375/Sf-LCC NPs exhibited pH-dependent drug release and cytotoxicity. *In vivo*, miR-375/Sf-LCC NPs increased miR-375 and Sorafenib uptake in tumor (2X compared with Lipofectamine 2000-miR-375 and 2–5 folds compared with free Sorafenib). This nano-formulation showed enhanced theranostic efficacy in an HCC xenograft model, suggesting that it may be a promising agent for the HCC theranostics.

FTY720, known as Fingolimod, is a new immunosuppressive agent with effective anticancer properties. Although it was recently confirmed that FTY720 inhibits cancer cell proliferation, it can also induce protective ATG and reduce cytotoxicity. Blocking ATG with Beclin-1 siRNA after treatment with FTY720 promoted apoptosis. Wu et al. (2018) enhanced the anticancer effect of FTY720 in HCC by the targeted co-delivery of FTY720 and Beclin-1 siRNA using calcium phosphate (CaP) NPs. The siRNA was encapsulated within the CaP core. To form an asymmetric lipid bilayer, an anionic lipid was used for the inner leaflet and a cationic lipid for the outer leaflet; after removing chloroform by rotary evaporation, these lipids were dispersed in a saline solution with FTY720. The NPs were analyzed by TEM, dynamic light scattering, and UV/VIS spectrophotometry. Cancer cell viability and cell death were analyzed by MTT assays, FACS, and immunoblotting. The *in vivo* effects of the NPs were investigated using an athymic nude mouse s.c. transplantation tumor model. When LCP-II NPs, were loaded with FTY720 and siRNA, they exhibited the expected size and were internalized by cells. These NPs were stable in systemic circulation. The cytotoxicity was enhanced when FTY20 and Beclin-1 siRNA were co-delivered as compared to free drug alone. Hence, a CaP NP system can be developed for the co-delivery of FTY720 and Beclin-1 siRNA to treat HCC as a novel theranostic strategy for HCC treatment. MGB1 is an important sepsis mediator when secreted and also functions as an inducer of ATG by binding to Beclin-1. Kim et al. (2018) studied the effect of Inflachromene (ICM), a novel HMGB1 secretion inhibitor, on ATG. ICM inhibited ATG by inhibiting the nucleocytoplasmic translocation of HMGB1 and by increasing Beclin-1 ubiquitylation for degradation by enhancing the interaction between Beclin-1 and E3 ubiquitin ligase RNF216, suggesting that ICM could be used as a potential ATG suppressor.

To mechanistically prove the concept of monocyte-mediated nano drug delivery in GBM, Wang et al. (2018b) conducted a study by developing nano-Dox-loaded monocytes (Nano-DOX-MC). Nano-DOX-MC were viable, crossed an artificial endothelial barrier, infiltrated GBM spheroids, and released the drug therein. GBM cells stimulated the unloading of Nano-DOX-MC and took up the unloaded drug and released damage-associated molecular patterns. In mice with orthotopic GBM xenografts, Nano-DOX-MC improved tumor drug delivery and damage-associated molecular emission. Nano-DOX sequestered in the lysosomes and induced ATG through lysosomal activation. Hence, Nano-DOX can be delivered by MC in GBM to induce cancer cell destruction.

Small-molecule inhibitors of the mTORC2 kinase (Torkinibs) have shown efficacy in early clinical trials. However, the Torkinibs also inhibit the other mTOR-containing complex mTORC1. While combined mTORC1/mTORC2 inhibition may be beneficial in cancer cells, recent reports described compensatory cell survival upon mTORC1 inhibition due to the loss of negative feedback on PI3K, increased ATG, and increased macropinocytosis. Genetic models suggested that selective mTORC2 inhibition would be effective in BCs, but the lack of selective small-molecule inhibitors of mTORC2 have precluded testing of this hypothesis. In this study, Werfel et al (2018) described that nanotheranostics inhibited the growth regulatory kinase mTORC2 in a preclinical model of BC. Werfel et al. (2018) reported the engineering of a NP-based RNAi theranostic that can silence the mTORC2 obligate cofactor Rictor. NP-based Rictor ablation in HER2-amplified breast tumors was achieved following intra-tumoral and i.v delivery, decreasing Akt phosphorylation and increasing tumor cell demise. Selective mTORC2 inhibition *in vivo*, combined with the HER2 inhibitor, Lapatinib, decreased the growth of HER2-amplified BCs to a greater extent than either agent alone, suggesting that mTORC2 promotes Lapatinib resistance, which can be attenuated by mTORC2 inhibition. The selective mTORC2 inhibition was effective in a TNBC model, decreasing Akt phosphorylation and tumor growth, consistent with the findings that Rictor mRNA correlates with worse outcome in patients with basal-like TNBC. These results conferred preclinical validation of a novel RNAi delivery platform for theranostic gene ablation in BC, and showed that mTORC2-selective targeting is feasible and efficacious in this disease. Li et al. (2017) developed a dual-target theranostic F_{671}, which exhibited synergetic anticancer effects for inhibiting the activities of glutathione S-transferase and the accumulation of HIF-1α. F_{671} undergoes self-immolative cleavage when exposed to GSTP1-1 in live cancer cells, facilitating the visualization of release and distribution, as well as confirming the ATG-induced apoptosis. The phosphinositide PtdIns(3)P plays an important role in ATG; however, the exact mechanism of its activity remains uncertain. Donia et al. (2019) used a Systematic Evolution of Ligands by EXponential enrichment (SELEX) screening to identify an RNA aptamer of 40 nucleotides that specifically recognizes and binds to lysosomal PtdIns(3)P. The binding occurred in a Mg^{2+} concentration- and pH-dependent manner, and inhibited ATG as determined by LC3-II/I conversion, p62 degradation, formation of LC3 puncta, and lysosomal accumulation of Phafin2, resulting in inhibited lysosomal acidification, and the hydrolytic activity of cathepsin D following ATG induction. Given the essential role of PtdIns(3)P as a key targeting molecule for ATG induction, PtdIns(3)P RNA aptamer confers novel opportunities for investigating the biological functions and mechanisms of phosphoinositides.

Jabłoński et al. (2017) reported the synthesis of four Cymantrene-5-Fluorouracil derivatives (1–4) and two Cymantrene-adenine derivatives (5 and 6). All of the compounds were characterized by spectroscopic methods and the crystal structure of two derivatives (1 and 6), together with the Cymantrene-adenine compound C was determined by X-ray crystallography. While the compounds 1 and 6 crystallized in the triclinic P-1 space group, compound C crystallized in the monoclinic $P2_1/m$ space group. The compounds 1–6 were tested together with the two cymantrene derivatives, B and C, for their *in vitro* anti-proliferative activity in seven cancer cell lines (MCF-7, MCF-7/DX, MDA-MB-231, SKOV-3, A549, HepG2m, and U-87-MG), five bacterial strains *Staphylococcus aureus* (Methicillin-sensitive, Methicillin-resistant, and Vancomycin-intermediate strains), *Staphylococcus epidermidis*, and *Escherichia coli*, including clinical isolates of *S. aureus* and *S. epidermidis*, as well as against the protozoan parasite *Trypanosoma brucei*. The most cytotoxic compounds were derivatives 2 and C for A549 and SKOV-3 cancer cell lines, respectively, with IC_{50} ~7 μM. The anticancer activity of the cymantrene compounds was determined by their ability to induce oxidative stress and trigger apoptosis and ATG in cancer cells. Three derivatives (1, 4, and 5) displayed promising antitrypanosomal activity, with GI_{50} 3–4 μM. The introduction of the 5-FU moiety in 1 enhanced trypanocidal activity. The antibacterial activity of cymantrene compounds 1 and C were within the range of 8–64 μg/mL and seemed to be the result of cell shrinking. Various pathophysiological barriers compromise effective airway drug delivery in cystic fibrosis (CF). Hence, Faraj et al. (2019) standardized the theranostic efficacy of the novel dendrimer-based CP/ATG-inducing the antioxidant drug, Cysteamine. Human primary-CF epithelial-cells, CFBE41o-cells, were used to standardize the efficacy of the dendrimer-Cystamine in correcting impaired-CP/ATG, rescuing ΔF508-CFTR and a Pseudomonas-aeruginosa (Pa) infection. They designed a novel Cystamine-core dendrimer formulation (G4-CYS) that increased membrane-ΔF508CFTR expression in CFBE41o-cells by forming its reduced-form Cysteamine, *in vivo*. G4-CYS treatment corrected ΔF508-CFTR-mediated impaired-CP/ATG as observed by a decrease in Ub-LC3-positive aggresome-bodies. In non-permeabilized CFBE41o-cells, G4-CYS induced ΔF508-CFTR's forward-trafficking to the plasma membrane. Cysteamine's known antibacterial and anti-biofilm properties against Pa were enhanced as their findings demonstrated that both G4-CYS and its control DAB-core dendrimer, G4-DAB, exhibited bactericidal-activity against Pa. Both G4-CYS and G4-DAB exhibited marked mucolytic-activity against porcine-mucus, suggesting that G4-CYS resolves CP/ATG-impairment by rescuing ΔF508-CFTR in CFBE41o-cells and corrects the phagocytosis defect, demonstrating the efficacy of novel Cystamine-dendrimer formulation in rescuing ΔF508-CFTR from the plasma membrane and inhibiting Pa bacterial-infection by augmenting CP/ATG in CF patients.

Presently available drugs for AD can only ameliorate the symptoms rather than reverse or prevent the AD progression. BBB impedes drug delivery from the blood circulation into the brain. Nanomedicine can be a safe, effective, and promising approach to treat AD. Ma et al. (2018) summarized the use of liposomes and NPs for targeted treatment of AD by searching MeSH Terms: "Alzheimer's disease; nanomedicine; NP; amyloid β peptide; tau protein; ATG". Nanomedicines have demonstrated superiority over conventional anti-AD drugs in AD because: (a) many unfavorable pharmaceutical properties of conventional anti-AD drugs can be overcome by nanomedicine; (b) nanomedicines trigger the efficient production of high-titer anti-Aβ antibodies following controlled release of antigens by them; (c) some apolipoprotein-based nanomedicines specifically bind to Aβ and augment the elimination of Aβ-induced ATG to facilitate the elimination of Aβ nanomedicine-induced inhibition of tau aggregation for the TSE-EBPT of AD. Graphene oxide (GO) is a nanomaterial with theranostic applications. CP/ATG is an intracellular degradation system that has been associated with the progression of NDDs. Jeong et al. (2017) showed that GO activates ATG flux in neuronal cells and confers a neuroprotection in prion protein(PrP)(106–126)-mediated neurotoxicity. GO can be detected in SK-N-SH neuronal cells, where it triggers ATG signaling. GO-induced ATG prevented PrP (106–126)-induced neurotoxicity in SK-N-SH cells. The inactivation of ATG blocked GO-induced neuroprotection in prion-mediated mitochondrial neurotoxicity demonstrating that GO regulates ATG in neuronal cells, and that the activation of ATG, induced by GO, plays a neuroprotective role in prion-mediated mitochondrial neurotoxicity involving CBMP, suggesting that GO may be used to activate CP/ATG as a neuroprotective strategy for the treatment of prion and other NDDs.

CQ-modified NPs as CP Regulators in Cancer Theranostics

Hydroxyethyl starch (HES) is a clinically-used polysaccharide colloidal plasma volume expander. Sleightholm et al. (2017) synthesized HES modified with HCQ as a novel polymeric drug which attenuates the invasive character of PC cells. HES was conjugated with HCQ using carbonyldiimidazole coupling to prepare CQ-modified HES (CQ-HES). CQ-HES with various degrees of HCQ substitution were synthesized and characterized. Atomic force microscopy was used to demonstrate a pH-dependent assembly of CQ-HES into NPs. CQ-HES have a similar toxicity profile as HCQ. Confocal microscopy revealed the propensity of CQ-HES to localize to lysosomes and confirmed that CQ-HES inhibits ATG in PC cells. The enhanced ability of CQ-HES to inhibit the migration and invasion of PC cells was observed as compared to HCQ. The enhanced inhibitory actions of CQ-HES compared to HCQ originated from the increased inhibition of ERK and Akt phosphorylation. Insignificant HCQ release from CQ-HES confirmed that the observed activity was due to the action of CQ-HES as a polymeric drug. Due to its ability to block cancer cell invasion and form NPs, CQ-HES has potential as a drug delivery platform for future development with chemotherapeutics to establish novel anti-metastatic treatments. Joshi et al. (2012) conjugated 11-mercaptoundecanoic acid-modified GNPs (~7 nm) with CQ to explore their application in cancer theranostics. The anticancer activity of CQ-GNP conjugates (GNP-Chl) was demonstrated in MCF-7 BC cells. The MCF-7 cells were treated with different concentrations of GNP-Chl conjugates, and the cell viability was assayed using Trypan blue. Flow cytometry analysis revealed that the major pathway of cell death was necrosis, which was mediated by ATG. The drug release kinetics of GNP-Chl conjugates revealed the release of CQ at an acidic pH, which was estimated using optical absorbance spectroscopy. The nature of stimuli-responsive drug release and the inhibition of cancer cell growth by GNP-Chl conjugates facilitated the design of combinatorial nanotheranostics for the treatment of cancer. A novel composite liposomal system co-encapsulating Paclitaxel (PTX) with CQ was designed for treating PTX-resistant carcinoma by Guo et al. (2018). Liposomal CQ sensitized PTX by ATG inhibition and was involved in competitively binding it with MDR transporters. The co-encapsulation of PTX and CQ in liposomes was superior to the mixture of PTX liposome plus CQ liposome due to the simultaneous delivery and synergetic effect of the two drugs. The composite liposome achieved superior anticancer efficacy *in vivo* than the PTX liposome plus CQ liposome mixture, indicating the significance of CQ and Palciteaxel co-delivery via liposome. Micelle may be the nano-carrier that is used due to its promising performance and technical simplicity. However, like the original drugs, micellar formulation may induce ATG that compromises their advantages for efficient drug delivery. Zhang et al. (2014b) showed that by using Docetaxel-loaded PEG-b-PLGA micelles as a micellar model, the micelles induce ATG and are subject to degradation through the endo-lysosome pathway. Co-administration of the micellar formulation with CQ enhanced their theranostic potential. The Docetaxel-loaded PEG-b-PLGA micelles were formulated by membrane dialysis, with 7.1% drug loading and 72.8% drug encapsulation efficiency in a size range of ~40 nm. The IC_{50} values of the drug formulated in the PEG-b-PLGA micelles after 24 hrs treatment of MCF-7 cancer cells with no ATG inhibitor or in combination with CQ were 22.30 ± 1.32 and 1.75 ± 0.43 µg/mL respectively, indicating 12X enhanced treatment with CQ. The *in vivo* study further confirmed the advantages of this nano-formulation, which may provide knowledge for the TSE-EBPT of chronic MDR diseases.

CONCLUSION

The conventional pegylation of CP/ATG antagonists-loaded NPs along with the co-delivery of routinely used chemotherapeutic agents is being clinically-attempted to enhance drug delivery, particularly to the cancer stem cells to improve selectivity, specificity, and targetability and to prevent their entrapment in the RE system including lungs, liver, and spleen and avoid unspecific and undesirable adverse effects of the new generation of anticancer drugs. Novel Cystamine-core dendrimer-formulations have been developed to rescue ΔF508-CFTR and inhibit Pseudomonas aeruginosa infection by CP/MTG/ATG modulation for the TSE-EBPT of CF patients.

REFERENCES

Ding, L., Q. Wang, M. Shen, Y. Sun, et al. 2017. Thermoresponsive nanocomposite gel for local drug delivery to suppress the growth of glioma by inducing autophagy. Autophagy 13: 1176–1190.

Donia, T., B. Jyoti, F. Suizu, N. Hirata, et al. 2019. Identification of RNA aptamer which specifically interacts with PtdIns(3)P. Biochem Biophys Res Commun 517: 146–154.

Duman, F.D., Y. Akkoc, G. Demirci, N. Bavili, et al. 2019. Bypassing pro-survival and resistance mechanisms of ATG in EGFR-positive lung cancer cells by targeted delivery of 5FU using theranostic Ag(2)S quantum dots. J Mater Chem B 7: 7363–7376.

Faraj, J., M. Bodas, G. Pehote, D. Swanson, et al. 2019. Novel cystamine-core dendrimer-formulation rescues ΔF508-CFTR and inhibits Pseudomonas aeruginosa infection by augmenting ATG. Expert Opin Drug Deliv 16: 177–186.

Gulumian, M. and C. Andraos. 2018. In search of a converging cellular mechanism in nanotoxicology and nanomedicine in the treatment of cancer. Toxicol Pathol 46: 4–13.

Guo, Z., V. Johnson, J. Barrera, M. Porras, et al. 2018. Targeting cytochrome P450-dependent cancer cell mitochondria: Cancer associated CYPs and where to find them. Cancer Metastasis Rev 37: 409–423.

Jabłoński, A., K. Matczak, A. Koceva-Chyła, K. Durka, et al. 2017. Cymantrenyl-nucleobases: Synthesis, anticancer, antitrypanosomal and antimicrobial activity studies. Molecules 22(12): 2220. doi:10.3390/molecules22122220.

Jeong, J.K., Y.J. Lee, S.Y. Jeong, S. Jeong, et al. 2017. Autophagic flux induced by graphene oxide has a neuroprotective effect against human prion protein fragments. Internat J Nanomed 12: 8143–8158.

Jiang, J., X. Che, Y. Qian, L. Wang, et al. 2020. Bismuth sulfide nanorods as efficient photothermal theranostic agents in cancer treatment. Front. Mater. 7: 234. doi: 10.3389/fmats.2020.00234

Kim, Y.H., M.S. Kwak, J.M. Shin and R.A. Hayuningtyas. 2018. Inflachromene inhibits ATG through modulation of Beclin 1 activity. J Cell Sci 131(4): 211201.

Kong, H., K. Xia, N. Ren, Y. Cui, et al. 2018. Serum protein corona-responsive ATG tuning in cells. Nanoscale 10: 18055–18063.

Li, Z., J. Ding, C. Chen, J. Chang, et al. 2017. Dual-target cancer theranostic for glutathione S-transferase and hypoxia-inducible factor-1α inhibition. Chem Commun (Camb) 53: 12406–12409.

Ma, T.J., J. Gao, Y. Liu, J.H. Zhuang, et al. 2018. Nanomedicine strategies for sustained, controlled and targeted treatment of Alzheimer's disease. Mini Rev Med Chem 18: 1035–1046.

Mei, L., X. Zhang and S.S. Feng. 2014. Autophagy inhibition strategy for advanced nanomedicine. Nanomedicine 9(3): 377–380.

Pelt, J., S. Busatto, M. Ferrari, E.A. Thompson, et al. 2018. Chloroquine and nanoparticle drug delivery: A promising combination. Pharmacol Ther 91: 43–49.

Sharma, S. 2014. Nanotheranostics in evidence based personalized medicine. Curr Drug Targets 15: 915–930.

Sipos, A., K.-J. Kim, R.H. Chow, P. Flodby, et al. 2018. Alveolar epithelial cell processing of nanoparticles activates autophagy and lysosomal exocytosis. Am J Physiol Lung Cell Mol Physiol 315: L286–L300.

Sleightholm, R., B. Yang, F. Yu, Y. Xie, et al. 2017. Chloroquine-modified hydroxyethyl starch as a polymeric drug for cancer therapy. Biomacromolecules 18: 2247–2257.

Song, Y., Z. Huang, X. Liu, Z. Pang, et al. 2019. Platelet membrane-coated NP-mediated targeting delivery of Rapamycin blocks atherosclerotic plaque development and stabilizes plaque in apolipoprotein E-deficient (ApoE–/–) mice. Nanomedicine 15: 13–24.

Thomas, M.B., D.P. Gnanadhas, P.K. Dash, J. Machhi, et al. 2018. Modulating cellular autophagy for controlled antiretroviral drug release. Nanomedicine (Lond) 13: 2139–2154.

Vercauteren, D., H. Deschout, K. Remaut, J.F. Engbersen, et al. 2011. Dynamic colocalization microscopy to characterize intracellular trafficking of nanomedicines. ACS nano 5: 7874–7884

Wang, F., X. Xia, C. Yang, J. Shen, et al. 2018a. $SMAD_4$ gene mutation renders pancreatic cancer resistance to radiotherapy through promotion of autophagy. Clin Cancer Res 24: 3176–3185.

Wang, C., K. Li, T. Li, Z. Chen, et al. 2018b. Monocyte-mediated chemotherapy drug delivery in glioblastoma. Nanomedicine (Lond) 13: 157–178.

Wei, W., Z.T. Rosenkrans, Q.Y. Luo, X. Lan, et al. 2019. Exploiting nanomaterial-mediated autophagy for cancer therapy. Small Methods 3(2): 1800365.

Werfel, T.A., S. Wang, M.A. Jackson, T.E. Kavanaugh, et al. 2018. Selective mTORC2 inhibitor therapeutically blocks breast cancer cell growth and survival. Cancer Res 78: 1845–1858.

Wu, J.Y., Z.-X. Wang, G. Zhang, X. Lu, et al. 2018. Targeted co-delivery of Beclin 1 siRNA and FTY720 to hepatocellular carcinoma by calcium phosphate nanoparticles for enhanced anticancer efficacy. Int J Nanomed 13: 1265–1280.

Yan, H., X. Duan, H. Pan, N. Holguin, et al. 2016. Suppression of NF-κB activity via nanoparticle-based siRNA delivery alters early cartilage responses to injury. PNAS 113(41): E6199–E6208. DOI: 10.1073/pnas.1608245113

Zhang, Y., C. Yu, G. Huang, C. Wang, et al. 2010. Nano rare-earth oxides induced size-dependent vacuolization: An independent pathway from ATG. Int J Nanomed 5: 601–9.

Zhang, X., Y. Dong, X. Zeng, X. Liang, et al. 2014. The effect of ATG inhibitors on drug delivery using biodegradable polymer NPs in cancer treatment. Biomaterials 35: 1932–1943.

Zhang, X., Y. Yang, X. Liang, X. Zeng, et al. 2014a. Enhancing therapeutic effects of docetaxel-loaded dendritic copolymer nanoparticles by co-treatment with autophagy inhibitor on breast cancer. Theranostics 4(11): 1085–1095.

Zhang, X., X. Zeng, X. Liang, Y. Yang, et al. 2014b. The chemotherapeutic potential of PEG-b-PLGA copolymer micelles that combine chloroquine as autophagy inhibitor and docetaxel as an anti-cancer drug. Biomaterials 35: 9144–9154.

Zhang, X., J. Du, Z. Guo, J. Yu, et al. 2018. Efficient infrared light triggered nitric oxide release nanocomposites for sensitizing mild photothermal therapy. Advanced Sci 6(3): 1801122.

Zhao, P., M. Li, Y. Wang, Y. Chen, et al. 2018. Enhancing anti-tumor efficiency in hepatocellular carcinoma through the autophagy inhibition by miR-375/sorafenib in lipid-coated calcium carbonate nanoparticles. Acta Biomater 72: 248–255.

Zheng, Y., C. Su, L. Zhao and Y. Shi. 2017. Chitosan nanoparticle-mediated co-delivery of shAtg-5 and gefitinib synergistically promoted the efficacy of chemotherapeutics through the modulation of autophagy. J Nanobiotechnol 15: 28.

Zhu, X., X. Ji, N. Kong and Y. Chen. 2018. Intracellular mechanistic understanding of 2D MoS2 nanosheets for anti-exocytosis-enhanced synergistic cancer therapy. ACS Nano 12: 2922–2938.

Index

A

Akt phosphorylation   21, 224, 419, 575, 577

Amyloid   15, 18, 38, 94, 117, 232, 237, 258, 360, 385, 387, 388, 389, 390, 528, 556, 576

Annexin   5, 170, 207, 289, 403, 404, 422, 423, 462, 533, 544, 547

Apolipoprotein E   218, 252, 387, 389

Argyrophilic nucleolar organizer   iv, v, 11, 62

Atherosclerosis   34, 103, 105, 250, 251, 298, 300, 307, 308, 347, 402, 510, 515, 540, 571, 572

Atomic force microscopy   23, 34, 40, 548, 577

Autophagy   iii, 1, 18, 45, 49, 64, 86, 307

B

Beclin-1   43, 52, 308, 413, 424, 425, 434, 446, 454, 470, 472, 473, 474, 538, 574, 575

Bioinformatics   iii, 33, 54, 64, 82, 109, 424

Blood brain barrier   19, 392, 571, 576

Burkitt cell lymphoma-2   48, 72, 84, 107, 167, 225, 310, 517, 520

Burkitt cell lymphoma-2/adenovirus E1B 19 kDa protein-interacting protein   3, 48, 51, 54, 60, 125, 131, 206, 223, 237, 245, 246, 273, 279, 280, 285, 289, 310, 311, 313, 314, 353, 360, 395, 417, 419, 434, 450, 505, 517

C

Caloric restriction mimetics   198, 200, 514

Cardiovascular diseases   iv, 16, 19, 36, 37, 42, 44, 53, 61, 65, 66, 68, 69, 91, 108, 110, 112, 199, 216, 236, 250, 251, 259, 315, 397, 461, 510, 513, 527, 528, 530, 554, 568, 572

Catechin   v, 66, 79, 107, 172, 461, 514

Chaperone-mediated autophagy   21, 42, 251, 307, 311, 369, 375, 401

Charnolopathies   3, 18, 83, 87, 108, 109, 110, 348, 366, 512, 530

Charnolopharmacotherapeutics   9, 87, 97

Charnolophagy index   53, 64, 67

Charnolosome   iii, 1, 5, 83, 86, 96, 99, 170

Charnoptosis   307, 569

Charnoly body   iii, 1, 6, 86

Charnoly body antagonists   4, 25, 66, 108, 387, 568

Charnoly body molecular pathogenesis antagonists   v, 66, 87

Charnolophagy regulators   iv, v, 16, 65, 66, 82, 110, 111, 257, 387, 458, 510, 514, 528, 530, 535, 541, 555, 577

Chronic obstructive pulmonary disease   26, 108, 286, 407, 505

Charnolosome stabilizers   v, 16, 65, 66, 77, 108, 387, 503, 530, 568

Corona (COVID-19) virus   iv, 3, 26, 110, 286, 473, 476, 570

Clustered regularly interspaced short palindromic repeats   40, 63, 172, 185, 277, 362, 419, 430, 432, 509

Curcumin   v, 19, 66, 79, 107, 396, 402, 413, 458, 475, 491

D

Danon Disease   22, 25, 163, 302, 339, 432

Delta Psi ($\Delta\psi$) collapse   13, 16, 27, 50, 62, 93, 457, 533, 543, 548, 550, 552, 553, 556, 557, 566

Deoxy ribonucleic acid methylation 6, 93, 507, 510

Dietary restriction iv, 42, 79

Diverse physicochemical injuries iii, 2, 6, 9, 16, 22, 41, 53, 54, 87, 516

Dynamin-related protein iv, 5, 6, 10, 11, 13, 29, 30, 53, 61, 62, 85, 98, 133, 192, 217, 223, 224, 279, 281, 288, 289, 291, 294, 305, 311, 313, 315, 323, 330, 348, 357, 370, 373, 374, 380, 389, 393, 396, 419, 430, 476, 483, 484, 518, 544

Drug delivery iv, v, 527, 528, 530, 531, 535, 553, 555, 567, 568, 570, 572, 575, 576, 577

E

Endocytosis iii, iv, v, 9, 15, 20, 54, 65, 85, 148, 182, 303, 387, 389, 418, 445, 495, 512, 532, 535, 539, 542, 544, 547, 554

Endoplasmic reticulum stress v, 18, 203, 208, 275, 545

Enhanced permeability and retention v, 404, 527, 572

Evidence-based personalized theranostics iv, 4, 86, 97, 527

Exocytosis iii, iv, v, 9, 15, 16, 21, 25, 26, 34, 39, 42, 54, 65, 77, 86, 102, 128, 157, 232, 372, 381, 387, 418, 444, 445, 446, 455, 456, 469, 503, 512, 530, 535, 552, 568, 569, 570, 574

F

Fluorescence 23, 29, 33, 35, 36, 38, 39, 40, 44, 53, 54, 64, 65, 259, 321, 341, 409, 421, 428, 448, 450, 452, 472, 476, 485, 490, 521, 532, 549, 550, 551, 570, 573

Free radicals 1, 6, 17, 61, 62, 83, 87, 556

G

Gaucher disease 20, 160, 173

Glutathione 133, 219, 241, 251, 517, 575

Graphene oxide-sliver nanoparticles 545

H

Histone acetylation 93, 387

Haplo-insufficiency 165, 169, 263, 363

8-Hydroxy, 2-deoxy guanosine 2, 10, 23, 35, 53, 84, 106, 569

Hypoxia-inducible factor 21, 44, 60, 62, 66, 107, 172, 341, 360, 417, 427, 434, 450, 455, 567, 569

I

Inclusionophagy 4, 320, 469

Inflammatory diseases 4, 45, 69, 168, 401, 404, 407, 408, 469, 471, 569, 570

Inflammasome 2, 26, 34, 42, 46, 85, 86, 212, 215, 216, 223, 244, 251, 259, 287, 401, 410, 469, 472, 551

Intramitochondrial detoxification iii, 17, 78, 86, 198, 508

Intracellular detoxification iii, 1, 3, 9, 15, 23, 41, 78, 87, 508

J

Jun nuclear kinase 43, 206, 224, 305, 311, 406, 447, 454, 460, 461, 485, 453, 557

K

Kyoto encyclopedia of genes and genomes (KEGG) pathway 303, 334, 428, 491

L

Light chain 3 (microtubule-associated) 53, 64, 261, 291, 308, 396, 397, 449, 548

Lipid droplets 1, 11, 78, 85, 209, 219, 470

Lipophagy 30, 104, 220, 259, 470, 493, 494, 569

Liposome 527, 528, 530, 531, 533, 535, 541, 566, 572, 576, 577

Lycopene v, 66, 79, 460, 514

Lysosome-associated membrane protein 21, 22, 302, 303, 376, 556

Lysosome storage diseases 10, 20, 28, 43, 53, 87, 107, 140, 157, 161, 323, 324, 351, 514

LysoTracker 35, 53, 302, 358, 431

M

Mechanistic target of Rapamycin 63, 163, 175, 203, 206, 236, 237, 272, 274, 277, 278, 279, 330, 419, 454, 460, 488, 571, 575

Melatonin v, 66, 79, 98, 147, 219, 241, 308, 333, 380

Metallothioneins 4, 16, 45, 87, 90, 98, 99, 107, 204, 238, 385, 418, 426, 477, 503, 512, 528, 529, 530, 570, 572

1-Methyl, 4-phenyl, 1,2,3,6-tetrahydropyridine 4, 41, 93, 366, 435

Micropinocytosis 535, 539, 554, 575

microRNA iii, 23, 106, 166, 233, 298, 421, 494, 528, 537, 570, 572

Middle east respiratory destress syndrome virus   3, 25, 473, 474, 475, 476,

Mitochondrial associated membranes   8, 28, 29, 61, 62, 63, 98, 367, 380, 507,

Mitochondrial bioenergetics   iii, iv, 2, 6, 26, 42, 48, 84, 259, 304, 505, 519

Mitochondrial DNA   iii, 1, 5, 6, 9, 17, 35, 49, 50, 51, 54, 60, 84, 87, 139, 147, 165, 182, 187, 238, 272, 286, 292, 370, 403, 404, 409, 410, 429, 446, 469, 478, 509, 515, 519, 569, 570

Mitochondrial miRNA   ii, 1, 54, 87, 106

Mitochondrial quality control   iii, 3, 7, 9, 30, 47, 198, 273, 338, 506, 508

Mitochondrial remodeling   iii, 2, 12, 54, 78, 86, 396, 397

Mitogen activated protein kinase   43, 49, 129, 219, 244, 278, 312, 334, 394, 395, 406, 424, 433, 449, 453, 454, 462, 486, 488, 491, 553, 554, 557

Mitofusin   iv, 6, 10, 53, 60, 61, 62, 85, 225, 246, 288, 289, 291, 305, 313, 325, 330, 358, 370, 372, 396, 427, 432

MitoTracker   35, 36, 48, 53, 321, 343, 353

Multidrug resistance (MDR) malignancies 2, 9, 15, 16, 19, 42, 65, 66, 68, 69, 418, 441, 456, 458, 461, 527, 528, 530, 531, 533, 569, 570.

Monoamine Oxidases   3, 84, 111, 373, 530

N

Nanoparticles   iv, v, 17, 222, 392, 527, 528, 529, 530, 536, 538, 539, 541, 542, 543, 544, 546, 547, 548, 550, 551, 552, 553, 554, 555, 556, 557, 558, 559, 568, 567, 571, 572, 573, 574

Nanotheranostics   4, 78, 112, 527, 528, 531, 533, 534, 536, 538, 552, 567, 572, 577,

Neurodegenerative diseases   iv, 15, 16, 19, 20, 25, 34, 37, 42, 43, 44, 46, 53, 61, 65, 66, 68, 69, 91, 112, 192, 277, 278, 389, 461, 476, 479, 512, 513, 518, 527, 528, 530, 553, 568, 570, 572

Neurodegenerative charnolopathies   348, 366, 512, 530

Nieman-Pick type disease   20, 28, 143, 160, 164, 175, 224

Nuclear deoxyribonucleic acid   iii, 1, 6, 54, 64, 429, 456, 469, 569, 570

O

Omics   iii, v, 23, 40, 63, 64, 172, 303, 304, 428, 446, 486, 496

P

Peroxisome proliferative activation receptor-γ (PPAR-γ)   30, 48, 66, 244, 247, 271

Polyunsaturated fatty acids   iv, 4, 10, 17, 110, 197, 475, 569

Pyroptosis   34, 210, 313, 341, 342, 409, 485, 551, 569

Q

Quercetin   v, 66, 79, 186, 190, 221, 412, 557, 566

R

Reactive oxygen and nitrogen species   2, 7, 9, 11, 54, 63, 86, 212, 219, 238, 302, 323, 405, 409, 450, 461, 512, 518, 545

Resveratrol   v, 66, 82, 237, 279, 315, 379, 402, 412, 459, 475, 506, 514

Reverse transcription-polymerase chain reaction   26, 40, 64, 166, 244, 303, 455, 473

S

Senotherapy   2, 520

Sequestosome   48, 61, 220, 229, 247, 340, 432

Severe acute respiratory destress syndrome virus   3, 25, 472, 473, 474, 475,

Short interfering ribonucleic acid   30, 35, 46, 52, 63, 113, 129, 130, 205, 208, 223, 259, 265, 288, 295, 306, 312, 323, 325, 393, 403, 404, 405, 421, 429, 434, 487, 528, 538, 539, 544, 550, 559, 571, 572, 574

Spermidine   196, 368, 475, 506, 507, 508, 514, 515

Surface plasmon resonance spectroscopy   23, 34, 40, 64

T

Theranostic potential   16, 20, 42, 65, 82, 94, 113, 234, 279, 315, 389, 411, 414, 476, 528, 530, 541, 543, 551, 555, 556, 557, 566, 567, 568, 570, 572, 577

Translocator protein (18 kDa)   2, 10, 26, 62, 84, 104, 435, 569

Triple negative breast cancer   421, 422, 424, 447, 454, 544, 575

U

Ubiquinone (CoQ$_{10}$)   4, 88, 93, 295, 303, 306, 516, 530

Ubiquitination   2, 10, 11, 18, 27, 37, 48, 60, 68, 84, 85, 163, 223, 225, 259, 362, 372, 373, 411, 420, 443, 468, 471, 472, 473, 474, 495

Unfolded protein response   20, 28, 197, 242, 424, 520

V

Verticillium   496, 498

W

Wortmannin   43, 265, 310, 313, 314, 393, 419, 490, 552

X

Xanthine oxidases   84, 103, 495

Y

Yes-associated protein-1   424, 454

Z

Zebrafish   35, 37, 152, 164, 250, 251, 264, 380, 435, 484, 540

About the Author

Sushil Sharma is Academic Dean, AISM, Georgetown, Guyana (Stone Mountain, Atlanta, USA). Prof. & Course Director, SJSM, Bonaire and St Vincent (2011-2017). Received Ph.D. (AIIMS, Delhi, India); Radiopharmaceutical Training (BARC, Bombay), GE, Siemens, Agilent Technologies, Cardinal Health (U.S.A), Royal Society Fellowship (U.K:1988-89); MHRC Post-Doctoral Fellowship (Canada:1989-91), 5 Gold Medals. Research Officer (AIIMS:1979-88); Research Officer (University of Montreal:1993-94); Research Associate (McGill University:1994-95); Senior Scientific Officer (IRCM, Montreal:1995-97); Scientist-E (DRDO, Delhi:1997); Scientist (U of M, Winnipeg:1997-99); Assist. Prof.2000-04; Assoc. Prof. Director, UND School of Medicine, Grand Forks:2004-08); Assoc. Prof. Director (Methodist Hospital), Scientist (TMC, Houston: 2008-11), Conference Organizer, Discovered Charnoly Body.

Printed and bound by CPI Group (UK) Ltd, Croydon, CR0 4YY

24/10/2024

01778292-0011